Basic Pharmacology in Medicine

Basic Pharmacology in Medicine Third Edition

Joseph R. DiPalma, M.D., D.Sc. (Hon.)

Professor Emeritus of Pharmacology and Medicine
Department of Pharmacology
Hahnemann University School of Medicine
Philadelphia, Pennsylvania

G. John DiGregorio, M.D., Ph.D.

Professor of Pharmacology and Medicine
Department of Pharmacology
Hahnemann University School of Medicine
Philadelphia, Pennsylvania

McGRAW-HILL PUBLISHING COMPANY
Health Professions Division

New York   St. Louis   San Francisco   Colorado Springs   Auckland   Bogotá
Caracas   Hamburg   Lisbon   London   Madrid   Mexico   Milan   Montreal
New Delhi   Paris   San Juan   São Paulo   Singapore   Sydney   Tokyo   Toronto

BASIC PHARMACOLOGY IN MEDICINE

Copyright © 1990, 1982, 1976 by McGraw-Hill, Inc. All rights
reserved. Printed in the United States of America. Except
as permitted under the United States Copyright Act of 1976,
no part of this publication may be reproduced or distributed
in any form or by any means, or stored in a data base or
retrieval system, without the prior written permission
of the publisher.

1 2 3 4 5 6 7 8 9 0   DOCDOC   8 9 4 3 2 1 0 9

ISBN   0-07-017013-4

This book was set in Plantin by York Graphic Services, Inc.
The editors were William Day and Muza Navrozov;
the production supervisor was Annette Mayeski;
the cover and text were designed by José Fonfrias.
R. R. Donnelley & Sons Company was printer and binder.

LIBRARY OF CONGRESS CATALOGING-IN-PUBLICATION DATA

Basic pharmacology in medicine / [edited by] Joseph R. DiPalma,
   G. John DiGregorio.—3rd ed.
      p.   cm.
   Includes bibliographies and index.
   ISBN 0-07-017013-4
   1. Pharmacology.   I. DiPalma, Joseph R.   II. DiGregorio, G. John.
   [DNLM: 1. Pharmacology.   QV 4 B311]
RM300.B29   1989
615′.7—dc20
DNLM/DLC
for Library of Congress   89-12326
                                     CIP

CONTENTS

PART III

LOCAL CONTROL SUBSTANCES

Section Editor Edward J. Barbieri

PART IV

CENTRAL NERVOUS SYSTEM DRUGS

Section Editor G. John DiGregorio

PART **V**

THE CARDIOVASCULAR AND RENAL AND RESPIRATORY SYSTEMS
Section Editor Joseph R. DiPalma

PART IX

ANTI-INFECTIVE AGENTS

Section Editor G. John DiGregorio

PART X

TOXICOLOGY

Section Editor Joseph R. DiPalma

CONTRIBUTORS

Martin W. Adler, Ph.D.
Professor of Pharmacology
Temple University School of Medicine
Philadelphia, Pennsylvania

Judith L. Albert, M.D.
Assistant Professor of Obstetrics and Gynecology
University of Pennsylvania School of Medicine
Philadelphia, Pennsylvania

Edward J. Barbieri, Ph.D.
Associate Professor of Pharmacology
Hahnemann University School of Medicine
Philadelphia, Pennsylvania

Carl Barsigian, Ph.D.
Assistant Professor of Pharmacology
Jefferson Medical College
Thomas Jefferson University
Cardeza Foundation for Hematologic Research
Philadelphia, Pennsylvania

Delphine B. Bartosik, M.D.
Associate Professor of Obstetrics and Gynecology
Hahnemann University School of Medicine
Philadelphia, Pennsylvania

Peter G. Bradford, Ph.D.
Assistant Professor of Pharmacology
Hahnemann University School of Medicine
Philadelphia, Pennsylvania

Isadore Brodsky, M.D.
Professor and Chairman
Department of Neoplastic Diseases
Hahnemann University School of Medicine
Philadelphia, Pennsylvania

David J. Brunswick, Ph.D.
Research Associate Professor
of Biochemistry in Psychiatry
University of Pennsylvania
Philadelphia, Pennsylvania

Benjamin Calesnick, M.D.
Professor Emeritus of Pharmacology and Medicine
Hahnemann University School of Medicine
Philadelphia, Pennsylvania

Pamela Crilley, D.O.
Senior Instructor of Oncology
Department of Neoplastic Diseases
Hahnemann University School of Medicine
Philadelphia, Pennsylvania

Domenic A. DeBias, Ph.D.
Professor and Chairman of Physiology
and Pharmacology
Philadelphia College of Osteopathic Medicine
Philadelphia, Pennsylvania

Raphael J. DeHoratius, M.D.
Professor of Medicine
Director, Division of Rheumatology
Hahnemann University School of Medicine
Philadelphia, Pennsylvania

G. John DiGregorio, M.D., Ph.D.
Professor of Pharmacology and Medicine
Hahnemann University School of Medicine
Philadelphia, Pennsylvania

Joseph R. DiPalma, M.D., D.Sc. (Hon.)
Professor Emeritus of Pharmacology and Medicine
Hahnemann University School of Medicine
Philadelphia, Pennsylvania

Andrew P. Ferko, Ph.D.
Associate Professor of Pharmacology
Hahnemann University School of Medicine
Philadelphia, Pennsylvania

Alan Frazer, Ph.D.
Professor of Pharmacology and Psychiatry
University of Pennsylvania School of Medicine
Philadelphia, Pennsylvania

Alexander Gero, Ph.D.
Professor Emeritus of Pharmacology
Hahnemann University School of Medicine
Philadelphia, Pennsylvania

Elizabeth L. Helfer, M.D.
Clinical Instructor in Medicine
Division of Endocrinology and Metabolism
Hahnemann University School of Medicine
Philadelphia, Pennsylvania

Henry W. Hitner, Ph.D.
Professor of Pharmacology
Philadelphia College of Osteopathic Medicine
Philadelphia, Pennsylvania

Jan C. Horrow, M.D.
Associate Professor of Clinical Anesthesiology
Hahnemann University School of Medicine
Philadelphia, Pennsylvania

Leonard S. Jacob, M.D., Ph.D.
Vice President, Clinical Development
  and Regulatory Affairs
Magainin Sciences, Inc.
Fort Washington, Pennsylvania

Sigmund B. Kahn, M.D.
Professor of Oncology
Department of Neoplastic Diseases
Hahnemann University School of Medicine
Philadelphia, Pennsylvania

George B. Koelle, M.D., Ph.D.
Distinguished Professor of Pharmacology
University of Pennsylvania School of Medicine
Philadelphia, Pennsylvania

Lawrence Levit, M.D.
Senior Instructor of Anesthesiology
Hahnemann University School of Medicine
Philadelphia, Pennsylvania

Jerry D. Levitt, M.D.
Associate Professor of Anesthesiology
Hahnemann University School of Medicine
Philadelphia, Pennsylvania

José Martinez, M.D.
Professor of Medicine
Associate Director for Research Education
Department of Medicine
Jefferson Medical College
  of Thomas Jefferson University
Cardeza Foundation for Hematologic Research
Philadelphia, Pennsylvania

Jeffrey L. Miller, M.D.
Associate Professor of Medicine
Division of Endocrinology and Metabolism
Hahnemann University School of Medicine
Philadelphia, Pennsylvania

Abdolghader Molavi, M.D.
Associate Professor of Medicine and Surgery
Director, Division of Infectious Diseases
Hahnemann University School of Medicine
Philadelphia, Pennsylvania

Benjamin Z. Ngwenya, Ph.D.
Associate Professor of Microbiology
Hahnemann University School of Medicine
Philadelphia, Pennsylvania

Charles O'Brien, M.D., Ph.D.
Professor of Psychiatry
University of Pennsylvania School of Medicine
Philadelphia, Pennsylvania

Raymond F. Orzechowski, Ph.D.
Professor of Pharmacology
Philadelphia College of Pharmacy and Science
Philadelphia, Pennsylvania

Ruby M. Padolina, M.D.
Assistant Professor of Anesthesiology
Hahnemann University School of Medicine
Philadelphia, Pennsylvania

David M. Ritchie, Ph.D.
Principal Scientist
Robert Wood Johnson Pharmaceutical
    Research Institute
Raritan, New Jersey

Leslie I. Rose, M.D.
Professor of Medicine
Director, Division of Endocrinology
    and Metabolism
Hahnemann University School of Medicine
Philadelphia, Pennsylvania

James M. Ross, M.D.
Clinical Instructor of Medicine
Hahnemann University School of Medicine
Philadelphia, Pennsylvania

Karl Salman, M.D.
Clinical Instructor of Medicine
Division of Endocrinology and Metabolism
Hahnemann University School of Medicine
Philadelphia, Pennsylvania

J. Bryan Smith, Ph.D.
Professor and Chairman of Pharmacology
Temple University School of Medicine
Philadelphia, Pennsylvania

Steven J. Sondheimer, M.D.
Associate Professor of Obstetrics and Gynecology
University of Pennsylvania School of Medicine
Philadelphia, Pennsylvania

Gerald H. Sterling, Ph.D.
Associate Professor of Pharmacology
Hahnemann University School of Medicine
Philadelphia, Pennsylvania

Neil M. Sussman, M.D.
Associate Professor of Neurology
Medical College of Pennsylvania
Director of Medical Research
Mid-Atlantic Regional Epilepsy Center
Philadelphia, Pennsylvania

Allen E. Lord Terzian, M.D.
Senior Instructor of Oncology
Department of Neoplastic Diseases
Hahnemann University School of Medicine
Philadelphia, Pennsylvania

William S. Thayer, Ph.D.
Associate Professor of Pathology
Hahnemann University School of Medicine
Philadelphia, Pennsylvania

David L. Topolsky, M.D.
Instructor of Oncology
Department of Neoplastic Diseases
Hahnemann University School of Medicine
Philadelphia, Pennsylvania

Michael P. Wachter, Ph.D.
Research Manager
Robert Wood Johnson Pharmaceutical
    Research Institute
Raritan, New Jersey

Martin A. Wasserman, Ph.D.
Director of Biomedical Evaluation
Division of Medical Affairs, Human Pharmacology
The Squibb Institute for Medical Research
Princeton, New Jersey

The following contributors, while not completing
individual chapters, aided materially in their
respective fields of discipline:

Bhavin R. Dave, M.D.
Research Associate in Pharmacology
Hahnemann University School of Medicine
Philadelphia, Pennsylvania

M. Mehdi Keykhah, M.D.
Professor of Clinical Anesthesiology
Hahnemann University School of Medicine
Philadelphia, Pennsylvania

Henry Rosenberg, M.D.
Professor and Chairman of Anesthesiology
Hahnemann University School of Medicine
Philadelphia, Pennsylvania

P R E F A C E

The third edition of this basic text of pharmacology represents not merely a revision but actually an entirely new text. The requirements of the new text have been dictated by the vast changes in science and technology, the changing attitudes of students and teachers toward medical education, and the new patterns and ethical considerations of health care delivery that have emerged since the last edition seven years ago.

First of all, a middle course has been followed between a huge comprehensive text and a core curriculum manual, which was the aim of the first and second editions. The present edition covers all the pharmacologic information that is pertinent for physicians and medical students who are to qualify for licensing or requalifying examinations to practice medicine in the United States. It is also of primary utility for scientists who desire pharmacologic information, students qualifying for advanced degrees in pharmacology, pharmacy students and practitioners, and of course other health care workers such as nurses and physicians' assistants.

One pattern that persists in this edition is concentration on the mechanisms of drug action. Thus the introductory chapters cover theory in depth, and the subsequent chapters on more practical aspects repeat and emphasize this information. A molecular biology approach has been applied wherever appropriate. Clinical pharmacology information is a standard part of each drug discussion. The information is designed to prepare the student for the therapy of disease. The toxicology section has been expanded.

Finally, the text has been divided into ten parts, with individual section editors. This was done to ensure as much uniformity as possible in a multiauthored text. In all cases references have been updated to provide the best and most recent information.

The editors are deeply grateful to their many collaborators. Most have come from Philadelphia medical schools or institutions. Their ready access to us has made our task easier. Our "computer gals" Linda Bush and Diane Ciamaichelo have shown extraordinary patience, for which we are especially thankful. Muza Navrozov, Area Editing Supervisor at McGraw-Hill, has rescued many a "dangling" participle, and her suggestions and criticisms have been most valuable. Emil Bobyock, Robert McMichael, and Eileen Ruch were of great help with the indexing.

JOSEPH R. DIPALMA
G. JOHN DIGREGORIO

Basic Pharmacology in Medicine

PART I

Modern Approaches to Pharmacology

SECTION EDITOR

Joseph R. DiPalma

The Drug-Receptor Interaction

Alexander Gero

A dictionary definition of the science of pharmacology is as follows: the study of the preparation, qualities, uses, and effects of drugs. Most modern textbooks define pharmacology broadly as "the effects of chemicals upon living systems." Medical pharmacology is limited to those chemicals that may influence the course of disease or that maintain well-being. It follows that any substance, usually a chemical of relatively small molecular size, that is found to have utility in the therapy or prevention of disease is defined as a *drug*. It may not be apparent now, but it is virtually impossible to separate nutritive chemicals (foods) from drugs.

At the present time, and in the immediate future, the bulk of knowledge and understanding of drug action will be concentrated in a molecular biology approach. Molecular pharmacology has provided the means of understanding the mechanisms of drug action that make possible the more accurate control of disease and indeed the development of new and superior drugs. It is permissible now to think of pharmacology as related mainly to *the action of chemicals on receptors in a living system*. What a receptor is and what the consequences of a drug-receptor interaction are will occupy the first two chapters of this text.

Of all the controllable variables in the investigation of drug action the dose is of crucial importance. In all instances the response of the drug-receptor interaction is dependent on the dose. Therefore, foresight would dictate that a logical approach to the understanding of the drug-receptor interaction would be the study of the language and the methods used to measure the re-

sponse in relationship to dose. Later, methods and theoretical implications of dealing with receptor quality and quantity may be defined.

DOSE-RESPONSE RELATIONSHIPS

The principle that the magnitude of the drug effect is related to the dose administered is, though self-evident, one of the most important in the science of pharmacology. Four variables enter into this relationship: time, biologic unit, dose of drug administered (or, with in vitro experiments, the drug concentration in the bath fluid), and the effect produced by the given quantity of drug. Thus only a four-dimensional representation would do justice to all the known factors influencing the dose-response relationship even in an isolated organ. Because we customarily write on two-dimensional surfaces, we arbitrarily select two variables and represent their functional relationship graphically, keeping the other two variables constant. Two choices of variables are in common use: *graded* dose-response plots, which represent the variation of the magnitude of the response as the dose varies, keeping the time and the biologic unit constant by using the same biologic object throughout the experiment and stipulating that measurements are to be made at the time when the system has come to equilibrium, i.e., when the effect has become constant as long as the drug concentration does not change; and *quantal* dose-response curves, representing the relationship between the dose of a drug and the proportion of biologic objects manifesting a specified pharmacologic effect.

Thus here the dose and the number of units are variable, and the magnitudes of the response and the time are constant.

Graded Dose-Response Curve

Graded dose-response curves generally look like that shown in Fig. 1-1. When the dose of a drug is gradually increased and the first noticeable effect is observed, the dose that produced this effect is called the *threshold* dose. Increments of drug administration result in larger effects; the curve obtained from the experiment is found to be a hyperbola and as such asymptomatically approaches the *ceiling* effect, where further increments of drug administration no longer change the response. The ceiling effect thus reveals the potency of the drug. However, representing the results on an arithmetic scale, as in Fig. 1-1, has its disadvantages: the data in the beginning of the curve are so crowded that drug doses responsible for different effects cannot be discerned; furthermore, a hyperbola is not a very informative display of data. It is customary, therefore, to plot the effect not against the dose of the drug (or its concentration) but against the logarithm of the dose (Fig. 1-2). Such *semilogarithmic* representation of the data results in a sigmoid (S-shaped) curve; it expands the lower part of the hyperbola (where the effect changes greatly with increasing drug dose) and compresses its upper part (where there is little change in effect). In addition, it has the advan-

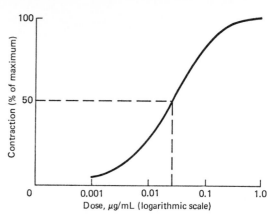

FIGURE 1-2 The same data as in Fig. 1-1 except that the dose is now plotted as a negative logarithm. The curve now becomes sigmoid in shape with a nearly linear central portion. This is far more convenient to interpret and has the advantage that the 50 percent maximal response may be easily determined. For these reasons the log-concentration curve has become the standard dose-response curve.

tage that the middle part of the sigmoid curve is very nearly a straight line. Mathematicians value straight lines in a plot because a straight line is uniquely defined by two easily observable parameters, its slope and its intersection with one axis of the coordinate system in which the results of the experiment are displayed. (The slope and the intercept together define the intercept on the other axis.)

Quantal Dose-Response Curve

Quantal (or all-or-none) dose-response curves, in which the time and the magnitude of the effect are constant and the variables are the drug dose and the number of individuals responding with the specified effect, are actually a statement on the population statistics of drug response. They show the proportion of a human or animal population, or of a population of isolated organs, that displays a specified response to a given drug dose. As a consequence of biologic variability, in a population of sufficient size there are always some few individuals so drug-sensitive that they respond to rather small doses, equally few so drug-insensitive that they require substantial doses, and the largest number responsive to a middle dose, with gradual transitions from the middle to the extremes. Hence a *Gaussian*, or *normal distribution*, *curve* (Fig. 1-3) will

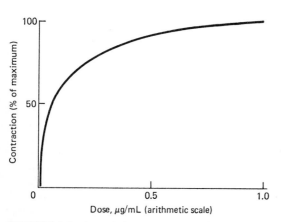

FIGURE 1-1 A graded response curve for increasing concentrations of a drug in a perfusion bath of a perfused isolated gut. Plotted on an arithmetic scale, the contraction response is hyperbolic as the concentration of the drug is increased until a ceiling effect is achieved.

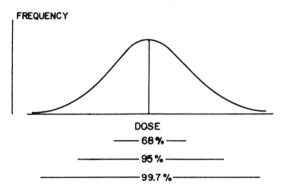

FIGURE 1-3 A graphic expression of the theoretical normal distribution of doses needed to elicit a quantal response in subjects from a large sample. The horizontal bars delineate the borders of plus or minus one, two, and three standard deviations from the mean dose, which is shown by the vertical bar. The proportion of subjects requiring doses within the boundaries is indicated as a percentage of the sample. The dose units are unspecified.

best represent the population statistics of drug response. In such a curve the drug dose is plotted on the abscissa and the frequency of response, i.e., the percentage of the population responding to each drug, on the ordinate. The curve is seen to be symmetric; hence the *mean* (or average) dose, the *median* dose (which bisects the total population into two equal parts), and the *mode* (the dose which draws the most frequent response) are all identical. Also, all the points on the curve deviate from the mean as much to the right (in a positive direction in the coordinate system) as to the left (in a negative direction), so that the sum of the deviations is zero. But the sum of their squares is a positive number because both positive and negative numbers have positive squares. Dividing the sum of the squares by the number of individual values that have been squared, we obtain the *variance*, and the square root of the variance is the *standard deviation*. This is an important parameter, which describes the width of the curve, that is, the scatter of individual points about the mean due to biologic variation. (It is to be distinguished from the *standard error*, which is a measure of the scatter of individual measurements due to experimental inaccuracy.) In the Gaussian curve one unit of standard deviation encompasses 34 percent of the total population, two units $47\frac{1}{2}$ percent, three units 49 percent, and so on. The two inflection points of the distribution curve occur at plus and minus one standard deviation.

In practice, distribution curves are seldom perfect because the sample may be too small for serviceable statistics, or the curve is *truncated* (one or the other end of the distribution curve is experimentally not available), or some extraneous influence or other experimental limitation opposes or modifies the drug action observed. In such cases the mean, the mode, and the median dose may differ. The situation can be improved by trying to eliminate disturbing influences, and, most importantly, by increasing the size of the population studied. But only an infinite population guarantees perfect results. Therefore all actual statistical findings have limited reliability, expressed as the *confidence limit*, a figure arrived at by known mathematical rules, which states the probability of some measured value being the true value. The statement that some particular value is, say, 0.63 to 0.65 with a confidence limit of 0.95 means that in 95 out of 100 experiments the value can be expected to be found between 0.63 and 0.65.

As in the case of graded dose-response curves, efforts have been made to convert the bell-shaped quantal dose-response curve to a form that is at least partially linear. To this end one may plot the results cumulatively, that is, instead of the number of individuals responding to some particular drug dose and not to lower ones, one records the total number of individuals who have responded up to that dose, as a percentage of the total population studied. This procedure transforms the bell-shaped Gaussian curve into a sigmoid one with a linear midsection (Fig. 1-4).

Therapeutic Index

The data provided by quantal dose-response plots can be utilized for a statement on the safety of a drug. Consider Fig. 1-4. It reports experiments conducted on a population of laboratory mice with a hypnotic drug, both parts of the figure showing two curves, sleep as the specified therapeutic effect in one curve and death—the ultimate toxic effect—in the other. Obviously, the farther apart the two curves are, the safer the drug. Numerically, the safety of the drug can be expressed as the *therapeutic index* TI_{50}, defined as the ratio of the median toxic dose TD_{50}, or the median lethal dose LD_{50}, to the median effective dose ED_{50}. But this information is insufficient: the TI_{50} is only a statement about the distance between the median effective and the median toxic dose in the plot. It says nothing about the standard deviations, i.e., the width of the two

Gaussian curves, and hence nothing about whether the lower end of the toxicity curve overlaps the upper end of the effect curve. If such an overlap occurs, then a dose of the drug, which is just the threshold dose for some individuals, is toxic and may even be lethal to others. (This is not a hypothetical problem: beverage alcohol is such a dangerous drug.) It is therefore customary to supplement the information given by the therapeutic index with the *standard safety margin*, which indicates the relative positions of the upper end of the effect curve and the lower end of the toxicity curve by a number which states by what percentage ED_{99}, the drug dose effective in 99 percent of the population, must be increased in order to equal TD_1, the dose that causes toxicity in 1 percent of the same population. (Instead of 99 percent and 1 percent, one may use, for example, 99.9 percent and 0.1 percent, or other values; this, of course, must be specified. See Table 1-1.)

Time-Action Curves

It was noted earlier that in choosing the two variables on which the graded and quantal dose-response curves are based one keeps the time variable constant by stipulating that observations are to be made when equilibrium—a constant effect at constant drug dose—has been attained. It may be desirable, however, to record

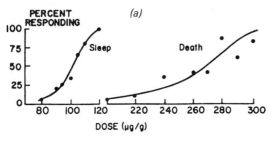

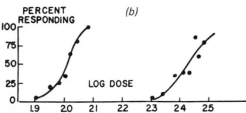

FIGURE   1-4 Cumulative quantal dose-response curves. Percent responding (*a*) against the drug dose and (*b*) against the logarithm of the dose. (See discussion in text.)

TABLE 1-1   Safety margin or therapeutic index calculated from the data in Fig. 1-4

Therapeutic index and symbol	Value of index
Median therapeutic index	2.62
$\dfrac{TD_{50}}{ED_{50}} = \dfrac{262\text{ mg}}{100\text{ mg}}$	
Standard safety margin	67%
$\left(\dfrac{TD_1}{ED_{99}} - 1\right) \times 100$	
Standard safety margin	8%
$\left(\dfrac{TD_{0.1}}{ED_{99.9}} - 1\right) \times 100$	

the time course of the appearance of the effect as well, both as a tool in the analysis of the mechanism of action of the drug and as clinical information for scheduling drug administration to patients. In order to avoid the need for a three-dimensional coordinate system, an array of curves in two dimensions can be used as seen in Fig. 1-5, which illustrates the three important phases of *time-action curves*: the time of onset (time interval from the moment of drug administration to the moment when the drug effect is first perceived), the time to peak effect (when the drug has reached all cells of the responsive tissue and has induced the maximum effect in all responsive cells, yet the physiologic factors antagonizing drug action have not yet diminished it perceptibly), and the duration of action (time from the onset to the disappearance of the effect). In some cases there are also residual effects, perceived only as increased potency of the same drug on readministration or as a modification in the activity of a different drug with which the first drug interacts positively or negatively.

DRUG ASSAYS

Drug assays may be performed to determine the amount of a drug in a particular pharmaceutical formulation or biologic specimen. Most drugs are assayed chemically, that is, by a chemical reaction involving the formation of a measurable end product.

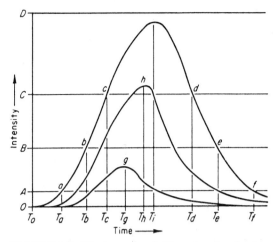

FIGURE 1-5   The intensity of effect related to the time of administration of a drug and the influence of dosage on the time-effect relationship. Three different doses of the same drug are given at time T_0. A is the threshold effect; B is the therapeutic effect; C is the toxic effect; D is the maximal effect of the drug. The peak effects of the three doses occur at times T_g, T_h, T_i. The other lowercase letters refer to other endpoints. For example, T_a = latency time; T_i = peak time; T_f = persistence time.

Some drugs are assayed by a biologic assay. *Bioassay* is defined as a determination of the potency of a physical, chemical, or biologic agent by means of a biologic indicator. Physical agents may include such forces as ionizing radiation; chemical and biologic agents include drugs, hormones, vitamins, toxins, and antitoxins. The indicators of biologic activity are the measurable responses provoked by these agents in a surviving organism or tissue. Numerous indicators exist: blood pressure, blood glucose level, muscle tension, and inhibition of microorganism growth are some examples. A variety of biologic objects supply the responses. These may be whole organisms, isolated organs, or tissue culture of cells. The objective of a bioassay is to establish the relative potency of a drug and to supply an estimate of the reliability of the potency.

A third approach to drug assay is *radioimmunoassay*. These are assays in which radioactively labeled haptens (drugs) compete with antigens or haptens in a biologic fluid for sites of antibodies. Radioimmunoassay permits determination of drugs in biologic fluids in quantities as small as a millionth or even a billionth of a milligram. It is also referred to as a *competitive protein-*

binding assay. The capacity of this method is impressive and permits detection of levels in body fluids hitherto considered impossible. Whereas before one considered micrograms (10^{-6}) to be the ultimate level of distinction, now even nanograms (10^{-9}) and picograms (10^{-12}) can be detected.

Biologic Assay versus Chemical Assay

The estimation of relative potency of a drug by bioassay generally is less precise than the determination of the quantity of a drug by chemical assay. Nevertheless, biologic assay is still the method of choice in the standardization of a substantial number of drugs, largely because of the following advantages of bioassay over chemical assay: (1) The active principle does not have to be known. (2) The active principle may be known, but its chemical composition does not have to be established. (3) The active principle does not have to be in a pure state. (4) The sensitivity of bioassay methods may be far greater than that of chemical methods; for example, in the microbiologic assay of vitamin B_{12} concentrations can be detected as low as 0.00002 $\mu g/mL$, whereas the chemical method requires 5 $\mu g/mL$, a 250,000-fold difference in sensitivity. (5) Drugs which are chemically pure but unstable may sometimes be bioassayed without loss of the drug activity. (6) Bioassay can often reveal the active isomer of a drug which has active and inactive isomers.

Biologic assay has the disadvantages of lower precision and costliness in time and animals. Wherever possible, chemical assay is preferred over biologic assay.

RECEPTORS

It is known from the study of physiology that signal transmission in the organism occurs by means of hormones and neurotransmitters that are bound by *receptors*, specialized proteins which, having bound such a ligand, trigger a physiologic response. The binding is made possible by a close structural complementarity between the receptor and the ligand. (The analogy with a lock-and-key relationship is often used.) If drugs can stimulate these same receptors to trigger a response, then the physiologic receptors are also pharmacologic receptors and such drugs are termed *agonists*. If, on the other hand, a drug molecule complexes with the receptor without evoking a response, that drug molecule will remove the receptor it occupies

from the total receptor pool available to the endogenous ligand or to an agonistic drug and function as an
antagonist.

Receptors and Acceptors

It should be noted that many binding agents in the
body, such as blood proteins, particularly serum albumin, can bind numerous compounds, including
drugs, but this binding does not result in drug action:
it is *silent binding*, and the binding agent is an *acceptor*
rather than a receptor. The ability to lead to an effect is
an integral part of the definition of a receptor; that is,
receptors are acceptors specialized to respond to certain molecules they bind by triggering a physiologic
response.

Experimental Study of Receptors

A number of receptors have been isolated, taking advantage of the discovery that solutions of nonionic de-
tergents can detach receptors from their natural habi-
tat. Sophisticated chromatography of the solution may
enrich and purify the receptors 200,000-fold in a single
step, and the receptors are then identified as proteins
and their structure elucidated by standard methods of
amino-acid sequencing and x-ray analysis.

Many receptors are located in cell membranes, held
in place by the compatibility of the cell membrane
with an accumulation of hydrophobic amino acid side
chains on the outside of that part of the receptor-
protein helix which is in contact with the membrane,
while hydrophilic portions of the helix protrude both
into the extracellular fluid and into the cytosol. The
outside hydrophilic portion contains the actual receptor site, a grouping of amino acids serving as the lock
which the ligand fits as the key. The stimulation of the
receptor by the ligand is then passed on by a complex
transduction system to a second messenger, cyclic
AMP or calcium ions, inside the cell. In the next chapter there are schematic pictures of such receptors
whose structure has been established. Other receptors, particularly those which respond to corticoid hormones and to thyroxin, are located in the cytosol
rather than in the cell membrane.

Furthermore, it is reasonable to consider the active
sites of the enzymes of intermediary metabolism as
possible drug receptors. If there is medical reason to
depress the activity of such an enzyme, this can be
done by means of a drug which functions as an inhibitor of the enzyme. Such a procedure is particularly
important in inhibiting the enzymes involved in the
metabolism or the reproductive function of harmful
cells, such as those of microbial invaders or of malignant cells of the organism. Another enzyme that functions as a drug receptor is prostaglandin synthetase. It
is inhibited by aspirin and related drugs, which therefore can counteract prostaglandin effects such as pain,
fever, and inflammation.

The Drug-Receptor Association

The forces involved in the drug-receptor interaction
are determined by the protein nature of the receptor
and by the requirement that the drug-receptor association must be reversible. This is not dictated by any law
of nature: chemical agents can attach themselves irreversibly to receptors, but except for rare cases, such as
nitrogen mustards (see Chap. 35) or organophosphorous insecticides (see Chap. 19), it is not usually
desired to inflict irreversible changes on any constituent of the organism. It is this practical consideration
which requires the drug-receptor association to be reversible.

It follows from this requirement that the forces
causing drug and receptor to associate must be ionic,
hydrophobic, or hydrogen bonds, all of which have
energies low enough to be broken under physiologic
conditions; they cannot be covalent bonds, which are
too strong. On the other hand, hydrogen bonds and,
even more, hydrophobic bonds are too weak and fall
off too fast with increasing distance to cause significant
binding unless there are many of them and unless the
bonded parts of drug and receptor molecules come in
very close contact. Hence the distribution of charges
and of potential hydrogen-bonding and hydrophobic-
binding groups in a receptor specifies structural features in a drug: in order to be able to attach itself to the
receptor, the drug must have charges and hydrogen-
bonding and hydrophilic-binding groups so arranged
that they fit corresponding groups in the receptor
closely.

This is the lock-and-key relationship mentioned
earlier. Therefore, certain structural characteristics
must be present in all drugs capable of interacting with
the same receptor, much as they must be present in all
substrates capable of interacting with the same enzymatic active site. (It will be noted later that receptors

are in many ways most similar to enzymes; in fact, enzymes might be defined as a class of receptors whose physiologic function is to catalyze chemical reactions.)

By similar reasoning, when a drug molecule is asymmetric, only one of its enantiomorphs will fit the receptor accurately; therefore drug-receptor interactions must be *sterospecific*. Examples illustrating this conclusion are found in drugs capable of interacting with receptors for epinephrine and norepinephrine (Chap. 7), for acetylcholine (Chap. 9), and for opiates (Chap. 22). Drugs acting on "adrenergic" receptors are, like the natural adrenergic agents epinephrine and norepinephrine, derivatives of phenylethylamine; and those among them which are asymmetric show sterospecificity. Thus the effect of natural $(-)$-epinephrine is 1000 times greater than that of the same dose of $(+)$-epinephrine; the effect of the alkaloid $(-)$-muscarine, a potent cholinergic agent, is 700 times greater than that of $(+)$-muscarine.

For another example, morphine and all other so-called opioid drugs are derivatives of γ-phenylpiperidine; and while the natural $(-)$-morphine is a powerful drug, the biologic activity of its $(+)$-enantiomorph is minimal.

Thus the nature of the forces which operate the drug-receptor interaction leads to the realization that, when drug action is based on receptors, a given pharmacologic activity hinges on a specific molecular structure of the drug. Conversely, when it is observed that some particular pharmacologic action is contingent on some particular chemical structure, this is evidence that the effect is mediated by receptors. The important principle of *structure-activity relationship* will be often illustrated in later chapters of this book.

THE PHYSICAL CHEMISTRY OF DRUG-RECEPTOR ASSOCIATION

If, as was explained in the foregoing, association of the drug D with the receptor R is reversible,

$$D + R \rightleftharpoons DR$$

then the law of mass action is applicable to it:

$$\frac{[D][R]}{[DR]} = K \qquad (1)$$

Noting that the presumably constant total receptor concentration $[R]_t$ is the sum of the concentrations of free receptor $[R]$ and drug-occupied receptor $[DR]$,

$$[R]_t = [R] + [DR]$$

one may substitute $[R]_t - [DR]$ for $[R]$ in Eq. (1):

$$\frac{[D]\,([R]_t - [DR])}{[DR]} = K \qquad (2)$$

which can be rearranged to

$$[DR] = \frac{[R]_t}{(K/[D]) + 1} \qquad (3)$$

This is an important equation because it is obvious that the magnitude of the drug effect E is a function of the concentration of the drug-receptor complex $[DR]$. Assuming that this functional dependence is a simple proportion with the proportionality constant α (for which the technical term is *intrinsic activity*),

$$E = \alpha[DR] = \frac{\alpha[R]_t}{(K/[D]) + 1} \qquad (4)$$

This equation is formally similar to a fundamental equation of enzyme kinetics: write V for E, k for α, K_m for K, enzyme for receptor, and substrate for drug, and Eq. (4) becomes the Michaelis-Menten equation. This is so because both Eq. (4) and the Michaelis-Menten equation are derived from the application of the law of mass action to the reversible association of two molecules followed by an observable consequence of the association. Like the Michaelis-Menten equation, Eq. (4) contains two variables, $[D]$ and E, both of which are measurable in favorable cases. Even though $\alpha[R]_t$ and K may not be known, it is enough to know that they are constants in order to make the statement (which follows from elementary algebra) that the effect depends hyperbolically on the drug concentration and that a plot of E versus log $[D]$ is the sigmoid curve discussed above, as indeed experiment shows that it is (Fig. 1-6).

Actually, it is possible to find the values of $[R]_t$ and K. Equation (2) can be rearranged, not only to Eq. (3), but also to

$$\frac{[DR]}{[D]} = \frac{1}{K}[R]_t - \frac{1}{K}[DR] \qquad (5)$$

This is a linear equation with the variables $[DR]$ and $[DR]/[D]$. $[D]$ is known, and if $[DR]$ can be determined, a plot can be drawn for the two variables (Scatchard plot) whose slope yields the value of K and

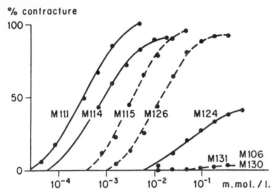

% contracture

FIGURE 1-6 Experimental dose-response curves: contraction of frog rectus abdominis muscle after administration of various quaternary ammonium compounds identified in the graph by code numbers.

whose intercept, knowing K, yields $[R]_t$. It is indeed possible to determine $[DR]$ by what is known as saturation analysis: the biologic material under study is incubated with a solution of a radioactive drug known to be a specific ligand for the receptor, and the amount bound is established by measuring the radioactivity of the biologic material after the incubation. If enough drug has been used, it will saturate all receptors and also the much more numerous acceptors. The experiment is then repeated, but this time in the presence of a very large excess of nonradioactive drug: as a result the relatively few receptors will be saturated, except for a very small fraction, by nonradioactive drug, and the modest amount of radioactivity found at the end of the experiment can be attributed to an equally small fraction of acceptor binding. The difference between the results of the two experiments therefore represents the receptor-bound radioactivity which, knowing the radioactivity of the administered drug, can be recalculated as $[DR]$. Hence saturation analysis and the Scatchard plot together permit to determine $[R]_t$, and knowing the number of cells involved in the experiments, one can calculate from the results that a typical cell bears 10,000 to 20,000 receptors on its surface and 10,000 to 100,000 receptors in the cytosol.

In enzyme kinetics, the reciprocal of the Michaelis-Menten equation results in the linear Lineweaver-Burk plot. Similarly, the reciprocal of Eq. (3)

$$\frac{1}{E} = \frac{K}{\alpha[R]_t}\frac{1}{[D]} + \frac{1}{\alpha[R]_t} \qquad (6)$$

shows that a double-reciprocal plot, i.e., a plot of the reciprocal value of the effect versus the reciprocal value of the drug concentration, must be linear. As Fig. 1-7 shows, it is. Dividing the slope of the linear plot $(K/\alpha[R]_t)$ by its intercept $(1/\alpha[R]_t)$, Eq. (6) thus provides another way to determine K.

The dissociation constant K is an important parameter of drug action in that its reciprocal, the *affinity constant* $1/K$, is a measure of the affinity of the drug for its receptor. The other important parameter is the intrinsic activity α. Between these two parameters the magnitude of the drug effect can be determined, as clearly shown by Eq. (4). A drug with high intrinsic activity and high affinity will be highly potent, but drugs with either low affinity or low intrinsic activity will have low potency, the former because relatively few drug molecules will be attached to receptors, the latter because, even though many receptors are occupied, they are not fully stimulated by the drug's low intrinsic activity.

It should be noted that other receptor theories are possible and in fact enjoy more favor among some pharmacologists. Still, the theory presented here is adequate and by far the simplest. For that reason it is used to introduce the reader to theoretical pharmacology.

A number of further conclusions may be derived from the rather self-evident assumptions about drug-receptor interaction made above. Some of these conclusions are illustrated in what follows below. The reader who wishes to find a full presentation of the theory and its algebraic derivations is referred to *Drill's Pharmacology in Medicine*, 4th ed., Chap. 5.

SIMULTANEOUS ACTION OF TWO DRUGS AND ITS THEORETICAL INTERPRETATION

Equation (4) describes the correlation of the effect E with the concentration $[D]$ of an agonist, that is, a drug which has an observable effect; and the correlation hinges on the magnitudes of the parameters K and α, both of which have to have finite magnitudes. If a drug has finite affinity for a receptor without having a measurable intrinsic activity, that is, if the drug has $\alpha = 0$, then from Eq. (4) it follows that this drug is not an agonist: it is an antagonist in the sense in which this term was introduced in the foregoing, and it will di-

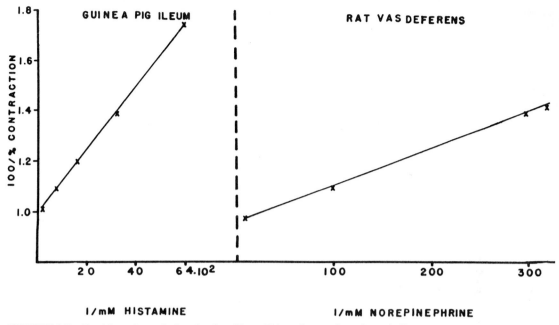

FIGURE 1-7   Double-reciprocal plots for the effect of histamine on the guinea pig ileum and of norepinephrine on the vas deferens of the rat.

minish the effect of an agonist present at the same time. This is again analogous to a situation in enzyme kinetics, namely, to *competitive antagonist* of an agonist acting on the same receptor. The theory predicts that, just as in the parallel situation in enzyme kinetics, when an agonist acts in the presence of a competitive antagonist, the log-dose-response curve of the agonist will be displaced to the right parallel to itself if the antagonist is present at a constant concentration. Double-reciprocal plots in the presence and absence of the competitive antagonist will have identical intercepts but different slopes. Figures 1-8 and 1-9 illustrate experimental examples complying with these predictions. It is seen that, even in the presence of the antagonist, a sufficiently large drug dose can overcome the antagonism, up to the maximum effect. The antagonist, in effect, removes part of the receptor pool, but a sufficient agonist concentration can take it back. That is the meaning of competition. From the algebra of competitive antagonism follows that IC_{50}, the antagonist concentration required to cut the effect of some particular agonist concentration in half, is equal to $K_A (1 + [D]/K)$, where K_A is the dissociation constant of the antagonist-receptor complex, so that,

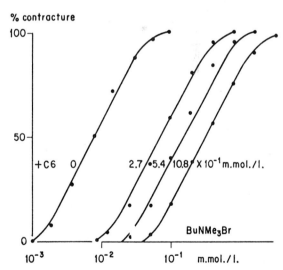

FIGURE 1-8   Experimental dose-response curves for combinations of several constant concentrations of hexamethonium (C_6) with varying concentrations of $BuN+Me_3 \cdot Br^-$.

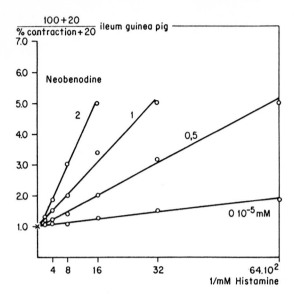

FIGURE 1-9 Double-reciprocal plots for the combination of several constant concentrations of a histamine antagonist with varying concentrations of histamine.

knowing the drug concentration and having determined K from Eq. (6) or from a Scatchard plot, we can also determine K_A.

Note that when the drug is a cation and the receptor the conjugate base of an acid, hydrogen ions will play the role of a competitive antagonist since they have finite affinity—expressed in the ionization constant of the receptor acid—for the same receptor with which the agonist associates. Figure 1-10 illustrates the validity of the theory applied to histamine as the drug.

Competitive antagonism is not the only way for the receptor pool to decrease. With many drugs it is observed that on repeated administration their effect diminishes. This phenomenon, to be discussed in some of the later chapters, has various names, such as drug resistance, tolerance, and tachyphylaxis, and various causes, such as fatigue (i.e., depletion of endogenous substances required for manifestation of the drug effect) and increased rate of biotransformation of the drug. What interests us in the present context is desensitization, interpreted as a change in the conformation of the receptor, which thereby loses its ability to provoke an effect. In recent years evidence has accumulated of a phenomenon termed *down-regulation*: some membrane receptors are removed by the drug from the membrane into the cytosol and later returned to the

membrane. Since the membrane is their locus of action, these receptors are unavailable while in the cytosol. Similarly *up-regulation* can occur by increased synthesis of receptors. In this instance the phenomenon is called sensitization. Note that there may be additional mechanisms of sensitization and desensitization.

When the antagonist is *noncompetitive*, that is, when it does not associate with the same receptor as the agonist does but lowers the intrinsic activity of the agonist instead, the result is a lower maximum effect and a double-reciprocal plot with altered slope and intercept. Figure 1-11 illustrates this phenomenon, papaverine being a noncompetitive antagonist of norepinephrine.

When both drugs are agonists, acting on the same target organ through different receptors (functional interaction), this may be diagnosed by means of isoboles, loci of identical effects of mixtures of the two

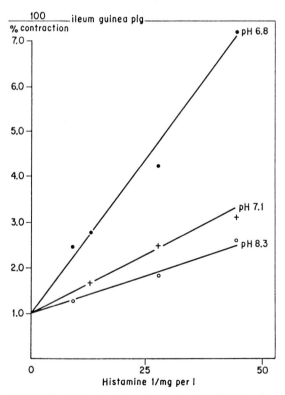

FIGURE 1-10 Double-reciprocal plot of histamine action as a function of pH.

drugs in varying proportions. The theory predicts that in this case the isobole must be hyperbolic. This case is illustrated by Fig. 1-12, the drugs being paredrinol and pentylenetetrazol, both of which act on the heart but by different mechanisms. Note that here the effect of the drug pair is greater than the sum of the separate effects of the component drugs, a phenomenon known as *synergism*, as opposed to additivity, where the total effect is equal to the sum of the separate effects. *Additivity* is observed when both drugs act on the same receptor; the isoboles in this case are linear.

The term *potentiation* is sometimes used as a synonym of synergism. More correctly, it applies to that special case of synergism where one of the two drugs has zero intrinsic activity, that is, where an inactive drug enhances the activity of the other. For example, the analgesic (pain-relieving) action of morphine is enhanced by the simultaneous administration of phenothiazines, which, by themselves, are not analgesic.

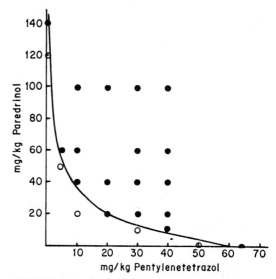

FIGURE 1-12 Isobole of the combination paredrinol and pentylenetetrazol showing synergism. ●=active combination; ○=inactive combination.

The phenomenon of two drugs acting on the same organ through independent receptors, but in opposite directions, is known as *physiologic antagonism*. An example is the drug pair epinephrine-carbamoylcholine. Both are agonists on the heart, but epinephrine accelerates the pulse by stimulating adrenergic receptors in the heart, while carbamoylcholine stimulates cholinergic receptors and slows the heartbeat.

Finally, *chemical antagonism* must be mentioned, in which a drug interferes chemically with another drug (or another poison). An example is a chelating agent used to sequester harmful metal ions, such as ethylenediaminetetraactic acid or dimercaprol in lead poisoning (Chap. 48).

From the point of view of therapy, competitive and physiologic antagonism are probably the most important mechanisms of drug interaction. Atropine, a competitive antagonist of acetylcholine, is widely used to block such parasympathetic actions as nasal and bronchial secretions, bradycardia, and peptic ulcer (Chap. 10); naloxone, a competitive antagonist of morphine, is the standard antidote in cases of morphine poisoning (Chap. 22); and antihistamines are utilized to block allergic conditions caused by the release of histamine from body stores (Chap.12). However, while histamine is also one of the causative agents of asthma, an

% contraction

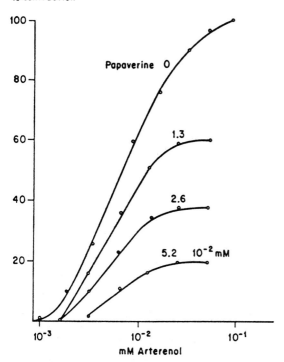

FIGURE 1-11 Experimental dose-response curves demonstrating noncompetitive antagonism of norepinephrine by papaverine.

acute asthmatic attack is better treated with isoproterenol, which dilates bronchioles by stimulating beta-adrenergic receptors while histamine constricts bronchioles by stimulating histamine receptors (see Chap. 8).

Nonspecific Drugs

Finally, drugs must be mentioned that do not act by way of receptors but rather by physical alteration of some essential part of the organism, for instance, cell membranes in the central nervous system. A number of drugs are soluble in the lipid cell membrane and, when so dissolved, inhibit the function of the membrane which is to carry messages by the mechanism known as *conduction*. The drugs that perform in this manner—for example, general anesthetics, sedative-hypnotics, heart muscle-depressant drugs—display no structure-activity relationship; what they have in common is the physical characteristic of solubility in cell membranes, and it has been found that their depressant potency is reasonably well correlated with the thermodynamic concentration c/c_s, where c is the actual concentration of the drug and c_s its saturation concentration (Ferguson's principle). The validity of this correlation is such that often when a series of drugs has equal potency at equal c/c_s, this has been considered as prima facie evidence that the action of those drugs is *nonspecific*, i.e., not mediated by receptors.

While the concept of nonspecific drug action is a useful and valid one, it must be admitted that in some instances a drug which was considered to be nonspecific as a result of new discoveries turns out to have a very specific receptor. An example is local anesthetics, which were considered to act nonspecifically on membranes but now are definitely assigned to interact with the sodium channels in membranes (Chap. 24). There is also the possibility that *lipids* may themselves act as receptors. For example the cholinergic ionophore has a lipid annulus which may have a profound effect on the protein structure.

Regarding the cell membrane as a receptor, there is a hypothesis that general anesthetics act by causing *fluidization* of the membrane, in other words, a transition of the lipid bilayer from a gel to a liquid-crystal form. While there is much indirect evidence of the validity of this hypothesis, including pressure reversal of anesthesia, it cannot be considered to be definitely proven.

The operation of Ferguson's principle leads to some interesting consequences when applied to a homologous series of organic compounds, e.g., aliphatic alcohols. The lowest alcohols (methanol and ethanol) are miscible with water; as we go up in the series, the alcohols become progressively less soluble in water, hence their saturation concentration c_s, decreases. But this means that the equipotent molar concentration c of the members of the series also must decrease on ascending the series, therefore their potency in terms of molar concentration increases. This, however, is only part of the story; it is the thermodynamic activity rather than the concentration of the solute that determines its behavior, and it is known that the activity coefficient decreases as the solute is increasingly different from the solvent. This is certainly true of alcohols in blood as one ascends a homologous series of alcohols. Hence, increasingly greater thermodynamic concentrations of alcohols are needed in order to attain the same thermodynamic activities. Sooner or later a point is reached at which the required absolute concentration is unattainable because it would be greater than the saturation concentration; in other words, from that point (the cutoff point) on all higher alcohols appear to be inactive.

TABLE 1-2 Comparison of the thermodynamic concentrations of normal primary alcohols required for 50 percent depression of the oxygen consumption of guinea pig lung

Alcohol	c/c_s	Relative potency
Methanol	0.071	1
Ethanol	0.085	2.05
Propanol	0.070	8.4
Butanol	0.117	20.6
Pentanol	0.145	72.6
Hexanol	0.208	210
Heptanol	0.497	252
Octanol		0

Source   H. P. Rang, *Br. J. Pharmacol.*, **15**:185–200 (1960).

Both of these conclusions, the apparent increasing potency and sudden cutoff of activity on ascending a homologous series, are borne out by experience; an example is shown in Table 1-2. The theory, therefore, appears to be as firmly based on the facts for nonspecific as for specific (receptor-requiring) drugs.

BIBLIOGRAPHY

DiPalma, J. R. (ed.): *Drill's Pharmacology in Medicine*, 4th ed., McGraw-Hill, New York, 1971.

Julius, D., MacDermott, A. B., Axel, R., Jessell, T. M.: "Molecular Characterization of a Functional cDNA Encoding the Serotonin IC Receptor," *Science*, **241**:558–564 (1988).

Kenakin, T. P.: *Pharmacologic Analysis of Drug-Receptor Interaction*, Raven Press, New York, 1987.

Kenakin, T. P.: "The Classification of Drugs and Drug Receptors in Isolated Tissues," *Pharmacol. Rev.*, **36**:122–165 (1984).

Leslie, F. M.: "Methods Used in the Study of Opioid Receptors," *Pharmacol. Rev.*, **39**:197–249 (1987).

Nogrady, T.: *Medicinal Chemistry, A Biochemical Approach*, 2d ed., Oxford University Press, New York, 1988.

C H A P T E R   **2**

Molecular Models of Receptors and Transduction Mechanisms

Peter G. Bradford

With few exceptions, the therapeutic benefit of drugs derives from their interaction with specific receptors within their target tissues. The binding of a drug to its receptor initiates or in some cases inhibits a series of biochemical reactions, which in sum account for the pharmacodynamic actions of the drug. In this context drug receptors may be broadly considered as to include not only classic hormone and neurotransmitter receptor proteins but also voltage-gated ion channels as well as many regulatory enzymes, which are the locus of action of specific drugs. The concept of a high-affinity molecular interaction of a drug with a target receptor is grounded in experimental observation and forms the centerpiece for current and future drug development. This chapter focuses on a molecular analysis of receptors, emphasizing common structural themes and mechanisms of receptor signal transduction. In this analysis the contributions of gene cloning and heterologous expression of receptor proteins to our current understanding of drug receptors are stressed, since these technologies constitute a promising new paradigm of drug development.

HISTORICAL PERSPECTIVE

Observations by Paul Ehrlich made more than a century ago established that pharmacologic agents must bind to their targets in order to be effective. In explaining the toxicity of certain arsenical compounds against strains of trypanosomes, Ehrlich noted that the effective congeners of a chemical series contained substituent domains that allowed their binding to the tar-

get cell. Ehrlich cited widespread evidence for this principle of fixation in antimicrobial chemotherapy and concluded that the parasite binding actions of drugs involved chemical connections of a specific nature and that these connections were essential for their parasiticidal activity. Although these observations supported the idea of specific receptors as the mediators of drug action, the nomenclature of a receptor was not used. The terminology of receptor or receptive substance was first used by J. N. Langley of Cambridge University, a contemporary of Ehrlich. Langley found that the chemical stimulation of frog gastrocnemius muscle by nicotine could be blocked by curare, the South American arrow poison. Likewise, the contractile response to electrical stimulation of the motor nerve was blocked by curare. However, direct electrical stimulation of the muscle could bypass the blockade, indicating that nicotine and curare act antagonistically at a common site or receptor that was neither nerve nor muscle. This receptor acted like a switch, enabling the chemical information of the neurohumor to be transduced into an active response within the muscle.

The realization that drug molecules interact specifically and reversibly with a small number of receptor sites in target tissues allowed the application of the law of mass action to drug dose-response relationships as originally proposed in the 1930s by A. J. Clark. With this approach the behavior of ligands and receptors was described in mathematical terms. These analyses have been applied almost universally in the study of drug receptors. A thorough discussion of the quantitative aspect of drug-receptor interaction stemming from the application of the law of mass action has been covered in Chap. 1. This quantitative approach has allowed a characterization of drugs within definitive classes and provided a means of categorizing individual receptors within larger families. Thus the concept that catecholamines regulate physiologic processes by their interaction with discrete cellular receptors enabled Ahlquist to classify these receptors as α- and β-adrenergic receptors. Vasoconstriction and other processes mediated by α-adrenergic receptors were activated by agonists in a relative potency order of epinephrine > norepinephrine > isoproterenol, whereas vasodilatation, myocardial excitation, and other responses defined as being mediated by β-adrenergic receptors had the rank order of isoproterenol > epinephrine > norepinephrine. Characterizations of other receptor subtypes have been made similarly based on end organ responses. However, with the advent of subcellular and molecular methods to assess the pharmacodynamic effects of drugs, receptor types have now been further defined and in some cases redefined in molecular terms. It is hoped that more selective new pharmaceuticals can be developed through such molecular studies of receptor proteins.

MECHANISMS OF RECEPTOR SIGNAL TRANSDUCTION

Receptors for both endogenous humoral substances and exogenous drugs can be catagorized into general classes based on the molecular mechanisms by which the receptors transduce signals. At least four distinct classes of receptors are identified on this basis: ion channel receptors, receptors linked to effector enzymes via guanine nucleotide binding proteins (G proteins), receptors with intrinsic tyrosine protein kinase activity, and receptors for steroid hormones. The activities of the first three types of receptors transduce information delivered extracellularly at the plasma membrane into ionic or biochemical signals within the cell, whereas the last receptor type is associated with the nuclear matrix and is activated by steroid hormones which permeate cells. Activated steroid hormone receptors interact with target DNA sequences and enhance genetic transcription. Within each class of signal transduction mechanism, individual receptor proteins conform to specific structural motifs.

ION CHANNEL RECEPTORS

The mechanism of action of several hormones and neurotransmitters is attributed directly to enhanced movement of ions across the plasma membrane. In some cases the hormone or neurotransmitter receptor is itself an ion channel. These systems are referred to as *ion channel receptors*. Included in this superfamily of receptors and considered here are the nicotinic acetylcholine receptor (nAChR), the $GABA_A$ receptor ($GABA_AR$), the glycine receptor (GlyR), and the glutamate receptors (GluRs) (Table 2-1). By and large these signaling systems are confined to excitable tissue of the central nervous system, the autonomic ganglia, and the neuromuscular junction. The ion channel receptors are activated by agonists on a millisecond time

TABLE 2-1   Characteristics of ion channel receptors

Receptor	Ion selectivity	Subunit structure (M_r)
Nicotinic ACh	Na, K (depolarize)	$\alpha_2\beta\gamma\delta$ (50, 55, 56, 57 kDa)
$GABA_A$	Cl (hyperpolarize)	$\alpha_2\beta_2$ (49, 51 kDa)
Glycine	Cl (hyperpolarize)	$\alpha_2\beta_2\gamma(?)$ (48, 58, 93 kDa)
Glutamate		
NMDA	Na, K, Ca (LT potentiation)	?
Quisqualate	Na, K (depolarize)	?
Kainate	Na, K (depolarize)	?

scale, and the resultant ion movements serve either to depolarize or hyperpolarize the electric charge across the membranes of postsynaptic neurons and muscle cells. As a class these receptor systems are involved in the rapid propagation of electric impulses and the transfer of information across synapses throughout the nervous system.

On a molecular level the ion channel receptors show marked similarity. All are multimeric proteins arranged across the membrane to contain an anion- or cation-selective channel whose conductivity is controlled by agonist binding to specific extracellular receptor sites. These receptor proteins have a common molecular mass of 250 to 300 kDa. Each receptor is composed of several nonidentical subunits of 50 to 60 kDa, or approximately 450 to 500 amino acid residues. The overall structure of the ion channel receptors, based on electron microscopy of the purified nAChR complex, indicates that these proteins are composed of multiple subunits arranged in a rosette around a central core of low election density, which forms the ion channel through the membrane (Fig. 2-1).

The primary structures of these receptor polypeptides have been deduced from the cloned complementary DNA sequences. The complete subunit sequences of the nAChR, the $GABA_A R$, and the GlyR have been determined, and all show a striking homology. This homology suggests that there are important structural features necessary to accommodate the function of a ligand-gated ion channel. The similarities among the gene sequences encoding the receptor subunits also indicate a common evolutionary origin and substantiate the identification of ion channel receptors as a superfamily of proteins.

The deduced amino acid sequence of the protein subunits includes a large extracellular N-terminal domain as well as four hydrophobic, α-helical domains (M1 to M4), each of which is predicted to span the plasma membrane. The ion channel receptor is composed of four or five of these similar subunits. Common features of the extracellular domain of each subunit are its length, invariably about 220 to 230 amino acids, the existence of multiple N-glycosylation sites, and the occurrence of a β-structural loop, which is formed by disulfide bonding between two conserved cysteine residues. This loop contains invariant amino acid residues and a conserved glycosylation site. This loop structure is found in the strychnine-binding subunit of the GlyR, in both the α and β subunits of the

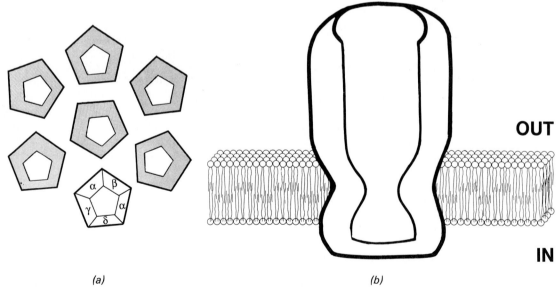

(a)   (b)

FIGURE 2-1   Schematic representations of ion channel receptors based upon high-resolution electron microscopy of the nicotinic acetylcholine receptor of electric ray, *Torpedo marmorata* [Toyoshima and Unwin, *Nature*, **336**:247 (1988)]. (*a*) Topographical image of the cytoplasmic face. (*b*) Axial section.

GABA$_A$R, and in all the known (20) subunits of the various nAChRs. The function of this highly conserved structural region is unknown, although it has been hypothesized to be involved in some stereotypical way either in the binding of agonist or in the intramolecular transduction of that signal. The second conserved structural feature among this class of receptors is the series of four hydrophobic segments (M1 to M4) common to all receptor subunits. Each segment is 20 to 26 amino acid residues long and adopts an energetically favorable α helix, which spans the width of the membrane. These segments orient with each other and with segments from other subunits to form the ion-selective channel through the membrane. The M2 segments are amphipathic; the hydrophobic side aligns with other hydrophobic segments, and the hydrophilic side lines the central channel rendering it conducive to ion flow. Despite these findings the precise molecular workings of the ion channel receptors in accommodating rapid synaptic transmission are not known.

Nicotinic Acetylcholine Receptor

The best studied of the ion channels receptors is the nicotinic acetylcholine receptor. This receptor mediates the action of acetylcholine at excitable synapses in all ganglia, both sympathetic and parasympathetic, at the neuromuscular junction, and at sites in the central nervous system. Activation of the nAChR depolarizes excitable membranes by increasing the permeability of the ion channel to sodium primarily but also to potassium. The ganglionic and neuromuscular nAChRs differ in their pharmacology, suggesting that they are distinct proteins. For example, nondepolarizing neuromuscular blocking drugs have variable effects in producing ganglionic blockade. Tubocurarine will block at both sites but acts predominantly as a true acetylcholine antagonist at the muscle nicotinic receptor and largely by noncompetitive channel blockade in the mammalian ganglia. Furthermore, α-bungarotoxin blocks the muscle receptor nearly irreversibly, whereas most neuronal receptors are unaffected.

Isolation of the nicotinic acetylcholine receptor was aided greatly by the use of α-bungarotoxin and other snake venom toxins, which bind selectively and with high affinity to the receptor. Equally important toward the ultimate purification of the protein was the use of the receptor-rich electric organs of the electric fish *Torpedo californica* and the electric eel *Electropho-rus electricus*. The electrocytes of these electric organs are derived ontogenetically from muscle cells, and it is not surprising, therefore, that the *T. californica* nAChR very much resembles that of the mammalian neuromuscular junction. The purified receptor has a pentameric structure composed of four distinct subunits with an $\alpha_2\beta\gamma\delta$ stoichiometry. Reconstitution studies in lipid vesicles and planar lipid bilayers show that agonist-controlled ion channel activity is wholly contained in this purified multimeric receptor complex. The subunits are of molecular masses ranging form 50 to 58 kDa and are arranged in the membrane in a quasi-fivefold symmetry surrounding a central channel. The receptor contains two acetylcholine binding sites that are important in both regulation of ion conduction and desensitization in response to agonist. The desensitization process is unusual in that it appears to be an intrinsic property of the receptor complex since it also can be demonstrated after reconstitution of the purified protein. The agonist binding sites are contained at least in part by the α subunits, since a competitive antagonist that can be photoactivated labels cysteines 192 and 193 of the α-subunit following irradiation. Similarly, noncompetitive blockers that can be photoactivated and that act by plugging the open ion channel have been used to label those subunit regions that form the channel. With these blockers photoirradiation labeled all four subunits. The labeled residues in each of the subunits were confined to the M2 hydrophobic α helices confirming that these regions are involved in agonist-stimulated ion conduction. When incorporated into lipid bilayers, synthetic 23 amino acid peptides that mimic the M2 segment of the *T. californica* delta subunit reconstitute discrete ion conductance. Energetic considerations indicate that an aggregate of five of these peptides forms the ion channel.

Comparison of the *T. californica* receptor genes with those encoding the acetylcholine receptor of the neuromuscular junction in several avian and mammalian species including human shows that these proteins are highly homologous. Overall similarities in sequence are seen even between unpaired subunits indicating that gene duplication was important in the evolution of nAChRs. An unusually high sequence homology (> 80 percent) is seen among the α subunits of the various species, stressing the importance of this subunit to receptor function. Greater sequence differences are seen between the receptors of the skeletal muscle end plate and of the postsynaptic neurons of autonomic ganglia in the same species. As indicated above, these receptors show pharmacologic differences as well.

Cloning studies and recombinant DNA techniques support the existence of a family of at least five members of mammalian nAChR proteins. Two types are found in muscle, and three others are in neuronal tissue. Muscle cells make both fetal and adult forms of the receptor, which differ in structure and in channel conductance. The ganglionic nAChR appears to differ from the muscle cell types and also from forms identified in the brain. In the brain, unique α-subunit clones identified two different mRNA molecules that encode proteins distinct from those found in muscle or ganglia. The physiology and pharmacology of these central nAChRs are unknown.

GABA$_A$ Receptor

γ-Aminobutyric acid (GABA) is the major inhibitory neurotransmitter in the mammalian brain. GABA-mediated neuronal hyperpolarization results from increased membrane chloride conductance and is attributed to the activation of an integral chloride channel. This chloride channel contains a specific GABA binding site and is the GABA$_A$ receptor. Less well characterized GABA$_B$ receptors exist, which have a pharmacology distinct from the GABA$_A$ receptor and may be coupled indirectly to cation-selective channels. GABA$_A$ receptors have binding sites for several pharmacologic agents which act allosterically to modulate chloride ion conduction. Benzodiazepines bind with high affinity to the receptor and increase GABA-stimulated ion current by increasing the frequency of channel opening. Barbiturates like pentobarbital and phenobarbital bind to a different site on the receptor and increase the mean open time of the chloride channel. The potentiation of GABA-mediated neuronal hyperpolarization by these drugs offers a compelling molecular explanation for their anxiolytic and depressant activites. The GABA binding site on the receptor recognizes other agonists like muscimol as well as competitive antagonists such as bicuculline. Certain convulsant drugs including picrotoxin bind to the GABA$_A$ receptor and inhibit chloride conductance either by direct channel block or by binding to a closely adjacent site which facilitates channel closure. Therapeutic advantages of these latter compounds have not yet been identified.

The GABA$_A$ receptor conforms to the superfamily of ligand-gated ion channels. The purified receptor is composed of two distinct but similarly sized glycoprotein subunits, and α subunit (M_r 53 kDa) and a β-subunit (M_r 58 kDa). Based on an overall molecular size of 230 kDa, the proposed GABA$_A$ receptor is a heterologous tetramer with stoichiometry $\alpha_2\beta_2$. The amino acid sequences of the receptor subunits have been deduced from full-length cDNA clones. The α-subunit clone has a coding region for 429 amino acids (M_r 48.8 kDa) and the β-subunit clone encodes 449 amino acids (M_r 51.4 kDa). The sequences and hydrophobicity patterns indicate a remarkable similarity of the subunits with extended regions showing greater than 60 percent homology. Expression of both the α- and β-subunit-specific mRNAs in *Xenopus laevis* oocytes is necessary and sufficient to reconstitute potent GABA-stimulated chloride conduction. Like the native ion channel, the conduction of the reconstituted channel is potentiated by chlorazepate and pentobarbital and is inhibited by bicuculline and picrotoxin. The structural and functional similarities of the receptor subunits are indicated by their individual expression in oocytes. When oocytes are injected singly with either α-subunit or β-subunit mRNA, GABA stimulates a normal chloride current which is increased by benzodiazepines and barbiturates. However, these responses require 100-fold greater GABA concentrations compared with those of eggs injected dually with both subunit mRNAs. Thus, both α and β subunits may recognize GABA, but the coordinate expression of both subunits is required for high-affinity agonist binding.

The GABA receptor protein subunits resemble each other and also the subunits of the nicotinic acetylcholine and glycine receptors. For example, overall sequence identity of the bovine GABA receptor compared with the α subunit of the bovine nicotinic receptor is 18 percent for the α subunit and 15 percent for the β subunit. Both subunits of the GABA receptor have large N-terminal hydrophilic domains containing the stereotypical β-structural loop. The subunits also contain the four hydrophobic α helices, which form the membrane-spanning region of the receptor. The GABA$_A$ receptor is distinctive in that there is a clustering of positively charged basic amino acids at both ends of the membrane-spanning helices. In contrast, these sites in the nAChR are either negatively charged or uncharged. It is likely that these charged regions may be involved in the anion and cation selectivity of the respective channels.

Glycine Receptor

Glycine is the principal inhibitory neurotransmitter in the mammalian spinal cord and brain stem. Like GABA, glycine inhibits neuronal firing by activating a chloride ion conductance which effectively hyperpolarizes excitable membranes. A glycine receptor (GlyR) has been affinity-purified, and when reconstituted in planar lipid bilayers, glycine-dependent ion conductances are observed. The convulsant alkaloid strychnine has been particularly useful in characterizing the pharmacology and molecular biology of the GlyR and its subunits. Strychnine acts as a competitive antagonist of glycine binding and inhibits glycine-mediated but not GABA-mediated chloride conductances. Strychnine binding to synaptic membranes is antagonized selectively by glycine and other GlyR agonists including the amino acids β-alanine and taurine.

The GlyR conforms to the superfamily of ion channel receptors. The affinity-purified GlyR contains three polypeptides; two of them, the 48- and 58-kDa subunits, are glycosylated integral membrane proteins, and the third, a 93-kDa subunit, is a peripheral protein associated with the cytoplasmic portion of the postsynaptic GlyR. The 48- and 58-kDa proteins are similar to each other and constitute the glycine-regulated chloride channel. The role of the 93-kDa protein in glycine-stimulated chloride conductance is not clear. Strychnine photoaffinity labels the 48-kDa subunit and to a lesser extent the 58-kDa subunit. The cloned and sequenced cDNA of the 48-kDa strychnine-binding subunit of the GlyR bears significant similarity to the subunit cDNAs of the nACh and GABA$_A$ receptors. The common structural features of the deduced polypeptides have been mentioned and support the functional similarity of these receptors.

Glutamate Receptors

The glutamate receptors, i. e., the excitatory amino acid receptors, are divided into the three subtypes based on pharmacologic agonist selectivity: the *N*-methyl-D-aspartate (NMDA) receptor, the quisqualate receptor, and the kainate receptor. The quisqualate and kainate receptors mediate conventional Na- and K-ion depolarizing conductances and are responsible for most fast excitatory postsynaptic potentials in the brain and spinal cord. In this way the quisqualate and kainate receptors resemble the nAChRs: receptor activation allows rapid ion flow, immediate depolarization, and sum to give an all-or-none activation of the postsynaptic cell. On the other hand, the NMDA receptor mediates not only monovalent cation but also calcium ion conductances, and these responses require both agonist binding and concurrent membrane depolarization. Depolarization is required because the ion channel is blocked under resting conditions in a voltage-dependent manner by magnesium. NMDA receptors are therefore not directly involved in fast synaptic transmission but in the modulation of postsynaptic neuronal activity. These properties of NMDA receptors support their proposed role in the complex phenomena of neuronal plasticity, long-term potentiation, and learning. Little is known about the molecular structures of the glutamate receptors except that separate genes and mRNAs encode the receptor subtypes. The purification, sequencing, and expression of the encoding mRNAs should indicate whether any or all of the glutamate receptors conform to the superfamily of ion channel receptors.

RECEPTOR-G PROTEIN-EFFECTOR SYSTEM

An emerging pattern of signal transduction involves receptors which activate cellular effector enzymes indirectly via interaction with guanine nucleotide binding proteins, the so-called G proteins. The three components of this transduction paradigm are receptors, G proteins, and effectors. Specific receptors in the plasma membrane recognize and bind ligands including hormones, neurotransmitters, sensory stimuli, and drugs. This signal is transmitted to G proteins on the cytoplasmic face of the membrane and results in the binding of guanosine triphosphate (GTP) to the G protein. Thus activated, the G protein functions as an allosteric regulator of other proteins capable of affecting cell responses.

Receptors Coupled to G Proteins

Dozens of pharmacologically important hormone and neurotransmitter receptors are dependent on G proteins to mediate their actions on cells. Included among these receptors are the adrenergic, muscarinic acetylcholine, serotonergic, and dopaminergic receptors as well as a multitude of peptide receptors. The genomic and deduced amino acid sequences of several of these receptors are now known (Table 2-2). The receptors are all monomeric proteins and the products of single gene transcripts. Analysis of these sequences indicates a remarkably conserved homology among these proteins. The most striking feature of these receptors is the conservation of seven stretches of 20 to 28 hydrophobic amino acids that likely represent membrane-spanning regions. Topographic analysis by high-resolution electron diffraction of the related bacteriorhodopsin indicates that these membrane-spanning regions exist and are arrayed in a bundle of α helices with a single central helix and six surrounding ones. It is likely that all the receptors in this class have

a similar topology. With an extracellular amino terminus and an odd number of transmembrane segments, this arrangement dictates that there are three extracellular connecting loops (EI-EIII), three cytosolic connecting loops (CI-CIII), and an intracellular carboxyl terminus (Figure 2-2).

The extracellular segments of these G-protein-coupled receptors contain sites for glycosylation but otherwise show weak sequence homology. The small intracellular loops (CI, CII) and the first two transmembranous regions exhibit the greatest similarity among the known sequences. It is therefore likely that these regions have less to do with specific properties of individual receptor types and more to do with processes basic to all G-protein-coupled receptors such as maintenance of the stereotypical receptor topography. In contrast, the regions with weakest homology and

TABLE 2-2   Cloned G-protein-coupled receptors

Receptor	AA residues/C-III segment	G protein	Effector
Rhodopsin	348/22	Gt1	cG-PDE
Color opsins	348/22	Gt2	cG-PDE
β-Adrenergic			
β_1	477/78	Gs	+AC
β_2	413/52	Gs	+AC
G21 protein	421/128	?	?
α-Adrenergic			
α_{1B} (muscle)	515/70	Gi4	PLC
α_{2A} (platelet)	450/156	Gil, $\beta\gamma$	−AC
Muscarinic ACh			
M1	460/155	Gi2	PLC
M2 (cardiac)	466/179	Gi3, Gil	K channel, −AC
m3 (neuronal)	479/173	Gil	−AC
m4 (pancreatic)	590/238	Gi4	PLC
Serotonin, 5HT1c	460/77	?	PLC
Substance K	384/32	?	PLC
Angiotensin (*mas*)	325/10	?	PLC

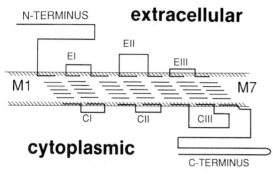

FIGURE 2-2 Schematic representation of G-protein-linked receptors showing hydrophobic helices (M1 to M7) in the membrane, extracellular N terminus and loops (EI-EIII), intracellular C terminus and loops (CI-CIII). [Structure based on Lefkowitz and Caron, *J. Biol. Chem.*, 263:4993 (1988).]

presumably involved in specific discrimination of closely related G proteins include the CIII cytosolic loop and the carboxy terminus. The CIII loop is smallest for the opsins, intermediate in size for the α_1- and β-adrenergic receptors, and largest for the α_2-adrenergic and muscarinic AChRs. Sequences of the C-terminal segments are quite varied although all are highly enriched in serines and threonines. These residues are sites of phosphorylation in the functioning receptors. The β-adrenergic receptors have an apparent insertion in this segment of 50 to 60 amino acid residues which is absent in the other receptors.

Several functional domains of G-protein-linked receptors can be identified in specific structural elements of the proteins. The seventh hydrophobic helix forms a central pocket in the protein structure and constitutes the ligand binding site of these receptors. This holds true for rhodopsin, in which retinal, the light-receptive chromophore, is covalently attached to a lysine residue of the seventh transmembranous segment. Likewise, the agonist and antagonist binding properties of the α_2- and β_2-adrenergic receptors have been localized to this region. Construction and expression of hybrid adrenergic receptor genes in which the stretch containing the EIII loop, the seventh transmembrane region and the C terminus of the β_2-receptor gene, was replaced with the α_2-receptor gene counterpart resulted in a hybrid protein with antagonist binding properties typical of the α_2-adrenergic receptor. An opposite construct with the sixth and seventh transmembranous domains contributed by the β_2-receptor gene conferred β-adrenergic ligand specificites to the hybrid protein. Although no experimental evidence exists, it is likely that the seventh transmembranous region will be important to the ligand binding properties of other G-protein-linked receptors.

The same studies of hybrid adrenergic receptors also showed that the fifth and sixth transmembranous regions and the connecting CIII loop determined whether these receptors could activate the associated G protein and, in turn, adenylate cyclase. The critical residues are in the transmembranous regions and the ten or so amino acids adjacent to these regions, since deletion of the rest of the CIII loop does not impair coupling to adenylate cyclase. Rhodopsin, which has exactly this small size of a CIII loop, is capable of efficiently activating purified preparations of various species of G proteins. Thus, the small CIII loop in rhodopsin and the opsins contains the minimum primary sequence capable of activating G proteins. The larger insertions in this cytoplasmic loop of other receptors may confer some ability to discriminate among the highly homologous G proteins and to affect coupling to distinct effectors.

G Proteins

G proteins are a family of homologous guanine nucleotide binding proteins which transduce signals of hormone receptor activation into stimulation of a series of effector enzymes and ion channels. The G proteins are on the cytoplasmic face of the plasma membrane, thus facilitating interaction with both membrane-bound proteins and soluble components (i.e., guanine nucleotides). The G proteins are heterotrimeric with α subunits (39 to 46 kDa), β subunits (35 to 36 kDa), and γ subunits (8 to 10 kDa). The α subunits bind guanine nucleotides and determine the specificity of receptor-effector coupling. The β and γ subunits form a tightly associated, highly hydrophobic complex and probably hold the more hydrophilic α subunit at the membrane.

The action of G protein involves a cycle of guanine nucleotide binding and hydrolysis. At rest, the G protein has guanosine diphosphate (GDP) bound to the nucleotide binding site of the α subunit. The agonist-occupied hormone receptor interacts with the G protein stimulating it to release GDP and subsequently bind GTP. The receptor-G protein complex dissociates at this point, releasing the $\beta\gamma$ complex and free α subunit with bound GTP. Free α-GTP directly regulates effector systems until an intrinsic GTPase activity converts bound GTP to GDP. The α-GDP unit reassociates with $\beta\gamma$, and the G protein complex is then available for another receptor-stimulated activation cycle. This scheme dictates that specificity for receptor-effector coupling lies within the nature of the α subunit. Indeed, there are 10 different classes of α subunits but only two highly related (90 percent amino acid identity) β subunits. Less is known of the smaller γ subunits.

All the α subunit classes have 350 to 400 amino acid residues. Sequence homologies are greatest in several regions which in the folded protein form the guanine nucleotide binding site (Fig. 2-3). Outside these regions variabilities exist and are concentrated in three "hot spots": at the amino terminus, in residues 120 to 150, and near the carboxy terminus. These regions likely encode specificity for receptor-G-protein and G-protein-effector interactions.

G proteins were initially distinguished for their functional interactions: transducin (Gt), which couples rhodopsin activation to cGMP phosphodiesterase

in retinal rods, and the G proteins (Gs and Gi), which mediated stimulation and inhibition of adenylate cyclase, respectively. Subsequently, a distinct, "other" G protein (Go) was isolated from brain, and several Gi-related proteins were identified that couple to effector systems other than adenylate cyclase. In not all cases have G proteins been unambiguously assigned to specific receptors and effectors. In some instances, it appears that a single G protein may couple to multiple effector systems, some systems being more potently activated than others.

A common property among G-protein α subunits is their susceptibility to covalent modification by specific bacterial toxins. Cholera toxin catalyzes the ADP-ribosylation of an arginine residue of Gs α, resulting in the inhibition of intrinsic GTPase activity and in the persistent activation of adenylate cyclase. This ADP-ribosylation site is in a highly conserved region of the G-protein α subunits; however, other α subunit types are either poor substrates or functionally unaffected by this modification. Pertussis toxin catalyzes the ADP-ribosylation of a cysteine residue which is located four amino acids residues from the α subunit carboxy terminus. All the known α subunits are substrates for this

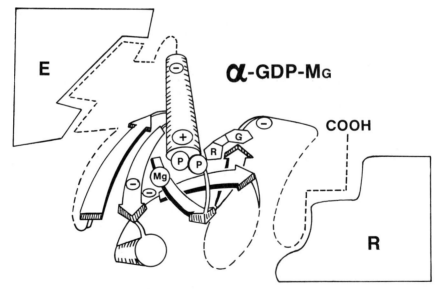

FIGURE 2-3   Schematic representation of G protein α subunit based on the x-ray crystallographic structure of *Escherichia coli* elongation factor Tu [F. Jurnak, *Science*, **230**:32 (1985)] as interpreted [H. Bourne, *Nature*, **321**:914 (1986)]. Cartoon shows the guanine nucleotide binding site, the receptor coupling region (R), and the effector coupling region (E).

toxin, except for $\alpha i4$, which lacks the susceptible cysteine residue, and αs, which has a tyrosine at this site. ADP-ribosylation by pertussis toxin blocks interactions between receptors and G proteins, thus inhibiting effector activities linked to these systems. This suggests that the *C*-terminal domain of G proteins is involved in receptor contacts. Support for this idea is seen in the *unc* mutant of the mouse S49 lymphoma cell line in which Gs cannot be activated by hormone receptors. The *unc* mutation encodes a variant αs with a single amino acid change six residues from the polypeptide carboxy terminus.

Effector Systems

Compared to the receptors and G proteins in this signal transduction class, the effector proteins are poorly characterized. The most thoroughly studied effector protein is adenylate cyclase. Enzymatic activity converts ATP to cyclic AMP. The rise in cyclic AMP levels and the resultant activation of cyclic AMP-dependent protein kinase initiate a cascade of substrate phosphorylations which adequately account for the cellular effects of cyclase-dependent hormones. Adenylate cyclase is stimulated and inhibited by distinct classes of G proteins. The GTP-liganded α subunit of Gs directly stimulates the enzyme. The inhibitory effect of activated Gi is less clear. There are indications that αi-GTP may be directly inhibitory, or alternatively the freed $\beta\alpha$ complex may accelerate the reassociation of any αs and thus remove the stimulatory influence on adenylate cyclase. Both mechanisms may be operative in this system and in other systems of G-protein-dependent functions. Effector systems under the control of G-protein-linked receptors are summarized in Table 2-3.

RECEPTOR TYROSINE KINASES

A third general mechanism by which signals are transduced at the plasma membrane involves receptors with intrinsic tyrosine-specific protein kinase activity. This pattern of signal transduction is evident in a number of receptors for growth factors and growth promoting hormones. Included in this class are the receptors for epidermal growth factor (EGF), insulin, macrophage colony stimulating factor (CSF-1), platelet derived growth factor (PDGF), and insulinlike growth factor

TABLE 2-3   G-protein-regulated effector system

Effector system	Proposed G protein
Adenylate cyclase (stimulation)	Gs
Adenylate cyclase (inhibition)	Gil,$\beta\gamma$?
cGMP-specific phosphodiesterase	Gtl,Gt2
PI-specific phospholipase C	Gi2,Gi4
PC, PE-specific phospholipase C	p21-ras?
Phospholipase A_2	?
Na/H antiporter	Gi?
K channel (atrial)	Gi3,$\beta\gamma$?
Ca channels (neuronal, inhibition)	Go?
Ca channels (vascular, stimulation)	?

(IGF-1). In addition to these receptors, analysis of viral oncogenes and their cellular homologs indicate that the *fms* oncogene, the *c-kit* gene, and the *neu* protooncogene encode membrane proteins with intrinsic tyrosine-specific protein kinase activity.

Structure

Analyses of cDNAs encoding receptor tyrosine kinases reveal a common structural organization. The deduced amino acid primary structure includes an amino terminal signal peptide and a single stretch of hydrophobic residues midway in the sequence. This dictates a protein structure with an extracellular amino terminal domain, a single transmembranous region, and an intracellular carboxy terminal domain (Fig. 2-4). The ligand-binding sites in all these receptors are in the extracellular region, whereas the tyrosine kinase domain is intracellular. Beyond this overall structural similarity, the receptors are grouped into three subclasses based on closer sequence specifics. Receptors of subclass I are characterized by two or three extracellular clusters of cysteine-rich regions and an uninterrupted intracellular tyrosine kinase domain. Subclass

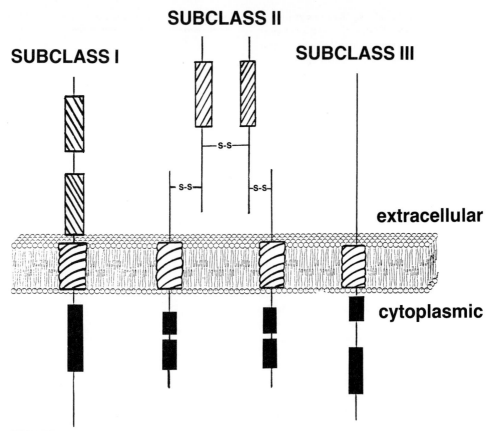

FIGURE 2-4   Schematic models of the structural subclasses of the receptor tyrosine kinase superfamily. Extracellular cysteine-rich domains are indicated by hatched areas. Tyrosine kinase domains are indicated by blackened boxed regions.

II receptors are heterotetrameric proteins with two extracellular α subunits disulfide-linked to two β subunits which traverse the membrane. The α and β subunits are encoded in a single gene which is transcribed and translated into a precursor protein that is glycosylated, dimerized, and then proteolytically processed to yield the mature receptor. Each α subunit contains a single cysteine-rich cluster, and each β subunit has an intact tyrosine kinase domain. Subclass III receptors are single polypeptides which lack extracellular cysteine clusters and have an interrupted cytoplasmic kinase domain. A 70 to 100 amino acid-long insertion in the catalytic domain separates the ATP-binding region from the major tyrosine acceptor site. The insertion shows no homology among receptors but is conserved among species. Known examples of each subclass of receptor tyrosine kinase are listed in Table 2-4.

Function

Receptor tyrosine kinases are critical proteins in the control of cell growth and differentiation. The activation of receptor tyrosine kinases induces a pleiotropic cellular response with both early and late events. Within minutes after agonist binding several events occur: the receptor undergoes autophosphorylation on specific tyrosine residues, there is an increase in tyrosine-specific phosphorylations on cytosolic substrates,

TABLE 2-4   Receptor tyrosine kinase family

Subclass I

Receptors (M_r): EGF (170 kDa), *HER2/neu* (138 kDa)
Characteristics: Single polypeptide chain
Two extracellular cysteine-rich regions
Uninterrupted tyrosine kinase domain

Subclass II

Receptors (M_r): Insulin (α,β: 135 kDa, 90 kDa),
IGF-1 (α,β: 135 kDa, 90 kDa)
Characteristics: Heterotetrameric structure ($\alpha_2\beta_2$)
One extracellular cysteine-rich region
Uninterrupted tyrosine kinase domain

Subclass III

Receptors (M_r): PDGF (180 kDa), CSF-1 (165 kDa), *c-kit*
Characteristics: Single polypeptide chain
No cysteine clusters
70–100 amino acid insertion in tyrosine kinase domain

and there is activation of cellular protein kinases and an enhanced transport of ions and nutrients across the plasma membrane. At a delayed time there is increased polyamine synthesis, an activation of ribosomes, and increased synthesis of protein, RNA, and DNA. Eventually, progression through the cell cycle may be seen. The mechanisms by which agonists stimulate receptor autophosphorylation and induce the myriad of associated metabolic events are uncertain. However, receptor autophosphorylation is critical to the induction of these events, since mutant receptors that do not bind ATP or that have altered autophosphorylation site are unable to stimulate typical metabolic responses. The molecular basis of agonist-induced autophosphorylation is difficult to envision for receptors whose extracellular and intracellular domains are connected by a single hydrophobic helix through the membrane. It is possible that a push-pull mechanism is operative or, alternatively, the response may require receptor dimerization. Aggregation can stimulate tyrosine kinase activity of the insulin receptor. In this regard it is significant that subclass II receptors are dimers, EGF receptors may dimerize during activation, and many polypeptide growth factors including PDGF are dimers.

The importance of this receptor family to normal growth and development is indicated by the great number of oncogenic viral analogs of these proteins. Thus a focus of cancer therapy is directed toward developing specific drugs which are inhibitors of tyrosine-specific protein kinases. Since this kinase activity is necessary for signal transduction of many growth factor receptors and their oncogenic analogs, its inhibition may slow down or stop tumor growth.

STEROID HORMONE RECEPTORS

Steroid hormones are important in the regulation of diverse developmental and homeostatic processes. These hormonal effects require increases in genetic transcription and protein synthesis. The mechanism of action of steroid hormones is attributable to their penetration into cells and their high affinity binding to intracellular receptors. The binding induces a structural change in the receptor, which facilitates its association with specific chromatin regions in the nucleus. These nuclear acceptor sites contain specific cis-acting nucleic acid regulatory sequences, which are upstream of inducible genes. Thus the interaction of the steroid-receptor complex with the 5'-flanking region of transcriptional initiation sites facilitates the binding of RNA polymerase and the expression of regulated genes.

The steroid hormone receptors are proteins associated with the nuclear matrix. In the absence of hormone this association is of low affinity, and upon cell homogenization the receptor species is recovered in the soluble fraction. Hormone binding allosterically alters the receptor so that it binds with high affinity to the nuclear acceptor sites. The availability of radiolabeled high-affinity steroid hormone analogs has allowed the purification, cDNA cloning, and ultimate sequencing of several of the steroid receptors. Included among these proteins are the human receptors for estrogen, glucocorticoids, progesterone, and 1,25-dihydroxy-vitamin D_3. Analysis of other cDNA sequences showed that the *v-erb-A* oncogene product of the avian erythroblastosis virus shows homology with the steroid receptors. Human *c-erb-A*, the cellular counterpart of the viral oncogene, encodes a receptor

for thyroid hormone. Thus the T3/T4 receptor must be considered in the superfamily of steroid hormone receptors.

Structure

There are several structural similarities and differences among the steroid hormone receptors, which are revealed by analysis of the corresponding cDNA sequences (Fig. 2-5). The proteins are single polypeptides which vary in size from 50 to 60 kDa for the vitamin D_3 and thyroid hormone receptors up to 90 to 100 kDa for the glucocorticoid and progesterone receptors. The estrogen receptor is intermediate in size at 65 kDa. These differences are contained solely in the variably sized amino termini. The function of this region is unknown. Adjacent to the amino terminus is the region of greatest identity. This includes a hydrophilic domain of 70 or so amino acids enriched in cysteine, lysine, and arginine residues. The positions of the nine cysteines are absolutely conserved among the receptors, suggesting a common functional role. Downstream from this region, and following an intervening nonconserved "hinge" area of 150 amino acids, is a second conserved region showing about 25 percent absolute identity among the receptors. This is followed by a more variable *C*-terminal region.

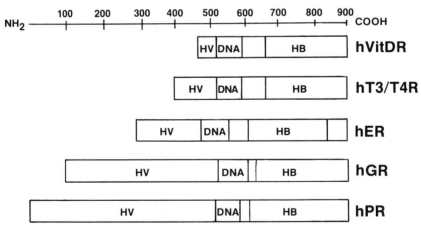

FIGURE 2-5 Representation of the domains of steroid and thyroid hormone receptors. Scale indicates length in amino acid residues. Indicated regions are the hypervariable (HV), DNA-binding (DNA), and hormone-binding (HB) domains. hVitDR = human vitamin D_3 receptor; hT3/T4r = human thyroid hormone receptor; hER = human estrogen receptor; hGR = human glucocorticoid receptor; hPR = human progesterone receptor.

Function

The DNA-binding function of the steroid hormone receptors is attributable to the highly conserved short 70-amino acid segment. This hydrophilic region is likely to be exposed on the receptor surface, and being rich in positively charged amino acid residues facilitates its binding to DNA. The secondary structure of this region is predicted to form two zinc-dependent "fingers," which are typical DNA binding motifs and are analogous to those found in certain transcriptional factors. A mutational change of a single amino acid in this region of the murine glucocorticoid receptor abolishes the nuclear association and function of the protein. The DNA-binding region of the steroid receptors recognizes a specific consensus oligogonucleotide sequence found in the 5'-flanking regions of transcriptional start sites.

A second common feature of steroid hormone receptors is the highly hydrophobic C-terminal region containing approximately 200 amino acid residues. Mutational analysis of this region indicates that it is the ligand binding domain. Among the known sequences, the lowest homology is with the *c-erb-A* gene product, the thyroid hormone receptor, which is consistent with the nonsteroid nature of the receptor agonist. The ligand-binding domain exerts a negative control on the upstream DNA-binding region. Receptor constructs in which the ligand-binding domain has been deleted are constitutively active in promoting transcription. Consideration of these structural and functional similarities among the steroid and thyroid hormone receptors allows them to be classified as regulatory elements of genetic transcription.

PROSPECTUS

Once the concept of drug receptors was established, it became apparent that these receptors could be classified on the basis of the variable effects of a series of agonists or antagonists. Thus, the cholinergic receptor systems can be subdivided into those whose actions are mimicked by the alkaloid muscarine and those mimicked by nicotine. Hence, the effects of acetylcholine are mediated by either muscarinic or nicotinic acetylcholine receptors. In another example, β-adrenergic receptors are defined as either β_1 or β_2 based on the relative affinities of epinephrine and norepinephrine. Similar distinctions within other receptor systems have been made based on the selective effects or rank order potencies of agonist or antagonist drugs.

The purification and analysis of the relevant proteins has substantiated the classification of receptor subtypes. Different subtypes are indeed different proteins. This is borne out at the genetic level as well. In fact, the screening of cDNA libraries at various levels of stringency has indicated that the diversity of genes encoding receptors is often greater than the number of recognized pharmacologic subtypes. For example, five distinct muscarinic receptor genes have been identified, whereas there are only two or three distinct pharmacologic subtypes.

Cloning and expression techniques offer the means of developing selective new pharmaceuticals. Specific in vitro-synthesized mRNA encoding receptors can be injected into *Xenopus laevis* oocytes or other expression systems. Each subtype identified from cDNA clones can be expressed individually, and pharmaceuticals can be identified that specifically affect only that subtype. This approach offers the advantage in not only being able to express individual receptor subtypes but also allowing the functional effects on signal transduction to be determined. G-protein coupling, activation of second messenger systems, and electrophysiologic events can all be assessed in this system.

A second approach to drug design is through structural analysis of the receptor site. It is now possible to think about the design of a drug molecule which will bind specifically to the active site as either an agonist or antagonist. Using structural information based on a wide range of biologically active molecules enables us to determine activity in terms of models of intermolecular interaction. The physical chemistry of drug-receptor recognition includes an analysis of hydrogen bonding, electrostatic interactions, van der Waals contact distances, solvent effects, and hydrophobic interactions. With the aid of computers, this information will yield predictions of the appropriate molecular shapes which effective agonists or antagonists must adopt. These approaches should enable chemists to tailor ligands so as to recognize specific subtypes of receptors. Out of these analysis, it is hoped that specific, effective therapeutic agents will be identified.

BIBLIOGRAPHY

Evans, R. M.: "The Steroid and Thyroid Hormone Receptor Superfamily," *Science*, **240**:889 (1988).

Gilman, A. G.: "G Proteins: Transducers of Receptor-Generated Signals," *Ann. Rev. Biochem.*, **56:**615 (1987).

Lefkowitz, R. J., and Caron, M. G.: "Adrenergic Receptors: Models for the Study of Receptors Coupled to Guanine Nucleotide Regulatory Proteins," *J. Biol. Chem.*, **263:**4993 (1988).

Lester, H. A.: "Heterologous Expression of Excitability Proteins: Routes to More Specific Drugs?" *Science*, **241:**1057 (1988).

Limbird, L. E.: *Cell Surface Receptors: A Short Course on Theory and Methods*, Martinus Nijhoff Publishing, Boston, 1986.

Putney, J. W., Jr. (ed.): *Phosphoinositides and Receptor Mechanisms, Receptor Biochemistry and Methodology, vol. 7* (J. C. Venter and L. C. Harrison, series eds.), Alan R. Liss; Inc., New York, 1986.

Strange, P. G.: "The Structure and Mechanism of Neurotransmitter Receptors: Implications for the Structure and Function of the Central Nervous System," *Biochem. J.*, **249:**309 (1988).

Yarden, Y., and Ullrich, A.: "Molecular Analysis of Signal Transduction by Growth Factors," *Biochem.*, **27:**3113 (1988).

Pharmacokinetics

Edward J. Barbieri

It is known that the intensity of the biologic response produced by a drug is related to the concentration of the drug at its site of action. As discussed in the previous chapter, an important factor in determining the magnitude of the response is the dose of drug administered; however, this dictates only the maximum amount of drug that can reach the site of action. The fraction of the dose that actually is attained at the active site(s) in the body is dependent on a multitude of factors, including the route of drug administration and the dosage form. It is advantageous to be able to select a route of administration, dose, and dosage form that place a drug at its site of action in a suitable concentration and maintain this concentration for a desired time. This goal can be attained for a considerable number of therapeutic agents if we understand the physiologic processes that influence drug concentrations throughout the body and the physical and chemical properties of drugs that determine their interactions with these processes.

Some of the physiologic factors that influence the concentration of a drug at its site of action (Fig. 3-1) are as follows: (1) absorption, i.e., the ability of a drug to enter the bloodstream; (2) distribution, i.e., the movement of a drug throughout the body to various tissue sites; (3) biotransformation, i.e., the alteration of the chemical structure of a drug; and (4) excretion, i.e., the ability of the living system to remove a drug and its biotransformation products from its internal environment. These vital biologic processes constitute *pharmacokinetics*, a subspecialty of pharmacology which describes the movement of drugs through the

body, but not their actions or effects. In a more restricted sense, the word *pharmacokinetics* refers to the mathematical analysis of drug absorption, distribution, biotransformation, and excretion and, therefore, is a detailed study of these processes in a quantitative and temporal fashion.

Pharmacodynamics is the study of mechanisms of action, the therapeutic and toxicologic effects of drugs, chemical structure-activity relationships, and many other drug-organism interactions. This discipline relies on and builds upon the subjects of biologic chemistry, physiology, microbiology, immunology, molecular biology, and pathology to both describe and quantitate drug actions and effects.

As shown in Fig. 3-2, the dose-response relationship, which was developed and explained in the previous chapter, can be divided into two parts, pharmacokinetics and pharmacodynamics. Both of these fields have been greatly aided by the development of technologies capable of measuring accurately even very minute quantities of drugs and their metabolites in body fluids and tissues. However, the measurement of drug concentrations in the plasma remains the most useful method of directly assessing pharmacokinetics and forecasting pharmacodynamics. For most drugs, changes in plasma concentrations are indicative of changes that occur at other tissues (including the active site) throughout the body. Analogous to the time-action curve, the time-plasma drug concentration curve (Fig. 3-3) is a useful device for monitoring the pharmacokinetics of a drug in relation to the therapeutic response of the patient. The goals in utilizing phar-

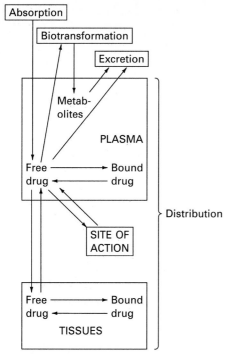

FIGURE 3-1 Factors affecting the concentration of a drug at its site of action.

macrokinetics are to maximize the time that plasma drug concentrations are within the therapeutic range, to minimize the time the drug concentrations are within the ineffective range, and to avoid toxic concentrations. A thorough understanding of the principles of pharmacokinetics provides for greater insight into the action of drugs and leads to more knowledgeable and rational drug selection and prescribing. Furthermore, many important drug-body and drug-drug interactions have been discovered by the application of these principles. This chapter provides the necessary information for a working knowledge of pharmacokinetics.

ABSORPTION

Absorption is the process by which a drug enters the bloodstream without being chemically altered. Various factors influence the rate of absorption, including types of transport, the physicochemical properties of the drug (e.g., lipid solubility, ionization), protein binding, the routes of administration, dosage forms, circulation at the site of absorption, and the concentration of the drug.

An important physiologic factor that determines the

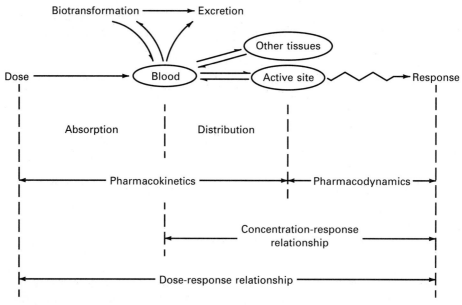

FIGURE 3-2 Interconnections among the dose-response relationship, the concentration-response relationship, pharmacokinetics and pharmacodynamics.

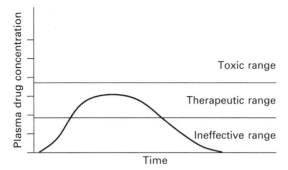

FIGURE 3-3 The time-plasma drug concentration curve showing the ineffective range, therapeutic range, and toxic range for a drug. These ranges are spaced according to arbitrary units of drug concentration for the purpose of illustration.

absorption of a drug, as well as its distribution and elimination, is the membranes that separate the biologic compartments. Electron microscopic studies of tissues suggest that all body membranes are composed of a fundamental structure called the *unit membrane*, or *plasma membrane*. This boundary, which is approximately 8 to 10 nm thick, surrounds single cells such as the erythrocyte, epithelial cell, and neuron, and also subcellular structures such as the mitochondrion and nucleus.

Cellular membranes appear to be composed of a bimolecular layer of phospholipids, with the hydrophilic heads facing the outer surfaces and the hydrocarbon chains pointing toward the interior and creating a continuous hydrophobic band within the membrane. *Integral proteins* (also called *intrinsic proteins*) of varying size appear to be interspersed, either singularly or as composites, in the lipoid matrix. The position of these within the membrane is determined by the distribution of hydrophilic and hydrophobic regions of the protein. Such proteins are found to extend through the entire lipid bilayer and are called *transmembrane proteins*. Other proteins are confined to either surface of the membrane and do not interact with the hydrophobic core of the membrane. These are known as *peripheral proteins* or *extrinsic proteins*.

The unit membrane is considered to be a constantly changing, dynamic structure. Phospholipids in the bilayer have lateral and rotational mobility, which allows the membrane to be flexible, pliable, and readily deformed (termed *fluidity*) while retaining relative impermeability to highly water-soluble compounds.

Intrinsic proteins can function as drug receptors, ionophores, enzymes, and regulatory substances. In addition these proteins may act in transporting drugs across the membrane. Extrinsic proteins appear to function largely as structural components of the membrane, although when associated with intrinsic proteins they may assist these molecules in their specific function.

While lipid-soluble substances penetrate the membrane by dissolving in the lipoid phase, many water-soluble molecules enter only if they are small enough to pass through small aqueous channels or pores. The cell membranes also possess specialized transport processes, and certain large water-soluble molecules, such as sugars and amino acids, can penetrate cells readily by these routes. The diverse ways in which drugs move across membranes can be grouped under two general headings: passive and specialized transport. The major difference between these is that specialized transport involves membrane-associated protein carriers for drugs and passive transport does not.

Passive Transport

Two main types of passive transport are recognized: filtration and simple diffusion. Neither of these processes is saturable, nor can they be inhibited by drugs.

Filtration is the process by which compounds cross membranes by hydrodynamic flow. In this passive process, when a hydrostatic or osmotic pressure difference exists across a membrane, water flows, in bulk, through the membrane pores, carrying with it any solute molecules whose dimensions are less than those of the pores. Solutes with molecular weights greater than 100 to 200 generally do not pass through membrane pores. Since most drugs often exceed this size limitation, they cannot filter through *cell* membranes. Furthermore, the filtration of highly ionized substances may be limited because of attraction to, or repulsion from, ionic charges which are carried on membrane surfaces or within the pores.

Filtration of drugs (by dissolving in the fluid that flows through *intercellular pores*) is the predominant process by which drugs cross most capillary endothelial membranes. With the exception of blood vessels in the central nervous system, where tight cellular junctions are numerous, capillary (and some epithelial) intercellular pores are large enough to permit the passage of most drugs. For example, the water that filters through the relatively large pores of the renal glomerular membrane is accompanied by all the solutes of plasma except the protein molecules.

Most drugs penetrate body membranes by *simple diffusion*; that is, their rate of transfer is directly proportional to their concentration gradient across the membrane. Some of the substances transverse the membrane as though it were a layer of lipoid material, the relative speed of passage being determined by the lipid solubility or, more precisely, the lipid-to-water partition coefficient of the substances. The higher the lipid-to-water partition coefficient, the greater the rate of transfer across the membrane. In contrast, a number of water-soluble (relatively lipid-insoluble) compounds of low molecular weight diffuse across the membrane as though it were a sieve made up of small aqueous channels, the smaller molecules crossing more rapidly than the larger ones. With water-soluble ions, however, the speed of transfer may be determined more by the ionic charge than by the molecular size; for example, in the red blood cell, anions penetrate much more rapidly than cations.

In considering the diffusion of drugs across membranes, it is necessary to take into account that most drugs are weak acids or weak bases which exist in solution as a mixture of the ionized and nonionized forms. This complicates the problem of describing the passage of drugs across a lipoid membrane, since usually only the nonionized species of the compound is sufficiently lipid-soluble and the ionized form of the molecule is too large to pass readily through the membrane channels. Accordingly, the nonionized component of a drug penetrates many cellular membranes at a rate related to its lipid-to-water partition coefficient and its concentration gradient across the membrane, whereas the ionized form penetrates at a very slow rate. This process is sometimes called *nonionic diffusion*.

The proportion of a drug in the nonionized form depends on the dissociation constant of the drug and on the pH of the medium in which it is dissolved, a relationship shown by the Henderson-Hasselbalch equation. Thus for a weak acid we have

$$pK_a = pH + \log \frac{\text{concentration of nonionized acid}}{\text{concentration of ionized acid}}$$

For a weak base:

$$pK_a = pH + \log \frac{\text{concentration of ionized base}}{\text{concentration of nonionized base}}$$

In these equations, the dissociation constant of both acids and bases is expressed as a pK_a, which is the negative logarithm of the acidic dissociation constant. From the equations, it can be determined that phenobarbital, a weak acid with a pK_a of 7.4, is approximately 91 percent ionized at pH 8.4, 50 percent ionized at pH 7.4, and 9 percent ionized at pH 6.4. Quinine, a weak base with a pK_a of 8.4, is about 91 percent ionized at pH 7.4, 50 percent ionized at pH 8.4, and 9 percent ionized at pH 9.4. While most drugs have pK_a values between 3 and 11 and are therefore partly ionized and partly nonionized over the range of physiologic pH values, some compounds are at the extreme ends of the scale. For instance, acetanilide, a weak base with a pK_a of 0.3, is almost completely nonionized at all body pH values. Sulfonic acids, with a pK_a below 1, are almost completely ionized at all pH values. Neutral molecules, e.g., ethanol, are always in the nonionized state, and quaternary compounds such as acetylcholine exist only as cations regardless of pH.

Drugs that penetrate a biologic membrane by simple diffusion become distributed across the membrane according to their degree of ionization, the charge of their ionized form, and the extent to which they are bound to proteins or other macromolecules in the solutions bathing the membrane. A difference in pH on the two sides of a membrane affects the distribution of a partly ionized substance because of the preferential permeability of membranes to the lipid-soluble, nonionized form of compounds. This is illustrated in Fig. 3-4, which shows the distribution of a weak acid ($pK_a = 6$) between solutions of pH 7 and 5; the solutions are separated by a membrane permeable only to the nonionized form of the compound. At equilibrium, the concentration of the nonionized solute is the same in both solutions, but the concentrations of the ionized form are unequal because of the difference in pH of the two fluids. Accordingly, the total concentration of solute (ionized plus nonionized) on both sides of the membrane is a function of the pH of the two fluids and the pK_a of the solute.

Specialized Transport

Although passive transfer across a lipoid boundary adequately describes the penetration of body membranes by most drugs and other foreign organic compounds, it does not explain the rapid penetration and peculiar kinetic behavior of certain large, lipid-insolu-

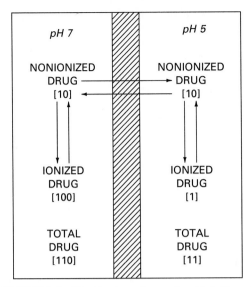

FIGURE 3-4 Distribution of a weak acid (pK_a = 6) between aqueous solutions of pH 7 and pH 5. The solutions are separated by a membrane that is permeable only to the nonionized form of the weak acid. Concentrations at the steady state are shown in brackets.

ble molecules and ions. For example, glucose and a number of other monosaccharides are readily absorbed from the small intestine and renal tubule and penetrate most cells at a rapid rate; moreover, the same is true of the highly ionized amino acids. In addition, a number of sulfonic acid anions and quaternary cations are rapidly transported across cell membranes of the liver, renal tubule, and choroid plexus. Not only are the rates of transport rapid, but in most cases the substances can move across membranes in an "uphill" direction, that is, from a solution of low concentration into one of higher concentration. The concept of membrane *carriers* offers an explanation for the unique permeability of membranes to these substances.

Membrane carriers are viewed as proteinaceous components of the unit membrane, which are capable of combining with a solute at one surface of the membrane. The carrier-solute complex moves across the membrane, the solute is released, and the carrier then returns to the original surface where it can combine with another molecule of solute.

Two main types of carrier-mediated transport are recognized: *active transport* and *facilitated diffusion*. Active transport signifies a process in which (1) the solute crosses the membrane against a concentration gradient, or, if the solute is an ion, it crosses against an electrochemical potential gradient; (2) the transport mechanism becomes saturated at high solute concentrations and thus shows a *transport maximum*; (3) the process is selective for certain ionic or structural configurations; (4) if two compounds are transported by the same mechanism, one will competitively inhibit the transport of the other; (5) the transport process can be inhibited noncompetitively by substances which interfere with cell metabolism. The term *facilitated diffusion* denotes a transport process that shows all the above characteristics except that the solute is *not* transferred against a concentration or electrochemical potential gradient and does *not* require energy.

Proteins and other macromolecules are transported across most membranes slowly, as compared with the rates of transfer of smaller lipid-soluble drugs and carrier-transported substances. A specialized transport process by which these large molecules (usually greater than 1000 daltons) can be transported to the interior of cells is by *pinocytosis*. In this complex process, the cell invaginates a small portion of the cellular membrane and engulfs a droplet of extracellular fluid containing the compound. The droplet becomes completely surrounded by a portion of the membrane, and the resulting vesicle buds off and moves into the cell cytoplasm where the transported compound is released. In many cases pinocytosis is initiated by complexation of the drug to a membrane receptor; it appears that the size and charge of the drug macromolecule are important factors in determining its degree of uptake.

SITES OF ABSORPTION, ROUTES OF ADMINISTRATION, AND DOSAGE FORMS

Alimentary Canal

The alimentary tract is by far the most common site of administration when a drug is intended for systemic action. The dosage forms include tablets, capsules, caplets, specially formulated tablets or capsules for prolonged or repeated action, powders, various flavored or unflavored liquids (syrups, solutions, suspensions, emulsions, tinctures, fluid extracts), and rectal suppositories.

Gastrointestinal Tract The passage of drugs and other foreign compounds across the epithelial lining of the oral cavity, stomach, small intestine, colon, and rectum is explainable, for the most part, in terms of simple diffusion across a lipoid membrane. Drugs in true solution are readily absorbed in their lipid-soluble nonionized forms; the relative rates of absorption are directly related to the lipid-to-water partition coefficients of the molecules.

The stomach is a significant site of absorption for many acidic and neutral compounds but not for basic compounds. For example, acidic drugs like the salicylates and barbiturates, which exist as nonionized lipid-soluble molecules in the acid gastric contents, are readily absorbed, whereas basic drugs like the plant alkaloids, which exist largely as ions, are hardly absorbed at all. In other portions of the alimentary tract where the intraluminal pH is closer to neutrality, many weak acids and bases are, to a considerable extent, nonionized and are absorbed at rates related to their lipid-to-water partition ratios. At all levels of the tract, slowest rates of absorption are found with completely ionized drugs, such as the quaternary ammonium compounds and sulfonic acids, and with lipid-insoluble neutral molecules, such as sulfaguanidine and mannitol. Certain quaternary amines may be absorbed in part in the form of chemical complexes.

The rate of absorption of most drugs is directly proportional to drug concentration in accordance with the process of simple diffusion. If the intraluminal concentration is raised threefold, 3 times as much drug will be absorbed per unit of time, the percentage absorption remaining constant.

The absorption of drugs is increased by changes in pH which increase the fraction of drug in the lipid-soluble nonionized form. For example, raising the gastric pH to 8 with sodium bicarbonate results in a markedly increased rate of absorption for many basic drugs; conversely, the gastric absorption of most acidic compounds is decreased at the elevated pH value. A similar relationship between pH and absorption rate occurs in the mouth, small and large intestines, and rectum.

In the small intestine, weak acids and bases become distributed between intestinal fluid of pH 6.6 and plasma of pH 7.4 (see Fig. 3-4) as though the intestinal pH were 5.3. Thus the pH at the absorption surface appears to be lower than that of the intestinal contents, and it is this lower pH value that may determine the degree of ionization and hence the rate of absorption of weak electrolytes. The colonic and rectal mucosae also show an apparent surface pH somewhat lower than that of the luminal contents.

While most drugs cross the intestinal boundary by a process of simple diffusion, a drug can be absorbed by specialized active transport if its chemical structure is similar enough to that of a substrate which is naturally transported; for example, the antitumor compound 5-fluorouracil is actively transported across the intestine by the process which transports the natural pyrimidines uracil and thymine. Macromolecules are absorbed from the small intestine in trace quantities. Examples include enzymes, food proteins, and bacterial toxins, and the absorption of these occurs via pinocytosis or diffusion through imperfections in the epithelium.

The oral route of administration is the safest, most convenient, and most economical. However, it has a number of disadvantages: (1) irritation to the gastric mucosa with resultant nausea or vomiting; (2) destruction of some drugs by gastric acid or digestive enzymes; (3) precipitation or insolubility of some drugs in gastrointestinal fluids; (4) formation of nonabsorbable complexes between drugs and food materials; (5) variable rates of absorption due to physiologic factors such as gastric emptying time, gastrointestinal motility, and mixing; (6) too slow an absorption rate for effectiveness in an emergency situation; (7) inability to use the oral route in an unconscious patient; and (8) the unpleasant taste of some drugs.

Some of the disadvantages of the oral route can be overcome in various ways. Gastric irritation, as well as the destruction, precipitation, or complexing of drugs in the stomach, can be avoided by using an enteric coated tablet or capsule which resists gastric acid but dissolves in the higher pH range of the intestine or in the presence of intestinal enzymes. In some cases, gastric irritation can be minimized or avoided simply by administering a drug at mealtime or immediately after a meal.

Conversely, for rapid and more complete absorption, some drugs should be taken with the stomach empty; a glass of water should accompany a solid dosage form to dissolve the drug and wash it into the intestine.

Prolonged-action dosage forms for oral administration have been developed with the idea of supplying in one capsule, or tablet, all the drug that will be needed over a period of many hours. For a particular drug, the objective might be to produce quickly a desired plasma concentration of drug and then supply additional drug to maintain this concentration for a number of hours. Or the objective might be to release various doses of one or more drugs at widely spaced intervals. Many names are used to describe these preparations, including *sustained-release*, *timed-release*, *repeat action*, and *long-acting*. A major obstacle to the use of these dosage forms is the high variability of physiologic factors in patients.

An important point to be emphasized in considering absorption after oral administration is that a drug must be dissolved before it can be absorbed. The drug administered in solid form will be absorbed at a rate limited by the rate at which it dissolves in the intestinal fluids. Many factors influence the dissolution rate; these include (1) solubility, particle size, crystalline form, and salt form of the drug; (2) the rate of disintegration of the solid-dosage form in the gastrointestinal lumina; and (3) gastrointestinal pH, motility, and food content.

Oral bioavailability is the measure of the rate and extent of drug absorption through the oral route. A drug is considered to be bioavailable once it reaches the systemic circulation. Therefore, oral bioavailability is decreased by a low rate and extent of absorption through the gastrointestinal mucosa and by biotransformation of the drug during its first passage through the portal circulation of the liver (the so-called *first pass effect* or *presystemic biotransformation*). Bioavailability is discussed in greater detail in the last section of this chapter.

Oral Mucosa Due to the extensive vascularity and relatively thin mucosal surfaces, many drugs are readily absorbed from the oral cavity. The *sublingual* route, in which a small tablet is placed under the tongue and allowed to dissolve, offers a simple, convenient method of administration. Drugs may also be given by the *buccal* route, in which the tablet is placed between the cheek and gingiva. Advantages of these routes include (1) delayed degradation of the drug by avoiding early passage through the liver and (2) avoidance of many of the disadvantages of oral administration. Disadvantages of the sublingual and buccal routes include the unpleasant taste and the local irritating effects of some drugs.

Rectal Mucosa Drugs can be administered rectally, for either local or systemic effect, in the form of suppositories which melt at body temperature. The rectal route is useful when unconsciousness or vomiting preclude use of the oral route. Approximately 50 to 60 percent of a drug dose, administered rectally, is absorbed directly into the general circulation (via the inferior and middle hemorrhoidal veins), avoiding the portal circulation and presystemic biotransformation. Local irritation to the rectal mucosa and inconvenience are major disadvantages of rectal administration; furthermore, as compared to other avenues of drug use, drug absorption from the rectum is slow and often erratic.

Injection Routes

The term *parenteral* literally means "by some other route than through the intestine" (the *enteral* route) and includes drug administration by injection, through the respiratory tract, and topical application to the skin, conjunctiva, urethra, and vagina. However, through common usage parenteral administration usually refers to the injection of drug by the subcutaneous, intramuscular, intravenous, intra-arterial, and intrathecal routes. In the follow discussion parenteral will be used in this more limited context. Each of the injection routes has its own merits and pitfalls, but a number of features are shared by all. Generally, parenteral administration produces a more prompt response than that obtained after oral administration, and more accurate dosage is usually attained. Injection routes are valuable when vomiting or unconsciousness preclude the use of the oral route.

Parenteral administration has several drawbacks. Because of the generally rapid rate of absorption, there often is not much time to combat adverse drug reactions and accidental overdoses. Moreover, parenteral administration requires sterile dosage forms and aseptic procedures; it may be painful; it is relatively expensive; and patients cannot readily administer the drug to themselves.

Subcutaneous Route Absorption of drugs from aqueous solutions injected at a subcutaneous site is rapid, occurs by simple diffusion, and depends mainly on the ease of penetration of the capillary wall, the area over which the solution has spread, and the rate of blood flow through the area. Accordingly, the rate of absorption can be influenced by a number of procedures. Absorption can be hastened by massage or application of heat to the injected area, or it can be slowed by reducing circulation to the injected area, for example, by local cooling or by inclusion of a vasoconstrictor, e.g., epinephrine, in the drug solution.

To obtain a slow, continuous rate of absorption from a subcutaneous site, drugs may be injected as a suspension of poorly soluble crystals (e.g., some insulin preparations) or implanted under the skin in the form of a compressed pellet (e.g., some sex hormones).

Irritating drugs should not be injected subcutaneously. They can produce severe pain, local necrosis, and sloughing.

Intramuscular Route   Drugs injected into skeletal muscle in the form of aqueous solutions are absorbed rapidly. As with the subcutaneous route, the rate of absorption is determined mainly by the speed of penetration of the capillary wall, the area of solution exposed to the circulation, and the rate of blood flow. For many drugs, the rates of absorption from muscle and subcutaneous sites are comparable.

The intramuscular route is often used for depot forms of drugs, for example, aqueous or oil suspensions of poorly soluble salts. In addition, some irritating medicinals that cannot be administered subcutaneously may be injected intramuscularly.

Intravenous Route   Injection of drugs directly into the bloodstream avoids all delays and variables of absorption. Penetration to the site of drug action is usually very rapid, and this is advantageous in emergency situations and in the continuous control of the degree of pharmacologic action, e.g., during general anesthesia, because the drug can be given slowly and the rate of administration varied as necessary. Other advantages of the intravenous route include (1) the greatest accuracy in drug dosage, (2) the ability to give large volumes of solutions over a long period of time, and (3) the ability to administer irritating, hypertonic, acidic, or alkaline solutions, since these become diluted in the large volume of circulating fluid when given slowly. However, it is important to avoid extravasation of these solutions into tissue surrounding the vein, which may result in pain and tissue necrosis.

The intravenous route is the most dangerous of all avenues of drug administration because of the speed of onset of pharmacologic action. An overdosage cannot be withdrawn, nor can its absorption be retarded. If a safe dose is given too rapidly, toxicity can result from the undesirable high drug concentration which initially perfuses reactive tissue sites.

Drugs which precipitate readily at the pH of blood and drugs suspended or dissolved in oily liquids should not be given intravenously because of the danger of embolism.

Intrathecal Route   Injection of drugs into the spinal subarachnoid space is used for producing spinal anesthesia with local anesthetic agents. It is also used for treating infections or tumors of brain and spinal tissues with drugs that do not penetrate well into the central nervous system.

Respiratory Tract

Due to the large surface area, many drugs and other chemicals are rapidly absorbed through the mucous membranes and pulmonary epithelium of the respiratory tract. Drugs may be administered as gases, sprays, aerosols, or powders. With the exception of oxygen and anesthetic gases, this route of absorption for systemic drug administration has had rather limited use in therapeutics. A major problem is the difficulty of administration and retention of exact quantities of drug. Physiologic variables may include respiratory tract infections and other pathologic states, ciliary action, and the mucous coating of the tract.

An *aerosol* is an air suspension of liquid or solid particles so small that they do not readily settle out under the force of gravity. Particles with a diameter greater than 10 μm become deposited mainly in the nasal passages, whereas particles smaller than 2 μm in diameter penetrate deeper into the respiratory tract before deposition occurs. For significant penetration into the alveolar ducts and sacs, it is probably necessary to have particles smaller than 1 μm in diameter.

Pulmonary administration of drugs for localized activity on the respiratory tree is a valuable dosing method. Certain sympathomimetics, for example, applied directly to the nasal mucosa are used as nasal decongestants; bronchodilators and other antiasthmatic compounds are inhaled as aerosols through the mouth for their effect in the lower portion of the respiratory tract.

Skin

For local effects on the skin, drugs are often applied in the form of ointments, creams, gels, lotions, liniments, and pastes. Drugs penetrate the skin much more slowly than through most other body membranes due to the relatively thick epithelial barrier and the reduced and less consistent blood perfusion. Lipid-soluble drugs are absorbed at greater rates than water-soluble compounds, and absorption can be enhanced by dissolving a drug in oil, an ointment base, or other organic solvents and rubbing it into the skin, a procedure known as *inunction.*

Although the skin is not ordinarily employed as a site for the systemic absorption of drugs, it has some useful applications. Nitroglycerin is slowly absorbed from ointments and is used in this form for the prophylaxis of nocturnal angina pectoris. In addition, a few drugs are commonly administered to the skin for systemic absorption via the *transdermal patch.* This is a unique bandagelike therapeutic system which provides for the continuous controlled release of the drug from a reservoir through a semipermeable membrane. The active compound gains access to the systemic circulation prior to any biotransformation in the liver, and a more consistent therapeutic plasma level is attained. However, systemic drug absorption through the skin is highly dependent on the site (e.g., thickness and vascularity) and its condition, i.e., intact versus broken and inflamed skin.

Other Routes of Administration

Drugs can be absorbed from sites other than those described above, for example, the conjunctiva, urethra, and vagina. Although medicinals are applied at these sites, the purpose is almost always for local action.

DISTRIBUTION

Once a drug enters the vascular space, its distribution to other tissues is assured; every tissue which has a blood supply eventually comes into equilibrium with the plasma concentration of the drug. The distribution of drugs will depend on the physicochemical properties of the drug (e.g., the lipid-to-water partition coefficient), cardiac output, blood flow to and capillary permeability in various tissues, binding to plasma proteins and other macromolecules, lipid content of the tissues, and tissue binding. Most drugs traverse the capillary wall by a combination of two processes, diffusion and filtration (hydrodynamic flow). In addition, most drugs, whether lipid-soluble or not, cross the capillary wall at rates which are extremely rapid in comparison with their rates of passage across many other body membranes. Thus, the supply of drugs to the various tissues may be limited more by the rate of blood flow than by the restraint imposed by the capillary endothelium.

The passage of drugs into and out of the central nervous system involves transfer between three major compartments: brain, cerebrospinal fluid (CSF), and blood. The boundary between blood and brain consists of several membranes: those of the capillary wall, the glial cells closely surrounding the capillary, and the neuron. The *blood-brain barrier,* which provides the main hindrance to the diffusion of drugs, is located at the capillary wall-glial cell region. After a drug penetrates this barrier and enters the extracellular fluid of the brain, it must then cross the neuronal cell membrane to enter nervous tissue. The *blood-CSF barrier* consists mainly of the epithelium of the choroid plexuses located within the cerebral ventricles.

Drugs pass from blood into brain and CSF at rates related to the lipid-to-water partition coefficients and degrees of ionization of the compounds. Lipid-soluble, nonionized substances penetrate readily, whereas water-soluble molecules and ions penetrate with great difficulty. For example, a highly lipid-soluble compound such as thiopental passes from blood into CSF thousands of times more rapidly than do certain quaternary ammonium compounds or sulfonic acids.

Although most drugs that enter the central nervous system do so by simple diffusion through the blood-brain barrier, specific carrier-mediated and receptor-mediated transport systems have been described (Table 3-1). Carrier-mediated systems appear to be involved predominantly in the transport of a variety of nutrients through the blood-brain barrier; however, the thyroid hormone, triiodothyronine, can also enter the brain via carrier-mediated transport. Moreover, drugs such as levodopa and methyldopa, which are structural derivatives of phenylalanine, cross the blood-brain barrier by the neutral amino acid transport system. Receptor-mediated transport (also known as *receptor-mediated transcytosis*) functions to allow certain peptides, e.g., insulin, to gain access to the brain. The awareness of these specialized transport

TABLE 3-1   Carrier-mediated and receptor-mediated transport systems of the blood-brain barrier

Transport system	Representative substrate
Carrier-mediated	
Hexose	Glucose
Amine	Choline
Basic amino acid	Arginine
Neutral amino acid	Phenylalanine
Monocarboxylic acid	Lactic acid
Purine	Adenine
Nucleoside	Adenosine
Thyroid hormone	Triiodothyronine
Receptor-mediated	
Insulin	Insulin
Transferrin	Transferrin
Growth factors	Insulin-like growth factors 1 and 2

systems in the blood-brain barrier has stimulated interest in using selected lipid-soluble prodrugs (i.e., inactive nutrient-drug complexes that can be transported into the brain and then split to release the active drug moiety) as a novel approach to drug delivery into the central nervous system.

The exit of drugs from the central nervous system involves more pathways than the entrance. Drugs can diffuse across the blood-brain and blood-CSF barriers in the reverse direction at rates determined by their lipid solubility and degree of ionization. Moreover, all drugs, whether lipid-soluble or not, pass from CSF into blood at similar rates as CSF drains into the dural blood sinuses by flowing through the wide channels of the arachnoid villi. In addition, certain organic anions and cations are rapidly transferred from CSF to blood by active transport across the choroid plexuses; anions such as penicillin are transported by one process, and

cations such as choline by another. Because of the ready removal of certain poorly lipid-soluble drugs from the CSF by active transport as well as by the CSF drainage mechanism, many of these substances never attain a concentration in CSF equal to that in plasma.

The ocular fluid is similar to CSF in regard to the entry and exit of drugs. Thus the blood-ocular fluid boundary, which consists mainly of the ciliary-body epithelium and the capillary walls and surrounding connective tissue of the iris, behaves as a lipoid barrier to most organic compounds.

Drugs applied to the corneal surface of the eye penetrate into the aqueous humor at rates related to the lipid-to-water partition coefficient of their nonionized form.

Protein and Macromolecule Binding

Binding of drugs to proteins and other macromolecules is known to occur in almost every tissue of the body. It has been demonstrated with albumin, mucopolysaccharides, nucleoproteins, and other substances.

Binding is generally a reversible process and, therefore, arrives at an equilibrium in which only the unbound (free) fraction of the drug is available to act and to be biotransformed and excreted, while the bound fraction functions as a depot from which the drug is released as the equilibrium is reestablished after removal of the free fraction. The forces responsible for the binding are weak bonds of the van der Waals, hydrogen, and ionic types. The position of the equilibrium and the rate at which the free fraction of the drug is removed by biotransformation and excretion determines the biologic half-life of the drug, which can vary widely.

Thus, the reversible binding of drugs to various intracellular and extracellular substances is important in determining how long a drug remains in the body. Without these storage pools, many drugs would be biotransformed and excreted so rapidly that they would hardly have time to exert their pharmacologic action.

Binding to Plasma Proteins

The plasma protein binding of drugs is usually expressed as the percent of total drug that is bound. Most drugs show some degree of binding in plasma, and much of this is due to binding with plasma albumin. Examples of highly bound compounds include phenylbutazone, warfarin, imipramine, and thiopental (80 to 98 percent bound); compounds with moderate degrees of binding include caffeine, phenobarbital, and terbutaline (20 to 50 percent bound). Drugs such as barbital, lithium, and tobramycin exhibit a low degree of plasma binding (1 to 8 percent).

Because albumin and other plasma proteins possess a limited number of binding sites and these sites are rather nonselective with respect to the drugs that will bind, two drugs with an affinity for the same site will compete with one another for binding. Furthermore, if one of the drugs is administered after the other, the second will displace a portion of the first from the binding sites, and the organism will be faced with a markedly increased plasma concentration of pharmacologically active compound. With a drug that is normally highly bound, the usual therapeutic dose may be toxic when followed by administration of a drug that displaces it from its storage sites.

Competition between drugs for binding sites can also bring about significant changes in the distribution of drugs between plasma and tissues. For example, one drug that has a high percentage binding to plasma proteins may displace another highly bound drug from plasma albumin; as a result, the free latter drug diffuses into tissues, thereby causing the (total) plasma concentration to decline.

The influence of protein binding on the passive transfer of drugs across membranes has already been mentioned. When binding to plasma proteins creates an equilibrium mixture of free and protein-bound drug, only the free fraction can diffuse across membranes. It is true that, as free drug is removed, more is liberated as the equilibrium is reestablished, but when the equilibrium is strongly influenced by binding, only a very small portion of the total drug may leave the blood on a single passage of the blood through an organ. This situation is modified when a drug is actively transported across a membrane or crosses by some other form of specialized transport. As an example, penicillin is tightly bound in plasma, but is actively transported into the urine by the renal tubular epithelium and is almost completely cleared from the plasma in one passage through the kidney. The speed of reversibility of the drug-protein interaction is apparently great enough to keep pace with the rapid removal of free drug from plasma by the membrane carriers.

Binding to Tissues

The binding of drugs to components of various tissues (other than plasma proteins) is difficult to measure quantitatively. Certain drugs show a much greater affinity for tissues than for plasma proteins, and in some instances, the affinity for one tissue is considerably greater than for another. Tetracycline has a high affinity for bone, digoxin for skeletal muscle, and guanethidine for cardiac muscle.

Redistribution

The pattern of distribution of drugs is governed by two factors: (1) the affinity of the drug for the various tissues, i.e., the equilibrium between the blood and each tissue, and (2) the rate of blood flow to each tissue. As mentioned previously, those tissues with the greatest blood flow come into equilibrium with the blood almost immediately; those with the poorest blood flow equilibrate very slowly. As a result, the tissues with good blood supply initially accumulate an inordinately high proportion of the total drug present, which is then gradually redistributed in the body as other tissues also come into equilibrium with the blood. The final situation, where all tissues are in equilibrium with each other by the intermediary of the blood which supplies them, may take many hours.

Thiopental, a highly lipid-soluble drug that penetrates all cells readily and has an especially high affinity for body fat, does not initially become localized in adipose tissue. Rather, after intravenous administration, it first reaches high concentrations in brain, liver, kidney, and other tissues that have high rates of blood flow (see Fig. 3-5). The concentration of drug in muscle rises slowly because of the slower rate of delivery to that tissue, and the concentration in the adipose rises even more slowly for the same reason. As thiopental is taken up by the large muscle mass of the body as well as by fat, the plasma concentration declines, and the drug begins to redistribute by diffusing out of the brain and other early sites of deposition.

ELIMINATION

Elimination includes all processes that terminate the presence of a drug in the body. The major processes are biotransformation, renal excretion, and biliary excretion. Minor elimination processes are elimination via saliva, sweat, milk, tears, feces, and exhaled air.

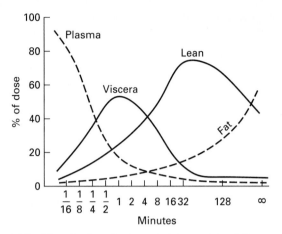

FIGURE 3-5 Distribution of thiopental in different body tissues at various times after intravenous injection. Time scale (in minutes) progresses geometrically. Final values are at infinity.

Biotransformation

Biotransformation is the process by which drugs or endogenous substances are altered chemically. It occurs mainly in the liver, but may occur in plasma or other tissues such as the lung or kidneys. This subject is discussed at length in Chap. 4; however, in the interest of continuity a brief discussion follows here.

There are four major biotransformation reactions that occur within the body; they are oxidation, reduction, hydrolysis, and conjugation. Drugs which undergo oxidative, reductive, or hydrolytic reactions may or may not be converted to a pharmacologically inactive product. However, once a drug has been conjugated as a result of the addition of another molecule (such as sulfate or glucuronic acid) to itself or its metabolite, the drug tends to be pharmacologically inert. In general, conjugation reactions follow oxidation, reduction, or hydrolytic reactions. A conjugated drug is generally more polar and therefore more water-soluble; this greatly enhances renal excretion of the compound.

Renal Excretion

The kidney serves as the major route of excretion of unchanged and biotransformed drugs. There are two

major renal routes of excretion: filtration and secretion. Filtered drugs are generally polar and water-soluble. They pass into Bowman's capsule and traverse the tubular lumen, and most reach the collecting duct without significant reabsorption. Drugs which are actively secreted into the tubular lumen by the proximal tubule generally are organic acids (such as penicillin, aspirin, and diuretics) or organic bases (such as quinine). Following its passage into the renal tubule, if a drug is nonionized, or becomes nonionized due to the acidic pH of the tubular filtrate, and possesses an appropriate molecular size, then reabsorption of the drug into the bloodstream at both the proximal and distal portions of the nephron may occur. As the renal tubular fluid becomes more concentrated, nonionized drug molecules are reabsorbed by diffusion across the tubular epithelium at rates related to their lipid-to-water partition coefficients. Accordingly, compounds of low lipid solubility, which are poorly reabsorbed, are excreted in the urine more readily than are compounds of high lipid solubility.

In accordance with the principles governing the distribution of weak electrolytes across a lipoid membrane, when the tubular urine is made alkaline, weak bases become less concentrated in the urine than in plasma and, as a result, are excreted more slowly; when the urine is made acidic, weak bases concentrate in the urine and are excreted more rapidly. Conversely, weak acids are excreted more readily in an alkaline urine and more slowly in an acidic urine.

Biliary Excretion

The hepatic parenchymal cell is readily penetrated by most drugs. In addition to the rapid penetration of many nonionized compounds, which presumably pass through lipoid areas as well as pores in the cell membrane, a wide variety of organic anions and cations are readily taken up by liver parenchymal cells by carrier-type transport processes.

The liver has at least three active transport processes for the biliary excretion of certain poorly lipid-soluble organic compounds. One process excretes a variety of organic anions including sulfonic acid dyes, bile acids, bilirubin, penicillin, and many drug biotransformation products such as glucuronides and other acidic conjugation substances. A second process is responsible for the biliary excretion of organic cations, including certain quaternary ammonium compounds and tertiary amines. A third process excretes a number of nonionic, poorly lipid-soluble cardioactive glycosides such as ouabain and lanatosides A and C. In each of these processes, compounds are transported from plasma into bile against a large concentration gradient, the excretion mechanism becomes saturated at high plasma levels of the compound, and substances that are excreted by the same process inhibit the transport of one another in a competitive manner.

In contrast, lipid-soluble, nonionized drugs do not appear in the bile in high concentrations. During their passage through the bile duct, reabsorption may occur whereby these molecules can diffuse readily across the bile duct epithelium and thus remain in equilibrium with the drug concentration in plasma.

After a drug has been excreted into the intestine via the bile, it may be partly reabsorbed and partly excreted in the feces. Glucuronides or other conjugated forms of drugs may be split within the intestinal lumina to release free, lipid-soluble drug molecules. Obviously the free drug is readily reabsorbed in the intestine, reconjugated in the liver, and again excreted into bile. This enterohepatic cycle can delay considerably the elimination of a drug from the body. Some drugs which undergo enterohepatic recirculation are glutethimide, digitoxin, morphine, and indomethacin.

Minor Elimination Processes

Drugs and their biotransformation products secreted into saliva, sweat, and mammary secretions tend to be lipid-soluble and nonionized. It is important to remember that the drugs pass into these fluids by simple diffusion and that only the free form of the drug or its metabolites can pass across the particular organs and their membranes. Of particular importance are mammary secretions in a nursing mother. Since the pH of milk is usually about 0.7 unit below that of plasma, basic drugs appear in milk in a concentration greater than that in plasma, and acidic drugs in a concentration less than that in plasma. Completely neutral substances, e.g., ethanol, become distributed equally between the two fluids. Breast-fed infants will thus become exposed to drugs ingested by the mother with consequent pharmacologic effects. Therefore, it is a good general rule to advise drug abstinence by the mother if she is breast-feeding her child.

FUNDAMENTAL MATHEMATICAL PRINCIPLES OF PHARMACOKINETICS

In order to simplify the discussion of the mathematical relationships in pharmacokinetics, we need to assume that the factors which influence drug absorption, distribution, and elimination in a single individual remain constant over a period of time. This assumption is made with the full realization that drug-drug interactions and changes in the function of the cardiovascular system, the liver, and the kidney may alter the pharmacokinetic pattern of a compound.

Pharmacokinetic Models and Compartments

As mentioned previously, the use of time-plasma drug concentration curves, as exemplified in Fig. 3-3, has become a useful standard device with which to monitor pharmacokinetics. Drugs are absorbed, distributed, biotransformed, and excreted at different rates. Since a variety of biologic and physicochemical processes influence how a particular drug is handled by the body, it would appear that a mathematical description of drug pharmacokinetics would be very complex and would vary for each drug. In contrast, owing to the equilibrium nature of drug disposition in the body, certain patterns, which tend to simplify pharmacokinetic analyses, emerge from using time-plasma drug concentration curves. These patterns, conceptualized into *pharmacokinetic models*, or *compartment models*, help to explain human pharmacokinetic data.

The simplest pharmacokinetic model, the *one-compartment model* (Fig. 3-6), assumes that after administration drugs are rapidly and homogenously distributed throughout all body fluids. This does not necessarily mean that the concentration of drug in plasma and other tissues is equal, rather, that the entire system is at equilibrium and changes in plasma drug concentrations quantitatively reflect changes in drug concentrations occurring in other fluids and tissues. Many drugs equilibrate between plasma and other tissues very rapidly. Furthermore, at the usual plasma sampling times, the one-compartment pharmacokinetic model adequately describes the data of time-plasma drug concentration curves (see Fig. 3-10). Therefore, this model, although the most elementary, is often the most appropriate pharmacokinetic model for many drugs.

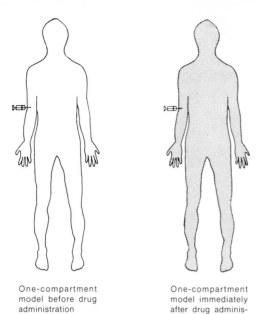

One-compartment model before drug administration

One-compartment model immediately after drug administration

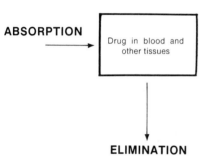

FIGURE 3-6 The one-compartment model before and after intravenous drug administration. [Modified from Dvorchik, B. H., and E. S. Vesell: *Clin. Chem.*, **22**:868 (1976).]

The *two-compartment model* (Fig. 3-7) considers the fact that drugs distribute to different tissues at rates related to the blood flow in each tissue, and therefore, divides tissues primarily upon vascularization. For example, tissues with high blood flow, i.e., adrenals, kidneys, heart, brain, and the blood vessels, may compose the "central compartment" and receive drugs rapidly. All other tissues (with lower blood flow) constitute the "peripheral compartment" and, therefore,

exchange drugs at a slower rate. If drug distribution throughout the body is relatively slow or if plasma sampling is performed frequently and quickly following drug administration, "two-phase" time-plasma drug concentration data can be seen (see Fig. 3-12). In this case, the two-compartment model describes drug disposition in the body. Three- and four-compartment models have been described but are rarely used. It is important to realize that these "compartments" have no real physiologic meaning; they vary in extent depending on the particular drug under consideration.

Kinetics

Kinetics is the study of rates of reactions. In general, drug absorption, distribution, and elimination (i.e., biotransformation and excretion) processes follow *first-order kinetics*. A first-order kinetic process is one in which a constant *fraction, or percentage,* of a drug is handled per unit of time. This is true for both passive processes (e.g., glomerular filtration) and active processes (e.g., renal tubular secretion) where drug concentrations do not saturate the enzyme or carrier system. In selected instances, drug concentrations may saturate the metabolic or transport system. When the capacity of those systems is exceeded, a constant *amount* of drug is handled per unit of time. This is known as *zero-order kinetics*.

First-Order Rate Equations   With first-order kinetics, the rate of an absorption, a biotransformation, a distribution, or an excretion process is directly proportional to the concentration of the substance remaining to be handled by the system at any given time. For example, if drug A is absorbed through the intestinal mucosa to the blood, then the rate of transfer of drug A from the intestinal lumen is proportional to the concentration of drug A in the intestine. The following relationships are applicable:

$$\text{Rate of transfer} \propto \ [\text{A}] \text{ in the intestine}$$

or

$$\text{Rate} = k[\text{A}]$$

where k is the proportionality constant or rate constant for the process. This is one form of the first-order rate equation.

For a biotransformation reaction where drug A is converted to its metabolite, drug B, the rate of reaction

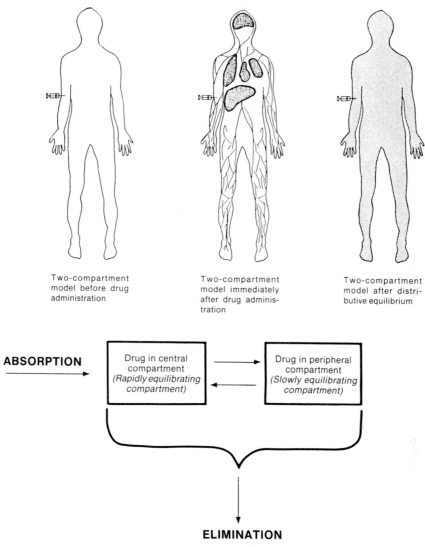

Two-compartment model before drug administration

Two-compartment model immediately after drug administration

Two-compartment model after distributive equilibrium

ABSORPTION

| Drug in central compartment (*Rapidly equilibrating compartment*) |

| Drug in peripheral compartment (*Slowly equilibrating compartment*) |

ELIMINATION

FIGURE 3-7 The two-compartment model before and after intravenous drug administration. [Modified from Dvorchik, B. H., and E. S. Vesell: *Clin. Chem.*, **22**:868 (1976).]

is also equal to $k[A]$. The rate of this reaction is the increase in the concentration of B with respect to time, $d[B]/dt$; therefore,

$$\text{Rate} = \frac{d[B]}{dt} = k[A]$$

The rate of the formation of B is equal to the rate of the biotransformation of A, or

$$\frac{d[B]}{dt} = \frac{-d[A]}{dt}$$

where the minus sign denotes that $[A]$ is decreasing with time. This provides another form of the first-order rate equation:

$$\text{Rate} = \frac{-d[A]}{dt} = k[A]$$

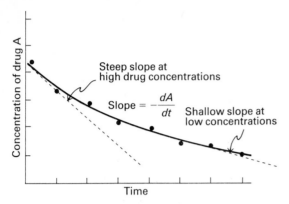

FIGURE 3-8   Arithmetic plot of drug concentration versus time for a first-order process.

which is plotted in Fig. 3-8. Note that the slope of the line reflects the rate of the reaction; at high [A], the rate is high (steep slope), and as the [A] decreases, so does the rate of the process (shallower slope). The same relationship holds for the gain or loss of a drug from a tissue or organ site, e.g., from gastric juice, plasma, or cerebrospinal fluid.

If we are interested in determining the rate constant k for absorption or elimination of a drug, the first-order rate equation as expressed graphically is difficult to analyze and leads to a considerable error in the estimate of k because of the constantly changing slope of the line. This equation can be converted mathematically (through rearrangement and integration) to

$$\ln [A] = \ln [A_0] - kt$$

where $\ln [A_0]$ is the natural logarithm of concentration of drug A before the process begins, or at time = 0, and $\ln [A]$ is the natural logarithm of the concentration of drug A at any subsequent time t. This equation, which is in a linear format, can also be written using common logarithms:

$$\ln [A] = \ln [A_0] - kt$$
$$\log [A] = \log [A_0] - \frac{k}{2.303} t$$
$$y = a + b\ x$$

The relationship between the log-concentration of drug A and time is shown in Fig. 3-9.

It is most useful to calculate the half-life ($t_{1/2}$) of a first-order process, which is the time necessary for the drug concentration to decrease to one-half of its origi-

nal value or the time required for the process to be half completed. At the half-life, $[A] = \frac{1}{2}[A_0]$; therefore

$$\log \tfrac{1}{2}[A_0] = \log [A_0] - \frac{k}{2.303} t_{1/2}$$

and

$$2.303 \log \frac{[A_0]}{\frac{1}{2}[A_0]} = kt_{1/2}$$

The left side of the equation equals 2.303 log 2, or 0.693. Therefore

$$t_{1/2} = \frac{0.693}{k}$$

which shows that the half-life for a first-order process is dependent only on k and is independent of the initial concentration of the drug. In addition, if the half-life is known, k can easily be calculated (see Fig. 3-10).

It is important to remember that k for any first-order pharmacokinetic process does not have a definitive value. It is a variable that depends on the individual patient's ability to handle a particular drug. Furthermore, when two or more first-order processes are involved in drug kinetics, the rate constants of each are additive. For example, in drug elimination which encompasses both hepatic biotransformation and renal excretion, the *systemic elimination rate constant* k_e is a composite of the rate constants for biotransformation and excretion. It follows that the *systemic half-life* of a

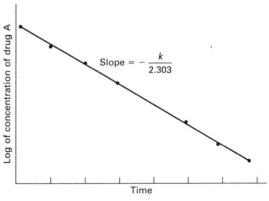

FIGURE 3-9   Logarithmic plot of drug concentration versus time for a first-order process.

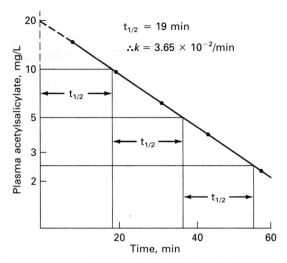

FIGURE 3-10 Logarithmic plot showing the rate of removal of acetylsalicylate from human plasma in vivo and the estimation of half-life ($t_{1/2}$). [Modified from Lamont-Havers, R. M., and B. M. Wagner (eds.): *Proceedings of the Conference on Effects of Chronic Salicylate Administration*, New York, June 13–14, 1966; U. S. Department of Health, Education and Welfare.]

For the one-compartment model, distribution of a drug is considered to be relatively rapid. Regardless of the rate at which distribution occurs, the extent of distribution varies widely among drugs. Some drugs are highly distributed throughout the body, others are largely confined to the plasma and therefore do not distribute well. The *apparent volume of distribution V_d* was developed as an index to compare the extent of drug distribution. V_d is defined as the volume of fluid into which a drug appears to distribute, with a concentration equal to that of plasma. Mathematically this is expressed as

$$V_d = \frac{\text{total amount of drug in the body}}{\text{concentration of drug in the plasma}}$$

An important question to consider is: How long after drug administration should the plasma concentration of a drug be measured? Time-plasma concentration curves vary for every drug in every patient, depending on the rates and extent of absorption, distribution, and elimination. Therefore, it is customary to use elimination data, i.e., plasma levels taken at various times following administration, and extrapolate back to the drug concentration of time = 0. For example, using data shown in Fig. 3-10, plasma acetylsalic-

drug equals $0.693/k_e$. It is the systemic half-life that is most useful clinically.

The Zero-Order Rate Equation Most enzyme-catalyzed processes in the body, such as facilitated diffusion, active transport, and biotransformation reactions, are saturable. That is, the drug in *too great a concentration* will overwhelm the capacity of the enzyme or carrier. In such a case, the rate of the process becomes independent of the drug concentration and dependent on only the rate constant k of the process. If the concentration of a drug (not the log) is plotted versus time, a linear plot results with the slope equal to $-k$. In zero-order kinetics a constant *amount* of drug is handled per unit of time; the clearance of ethanol from the plasma provides an excellent example of zero-order kinetics (see Fig. 3-11).

Apparent Volume of Distribution Every drug has a characteristic distribution pattern which depends on the physicochemical properties of the drug as well as the inherent biologic variability of the organism.

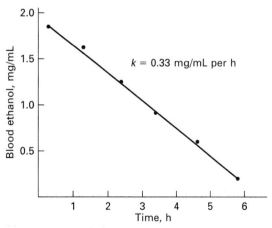

FIGURE 3-11 Arithmetic plot of the changes in blood ethanol concentrations with respect to time following intraperitoneal injection of ethanol to rats. [Modified from Ferko, A. P., and Bobyock, E.: *Toxicol Appl. Pharmacol.* **46**:235–248 (1978).]

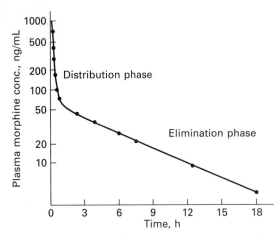

FIGURE 3-12 Logarithmic plot of plasma morphine concentrations following intravenous administration of morphine to a patient. Note that the first phase of the curve (distribution phase, or the α phase) shows a rapid decline. This is due to prompt distribution into the slowly equilibrating tissues. After this phase, the body is at equilibrium and the elimination phase (or the β phase) proceeds more slowly. [Modified from Stanski, D. R., et al.: *Clin. Pharmacol. Ther.*, **24**:52–59 (1978).]

ylate concentrations were taken at various times following IV administration of 200 mg of the drug. Extrapolation of the linear elimination data to time = 0 gives the acetylsalicylate concentration of 20 mg/L. This would be the plasma concentration if absorption and distribution of the drug were rapid enough to be essentially instantaneous. In this example, $V_d = (200 \text{ mg})/(20 \text{ mg/L})$, or 10 L.

If drug data appear to follow a two-compartment model, the distribution phase is ignored in estimating the plasma concentration at time = 0 for calculating V_d. This is because V_d describes drug distribution after *equilibrium has occurred*, which is not until the elimination phase is observed. Using the data in Fig. 3-12 for calculating V_d, the plasma concentration of morphine at time = 0 would be 50 ng/mL.

V_d is a theoretical concept that provides some indication of the extent of drug distribution; it is generally a characteristic of the drug rather than the biologic system (however, biologic variability affects patient V_d values to some extent). Most drugs have a V_d between 0.1 and 6 L/kg. Often V_d is expressed in liters per 70 kg or simply liters (which assumes a 70-kg weight). A low V_d indicates that the drug remains largely within the plasma and does not readily distribute to other tissues. This may be due to a high degree of drug binding to plasma proteins or a very low lipid-to-water partition coefficient and low penetrability through membranes and storage in adipose tissue. A high V_d is indicative of significant uptake by many tissues and widespread distribution of the compound. In addition to providing insight into the distribution of a drug, V_d is useful for estimating the plasma concentration after a dose of the drug or in calculating the total amount of drug in the body when the plasma concentration is known.

Clearance Clearance is defined as the apparent volume of a biologic fluid from which a drug is removed by elimination processes per unit of time. Clearance is *not* a measure of the quantity of drug being eliminated; it provides an indication of the *volume of fluid* from which the drug is eliminated. For example, if drug A is biotransformed in the liver to metabolite B and has a hepatic clearance of 1 mL/min/kg (or 70 mL/min), this means that as blood flows through the liver containing drug A, every minute 70 mL of blood leaves the organ containing only drug B (i.e., completely cleared of drug A).

Organ clearance CL_{organ} is dependent on the blood flow through the organ Q and the maximum ability of the organ to remove the free drug from the circulation, known as the *intrinsic clearance*, or the *extraction efficiency E*. Therefore

$$CL_{organ} = Q \times E$$

The extraction efficiency is determined by the difference between the arterial drug concentrations C_A and venous drug concentrations C_V divided by the arterial drug concentration, or

$$E = \frac{C_A - C_V}{C_A}$$

Therefore

$$CL_{organ} = Q \times E = Q \times \frac{C_A - C_V}{C_A}$$

One generally discusses clearance of a drug from the plasma (or blood) by elimination processes that affect the whole body. Total body clearance CL_{total} is the rate of removal of a drug from the body and represents the sum total of all the organs that eliminate a drug, i.e.,

$$CL_{total} = CL_{liver} + CL_{kidney} + CL_{saliva} + CL_{lung} + \cdots$$

Total body clearance is influenced by the apparent volume of distribution V_d and the elimination rate constant k_e. Kinetically,

$$CL_{total} = V_d \times k_e = \frac{0.693 \times V_d}{t_{1/2}}$$

or expressed in terms of half-life,

$$t_{1/2} = \frac{0.693 \times V_d}{CL_{total}}$$

Therefore, the elimination half-life of a drug is dependent on how widely a drug is distributed throughout the body and its rate of clearance.

DOSAGE REGIMENS AND PHARMACOKINETIC PROFILES

Single Doses

Intravenous Administration After intravenous injection of a drug as a bolus, the compound mixes with and becomes diluted by circulating blood. Even though distribution within the circulation and to other tissues begins to occur rapidly, uniform systemic distribution is not established for several minutes after drug administration. As distribution equilibrates, plasma concentrations of the drug decrease rapidly; following this distribution phase, drug elimination from the plasma takes the form of a first-order process.

If plasma concentrations of the drug are measured quickly enough following intravenous bolus administration and at various times thereafter, time-plasma drug concentration data will resemble those shown in Fig. 3-12 and will appear to follow a two-compartment model. If, on the other hand, the rate of drug distribution is more rapid than the ability to quantitate the initial plasma concentrations, then the data for the distribution phase will be lost, only the elimination phase will be observed (see Fig. 3-10), and the data will appear to follow a one-compartment model.

Oral Administration Oral dosing of a substance introduces absorption as a significant variable factor.

In addition to the inherent biologic variations in rates of drug absorption, differences in dosage forms, formulations of a dosage form, or salts of a drug may dramatically alter the pharmacokinetic pattern of a compound. These problems relate to bioavailability of drugs and bioequivalence of drug products.

As discussed earlier, due to the ability of drugs to traverse membranes, once within the systemic circulation, they become *available* to the tissues of the body. The term used to describe the amount of drug that is delivered the general circulation and the rate at which this occurs is *bioavailability*. If a drug is injected by the intravenous route, it is at once completely bioavailable. All other avenues of drug administration usually result in incomplete bioavailability due to (1) incomplete absorption, (2) biotransformation of some of the drug prior to reaching the systemic circulation, or (3) both. Therefore, bioavailability F is a measure of the fraction of an administered dose that reaches the general circulation.

The area under the time-plasma drug concentration curve, or simply the *area under the curve* (AUC) for any drug represents the total amount of that drug delivered to the circulation (during the time period of measurement) following administration. Using IV dosing as the basis of comparison and assuming no changes in drug distribution or elimination, the bioavailability of a drug (given by any route) can be calculated by the AUCs according to the following:

$$F = \frac{AUC \times dose_{IV}}{AUC_{IV} \times dose}$$

If the doses are equal, the relationship simplifies to the ratio of AUC values only. In this context, the bioavailability of a drug by any route is the *absolute bioavailability*. Usually oral bioavailability of drugs is of most interest, since the oral route is the most common method of drug administration. As an example, the antimicrobial drug penicillin G has an oral bioavailability of approximately 20 percent, i.e., only about 20 percent of an oral dose reaches the systemic circulation. A compound with similar antimicrobial activity and potency, penicillin V, has an oral bioavailability of over 80 percent and would be preferred to penicillin G for oral use since more drug would reach the bloodstream at equivalent oral doses.

When bioavailability comparisons are made between two different drug preparations, e.g., capsules versus tablets, or between two different manufacturers of the same preparation and the dose and route of administration are the same, the AUC ratio refers to the *relative bioavailability*.

Multiple Doses

It is rare that a drug will be used in a single-dose regimen; in most therapeutic situations, including the treatment of acute illnesses, drugs are usually given in multiple doses. Regardless of the route of administration, if these doses are spaced far enough apart, complete elimination of the first dose may occur prior to the administration of the second dose; the second dose will be completely eliminated prior to the third dose, etc.; the time-plasma drug concentration curves resulting from this schedule of drug administration will resemble individual single doses, separated by the dosing interval (Fig. 3-13). Pharmacokinetic data may be calculated for each dose using the concepts and equations developed previously in this chapter.

Repeated administration of a drug at intervals selected so that complete elimination of the compound has not occurred, will result in drug accumulation. Plasma concentrations will fluctuate in response to the inherent pharmacokinetics of the drug and in proportion to the dosage interval selected. Accumulation of the compound within the body will continue to occur

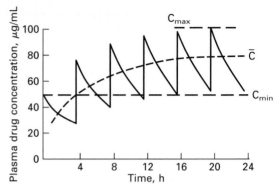

FIGURE 3-14   Arithmetic plot of plasma drug concentration versus time following multiple intravenous injections given every 4 h. Since the drug is not completely eliminated prior to each succeeding dose, drug accumulation will occur. Eventually, plasma drug concentrations will attain the steady state, fluctuating between the maximal (C_{max}) and minimal (C_{min}) drug concentrations at the beginning and end of each dosing interval, respectively.

until the amount of drug eliminated per dose interval equals the amount of drug absorbed per dose. When this condition is attained, the plasma level will be at the *plateau* or *steady state*.

Multiple Intravenous Administration   Figure 3-13 shows the time-plasma drug concentration curve of a drug with a 4-h half-life given by IV injection every 24 h. If this drug were administered in more closely spaced intervals, e.g., once every half-life (4 h), the data would appear as shown in Fig. 3-14. The plasma drug concentration will continue to increase until the steady state is attained, at which time the drug concentration will fluctuate between a minimum C_{min} and maximum C_{max} during each dosing interval.

The average plasma concentration at the steady state $\bar{C}$ during multiple IV administration can be calculated by

$$\bar{C} = \frac{D}{V_d \times k_e \times T} = \frac{D}{CL_{total} \times T}$$

where D is the dose, V_d the apparent volume of distribution, k_e the elimination rate constant, CL_{total} the total body clearance, and T the dosing interval. Therefore, given some pharmacokinetic data following a sin-

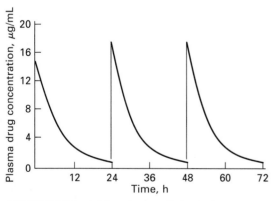

FIGURE 3-13   Arithmetic plot of plasma drug concentration versus time following multiple intravenous bolus injections given every 12 h. There is no accumulation of the drug since the doses are widely separated and each dose is almost completely eliminated prior to the next injection.

gle dose of a drug, one can estimate the plasma concentration at the steady state with a variety of dosage regimens.

Continuous Intravenous Infusion This can be considered as a variation of multiple IV injections where the dosing interval is infinitely small. Instead of many small single IV doses, a suitable constant rate of drug infusion and duration of infusion is chosen. If the infusion is continued indefinitely, the plasma concentration will increase until the rate of elimination (which increases as drug concentration increases) becomes equal to the rate of infusion. At this point a steady-state plasma concentration will be achieved (Fig. 3-15). With this form of drug administration, the infusion rate = dose/T, and therefore

$$\bar{C} = \frac{\text{infusion rate}}{\text{CL}_{\text{total}}}$$

Multiple Oral Dosing Similar to the case of multiple IV injections, the average plasma concentration $\bar{C}$ is related to the dose, dosage interval, and clearance of the compound, but is complicated by the inclusion of a first-order absorption step. Therefore the dose administered is reduced by the oral bioavailability F, and the equation for calculating $\bar{C}$ becomes

$$\bar{C} = \frac{F \times D}{V_d \times k_e \times T} = \frac{F \times D}{\text{CL}_{\text{total}} \times T}$$

Using this relationship, a uniform maintenance dose and dosage interval can be selected for any drug in order to achieve any average steady-state plasma concentration that is desired. This works well when patients are instructed to take a medication with a uniform dosing interval, for example, four times a day around the clock, i.e., every 6 h. Unfortunately, in practice uniform dosing regimens such as this are seldom used and rarely adhered to by the patient. Thus drug plasma levels often tend to fluctuate more than desired, leading to ineffective therapy, and/or unwanted adverse drug effects.

BIBLIOGRAPHY

Azarnoff, D. L., and D. H. Huffman: "Therapeutic Implications of Bioavailability," *Annu. Rev. Pharmacol. Toxicol.*, **16**:53–66 (1976).

Bend, J. R., C. J. Serabjit-Singh, and R. M. Philpot: "The Pulmonary Uptake, Accumulation and Metabolism of Xenobiotics," *Annu. Rev. Pharmacol. Toxicol.*, **25**:97–125 (1985).

Benet, L. Z., N. Massoud, and L. G. Gambertoglio: *Pharmacokinetic Basis for Drug Treatment*, Raven, New York, 1984.

Bochner, F., G. Carrothers, J. Kampmann, and J. Steiner: *Handbook of Clinical Pharmacology*, Little, Brown, Boston, 1983.

Creasey, W. A.: *Drug Disposition in Humans*, Oxford, London, 1979.

Gladtke, E., and H. M. vonHattingberg: *Pharmacokinetics, An Introduction*, Springer-Verlag, New York, 1979.

Greenblatt, D. J., and R. I. Shader: *Pharmacokinetics in Clinical Practice*, Saunders, Philadelphia, 1985.

Ladua, B. N., H. G. Mandel, and E. L. Way (eds): *Fundamentals of Drug Metabolism and Drug Disposition*, Williams & Wilkins, Baltimore, 1971.

Levine, R. R.: *Pharmacology: Drugs Actions and Reactions*, 3d ed., Little, Brown, Boston, 1983.

Partridge, W. M.: "Recent Advances in Blood-Brain Barrier Transport," *Annu. Rev. Pharmacol. Toxicol.*, **28**:25–39 (1988).

Ther, L., and D. Winner: "Drug Absorption," *Annu. Rev. Pharmacol.*, **11**:57–70 (1971).

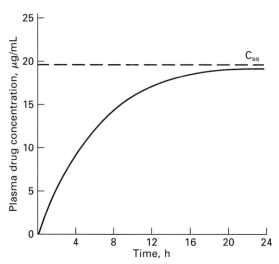

FIGURE 3-15 Arithmetic plot of plasma drug concentration versus time following continuous intravenous infusion. The plasma drug concentration will, in time, reach the steady state (C_{ss}) concentration.

Biotransformation

William S. Thayer

The chemical changes undergone by a drug within the body are referred to as *drug biotransformation*. The majority of these chemical alterations result from the interaction of drugs with endogenous enzyme systems, although nonenzymatic reactions may also be involved. Many of the enzymes exhibit broad substrate specificity and thus catalyze reactions involving a wide range of foreign chemicals known as xenobiotics. Pharmacologic agents, or drugs, represent a particular type of xenobiotic.

The liver is the major organ responsible for the biotransformation of drugs or other xenobiotics. The smooth endoplasmic reticulum, a subcellular membrane system rich in enzymes for xenobiotic metabolism, is especially prominent in hepatic tissue. When liver is homogenized, the endoplasmic reticulum forms small membrane vesicles which can be isolated by differential centrifugation and are known as *microsomes*. Thus, the group of enzymes associated with the smooth endoplasmic reticulum is often termed the *drug-metabolizing microsomal system* (DMMS). Extrahepatic metabolism, involving similar enzymes, can also be important for many drugs and occurs mainly in kidney, lung, and intestine.

TYPES OF BIOTRANSFORMATION REACTIONS

Lipid-soluble xenobiotics introduced into the body are usually not excreted until they undergo chemical changes that result in an increase in polarity. Since many drugs are lipophilic, biotransformation increases their water solubility. This solubility change restricts further penetration of the drug through cellular membranes, reduces systemic distribution, and promotes elimination through excretory systems such as the kidney. Therefore, biotransformation of a drug usually limits its pharmacologic activity.

Traditionally, drug biotransformation reactions have been regarded as occurring in two general phases. Phase I reactions consist of oxidations, reductions, and hydrolyses which introduce new functional groups to the parent drug molecule. Phase I reactions often alter the chemical reactivity of a drug and increase its aqueous solubility. Phase II reactions consist of conjugation (synthetic) reactions in which an endogenous substrate, such as glucuronic acid, sulfate, or glutathione, is coupled to the drug molecule. Conjugation reactions generally involve the new chemical groups introduced during phase I reactions. Phase II reactions further increase the water solubility of the drug molecule, thus promoting its elimination.

Phase I and phase II reactions may occur either sequentially or simultaneously and often involve multiple functional groups on the drug molecule. Phase I reactions usually precede phase II reactions, but in some cases phase II reactions occur prior to those of phase I. Alternatively, a given drug may undergo only phase II reactions. The pattern of drug biotransformation reactions, as well as the pattern of metabolites, is determined by the chemical structure and reactivity of each particular drug.

It is important to recognize that biotransformation can result in conversion of (1) a pharmacologically active drug to an inactive metabolite, (2) an active drug to an active metabolite, or (3) an inactive agent to an active metabolite.

As an example of the first case, phase I biotransformation of phenytoin by hydroxylation leads to its inactivation:

Phenytoin [active] $\longrightarrow$ hydroxyphenytoin [inactive]

In the second case, a metabolite of a drug retains pharmacologic activity similar to the parent drug. An example is provided by the phase I dealkylation of diazepam:

Diazepam [active] $\longrightarrow$ desmethyldiazepam [active]

When an inactive precursor is metabolized to a pharmacologically active drug, the parent compound is known as *prodrug*. An example is

Sulindac (sulfoxide) [inactive] $\longrightarrow$
sulindac sulfide [active]

A corollary is that a metabolite can exhibit greater toxicity than its precursor. This may be especially important during carcinogenesis, for example, where a xenobiotic is converted to a more reactive metabolite (e.g., an electrophile) capable of inducing a modification in the genome (DNA). An example of this is the metabolism of benzo[a]pyrene to a highly reactive epoxide:

Benzo[a]pyrene $\longrightarrow$ benzo[a]pyrene epoxide

Phase I and phase II biotransformation reactions are mediated by enzymes located in various subcellular compartments, such as cytoplasm, mitochondria, lysosomes, and microsomes. In general, highly lipid-soluble foreign chemicals that do not resemble endogenous metabolic intermediates tend to be metabolized through the microsomal enzyme systems. On the other hand, drugs that are structural analogs of endogenous compounds compete with the latter and thus may be metabolized by nonmicrosomal enzymes.

STRUCTURE AND FUNCTION OF MICROSOMAL CYTOCHROMES P-450

The most important and widespread enzyme system active in biotransformation reactions is that of microsomal cytochromes P-450. These electron transfer proteins contain a prosthetic group having a single iron atom coordinated to protoporphyrin IX. The prosthetic group, termed *heme*, undergoes reduction and oxidation during the catalytic cycle of the enzyme. The noncovalent binding of the heme prosthetic group with the apoprotein forms an enzyme active in oxidation-reduction reactions known as a *cytochrome*. It functions to activate molecular oxygen to a form capable of insertion into various types of chemical bonds on organic substrates. Because it is an oxygen-binding hemoprotein, cytochrome P-450 is inhibited by carbon monoxide (CO), an electronic analog of molecular oxygen. The name *P-450* derives from the spectral position of the distinctive absorbance maximum observed when the reduced enzyme is mixed with CO. Under such conditions, a maximum, or peak, is seen at 450 nm.

Cytochrome P-450 is now known to be a group of closely related proteins, rather than a single protein, which catalyze a diverse number of oxidative reactions involved in metabolism of drugs and other xenobiotics. Cytochromes P-450 and other enzymes of the drug-metabolizing microsomal system are encoded by a supergene cluster on mammalian nuclear DNA. Several distinct isoenzymes (isozymes) of cytochrome P-450 exist within the microsomal membrane. These exhibit broad and partially overlapping substrate specificities but are unique by immunologic criteria. The mix of particular cytochrome P-450 isozymes present within the microsomal membrane is subject to complex genetic and environmental regulatory influences. Effectors operate at the level of transcription through both induction and repression mechanisms, leading to alterations in membrane enzyme composition.

From a practical view, this means that metabolism of a given drug can be influenced by factors such as nutrition, age, presence of disease, or prior exposure to structurally related drugs. For example, such physiologic and environmental factors may cause microsomal enzyme induction resulting in more rapid metabolism of the drug. Consequently, the duration and intensity of pharmacologic action may be curtailed.

MICROSOMAL OXIDATION REACTIONS IN DRUG BIOTRANSFORMATION

Many of the reactions catalyzed by the microsomal drug metabolizing enzyme system may be classified as oxidations. These include oxygenation or hydroxylation reactions, and dealkylation reactions at both carbon and nitrogen atoms, as well as a number of other types of reactions (Table 4-1). Microsomal enzymes act on a broad spectrum of aliphatic and aromatic structures. These diverse oxidations are catalyzed by cytochromes P-450, which activate molecular oxygen using reducing equivalents derived from NADPH. The reducing equivalents are transferred to a cytochrome P-450 through a flavoprotein known as NADPH-cytochrome P-450 reductase. These proteins are embedded within a lipid membrane which is relatively fluid, thus permitting the enzymes and lipophilic substrates to interact by diffusion.

In microsomal monooxygenase or "mixed-function oxidase" reactions, reducing equivalents from NADPH are utilized to activate molecular oxygen, which is then incorporated into the drug substrate (e.g., as a hydroxyl group). The general stoichiometry for cytochrome P-450-linked monooxygenase reactions is

$$RH + NADPH + O_2 + H^+ \longrightarrow ROH + NADP^+ + H_2O$$

The catalytic cycle for activation of molecular oxygen by cytochrome P-450 includes several steps and is outlined in Fig. 4-1. Reducing equivalents are delivered

TABLE 4-1   Types of microsomal cytochrome P-450-dependent oxidation reactions

Reaction type	Chemical change	Examples
Aliphatic hydroxylation	$R \longrightarrow R{-}OH$	Pentobarbital Phenylbutazone
Aromatic hydroxylation	$Ar \longrightarrow Ar{-}OH$	Phenytoin
Epoxidation	$R_1{-}CH{=}CH{-}R_2 \longrightarrow R_1{-}\overset{\displaystyle O}{\overset{\diagup\diagdown}{CH{-}CH}}{-}R_2$	Benzo[a]pyrene Aflatoxin
N-Dealkylation	$R_1{-}\underset{\underset{\displaystyle CH_3}{\|}}{N}{-}R_2 \longrightarrow R_1{-}\underset{\underset{\displaystyle H}{\|}}{N}{-}R_2$	Diazepam Prazepam Methadone
O-Dealkylation	$R{-}O{-}CH_3 \longrightarrow R{-}OH$	Codeine
S-Dealkylation	$R{-}S{-}CH_3 \longrightarrow R{-}SH$	Methylthiopurine
N-Hydroxylation	$R_1{-}\underset{\underset{\displaystyle H}{\|}}{N}{-}R_2 \longrightarrow R_1{-}\underset{\underset{\displaystyle OH}{\|}}{N}{-}R_2$	2-Acetylaminofluorene
Sulfoxidation	$R_1{-}S{-}R_2 \longrightarrow R_1{-}\overset{\overset{\displaystyle O}{\|}}{S}{-}R_2$	Chlorpromazine
Desulfuration	$R_1{-}\overset{\overset{\displaystyle S}{\|}}{P}{-}R_2 \longrightarrow R_1{-}\overset{\overset{\displaystyle O}{\|}}{P}{-}R_2$	Parathion
Dehalogenation	$R_1{-}\underset{\underset{\displaystyle X}{\|}}{\overset{\overset{\displaystyle H}{\|}}{C}}{-}R_2 \longrightarrow R_1{-}\underset{\underset{\displaystyle OH}{\|}}{\overset{\overset{\displaystyle H}{\|}}{C}}{-}R_2 + XH$	Halothane

Note   R,R_1,R_2, etc., can be alkyl, aryl, or hydrogen groups for most reaction types. Additional oxidation reactions, such as oxidative deamination, are catalyzed by FAD-containing monooxygenase.

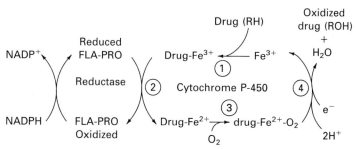

FIGURE 4-1 Catalytic cycle for cytochrome P-450-dependent monooxygenase reactions. The sequence of steps in the hydroxylation of a drug substrate (RH) is illustrated (flavoproteins = FLA-PRO). (1) Drug binds to the oxidized heme of the enzyme; (2) the first electron from NADPH-cytochrome P-450 reductase reduces the drug-enzyme complex; (3) oxygen binds to the reduced enzyme-drug complex; (4) an intramolecular oxidation-reduction reaction forms "activated oxygen" concomitant with entry of the second electron from the reductase. This activated oxygen is inserted into the drug substrate, and the hydroxylated product (ROH) is released, regenerating the oxidized enzyme. [Adapted from R. E. White and M. J. Coon, *Ann. Rev. Biochem.*, **49**:315–356 (1980).]

in two separate one-electron transfer reactions from NADPH-cytochrome P-450 reductase. An enzyme-bound activated species of oxygen, possibly a free radical, is an intermediate in the cycle.

An alternative branch of the microsomal electron transport system consists of a distinct NADH-cytochrome b_5 flavoprotein reductase and cytochrome b_5. This branch of the microsomal electron transport system normally functions in fatty acid desaturation, the synthesis of long-chain unsaturated fatty acids from saturated precursors. Fatty acid desaturation requires oxygen. It can be inhibited by cyanide, but not by CO, indicating that it proceeds independently of cytochromes P-450. With certain xenobiotic substrates, however, the second electron required in the P-450 catalytic cycle can be provided by NADH, rather than NADPH, through the NADH-cytochrome b_5 reductase/cytochrome b_5 system.

The hepatic microsomal electron transport system also contains a third distinct flavoprotein known as FAD-containing monooxygenase. This enzyme, formerly known as amine oxidase, catalyzes the oxidative deamination of substituted amines, such as amphetamine, to the corresponding ketones plus ammonia. Microsomal FAD-containing monooxygenase requires oxygen and NADPH but acts independently of cytochromes P-450. It is not inhibited by CO. This enzyme also functions as a sulfur oxidase, converting thioethers to sulfoxides and sulfones. The flow of re-

ducing equivalents through the microsomal electron transport system is shown in Fig. 4-2.

The utilization of oxygen by the drug-metabolizing microsomal system outlined above is mechanistically different from that of mitochondria. Microsomal electron transport results in conversion of molecular oxygen to a chemically more reactive form that is capable of condensing with an organic substrate. In mitochondrial respiration, reducing equivalents (hydrogen atoms) from substrates such as glutamate or succinate are transferred through sequential oxidation-reduction reactions to molecular oxygen, which is reduced to water. The stepwise transfer of reducing equivalents through the mitochondrial respiratory chain catalyzed by hydrogen and electron carriers (e.g., cytochromes) is coupled to the synthesis of adenosine triphosphate (ATP) by means of an intermediate transmembrane electrochemical proton gradient. In this way, the energy of substrate oxidation is conserved as ATP. By contrast, microsomal electron transport is not coupled to ATP synthesis and thus does not conserve energy.

NONMICROSOMAL OXIDATION REACTIONS IN DRUG BIOTRANSFORMATION

Enzymes localized in subcellular compartments other than the endoplasmic reticulum also play a role in drug biotransformation. For the most part, these enzymes tend to have broad substrate specificities (Table 4-2).

1. *Alcohol oxidation* The oxidation of primary and secondary alcohols to the corresponding aldehydes is catalyzed by NAD-linked alcohol dehydrogenase. This enzyme is localized in the cytoplasm and is found predominantly in liver, with lesser amounts in kidney and lung. Hepatic alcohol dehydrogenase is responsible for the bulk of ethanol metabolism following consumption of alcoholic beverages. The enzyme exhibits reactivity with a variety of alcohols. Retinol has been suggested to be its natural endogenous substrate.

2. *Aldehyde oxidation* The oxidation of aliphatic aldehydes to carboxylic acids is catalyzed by NAD-linked aldehyde dehydrogenase. Several isozymes with different substrate preferences exist. An intramitochondrial isozyme having a high affinity for acetaldehyde is primarily involved in metabolism of ethanol-derived acetaldehyde, while a low affinity cytoplasmic isozyme is active in catabolism of aldehydes derived from biogenic amines and xenobiotics.

3. *Monoamine and diamine oxidation* Monoamine oxidase (MAO), a flavoprotein localized on the outer mitochondrial membrane, oxidatively deaminates short-chain monoamines (e.g., catecholamines and tyramine) to aldehydes. Short-

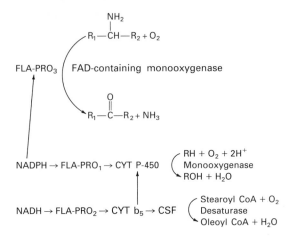

FIGURE 4-2 Pathways for microsomal electron transport. Flow of reducing equivalents (electrons) through branches of the microsomal electron transport chain is indicated by the arrows. The various microsomal flavoproteins are designated by the abbreviation FLA-PRO. $FLA\text{-}PRO_1$ = NADPH-cytochrome P-450 reductase; $FLA\text{-}PRO_2$ = NADH-cytochrome b_5 reductase; $FLA\text{-}PRO_3$ = FAD-containing monooxygenase (amine oxidase); CSF = cyanide-sensitive factor of the fatty acid desaturase complex. With some cytochrome (Cyt) P-450-dependent substrates, the second electron of the catalytic cycle (Fig. 4-1) can be derived from NADH, rather than NADPH, by way of cytochrome b_5.

TABLE 4-2   **Nonmicrosomal oxidative reactions in biotransformation**

Reaction type	Chemical change	Examples
Alcohol oxidation	$RCH_2OH + NAD^+ \longrightarrow RCHO + NADH$	Ethanol Retinol
Aldehyde oxidation	$RCHO + NAD^+ \longrightarrow RCOOH + NADH$	Acetaldehyde
Monoamine oxidation	$RCH_2NH_2 + O_2 \longrightarrow RCHO + NH_3$	Tyramine Epinephrine Norephinephrine Dopamine Serotonin
Diamine oxidation	$NH_2RCH_2NH_2 + O_2 \longrightarrow NH_2RCHO + NH_3$	Histamine
Purine oxidation	$Ar(N) \longrightarrow Ar(O)$	Xanthine Theophylline

chain amines having a methyl group on the adjacent carbon, such as amphetamine, are not substrates for MAO and are oxidized instead by the microsomal enzyme system. A distinct diamine oxidase acts on short-chain unsubstituted diamines such as histamine.

4. *Purine oxidation* Xanthine oxidase, a flavoprotein found in the cytosol, catalyzes the oxidation of xanthine to uric acid. It is also active with a number of purine derivatives, including theophylline and caffeine.

REDUCTION REACTIONS IN DRUG BIOTRANSFORMATION

Reductions are less common in biotransformation than are oxidations. Table 4-3 provides some pharmacologically important examples. Reductions of nitro and azo groups are involved in the biotransformation of drugs such as chloramphenicol and prontosil, respectively. Microsomal cytochromes P-450-linked reductions can occur under conditions of low oxygen tension. Reductive dehalogenation reactions catalyzed by cytochromes P-450 are implicated in the toxicities of carbon tetrachloride and the pesticide DDT.

The most important microsomal reduction reactions involve NADPH-cytochrome P-450 reductase. Many quinone-containing drugs can function as electron acceptors with this flavoprotein. These drugs become reduced by a single electron to give unstable semiquinone species. The latter autooxidize with molecular oxygen, forming free radicals which can potentially initiate pathologic processes, and regenerate the parent drug. Such a sequence of enzymatic reduction followed by autooxidation provides a mechanism for catalytic amplification of oxygen radical production by the drug itself. This process is referred to as redox cycling (Fig. 4-3). Cytotoxicity of the anticancer agents doxorubicin and mitomycin C may involve such a sequence of reactions.

Alcohol dehydrogenase, a reversible enzyme, can catalyze the reduction of chloral hydrate to trichloroethanol. Quinone reductase, a flavoprotein found in the cytoplasm of hepatocytes and formerly known as diaphorase, catalyzes the NADPH-dependent two-electron reduction of menadione (vitamin K_3) and several quinone-containing xenobiotics. Other carbonyl reductases catalyze reduction of certain aldehydic sugars (aldoses) and prostaglandins.

TABLE 4-3   Reduction reactions in biotransformation

Reaction type	Chemical change	Examples
Microsomal		
Nitro reduction	$Ar{-}NO_2 \longrightarrow Ar{-}NH_2$	Chloramphenicol Clonazepam
Azo reduction	$Ar_1{-}N{=}N{-}Ar_2 \longrightarrow Ar_1NH_2 + Ar_2NH_2$	Prontosil
Reductive dehalogenation	$RCCl_3 \longrightarrow RCHCl_2$	Carbon tetrachloride DDT
Nonmicrosomal		
Aldehyde reduction	$RCHO + NADH \longrightarrow RCH_2OH + NAD^+$	Chloral hydrate
Ketone reduction	$R_1{-}\overset{\displaystyle O}{\overset{\|}{C}}{-}R_2 + NADPH \longrightarrow R_1{-}\overset{\displaystyle OH}{\overset{\|}{C}H}{-}R_2 + NADP^+$	Naloxone
Quinone reduction	$Q + NADPH \longrightarrow QH_2 + NADP^+$	Menadione

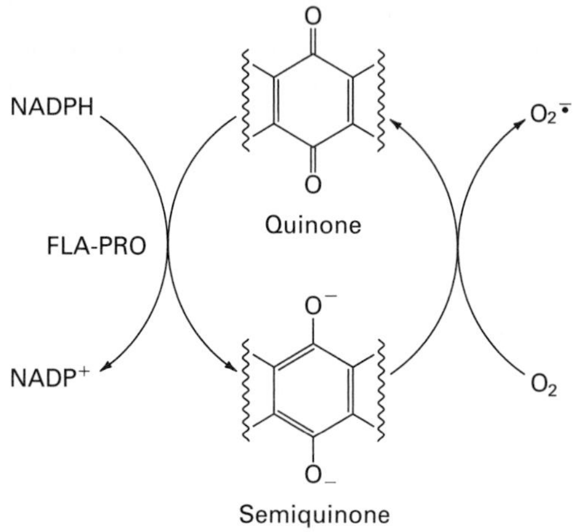

FIGURE 4-3 Redox cycling by a quinone-containing drug. Enzymatic one-electron reduction of a quinone-containing xenobiotic catalyzed by a flavoprotein (FLA-PRO), such as NADPH-cytochrome P-450 reductase, forms an unstable semiquinone. The semiquinone undergoes autooxidation with molecular oxygen in a spontaneous nonenzymatic reaction, forming an oxygen radical (superoxide anion O_2^-) and regenerating the parent quinone. The quinone thus acts catalytically to promote the formation of oxygen free radicals which are potentially toxic. A quinone can also undergo two-electron reduction to a hydroquinone, which is often more stable than the corresponding semiquinone species. The relative formation of semiquinone and hydroquinone species is dependent on both the oxidation-reduction chemistry of the quinone itself and the catalytic mechanism of the flavoenzyme catalyzing the reduction. Redox cycling mechanisms have been demonstrated in vitro with the anticancer drug doxorubicin and the xenobiotic paraquat.

HYDROLYSIS REACTIONS IN DRUG BIOTRANSFORMATION

Esterases and amidases hydrolyze ester and amide groups, respectively, producing carboxylic acids (Table 4-4). These enzymes typically exhibit low substrate selectivity. They are widely distributed throughout mammalian cells and in the plasma. Recent studies have indicated that both types of hydrolytic activities are often catalyzed by the same enzyme. In most cases, amides are hydrolyzed at a slower rate than the corresponding esters.

CONJUGATION REACTIONS IN PHASE II BIOTRANSFORMATION

The coupling of endogenous small molecules with polar functional groups on a xenobiotic is termed *conjugation*. In humans, the synthesis of glucuronides is the most important type of conjugation in drug biotransformation. Glucose 1-phosphate is first activated by condensing with uridine triphosphate (UTP) to form uridine diphosphoglucose (UDPG), a normal intermediate in the synthesis of glycogen. UDPG is subsequently oxidized to uridine diphosphoglucuronic acid (UDPGA) in an NAD-dependent reaction catalyzed by a specific dehydrogenase. Both of these reactions are accomplished by cytoplasmic enzymes. A microsomal glucuronyl transferase then catalyzes transfer of the glucuronic acid moiety to a polar group (often hydroxyl) on the drug molecule.

$$\text{Glucose 1-P} + \text{UTP} \longrightarrow \text{UDPG} + \text{PP}_i$$
$$\text{UDPG} + 2\text{NAD}^+ \longrightarrow \text{UDPGA} + 2\text{NADH}$$
$$\text{UDPGA} + \text{ROH} \longrightarrow \text{RO-glucuronide} + \text{UDP}$$

The polar nature of the glucuronic acid residue renders the conjugated molecule more readily excretable than the parent drug. Glucuronyl transferase, like other microsomal enzymes, is inducible by various drugs or xenobiotics which cause proliferation of endoplasmic reticulum.

Other important, but less frequent, routes of phase II biotransformation in humans include sulfate ester synthesis, methylation, acylation, and conjugation with glutathione (Table 4-5). These reactions are catalyzed mainly by nonmicrosomal enzymes. Sulfate groups are transferred by means of an activated intermediate form, 3'-phosphoadenosine-5'-phosphosulfate, synthesized by an ATP-dependent enzyme. Sulfate is typically conjugated to hydroxyl groups on a drug molecule by a cytoplasmic sulfotransferase. Sulfation is less common than glucuronide formation in biotransformation owing to the limited availability of inorganic sulfate.

Methyl groups are transferred in the form of S-adenosyl methionine to various functional groups on xenobiotics. Nonspecific N-, O-, and S-methyl transferase enzymes, found mainly in the cytosol, are responsible for these conjugations. By contrast with other phase II reactions, methylation tends to decrease the polarity of the xenobiotic molecule.

TABLE 4-4   Hydrolysis reactions in biotransformation

Reaction type	Chemical change	Examples
Ester hydrolysis	$$R_1-\overset{\overset{\displaystyle O}{\|\|}}{C}-OR_2 + H_2O \longrightarrow R_1-\overset{\overset{\displaystyle O}{\|\|}}{C}-OH + R_2OH$$	Acetylcholine Succinylcholine Aspirin Procaine
Amide hydrolysis	$$R_1-\overset{\overset{\displaystyle O}{\|\|}}{C}-NH-R_2 + H_2O \longrightarrow R_1-\overset{\overset{\displaystyle O}{\|\|}}{C}-OH + R_2NH_2$$	Procainamide Lidocaine Indomethacin
Peptide hydrolysis	$$-R_1-\overset{\overset{\displaystyle O}{\|\|}}{C}-NH-R_2^- + H_2O \longrightarrow -R_1-\overset{\overset{\displaystyle O}{\|\|}}{C}-OH + -R_2NH_2$$	Proinsulin

Acylation reactions utilize coenzyme A esters as acyl donors and commonly result in transfer of the acyl group to an amine functional group on the drug. This reaction is catalyzed by various acyl transferase enzymes. Drug acyl CoA derivatives are subsequently conjugated with amino acids such as glycine or glu-

TABLE 4-5   Conjugation reactions in biotransformation

Reaction type	Enzyme	Examples
Glucuronidation	UDP-glucuronyl transferase	Bilirubin Chloramphenicol Diazepam
Sulfation	Sulfotransferases	Estrone Androsterone Acetaminophen
Acetylation	Acyl CoA transferases	Isoniazid Sulfonamides
Methylation	Methyl transferases	Norepinephrine Thiouracil
Glutathione conjugation	GSH transferases	Bromobenzene Ethacrynic acid

tamic acid prior to excretion, regenerating free coenzyme A in the process.

Coupling of glutathione, the principal sulfhydryl buffer of mammalian cells, with a drug functional group leads to the formation of thioether compounds. This reaction is catalyzed by broad-specificity glutathione-S-transferases present in liver and, to a less extent, in other tissues. The glutathione conjugates are subsequently hydrolyzed to cysteine derivatives by enzymes in the kidney. The latter are then acetylated to form N-acetylcysteine conjugates, known as mercapturic acids, which are readily excreted into the urine. Mercapturic acid formation is a frequent route for detoxication of electrophilic metabolites of xenobiotics. Conjugation reactions with glutathione are also involved in the synthesis of leukotrienes from endogenous arachidonic acid.

DRUGS WITH LIMITED BIOTRANSFORMATION

Highly polar and charged compounds, such as moderately strong acids and bases, have restricted permeability through lipid membranes and thus are usually not metabolized to a significant extent. Hexamethonium is an example of a polar compound that is not biotransformed prior to excretion. Likewise, nonpolar compounds which are relatively inert and chemically unreactive are not biotransformed to any significant extent. Examples are some gaseous anesthetics such as isoflurane and halothane. These anesthetic agents are mainly excreted unchanged via the lungs, although minor amounts are metabolized through the hepatic microsomal system.

INDUCTION OF THE DRUG-METABOLIZING MICROSOMAL SYSTEM

The level of activity of the drug-metabolizing microsomal system determines the duration and intensity of pharmacologic action of many drugs owing to its predominance in biotransformation reactions. One of the most important aspects of the microsomal enzyme system is its ability to be induced, or increase its activity, in response to various physiologic and environmental factors. Molecular biology has begun to unravel the mechanisms responsible for this phenomenon. As mentioned earlier, cytochrome P-450 is now known to be a group of closely related hemeproteins with overlapping substrate specificities. At least 10 species of cytochrome P-450 have been identified on the basis of DNA coding sequences as well as by immunologic and enzymatic criteria. Unique cytochrome P-450 species are involved in reactions with several aliphatic and aromatic hydrocarbons, steroids, fatty acids, ethanol, and a variety of drugs and xenobiotics.

The two most thoroughly studied inducers of microsomal drug-metabolizing enzymes are phenobarbital and 3-methylcholanthrene. These are representative of barbiturates and polycylic aromatic hydrocarbons, respectively. Administration of phenobarbital causes proliferation of the liver endoplasmic reticulum, an increase in the microsomal content (nanomoles per milligram of protein) of cytochromes P-450, and enhancement of the metabolism of a variety of xenobiotic substrates. Methylcholanthrene induces a distinct isozyme of cytochrome P-450 and elicits a different pattern of enhancement of microsomal enzyme activities compared to phenobarbital. Chronic ethanol consumption likewise induces a unique form of cytochrome P-450 which is involved in ethanol metabolism.

The molecular mechanism by which activity is induced is thought to involve binding of an inducer, commonly the substrate or drug, to a specific receptor molecule in the cytoplasm of the hepatocyte. The receptor-inducer complex is then translocated into the nucleus whereupon it activates transcription of specific genes through an interaction with DNA. The mRNA transcribed from DNA is subsequently translated, leading to synthesis and incorporation of new cytochrome P-450 species into the membrane of the smooth endoplasmic reticulum. In addition, a regulatory control site, termed the A_h locus, is present on the DNA. This site controls transcription of several genes for related microsomal enzymes, particularly NADPH-cytochrome P-450 reductase and UDP-glucuronyl transferase, as well as the cytochrome P-450 genes themselves. Thus the induction sequence involves interaction of the receptor-inducer complex with the A_h locus and leads to increased amounts of the complement of microsomal enzymes. For this reason, factors such as sex (hormonal status), age, nutrition, and prior exposure to related xenobiotics can alter metabolism of a drug by changing the amount or relative composition of the enzymes present in the microsomal membrane. By far the most important factor, however, is prior exposure to the drug itself. This often results in preinduction of the microsomal enzymes responsible for its biotransformation, thus altering its pharmacokinetics. When the enzymes responsible for biotransformation of a drug are induced, the administered drug will be metabolized more rapidly. Consequently, a normally effective dose may be completely ineffective.

ROLE OF METABOLIC EFFECTS IN DRUG-DRUG INTERACTIONS

The overlapping substrate specificities of the cytochrome P-450 enzymes and the phenomenon of enzyme induction play roles in drug-drug interactions. Exposure to one drug sometimes alters the pharmacology of a second, often structurally unrelated, drug. Induction of the microsomal drug-metabolizing system provides a molecular mechanism which can account for such a situation. That is, alteration of the content of enzymes involved in biotransformation of the second drug as a consequence of enzyme induction caused by the first drug will modify the pharmacokinetics of the second drug. A clinically important example of this concerns the action of barbiturates in alcoholics. Chronic alcohol abusers, in the absence of ethanol, show a decreased sedative effect following administration of barbiturates, due in part to an enhanced rate of barbiturate metabolism through the cytochrome P-450 system. On the other hand, non-alcoholics who become acutely intoxicated by the concomitant use of both ethanol and barbiturates show enhanced central nervous system depression. This arises from an additive sedative effect plus decreased biotransformation of the barbiturate. In this case, competition between ethanol and the barbiturate for metabolism through the microsomal system, as well as competition for reducing equivalents, slows the inactivation and elimination of both agents.

ENVIRONMENTAL FACTORS IN REGULATION OF BIOTRANSFORMATION

The commonality of the enzymatic pathways involved in biotransformation of drugs and other xenobiotics may account for many drug-drug interactions observed clinically. Both direct effects, such as two agents acting as substrates for the same enzyme, and indirect effects, such as enzyme induction, can be important factors. In addition to drugs, many chemicals present in the environment are known to stimulate the activity of the hepatic microsomal system. Polychlorinated biphenyls (PCBs), a group of chemicals widely employed in manufacturing and electrical industries, are potent inducers of the microsomal drug-metabolizing system. Likewise, many pesticides and herbicides used in agriculture and many organic solvents used in industry are metabolized via the microsomal enzyme systems. These can function as both inducers and inhibitors of microsomal enzyme activities.

Tobacco smoke, which contains a complex mixture of hydrocarbons, including benzo[a]pyrene, and gases such as CO, also affects microsomal enzyme activities. For this reason, smokers may exhibit markedly different pharmacokinetic profiles as compared to non-smokers with respect to drugs biotransformed via microsomal enzymes. Most often, smokers demonstrate enhanced rates of drug biotransformation owing to preinduction of the microsomal enzymes.

PHYSIOLOGIC FACTORS IN REGULATION OF BIOTRANSFORMATION

Physiologic factors are also important clinically for modulating drug actions. For example, newborns have low levels of drug-metabolizing enzymes and thus may be more sensitive to drugs. Likewise, liver damage makes individuals more sensitive to a variety of drugs. Obstructive jaundice, hepatitis, and cirrhosis impair the formation of glucuronide and sulfate conjugates. Thus caution should be taken in prescribing drugs for such patients.

PHARMACOGENETIC VARIANTS IN BIOTRANSFORMATION

Many enzymes involved in biotransformation exhibit substantial variation in activity levels between individuals. This phenomenon was first identified with respect to acylation reactions involved in metabolism of the antitubercular drug isoniazid. Measurements of the rate of acylation of isoniazid in various populations have demonstrated a bimodal distribution of "slow" and "fast" acetylators. Genetic studies have established that slow acetylation is inherited as an autosomal recessive trait. Genetic polymorphism has also been found for cytochrome P-450-dependent hydroxylation of debrisoquine and related drugs.

The existence of pharmacogenetic variants can account for markedly different pharmacokinetic profiles between individuals. Such genetic differences illustrate the central role of biotransformation in governing pharmacologic activity. Likewise, genetic differences may result in altered metabolite profiles between individuals. Pharmacogenetic variations may also underlie, at least in part, idiosyncratic drug toxicities. For example, the trait of rapid acetylation of procainamide has been associated with the development of systemic lupus erythematosus-like conditions in some patients.

In summary, an awareness of the basic metabolic patterns involved in drug biotransformation allows the physician to employ the full spectrum of modern pharmaceutical agents to greatest advantage in treatment of disease.

BIBLIOGRAPHY

Creasey, W. A.: *Drug Disposition in Humans*, Oxford, Oxford, England, 1979.

Gibson, G. G., and P. Skett: *Introduction to Drug Metabolism*, Chapman and Hall, London, 1986.

Gram, T. E., L. K., Okine, and R. A. Gram: "The Metabolism of Xenobiotics by Certain Extrahepatic Organs and Its

Relation to Toxicity," *Ann. Rev. Pharmacol. Toxicol.*, **26**:259–291 (1986).

Greenblatt, D., and R. I., Shader: *Pharmacokinetics in Clinical Practice*, Saunders, Philadelphia, 1985.

Hodgson, E.: "Metabolism of Toxicants," in E., Hodgson, and P. E. Levi (eds.), *A Textbook of Modern Toxicology*, pp. 51–84, Elsevier Science Publishing, New York 1987.

Kappus, H.: "Overview of Enzyme Systems Involved in Bioreduction of Drugs and in Redox Cycling," *Biochem. Pharmacol.*, **35**:1–6 (1986).

Kupfer, A.: "Genetic Differences of Drug Metabolism in Man: Polymorphic Drug Oxidation," in G. Siest (ed.), *Drug Metabolism: Molecular Approaches and Pharmacological Implications*, pp. 25–33, Pergamon, Oxford, England, 1985.

Nebert, D. W., and F. J. Gonzalez: "P450 Genes: Structure, Evolution, and Regulation," *Ann. Rev. Biochem.*, **56**:945–993 (1987).

Waterman, M. R., and R. W. Estabrook: "The Induction of Microsomal Electron Transport Enzymes," *Molec. Cell. Biochem.*, **53/54**:267–278 (1983).

Sipes, I. G., and A. J. Gandolfi: "Biotransformation of Toxicants," in C. D., Klaassen, M. D., Amdur, and J. Doull (eds.), *Casarett and Doull's Toxicology*, 3d ed., pp. 64–98, Macmillan, New York, 1986.

White, R. E., and M. J. Coon: "Oxygen Activation by Cytochrome P-450," *Ann. Rev. Biochem.*, **49**:315–356 (1980).

Whitlock, J. P.: "The Regulation of Cytochrome P-450 Gene Expression," *Ann. Rev. Pharmacol. Toxicol.*, **26**:333–369 (1986).

C H A P T E R   5

Clinical Pharmacology

Joseph R. DiPalma

Clinical pharmacology is that branch of the medical sciences which is most concerned with the rational development, the effecive and safe use, and the proper evaluation of drugs and other chemical entities in humans for the diagnosis, prevention, alleviation, and cure of disease and disease syndromes. Alternative definitions, which are less specific and satisfactory, identify clinical pharmacology as the science of the development of new drugs, the scientific basis of therapeutics, or the science of pharmacology applied to humans. There is obviously merit in each of these latter definitions, but it is also true that clinical pharmacology is not solely confined to the development of new drugs, that therapeutics is a distinct branch of medical practice, and that clinical pharmacology is pharmacology and deals with the use of drugs with safety not restricted to any animal species. The laws of clinical pharmacology apply to veterinary medicine as well as human medicine.

ORGANIZATION

There are three organizations devoted to fostering and promoting the discipline. The oldest and largest is the *American Society of Clinical Pharmacology and Therapeutics*, which publishes the journal *Clinical Pharmacology and Therapeutics*. *The American College of Clinical Pharmacology*, the second organization completely devoted to this speciality, publishes the journal *Clinical Pharmacology*. The third organization is the Clini-

cal Pharmacology Section of the *American Society for Pharmacology and Experimental Therapeutics*.

Pharmacy, formerly devoted almost entirely to dispensing drugs, has its counterpart in clinical pharmacology. This concerns the development of the Phar.D., or clinical pharmacist. Most pharmacy schools now offer this advanced degree, which trains pharmacists in a clinical setting such as hospitals or ambulatory clinics. Phar.D.s have contributed in the areas of pharmacokinetics, adverse drug reactions, drug interactions, and in the development of new drugs and therapies.

All large medical centers employ both M.D. clinical pharmacologists and Phar.D.s to manage the complex problems of modern drug therapy. The drug industry also employs large numbers of these specialists to develop and market drugs. Many others are employed by the government for research and drug control. There has been a movement to form a speciality board for clinical pharmacology. Encouragement from all three aforementioned societies appears to ensure its institution.

This chapter is devoted to those areas in pharmacology which are the special province of clinical pharmacology and therapeutics. All physicians, since they prescribe drugs, must know clinical pharmacologic principles. For this reason a modern text of medical pharmacology is also a text of clinical pharmacology. Most medical schools now have instructional hours in clinical pharmacology in the third and fourth years.

PREDICTION OF BENEFICIAL AND ADVERSE EFFECTS

When drugs cause effects which are undesired, they are known as *adverse reactions* or *side effects*. In most cases they are extensions of the pharmacologic actions of the drug. For example, atropine used to reduce gastric secretions may also cause dryness of the mouth. Adverse reactions may in some instances be caused by a biotransformation product. Less common adverse reactions occur when the individual has a hypersensitivity or allergy to the drug or has a genetic constitution which may cause the drug to be biotransformed in an unusual fashion or to interact with an abnormal body component. The latter reactions are ordinarily termed *idiosyncratic*. Finally in many cases minor adverse reactions such as nausea, headache, and dizziness usually disappear with continued use of the drug, and the mechanism of these side effects in most cases is obscure. They, nevertheless, are of importance because they affect the acceptability of the drug by the patient.

Some drugs are specifically toxic to certain tissues, and this extends beyond their pharmacologic actions. Thus the analgesic phenacetin may, after extended use, cause renal damage, and tetracycline, an antibiotic, causes staining of the teeth when given to children. Unfortunately, not all toxic effects can be predicted by in vitro or animal studies. However, it is quite certain that if a toxicity occurs in two animal species such as rats and dogs it is very likely to occur also in humans. It follows that the same general rules apply to the prediction of beneficial actions.

STATISTICS

A mandatory feature of the design of any protocol for drug investigation is the assurance of the statistical validity of the results. This starts with insistence on *random selection* of subjects and the enrollment of appropriate number of individuals based on the estimated probability of securing a statistically valid result. In an all-or-none situation (cure of a bacterial infection which is ordinarily incurable) one or two subjects would suffice. In the study of an analgesic which relieves pain in only 20 percent of patients, many hundreds of subjects might be needed to prove efficacy. In epidemiologic studies of a drug to prevent coronary thrombosis, thousands of subjects and years of study would be required to secure conclusive results. Large and complex studies, as a consequence, require that a statistician be part of the research team.

BIOAVAILABILITY AND BIOEQUIVALENCE

Bioavailability applies particularly to orally administered drugs and less frequently to other routes of administration. It takes into consideration the fact that not all the administered drug is absorbed. Measurements of bioavailability are best done in humans and determined by the amount that reaches the general circulation (or excreted in the urine) compared with the amount administered. Many factors contribute to availability, such as solubility, particle size, excipients, local factors in the gut, rapid metabolism in the liver (first-pass effect), and many other elements. Seemingly minor differences in product formulation of the same drug sometimes cause wide differences in bioavailability. Two drugs may be chemically identical but may not produce the same blood levels after oral administration because of formulation differences. In this case they are not *bioequivalent* because they have different bioavailability.

PLACEBO EFFECT

Early in this century it was realized that certain drugs which had been used for years for specific conditions actually had no pharmacologic effect when studied objectively. Distinction must be made between the placebo and the placebo effect. *Placebo* is a Latin verb meaning "I shall please"; *placebo effect* may or may not occur and is defined as the psychologic or physiologic effect of a therapeutic drug or procedure which is not related to its specific pharmacologic activity. Most observers believe placebo effect can be explained by a psychologic mechanism. Experienced clinicians are well aware that many therapeutic effects are the results of a good sales talk and a pat on the back.

In any population some individuals are more susceptible to placebos than others. It must also be pointed out that while a greater number respond to a placebo with positive effects there are a minority who react negatively. Double-blind and blind studies help to identify placebo effects because the patient does not know when he or she is receiving the active ingredient or the placebo.

DRUG INTERACTIONS

It is rare for a patient to receive only one drug. As the number of drugs administered concomitantly increases beyond two, the probability of interaction of one drug with another increases. It is estimated for example that a hospitalized patient receives on the average 10 or more drugs. Most drug interactions probably are mild and escape notice by patient or clinicians; but there still are many which seriously affect the effectiveness and safety of the therapy, and some are even fatal.

The mechanisms of drug interactions are complex and varied. Any classification suffers from oversimplification. Most interactions are mainly involved with pharmacokinetic modalities such as the effect of one drug upon a second with respect to gastrointestinal absorption, plasma protein binding, increased or decreased drug biotransformation, and factors affecting excretion such as urinary pH. Drugs may also have synergistic and additive effects which exaggerate responses. Conversely they may antagonize each other by various mechanisms involving either the same or different receptors. The best approach to an understanding of drug interaction is to have a working knowledge of the major mechanisms and to realize which drugs are likely to be involved.

Enzyme Stimulation (Induction)

It is now known that many drugs and chemicals are capable of causing a proliferation both in activity and quantity of certain enzyme systems. Thus barbiturates, for example, induce the hepatic microsomal enzyme system. This may result in an accelerated biotransformation of the barbiturate itself or other drugs which are handled by this system. Thus, a cardiac patient might well be receiving both a barbiturate for sedation and an anticoagulant such as warfarin to prevent thromboembolic accidents. The dose of anticoagulant must be controlled carefully and is monitored by the prothrombin time. Since it is also inactivated by the hepatic microsomal enzyme system, the addition of barbiturate causes increased biotransformation, which in turn requires that a higher dose of anticoagulants be administered to prolong the prothrombin time, or else intravascular thrombosis might occur. Furthermore, when the barbiturate is withdrawn, the anticoagulant is not biotransformed as readily, and if the dose is not promptly lowered, it might cause excessive and even fatal bleeding episodes. (See Chap. 4 for a discussion of the drug-metabolizing microsomal system, also called the *microsomal mixed-function oxidase system.*)

Enzyme Inhibition

It is well known that drugs may inhibit or impede the usual functions of an enzyme or enzyme system. In fact some drugs, such as monoamine oxidase inhibitors (MAOI), are primarily used for this purpose. Monoamine oxidase inhibitors reduce the biotransformation of sympathomimetic amines, and thus they may have an exaggerated response. This is the basis of certain drug interactions; for example, the tyramine in food (aged cheese or wine) may cause a hypertensive crisis (see below).

Gastrointestinal Absorption

Insoluble complexes may be formed when two drugs are given simultaneously, for example, an antacid which chelates tetracycline and prevents its absorption. Antacids may also prevent the absorption of drugs which depend on an acid pH to exist in an unionized form. Other drugs such as anticholinergics may affect gastrointestinal motility, which may actually increase absorption in some cases and decrease absorption in other cases. Phenytoin may inhibit the activity of conjugase enzymes, which in time may prevent the conversion of folic acid to an absorbable form, eventually causing megaloblastic anemia. Other mechanisms may involve changes in intestinal flora and inhibition of vitamin K synthesis or absorption, thus influencing anticoagulant therapy.

Protein Binding

Drugs do not exist in a free form in body fluids. The blood proteins bind nearly all drugs to a varying degree, and there is therefore a competition between this site and the receptor site. A second drug which has a greater affinity for binding to plasma proteins may displace the first drug, and this leads to a greater effect than might be expected from a particular dose. An example might be displacement of coumarin anticoagulants by clofibrate, leading to enhanced antiprothrombin effect and perhaps bleeding tendencies.

Another example is the displacement of methotrexate from plasma protein by salicylates. This has caused increased methotrexate toxicity.

Adrenergic Mechanisms

Many active drugs resemble sympathomimetic amines and may interact with the adrenergic receptor so as to displace norepinephrine and prevent its reabsorption at the adrenergic site, or they may cause its release from a storage site. Tricyclic antidepressants block the uptake of norepinephrine. Some drugs may compete for the receptor site for norepinephrine and thus become antagonists or blockers.

Another major adrenergic mechanism involves catecholamine metabolism by monoamine oxidase (MAO). Inhibition of MAO results in accumulation of norepinephrine in adrenergic neurons. Administration of indirect-acting sympathomimetic amines such as tyramine (old wine, cheese) can result in an exaggerated hypertensive response.

Thus a great many interactions are possible at the adrenergic neuron. These may involve drugs such as guanethidine (an antihypertensive), tolbutamide (a hypoglycemic), propranolol (a beta-adrenergic-receptor blocking agent), and many others.

Cholinergic Mechanisms

Many commonly used drugs have anticholinergic actions in addition to their major pharmacologic action. Examples are meperidine, tricyclic antidepressants, diphenhydramine, and phenothiazines. When given in conjunction with a standard anticholinergic such as atropine, excessive anticholinergic effects may be noted.

Neuromuscular Junction

Antibiotics such as neomycin and kanamycin have a blocking action on the neuromuscular junction, aside from their antibiotic effect. When used together with anesthetics such as ether, halothane, or methoxyflurane, excessive and prolonged muscle paralysis might occur. Quinidine, another drug with a blocking action at the neuromuscular junction, is capable of intensifying the effects of tubocurarine, gallamine, and other standard neuromuscular blocking agents. Anticholinesterase agents may prolong the action of succinylcholine.

Drug Biotransformation

The term *drug interaction* arose from studies which implicated the potential of one drug to influence greatly the biotransformation of another through an intermediary mechanism. It was observed that phenobarbital and other highly lipophilic drugs caused induction of the microsomal enzyme system of the liver. This increased the amount and activity of this enzyme system. In consequence, a second drug given during the course of phenobarbital therapy would be rapidly biotransformed and thus be relatively less effective for a given dose. An anticoagulant, for example, would be rapidly biotransformed under these circumstances, and the attending physician would consequently increase the dose. If phenobarbital therapy were then terminated, the anticoagulant might cause fatal bleeding.

Many examples of this type of interaction have been established experimentally and clinically. In some instances biotransformation of the second drug is inhibited instead of enhanced. Some cases are rarely significant clinically, but it is always a mechanism to be kept in mind, since it might be exaggerated in such unusual circumstances as a primary defect in an enzyme.

Renal Tubular Transport

Some drugs inhibit the excretion of a second drug at the renal tubular level. One of the classic drug interactions is that of probenecid and its blockade of penicillin secretion. This is an example of drug interaction which may be used to achieve a useful purpose—to increase and prolong the therapeutic blood level of an antibiotic. On the other hand, there are instances where probenecid has produced toxic effects by causing the accumulation of a second drug. Indomethacin secretion, for example, is blocked by probenecid.

There are many other drugs which act on the renal tubule. It should be mentioned that dicumarol (bishydroxycoumarin), phenylbutazone, and salicylates inhibit the excretion of oral hypoglycemic drugs, causing an excessive hypoglycemic effect.

Urinary pH and Drug Excretion

Altering the pH of the urine has a profound effect on the rate of excretion of many drugs. Creation of an alkaline urine by diet or drug therapy will cause an increased excretion of phenobarbital, salicylic acid, and some sulfonamides. In fact, the excretion of all drugs that are weak acids (pK_a 3.0 to 7.5) will be increased; conversely, in acid urine their excretion will be decreased.

On the other hand, many drugs which are weak bases (pK_a 7.5 to 10.5) will demonstrate an increased excretion in acid urine and decreased excretion in alkaline urine. Examples of these drugs are amphetamine, meperidine, and quinidine.

There are other mechanisms of drug interactions which are mentioned throughout this text. The above cited are the ones most frequently encountered. Fortunately, there are now many sources of drug interaction information (see Bibliography).

FACTORS AFFECTING DRUG DOSAGE

Once a particular drug is selected for a disease or disease syndrome, the determination of the dosage regimen is the next important consideration. Most dosage ranges given in standard texts are for average adults. The vast majority of all patients are well served by such ranges, but there are important modifications in particular cases that are, for the most part, dictated by factors of age, sex, pregnancy, lactation, and renal and hepatic disease.

Age, Sex, and Weight

Recommended doses such as those in the *United States Pharmacopeia* (USP) are generally oral and intended for an adult who weighs in the neighborhood of 70 kg. It follows that a dose for an infant or child should be smaller. If weight alone is to be considered, one can easily calculate that a 3-month-old infant weighing 9.5 kg should receive only 13.5 percent of the adult dose. Unfortunately, weight is not the only factor. Rate of biotransformation is higher in the young, and it is more closely related to surface area than to weight. Also there is active growth and proliferation of tissues, as well as different hormonal balances, in the process of development. The very young are more easily dehydrated and demineralized than the adult. Some enzyme systems are not developed until 6 months or even a year of life. Fortunately, exact doses on a milligram per kilogram basis are available for drugs used in pediatrics, and the physician very rarely has to estimate dosage. Formulas which have been developed for pediatric dosage are generally not reliable in all instances, and it is better to rely on specific information about particular drugs.

There is some evidence that the elderly may require a smaller dose for a given effect as compared with younger individuals. Evidence has been advanced that many enzyme systems show a decline with age and that the reserve functions of the kidney and liver are markedly diminished. However, there is every indication that *ordinary* doses of *most* drugs are handled quite the same pharmacokinetically by the elderly as by younger adults. Degenerative disease of the CNS may require great caution with narcotics, and cardiovascular disease may greatly restrict the dose of cardiogenic agents. Good sense would dictate that where frailty, debility, and weight loss are an accompaniment of old age the adult dose should be reduced by one-third or even one-half.

Sex is a factor to consider in the determination of doses of some drugs. For example, the differences in the actions of sex hormones in females as contrasted with males are quite marked. But for the great majority of drugs, sex seems to make little difference in the adult dose requirements. On a milligram per kilogram basis, which is how all drugs should be prescribed, there is little reason to administer differently to a female than to a male. Certainly a frail 40-kg female should not receive the same dose as a robust 80-kg male.

Pregnancy and Lactation

In pregnancy there is the consideration that any drug administered to the mother is also administered to the developing fetus because many drugs cross the placental barrier. Most drugs now carry the warning "not recommended in pregnant females." Since the thalidomide episode of 1962, all drugs are suspected of being capable of causing birth defects. This is of particular importance in the first trimester of pregnancy, as it is now recognized that many drugs, including hormones and cancer chemotherapeutic agents, are definitely teratogenic. It is extremely difficult to prove that any drug is completely safe in the first trimester of pregnancy, and drug manufacturers, encouraged by the Food and Drug Administration (FDA), always label their drugs as contraindicated especially in the first trimester of pregnancy. Few would dare to argue with this dictum, but on occasion, e.g., in problems of cancer chemotherapy and other serious disease syndromes, the physician must wrestle with the problem of treating the mother with obvious risk to the fetus. Certainly, there is a choice of not prescribing antinausea or sedative agents in the first trimester of pregnancy.

During lactation most drugs will be secreted in the milk. The risk here is that treatment of the mother will also result in the drug reaching the nursing child. For example, morphine easily enters the milk supply, and an addicted mother will have an addicted nursing child. The safest rule is that any mother who needs continuing drug therapy of any type, but especially lithium or tricyclic antidepressants, should stop nursing her child. Aspirin, barbiturates, and antibiotics may be prescribed to the nursing mother in modest doses for limited periods of time without much danger. However if serious antipsychotic therapy is to be undertaken, it would be wiser to stop the nursing.

Renal Disease, Uremia

Impairment of renal function profoundly affects considerations of dosage to achieve a therapeutic effect while avoiding toxicity. Obviously, the most important factor is diminished glomerular filtration and tubular secretion of unchanged drug and active biotransformation products. However, delayed absorption, altered protein binding, impaired biotransformation, and abnormalities of distribution of drugs in the body all play a role in the increased incidence of adverse drug reactions observed to occur in uremic states.

Many ingenious approaches to this problem have been advanced. The most practical of these relates the dosage adjustment to the estimated decrease of excretion of the unchanged drug in the impaired kidney as compared with the normal kidney. The degree of impairment of the diseased kidney is calculated from the reduction of creatinine clearance (normal 120 mL/min). This may be calculated from serum creatinine levels using available nomograms. Tables of dosage adjustments of common drugs necessary in various degrees of renal failure as measured by serum creatinine levels are also available. Package inserts also carry this information where pertinent.

It is also evident that the uremic patient can benefit from more frequent measurement of serum blood levels. This is especially true for drugs which have a small benefit/risk ratio margin such as digitalis or aminoglycosides.

Considerations of potential toxicity require that spe-

cial care be taken regarding dosage with particular drugs. In uremia, for example, anticoagulants are especially prone to cause bleeding tendencies, salicylates and other analgesics have an increased incidence of gastric ulceration, and drugs which affect potassium, such as spironolactone, may cause hyperkalemia. Such drugs as gold, animoglycosides, and amphotericin B, among others, are apt to be more toxic even in smaller doses to the uremic kidney.

Hepatic Disease

It appears reasonable to assume that a loss of liver parenchyma would lead to a decrease in the capacity of this organ to biotransform drugs. This is true only in certain instances, and it turns out in practice that such factors as protein binding and changes in distribution may be more important. The influence of liver disease on various sample drugs is shown in Table 5-1.

It turns out that the rate of blood flow through the liver becomes of crucial importance in first-pass drugs (see Chap. 4). Thus in heart failure or advanced cirrhosis of the liver, where blood flow through this organ is markedly impaired, drugs such as meperidine, propranolol, propoxyphene, and lidocaine may have a markedly reduced clearance. On the other hand, drugs with a much lower extraction ratio, such as warfarin and phenytoin, may not be affected very much.

One of the problems which remains to be solved is an accurate measure of liver function comparable to creatinine clearance in the kidney. Unfortunately, available liver-function tests correlate poorly with impairment of drug-biotransformation capacity. Unless the liver is markedly impaired, drug-biotransformation capacity does not seem to be decreased. Even

TABLE 5-1   Serum half-life of sample drugs as affected by parenchymal liver disease

Prolonged $t_{1/2}$	Unchanged $t_{1/2}$
Carbenicillin	Chlorpromazine
Chloramphenicol	Phenytoin
Diazepam	Dicumarol
Lidocaine	Salicylic acid
Meperidine	
Prednisone	

so, a modest decrease in biotransformation capacity may not show any distinct changes clinically.

It is also important to consider that many drugs are inherently toxic to the liver, such as ethanol, tetracyclines, dactinomycin, and isoniazid. These drugs as well as those drugs which cause hypersensitivity like reactions in the liver, such as halothane, long-acting sulfonamides, phenytoin, and phenylbutazone, should be avoided wherever possible when impaired liver function is present.

It appears most practical to measure serum blood levels of drugs in advanced liver disease in an attempt to avoid overt toxicity. Observation of clinical effect in relationship to blood level is most important as a means to adjust the dose to a satisfactory level.

Pharmacogenetics

There are hereditary factors which influence the dosage of drugs. In fact the explanation of idiosyncratic and hypersensitivity reactions resides in the different genetic constitution of individuals. Often the difference lies in an altered rate of biotransformation because of the lack of, or excess amount of, a certain critical enzyme. Some of the classical genetic defects which change drug biotransformation are listed in Table 5-2.

DEVELOPMENT OF NEW DRUGS

Once a new chemical or an old drug with a new indication has been studied in animals and a distinctly favorable benefit/risk ratio is anticipated with the expectancy of small toxicity, it is desirable to study it in humans. How to do this safely has been the subject of much investigation. Furthermore, the study in humans must be performed in a meaningful and statistically valid manner. Some technologies have been designed which lessen the risk and make the probability of useful results more likely.

Animal versus Human Dose

One of the main problems in the initial human studies is to extrapolate the first dose to be used from the data obtained in lower animals. These data predict the quantitative and qualitative effects that may be expected from a compound. Although there is no set of rules here, the basis of extrapolation must include a comparison of animal species, body weights, metabolic rates, and rates of drug metabolism. One should be conservative in determining the first dose to be administered to people because of possible unexpected reactions. These include idiosyncrasy, hypersensitivity, effects on special brain centers, blood and bone marrow disturbances, and unusual metabolic actions.

Based on the data from acute animal toxicity studies, logarithmically increasing doses of the agent are administered to the selected animal to obtain the minimum effective dose. From these data are made estimates of the therapeutic index and therapeutic range. For example, perhaps a parasympathomimetic agent is studied in a group of animals and the dose-response relationship is as follows:

mg/kg	Pharmacologic response
2.5	No effect
5.0	Mild diarrhea
7.5	Bradycardia
10.0	Hyperpyrexia and achromodacryorrhea

The initial single human dose would be a fraction of the minimum effective dose, which in this example is 5.0 mg. If the rat were the test animal, a safe arbitrary suggestion might be $\frac{1}{200}$ of this dose as the total single initial dose for an average-size human, using the same route of administration. If the dog were the test animal, then $\frac{1}{10}$ of this minimum effective dose might be used.

Although mice, rats, rabbits, cats, and dogs are the animal species generally used, it is highly desirable to study nonhuman (monkey) and subhuman (orangutan or baboon) primates because of their physiologic similarity to humans. Here, one-half the minimum effective dose might be used in the initial human studies.

If an atropine-like agent is studied in certain rodents, a much smaller fraction of the minimum effective dose would be used in humans, since the rodent is resistant to compounds having atropine-like structures, and consequently, humans can be expected to be more sensitive. Such preclinical evaluations are important considerations.

TABLE 5-2   Some examples of genetic defects which modify drug biotransformation

Enzymatic reaction	Examples of drugs involved	Effect
1 Glucose-6-phosphate dehydrogenase deficiency in erythrocytes	Acetylsalicylic acid Acetophenetidin Nitrofurans p-Aminosalicylic acid Primaquine and others 8-Aminoquinolines Quinidine Sulfonamides	Acute hemolytic anemia
2 Glucuronyl transferase deficiency (found in Crigler-Najjar syndrome and newborn infants)	Acetophenetidin Chloral hydrate Codeine Chloramphenicol Indomethacin Morphine Nicotinic acid Probenecid	Exaggerated drug toxicity
3 γ-Aminolevulinic acid (ALA) synthetase stimulation	Barbiturates Chloroquine Estrogens Griseofulvin Sulfonamides	Acute intermittent porphyria
4 Pseudocholinesterase abnormality or deficiency	Succinylcholine	Prolonged apnea
5 Acetylase deficiency	Isoniazid	Peripheral neuropathy
6 Methemoglobin reductase deficiency	Chloroquine Diaminodiphenylsulfone (DDS) Primaquine	Methemoglobinemia

Single-Dose Methodology

When there is no detectable response in the human to the initial dose (based on the estimated dose suggested by the preceding considerations), the dose is slowly increased until a response appears. The response may or may not be the anticipated one, but all subjective and objective reactions are recorded. A second subject is given the same dose, and the reactions are again observed. When there is no response to these initial human trials using the estimated dosage, the dose is slowly increased until drug activity is manifested. Once this minimum effective dose has been determined, the dose is further increased to establish the *maximum tolerated dose,* or the dose which does not elicit undesirable effects. No individual should be exposed to more than a single dose in a short period of time. Usually a rest period of at least 1 week is allowed to prevent cumulative effects.

Blind and Double-Blind Studies

When evaluation of drug efficacy involves personal judgment, either subjective on the part of the patient or objective on the part of the investigator, further controls are necessary to prevent bias. This is particularly true for such drugs as analgesics, sedatives, antianginals, or tranquilizers, which are usually evaluated by their subjective effects. Even in diseases with such objective signs as hypertension, patient reassurance alone may produce a therapeutic effect and thereby mask the effect of the test substance. Because of psychologic influences, proper control is often difficult to achieve. Transference and countertransference between the enthusiastic investigator and subject or patient may lead to a variety of results. To avoid these bias factors, statistical techniques are resorted to, and *blinding* becomes necessary. In *single-blind* trials, the physician and associates—but not the patient—know the substance being used. When a completely dispassionate evaluation is needed, a *double-blind* trial is performed. Here, neither the individual administering the compound nor the patient knows the identity of the substance. All material is coded, including the test substance and a placebo and, if possible, an already known active substance therapeutically similar to the one being tested (standard reference or positive control). Occasionally, negative controls are used to duplicate certain side effects to prevent identification of the test substance. For example, quinine may be used to mimic the taste of a bitter substance. Obviously, the physical appearance and manner of handling the materials should render them indistinguishable.

A particularly valuable technique to ensure reliability of results is the *crossover*. Here the experimental and the control groups are exchanged once a therapeutic endpoint has been obtained. Thus each subject serves as his or her own control in addition to comparison with the whole group.

THE FOOD AND DRUG ADMINISTRATION

In the United States, the Food and Drug Administration (FDA) is responsible for monitoring investigational studies in humans and for determining the adequacy of pharmacologic, animal-toxicologic, and manufacturing-control information before and during clinical trials. In addition, the FDA must decide whether the design of clinical trials is appropriate in relation to the questions asked in the studies.

No new drug may be distributed interstate unless an investigational new drug (IND) application containing all the above information has been submitted to the FDA. For the purposes of the IND application, a new drug is defined as one not previously approved for marketing in the United States.

Once a drug has received full clinical investigation and it is desired to market it, a new drug application (NDA) must be made to the FDA. This application must contain full reports of pharmacologic and clinical trials, manufacturing data, and labeling information. Only after approval by the FDA may the drug be marketed.

Each IND and NDA application is reviewed by FDA scientists, including a physician, a pharmacologist, a chemist, a pharmacokineticist, a biometrician, and, where applicable, a microbiologist. In important or difficult cases the application may be presented to an advisory committee consisting of extramural experts. These committees may or may not approve a drug for marketing, or they may suggest additional studies to be done or special labeling.

The protocol for the study of a drug in humans differs, depending on the agent and its purported activity. Generally, the protocol allows for four phases of study which overlap each other but which are designed to progressively reveal the drug's beneficial and adverse properties.

Phase I Studies

In this phase small numbers of human volunteers, usually healthy with no disease syndrome, are given single doses of the drug. Careful pharmacodynamic and pharmacokinetic studies are done. The aim is to establish a minimum effective dose to achieve activity without significant adverse reactions. If the drug is one which is likely to be used chronically, then after single-dose parameters have been established, it may be given chronically to simulate the therapy of a disease situation and thus to determine its feasibility for chronic usage. If after these studies the drug shows promise and no adverse reactions become evident, then with the approval of the FDA the studies may proceed to phase II.

Phase II Studies

In phase II, small numbers of patients are selected with the symptoms or diseases for which the drug is purported to be effective. A design protocol is established which aims to demonstrate conclusively efficacy in relation to safety. Again the design may follow a single-blind, a double-blind, or indeed any rational approach indicated for a particular drug or disease. As new data accumulate, it is usually advisable to do chronic toxicity studies in animals. Additional metabolic and pharmacokinetic studies may also be indicated. If the drug is to be used for long periods of time in females, special studies of its effects on reproduction and fertility are necessary to forestall teratogenic effects. Usually there will be a late stage in phase II where findings are finalized and any additional observations are performed which are believed to be important.

Phase III Studies

If the drug survives phase II, then—with the approval of the FDA—phase III may be performed. This is actually a broad clinical trial on a large sample of specified patients. Here the attempt is to prove efficacy in the field; the investigation is usually performed by a number of different clinicians in different centers or even under actual medical practice conditions. The protocol of the investigation is designed to be more restrictive about the variability of what can be done. Dosage forms, methods, and routes of administration are clearly defined. The protocol must be approved by the FDA, and any toxicity must be immediately reported. Phase III studies usually require from 1 to 3 years. Following the collection and documentation of all data in humans, the FDA may allow the drug to be marketed for specified therapeutic purposes and applications. In most instances, clear proof must be advanced that the new drug is superior to an established product.

Phase IV Studies

FDA approval may be conditional and require monitoring. This constitutes, in practice, phase IV. Relatively small numbers of patients under conditions of actual use are followed in selected medical centers under the guidance of qualified physicians. The purpose is to further establish usefulness and safety. Some drugs will require postmarketing surveillance. In many cases adverse reactions become demonstrated only after the drug is used in large numbers of patients under environmental circumstances. Continual vigilance is required to collect data which establish the safety of drugs and document the beneficial action. Table 5-3 is a flowchart which summarizes the controlled clinical trial. It is evident that from 5 to 10 years is required to introduce a new drug for use in humans. The cost varies with the complexity of the study but is on the average in the vicinity of $7 to $10 million or more. A recently developed fibrinolytic drug is reported to have cost $200 million to bring it to a marketing level. This has given rise to criticism that there is a drug lag in the United States as compared with other countries because of the more stringent requirements of the FDA in this country. It is not likely, however, that there will be a lessening of vigilance in the control of the introduction of new drugs.

ETHICS OF DRUG INVESTIGATION IN HUMANS

In view of the inevitable toxicity of drugs, it might well be asked, "What are the moral and humanistic aspects of human investigation?" Obviously, when the only object of administering a drug is an attempt to alter a course of a usually fatal disease, considerable toxicity may be justified, for example, in cancer chemotherapy. However, systematic medical research may not have as its sole or even major aim the cure of immediate disease but the explanation of mechanisms which may later lead to beneficial therapeutic agents. Under what conditions may an individual then serve as "guinea pig"? The code laid down in 1947 by the Nuremberg judges following the atrocities of World War II still stands as a classic document. It clearly states the principles which are still followed today.

1. The voluntary consent of the human subject is absolutely essential.
    a. This means that the person involved should have legal capacity to give consent; should be so situated as to be able to exercise free power of choice, without the intervention of any element of force, fraud, deceit, duress, overreaching, or other ulterior form and constraint or coercion; and should have sufficient knowledge and comprehension of the elements of the

TABLE 5-3 The controlled clinical trial as a means of developing a new drug in humans

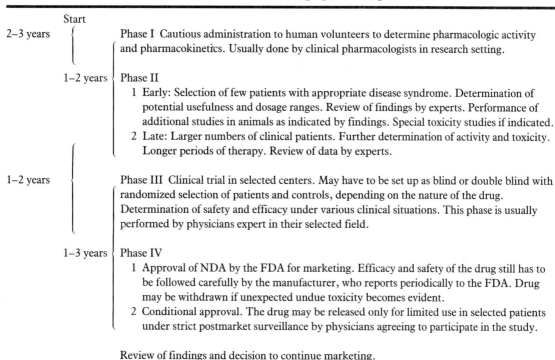

	Start	
2–3 years		Phase I Cautious administration to human volunteers to determine pharmacologic activity and pharmacokinetics. Usually done by clinical pharmacologists in research setting.

1–2 years { Phase II

    1 Early: Selection of few patients with appropriate disease syndrome. Determination of potential usefulness and dosage ranges. Review of findings by experts. Performance of additional studies in animals as indicated by findings. Special toxicity studies if indicated.

    2 Late: Larger numbers of clinical patients. Further determination of activity and toxicity. Longer periods of therapy. Review of data by experts.

1–2 years { Phase III Clinical trial in selected centers. May have to be set up as blind or double blind with randomized selection of patients and controls, depending on the nature of the drug. Determination of safety and efficacy under various clinical situations. This phase is usually performed by physicians expert in their selected field.

1–3 years { Phase IV

    1 Approval of NDA by the FDA for marketing. Efficacy and safety of the drug still has to be followed carefully by the manufacturer, who reports periodically to the FDA. Drug may be withdrawn if unexpected undue toxicity becomes evident.

    2 Conditional approval. The drug may be released only for limited use in selected patients under strict postmarket surveillance by physicians agreeing to participate in the study.

           Review of findings and decision to continue marketing.

---

subject matter involved to enable him to make an understanding and enlightened decision. The latter element requires that before the acceptance of an affirmative decision by the experimental subject, there should be made known to him the nature, duration, and purpose of the experiment; the method and means by which it is to be conducted; all inconveniences and hazards reasonably to be expected; and the effects upon his health or person which may possibly come from his participation in the experiment.

  b. The consent of the human subject shall be in writing; his signature shall be affixed to a written instrument setting forth substantially the aforementioned requirements which shall be signed in the presence of at least one witness who shall attest to such signature in writing.

  c. The duty and responsibility for ascertaining the quality of the consent rests upon each individual who initiates, directs, or engages in the experiment. It is a personal duty and responsibility which may not be delegated to another with impunity.

2. The experiment should be such as to yield fruitful results for the good of society, unprocurable by other methods or means of study, and not random and unnecessary in nature.

3. The number of volunteers used shall be kept at a minimum.

4. The experiment should be so designed and based on the results of animal experimentation and a knowledge of the natural history of the disease or other problem under study that the anticipated results will justify the performance of the experiment.

5. The experiment should be so conducted as to avoid all unnecessary physical and mental suffering and injury.

6. No experiment should be conducted where there is a priori reason to believe that death or disability injury will occur.

Since this code was promulgated, other declarations have been published. The AMA affirmed the concepts of consent, competence, and care. The British Medical Association, the Medical Research Council, and the World Medical Association have issued guidelines for conduct of experimentation not essentially different in principle.

The World Medical Association approved the Helsinki declaration in 1964, which established:

> In the field of clinical research, a fundamental distinction must be recognized between clinical research in which the aim is essentially therapeutic for a patient, and clinical research, the essential object of which is purely scientific and without therapeutic value to the person subjected to the research.

The declaration asserts that where research is combined with professional care

> If at all possible, consistent with patient psychology, the doctor should obtain the patient's freely given consent after the patient has been given a full explanation.

The Helsinki declaration is the current vade mecum to guide us through the ethical maze.

In addition, there is the "consent clause" of the FDA law. This statute states that investigators must inform any human being used in the tests or controls that the agent is being used for investigational purposes; it also states that investigators will obtain the informed consent of such individuals or their representatives, except where it is deemed not feasible or, in their professional judgment, contrary to the best interests of the individual.

In all human drug studies performed under a government contract or grant (for example, the National Institutes of Health), and in order to comply with the more recent regulations of the FDA, there is the additional requirement that the study be approved by a human research review committee often called *Institutional Review Board* (IRB). Such a committee must be composed of impartial scientists, clinicians, lay people from the community, including, at the least, a lawyer and a member of the clergy. Full disclosure of the drug's chemical and biologic background is required. The risks to the human subjects involved are estimated, the responsibility of the investigation is established, and it is determined that the facilities available for the investigation are adequate and ensure safety.

The use of consultants is often made a requirement. Disclosure of the risk involved to the volunteer is mandatory, and informed consent is supervised. The protocol of the investigation is carefully reviewed. Reports of any toxicity are to be immediately reported to the committee. A more recent requirement is the surveillance of the conduct of the investigation and the facility in which it is performed. The work of IRBs becomes more difficult as ethical questions arise which in the past were not even considered. For example, who pays for therapies and diagnostics which are clearly experimental? Is it ethical to have a washout period in testing a new antiarrhythmic when the standard drug is effective and the arrhythmia might be lethal? Should the IRB review advertising for recruits? What is the appropriate pay of volunteer subjects not to encourage them unduly to submit to dangerous drugs and procedures? When a tissue is obtained from a donor, who owns it? This is especially important when a useful and profitable agent is developed from this tissue.

These and other issues plague clinical investigation. With the rising cost of health care the public seriously questions the increasing cost of drug development. In addition ligation over drug toxicity is growing. It is estimated that from 5 to 30 percent of all hospital admissions are attributable to drug toxic reactions. Thus the societal function of clinical pharmacology is not only the development of new and better drugs but also to contain their cost and most of all to ensure their safety.

FATE OF MARKETED DRUGS

Results of the experimental and clinical evaluation of new drugs ofen become well publicized and may have a tremendous influence on sales; however, the results then obtained by practicing physicians may not be the same as those obtained under experimental conditions. Since the new drug may offer no advantage over the drug already being prescribed, physicians may become reluctant to use the new product, so that its sale diminishes rapidly. On the other hand, because of keen competition among over 1000 companies in the pharmaceutical industry, research programs will be either initiated or intensified to develop a competitive product. Thus, the natural history of many new drug products may be divided into four phases: (1) enthusiastic reception; (2) qualified use; (3) declining use due to ineffectiveness, side effects, or competitive drugs; and (4) obsolescence.

BIBLIOGRAPHY

AMA Drug Evaluations, 6th ed., Saunders, Philadelphia, 1986.

Bennett, W. M., and T. A. Golfer: In E. Rubenstein and D. D. Federman (eds.), *Drug therapy in renal disease in Scientific American Medicine*, appendix A, *Scientific American*, New York, 1988.

Blaschke, T. F.: In E. Rubenstein and D. D. Federman (eds.), *Pharmacokinetics and Pharmacoepidemiology in Scientific American Medicine*, appendix A, *Scientific American*, New York, 1988.

Branch, R. A. and R. Johnston: "Therapeutic Advisory Program: An opportunity for clinical pharmacology," *Clin. Pharmacol. Ther.*, **43**:223–227 (1988).

DiPalma, J. R.: "The Case for Boards in Clinical Pharmacology," *JAMA*, **243**:1918–1920 (1980).

Dollery, C. T.: "The Future of Clinical Pharmacology and Therapeutics," *Clin. Pharmacol. Ther.*, **41**:1–2 (1987).

Spector, R., G. D. Park, G. F. Johnston, and E. S. Vessell: "Therapeutic Drug Monitoring," *Clin. Pharmacol. Ther.*, **48**:345–353 (1988).

Lind, S. E., "Can Patients Be Asked to Pay for Experimental Treatment?" *Clin. Res.*, **32**:393–398 (1984).

Kaitin, K. I., B. W. Richard, and L. Lasagna: "Trends in Drug Development: The 1985–86 New Drug Approvals," *J. Clin. Pharmacol.*, **27**:542–548 (1987).

Maloney, D. M. (ed.): "Federal Agency Reorganizes to Monitor Research Better" *Human Research Report* **2**:8 (August 1987), Deem Corporation, P.O. Box 44069, Omaha, Nebraska.

McMahon, G. F.: "Does Your Institutional Review Board Review Advertising for Recruits?" *Clin. Pharmacol. Ther.*, **43**:1–3 (1988).

Niabyl, J. R.: *Drug Use in Pregnancy*, 2d ed., Lea & Febiger, Philadelphia, 1988.

Nisenberg, D. W.: "Clinical Pharmacology Instruction for All Medical Students," *Clin. Pharmacol. Ther.*, **40**:484–487 (1986).

Olin, B. (ed.): *Facts and Comparisons*, Facts and Comparisons Division, Lippincott, St. Louis, Missouri, 1988 (update monthly).

Riedenberg, M. M.: "The Discipline of Clinical Pharmacology," *Clin. Pharmacol. Ther.*, **38**:2–5 (1985).

Speight, T. M. "Principles and Practice of Clinical Pharmacology and Therapeutics," *Avery's Drug Treatment*, 3d ed., Adis Press, Williams and Williams, Baltimore, 1987.

Vesell, E. S.: "Clinical Pharmacology: A Personal Perspective," *Clin. Pharmacol. Ther.*, **38**:603–612 (1985).

Weinshilbaum, R. M.: "The Therapeutic Revolution," *Clin. Pharmacol. Ther.*, **42**:481–484 (1987).

PART II

The Autonomic Nervous System

SECTION EDITOR

Edward J. Barbieri

C H A P T E R   6

Introduction to the Autonomic Nervous System

Domenic A. DeBias

GENERAL CONSIDERATIONS

The autonomic nervous system provides an important means whereby major visceral functions are regulated so that the limits for survival are not surpassed. The system is organized into two specialized subsystems, the parasympathetic and the sympathetic. In controlling bodily function under normal physiologic conditions, such as rest and/or restoration, the parasympathetic nervous system usually predominates; the sympathetic nervous system generally directs the response of the organism to various environmental stresses. When mammals are confronted with danger, the heart beats more rapidly and more forcefully, the pupils dilate to permit more light to reach the retina, blood flow through skeletal muscles is enhanced, blood sugar is elevated, the sphincters of the alimentary tract close, and the mind becomes more alert. Each of these responses is achieved by activation of the sympathetic nervous system through various somatic and visceral afferent (sensory) fibers. The autonomic nervous system consists of spinal and supraspinal peripheral components. Excitation of many autonomic reflexes can occur at the spinal level, whereas integration of several autonomic activities occurs at supraspinal levels.

ANATOMIC CONSIDERATIONS

The efferent pathways of each of the two major subdivisions of the autonomic nervous system consist of two neurons (Fig. 6-1). The cell body of the first is found in the brain or spinal cord, and its neural endings synapse with the cell body of the second outside the central nervous system (CNS), either in discrete ganglia or within the innervated organ. With few exceptions, the preganglionic fibers are myelinated, and the postganglionic fibers are nonmyelinated.

The *parasympathetic division* of the autonomic nervous system, with its preganglionic cell bodies in the brain stem (tectobulbar) and the sacral cord, is also called the *craniosacral division* (or tectobulbosacral division). The cells of the postganglionic fibers are near, on, or within the innervated organ. The cranial division of the parasympathetic nervous system distributes fibers through the oculomotor (III), facial (VII), glossopharyngeal (IX), and vagal (X) nerves to terminal ganglia. Fibers from these innervate structures of the head, neck, thorax, and abdominal viscera; exceptions are the descending colon and the pelvic viscera, which are innervated by the sacral division. The sacral division arises from the sacral cord (S2–S4) and forms the pelvic nerve (*nervus erigens*), which synapses in terminal ganglia near, on, or within the innervated organs. Only in the head are there discrete parasympathetic ganglia separated from the innervated structure.

The *sympathetic division* of the autonomic nervous system, with its preganglionic cell bodies in the intermediomedial or intermediolateral column of the thoracic and upper lumbar (T1–L2 or L3) spinal cord, is called the *thoracolumbar division*. Sympathetic preganglionic fibers pass out of the spinal cord with the ventral root and into the chain ganglia through the *white rami communicantes*. The cells of origin of the postgan-

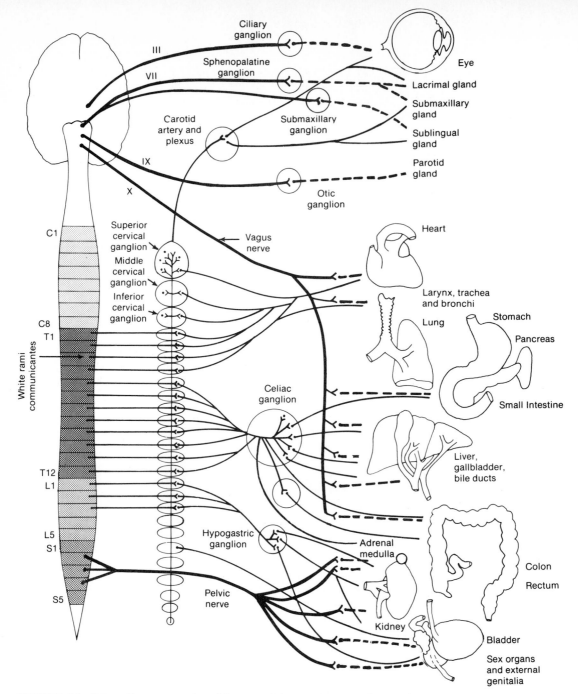

FIGURE 6-1 Schematic representation of the autonomic nervous system. Innervation to various effector organs is shown for both the parasympathetic nervous system (———<— — —) and the sympathetic nervous system (———————<———). The parasympathetic nervous system distributes fibers from cranial nerves (III, VII, IX, and X) and from the sacral cord (▨); sympathetic fibers originate from the thoracic (▨) and lumbar (▨) spinal cord through the white rami communicantes. Autonomic fibers do not originate from the cervical (▨) spinal cord.

glionic sympathetic nerves are in autonomic ganglia of three types: (1) chain, or paravertebral; (2) collateral, or prevertebral; (3) terminal, or peripheral. The synapses of sympathetic nerves occur in the first two ganglia, but occasionally sympathetic nerves synapse in terminal ganglia.

Autonomic ganglia consist of small preganglionic nerve terminals, the ganglionic cells and their associated dendritic processes, and satellite or glial cells. In mammalian sympathetic ganglia, the ratio of preganglionic to postganglionic fibers is of the order of 1:20; mammalian parasympathetic ganglia usually have a ratio of 1:1 or 1:2 (e.g., ciliary ganglion). The differences between sympathetic and parasympathetic ganglia, together with the widespread distribution of postganglionic sympathetic fibers, as compared with localized postganglionic parasympathetic fibers, is often regarded as the anatomic basis for the different physiologic characteristics of the two divisions of the autonomic nervous system. While activation of the sympathetic division results in a generalized response of many organ systems, activation of the parasympathetic division results in a more localized and discrete response. The organization of parasympathetic innervation by the vagus nerve is a notable exception to this generalization. The ratio of preganglionic vagal fibers to postganglionic fibers in the plexuses of Auerbach and Meissner is about 1:8000.

PHYSIOLOGIC CONSIDERATIONS

The actions of the various autonomic nerves on effector cells are summarized in Table 6-1 and require little additional comment. Many organs receive both sympathetic and parasympathetic fibers and are influenced in opposite ways by the two divisions of the autonomic nervous system. In some instances, e.g., heart and intestine, the organs are endowed with intrinsic activity and require dual innervation with opposing actions in order to elevate or suppress this inherent activity when appropriate. In other instances, control of function is regulated by opposing actions on different effector cells. For example, pupillary constriction occurs following the activation of parasympathetic nerves to the circular muscles of the iris or following the inactivation of sympathetic nerves to the radial muscles of the iris. Conversely, pupillary dilation occurs following activation of sympathetic fibers to the radial muscles or the inactivation of parasympa-

thetic fibers to the circular muscles. Stated in other terms, the circular muscles of the iris are under the control of parasympathetic nerves and the radial muscles are under sympathetic control, with pupil size determined by the interplay between the sympathetic and parasympathetic nerves. Parallel action of sympathetic and parasympathetic innervation to effector cells is illustrated by the increase in conduction velocity in atrial fibers following either sympathetic or vagal stimulation. However, the increase in atrial conduction by vagal stimulation is not a constant finding.

It follows from these considerations that the activity of most organ systems reflects a balance of modulating influences between the sympathetic and parasympathetic nervous systems. Blockade of the sympathetic nervous system by drugs can be expected to result in an exaggeration of parasympathetic activity. Conversely, blockade of parasympathetic activity results in the exaggeration of sympathetic activity. When both pathways are blocked, the effect on the organ system depends on its inherent activity and on the pathway that normally dominates the organ system.

SYNAPTIC TRANSMISSION

The release of neurotransmitter substances from the small, unmyelinated neuronal endings is initiated by nerve action potentials (Figs. 6-2 and 6-3). Obviously, drugs or procedures modifying conduction of impulses in neuronal terminals can be expected to produce corresponding changes in the release of the synaptic transmitter.

Vesicular organelles, which contain transmitter substances, are present in synaptic neuronal terminals and move toward the terminal membrane to discharge their contents into the junctional cleft during nervous activity. Release of transmitter occurs when an action potential, propagated down the axon by activation of voltage-sensitive sodium channels, terminates at the nerve ending. As the membrane depolarizes, voltage-sensitive calcium channels in the membrane open, allowing an influx of ionic calcium. The increase in intracellular calcium facilitates fusion of the vesicular membrane with the neuronal membrane resulting in exocytotic release of neurotransmitter into the junctional cleft.

The neurotransmitter diffuses through the synaptic cleft and attaches reversibly with the receptors on the postsynaptic membrane at a rapid rate, causing

TABLE 6-1   Major effector responses to autonomic nervous system activity

Effector	Sympathetic		Parasympathetic	
	Receptor	**Response**	**Receptor**	**Response**
Eye				
Iris				
Radial muscle	α_1	Contraction	—[a]	—
Sphincter muscle	—	—	M	Contraction
Ciliary muscle	β	Relaxation	M	Contraction
Glands				
Sweat	α/M	Secretion[b]	M	Secretion
Salivary	α_1	Potassium and water secretion	M	Potassium and water secretion
	β	Amylase secretion		
Lacrimal	—	—	M	Secretion
Nasopharyngeal	—	—	M	Secretion
Gastrointestinal tract	—	—	M	Secretion
Skin				
Pilomotor muscles	α	Contraction	—	—
Lung				
Tracheal muscle	β_2	Relaxation	M	Contraction
Bronchial muscle	β_2	Relaxation	M	Contraction
Heart				
S-A node	β_1	Increase in rate	M	Decrease in rate
Atria	β_1	Increase in contractility and conduction velocity	M	Decrease in contractility; usual: increased conduction velocity
A-V node	β_1	Increase in conduction velocity	M	Decrease in conduction velocity
His-Purkinje system	β_1	Increase in conduction velocity	—	—
Ventricles	β_1	Increase in contractility and conduction velocity	—	—
Arterioles				
Coronary	α	Constriction[c]	—	—
Skin and mucosa	α	Constriction	—	—
Skeletal muscle	β_2	Dilation[d]	—	—
Pulmonary	α	Constriction[c]	—	—
Abdominal viscera	α	Constriction	—	—
Salivary glands	α	Constriction	M	Dilation
Renal	α	Constriction	—	—

TABLE 6-1 *(continued)*   **Major effector responses to autonomic nervous system activity**

Effector	Sympathetic		Parasympathetic	
	Receptor	**Response**	**Receptor**	**Response**
Veins (systemic)	α	Constriction	—	—
	β_2	Dilation		
Gastrointestinal tract				
Longitudinal muscle (tone and motility)	α_2, β_2	Decrease	M	Increase
Sphincters	α	Contraction	M	Relaxation
Urinary bladder				
Detrusor	β_2	Relaxation	M	Contraction
Trigone and sphincter	α	Contraction	M	Relaxation
Adrenal medulla	N-I	Secretion[e]	—	—
Uterus				
Nonpregnant	β_2	Relaxation	M	Variable[f]
Pregnant	α	Contraction	M	Variable[f]
	β_2	Relaxation		
Male sex organs	α	Ejaculation	M	Erection
Spleen Capsule	α	Contraction	—	—
Liver	α/β_2[g]	Glycogenolysis and gluconeogenesis		
Pancreas				
Acini	α	Decreased secretion	M	Secretion
Islets (β cells)	α_2	Decreased secretion	—	—
	β_2	Increased secretion	—	—
Fat cells	β_1	Lipolysis	—	—
Pineal gland	β	Melatonin synthesis	—	—

[a] No known functional innervation.
[b] Thermoregulatory sweat (cholinergic); apocrine [stress] activation sweat (adrenergic).
[c] β_2-Receptor-mediated dilation observed in situ (autoregulatory phenomenon).
[d] Predominant effect over α-receptor-mediated constriction.
[e] Secretion of epinephrine and norepinephrine in response to sympathetic preganglionic cholinergic fibers.
[f] Depends on the phase of the ovulatory cycle and amounts of estrogen and progesterone circulating.
[g] Species-dependent.

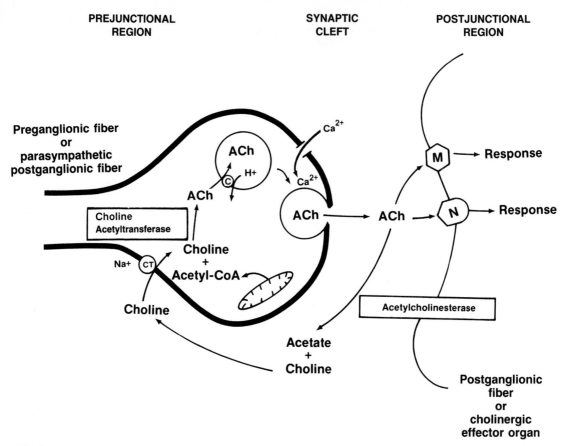

FIGURE 6-2 Schematic representation of neurohumoral transmission at cholinergic nerve endings. Choline is taken up into the neuron by a Na^+-dependent carrier transport (CT) and is combined with acetyl CoA, released by mitochondria, to form acetylcholine (ACh). Synthesized ACh is transported into storage vehicles by a carrier which utilizes effluxing protons as a source of energy. Influx of ionic calcium (Ca^{2+}) through Ca^{2+} channels causes fusion of the vesicular and neuronal membranes and liberation of ACh into the synaptic cleft. ACh will interact with muscarinic (M) and/or nicotinic (N) receptors on the postjunctional tissue and can be hydrolyzed by acetylcholinesterase to acetate and choline.

changes in membrane activity. At many junctions, the dissociation of the transmitter and receptor must occur at a rapid rate for synaptic activity to remain responsive to succeeding incoming impulses. Equally important, mechanisms must be available for the elimination of the transmitter from the junctional region in order to prevent the accumulation within the synapse of concentrations of transmitter, which may interfere with further synaptic activity. Termination of transmitter activity can occur by a variety of means. After

dissociation of the transmitter from the postsynaptic receptor, the transmitter may (1) diffuse away from the synapse, (2) be converted to inactive degradation products by metabolic means, or (3) be taken up (re-uptake) into neuronal terminals from the extracellular space. At cholinergic junctions, a significant portion of the neurotransmitter is eliminated by enzymatic means; at adrenergic junctions, re-uptake of the transmitter by nerve endings is the major route of inactivation.

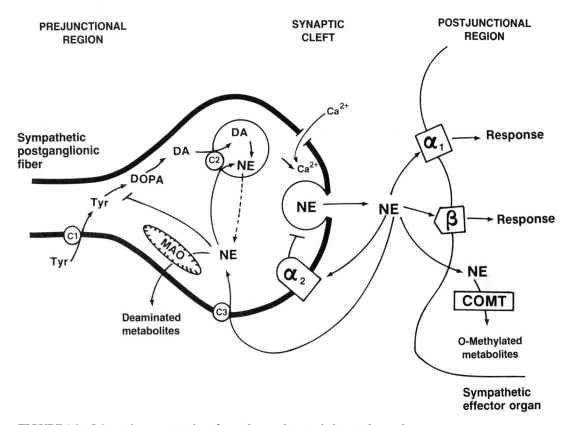

FIGURE 6-3 Schematic representation of neurohumoral transmission at adrenergic nerve endings. Tyrosine (Tyr) enters sympathetic postganglionic neurons by an active carrier transport (C1) system. Dopamine (DA), formed from DOPA in the cytoplasm is transported into the storage vesicle by another active transport mechanism (C2); norepinephrine (NE) is synthesized from DA within the vesicles and stored for release. Influx of ionic calcium (Ca^{2+}) through Ca^{2+} channels causes fusion of the vesicular and neuronal membranes and liberation of NE into the synaptic cleft. NE will (1) complex with postjunctional α_1- and β-adrenergic receptors and initiate a physiologic tissue response, (2) bind to neuronal α_2-adrenergic receptors and inhibit further NE release from neurons, and (3) be inactivated by carrier transport (C3) mediated re-uptake into the neuron (uptake 1) and effector tissue (uptake 2). Cytoplasmic NE will (1) be transported back into the storage vesicle, by the same active transport mechanism (C2) that transports DA, (2) be metabolized by mitochondrial monoamine oxidase (MAO), and (3) inhibit the formation of DOPA. NE that is accumulated in effector tissues will be metabolized by catechol-O-methyl transferase (COMT).

Cholinergic Transmission

The transmission of impulses at preganglionic nerve endings, postganglionic parasympathetic and some postganglionic sympathetic nerve endings, as well as somatic nerve endings, occurs by means of acetylcholine (ACh) that is synthesized in the axonal terminal and is liberated from storage vesicles within the nerve terminals (Fig. 6-2).

The chemical process involved in the formation of ACh within the nerves are complex; however, the major step in the biosynthetic process is the acetylation of choline catalytically by choline acetyltransferase. This reaction requires the presence of acetyl coenzyme A (CoA) and choline. Acetyl CoA is formed by and released from mitochondria, found in large numbers in axonal terminals. Choline is taken up into the axoplasm from the extracellular fluid by active transport, a process which is Na^+-dependent and can be inhibited by hemicholinium (a congener of choline).

$$\text{Acetyl CoA + choline} \xrightarrow{\text{choline acetyltransferase}} \text{ACh + CoA}$$

Following its formation in the cytoplasm, ACh is stored in vesicles that accumulate at neuronal endings and range in diameter from 20 to 40 nm. Among the inorganic ions present in nerve tissue, calcium plays a prominent role in the release mechanism. As previously mentioned, depolarization of the axonal terminal results in calcium ion influx through voltage-sensitive calcium channels. Ionic calcium binds to negative charges on the internal surface of the neuronal membrane, an interaction which promotes fusion of the neuronal and vesicular membranes, resulting in ACh release into the synaptic cleft. In addition to the marked hyperirritability of neural structures associated with calcium deficiency, there is a profound reduction in the output of ACh from cholinergic nerves resulting in the failure of transmission. Conversely, an elevation in the concentration of calcium ions bathing the nerve terminals enhances the output of the neurotransmitter.

Acetylcholine is subjected to a number of inactivation processes following its release from the nerve endings. These include diffusion from the site of release, dilution in extracellular fluids, binding to nonspecific sites, and enzymatic destruction. For most cholinergic junctions, the most important inactivation process is the enzymatic hydrolysis of ACh to acetate and choline. This reaction is catalyzed by the enzyme acetylcholinesterase and occurs at a rate sufficiently rapid to prevent the accumulation of ACh in the synaptic cleft.

Acetylcholinesterase is one of a family of enzymes which catalyze the hydrolysis of ester linkages. It differs from other members of the family in being almost completely specific for ACh, which it hydrolyzes with great efficiency. For this reason it is also termed *true*, or *specific*, *cholinesterase*. Apart from neural structures, it also occurs in red blood cells, in the placenta, and in the motor end plate of skeletal muscle. Another member of this family of enzymes is butyrylcholinesterase (also called *nonspecific cholinesterase*, or *pseudocholinesterase*), which is not specific for ACh but hydrolyzes a great variety of esters in addition to acetylcholine. This enzyme is found in the plasma in the liver, and in glial and other cells associated with nerve tissues.

Adrenergic Transmission

The transmission of impulses at adrenergic nerve endings occurs by means of norepinephrine liberated from storage granules within the nerve terminals (Fig. 6-3). Norepinephrine is one of several naturally occurring biogenic catecholamines; other important catecholamines are epinephrine, which is found in high concentrations in the adrenal medulla and other chromaffin cells, and dopamine, a precursor of both norepinephrine and epinephrine found in adrenergic nerve endings and in some areas of the CNS.

The synthetic pathway for norepinephrine in adrenergic neurons, appropriate cells of the CNS, and chromaffin tissue involves a complex series of enzymatic steps (Fig. 6-4). At adrenergic nerve endings the amino acid tyrosine is transported from the extracellular fluid to the intraneuronal cytoplasm by metabolically dependent processes. In the first step of the enzymatic series, tyrosine undergoes hydroxylation to form dopa. This cytoplasmic reaction is catalyzed by the enzyme tyrosine hydroxylase and requires tetrahydrobiopterin as a cofactor. When compared with other enzymes involved in the formation of catecholamines, the activity of tyrosine hydoxylase is the lowest. Therefore, the hydroxylation of tyrosine is the primary rate-limiting step in the series of reactions. Inhibition of tyrosine hydroxylase by analogs of tyrosine results in a depletion of catecholamine stores in the brain and adrenergic nerves and is the most effective mechanism for impairing the synthetic pathway for catecholamines. In addition, this step is subject to end-product (norepinephrine) feedback inhibition. The second step in the pathway results in the conversion of dopa to dopamine by a decarboxylation reaction catalyzed by dopa decarboxylase (aromatic l-amino acid decarboxylase) with the cofactor pyridoxal phosphate. The enzyme is not specific for dopa and will bring about the decarboxylation of histidine, tyrosine, and 5-hydroxytryptophan. In addition, the enzyme is present in many nonnervous tissues. Dopamine is actively transported into vesicles; the transport

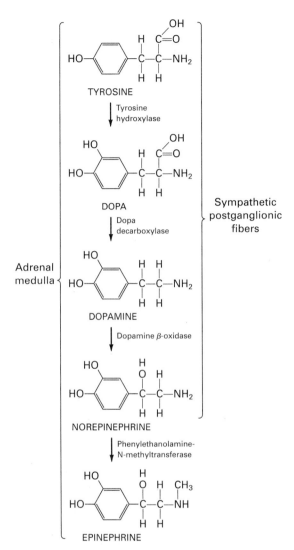

FIGURE 6-4 Metabolic syntheses of norepinephrine and epinephrine from tyrosine. Since postganglionic sympathetic neurons do not contain significant amounts of the enzyme phenylethanolamine-*N*-methyltransferase (PNMT), the synthetic pathway terminates with production of norepinephrine. PNMT is present in the adrenal medulla and continues the synthetic pathway to the biosynthesis of epinephrine. For this reason the adrenal medulla secretes both epinephrine and norepinephrine directly into the blood, whereas adrenergic resources secrete only norepinephrine into the synaptic cleft.

system requires Mg^{2+} and is driven by pH and potential gradients through an ATP-dependent proton translocase. In the vesicle the hydroxylation of the β carbon of dopamine to form norepinephrine takes place under the control of the enzyme dopamine-β-oxidase. This enzyme has been isolated from the chromaffin granules of the adrenal medulla and the synaptic vesicles of adrenergic nerves. The vesicles also contain relatively high concentrations of ATP (in a ratio of ATP to norepinephrine of 1:4), proteins known as chromogranins, certain peptides (e.g., enkephalin precursors), and ascorbic acid (a cofactor for dopamine-β-oxidase). These electron-dense vesicles range in size from 40 to 130 nm and have the capacity to concentrate norepinephrine from the cytoplasm. The formation of epinephrine from norepinephrine is confined primarily to the adrenal medulla (and similar tissues), and the enzyme catalyzing the conversion, phenylethanolamine-*N*-methyltransferase, is localized in those tissues.

Similar to cholinergic neurons, calcium ions appear to be the required link between membrane excitation and the release of catecholamines from adrenergic neurons and adrenal medullary cells. At both sites calcium deprivation causes a failure of the release mechanisms, and at both sites there is an influx of calcium ions during the release of the catecholamines. The mechanism whereby calcium brings about the release of norepinephrine is exocytosis. The vesicular membrane fuses with the neuronal membrane, and the entire contents of the vesicle (including norepinephrine, dopamine, dopamine-β-oxidase, ATP, etc.) are discharged into the synaptic cleft.

By comparing the depletion of catecholamine stores produced by nerve stimulation and chemical agents such as tyramine and reserpine, it is apparent that the intraneuronal distribution, binding, and release of catecholamines are heterogeneous. As determined by isotopically labeled norepinephrine, there are two major neuronal compartments for the storage of catecholamines. The first compartment (pool I) contains norepinephrine, which undergoes rapid turnover (half-life of approximately 2 h). The second compartment (pool II) contains a storage form of norepinephrine with a slower turnover rate (half-life of about 24 h) and may represent a neuronal transmitter reserve. Norepinephrine released into the synaptic cleft from the first compartment is metabolized by the enzyme catechol-O-methyltransferase (COMT). The norepinephrine released into the neuronal cytoplasm from the second compartment is metabolized by monoamine oxidase (MAO).

The activity of norepinephrine released from adrenergic neurons can be terminated by (1) re-uptake into the neuron (uptake 1), (2) enzymatic inactivation, and (3) diffusion away from the synapse and uptake at extraneuronal sites (uptake 2). Re-uptake (both uptake 1 and uptake 2) is the most important method of terminating neuronally released norepinephrine as well as circulating norepinephrine and epinephrine, i.e., catecholamines present in the blood as a consequence of sympathetic nerve activity, release from the adrenal medulla, and/or release from chromaffin tissues. *Neuronal re-uptake* is a Na^+-dependent active process which transports catecholamines from the junctional extracellular fluid, across the neuronal membrane, into the cytoplasm. *Vesicular transport* involves the transfer of the compound from the cytoplasm, across the membrane of the vesicle, into the storage vesicle and appears identical to the active transport of dopamine into the vesicle during norepinephrine synthesis.

There are two major enzyme systems involved in the transformation of the catecholamines to inactive degradation products (Fig. 6-5). Oxidative deamination of epinephrine and norepinephrine is catalyzed by MAO. Adrenergic nerve endings contain large quantities of the enzyme, which is localized on the outer surface of mitochondrial membranes. Apparently, because of its intraneuronal localization, MAO plays more of a role in the regulation of the intraneuronal disposition of catecholamines than the destruction of circulating biogenic amines, which takes place in the liver. Inhibition of MAO leads to an increase in the tissue concentration of the catecholamines but has no appreciable effect on the responses to injected epinephrine or norepinephrine.

The second major enzyme involved in the metabolism of the catecholamines is COMT. This enzyme is responsible for the inactivation of circulating catecholamines. Although the enzyme is widely distributed, highest concentrations are found in the liver and kidneys; lesser amounts are localized in the neuroeffector junction, especially in the tissues served by the adrenergic nerves. Sympathetic nerves contain very little COMT activity. The metabolic conversion by O-methyltransferase of the catecholamines to inactive forms is due to the transfer of a methyl group from

"activated" methionine to the 3-hydroxyl group of the phenyl ring. Part of the norepinephrine released from adrenergic nerves during nerve stimulation as well as circulating catecholamines, is taken up by the effector cells (uptake 2) and acted upon by COMT.

NEURONAL COTRANSMITTERS

Although junctional transmission is currently conceived as involving a single transmitter from each neuron, there is evidence that more than one transmitter is released from a single neuron. Enkephalins can be demonstrated to be present in preganglionic neurons, postganglionic sympathetic neurons, and adrenal medullary cells. Vasoactive intestinal polypeptide (VIP) can also be found in peripheral cholinergic nerves to exocrine glands. Stimulation of the preganglionic sympathetic nerve to the adrenal medulla results in a release of substance P along with acetylcholine. The vesicles in autonomic nerve terminals contain ATP which is also released with the neurotransmitter. Therefore there appears to be an association of neuropeptides with the more familiar cholinergic and adrenergic neurotransmitters. Although specific receptors and antagonists are readily discernible for many of the neuropeptides, data to substantiate their roles as neurotransmitters are not presently conclusive.

RECEPTORS

Virtually all hormones and drugs initiate their physiologic or pharmacologic actions by binding to specific cellular sites referred to as *receptors*. Receptor binding initiates alterations of cellular metabolic events such as enzyme activities, ion fluxes, glandular secretions, muscle contractions, and other activities characteristically expressed as physiologic or pharmacologic.

Exogenously administered drugs, such as epinephrine and acetylcholine, mimic the effects of autonomic nervous activity and produce their characteristic effects on suitably denervated structures; thus, these drugs react directly with specific receptors on the effector cell rather than on the nerve endings.

In effector cells innervated by sympathetic and/or parasympathetic fibers, the responses to the neurotransmitter upon activation of the nerve fiber or to the

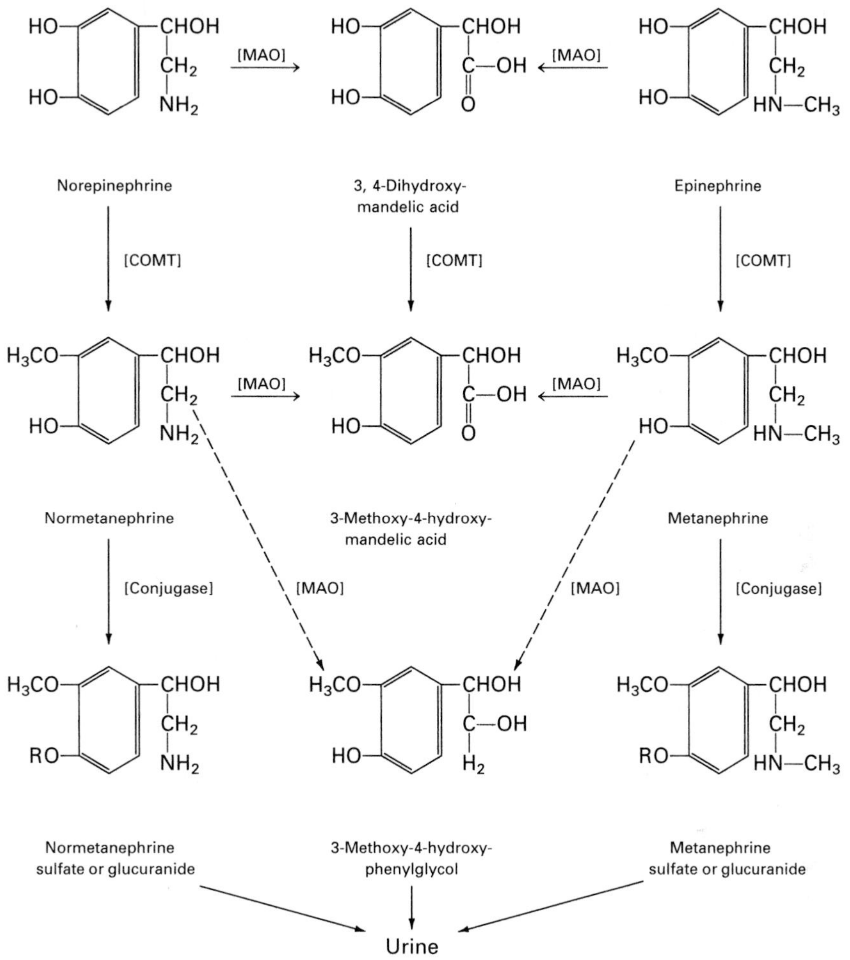

FIGURE 6-5 Metabolic pathways showing the inactivation of norepinephrine and epinephrine by various enzyme systems.

administered mimetic agent are similar. It is therefore postulated that responding cells possess receptors for acetylcholine and other receptors for norepinephrine. These two general classes of receptors are often referred to as *cholinergic receptors* and *adrenergic receptors,* respectively (Table 6-2). Additionally, it should be noted that specific dopamine receptors are found in certain renal and mesenteric blood vessels.

The receptor concept is based on the presence of distinct cellular macromolecules which are capable of binding with the biologically active agonists or their functionally inert antagonists. The molecular structure of the ligand-binding site determines the specificity of the physiologic or pharmacologic action characteristic of the tissue. The specific binding of an agonist with the receptor must therefore activate a biologic process which terminates in a response such as glandular secretion, muscle contraction, ion channel regulation, and other such actions. Receptor-effector coupling mechanisms are discussed in detail in Chap. 2.

TABLE 6-2   **Autonomic receptors**

Designation	Typical locations
Cholinoceptors	
Muscarinic (M)	
M_1	Parasympathetic effector cells (e.g., gastric mucosa), neurons (e.g., cerebral cortex, ganglia)
M_2	Parasympathetic effector cells (e.g., intestinal smooth muscle, cardiac muscle, exocrine glands)
Nicotinic (N)	
N I	Autonomic ganglia, both parasympathetic and sympathetic
N II	Skeletal muscle end plate
Adrenoceptors	
Alpha (α)	
α_1	Postsynaptic effector cells (e.g., vascular smooth muscle)
α_2	Adrenergic nerve terminals (presynaptic) and smooth muscle (postsynaptic); also nonsynaptic sites (e.g., platelets, lipocytes)
Beta (β)	
β_1	Postsynaptic effector cells (especially heart and kidney); also nonsynaptic sites (e.g., lipocytes)
β_2	Postsynaptic effector cells (e.g., smooth muscle)

Cholinergic Receptors

There are many peripheral efferent nerves which are cholinergic. It is convenient and empirically useful to group them into three categories: (1) preganglionic fibers of the autonomic nervous system, (2) postganglionic fibers of the parasympathetic division and some postganglionic fibers of the sympathetic division, and (3) somatic motor nerves (Fig. 6-6). Although each of these nerves transmits to a cell which contains receptors for ACh (cholinergic receptors, cholinoceptive sites) and each of these cells responds to properly applied exogenous ACh, the pharmacologic characteristics of the receptors at the three sites are different in significant ways. Drugs that strongly mimic the effects of ACh at one cholinergic junction may have a markedly reduced effect at another. Similarly, drugs that block cholinergic transmission at one site may have no effect on cholinergic transmission at another site.

All three groups of cholinergic receptors respond to ACh; the differences among the receptors have been determined by using drugs which act like ACh (cholinomimetic) or which antagonize the effects of ACh (anticholinergic). The cholinergic effects of *muscarine* and *nicotine* have long been known and form the basis for classifying the cholinergic receptors. The alkaloid muscarine produces all the effects of postganglionic parasympathetic nerve stimulation and also induces sweating (a response produced by cholinergic sympathetic postganglionic fibers). The effects of muscarine are readily suppressed by atropine, as are those of ACh on these same responses. On this basis, the receptors for ACh on effector cells innervated by postganglionic cholinergic fibers (all parasympathetic and certain sympathetic postganglionic fibers) may be called *muscarinic receptors* or *atropine-sensitive receptors*. Drugs with the same pattern of activity as muscarine have been termed *muscarinic agents* or *parasympathomimetic drugs*. Muscarinic cholinoceptive sites are also found in some tissues that are not innervated; most arterioles do not receive parasympathetic innervation but are extremely sensitive to the actions of muscarine and muscarine-like drugs.

Based on the selectivity of certain agonists and antagonists, muscarinic receptors have been subclassified as M_1 and M_2. Although muscarinic receptor subtypes have been associated with different effector structures (Table 6-2), to date the important functional differences of M_1 and M_2 receptors have not been elucidated.

The cholinergic receptors in autonomic ganglia and at the neuromuscular junction are responsive to low concentrations of nicotine and to ACh applied in ade-

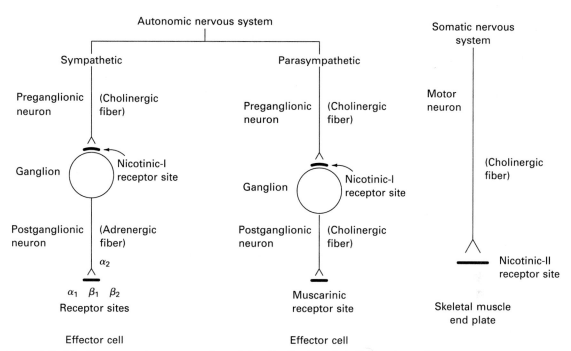

FIGURE 6-6 Diagrammatic representation of the distribution of cholinoceptive and adrenoceptive sites in the autonomic nervous system and the somatic nervous system.

quate concentrations by an appropriate route of administration. The responses to ACh at these sites are called *nicotinic effects,* and the respective cholinoceptive sites *nicotinic receptors.* The nicotinic receptors for ACh are further subdivided into two groups: nicotinic I (found mainly in autonomic ganglia) and nicotinic II (located at the skeletal muscle end plate). There are drugs which selectively interfere with transmission in autonomic ganglia (*ganglionic blocking agents*) and others that selectively interfere with neuromuscular transmission (*neuromuscular blocking drugs*). It is important to remember that cholinergic fibers to skeletal muscle and the nicotinic II receptors associated with the muscle end plate are part of the somatic nervous system, not the autonomic nervous system.

Adrenergic Receptors.

The organs innervated by adrenergic nerves respond to exogenous epinephrine or norepinephrine in a manner which qualitatively mimics the effects of sympathetic nerve stimulation; drugs which act in this manner are termed *sympathomimetic agents.* The primary reaction between norepinephrine or epinephrine and the effector cell is mediated by *adrenergic receptors* (*adrenoceptive sites*).

A careful study of the relative potencies of several sympathomimetic amines for producing the characteristic sympathetic response in several tissues has suggested that adrenergic receptors could be grouped into two major classes: alpha (α) and beta (β) receptors (Table 6-2). The synthesis of selective blocking agents has allowed a further subdivision of β-adrenergic receptors into β_1 (chiefly at cardiac and renal sites) and β_2 (most other sites). More recently, α-adrenergic receptors have been subdivided into α_1 (found mainly on effector organs) and α_2 (located on adrenergic neurons at presynaptic sites and to a lesser extent on effector tissues).

Although there are exceptions, activation of α_1 receptors generally results in an excitatory response; activation of β_2 receptors generally results in tissue relaxation or an inhibitory response. Activation of β_1 receptors results in a stimulatory effect on the heart and kidney, and activation of *presynaptic* α_2-adrenergic receptors appears to constitute a mechanism for presynaptic feedback inhibition of neuronal release of norepinephrine, while stimulation of *postsynaptic* α_2 receptors, similar to α_1 receptors, mediates tissue excitation.

Effector organ response to epinephrine and/or norepinephrine is primarily determined by the type of adrenoceptor as well as the proportion of α-adrenergic and β-adrenergic receptors. The radial muscle of the eye will contract in response to epinephrine and norepinephrine because the receptor mediating this effect is α_1; since both epinephrine and norepinephrine are capable of activating α_1 receptors, mydriasis will be a consistent response. Blood vessels of striated muscle have both α_1, and β_2 receptors, but β_2 receptors predominate; in response to circulating epinephrine these blood vessels dilate as β_2-adrenergic receptors are activated; norepinephrine resulting from sympathetic discharge has little effect on these blood vessels because of the low density of α_1 receptors. Conversely, cutaneous blood vessels contain predominantly α_1 receptors and will respond to both epinephrine and norepinephrine with vasoconstriction.

The catecholamines cause striking changes in the metabolism of most organs. An increase in oxygen consumption, a breakdown of glycogen, an increase in the formation of lactic acid, and an increase in the mobilization of free fatty acids represent the major metabolic effects. In mammals, the metabolic effects of epinephrine include hyperglycemia, the release of free fatty acids, and an increase in plasma lactic acid. These effects are produced by the action of epinephrine on β-adrenergic receptors and the subsequent increase in the formation of cyclic AMP by the adenylate cyclase enzyme system (see Chap. 2).

PHYSIOLOGIC REGULATION OF RECEPTORS

A diminution of responsiveness to pharmacologic action with time is a fundamental mechanism of cellular adaptation which is known as *desensitization* (toler-ance, tachyphylaxis, refractoriness). Desensitization markedly limits the therapeutic efficacy of drugs, including parasympathomimetic and sympathomimetic agents; the refractoriness to bronchodilators administered to asthma patients is a classic example. Detailed information concerning desensitization phenomena is given in Chap. 2.

BIBLIOGRAPHY

Brimblecombe, R. W.: "Drug Actions on Cholinergic Systems," in P. B. Bradley (ed.), *Pharmacology Monographs*, University Park, Baltimore, 1974.

Higgins, C. B., S. F. Vatner, and E. Braunwald: "Parasympathetic Control of the Heart," *Pharmacol. Rev.*, 25:119–155 (1973).

Hoffman, B. B., and R. J. Lefkowitz: "Radioligand Binding Studies of Adrenergic Receptors: New Insights Into Molecular and Physiological Regulation," *Annu. Rev. Pharmacol. Toxicol.*, 20:581–608 (1980).

Hoffman, B. B., R. J. Lefkowitz: "Alpha-adrenergic Receptor Subtypes," *N. Engl. J. Med.*, 302:1390–1396 (1980).

Kunos, G.: "Adrenoceptors," *Annu. Rev. Pharmacol. Toxicol.*, 18:219–311 (1978).

Lefkowitz, R. J., M. G. Caron, and G. L. Stiles: "Mechanisms of Membrane-Receptor Regulation," *N. Engl. J. Med.*, 310:1570–1579 (1984).

Levitzki, A.: "β-Adrenergic Receptors and Their Mode of Coupling to Adenylate Cyclase," *Physiol. Rev.*, 66:819–854 (1986).

Moreland, R. S., and D. F. Bohr: "Adrenergic Control of Coronary Arteries," *Fed. Proc.*, 43:2858–2861 (1984).

Patil, P. N., D. D. Miller, and U. Trendelenburg: "Molecular Geometry and Adrenergic Drug Activity," *Pharmacol. Rev.*, 26:323–392 (1974).

Ruffolo, R. R.: "Interactions of Agonists with Peripheral α-Adrenergic Receptors," *Fed. Proc.*, 43:2910–2916 (1984).

Shore, P. A.: "Transport and Storage of Biogenic Amines," *Annu. Rev. Pharmacol.*, 12:209–226 (1972).

Triggle, D. J.: "Adrenergic Receptors," *Annu. Rev. Pharmacol.*, 12:185–196 (1972).

Volle, R. L.: "Ganglionic Transmission," *Annu. Rev. Pharmacol.*, 9:135–146 (1969).

Wolfe, B. B., T. K. Harden, and P. B. Molinoff: "In Vitro Study of β-Adrenergic Receptors," *Annu. Rev. Pharmaol. Toxicol.*, 17:575–604 (1977).

Adrenergic Drugs

Raymond F. Orzechowski

Adrenergic drugs and *sympathomimetic amines* are conventional terms used in reference to a class of chemicals that evoke responses in the living organism which simulate the functional consequences of sympathetic nerve activation or the hormonal secretion of epinephrine by the adrenal glands. Both naturally occurring and synthetic compounds make up this diverse group of substances. Indeed, three *endogenous catecholamines*—epinephrine, norepinephrine, and dopamine—are clinically useful as sympathomimetic drugs.

Epinephrine is recognized as a hormonal substance synthesized and released into the systemic circulation from chromaffin cells of the adrenal medulla during the defensive "fight or flight" reaction. Relatively small amounts of epinephrine also occur in some regions of the brain, where it apparently functions as a neurotransmitter or neuromodulator. Norepinephrine and dopamine are released from neurons in the brain and periphery; their physiologic roles as neurotransmitter molecules have been extensively studied. Norepinephrine is considered to be the principal neurotransmitter of the sympathetic division of the autonomic nervous system.

Sympathetic neurons exert a prominent regulatory influence on the heart and vasculature. Thus, many therapeutic uses of sympathomimetic drugs are based on their ability to alter the cardiovascular status of the organism.

Some typical and important pharmacologic actions of adrenergic drugs include the following:

Cardiac stimulation Increased heart rate and myocardial contractile force

Vasomotor changes Vasoconstriction and/or vasodilation

Bronchodilation and a "decongestant" action on mucous membranes

Regulation of endocrine status Modulation of insulin, renin, and pituitary hormones

Regulation of metabolic status Enhanced glycogenolysis in liver and muscle and liberation of free fatty acids from adipose tissue

Behavioral changes Complex stimulatory or "alerting" effects in the central nervous system

The spectrum of cardiovascular, respiratory, hormonal, metabolic, and neuropsychic responses that may be elicited by adrenergic drugs in general clearly resembles many of the systemic adaptive reactions to increased physical activity and psychic stress. Both pharmacodynamic and pharmacokinetic distinctions among the drugs included in this broad classification scheme provide the rationale for their specific therapeutic applications. Considered individually, adrenergic drugs exhibit notable quantitative and qualitative differences with respect to their potencies and most prominent actions. The variation in responses to subclasses of adrenergic drugs is largely based on their relative selectivity of interaction with populations of receptor molecules that are differentially distributed in effector structures (heart, vasculature, lungs, brain, peripheral nerves, etc.) throughout the body.

SITES AND MODE OF ACTION

Conceptually, sympathomimetic drugs induce their effects:

1. By binding directly to and thereby activating adrenergic receptors on the cell membranes of target tissues. The term *direct-acting agonist* is descriptively used for such drugs. Examples include epinephrine, phenylephrine, and isoproterenol.
2. By evoking the neuronal release of stored catecholamines, which then bind to and activate adrenergic receptors. The sympathomimetic activity of the drug is therefore dependent on the presence of endogenous catecholamines. The phrase *indirect-acting agent* is used with reference to this mode of action. Tyramine, a compound used as an experimental tool, is an example of an indirect-acting sympathomimetic.
3. By a combination of direct adrenergic receptor activation and indirect catecholamine-releasing actions. Drugs with this duality of action are referred to as *mixed-acting* and are exemplified by ephedrine, amphetamine, and dopamine.

Figure 7-1 depicts direct and indirect-acting modes of action of sympathomimetic agents.

Adrenergic receptors (adrenoceptors) exist throughout the body—in the brain, peripheral nerves, and non-neural cells (muscles, glands, blood cells). From a molecular perspective, the binding of an adrenergic agonist drug to a complementary receptor on the cell membrane regulates a cascade of biochemical reactions within the cell ultimately to alter its intrinsic metabolic status. The drug (or an endogenous neurotransmitter or hormone) thus provides an informational message which is transduced into the cell interior and subsequently amplified (see Chap. 2). From a macroscopic perspective, altered cellular activity elicits a measurable effect at the tissue or organ level. Two major classes of adrenergic drug-binding receptor proteins have been historically designated as *alpha* (α) and *beta* (β). Several subtypes of these two classes have been characterized on the basis of anatomic, pharmacologic, biochemical, and molecular criteria. Currently, four subtypes are widely recognized and designated as α_1, α_2, β_1, and β_2. This classification of adrenergic receptor subtypes may yield to modified schemes as detailed structural and functional charac-

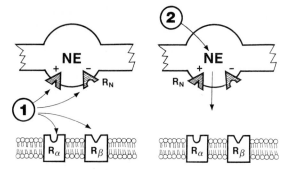

FIGURE 7-1 Diagrammatic illustration of direct and indirect actions of sympathomimetic drugs. (1) *Direct-acting agonists* activate adrenergic receptors (R_α, R_β) on the target cell membrane (i.e., postsynaptic site) and on presynaptic neuronal receptors (R_N) located on the neurilemma. Presynaptic "autoregulatory" receptors modulate [enhance $(+)$ or reduce $(-)$] release of the endogenous neurotransmitter [norepinephrine (NE)]; presynaptic receptors can be inhibitory (α_2-adrenergic) or excitatory (β-adrenergic). Examples of direct-acting drugs: phenylephrine (selectivity for α_1 receptors) and isoproterenol (selectivity for β receptors). (2) *Indirect-acting compounds* promote the release of the neurotransmitter (NE) from the sympathetic neuron. Examples of indirect-acting drugs: tyramine and hydroxyamphetamine. *Note:* The distinction between actions 1 and 2 is not necessarily absolute; many "mixed-acting" adrenergic drugs combine both actions. Examples of mixed-acting sympathomimetic drugs: dopamine, ephedrine, and amphetamines.

terization is accomplished, especially in the case of the α-adrenergic receptors.

Drugs such as epinephrine, norepinephrine, and isoproterenol are nonselective adrenergic agonists, i. e., they stimulate both subtypes of α- and/or β-adrenergic receptors. Several examples serve to illustrate the variation in pharmacologic effects of drugs that *selectively* activate subpopulations of adrenergic receptors.

The activation of α-adrenergic receptors in vascular smooth muscle elicits vasoconstriction. Consequently, drugs with α-adrenergic agonist activity increase vascular resistance and thereby elevate arterial blood pressure. Phenylephrine is a representative vasopressor drug with highly selective α_1-adrenergic agonist activity. The term *vasopressor amine* refers to the ability of many, but not all, sympathomimetic drugs to elicit a rise in arterial blood pressure.

The activation of *presynaptic* α_2 "autoreceptors" located on peripheral postganglionic sympathetic neurons causes a reduced amount of norepinephrine to be released in response to electrical stimulation of the nerve. *Postsynaptic* α_2-adrenergic receptors also exist in target tissues such as blood vessels, where their activation results in vasoconstriction. When α_2-adrenergic receptors located on blood platelets are activated, enhanced platelet aggregation occurs. α_2 Receptors in the brain stem modulate sympathetic neural outflow to peripheral organs. Clonidine and guanfacine are centrally active α_2-adrenergic agonists which lower systemic blood pressure and heart rate.

β_1-Adrenergic receptors in the heart regulate myocardial contractility, heart rate, and the electrophysiologic characteristics of cardiac cells. β_2-Adrenergic receptors in the trachea and bronchi of the lungs modulate the contractile state of airway smooth muscle. Isoproterenol, a potent selective agonist on β-adrenergic receptors, is a powerful myocardial stimulant (β_1-adrenergic receptors) and bronchodilator (β_2-adrenergic receptors). Sympathomimetic drugs that can activate pulmonary β_2 receptors in preference to cardiac β_1 receptors, e. g., terbutaline, albuterol, metaproterenol, and isoetharine, are widely used as bronchodilators to treat bronchospastic disorders.

The terms *desensitization* and *down-regulation* are used to describe certain biochemical phenomena, associated with reduced functional responsiveness, which have been noted when target tissues are continually exposed to drugs that activate adrenoceptors. Desensitization refers to cellular events possible following relatively brief periods of tissue exposure to adrenergic drugs, such as a redistribution of receptors on the cell membrane, uncoupling of the receptor from distal regulatory components, internalization of receptors within the cell cytosol, and possibly, receptor phosphorylation. Down-regulation refers to a reduction in number of adrenoceptors, i. e., lowered receptor density, following longer periods of contact with adrenergic drugs. Such phenomena have been more thoroughly documented for β-adrenergic receptors than for α-adrenergic receptors. They offer several plausible mechanistic explanations for observations—variously described as refractoriness, tolerance, and tachyphylaxis—of diminished effectiveness of an adrenergic drug during prolonged, continuous, or repeated administration. The possible relevance of these dynamic aspects of adrenergic receptor proteins to clinical pathologic states is under investigation.

CHEMISTRY AND STRUCTURE-ACTIVITY RELATIONSHIPS

Figure 7-2 shows some key structural features of several representative adrenergic drugs. The physiologic catecholamines and most synthetic sympathomimetic drugs are viewed as substituted β-phenethylamines. It is noteworthy that substituted imidazolines and some aliphatic amines also possess sympathomimetic activity. The sympathomimetic characteristics of substituted β-phenethylamines are, to some extent, predictable from an inspection of their structural differences. Several general statements can be made about such correlations between molecular structure and biologic activity:

1. Sympathomimetic activity is maximal when two carbon atoms separate the aromatic ring from the amino group.
2. The lesser the degree of substitution on the amino group, the greater is the selectivity for activating α-adrenergic receptors. Conversely, increasing the bulk of substituents on the primary amino group confers greater selectivity for β-adrenergic receptors.
3. Maximal activity (potency) depends on the presence of hydroxyl groups at positions 3 and 4 on the aromatic ring, i. e., the catecholamines. This holds for both α- and β-adrenergic receptor activation.
4. Noncatecholamines elicit more prominent central nervous system stimulatory effects than catecholamines.
5. Substitution on the α carbon atom blocks oxidative inactivation of the molecule by monoamine oxidase and thus greatly prolongs the duration of activity. α-Carbon substitution also enhances the ability of the molecule to release endogenous catecholamines from neuronal storage sites.
6. Compounds with only a 3-hydroxy substitution on the aromatic ring yield a high ratio of direct/indirect agonist activity, as exemplified by phenyleph-

Many adrenergic drugs can be considered as substituted derivatives of β-phenethylamine:

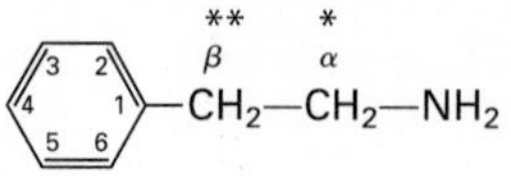

$$\text{—CH}_2\text{—CH}_2\text{—NH}_2$$

*Designates the "alpha" carbon atom of the molecule.
**Designates the "beta" carbon atom of the molecule.

REPRESENTATIVE CATECHOLAMINES

Norepinephrine

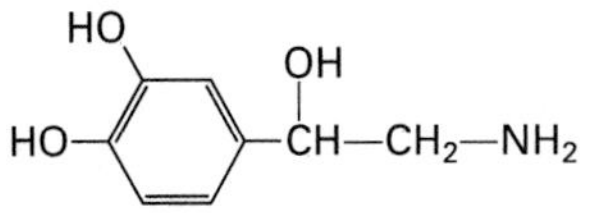

$$\text{—CH—CH}_2\text{—NH}_2$$

Epinephrine

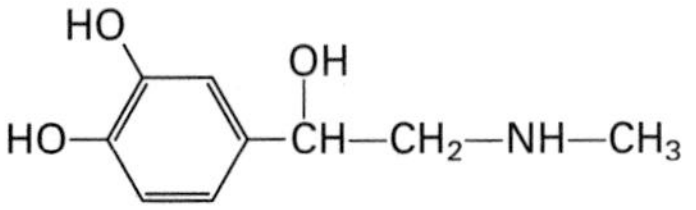

$$\text{—CH—CH}_2\text{—NH—CH}_3$$

Isoproterenol

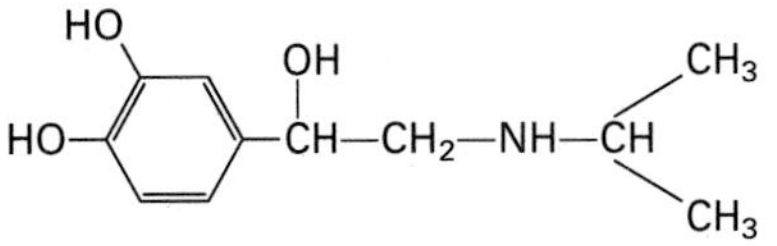

$$\text{—CH—CH}_2\text{—NH—CH}\big(\text{CH}_3\big)_2$$

Dobutamine

$$\text{—CH}_2\text{—CH}_2\text{—NH—}$$
$$\text{—CH}_2\text{—CH}_2\text{—CH—CH}_3$$

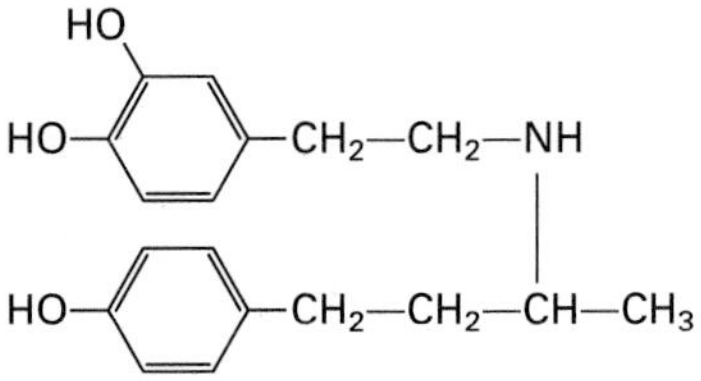

REPRESENTATIVE NONCATECHOLAMINES

Phenylephrine

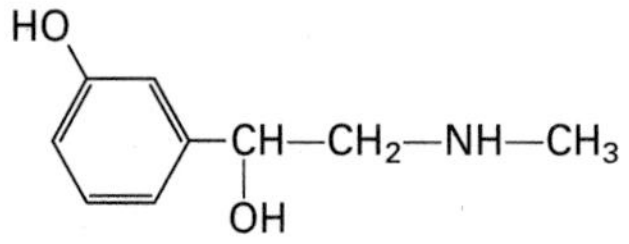

$$\text{—CH—CH}_2\text{—NH—CH}_3$$

Phenylpropanolamine

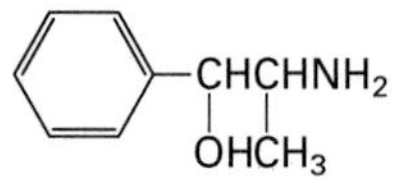

$$\text{—CHCHNH}_2$$
$$\text{OHCH}_3$$

Amphetamine

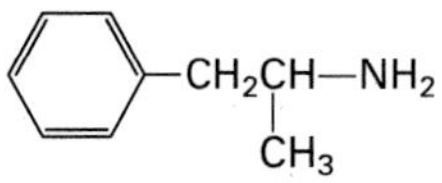

$$\text{—CH}_2\text{CH—NH}_2$$
$$\text{CH}_3$$

Ephedrine

$$\text{—CHCHNH—CH}_3$$
$$\text{OHCH}_3$$

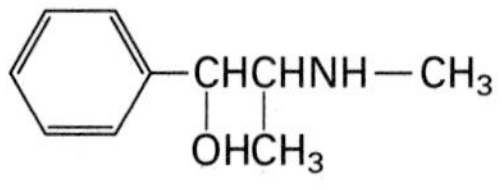

Tetrahydrozoline
(an imidazoline derivative)

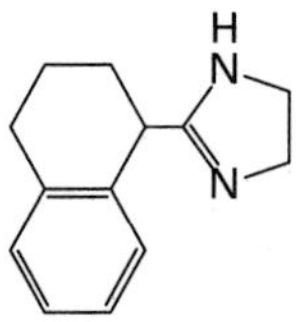

Albuterol

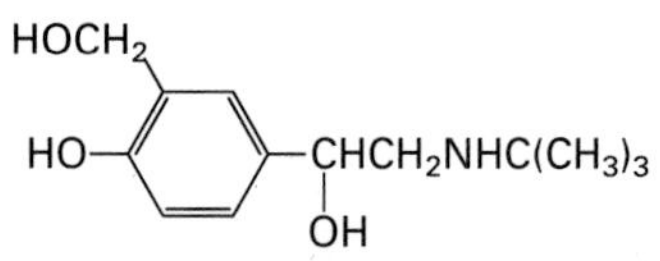

$$\text{—CHCH}_2\text{NHC(CH}_3)_3$$
$$\text{OH}$$

FIGURE 7-2 Structural aspects of adrenergic drugs.

rine. Compounds with only a 4-hydroxy substitution on the aromatic ring yield a high ratio of indirect/direct activity, as exemplified by tyramine.

DIRECT-ACTING AGONISTS

Epinephrine

This endogenous catecholamine is also known by its official British name *adrenaline*. Epinephrine is a potent agonist on both α- and β-adrenergic receptors. Its actions are complex, being dependent not only on the relative distribution of adrenergic receptive sites in various tissues and organs but also on the conditions of dosage and route of administration. The natural $(-)$ isomer of epinephrine is up to 50 times more biologically active than the $(+)$ isomer. Although prominent pharmacologic actions are exerted on the cardiovascular and respiratory systems, the full profile of its effects throughout the body reflects its physiologic importance as a systemic neurohormone involved in "defense activation." Since it can represent the prototype of many adrenergic drugs reviewed in this chapter, the pharmacodynamic characteristics of epinephrine on several organ systems are presented below in some detail.

Effects on Organ Systems

Cardiovascular System   The typical cardiovascular response to an intravenous injection or infusion of epinephrine is an immediate rise in systemic arterial blood pressure. Systolic pressure is usually elevated to a greater degree than diastolic pressure; thus, pulse pressure is increased (Fig. 7-3). This pressor response to epinephrine is due to the combined actions of (1) vasoconstriction in many, but not all, vascular beds and (2) myocardial stimulation, i. e., increased contractile force and heart rate.

Significant differences in reactivity to epinephrine are observed among the regional vascular networks of the body. Such variations in response have been shown to be related to the distribution of adrenergic receptor types in different blood vessels. The vasoconstrictive action of epinephrine results from activation of α-adrenergic receptors and is principally exerted on small arterioles and precapillary sphincters (i. e., resistance vessels) and also on veins (i. e., capacitance vessels). Vascular constriction is particularly marked in blood vessels supplying the skin and mucous mem-

branes, in the splanchnic circulation and in the kidneys. Although *vasopressor amine* is an appropriate reference to the vasoconstrictor action, small doses of epinephrine can sometimes evoke a fall in diastolic blood pressure. This vasodepressor component is a consequence of regional vasodilatation in blood vessels supplying skeletal muscle because of the activation by epinephrine of vascular β_2-adrenergic receptors which subserve vasodilation. Depending on dose and route of administration, the total peripheral vascular resistance may be increased, decreased, or relatively unchanged, as determined by the net combined vasoconstrictive (α-adrenergic) and vasodilatory (β_2-adrenergic receptor) regional vascular responses.

Cardiostimulation is primarily mediated via the activation of β_1-adrenergic receptors, and is coupled to an elevated intracellular concentration of cyclic AMP and augmented influx of calcium into cardiac cells. Epinephrine alters both the mechanical (contractile) and electrophysiologic (rhythmic) properties of the heart. The increase in myocardial contractility is referred to as a positive inotropic action. Functional components of this direct myocardial action of epinephrine are observed in isolated cardiac tissue preparations as (1) an accelerated rate of isometric tension development, (2) increased peak contractile force, and (3) an enhanced rate of relaxation. In the intact organism, myocardial work, cardiac output, coronary blood flow, and myocardial oxygen consumption are increased (Fig. 7-4).

Epinephrine elevates heart rate (a positive chronotropic action) by increasing the rate of depolarization of pacemaker cells in the sinoatrial node. However, depending on the dosing conditions in vivo, baroreceptor reflexes triggered by a rapidly elevated arterial blood pressure may elicit vagal discharge, and thus avert any significant appearance of tachycardia, or result in reflex bradycardia. Blockade of this vagal cholinergic effect by the administration of atropine unmasks the direct cardioaccelerating effect of epinephrine. Large doses of epinephrine can activate latent, i. e., abnormal, pacemaker cells, induce complex changes in impulse formation and conduction characteristics, and thereby precipitate various cardiac arrhythmias such as premature ventricular systoles, ventricular tachycardia, and fibrillation. Accidental intravenous and even conventional subcutaneous doses of epinephrine have the potential to cause lethal arrhythmias.

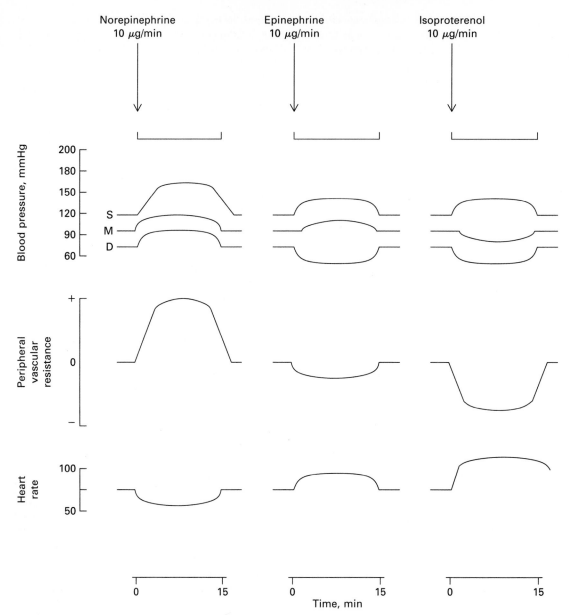

FIGURE 7-3   The cardiovascular effects of IV administration of norepinephrine, epinephrine, and isoproterenol. Under blood pressure: S = systolic pressure; M = mean blood pressure; D = diastolic pressure. [Modified from M. J. Allwood et al., *Br. Med. Bull.*, **19**:132–136 (1963).]

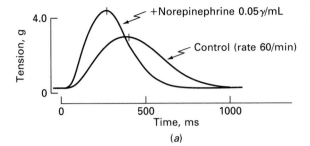

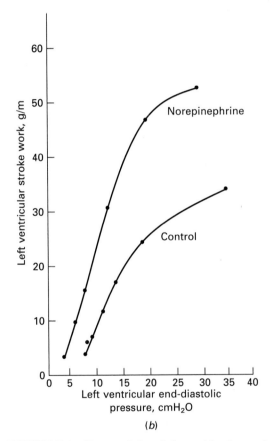

FIGURE 7-4 Characteristics of the positive inotropic action of catecholamines. (*a*) Effect of norepinephrine on isometric contractions in papillary muscle in vitro. [From E. Sonnenblick, *Fed. Proc.*, 21:975–990 (1962).] (*b*) Effect of norepinephrine on the relationship between left ventricular end-diastolic pressure and stroke work in vivo. [From S. J. Sarnoff, et al., *Circ. Res.*, 8:1108–1122 (1960).]

Respiratory System β_2-Adrenergic receptors which mediate relaxation are found in the smooth muscle of the bronchi. Epinephrine and other sympathomimetic drugs with β_2-adrenergic agonist properties are thus capable of relaxing bronchial muscle and evoking bronchodilation. This therapeutically important action is most pronounced in circumstances when the bronchial muscle is abnormally constricted. Examples of such conditions include bronchial asthma, the administration of bronchoconstrictive drugs, and the release of autacoids (e. g., histamine) during an allergic reaction. Additionally, the α-adrenergic agonist activity of epinephrine contributes to pulmonary vasoconstriction and a respiratory mucosal decongestant effect. The combined bronchodilatation and relief of airway congestion result in an improved vital capacity in bronchospastic states. These effects of epinephrine are attainable when the drug is given systemically by subcutaneous injection, or by inhalation in the form of an aerosolized solution. The respiratory actions of epinephrine are rapid in onset and rather brief in duration and may be accompanied by adverse cardiovascular reactions and other sympathomimetic side effects.

Although epinephrine is clearly valuable in acute bronchospastic states, the use of this catecholamine as a primary medication in the chronic treatment of asthma has waned as longer acting and safer β_2-selective adrenergic agonists have been developed. Members of this subgroup of adrenergic agonists are discussed in another section of this chapter.

Ocular Effects Epinephrine and other α-adrenergic agonists, e. g., phenylephrine, contract the radial muscle of the iris to produce mydriasis. The mydriatic effect of topically applied epinephrine is weaker than that of the more selective α-adrenergic agonists. Of greater therapeutic importance is the reduction of intraocular pressure that occurs upon local administration of epinephrine in patients with open-angle glaucoma. The precise mechanism by which epinephrine evokes ocular hypotension is not fully understood but is probably caused by facilitating the outflow of aqueous humor through the ocular drainage network (the trabecular meshwork and Schlemm's canal). Instillation of epinephrine into the eyes can reduce intraocular tension for 12 to 24 h. Dipivefrine hydrochloride (dipivalyl epinephrine), a lipophilic analog of epinephrine, penetrates the tissues of the eye more readily. It is employed for its ocular hypotensive action in chronic glaucomas. Dipivefrine, a prodrug, is hydrolyzed into active epinephrine by esterase enzymes in ocular tissues.

Gastrointestinal System Smooth muscle of the gastrointestinal tract contains α- and β-adrenergic receptors, both of which subserve relaxation. Thus epinephrine and other sympathomimetic drugs may reduce gastric and intestinal contractions, but the magnitude of this inhibitory action depends on the preexisting tone of the muscle. There is also evidence that sympathomimetic agents activate inhibitory presynaptic adrenergic receptors located on cholinergic neurons in the gastrointestinal tract to suppress the release of acetylcholine. These inhibitory effects of sympathomimetic amines on gastrointestinal function are considered to be of minor therapeutic importance.

Genitourinary System Epinephrine and other sympathomimetics relax the urinary bladder detrusor muscle (mediated by β-adrenergic receptors), constrict the trigone and urethral sphincter (mediated by α-adrenergic receptors), and thus promote bladder continence. The reactivity of uterine smooth muscle to adrenergic drugs is influenced by several factors: species, stage of the estrus cycle, and pregnancy. In pregnant women, uterine relaxation occurs upon activation of myometrial β_2-adrenergic receptors. This effect provides the basis for the use of selective β_2-receptor agonists in the prevention of premature delivery. In males, sympathetic control of ejaculation is accomplished via α-adrenergic receptors. Inhibition of ejaculation is a relatively common side effect of drugs with α-adrenergic antagonist activity.

Metabolic Effects Epinephrine has prominent and complex actions on several key aspects of intermediary metabolism. Following injections of epinephrine, glycogenolysis in liver and skeletal muscle is enhanced, and lipolysis in adipose tissue is accelerated. Elevated plasma concentrations of glucose (hyperglycemia), lactate (hyperlactacidemia), and free fatty acids (hyperlipidemia) occur. For the most part, these metabolic stimulatory effects of epinephrine result from activation of β-adrenergic receptors with the associated increase in intracellular cyclic AMP. Epinephrine inhibits the pancreatic secretion of insulin and augments glucagon secretion. Liberation of potassium from the liver leads to a transient hyperkalemia, which

is followed by a more prolonged hypokalemia as potassium is taken up by muscle cells. A calorigenic action of epinephrine is manifested by an increase in oxygen consumption and elevated body temperature. These metabolic actions of epinephrine represent an integrated mobilization of energy reserves. In contrast, norepinephrine is significantly less potent in evoking these metabolic alterations.

Central Nervous System Following their peripheral systemic administration, the polar nature of catecholamines greatly limits their access into the brain. Nevertheless, in some patients epinephrine may provoke reactions such as headache, anxiety, restlessness, confusion, and skeletal muscle tremor. Many of these untoward reactions may be secondary to the marked peripheral cardiorespiratory and metabolic actions of epinephrine. The more lipid-soluble noncatecholamines, particularly amphetamine and its congeners, are capable of inducing much more pronounced central stimulatory effects.

Pharmacokinetics Parenteral administration is required to elicit the systemic effects of epinephrine and other catecholamines; little or no actions are observable if these drugs are given orally. Several factors accounting for this lack of oral activity include: (1) inactivation by digestive secretions, (2) poor absorption due to a low lipid-to-water partition coefficient, (3) local vasoconstriction which diminishes blood flow and absorptive ability of mucous membranes, and (4) rapid enzymatic inactivation in the intestines and liver. The usual routes of parenteral administration of epinephrine are by subcutaneous or intramuscular injection. Intravenous infusion is uncommon in the clinical setting and potentially hazardous.

Solutions of epinephrine may be topically applied to mucous membranes for control of capillary bleeding. Epinephrine and other vasoconstrictive sympathomimetics may be combined with local anesthetics to reduce systemic absorption of the local anesthetic from the injection site.

In bronchial asthma, epinephrine solution is aerosolized in a suitable nebulizer, and the fine mist is inhaled through the mouth. Adverse reactions due to systemic absorption may occur; the risk of toxicity is higher in geriatric patients and in patients with longstanding chronic lung disease.

The metabolism of catecholamines is based on an interplay of several biochemical reactions, including oxidative deamination, methylation, and conjugation. Only a minute fraction of circulating epinephrine and norepinephrine are excreted unchanged. Two key enzyme systems—monoamine oxidase (MAO) and catechol-O-methyltransferase (COMT)—participate in the degradation of catecholamines, and the group of metabolic products resulting from the actions of both enzymes is excreted in the urine. An estimate of catecholamine turnover can be obtained from analysis of the urinary concentrations of these metabolites.

The metabolism of these compounds, as well as important tissue re-uptake processes which are involved in terminating the activity of neurally released catecholamines are discussed in Chap. 6.

Adverse Reactions Many untoward reactions from epinephrine and related catecholamines are predictable extensions of their sympathomimetic effects resulting from α- and β-adrenergic receptor activation. Owing to the transient duration of activity of the catecholamines, palpitations, mild tachycardia, hypertension, anxiety, headache, and tremor may not represent serious complications. However, increased cardiac work with an attendant increase in myocardial oxygen requirement may precipitate angina pectoris or myocardial infarction. Excessive or inappropriate dosing with catecholamines can promote convulsive seizures, extremely high arterial pressure resulting in cerebrovascular hemorrhage, and life-threatening ventricular arrhythmias. The halogenated volatile general anesthetics, e. g., halothane, are well known to sensitize the myocardium to the arrhythmogenic actions of the catecholamines.

General contraindications to the use of epinephrine include hypertension, hyperthyroidism, ischemic heart disease, cerebrovascular insufficiency, organic brain damage, and predisposition to narrow angle glaucoma. Because of cardiac stimulation and vasoconstriction, pulmonary hypertension leading to pulmonary edema may be a cause of fatality.

Several important drug interactions are possible with epinephrine. The cardiovascular effects of epinephrine may be potentiated to a dangerous degree in patients receiving monoamine oxidase inhibitors, tricyclic antidepressants, thyroxine, or other sympathomimetic agents (e. g., vasoconstrictors and nasal decongestants). Propranolol and other β-adrenergic blockers antagonize the cardiostimulatory and bronchodilator effects, and intensify the pressor effect of epinephrine. Dosage adjustments of insulin or oral hypoglycemic drugs may be necessitated because of the hyperglycemic effect of epinephrine. Fatal cardiac arrhythmias can occur in digitalized patients receiving epinephrine.

Therapeutic Uses Epinephrine, given by subcutaneous injection, can be lifesaving and is the drug of choice in the treatment of anaphylactic shock and related acute hypersensitivity reactions. By its combined cardiorespiratory actions on α-, β_1-, and β_2-adrenergic receptors, it is able to reverse the syndrome of cardiovascular collapse, bronchospasm, airway congestion, and angioedema.

The use of epinephrine by aerosol as a bronchodilator and pulmonary decongestant in the treatment of bronchial asthma has been previously described, as was its value in lowering intraocular tension in the treatment of simple, wide-angle glaucoma. Other ophthalmic indications are based on its decongestant (vasoconstrictive) and mydriatic actions in the eye. Similarly, the use of epinephrine as a topical hemostatic to control superficial bleeding and its combination with local anesthetics to prolong their action are based on a local vasoconstrictive effect. Epinephrine and other cardiostimulatory catecholamines have been used in the emergency treatment of complete heart block and cardiac arrest.

Norepinephrine

Norepinephrine, the principal neurotransmitter produced and released by adrenergic neurons, is also known as ($-$)-*noradrenaline* and *levarterenol*. This vasopressor catecholamine constricts both resistance and capacitance blood vessels (by stimulating α-adrenergic receptors) and has direct cardiostimulatory actions on the heart (mediated through β_1-adrenergic receptor activation). Norepinephrine has significantly weaker effects than epinephrine on vascular β_2-adrenergic receptors mediating vasodilation. The typical response to intravenous infusion of this drug consists of a rise in both systolic and diastolic arterial blood pressure resulting from an increased peripheral vascular resistance, accompanied by bradycardia. Thus, the direct chronotropic action on the heart is overshadowed by vagal reflexes. Norepinephrine may be used by intravenous infusion in acute hypotensive states when a potent vasoconstrictor is needed to maintain tissue perfusion. It can cause ischemic tissue necrosis at the infusion site. In contrast to epinephrine, norepinephrine has little or no stimulatory effect on carbohydrate and lipid metabolism.

Isoproterenol

This synthetic catecholamine is representative of a sympathomimetic drug with high selectivity for β-adrenergic receptors. Substitution of a bulky alkyl group (e. g., isopropyl or tertiary butyl) on the amino nitrogen atom of the β-phenethylamine skeleton confers greater affinity for β-adrenergic receptor sites than for α-adrenergic sites. Thus, isoproterenol lacks significant α-adrenergic agonist actions.

The activation by isoproterenol of β_1-adrenergic receptors in the heart evokes positive chronotropic and inotropic actions. Peripheral vascular resistance is reduced via β_2-adrenergic-mediated vasodilation, principally in skeletal muscle but also in the renal and mesenteric circulations. These combined cardiostimulatory and vasodilatory effects result in a marked increase in stroke volume and cardiac output. Since the drug does not activate α-adrenergic receptors, isoproterenol lacks a vasoconstrictive action and does not elevate systemic arterial blood pressure as do norepinephrine and epinephrine. Arterial pulse pressure increases as a consequence of increased stroke volume in the face of reduced peripheral vascular resistance. Large doses of isoproterenol can produce a significant fall in systemic blood pressure. Figure 7-3 illustrates the differential profiles of three representative sympathomimetic catecholamines exhibiting relatively selective α-adrenergic agonist (norepinephrine), β-adrenergic agonist (isoproterenol), or both α- and β-adrenergic agonist (epinephrine) actions on the cardiovascular system.

Bronchodilation is another priminent action of isoproterenol, resulting from activation of pulmonary β_2-adrenergic receptors. Inhalation of a mist of isoproterenol can prevent and relieve bronchoconstriction in asthmatics but is usually accompanied by cardiac stimulation. The use of isoproterenol as a bronchodilator has decreased as newer β_2-selective adrenergic agonists have become available. When compared to isoproterenol, this latter group of drugs has an advantage of causing fewer cardiac side effects (palpitations, tachycardia, arrhythmias) at doses that are equally bronchodilatory.

Phenylephrine

This synthetic drug is a noncatecholamine but is related both in chemical structure (see Fig. 7-2) and pharmacologic activity to norepinephrine. The characteristic feature of phenylephrine is its marked selectivity for α-adrenergic receptors (specifically, α_1). Thus, phenylephrine evokes vasoconstriction but little or no cardiostimulation. Parenteral administration results in elevated arterial blood pressure, accompanied by reflex bradycardia. Blood vessels in mucous membranes are constricted. Topical application to the nasal mucosa of patients with infectious or allergic rhinitis promotes a local decongestant effect by reducing blood flow to engorged, edematous tissue. Central stimulatory effects are minimal with phenylephrine.

Other Sympathomimetic Decongestants

Phenylephrine and *phenylpropanolamine* (see below) are among the most popular sympathomimetic drugs used for their mucosal decongestant action. Drugs such as *naphazoline, oxymetazoline, tetrahydrozoline,* and *xylometazoline* are chemically related imidazolines (see Fig. 7-2) used topically as mucosal decongestants. These are all α-adrenergic agonists which cause a "drying" effect when applied to congested membranes by constricting nasal mucosal blood vessels. Oxymetazoline is somewhat longer acting than the others. The onset of effects is less than 10 min, and duration of action may be longer than 5 h.

Continued use of topical decongestant drugs can result in rebound congestion. As the drug effect wanes, the congestion returns with increased severity and encourages further use of the medication. Prolonged use over several days may lead to rhinitis medicamentosa, a disorder characterized by chronic swelling and a red, boggy edematous appearance of the mucosa.

Clonidine

As previously mentioned, this drug is a selective α_2-adrenergic agonist. Clonidine, methyldopa, and guanfacine alllower systemic blood pressure and heart rate by stimulating α_2-adrenergic receptors in certain areas of the central nervous system and are used primarily as antihypertensive drugs. The pharmacology of these compounds is discussed in Chap. 31.

Dobutamine

The increased myocardial contractility produced by intravenous infusion of this synthetic catecholamine has been attributed to selective activation of cardiac β_1-adrenergic receptors. However, the mechanism of action of this compound is more complex since dobutamine can also activate α_1-adrenoceptors in the myocardium and vascular β_2-adrenoceptors. In moderate doses, dobutamine increases cardiac output without greatly increasing heart rate and tends to lower peripheral vascular resistance. Higher doses elevate blood pressure and increase heart rate.

The onset of action of dobutamine occurs within 2 min of intravenous infusion; peak activity usually occurs within 10 min. Dobutamine is not effective by the oral route. The plasma half-life of a single intravenous injection is 2 min. Biotransformation of this compound is primarily via methylation of the catechol group and subsequent conjugation (see Fig. 7-2). Conjugates of 3-O-methyl dobutamine, an inactive biotransformation product, and the parent compound are the major urinary excretion products.

Dobutamine is used to improve myocardial function in patients with severe refractory cardiac failure and to provide inotropic support following cardiac surgery. A greater improvement in cardiac performance may be attained when dobutamine is used in combination with intravenously administered vasodilators such as nitroprusside and nitroglycerin.

Hypertension, tachycardia, and ventricular arrhythmias are the most commonly encountered adverse effects. More rarely, nausea, headache, anginal pain, palpitations, and shortness of breath may occur. Dobutamine may also accelerate AV conduction. Untoward cardiovascular reactions to this drug can usually be controlled by reducing the dose.

Terbutaline

Terbutaline

Terbutaline, a synthetic noncatecholamine sympathomimetic amine, is a direct-acting β-adrenergic receptor agonist. In therapeutic doses, terbutaline selectively stimulates the β_2-adrenoceptors found in bronchial smooth muscle with relatively little activity on the cardiac β_1-adrenergic receptors. Although this drug is one of the more selective β_2-adrenergic receptor stimulants, the degree of selectivity of terbutaline and similar agents will vary with dose and cardiovascular effects have been reported.

Terbutaline can be administered orally, by inhalation or by subcutaneous injection. Since it is not a catecholamine, it is less susceptible to enzymatic degradation by sulfatase and COMT than catecholamines. Thus, its duration of action is considerably longer than that of isoproterenol and epinephrine. By the oral route the onset is within 30 min and the duration of effect up to 8 h; by inhalation the duration of the drug is somewhat shorter (Table 7-1).

Terbutaline is used in the treatment of bronchiolar spasm such as occurs in chronic obstructive pulmonary diseases, e. g., bronchitis and emphysema, and as a bronchodilator in asthma.

Adverse reactions produced by terbutaline are those commonly associated with other sympathomimetic amines, and include tremors, nervousness, and more rarely headache, tachycardia, palpitations, sweating, drowsiness, nausea, and vomiting. Tolerance appears to develop to these untoward effects as therapy with terbutaline continues.

Albuterol

Albuterol

Albuterol is another noncatecholamine selective β_2-adrenergic sympathomimetic with pharmacologic characteristics similar to terbutaline and several other adrenergic bronchodilators. It is widely used in acute and chronic bronchial asthma, bronchitis, and other chronic obstructive pulmonary diseases. When administered by the inhalation route, significant bronchodilation occurs within 15 min and lasts for 3 to 4 h (Table 7-1). Following oral administration, albuterol is conjugated in the intestinal mucosa and liver; uri-

TABLE 7-1 Beta₂-adrenergic receptor selectivity and pharmacokinetic properties of some adrenergic bronchodilators

Drug	β_2-Receptor selectivity[a]	Inhalation		Oral	
		Onset, min	Duration, h	Onset, min	Duration, h
Epinephrine	0	3–5	1–2	—[b]	—[b]
Isoproterenol	0	2–5	1–2	15–30[c]	1–2[c]
Isoetharine	+	1–5	1–3	—[b]	—[b]
Metaproterenol	++	1–5	3–4	15–30	4–5
Terbutaline	+++	5–30	3–6	15–30	4–8
Albuterol	+++	5–15	3–4	15–30	4–8

[a] High selectivity (+++), moderate selectivity (++), low selectivity (+), or no selectivity (0) for β_2-adrenergic receptors.
[b] Not used by the oral route.
[c] Tablets for sublingual use; not generally recommended.

nary excretion of both the unchanged drug and sulfate conjugates occurs. Greater separation of β_2 effects (bronchodilation) from β_1 effects (cardiostimulation) can be achieved when the drug is used by inhalation than by systemic administration.

Similar to other selective β_2 agonists, a common side effect of albuterol is skeletal muscle tremor, more frequently encountered during oral dosing regimens. Fine finger tremors may interfere with manual activities. Disturbances in cardiac rate and rhythm may also occur but are less problematic than with epinephrine or isoproterenol. The incidence of nervousness, insomnia, and other CNS effects is less frequent than with ephedrine. Excessive use may lead to a state of tolerance and refractoriness to the bronchodilatory ef-

fect. A paradoxical bronchoconstrictive reaction has been rarely reported with some of these selective β_2-adrenergic agonists.

Metaproterenol is less selective than terbutaline and albuterol as a β_2-adrenergic stimulant, but is still useful in the treatment of chronic obstructive airway diseases; it can be administered by either the oral or inhalational route. The drug is adequately absorbed (40 percent) following oral dosing. It is not biotransformed by COMT as is the case with the catecholamines but is excreted primarily as glucuronide conjugates via the kidney. Duration of action is approximately 4 h following a single dose. Adverse reactions are similar to the other aforementioned drugs.

Metaproterenol

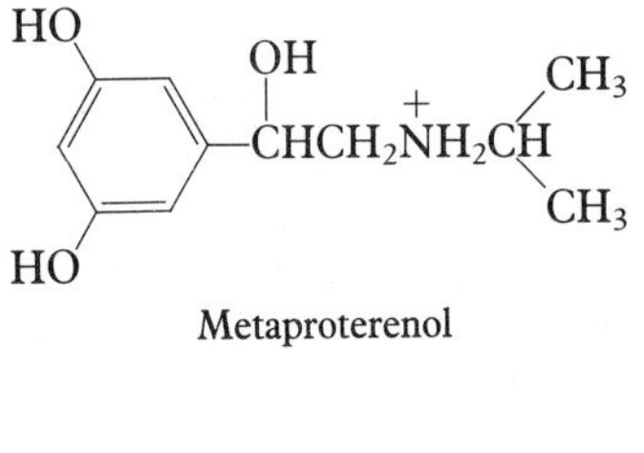

Metaproterenol

Isoetharine

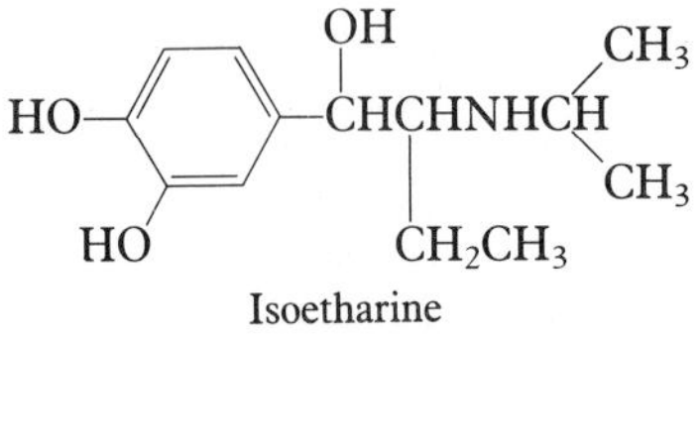

Isoetharine

Isoetharine is a direct-acting sympathomimetic with relatively low selectivity for β_2-adrenergic receptor sites. However, this drug produces more rapid relief of bronchiolar spasms than the more selective bronchodilator agonists. Isoetharine is a catecholamine, metabolized by COMT and is effective only by inhalation. As with other sympathomimetic amines administered by inhalation, tolerance may develop with prolonged continuous use of isoetharine.

Ritodrine

This selective β_2-adrenergic agonist is approved for use both intravenously and orally in carefully selected patients as a uterine relaxant for the prevention of premature labor. Other selective β_2 agents, especially terbutaline and albuterol have been reported to arrest premature labor but are as yet unapproved for this use in the United States. Intravenous therapy with ritodrine is initiated when contraindications have been ruled out; if successful, oral maintenance dosing is then instituted. Cardiovascular and metabolic reactions, i.e., hypokalemia and diabetogenic effects, have been noted in both mother and fetus, especially during intravenous infusion of this drug. Ritodrine therapy has largely replaced the previous use of intravenous alcohol to inhibit premature labor.

INDIRECT-ACTING AGENT

The only indirect-acting compound that will be mentioned here is tyramine, which exerts its sympathomimetic effect by causing the release of endogenous norepinephrine from storage vesicles in the adrenergic neuron. Tyramine has no other action, and because its effectiveness is limited by the extent of neuronal norepinephrine stores and it is rapidly inactivated by intraneuronal monoamine oxidase, it is of no clinical value. Tyramine is, however, important as an experimental laboratory tool and has toxicologic importance with some types of antidepressant drugs (see Chap. 20).

MIXED-ACTING AGENTS

The mixed-acting sympathomimetic drugs discussed below all possess, to some extent, a tyramine-like indirect action in addition to direct adrenergic receptor activation.

Dopamine

Dopamine

Dopamine is one of the intermediate products in the synthesis of norepinephrine and is formed by the decarboxylation of DOPA. Dopamine has been found in all sympathetic neurons and ganglia and in the CNS.

As a drug, dopamine stimulates both α- and β_1-adrenoceptors in addition to dopaminergic receptors; it has little activity on β_2-adrenoceptors. Dopamine can also release norepinephrine from tissue storage sites. Although dopamine has activity at central dopamine receptors, the drug does not cross the blood-brain barrier to any significant extent and only the administration of levodopa will elicit a central response.

Dopamine exerts its major effects on the cardiovascular system and on renal and mesenteric vasculature. Intravenous infusion of this endogenous catecholamine evokes a unique complex of hemodynamic actions which is dependent on the dose administered. Small doses [less than 5 (μg/kg)/min] produce increases in renal and mesenteric blood flow by activating dopaminergic receptors which mediate vasodilation in these areas. Somewhat greater doses [5 to 10 (μg/kg)/min] additionally stimulate the heart via β_1-adrenergic receptor activation; cardiac output is increased without markedly increasing heart rate or blood pressure and with less oxygen consumption than occurs with the catecholamines. Larger doses [more than 10 (μg/kg)/min] of dopamine evoke vasoconstriction (an α-adrenergic receptor-mediated effect) resulting in elevated systolic and diastolic blood pressure.

Dopamine is commonly used as a temporary adjunct in treating hypotension and circulatory shock caused by myocardial infarction, trauma, renal failure, and endotoxic septicemia. Because of its renal vasodilatory action, it may be more beneficial than other sympathomimetic amines (e.g., norepinephrine, metaraminol) in patients with impaired renal function. However, excessive doses can decrease renal blood flow and urine output. Dopamine is a more potent vasopressor agent than dobutamine.

The most common adverse reactions to dopamine include nausea, vomiting, CNS disturbances, and a variety of cardiovascular manifestations: tachyarrhythmias, palpitations, hypotension, vasoconstriction, and anginal pain. An improvement in hemodynamic status may be accompanied by increased myocardial oxygen demand. Large doses or long infusion periods have resulted in peripheral ischemia and gangrene. Since dopamine is metabolized by monoamine oxidase, a tenfold reduction in dosage is warranted if the drug is administered to patients receiving monoamine oxidase inhibitors.

Ephedrine

Ephedrine, an alkaloid which occurs in certain species of the plant genus *Ephedra*, is now produced by synthetic means (see Fig. 7-2). Since the molecule contains two asymmetric carbon atoms, four isomeric forms exist. *Pseudoephedrine* (*d*-isoephedrine) is a stereoisomer with pharmacologic actions only subtly different from ephedrine. Lacking the catechol moiety, ephedrine is distinguished from epinephrine and norepinephrine by its oral efficacy, longer duration of effect, more pronounced actions on the CNS, and significantly lower potency.

The pharmacologic profile of ephedrine is presented as typical of a "mixed-acting" noncatecholamine sympathomimetic agent. The drug directly stimulates both α- and β-adrenergic receptors and also causes the release of norepinephrine from sympathetic neurons. Two principal uses of ephedrine as a mucosal decongestant and bronchodilator are consequences of activating α- and β-adrenergic receptors, respectively.

Effects on Organ Systems

Cardiovascular System   If given intravenously, ephedrine produces cardiovascular effects similar to those of epinephrine. Systemic arterial blood pressure rises (both systolic and diastolic) and reflexly mediated cardiac slowing occurs. If vagal reflexes are blocked, heart rate is seen to increase. The hypertensive response is due to a combination increased vascular resistance resulting from vasoconstriction and an increase in cardiac output resulting from cardiac stimulation. In comparison with epinephrine, the pressor response to ephedrine is slower in onset, lasts considerably longer, and requires a much higher dose (approximately 100-fold more) to obtain an equivalent pressure elevation. If a second identical intravenous dose of ephedrine is administered shortly thereafter,

the ensuing pressor response proves weaker than that following the first dose. This phenomenon, known as *tachyphylaxis* (i.e., "rapid tolerance"), is a characteristic of sympathomimetic amines with an indirect-acting component that liberate norepinephrine from storage sites in the body. Tachyphylaxis is not observed with norepinephrine, epinephrine, and other direct-acting sympathomimetic amines. One explanation which has been given for this phenomenon is neuronal depletion of the neurotransmitter following repetitive exposure to the indirect-acting compound.

Bronchi   The smooth muscle of the bronchial tree is relaxed by ephedrine as a result of activating bronchopulmonary β_2-adrenergic receptors. Compared to epinephrine, this bronchodilatory effect of ephedrine is significantly weaker and is slower in onset but more sustained.

Eye   Pupillary dilation, i.e., mydriasis, occurs when ephedrine is instilled into the conjunctival sac. Reflexes to light and accommodative ability are unaffected, and intraocular pressure is unchanged. Heavily pigmented irises are significantly less responsive to the mydriatic action of ephedrine than are lightly colored ones. Ephedrine is rarely used today for its ocular effects.

Other Smooth Muscles and Glands   In general, ephedrine has effects on smooth muscle and glands that are qualitatively similar to epinephrine. Inhibition of the intact gastrointestinal musculature and contraction of the splenic capsule and of pilomotor muscles may be produced. The actions of ephedrine on the human myometrium and urinary bladder resemble those of epinephrine. Hyperglycemia can occur but is less pronounced than following administration of epinephrine.

Central Nervous System   Ephedrine passes the blood-brain barrier and is a corticomedullary stimulant, as are other sympathomimetic amines with structural features of an unsubstituted phenyl ring and a methyl group on the alpha carbon. The mental "alerting" activity of ephedrine is less pronounced than that of adrenergic drugs such as amphetamine and methamphetamine and is accompanied by the significant cardiovascular effects noted above. Depending on the dose, ephedrine can produce insomnia, restlessness, anxiety, agitation, and tremor. Sedative drugs can counteract the central stimulatory effects of ephedrine; for example, phenobarbital is included in some fixed-combination products containing ephedrine.

Pharmacokinetics Ephedrine is readily and completely absorbed after oral administration. If given subcutaneously or intramuscularly, local vasoconstriction at the injection site is not significant enough to prevent systemic absorption. Ephedrine resists oxidative deamination by monoamine oxidase (MAO), but deamination and conjugation do occur to some extent via the hepatic microsomal system. Up to 40 percent of an administered dose of the drug may be excreted unchanged in the urine. The pharmacologic activity of a single dose persists for several hours. For continuous effects, small doses of ephedrine are administered at 4-h intervals.

Ephedrine is usually administered orally in tablet, capsule, or liquid forms. Sterile solutions can be given by the subcutaneous, intramuscular, and intravenous routes, but the parenteral use of the drug is relatively uncommon. For local decongestion of the nasal mucosa, ephedrine solutions are applied directly by drops or as a spray.

Therapeutic Uses Ephedrine is an orally effective, long-acting sympathomimetic agent. Its clinical applications include allergic disorders, nasal congestion, and bronchial asthma; the drug is not useful for severe attacks of bronchial asthma because of its limited potency, but it is widely employed in numerous oral medications as a mild bronchodilator. Unfortunately, tolerance develops during prolonged administration. Both ephedrine and pseudoephedrine are popular ingredients of many proprietary decongestants and cough and cold formulations. Ephedrine can also be used as a pressor agent in spinal anesthesia, for mydriasis, and occasionally as a CNS stimulant.

Adverse Reactions Untoward reactions from ephedrine such as nervousness, insomnia, nausea, vertigo, and tremor are related to its actions on the central nervous system. Cardiovascular complications are similar to those possible with epinephrine. Many nonprescription drug products for the symptomatic relief of allergies and upper respiratory infections contain ephedrine or related sympathomimetic drugs such as phenylpropanolamine. Patients with hypertension,

cardiac problems, hyperthyroidism, and diabetes mellitus should be warned of the potential risks entailed by injudicious use of these products. Prolonged and continuous use of ephedrine can result in tolerance. The abuse of drug products containing ephedrine is known to occur; there are case reports in the medical literature of psychiatric disturbances induced by ephedrine abuse.

Phenylpropanolamine

The pharmacologic actions of phenylpropanolamine are similar to those of ephedrine. This sympathomimetic agent can cause transient elevations of blood pressure and is used for its nasal decongestant activity. A weak central stimulant, phenylpropanolamine has anorexigenic properties similar to but weaker than those of the amphetamines (see next section). It is currently available in nonprescription drug products promoted for short-term use as an adjunctive drug in weight control programs. The appetite suppressant effect of phenylpropanolamine is probably mediated at adrenergic neurotransmission sites in the brain stem. Adverse effects can include both cardiovascular and CNS reactions such as hypertension, stroke, nausea, nervousness, insomnia, and neuropsychiatric problems. The incidence of such adverse reactions is relatively low when used at recommended oral therapeutic doses, but there appear to be individuals who are highly sensitive to the drug. Contraindications to the use of phenylpropanolamine are the same as those of epinephrine.

Amphetamines

This term is customarily used in reference to racemic amphetamine, dextroamphetamine, and methamphetamine. As mixed-acting drugs, the amphetamines activate adrenergic receptors and also release endogenous catecholamines (norepinephrine and dopamine) from neurons in the brain and periphery. Their peripheral sympathomimetic properties closely resemble ephedrine. Oral administration raises systolic and diastolic blood pressure often with reflex cardiac slowing, but bronchodilatation is a less prominent effect. The most distinguishing characteristic of the amphetamines relates to their psychic stimulatory activity. Dextroamphetamine, the (+)-isomer of racemic amphetamine, is 3 to 4 times more potent than the (−)-isomer in evoking CNS excitatory effects. The stimulatory actions of amphetamines result in increased alertness, elevated mood states, insomnia, irritability, and dizziness. Large doses can induce hallucinations, violent behavior, and a psychotic state that clinically resembles paranoid schizophrenia.

Amphetamines are biotransformation by oxidative deamination in the drug-metabolizing microsomal system, and their metabolic fate may be affected by agents which alter the response of this system.

Amphetamines were the first drugs widely prescribed for appetite suppression in treating obesity. They are no longer recommended for use as anorexiants because of their striking psychic and physical dependence liability. Tolerance to the anorexic effect (and euphoric "high") can develop quite rapidly, and progressively larger doses must be taken to obtain the desired psychic response. A few states and Canada have prohibited their use for weight control. Based on its central actions, dextroamphetamine has been used in treating narcolepsy, urinary incontinence, and attention-deficit disorder in children. Prolonged use in children can impair linear growth and reduce weight gain.

Several substituted phenethylamines possess anorexiant and CNS stimulant properties similar to those of amphetamine, although they differ in potency and other actions. *Diethylpropion, phenmetrazine,* and *phenteramine* are representative of this group of "non-amphetamines." *Fenfluramine* has anorexiant actions but differs somewhat in that it depresses rather than stimulates the CNS. Drowsiness is frequently encountered. *Mazindol* is atypical in that it is not a substituted phenethylamine, does not appear to produce euphoria, and may therefore have less abuse potential.

The use of an amphetamine or an amphetamine-like sympathomimetic drug is contraindicated in patients with cardiovascular disease, hypertension, hyperthyroidism, glaucoma, and pregnancy. Persons with a history of emotional disorders or drug abuse should not receive these agents.

Metaraminol

Metaraminol is a sympathomimetic amine that has both direct and indirect actions and has hemodynamic characteristics similar to those of norepinephrine. Because of its prominent α-adrenergic agonist activity it may be useful parenterally as a vasoconstrictor, e.g., in treating acute hypotensive states during spinal anesthesia.

SUMMARIZED USES OF ADRENERGIC DRUGS

Cardiovascular Uses

The positive inotropic effect of adrenergic agents with β-adrenoceptor agonist properties provides a basis for their use in conditions in which myocardial stimulation and increased cardiac output are desired. Cardiostimulatory sympathomimetics have been used in circulatory and cardiogenic shock, for the short-term therapy of severe congestive heart failure, and in the emergency management of complete heart block and cardiac arrest.

Vasoconstrictor agents may convert episodes of paroxysmal atrial tachycardia to a sinus rhythm by elevating arterial blood pressure and thereby activating vagal cholinergic reflexes. Alternative therapies (i.e., other drug classes, electrical cardioversion) exist for some of these indications. Regional vasoconstriction may be desirable to control hemorrhage in surgical procedures and to reduce diffusion of local anesthetics from their site of injection. Vasoconstriction in mucous membranes forms the basis of use of sympathomimetics as nasal, bronchopulmonary, and ocular decongestants.

Bronchopulmonary Uses

β-Adrenergic agonists, and in particular the selective β_2 receptor agonists, are an important class of drugs used in both acute and chronic therapy of bronchial asthma and certain other obstructive respiratory diseases. Their efficacy is primarily based on their ability to reverse bronchoconstriction, but evidence also exists that they can inhibit the release of chemical mediators of inflammation and increase the rate of mucociliary clearance. Other classes of drugs used in bronchial disorders are described in Chap. 32.

Central Nervous System Uses

Sympathomimetic drugs with central stimulatory actions, i.e., the amphetamines, have been used as anorexiants in obesity, in psychogenic reactive depression, in the treatment of narcolepsy, and in children diagnosed with attention deficit disorder. Methylphenidate, another central stimulant, is also used in the latter two conditions. The clinical efficacy of amphetamines in many of these neuropsychiatric applications is not well proven and controversial. Physical dependence and addiction to amphetamines severely limits their therapeutic value. The illicit sale of amphetamine-like stimulants and their widespread abuse for "antifatigue" and euphoric effects is a major social problem. Their legitimate use in medicine for trivial purposes is unwarranted.

Other Uses

Ophthalmic uses of sympathomimetics are based on their mydriatic and decongestant properties and their ability to reduce intraocular pressure in open-angle glaucoma. The use of β_2-adrenergic agonists (specifically ritodrine) for their uterine relaxant activity is replacing older therapies in suppressing premature labor.

BIBLIOGRAPHY

Allwood, M. J., A. F. Cobbold, and J. Ginsburg: "Peripheral Vascular Effects of Noradrenaline, Isopropylnoradrenaline and Dopamine," *Br. Med. Bull.*, **19**:132–136 (1963).

Axelrod, J., and T. Reisine: "Stress Hormones: Their Interaction and Regulation," *Science*, **224**:452–459 (1984).

Barach, E. M., R. M. Nowak, G. L. Tennyson, and M. C. Tomlanovich: "Epinephrine for Treatment of Anaphylactic Shock," *J. Am. Med. Assoc.*, **251**:2118–2122 (1984).

Bilezikian, J. P.: "Defining the Role of Adrenergic Receptors in Human Physiology," in P. A. Insel (ed.), *Adrenergic Receptors in Man*, Marcel Dekker, New York, 1987, pp. 37–68.

Bravo, E. L.: "Phenylpropanolamine and Other Over-the-Counter Vasoactive Compounds," *Hypertension*, **Mar 11 (3 Pt 2)**:II 7–10 (1988).

Bulbring, E., and T. Tomita: "Catecholamine Action on Smooth Muscle," *Pharmacol. Rev.*, **39(1)**:49–96 (1987).

Dohlman, H. G., M. G. Caron, and R. J. Lefkowitz: "A Family of Receptors Coupled to Guanine Nucleotide Regulatory Proteins," *Biochemistry*, **26**:2657–2664 (1987).

Drug Evaluations, 6th ed., prepared by the American Medical Association Department of Drugs, Division of Drugs and Technology, Saunders, Philadelphia, 1986.

Dwyer, J. M.: "Pharmacologic Approach to Management of Asthma," *Ration. Drug Ther.*, **18**:1–8 (1984).

Feldman, R., and L. E. Limbird: "Biochemical Characterization of Human Adrenergic Receptors, in P. A. Insel (ed.), *Adrenergic Receptors in Man*, Marcel Dekker, New York, 1987, pp. 161–200.

Goldberg, L. I.: "Dopamine: Clinical Uses of an Endogenous Catecholamine," *N. Engl. J. Med.*, **291**:707–710 (1974).

Kopin, I. J.: "Catecholamine Metabolism: Basic Aspects and Clinical Significance," *Pharmacol. Rev.*, **37**:333–364 (1985).

Lefkowitz, R. J., and M. C. Caron: "Molecular and Regulatory Properties of Adrenergic Receptors," *Recent Prog. Horm. Res.*, **43**:469–487 (1987).

Minneman, K. P.: "α_1-Adrenergic Receptor Subtypes, Inositol Phosphates, and Sources of Cell Ca^{2+}," *Pharmacol. Rev.*, **40**:87–119 (1988.)

Ruffolo, R. R., Jr.: "The Pharmacology of Dobutamine," *Am. J. Med. Sci.*, **294**:244–248 (1987).

Sarnoff, S. J., S. K. Brockman, J. P. Gilmore, R. J. Linden, and J. H. Mitchell: "Regulation of Ventricular Contraction. Influence of Cardiac Sympathetic and Vagal Nerve Stimulation on Atrial and Ventricular Dynamics," *Circ. Res.*, **8**:1108–1122 (1960).

Sonneblick, E. H.: "Implications of Muscle Mechanics in the Heart," *Fed. Proc.*, **21**:975–990 (1962).

Weiner, N.: "Norepinephrine, Epinephrine, and the Sympathomimetic Amines," in A. G. Gilman, L. S. Goodman, T. W. Rall, and F. Murad (eds.), *Goodman and Gilman's The Pharmacological Basis of Therapeutics*, 7th ed., Macmillan, New York, 1985, pp. 145–180.

Whitehouse, A. M., and J. M. Duncan: "Ephedrine Psychosis Rediscovered," *Br. J. Psychiatry*, **150**:258–261 (February 1987).

Adrenergic Blocking and Neuronal Blocking Drugs

Andrew P. Ferko and G. John DiGregorio

Over the years the drugs that attenuate the effects of the sympathetic nervous system have attained importance. There is a wide use of these agents in many disease conditions in which the adrenergic nervous system has a pathogenic role. In addition to drugs which have been in use for many years and appear to block all alpha (α)- or beta (β)-adrenergic receptors, newer agents are being developed which show selective blockade for the subgroups of α- and β-adrenergic receptors. *Adrenergic blockade* refers to the capacity of a drug to antagonize the effects elicited by either sympathetic nerve stimulation or the administration of adrenergic drugs. The drugs in this chapter are classified into three general groups: *β-adrenergic blocking agents*, *α-adrenergic blocking agents*, and *adrenergic neuronal blocking drugs*.

The first group, drugs which block β-adrenergic receptor sites, is divided into nonselective and selective blockers. The nonselective β-adrenergic blocking agents have affinity for both β_1- and β_2-adrenergic receptor sites. Drugs such as propranolol, nadolol, timolol, and labetalol are in this category. The selective β-adrenergic blocking agents preferentially attach to the β_1-adrenergic receptor sites at therapeutic doses. Compounds with selectivity for the β_1-adrenergic receptor are acebutolol, atenolol, esmolol, and metoprolol. To date there are no therapeutically useful β_2-adrenergic blockers, although a number of experimental compounds exist.

The second group of drugs block α-adrenergic receptors. These agents are also divided into nonselective and selective blockers. The nonselective α-adrenergic blocking agents bind to both α_1- and α_2-adrenergic receptors. Examples of drugs in this classification include phentolamine and phenoxybenzamine. Also contained in this category are ergotamine and ergonovine, which belong to a group of compounds called the *ergot alkaloids*. Although the reason for the therapeutic use of ergotamine and ergonovine in medicine today is unrelated to α-adrenergic blockade, they are included in this section from a historical standpoint. The ergot alkaloids were the first adrenergic blocking drugs to be investigated. The selective α-adrenergic blocking agents exhibit, at therapeutic doses, a high degree of affinity for either the α_1-adrenergic site (e. g., prazosin and terazosin) or the α_2-adrenergic site (e. g., yohimbine).

The final group of adrenergic blocking drugs include those which act primarily in the nerve terminal to impair biogenic amine (norepinephrine, dopamine, or serotonin) synthesis, storage, or release. These drugs are termed *adrenergic neuronal blocking agents*. Examples of drugs in this group are reserpine, guanadrel, guanethidine, and metyrosine. Figure 8-1 illustrates the sites of action of the various adrenergic blocking drugs.

BETA-ADRENERGIC BLOCKING DRUGS

The introduction of the β-adrenergic blocking drugs has been one of the major advances in cardiovascular pharmacology. Initially these drugs had been utilized only in the treatment of essential hypertension; pres-

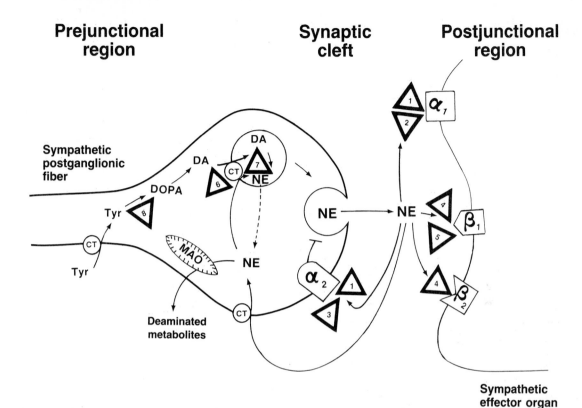

FIGURE 8-1   Sites of action of adrenergic blocking drugs and adrenergic neuronal block-ers. The diagram illustrates an adrenergic synapse, which shows the synthesis of norepi-nephrine, its storage in intraneuronal vesicles or granules, and its release into the synaptic cleft. The location of α_1, α_2, β_1, and β_2 adrenergic receptors is shown. Numbered triangles represent the blocking drugs: (1) phentolamine and phenoxybenzamine, (2) prazosin and terazosin, (3) yohimbine, (4) nonselective β-adrenergic blockers (5) selective β-adrenergic blockers, (6) reserpine, (7) guanethidine and guanadrel, and (8) metyrosine. Abbrev-iations: Tyr = tyrosine; DOPA = dihydroxyphenylalanine; DA = dopamine; NE = nor-epinephrine; MAO = monoamine oxidase; CT = catecholamine transport (uptake).

ently they are being used in a wide variety of clinical situations such as angina pectoris, supraventricular and ventricular arrhythmias, migraine headaches, glaucoma, and the hyperactive phase of myocardial infarction. Their effectiveness in many diseases is based primarily on the competitive blockade of the β-adrenergic receptors within the autonomic nervous system that occurs with all of these drugs. Included in this group of compounds are propranolol, metoprolol, nadolol, atenolol, timolol, acebutolol, pindolol, es-molol, and labetalol.

Chemistry

The chemical structures of the β-adrenergic blockers are shown in Fig. 8-2. There are several structural fea-tures that are common to these drugs: (1) a substituted or unsubstituted aromatic or heterocyclic group, (2) a methoxy linkage ($-OCH_2-$), and (3) a substituted ethanolamine side chain [$-CH(OH)-CH_2-NH-$] with either a tertiary butyl group (as in nadolol and timolol) or an isopropyl group (all others) on the termi-nal nitrogen. The substituted ethanolamine group is similar to that found in many compounds with β-

Acebutolol

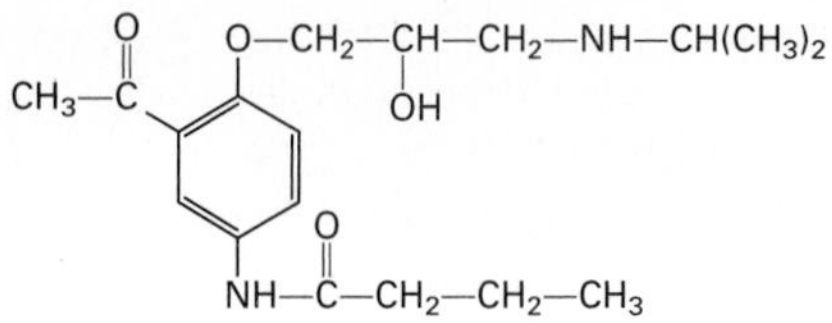

Atenolol

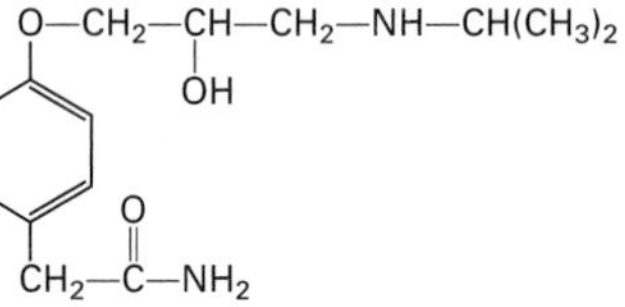

Esmolol

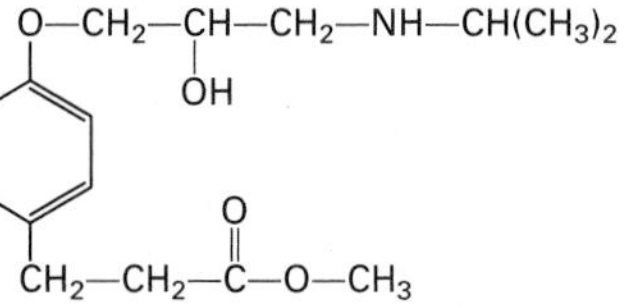

Metoprolol

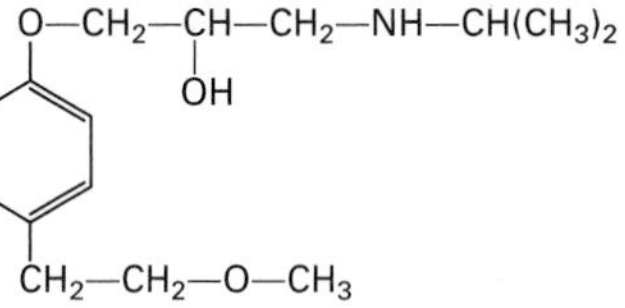

Nadolol

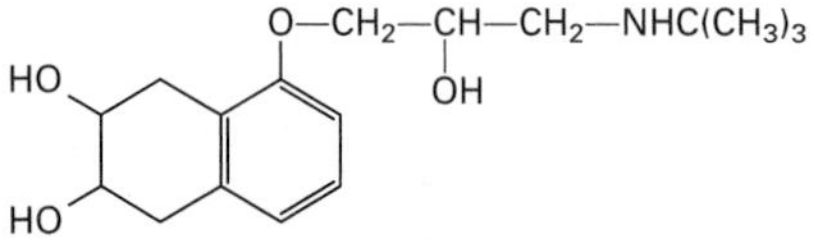

Pindolol

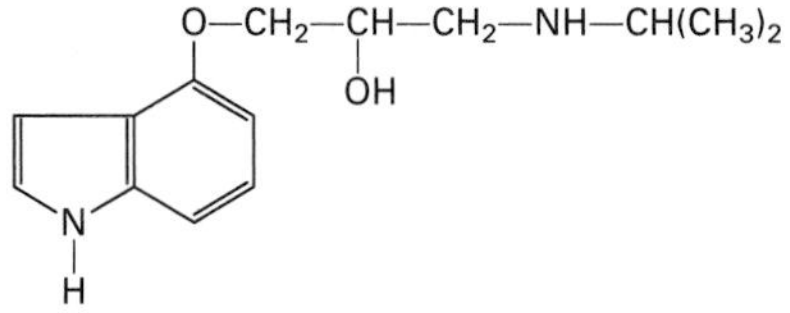

Propranolol

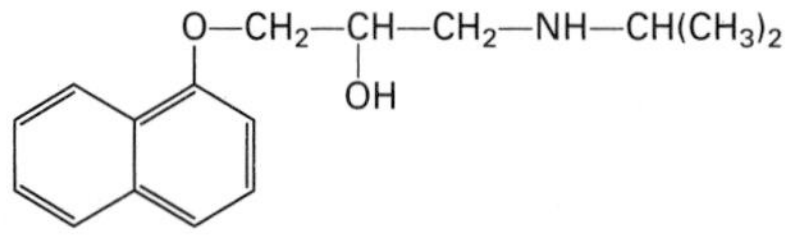

Timolol

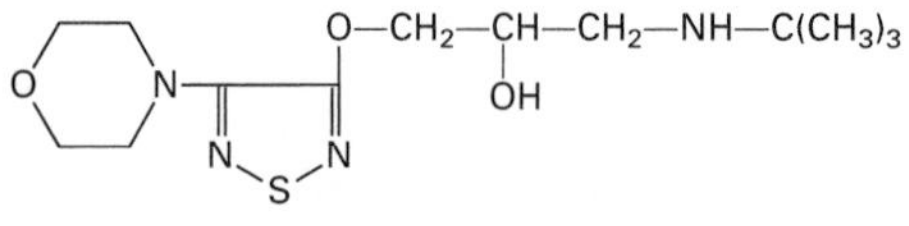

FIGURE 8-2 Structures of some β-adrenergic blocking drugs.

adrenergic receptor agonist activity (e. g., isoproterenol and albuterol, see Fig. 7-2), and believed to be responsible for the high affinity of these blocking agents for binding to β-adrenergic receptors. The levorotatory stereoisomers of these drugs are much more potent with respect to their β-adrenoceptor blocking activity than the dextrorotatory isomers; however, all these compounds are marketed as racemic mixtures.

Mechanism of Action

These drugs attach reversibly to β-adrenergic receptor sites and competively prevent the activation of these receptors by catecholamines released via the sympathetic nervous system or by exogenously administered sympathomimetics (Fig. 8-1). β-Adrenergic receptors are divided into β_1 receptors (located mainly in cardiac muscle) and β_2 receptors (located mainly in bronchial and vascular musculature) (see Chap. 6 for more details). The β-adrenergic blocking drugs may be classified according to their selectivity toward these receptors. Those drugs that have approximately equal affinity for both β_1- and β_2-adrenoceptors, independent of dose, are referred to as *nonselective* blocking

agents and include nadolol, pindolol, propranolol, timolol, and labetalol. Those agents that have a higher affinity for the β_1 receptors than the β_2 receptors (at therapeutic doses), e. g., acebutolol, atenolol, metoprolol, and esmolol, are classified as *selective* (or *cardioselective*) β-adrenergic blockers. It is important to remember, however, that this receptor selectivity is not absolute; rather, it is dose-dependent, i. e., the selective blocking agents, administered at high therapeutic doses, will loose their selectivity and inhibit both the β-adrenergic receptor subtypes equally.

In addition to blocking β-adrenoceptors, these drugs have other properties which result in certain cardiovascular effects (Table 8-1). Propranolol, acebutolol, metoprolol, and pindolol have a nonspecific myocardial depressant effect [also known as a *quinidine-like effect* or *membrane stabilizing activity (MSA)*], which usually occurs at higher dose regimens and has been suggested as being partly responsible for the antiarrhythmic properties of certain β-adrenergic blockers. There are, however, β-receptor blocking drugs which lack this property but still possess certain antiarrhythmic activities.

Pindolol and, to a lesser extent, acebutolol and la-

TABLE 8-1   Comparison of some pharmacodynamic properties of beta-adrenergic blocking drugs

	β_1-Adrenoceptor selectivity	Intrinsic sympathomimetic activity (ISA)	Membrane stabilizing activity (MSA)
Acebutolol	Yes	+	+
Atenolol	Yes	−	−
Esmolol	Yes	−	−
Labetalol	No	−	+
Metoprolol	Yes	−	+
Nadolol	No	−	−
Pindolol	No	+ +	+
Propranolol	No	−	+ +
Timolol	No	−	−

betalol possess partial agonist activity, also known as *intrinsic sympathomimetic activity (ISA)* (Table 8-1). ISA is most often manifested at the β_1-adrenergic receptor site resulting in less of a depression of heart rate and cardiac output than drugs lacking this property.

Propranolol

Propranolol is the oldest and most widely used of the clinically useful β-adrenergic blocking agents. Therefore it is considered the prototypical drug in this category and will be discussed in greatest detail.

Pharmacodynamics

Effects on the Cardiovascular System Propranolol is a cardiac depressant which can affect the mechanical and electrophysiologic properties of the myocardium. It can block atrioventricular conduction and automaticity of cardiac pacemaker potentials and the adrenergic stimulation induced by catecholamines; therefore, the drug lowers myocardial contractility, heart rate, blood pressure, cardiac work, and myocardial oxygen demand. Because of these effects, propranolol and other β-adrenergic blockers are useful as antiarrhythmic agents (see Chap. 27) and as antianginal drugs (see Chap. 28).

Propranolol reduces the blood pressure of most patients with essential hypertension without causing orthostatic hypotension. The antihypertensive effect of propranolol may be the result of a number of proposed mechanisms: (1) *Reduced cardiac output.* As mentioned, the blockade of adrenergic stimulation to the heart, reduces heart rate and cardiac output. These effects are more pronounced during exercise and are a potential problem in active individuals. (2) *Inhibition of renin release.* By decreasing the release of renin from the juxtaglomerular cells in the nephron, a reduction in serum angiotensin II (a potent vasoconstrictor) occurs. (3) *Decreased sympathetic outflow from the central nervous system.* This mechanism effectively lowers sympathetic tone to the heart, kidney, and vasculature. (4) *Inhibition of norepinephrine release from sympathetic postganglionic neurons.* In addition to blocking postsynaptic β-adrenergic receptors, it has been suggested that presynaptic β-adrenoceptors enhance neurotransmitter release from sympathetic neurons; blockade of these receptors would reduce sympathetic activity to the heart and vascular smooth muscle. None of these mechanisms adequately ex-

plains the antihypertensive activity of propranolol and the other β-adrenergic blocking drugs. For example, some of these drugs (e. g., nadolol and atenolol) do not enter the CNS very readily, yet these are no less effective as antihypertensive drugs than propranolol.

A mild increase in peripheral vascular resistance is associated with propranolol and the other nonselective β-adrenergic blockers. This is due to inhibition of peripheral β_2 receptors, resulting in an α-adrenergic receptor effect (i. e., vasoconstriction) which will be unopposed by reduced β-adrenergic receptor-mediated vasodilatation. During chronic administration of these drugs, the antihypertensive effect predominates and the increased peripheral vascular resistance returns to the pretreatment level and does not significantly affect systemic blood pressure.

Effects on the Respiratory System Due to β_2-adrenergic receptor blockade throughout the pulmonary system, the resting bronchiolar smooth muscles become hypersensitive to agents which increase airway resistance and induce bronchoconstriction. This is of little or no consequence in patients with normal respiratory function; however, in susceptible individuals an asthmatic attack can be precipitated. Bronchoconstriction is less evident with the selective β_1-adrenergic blocking agents.

Metabolic Effects Propranolol has effects on carbohydrate and fat metabolism which are a result of the blocking activity of these drugs on catecholamine-induced β-adrenergic receptor-mediated responses.

The action of propranolol and the other β-adrenergic blockers on carbohydrate metabolism is complicated. Glycogenolysis can be inhibited in the heart and skeletal muscle resulting in the depression of blood glucose levels. Hypoglycemia is not common, however, but may present difficulty should it occur in a diabetic patient since propranolol may mask some of the premonitory signs of acute hypoglycemia, e. g., tachycardia. In addition, propranolol may delay the recovery of blood glucose to normal levels following insulin-induced hypoglycemia in a diabetic patient.

Propranolol will also inhibit the rise in plasma free fatty acids induced by sympathomimetic agents such as epinephrine and will subsequently inhibit the lipolytic action of the sympathetic nervous system. Serum triglyceride levels generally increase with β-receptor blockade; however, these drugs generally do not significantly alter serum cholesterol levels. In some specific cases, propranolol may decrease high density lipoproteins, whereas drugs with a high degree of intrinsic sympathomimetic activity (ISA) may increase this serum lipoprotein.

Pharmacokinetics Propranolol is well absorbed after oral administration, but the systemic bioavailability is low due to high first-pass biotransformation (Table 8-2). Of all the β-adrenergic blockers propranolol has the highest lipid solubility, which results in the greatest penetration into the CNS. In addition this drug has the highest degree of binding to plasma proteins, mainly albumin and α_1-acid glycoprotein.

Propranolol is converted by the hepatic mixed function oxidase system to 4-hydroxypropranolol, an active metabolite; the $t_{1/2}$ of the 4-hydroxy derivative is short (approximately 2 h) and does not account for the major effects of propranolol during chronic oral therapy. Propranolol can also be biotransformed to a number of inactive products; these and the small amounts of the parent compound are all excreted in the urine.

The pharmacokinetic profile of propranolol is complex and depends to a great extent on the route of administration. β-Adrenergic blockade usually develops within 30 min following oral ingestion and is maintained for approximately 3 to 8 h. The duration is about 12 to 24 h following a single oral dose. When administered by the intravenous route, the onset of action occurs within 2 min and reaches a peak effect in 3 to 5 min; the duration of effect is 2 to 4 h. The $t_{1/2}$ has been estimated at 3 h after IV use and 4 to 6 h following oral administration. Plasma levels of propranolol and many other drugs in this group are not closely correlated with therapeutic responses.

There are certain factors, such as genetics, age, and various disease states, that can influence the pharmacokinetics of propranolol and other β-adrenergic blockers. The biotransformation of the drugs may be influenced by genetic differences in oxidation or by disease. Hence patients having gene characteristics which result in poor oxidative metabolism, or individuals with liver disease, may acquire higher plasma concentrations of β-adrenergic blockers, which may lead

TABLE 8-2 Physicochemical and pharmacokinetic properties of beta-adrenergic blockers

	Lipid solubility	Plasma protein binding, %	Elimination half-life, h	Excreted unchanged, %	Major metabolic process	Active metabolites
Acebutolol	Low	25	3–7	20	Acetylation	N-acetyl acebutolol (diacetolol)
Atenolol	Low	5–15	6–7	100	None	None
Esmolol	Low	55	0.16	1	Hydrolysis	None
Labetalol	Moderate	50	5–8	20	Conjugation	None
Metoprolol	Moderate	10	3–4	5	Oxidation	Yes
Nadolol	Low	30	20–24	100	None	None
Pindolol	Moderate	50–70	3–4	40	Oxidation and conjugation	None
Propranolol	High	90–95	3–4	1	Oxidation	4-Hydroxy propranolol
Timolol	Low	25–60	3–5	20	Oxidation	None

to drug toxicity. In the neonate and the elderly patient, the renal excretion of the drugs may be delayed due to decreased renal function.

Therapeutic Uses Propranolol is indicated in the management of hypertension, angina pectoris, supraventricular arrhythmias, ventricular tachycardias, migraine headache, hypertrophic subaortic stenosis, and pheochromocytoma. It is also indicated to reduce cardiovascular mortality in the post-acute phase of myocardial infarction. Additional information concerning the use of propranolol in arrhythmias, angina, and essential hypertension is found in Chaps. 27, 28, and 31, respectively.

Adverse Reactions Propranolol produces mild and transient side effects that rarely require cessation of therapy. Some of these include nausea, vomiting, anorexia, gastric pain, flatulence, dizziness, vertigo, fatigue, insomnia, depression, hallucinations, visual disturbances, mild diarrhea or constipation, and cutaneous eruptions such as rash and pruritus. Agranulocytosis and thrombocytopenic purpura are very rare, as is the development of antinuclear antibodies.

Serious adverse effects resulting from the pharmacologic action of β-adrenergic blockade include severe hypotension, bradycardia, atrioventricular conduction delay, which may lead to heart block, and congestive heart failure especially in patients that require an active sympathetic nervous system for their myocardial drive. Other adverse effects associated with β-receptor blockade include decrease in exercise tolerance, bronchoconstriction, and the induction of Raynaud's phenomenon. Following abrupt cessation of propranolol, as well as the other β-adrenergic blocking drugs, episodes of angina and myocardial infarction have occurred. This effect is probably related to the increase in the β-adrenoceptor population after chronic β-adrenergic blocker use. When administration of the antagonist is suddenly stopped, there is an overabundance of β-adrenoceptors available to interact with endogenous catecholamines causing increased cardiac activity.

Since propranolol may precipitate an acute, severe crisis in asthmatic patients and since these patients may respond poorly to β-adrenergic bronchodilators, propranolol is contraindicated in the presence of bronchial asthma. This drug must also be given with extreme caution to patients with borderline cardiac re-

serve or frank congestive heart failure, unless the failure is due to an arrhythmia that may be controlled by propranolol.

The drug should also be used with caution in diabetics and patients subject to hypoglycemia, since propranolol may mask some of the symptoms of acute hypoglycemia reactions, e. g., tachycardia.

Drug Interactions Since β-adrenergic blockers are widely coadministered with other drugs, the occurrence of drug interactions is not uncommon. Table 8-3 lists some of the important drug interactions and the possible mechanisms. The most important drug interactions are those that occur between the β blockers and other drugs associated with the myocardium. For example, both digoxin and verapamil will decrease heart rate and decrease conduction across the AV node; if administered with propranolol, then a serious bradycardia may occur.

Preparations Propranolol hydrochloride (Inderal) is available in tablets of 10, 20, 40, 60, 80, and 90 mg.

TABLE 8-3 **Drug interactions of beta-adrenergic blockers**

Drug	Response with β-adrenergic blocker
Antacids	Decreases absorption of beta blockers
Cardiac glycosides	Increased bradycardia
Lidocaine	Increased lidocaine blood levels
Phenytoin	Additive cardiac depression
Quinidine	Additive cardiac depression
Tricyclic antidepressants	Inhibits negative inotropic and chronotropic effects of beta blockers
Tubocurarine	Enhanced neuromuscular blockade
Verapamil	Potentiation of bradycardia and myocardial depression

A solution (1 mg/mL) for intravenous administration is available as well as sustained release capsules (Inderal LA) of 60, 80, 120, and 160 mg.

Metoprolol

Unlike propranolol, which blocks both β_1- and β_2-adrenergic receptors, metoprolol has a cardioselective action, i. e., in therapeutic doses metoprolol will block β_1-adrenoceptors with little effect on β_2-adrenergic receptors (Table 8-1). Metoprolol is *less likely* to induce bronchoconstriction and does not compromise bronchodilation provided by isoproterenol, albuterol, etc. The drug has no ISA and only weak membrane-stabilizing activity (MSA).

Metoprolol is rapidly and completely absorbed from the gastrointestinal tract following oral administration; however, like propranolol, its systemic bioavailability is reduced significantly due to high first-pass biotransformation (Table 8-2). Only about 10 percent of metoprolol is bound to plasma proteins, resulting in a relatively high apparent volume of distribution (4.2 L/kg); the elimination $t_{1/2}$ is 3 to 4 h. The drug is biotransformed to a small extent to an active oxidation product (which has no clinical significance) and to inactive products, all of which are eliminated in the urine.

Metoprolol is indicated for essential hypertension and angina pectoris and appears comparable to propranolol in these diseases. It is also indicated for use in the post-myocardial infarcted patient. The adverse reactions of this drug are similar to propranolol.

Preparations Metoprolol tartrate (Lopressor) is available as tablets of 50 and 100 mg for oral administration and as a solution (1 mg/mL) in ampuls and prefilled syringes for intravenous use.

Other Beta-Adrenergic Blockers

The other β-adrenergic blocking agents are very similar to propranolol and metoprolol in their pharmacology. The *nonselective* blocking agents like propranolol are nadolol, pindolol, and timolol; those agents that have a higher affinity for the β_1 receptors than the β_2 receptors, the *cardioselective* β-adrenergic blockers, are acebutolol, atenolol, and esmolol (Table 8-1). All the effects of these drugs are similar to propranolol; labetalol has one different property and is discussed separately below.

The major difference with respect to these drugs resides in their pharmacokinetics, and some of these properties are outlined in Table 8-2. With the exception of esmolol, all these compounds are absorbed from the gastrointestinal tract; nadolol and atenolol are absorbed to the extent of 30 and 50 percent, respectively, while all the others are absorbed greater than 90 percent. Once absorbed, acebutolol and timolol, like propranolol, undergo a high first-pass metabolism within the liver. Pindolol, atenolol, and nadolol have a high systemic bioavailability because they escape this initial hepatic inactivation; in fact, atenolol and nadolol are not biotransformed and are excreted in the urine unchanged. The remaining β-adrenergic blockers are metabolized quite extensively in the liver to either active or inactive metabolites. All the resulting metabolites and parent compounds are excreted primarily in the urine. The elimination $t_{1/2}$ of these drugs ranges from 3 to 24 h; the two compounds that are not biotransformed (atenolol and nadolol) remain in the body the longest. Plasma protein binding to both albumin and α_1-acid glycoprotein ranges from 5 to 95 percent.

With respect to pharmacokinetics, esmolol is unique. It is an ester that is metabolized rapidly by hydrolysis of the ester linkage, chiefly by esterases in the cytosol of erythrocytes (not by plasma cholinesterase or red cell membrane acetylcholinesterase) to an inactive product, resulting in a compound with an elimination $t_{1/2}$ of approximately 10 min. Less than 2 percent of the drug is excreted unchanged in the urine.

These drugs are used for a wide variety of clinical conditions. Each drug or preparation has a specific FDA-approved indication. Acebutolol is indicated for the treatment of essential hypertension and ventricular arrhythmias. Atenolol and nadolol are indicated for the treatment of hypertension and long-term management of patients with angina pectoris. Esmolol is indicated for the rapid control of ventricular rate in patients with atrial fibrillation or atrial flutter in perioperative, postoperative, or other emergency circumstances where short-term control of ventricular rate is necessary. Pindolol is indicated only for the management of hypertension. Timolol is indicated for the treatment of hypertension and to reduce the cardiovascular mortality and the risk of reinfarction after an acute phase of a myocardial infarction. Timolol, administered topically to the eye, is also useful in chronic open angle glaucoma and in secondary glaucoma.

Preparations   Acebutolol hydrochloride (Sectral) is available as capsules of 200 and 400 mg. Atenolol (Tenormin) is available as tablets of 50 and 100 mg. Esmolol hydrochloride (Brevibloc) is available for intravenous infusion as a solution (250 mg/mL) in ampuls. Nadolol (Corgard) is available as tablets of 20, 40, 80, 120, and 160 mg. Pindolol (Visken) is available as tablets of 5 and 10 mg. Timolol maleate (Blocadren) is available as tablets of 5, 10, and 20 mg for systemic administration and as ophthalmic solutions (Timoptic) of 0.25 and 0.5 percent.

Labetalol

Chemically, labetalol differs somewhat from other β-adrenergic blockers in that it is a substituted phenylpropylamino salicylamide derivative.

Labetalol also differs in its pharmacologic properties; it is a competitive blocker of both α- and β-adrenergic receptors. The drug will selectively block α_1-adrenergic receptors and nonselectively block β_1-

Labetalol

and β_2-adrenergic receptors; the potency ratios for $\alpha{:}\beta$ blockade is 1:3 for the oral route and 1:7 following intravenous administration.

Labetalol will block cardiac β_1-adrenoceptor sites resulting in a decreased heart rate. There appears to be little or no effect on intraventricular conduction or QRS duration; a mild prolongation of the AV conduction time has been observed in some patients. Peripheral vascular resistance will decrease slightly due to both α- and β-adrenergic blocking action, and both of these actions of labetalol contribute to the decrease in blood pressure in hypertensive patients. Because of the α_1-adrenergic blocking activity, blood pressure is decreased more in the standing than in the supine position, and symptoms of postural hypotension can occur. Labetalol lowers blood pressure without significant reflex tachycardia. As with the other β-adrenergic blockers, abrupt withdrawal of the drug

may lead to an exacerbation of angina and, in some cases, myocardial infarction.

Following oral administration, labetalol is subjected to a high first-pass effect resulting in an oral bioavailability of only 25 percent. Plasma protein binding is approximately 50 percent. The elimination $t_{1/2}$ of the drug is about 5.5 h after intravenous use and 6 to 8 h following oral administration. Total body clearance is estimated at about 33 mL/min/kg. Metabolism of labetalol is via the drug-metabolizing microsomal system with the production of glucuronide conjugates. Approximately 55 to 60 percent of the dose appears in the urine as conjugates or unchanged drug within the first 24 h of dosing.

Labetalol is usually well tolerated. The most common adverse reactions include dizziness, fatigue, nausea, vomiting, nasal stuffiness, impotence, and edema.

The only indication for labetalol is in the treatment of essential hypertension. Labetalol hydrochloride (Normodyne, Trandate) is supplied as tablets of 100, 200, and 300 mg and as a solution for injection in vials of 5 mg/mL.

NONSELECTIVE ALPHA-ADRENERGIC BLOCKING AGENTS

These adrenergic blocking drugs include a structurally heterogeneous group of compounds which possess varied pharmacologic effects. All these drugs have one common property: the ability to block α_1- and α_2-adrenergic receptors.

Phentolamine

Phentolamine

Chemistry   Phentolamine is an imidazoline derivative which has α-adrenergic blocking, direct smooth muscle relaxant, cholinomimetic, histaminic, and sympathomimetic activity. The drug is one of a group of substituted imidazolines which share these properties. Structural changes make some actions more prominent. For example, tolazoline, a structural congener of phentolamine, has greater smooth muscle relaxant and histaminic action than phentolamine, but less α-receptor blocking activity.

Mechanism of Action As discussed in Chap. 6, norepinephrine is released from sympathetic nerve terminals during neuronal activity; it diffuses across the synaptic space, binds to adrenergic receptors on the effector cells of smooth muscle, cardiac muscle, or exocrine glands, and a response occurs. Circulating catecholamines elicit similar responses by stimulating the same effectors.

Phentolamine exerts its action by competing for α-adrenergic receptors and therefore is termed a *competitive blocking agent*, which has high affinity but little intrinsic activity at these receptor sites. Such drug-receptor combinations reduce the availability of the α-adrenergic receptors for reaction with sympathomimetic amines and therefore reduce the magnitude of the response elicited either from endogenous or administered amines. The duration of the blockade of the α-adrenergic receptor by phentolamine is relatively short when compared with phenoxybenzamine.

Pharmacodynamics Phentolamine produces a moderately effective, transient, competitive α-adrenergic blockade; in addition, it has a direct relaxant (musculotropic spasmolytic) effect on vascular smooth muscle. The vasodilatation and reduced blood pressure which occur are due to the direct relaxant effect on the vasculature (in low doses) and to α-adrenergic blockade (at therapeutic doses).

The physiologic responses of the heart to epinephrine and norepinephrine are not effectively blocked by phentolamine or by other α-adrenergic blocking agents, since the cardiac response to these drugs is mediated by β_1-adrenergic receptors, and therefore α-adrenergic blockers have little effect on arrythmias induced by adrenergic stimuli. Tachycardia and increased cardiac output may result as reflex responses to the decreased blood pressure induced by phentolamine. In addition phentolamine has a sympathomimetic action on the heart, which appears to be the result of increased endogenous norepinephrine release due to blockade of presynaptic α_2-adrenergic receptors and a reduction in negative feedback inhibition of neurotransmitter release. Therefore, cardiac stimula-

tion resulting from therapeutic doses of the drug is more than just a reflex response to the vasodilatation and hypotension.

In addition to the ability of phentolamine to antagonize α-adrenergic receptors, this compound has activity at other receptor sites. Phentolamine can block the effects of serotonin. At the H_1 and H_2 histamine receptor sites phentolamine has both affinity and intrinsic activity. This is observed as a histamine-like effect on the stomach, causing secretion of both acid and pepsin. Phentolamine increases the motility of the intestine by a cholinomimetic action, which is the result of a direct effect on muscarinic receptors and unrelated to its α-adrenergic blockade.

Pharmacokinetics Phentolamine has low bioavailability when it is given by the oral route. Upon intravenous administration the compound has a half-life of 19 min, and approximately 10 percent of an injected dose is found in the urine unchanged. The actual biotransformation reactions that phentolamine undergoes in the body are unknown.

Adverse Reactions Adverse effects are common with phentolamine and are attributable to cardiac and gastrointestinal stimulation. Tachycardia, anginal pain, cardiac arrhythmias, and episodes of hypotension may occur, especially after parenteral administration. Gastrointestinal stimulation may produce nausea, vomiting, abdominal pain, diarrhea, and exacerbation of peptic ulceration.

Clinical Uses Although the drug causes hypotension, phentolamine is not useful in the treatment of essential hypertension because of the frequency of adverse reactions and the development of tolerance. However, phentolamine is of use in controlling severe acute hypertensive crises due to an excess in circulating catecholamines from pheochromocytoma or drug interactions involving monoamine oxidase inhibitors. Its use is based on the fact that the α-adrenergic receptor effects of circulating catecholamines, e. g., vasoconstriction, are readily blocked by phentolamine. In pheochromocytoma phentolamine is indicated both preoperatively and during surgical removal of the tumor to prevent or control excessive elevation of blood pressure.

This α-adrenergic receptor blocking agent is also indicated in the diagnosis of pheochromocytoma. In patients with this tumor the administration of phentol-amine may cause a reduction in the sustained or parox-ysmal hypertension that is present. However, many false-positive responses can occur with this test; there-fore, measurement of urinary concentrations of cate-cholamine metabolites (e. g., vanillymandelic acid, VMA) is a more reliable diagnostic procedure.

In addition, during the treatment of arteriolar hypo-tension and shock with intravenous norepinephrine, small doses of phentolamine have been added to the infusion to prevent local tissue necrosis following ex-travasation of the catecholamine.

Preparation   Phentolamine mesylate (Regitine) is available as a lyophilized powder for injection in 5-mg vials.

Phenoxybenzamine

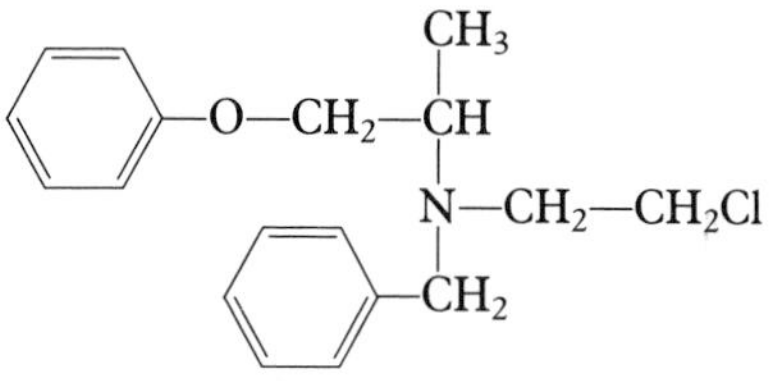

Phenoxybenzamine

Chemistry   Phenoxybenzamine is a haloalkylamine that is structurally related to the nitrogen mustard al-kylating agents used in cancer chemotherapy. The chemical mechanism responsible for the long-lasting α-adrenergic receptor blockade appears to be related to alkylation of the receptors.

Mechanism of Action   Phenoxybenzamine pro-duces an initial reversible competitive antagonism of adrenergic agonists at both α_1 and α_2 receptors that is similar to phentolamine. After the initial competitive phase which is relatively short, the receptor blockade by phenoxybenzamine becomes more fully developed and leads to a persistent ("irreversible") α-adrenergic receptor blockade.

Chemically it appears that the terminal N-C-C moi-ety cyclizes at the alkaline pH of body fluids to form an ethylenimonium intermediate (Fig. 8-3). The drug, as a highly reactive carbonium ion, produced when the unstable cyclic structure opens, forms a stable cova-lent bond with the receptor. This antagonist-receptor complex cannot be affected by even large concentra-

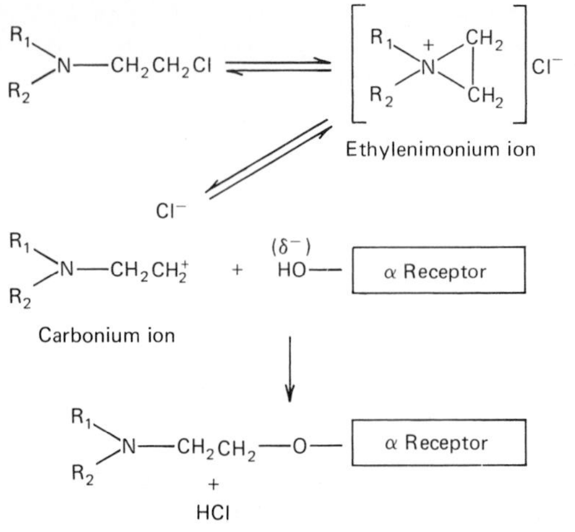

FIGURE 8-3   Schematic representation of the mecha-nism by which α-adrenergic receptors are alkylated by phenoxybenzamine.

tions of α-receptor agonists. Therefore the blockade is no longer reversible and is referred to as *nonequilibrium receptor blockade.*

In addition to the blockade of α-adrenergic recep-tors, high doses of phenoxybenzamine can inhibit re-sponses to serotonin, acetylcholine, and histamine.

Pharmacodynamics   Most actions of phenoxy-benzamine, as well as other α-adrenergic blockers, are dependent on the normal level of adrenergic tone, i. e., the greater the sympathetic tone the greater the ob-served effect of the drug that is due to receptor block-ade. For example, phenoxybenzamine has little effect on blood pressure in normal, recumbent subjects. However, hypotension may result in any situation in-volving compensatory sympathetic vasoconstriction, such as an upright posture. Therefore, *postural (ortho-static) hypotension* is a prominent effect of α-adrenergic receptor blockade of the vascular system. As a reflex response to the hypotension produced by phenoxy-benzamine, tachycardia is generally observed.

In addition to blocking the vascular effects of en-dogenous norepinephrine, small doses of phenoxy-benzamine will diminish the pressor responses to ex-ogenously administered epinephrine, norepinephrine, and other adrenergic drugs. Large doses of phenoxy-benzamine "reverse" the pressor action of epinephrine, so that a depressor response is the prominent effect (Fig. 8-4). These larger doses antagonize the pressor responses to injected norepinephrine or sympathetic vasoconstrictor nerve stimulation but do not reverse them. *Epinephrine vasomotor reversal*, as it is commonly called, is best understood by remembering that epinephrine has pronounced β_2-adrenergic receptor stimulant activity, notably in skeletal muscle vasculature, which is not blocked by α-adrenergic blocking agents. As would be expected, α-adrenergic blocking agents have no effect on the vasodepressor action of isoproterenol, since isoproterenol is predominantly a potent stimulant of β-receptor mediated responses.

Phenoxybenzamine has a negligible effect on the gastrointestinal tract. The drug can affect the CNS and cause nausea, vomiting, and sedation.

Pharmacokinetics Although phenoxybenzamine has a low bioavailability, the drug is sufficiently absorbed from the gastrointestinal tract to provide a therapeutic effect. Little information is known about its biotransformation and excretion from the body.

Adverse Reactions The use of this drug is generally limited by the frequent occurrence of adverse reactions; nasal congestion, miosis, inhibition of ejaculation, and severe hypotension with reflex tachycardia may occur. These adverse reactions are manifestations of adrenergic blockade and vary according to the degree of blockade.

Therapeutic Uses Phenoxybenzamine is effective in the treatment of pheochromocytoma. The drug is indicated preoperatively or chronically in patients with inoperable tumors of pheochromocytoma. The drug has also been employed in vasospastic peripheral vascular diseases associated with increased α-adrenergic activity, e. g., Raynaud's syndrome, and in cases of endotoxin-induced shock where the vasoconstrictor effect of endotoxin is mediated by release of epinephrine and norepinephrine. Phenoxybenzamine has found some usefulness in patients with urinary retention caused by a spastic detrusor.

Preparation Phenoxybenzamine hydrochloride (Dibenzyline) is available in capsules of 10 mg.

Ergot Alkaloids

Ergotamine, ergonovine, and a variety of other alkaloids were isolated from ergot, which is a product of a fungal infestation of grains, particularly rye. In the early history of civilization and during the Middle Ages the consumption of grain contaminated with ergot resulted in gangrene of the extremities, abortions, and convulsions. In the Middle Ages ergot poisoning was known as *St. Anthony's fire*. In the early 1900s the ergot alkaloids were the first adrenergic blocking drugs to be investigated. Although most of

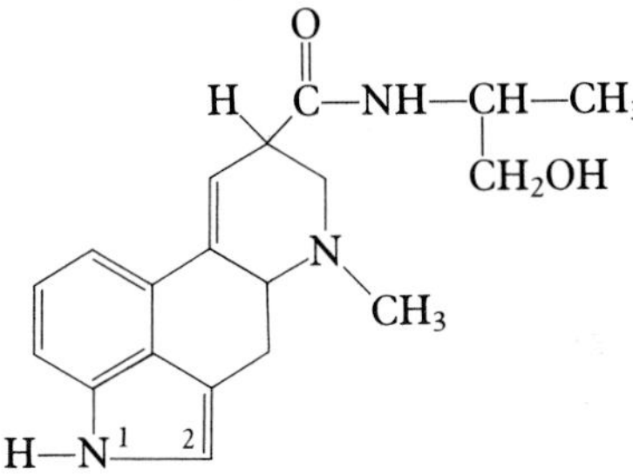

Ergotamine

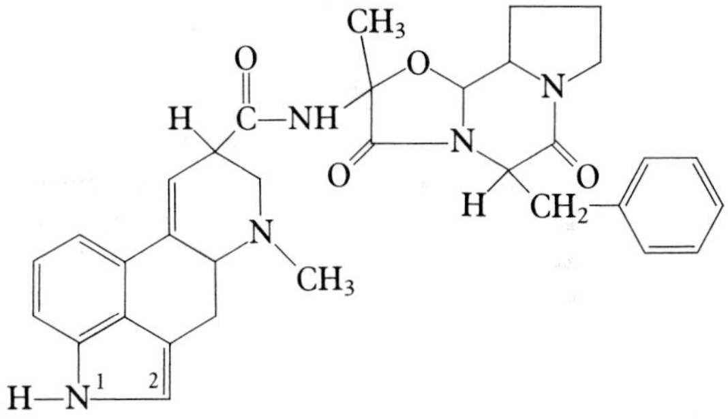

Ergonovine

the ergot alkaloids possess α-adrenergic blocking activity, their pharmacology is somewhat diversified. Chemically, ergotamine and ergonovine are related to *d*-lysergic acid (see Chap. 18).

Ergotamine

Ergotamine possesses α-adrenergic blocking activity, a direct vasoconstrictor effect, and a degree of oxytoxic action. The drug is used in therapy because of its ability to produce vasoconstriction. Ergotamine is used to terminate the acute attacks of a migraine headache. The migraine headache appears to be due to vasodila-

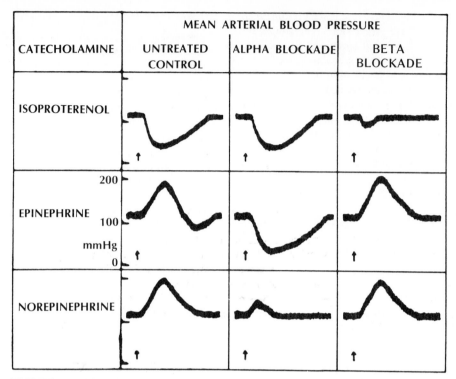

FIGURE 8-4   The influence of α- and β-adrenergic blocking agents on the idealized responses of the mean arterial pressure to intravenous injections of three catecholamines. The direction of the blood pressure response is largely determined by the influence the amines exert on total peripheral resistance. In the first column the responses in untreated animals are presented. Isoproterenol, which is predominantly an evoker of β-adrenergic responses, dilates the arterioles and pressure falls. Epinephrine, which is a potent stimulant of both α- and β-adrenoceptor responses, tends to constrict and dilate simultaneously. The algebraic summation of these opposing effects on peripheral vascular resistance frequently yields a biphasic effect on blood pressure. Pressure is first greatly increased, then falls somewhat below control level before recovering. Norepinephrine, which predominantly evokes α-adrenergic responses, constricts the resistance vessels, and only a pressor response is observed.

In the presence of an effective dose of an α-blocking agent, catecholamine-induced vasoconstriction is inhibited. Isoproterenol exerts its full depressor activity, epinephrine is purely depressor, and norepinephrine exerts only slight or no pressor effect. In the presence of an effective dose of a β-blocking agent, catecholamine-induced vasodilation is inhibited. Isoproterenol has only slight or no depressor activity. Epinephrine is purely pressor, and the magnitude of the response is increased. Norepinephrine retains its usual pressor effect.

Arrows indicate time at which the catecholamine is injected intravenously (abscissa is time).

tion of cranial arteries. The unilateral pain sensation is related to increased pulsation in the arteries and cranial nerve stimulation that is produced by edema and swelling of the blood vessels. Although ergotamine possesses several pharmacologic properties such as α-adrenergic blockade, its mechanism of action in treating migraine headaches is primarily related to its direct vasoconstrictor action and its agonistic interaction with serotonin receptors.

Absorption of ergotamine from the gastrointestinal tract is poor. To achieve a therapeutic effect by oral administration, ergotamine is combined with caffeine, which appears to enhance its absorption. In addition the vasoconstrictor effect of caffeine on cranial blood vessels may contribute to the desired therapeutic effect. Other routes of administration of ergotamine in the treatment of migraine headaches are inhalation and sublingual. Suppositories which contain ergotamine and caffeine may also be used. In addition ergotamine may have value in the treatment of acute attacks of cluster headache.

Adverse reactions of ergotamine may include nausea, vomiting, diarrhea, paresthesia of limbs, and cramps. In the absence of peripheral vascular disease, gangrene is rare. The drug is contraindicated in severe hypertension, peripheral vascular disease, ischemic heart disease, and pregnancy.

Ergotamine cannot be used for the chronic or prophylactic treatment of migraines because of its potential adverse reactions such as the induction of gangrene. Drugs such as propranolol, methysergide, and clonidine may be used on a prophylactic basis to prevent or reduce the incidence of migraine headaches in patients. Calcium channel blockers may also be of some value.

Ergotamine tartrate (Ergomar, Ergostat) is available as 2-mg tablets for sublingual administration, and as an aerosol for inhalation (Medihaler Ergotamine) which contains 9 mg/mL in a 2.5-mL container. Ergotamine tartrate (1 mg) and caffeine (100 mg) tablets (Cafergot) are also available.

Ergonovine

This ergot alkaloid is used in the treatment of postpartum bleeding. The mechanism of action for the uterine-stimulating activity of ergonovine seems to be related to a direct musculotropic spasmogenic effect on the uterus (oxytocic effect) and possibly to agonistic properties at serotonin and α-adrenergic receptor sites. Although ergonovine is an ergot alkaloid, it does not possess significant α-adrenergic blocking properties.

Upon oral administration ergonovine has adequate bioavailability in contrast to ergotamine. In addition the drug may be injected by the intramuscular and intravenous routes. The intravenous route is used for emergency situations of excessive postpartum bleeding.

Adverse reactions of ergonovine that may occur are nausea, vomiting, blurred vision, headache, hypertension, and convulsions. The use of ergonovine is contraindicated in pregnant women.

A semisynthetic compound, methylergonovine, which has similar pharmacologic effects to ergonovine, is also indicated in the treatment of postpartum bleeding.

Ergonovine maleate and methylergonovine maleate (Methergine) are available in 0.2-mg tablets or as a solution of 0.2 mg/mL for injection.

SELECTIVE ALPHA-ADRENERGIC BLOCKING AGENTS

Prazosin and Terazosin

These drugs are peripheral vasodilators which have been found to possess significant α-adrenergic receptor blocking activity. Prazosin and terazosin differ from the aforementioned α-adrenergic blocking drugs in their selectivity for certain α-adrenergic receptors.

Prazosin and terazosin, unlike phentolamine and phenoxybenzamine, appear to selectively block postsynaptic α_1-adrenergic receptors with little affinity for presynaptic α_2-adrenergic receptors. It has been shown that norepinephrine regulates its own release from adrenergic neuronal terminals via a negative feedback mechanism mediated by α_2-adrenergic receptors located on the presynaptic membrane. Since prazosin and terzosin do not block α_2-adrenergic receptor sites at therapeutic doses, feedback inhibition of norepinephrine release is not greatly affected, which may account for the low degree of tachycardia with these drugs (Fig. 8-5). Prazosin and terazosin are employed for the treatment of hypertension and are discussed in greater detail in Chap. 31.

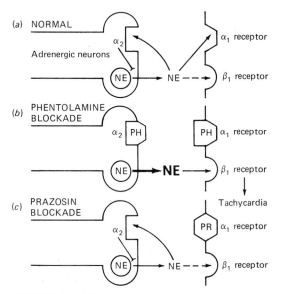

FIGURE 8-5 Diagrammatic representation of the mechanism of action of certain α-adrenergic receptor blocking agents. (*a*) Normal autoregulation of norepinephrine (NE) release from adrenergic neurons via α_2-adrenergic receptor stimulation. (*b*) Blockade of α_1- and α_2-adrenoceptors by classic α-adrenergic blocking drugs, e. g., phentolamine (PH), leads to a reduction in the negative feedback inhibition of NE release. Greater NE release from the cardioaccelerator neurons in the heart allows for greater cardiac β-receptor activation and greater tachycardia. (*c*) Selective α_1-adrenergic blockade by prazosin (PR) does not significantly effect α_2-adrenergic receptors; NE release is controlled, and tachycardia is minimal.

Yohimbine

Yohimbine is a selective α_2-adrenergic antagonist. Chemically this compound resembles the alkaloid reserpine in that it is an indolealkylamine. Since yohimbine can block α_2-adrenergic receptor sites on the nerve terminal, it can attenuate the negative feedback mechanism on the release of norepinephrine.

There is evidence that this drug possesses some sympathomimetic effects. In addition other studies indicate that yohimbine can promote a sympatholytic effect, which can result in an enhanced parasympathetic activity. It appears that further research is needed to more clearly delineate the pharmacologic actions of this drug. In clinical studies yohimbine has

been used to treat certain types of male erectile impotence and to treat orthostatic hypotension. At the present time there are no approved FDA indications for this drug.

ADRENERGIC NEURONAL BLOCKING DRUGS

The adrenergic neuronal blocking agents cause a depletion of biogenic amines in neuronal terminals. These drugs may interfere with the synthesis, storage, or release of norepinephrine, dopamine, and serotonin.

Reserpine

Resepine is the principal alkaloid found in the roots of *Rauwolfia serpentina* and is presently isolated from the plant for medical purposes. Other *Rauwolfia* alkaloids related structurally and pharmacologically to resepine are deserpidine, rescinnamine, and alseroxylon. In the following discussion, reserpine is used as the prototype compound of the *Rauwolfia* alkaloids.

Reserpine

Mechanism of Action   Resepine causes depletion of central and peripheral stores of norepinephrine, dopamine, and serotonin at neuronal terminals (see Fig. 8-1). It impairs intracellular biogenic amine uptake and reduces storage in vesicles (granules). Reserpine appears to act on the membranes of vesicles to irreversibly inhibit the ATP-Mg^{2+}-dependent transport process that is responsible for uptake of biogenic amines into intraneuronal vesicles. Catecholamine depletion results in decreased sympathetic predominance. A reduction in intraneuronal serotonin and dopamine produces an attenuation of serotonergic and dopaminergic activity, respectively.

Pharmacodynamics   Reserpine acts in the central nervous system to produce sedation and tranquilization. It is believed that these effects are due to depletion of stores of catecholamines and serotonin centrally. Large doses cause hypothermia and respiratory depression.

The cardiovascular effects of reserpine include hypotension and reduced heart rate and cardiac output. The hypotensive response to the drug is due to impairment of adrenergic transmission both centrally (inhibition of vasomotor and cardioaccelerator centers of the hypothalamus) and peripherally (arteriolar dilatation, decreased peripheral resistance). Reflex tachycardia is effectively blocked.

Adverse Reactions   The use of the *Rauwolfia* alkaloids has been limited, largely because of the adverse reactions which commonly occur.

Central nervous system effects include drowsiness, lethargy, depression, and nightmares. The most serious adverse effect is depression, which may require hospitalization and may persist for several months after the drug has been withdrawn. Therefore, the drug should be used with extreme caution in patients with a history of depressive episodes. On occasion parkinsonian and other extrapyramidal reactions may be observed.

Parasympathetic predominance due to reduced sympathetic function may occur, and results in nasal congestion, bradycardia, salivation, and diarrhea. Increased gastric secretion with aggravation of peptic ulcer frequently occurs.

Endocrinologic disturbances have been reported. Reserpine inhibits ovulation and menstruation, probably through an action on the hypothalamus which alters the secretion of regulatory hormones. Gynecomastia in males has also been observed.

Therapeutic Uses   Reserpine is employed in the treatment of hypertension because of its cardiovascular effects. It is not a drug of choice, principally because of the high incidence of adverse reactions, but it may be combined with more effective, less toxic antihypertensive drugs such as diuretic agents. Reserpine is also indicated in the chronic treatment of Raynaud's

disease and may be of some value in the initial treatment of tardive dyskinesia.

Preparations   Reserpine (Serpasil) is available as tablets of 0.1, 0.25, and 1 mg.

Guanethidine

The structure of guanethidine is

Guanethidine

Mechanism of Action   The terminals of the sympathetic neurons contain vesicles of norepinephrine. In the vesicles norepinephrine appears to be bound to adenosine triphosphate (ATP) in a ratio of 4 molecules of norepinephrine to 1 ATP molecule. Upon nerve stimulation the vesicle fuses with the presynaptic membrane and releases the adrenergic neurotransmitter. The released norepinephrine impinges on the effector cells, which are adjacent to the nerve ending.

Guanethidine does not act on the effector cells, as do adrenergic blocking agents. It acts on the terminal ramifications of the peripheral sympathetic nerve fibers. Guanethidine enters into the neuron by the same re-uptake mechanism that returns norepinephrine to the terminal portion of the neuron from the synaptic area (see Fig. 8-1). Inside the neuron guanethidine is actively transported into the adrenergic storage granule where it accumulates. Guanethidine and norepinephrine compete for the same storage sites in the granule. As guanethidine increases in concentration, norepinephrine is displaced and there is a decrease in the transmitter available for release. Guanethidine itself may be released by nerve stimulation but is ineffective as an adrenergic-receptor stimulant. In addition to depletion of catecholamine stores from adrenergic nerve endings, it readily acts on catecholamine stores in organs such as the heart, spleen, and aorta. Guanethidine does not affect central sympathetic neurons, since the drug does not readily cross the blood-brain barrier.

Pharmacodynamics   Guanethidine may produce an initial pressor response that is followed by decreased mean blood pressure as a result of decreased peripheral vascular resistance, bradycardia, and decreased cardiac output. The initial pressor response is due to displacement of large amounts of norepinephrine; this effect is generally observed after intravenous administration of the drug. The drug has considerably greater hypotensive effects when patients are in the standing position than when patients are supine. Such postural hypotension is a characteristic response to agents which block the sympathetic nervous system. The hypotension is presumably due to a reduction in the capacity of vasoconstrictor fibers to bring about the usual reflex compensations upon standing.

Pharmacokinetics Guanethidine is incompletely but predictably absorbed from the gastrointestinal tract. Approximately 40 percent of an oral dose is biotransformed to several inactive metabolites. The parent compound and its metabolites are excreted into the urine via glomerular filtration and tubular secretion.

Adverse Reactions Orthostatic hypotension can occur frequently. Additionally, dizziness, weakness, lassitude, syncope, bradycardia, diarrhea, inhibition of ejaculation, fluid retention, and edema are common side effects. Severe organ toxicity is very rare with this drug. Unlike reserpine, guanethidine does not produce any central adverse reactions.

Therapeutic Uses Guanethidine is indicated in the treatment of severe hypertension in which other more commonly used therapeutic agents have not been successful in patients. This drug reduces elevated arterial pressure in short-term therapy and is also effective in long-term management of hypertension. In addition guanethidine may be useful in the treatment of Raynaud's disease, a vasospastic disorder.

Guanethidine is a very potent and long-lasting anithypertensive agent with a slow onset of activity. It primarily causes postural hypotension. The antihypertensive effect of guanethidine is usually delayed for 2 or 3 days following oral administration of an effective dose. The ensuing pressure reduction is sustained for several days. Because of its long duration of action, the drug can be administered effectively in a single daily dose or a dose every other day.

Preparations Guanethidine sulfate (Ismelin) is available in 10- and 25-mg tablets.

Guanadrel

Guanadrel is an adrenergic neuronal blocking agent that is used in the treatment of essential hypertension. Its mechanism of action and adverse reactions are similar to those of guanethidine. The drug is well absorbed from the gastrointestinal tract but does not readily enter the central nervous system. Guanadrel appears to be somewhat more useful than guanethidine in the treatment of essential hypertension and may produce less of an incidence of diarrhea, morning orthostatic hypotension on arising, and impaired ejaculation. The drug, as the sulfate (Hylorel), is available in 10- and 25-mg tablets.

Metyrosine

Metyrosine is the alpha-methylated derivative of tyrosine. This drug competitively inhibits the action of tyrosine hydroxylase and thus decreases the endogenous formation of epinephrine and norepinephrine (see Fig. 8-1). Metyrosine is used in patients with pheochromocytoma who produce excessive quantities of these catecholamines, which results in hypertension. The drug is not recommended for the control of essential hypertension.

The drug is well absorbed from the gastrointestinal tract. Approximately 30 percent of an oral dose is biotransformed to methyldopa, methyldopamine, and methylnorepinephrine; the remainder is excreted unchanged in the urine. Metyrosine (Demser) is available in capsules of 250 mg.

Adverse reactions include sedation, extrapyramidal symptoms, anxiety, depression, nausea, vomiting, diarrhea, abdominal pain, and nasal stuffiness. Crystalluria and transient dysuria have been observed in a few patients.

BIBLIOGRAPHY

Bravo, E. L., and R. W. Gifford, Jr.: "Pheochromocytoma: Diagnosis, Localization and Management," *N. Engl. J. Med.*, **311**:1298–1303 (1984).

Frishman, W. H.: "β-Adrenergic Blockers," *Medical Clin. North Am.*, **72**:37–81 (1988).

Hoffmann, B. B., and R. J. Lefkowitz: "Alpha-Adrenergic Receptor Subtypes," *N. Engl. J. Med.*, **302**:1390–1396 (1980).

Ibraheem, J. J., L. Paalzow, and P. Tfelt-Hansen: "Low Bioavailability of Ergotamine Tartrate After Oral and Rectal Administration in Migraine Sufferers," *Br. J. Clin. Pharmacol.*, **16**:695–699 (1983).

Kincaid-Smith, P. S.: "Alpha Blockade. An Overview of Efficacy Data," *Am. J. Med.*, **82**:21–25 (1987).

McDevitt, D. G.: "Pharmacological Characteristics of β-Blockers and Their Role in Clinical Practice," *J. Cardiovasc. Pharmacol.*, **8(suppl. 6)**:S5–11 (1986).

McNeil, J. J., O. H. Drummer, E. L. Conway, B. S. Workman, and W. J. Louis: "Effect of Age on Pharmacokinetics of and Blood Pressure Responses to Prazosin and Terazosin," *J. Cardiovascular Pharmacol.*, **10**:168–175 (1987).

Prichard, B. N. C.: "Pharmacologic Aspects of Intrinsic Sympathomimetic Activity in Beta-Blocking Drugs," *Am. J. Cardiol.*, **59**:13F–17F (1987).

Riddell, J. G., D. W. G. Harron, and R. G. Shanks: "Clinical Pharmacokinetics of β-Adrenoreceptor Antagonists," *Clin. Pharmacokinetics*, **12**:305–320 (1987).

Singh, B., and A. R. Laddu: "Esmolol: A Novel Ultra-short Acting β-Adrenoreceptor Blocking Agent," *Rational Drug Therapy*, **20**:1–7 (1986).

Titmarsh, S.: "Terazosin. A Review of Its Pharmacodynamics and Pharmacokinetic Properties and Therapeutic Efficacy in Essential Hypertension," *Drugs*, **33**:461–477 (1987).

C H A P T E R 9

Cholinomimetic Agents

Gerald H. Sterling

Cholinomimetic agents are drugs which evoke responses similar to both those produced by acetylcholine and those which result from activation of all ganglia and the parasympathetic nervous system. These drugs *mimic* the actions of acetylcholine released endogenously. Those drugs that act primarily on muscarinic receptors and mimic stimulation of the parasympathetic nervous system are called *parasympathomimetics*. Cholinomimetic agents produce their effects through two mechanisms: (1) direct stimulation of cholinergic receptors and (2) indirectly, through inhibition of acetylcholinesterase, the enzyme responsible for the chemical destruction of acetylcholine at its site of action. The primary mechanism of action of each drug can be used to classify the agents.

DIRECT ACTING CHOLINOMIMETIC AGENTS

The direct-acting cholinomimetic agents are those drugs which act by direct stimulation of cholinergic receptors. The drugs can be subdivided based on their selectivity in stimulating muscarinic or nicotinic receptors. A description of these receptors including their location and major effects elicited by receptor activation is found in Chap. 6. Those drugs whose effectiveness is based primarily on their stimulation of muscarinic receptors include (1) choline esters consisting of acetylcholine and structural analogs and (2) the naturally occurring alkaloids, muscarine and pilocar-

pine. Drugs whose actions are based primarily on their stimulation of nicotinic receptors include nicotine and lobeline.

Choline Esters

Drugs in this class consist of acetylcholine and its structural analogs, methacholine (acetyl-β-methylcholine), bethanechol, and carbachol (carbamylcholine) (Fig. 9-1). Although these compounds have the ability to directly stimulate all cholinergic receptors, their therapeutic effectiveness is due to their action on muscarinic receptors (e.g., subtypes M_1 and M_2). The compounds differ only in the duration of their effects and, to some degree, in their selectivity for receptors. Acetylcholine is the prototype for the group. No selective M_1 or M_2 receptor agonists are currently available for therapeutic use. A detailed description of muscarinic receptors is found in Chap. 2.

Acetylcholine Acetylcholine is composed of a molecule of choline with an acetyl functional group connected by an ester linkage (Fig. 9-1). Because of its highly polar, positively charged ammonium group, acetylcholine does not readily cross lipid membranes. For that reason, the exogenously administered drug is confined to extracellular spaces of the body and does not cross the blood-brain barrier. To obtain systemic effects, acetylcholine must be administered intravenously; oral bioavailability is extremely low.

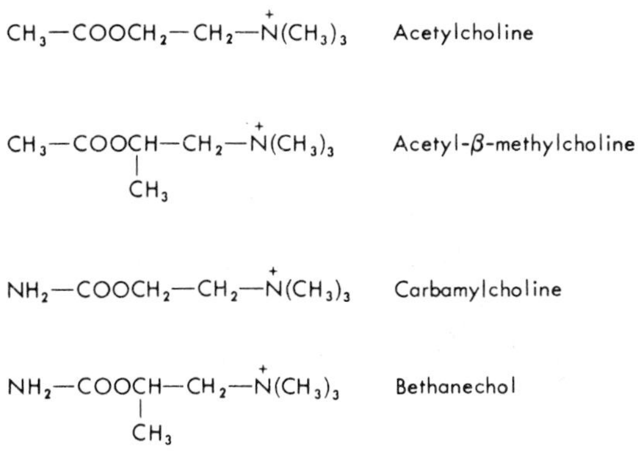

$$CH_3-COOCH_2-CH_2-\overset{+}{N}(CH_3)_3 \qquad \text{Acetylcholine}$$

$$CH_3-COOCH-CH_2-\overset{+}{N}(CH_3)_3 \qquad \text{Acetyl-}\beta\text{-methylcholine}$$
$$\underset{CH_3}{|}$$

$$NH_2-COOCH_2-CH_2-\overset{+}{N}(CH_3)_3 \qquad \text{Carbamylcholine}$$

$$NH_2-COOCH-CH_2-\overset{+}{N}(CH_3)_3 \qquad \text{Bethanechol}$$
$$\underset{CH_3}{|}$$

FIGURE 9-1   Structures of choline esters.

Moreover, being an ester, this compound is readily hydrolyzed and inactivated by acetyl- and plasma cholinesterases. Even large intravenous doses would produce effects with a very brief duration.

Pharmacodynamics   *Cardiovascular system*   The cardiovascular system is affected more profoundly than any other organ system following intravenous administration. At low doses, acetylcholine produces vasodilatation in essentially all vascular beds, including cutaneous, cerebral, pulmonary, and coronary vessels. Although these blood vessels are not innervated by cholinergic vasodilator fibers, they do contain cholinergic (muscarinic) receptors which can be stimulated by exogenously administered drugs. The vasodilatation may be accompanied by reflex tachycardia; this would usually be masked by direct actions on cardiac tissue.

Acetylcholine has prominent direct actions on cardiac rhythm, conduction processes of the heart, and the atrial myocardium; these actions parallel almost exactly those produced by stimulation of the vagus nerve. Acetylcholine reduces heart rate by slowing the rate of firing of the sinoatrial node, an effect which is associated with hyperpolarization of the pacemaker membrane. Acetylcholine also slows conduction velocity across the AV node. The His bundle and Purkinje system appear to be relatively resistant to these effects of the compound. Atrial fibers are also inhibited by acetylcholine, causing a decrease in the force of contraction of atrial muscle. Ventricular fibers, which are not innervated by cholinergic neurons, are resist-

ant to stimulation by the vagus. However, exogenously administered acetylcholine will slightly reduce the force of contraction of ventricular muscle fibers due to the presence of some muscarinic receptors.

In addition to the changes in cardiac activity, the local application of acetylcholine can also induce atrial fibrillation. The fibrillation is not due to an increase in the sinus rate but appears to be due to a phenomenon called *reexcitation by reentry*. This phenomenon results from the circular movement of excitation and the reexcitation of fibers which have already passed through their refractory periods. It is favored by (1) a restriction of normal pathways as a result of local block, (2) a reduced refractory period, and (3) reduced conduction velocity. In addition to producing various degrees of blockade, both vagal stimulation and acetylcholine reduce the refractory period of atrial fibers by shortening the duration of the action potentials. Thus, two of the conditions which predispose the atrium to fibrillation are produced by acetylcholine and stimulation of the vagus nerve. All the direct effects of this drug on the heart are reversed by atropine, a muscarinic antagonist, and enhanced by cholinesterase inhibitors.

Smooth muscle cells   In contrast with vascular smooth muscle cells, those of most other organs respond to acetylcholine with an increase in tone. By direct stimulation of muscarinic receptors, acetylcholine causes contraction of smooth muscle cells of the (1) bronchioles causing bronchoconstriction, (2) gastrointestinal tract increasing motility, (3) bladder and ureters increasing the frequency of urination, (4) uterus, and (5) iris sphincter and ciliary muscle of the eye, causing miosis and accommodation for near vision, respectively. The contraction of smooth muscle is antagonized by atropine and enhanced by cholinesterase inhibitors.

Glands   All glands which are innervated by cholinergic neurons are stimulated by exogenous administration of acetylcholine. This causes increased salivation, lacrimation, and sweating, in addition to increases in gastrointestinal, pancreatic, and bronchial secretions. These are also muscarinic effects, antagonized by atropine.

Neuromuscular junction   Although acetylcholine is the primary neurotransmitter at the neuromuscular junction, the exogenous administration of this drug causes little contraction of skeletal muscle. This is because acetylcholine, a quaternary compound, cannot readily get to its site of action, which is surrounded by lipoid membranes. Higher doses, however, will cause some contraction of skeletal muscle. Intravenously administered acetylcholine also does not penetrate very well to the autonomic ganglia. The effects of acetylcholine at the ganglia and neuromuscular junction are due to stimulation of nicotinic receptors, and these would not be antagonized by the administration of atropine.

Therapeutic Use   Acetylcholine has no therapeutic effectiveness by intravenous administration. This is due to its diffuse action and rapid inactivation by cholinesterases. It is, however, used as a sterile solution for intraocular administration to produce miosis during cataract surgery. Its short duration of action is advantageous, allowing rapid recovery postoperatively.

Adverse Reactions   Administered locally in the eye, acetylcholine only rarely produces systemic side effects. Reactions may include hypotension, bradycardia, flushing, sweating, and dyspnea. No local toxic reactions have been reported.

Methacholine   (Acetyl-β-Methylcholine)   As shown in Fig. 9-1 this compound differs from acetylcholine only by the addition of a methyl group to the β carbon of choline. This structural change results in

two important alterations in the pharmacologic properties of the molecule (Table 9-1). Unlike acetylcholine, methacholine is hydrolyzed only by acetylcholinesterase, and the rate of hydrolysis of methacholine is considerably slower than that of acetylcholine. Thus the actions of methacholine are more persistent than those of acetylcholine. The introduction of the methyl group to the β carbon also endows the compound with more selectivity. Methacholine acts primarily on muscarinic receptors in smooth muscle, glands, and the heart and has very little activity on nicotinic receptors at the autonomia ganglia and skeletal muscle. These two features, duration of response and improved selectivity, represent the primary differences between the pharmacologic actions of methacholine and acetylcholine.

The actions of methacholine on the cardiovascular system are the same qualitatively as those described above for acetylcholine. Its clinical use in selected cases of atrial tachycardia not responding to other forms of therapy has been replaced by other modalities. Methacholine is currently used in the diagnosis of bronchial hyperreactivity in patients who do not have clinically apparent asthma.

Carbachol (Carbamylcholine)   In contrast to acetylcholine and methacholine, carbachol contains a carbamic rather than esteratic functional group (Fig. 9-1). The carbamate group is not readily susceptible to hydrolysis by cholinesterases. Although enzymatic

TABLE 9-1   Comparison of the pharmacologic properties of choline esters[a]

	Susceptibility to cholinesterases	Muscarinic effects	Nicotinic effects	Therapeutic use
Acetylcholine	+4	+3	+3	Miotic
Methacholine	+1	+4	+1	Diagnosis of bronchial hyperreactivity
Carbachol	0	+2	+3	Miotic
Bethanechol	0	+2[b]	0	Nonobstructive urinary retention

[a] 0 to +4 indicates increasing activity, where 0 is no effect and +4 is the greatest effect.
[b] Bethanechol has more selectivity for muscarinic receptors of the gastrointestinal tract and urinary bladder than do other choline esters.

destruction has been demonstrated in vitro, the rate of hydrolysis is too slow to be of any practical significance.

Carbachol is a potent choline ester, stimulating both muscarinic and nicotinic receptors. It therefore possesses all the pharmacodynamic properties of acetylcholine. In addition to producing vasodilatation, reduced heart rate, increased tone and contraction of smooth muscle and stimulation of salivary, lacrimal, and sweat glands, carbachol also stimulates autonomic ganglia and skeletal muscle.

Carbachol has a limited place in therapy due to its lack of receptor selectivity and potency. At present, the principal use of carbachol is in ophthalmology as a miotic agent. The drug is applied topically to the conjunctiva, producing prolonged miosis during ocular surgery.

Bethanechol Bethanechol combines the structural features of methacholine and carbachol, containing both beta-methyl and carbamate functional groups (Fig. 9-1), and therefore has pharmacologic properties of both drugs. Bethanechol, like carbachol, is resistant to hydrolysis by acetyl- and plasma cholinesterases. Similar to methacholine, bethanechol has very little action at nicotinic receptors of autonomic ganglia or neuromuscular junctions.

Bethanechol has a more selective action at muscarinic receptors of the gastrointestinal tract and urinary bladder than do the other choline esters. Its therapeutic application is based on these actions; the primary use of bethanechol is in treatment of postoperative nonobstructive urinary retention and neurogenic atony of the bladder. It was also used in the past for treatment of gastrointestinal disorders including postoperative abdominal distention, but this has been largely replaced by other agents. Bethanechol has also been used with very limited success in the treatment of Alzheimer's disease.

Bethanechol is available for both oral and subcutaneous administration; it is readily absorbed from either route. Following oral administration, onset of action is approximately 30 min with peak effects in 1 to 1.5 h; its duration is about 2 to 2.5 h. Subcutaneous administration provides a more rapid onset (15 to 30 min) with a duration of about 2 h.

Adverse effects of bethanechol are due to overstimulation of the parasympathetic nervous system and include gastrointestinal distress, abdominal cramping,

sweating, flushing, hypotension, and bronchoconstriction. Reactions are less likely to occur following oral administration than after dosing by the subcutaneous route. Bethanechol is contraindicated in patients with peptic ulcer, bronchial asthma, pronounced bradycardia, hyperthyroidism, coronary artery disease and parkinsonism (although very little crosses the blood-brain barrier).

Naturally Occurring Muscarinic Alkaloids

Muscarine Muscarine (Fig. 9-2) is an alkaloid present in various wild mushrooms with wide geographic distribution (Europe, Asia, North and South America, and South Africa). *Amanita muscaria*, in which muscarine was first identified, contains low concentrations of the compound; much higher levels are found in *Clitocybe inocybe*. Although it is not useful as a therapeutic agent, muscarine is of interest because of its toxic properties and because historically it was one of the first cholinomimetic drugs to be systematically

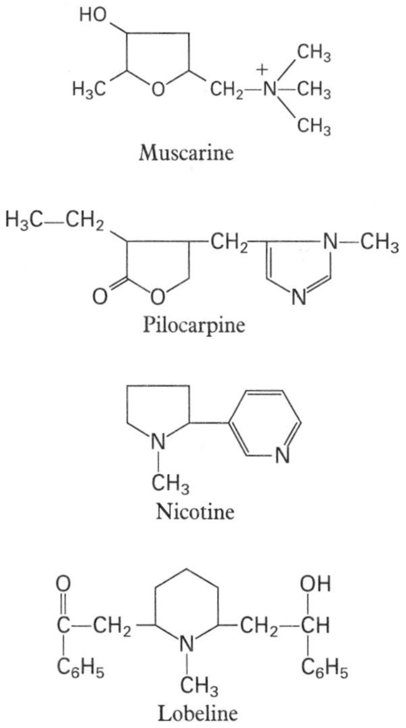

FIGURE 9-2 Structures of naturally occurring akaloids and a synthetic analog.

studied. The compound has provided the basis for classification of cholinergic *muscarinic* receptors. The actions of muscarine are similar to those of acetylcholine on peripheral autonomic effector organs and are antagonized by atropine. Unlike acetylcholine, muscarine has no effects on nicotinic receptors.

Mushroom poisoning is still fairly common and may constitute a serious medical emergency, requiring intensive supportive therapy. Muscarine is well absorbed from the gastrointestinal tract, and therefore ingestion can lead to accidental intoxication. It is much more potent than acetylcholine, probably as a result of its greater stability; not being an ester, muscarine is resistant to hydrolysis by cholinesterases. It is important that a physician be able to differentiate the symptoms of muscarine intoxication (overstimulation of the parasympathetic nervous system) from that of other toxins found in mushrooms so that proper treatment can be started. Muscarine poisoning is treated with atropine sulfate, a muscarinic-blocking drug.

Pilocarpine Pilocarpine is an alkaloid obtained from the leaf of the tropical American shrub *Pilocarpus jaborandi*. Its actions are primarily due to stimulation of muscarinic receptors and, therefore, given systemically are similar to acetylcholine. The compound differs from acetylcholine in that it does not have any effects on nicotinic receptors, and since it is a tertiary amine (Fig. 9-2), it can produce central nervous system stimulation. All these effects are blocked by atropine.

The primary therapeutic use of pilocarpine is in ophthalmology as a miotic. Pilocarpine is an important drug for initial and long-term treatment of various types of glaucoma, i.e., primary open-angle glaucoma, other chronic glaucomas, and emergency therapy of acute angle closure glaucoma. Topical administration produces miosis by contracting the circular muscle of the iris. It also causes contraction of the ciliary muscle, leading to an increased opening of the trabecular space and hence an increase in the outflow of aqueous humor, which reduces intraocular pressure. The drug has an onset of action of 15 to 30 min and a duration of 4 to 8 h. It can be used alone or in combination with other agents such as epinephrine or physostigmine. Pilocarpine is available for treatment of chronic glaucoma in a specialized drug delivery system (Ocusert); this is placed directly in the conjunctival sac, allowing for continuous release of the drug.

Although pilocarpine is generally well tolerated, it can produce local burning and irritation. Systemic cholinergic effects following topical administration are uncommon.

Naturally Occurring Nicotinic Alkaloids

Nicotine Nicotine has been extensively studied for several reasons. First, the chemical was used experimentally to characterize cholinergic *nicotinic* receptors and to simulate or block the autonomic ganglia. Second, the inherent toxicity of nicotine has been applied in the control of insects and is of concern because of the possibility of accidental poisoning. Today, nicotine is also important owing to its presence in tobacco products and the link of habitual cigarette smoking to cancer of the lung, mouth, larynx, and esophagus. Chronic bronchitis and emphysema are common in smokers. Nicotine is also a risk factor for coronary artery disease, arteriosclerosis, and hypertension.

Source and Chemistry Nicotine (Fig. 9-2) occurs as an alkaloid in the dried leaves of *Nicotiana tabacum* and *N. rustica* to the extent of 2 to 8 percent. The nicotine content varies from about 2 percent in the average cigarette to about 1 percent in so-called denicotinized preparations.

Mechanism of Action Nicotine acts by interacting with the peripheral cholinergic nicotinic receptors at the postsynaptic membrane in the autonomic ganglion (N-I) and neuromuscular junction (N-II) as well as nicotinic receptors in the central nervous system. At low doses (such as obtained in cigarette smoking) or initially at high doses, nicotine stimulates the receptors causing depolarization of the membrane and influx of sodium and calcium. If large doses are used, the stimulation is followed by a prolonged blockade of repolarization. This makes the receptor refractory to subsequent stimulation by acetylcholine released from the preganglionic cholinergic fibers and, therefore, there is a block of transmission. This is referred to as a *depolarizing ganglionic blockade,* in which the actions of all nicotinic agonists, including the endogenous neurotransmitter, acetylcholine, is blocked.

Pharmacodynamics *Central nervous system* The effects of nicotine on the CNS are both stimulatory and depressive. Nicotine causes excitation of the motor cortex leading to tremors and even convulsions at toxic doses. The tremors are also due to peripheral stimulation of the neuromuscular junction. Nicotine stimulates release of antidiuretic hormone, possibly causing a temporary antidiuresis following cigarette smoking. Nausea and vomiting are frequent effects on first exposure to nicotine due to stimulation of the chemoreceptor trigger zone in the area postrema as well as vagal and spinal afferent nerves. Respiration can be stimulated or depressed. Tolerance develops fairly rapidly to these effects.

Autonomic nervous system   Actions of nicotine extend to all autonomic ganglia, both sympathetic and parasympathetic. These manifestations are further complicated by actions of nicotine outside the autonomic ganglia, namely, the release of epinephrine from the adrenal medulla, and activation of visceral receptors with resulting reflex actions. The combined picture is an increase in sympathetic activity of some organs (heart, blood vessels, pupil) and in parasympathetic activity of others (salivary glands, gastrointestinal tract).

Respiratory system   Nicotine initially stimulates respiration; with increasing doses the stimulation is followed by respiratory depression. The initial increase in rate and depth of respiration from small doses is due to stimulation of chemoreceptors in the carotid body and aortic arch. Larger doses cause direct stimulation of the medullary pontine respiratory center. At toxic levels, respiratory depression is caused by (1) depression of the respiratory center and (2) blockade of nicotinic receptors in skeletal muscles (i.e., intercostals and diaphragm).

An intravenous injection of nicotine would elicit respiratory stimulation, but this is often preceded by a brief period of apnea, which arises from stimulation of receptors in the lungs. From the toxicologic standpoint, the reflex apnea is not so important as the paralysis of respiratory muscles brought about by a direct action of nicotine on the neuromuscular junction.

Cardiovascular system   The effects of nicotine on the cardiovascular system are complex and a summation of its actions at multiple sites: sympathetic and parasympathetic ganglia and the adrenal medulla. Chronic smokers (as well as occasional smokers) show an increase in pulse rate from a few to over 50 beats per minute. Nicotine-induced increases in heart rate may be accompanied by a rise in cardiac output and an increase in total peripheral resistance, both contributing to an increase in blood pressure. These effects can exacerbate cardiovascular disease and hypertension.

Pharmacokinetics   Nicotine is highly lipid-soluble and is readily absorbed through all mucosal membranes and also via the intact skin. When administered by mouth, nicotine is absorbed through the buccal mucosa, the stomach, and the intestine. Nicotine is rapidly distributed throughout the body, readily crossing the blood-brain barrier, placenta, and also accumulating in breast milk. Approximately 80 to 90 percent of the drug is oxidized in the liver, lung, and kidney to the inactive products cotinine and nicotine-N-oxide, which are excreted in the urine.

Therapeutic Use   The only therapeutic use of nicotine is as a temporary aid to an individual attempting to quit smoking. Nicotine is available as a chewing gum, bound to an ion exchange resin. The drug has proven effective but should only be used for periods shorter than 3 months. Though abuse potential is considered minimal, nicotine gum does maintain the patient's addiction and should be withdrawn gradually.

Adverse Reactions   The adverse reactions associated with the use of nicotine are generally mild. Gastrointestinal distress, nausea, and vomiting are most common. Headache, dizziness, insomnia, and irritability occur in 1 to 2 percent of patients. Nicotine-induced hiccups have also been reported.

Poisoning may occur from the accidental exposure to large doses of this compound, i.e., ingestion of tobacco products in children or the extensive contact with an insecticide spray containing nicotine. The symptoms of nicotine poisoning which appear immediately include salivation, nausea or vomiting, abdominal pain and diarrhea, mental confusion, and marked weakness. The pupils become constricted and later dilated; pulse rate is at first slow and then rapid; blood pressure rises and then falls. Respiration becomes irregular when convulsions appear. Death results from respiratory paralysis followed by cardiovascular collapse. Therapy for acute poisoning should include vomiting induced by syrup of ipecac or gastric lavage with activated charcoal. Respiratory and cardiovascular support may be necessary. There is no specific antidote for nicotine.

Chronic toxicity to nicotine is a major problem owing to the large number of people exposed through smoking of cigarettes, cigars, and pipes. There is a causal connection between chronic smoking and cardiovascular disease and lung cancer. Cardiovascular diseases associated with tobacco smoking include peripheral vascular disease, cerebrovascular disease, and coronary artery disease. These are due not only to nicotine but also to other constituents of tobacco smoke.

Tolerance and Dependence Tolerance does develop to some of the effects of nicotine following chronic smoking. The dizziness, nausea, and vomiting experienced by first-time smokers usually are not observed in the chronic smoker. However tolerance does not appear to develop to the hand tremor, increase in blood pressure and pulse rate, and increased secretion of certain hormones. The mechanism for tolerance appears to be pharmacodynamic, although chronic smokers also biotransform nicotine more rapidly than nonsmokers owing to the induction of the drug-metabolizing microsomal system.

An abstinence syndrome may occur on cessation of chronic smoking. Symptoms may include irritability, restlessness, anxiety, headache, insomnia, gastrointestinal upset, increased appetite, and a craving to start smoking again. Symptoms may begin within 24 h, with some persisting for several weeks or months.

Lobeline Lobeline (α-lobeline; L-lobeline; inflatine) is the principal alkaloid of the dried leaves and tops of *Lobelia inflata*. The actions of lobeline are in many respects similar to those of nicotine, but lobeline has a potency of 1/50 to 1/100 that of nicotine. Like nicotine, lobeline is a primary stimulant and secondary depressant to the sympathetic ganglia, parasympathetic ganglia, adrenal medulla, central medullary centers (especially the emetic centers), neuromuscular junction, and chemoreceptors in the carotid body and aortic arch. Lobeline is used therapeutically as a smoking deterrent to aid an individual to give up cigarette smoking. It is not to be used for longer than 6 weeks. Adverse reactions including nausea, vomiting, heartburn, belching, epigastric pain, and dizziness.

INDIRECT ACTING CHOLINOMIMETIC AGENTS

As a class, the cholinesterase inhibitors (anticholinesterases) are very important members of the cholinomimetic family of drugs. In addition to their importance therapeutically, some compounds are widely used as agricultural pesticides and others are extremely toxic chemical warfare agents. All uses of these compounds are based on the changes which occur following inactivation of cholinesterases, i.e., the effects observed are due to the accumulation and action of acetylcholine at the neuronal-effector junctions. Before discussing the pharmacologic effects of the individual agents, some of the characteristics of the cholinesterases and the inhibitors will be considered.

Acetylcholinesterase is depicted schematically as shown in Fig. 9-3. Acetylcholine binds to the enzyme, orienting the molecule for enzymatic hydrolysis of the ester linkage. The nitrogen atom of acetylcholine binds ionically to the anionic site of the enzyme, whereas the carbonyl group of the acetyl portion of the substrate forms a covalent bond at the esteratic site. This substrate-enzyme complex results in acetylation of the enzyme, destruction of the ester linkage, and removal of the choline. The acetylated enzyme then reacts with water to form acetate and a regenerated enzyme. Acetylcholine is cleaved within 100 to 150 μs. Plasma cholinesterase (or pseudocholinesterase) acts in a similar manner to hydrolyze acetylcholine. It is, however, less specific for acetylcholine and biotransforms other aliphatic and aromatic esters as well.

The cholinesterase inhibitors can inhibit both cholinesterases. They are divided based either on their chemical structure or their chemical interaction with the enzyme which determines their time course of action. There are three broad chemical classes of cholinesterase inhibitors (Fig. 9-4): (1) carbamates, e.g., physostigmine, neostigmine, pyridostigmine, and several insecticides represented by carbaryl; (2) quaternary amines, e.g.; edrophonium, ambenonium, and demecarium; and (3) organophosphates, e.g., isofluorophate, echothiophate, insecticides represented by malathion and parathion, and toxins represented by soman. Based on differences in their time course of inhibition, cholinesterase inhibitors can also be classified as reversible and irreversible inhibitors. The reversible inhibitors comprise the carbamates and quaternary amines; the organophosphates are irreversible inhibitors of the cholinesterases.

Reversible Cholinesterase Inhibitors

As the name implies, the reversible cholinesterase inhibitors form a transient complex with the enzyme, in much the same way as does acetylcholine. These compounds compete with acetylcholine for binding at the active site of the enzyme. The chemical structure of

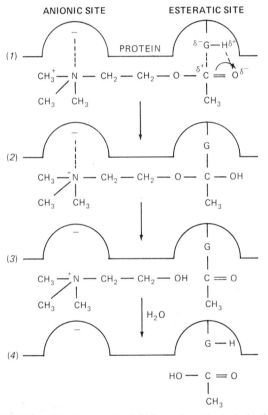

FIGURE 9-3   Steps in the AChE-catalyzed hydrolysis of ACh: (1) Attachment of ACh to the anionic site ($-$) and esteratic site (G—H) of the enzyme. (2) Formation of a covalent bond to the esteratic site, with loss of the resonance energy of the C=O group. (3) Cleavage of the ACh-enzyme complex into choline and acetyl AChE. (4) Very rapid hydrolysis of the acetyl-AChE and regeneration of the enzyme.

the classic reversible inhibitors physostigmine and neostigmine suggests a similarity to acetylcholine. Like the carbonyl moiety of acetylcholine, the carbonyl group of physostigmine and neostigmine attaches to the esteratic site of the enzyme. In addition, neostigmine also forms an ionic bond between its quaternary nitrogen and the anionic site of the enzyme, thus forming a two-point attachment to the enzyme. Edrophonium, also a potent reversible inhibitor (but not a carbamate), binds primarily to the anionic site, with hydrogen bonding to the esteratic site. While these compounds have high affinity for the enzyme, the inhibition of the enzyme is reversible. These inhibitors differ from acetylcholine, in that they are not readily degraded by the enzyme; the enzyme is reactivated much more slowly than following hydrolysis of acetylcholine. Therefore, the pharmacologic effects produced by these agents are reversible.

Physostigmine   Physostigmine is an alkaloid extracted from the calabar bean, the dried ripe seed of a wood vine *Physostigma venenosum* that grows in tropical West Africa. Unlike most other reversible cholinesterase inhibitors, physostigmine is a tertiary amine (Fig. 9-4); thus physostigmine is readily absorbed from the gastrointestinal tract and from other mucous membranes, but it is not used by the oral route. It is available for topical and parenteral administration. Once physostigmine enters the bloodstream, the drug is widely distributed throughout the organism, readily crossing the blood-brain barrier. The drug is inactivated by plasma cholinesterases. Renal impairment has no effect on drug elimination. Following intravenous administration, the duration of action is approximately 0.5 to 2 h, depending on the dose.

All those systems which normally produce and respond to acetylcholine are affected by physostigmine. At each of these sites, following the administration of adequate amounts, the resultant accumulation of acetylcholine gives rise to marked cholinergic stimulation. Physostigmine has minimal direct effects on cholinergic receptors. Since the responses to physostigmine are essentially the same as mentioned for acetylcholine and those described in Table 9-2, they will not be described here except as they relate to the therapeutic uses of physostigmine. In ophthalmology, physostigmine is useful topically in the treatment of glaucoma. It lowers intraocular pressure by increas-

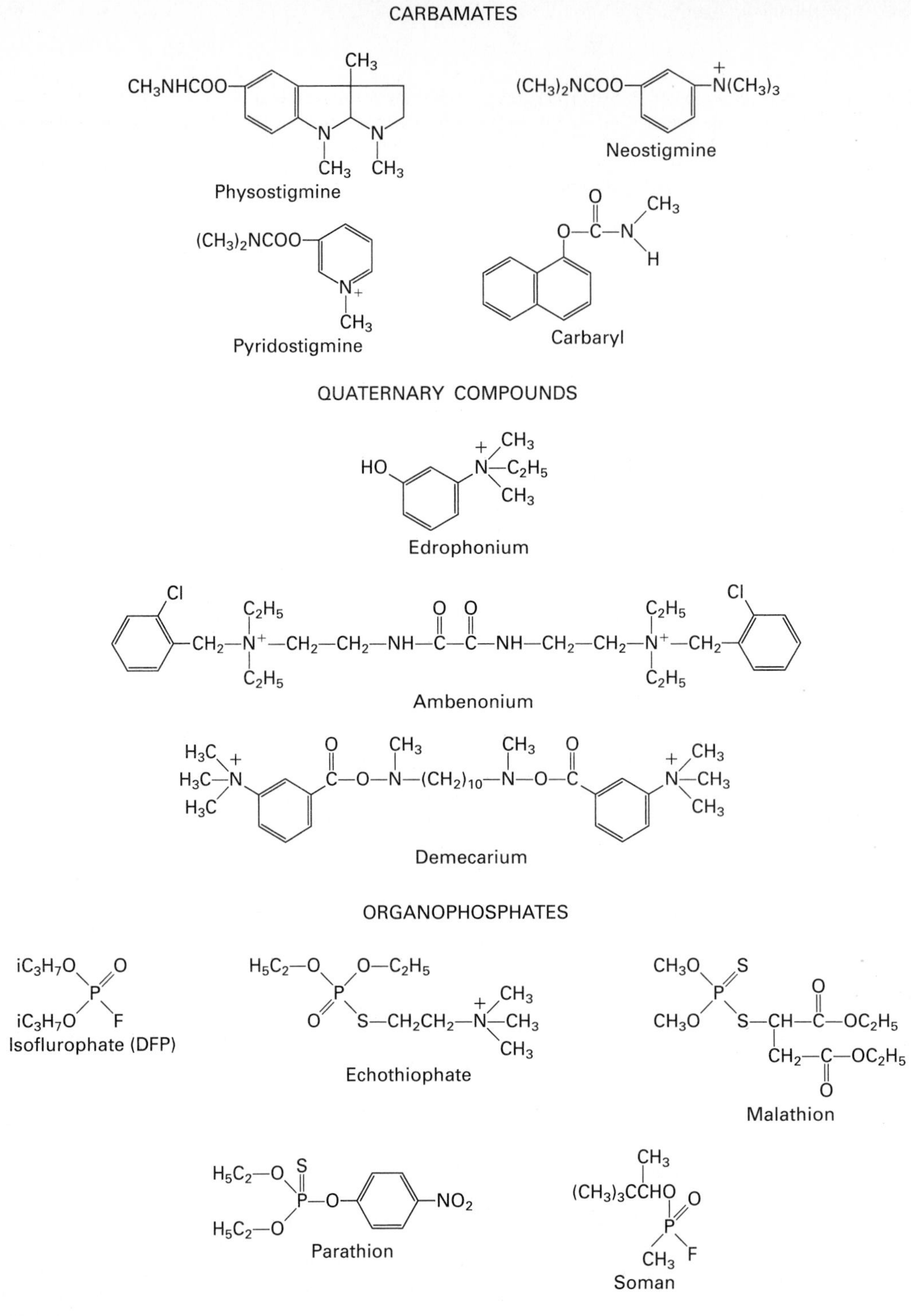

FIGURE 9-4 Structures of representative cholinesterase inhibitors.

TABLE 9-2 Signs and symptoms produced in humans by anticholinesterase agents

Site of action	Signs and symptoms
Following local exposure	
Pupils	Miosis, marked, usually maximal (pinpoint), sometimes unequal
Ciliary body	Frontal headache, eye pain on focusing, slight dimness of vision, occasional nausea and vomiting
Conjunctiva	Hyperemia
Nasal mucous membranes	Rhinorrhea, hyperemia
Bronchial tree	Tightness in chest, sometimes with prolonged wheezing expiration suggestive of bronchoconstriction or increased secretion, cough
Sweat glands	Sweating at site of exposure to liquid
Striated muscle	Fasciculation at site of exposure to liquid
Following systemic absorption	
Bronchial tree	Tightness in chest, with prolonged wheezing expiration suggestive of bronchoconstriction or increased secretion, dyspnea, slight pain in chest, increased bronchial secretion, cough
Gastrointestinal system	Anorexia, nausea, vomiting, abdominal cramps, epigastric and substernal tightness (cardiospasm?) with "heartburn" and eructation, diarrhea, tenesmus, involuntary defecation
Sweat glands	Increased sweating
Salivary glands	Increased salivation
Lacrimal glands	Increased lacrimation
Heart	Slight bradycardia
Pupils	Slight miosis, occasionally unequal, later more marked miosis
Ciliary body	Blurring of vision
Bladder	Frequency, involuntary micturition
Striated muscle	Easy fatigue, mild weakness, muscular twitching, fasciculations, cramps, generalized weakness, including muscles of respiration, with dyspnea and cyanosis

TABLE 9-2 (*continued*) **Signs and symptoms produced in humans by anticholinesterase agents**

Site of action	Signs and symptoms
Sympathetic ganglia	Pallor, occasional elevation of blood pressure
Central nervous system	Giddiness; tension; anxiety; jitteriness; restlessness; emotional lability; excessive dreaming; insomnia; nightmares; headache; tremor; apathy; withdrawal and depression; bursts of slow waves of elevated voltage in EEG, especially on overventilation; drowsiness; difficulty in concentrating, slowness of recall; confusion; slurred speech; ataxia; generalized weakness; coma, with absence of reflexes; Cheyne-Stokes respiration; convulsions; depression of respiratory and circulatory centers with dyspnea, cyanosis, and fall in blood pressure

ing the outflow of aqueous humor. As mentioned before, it can be used in conjunction with pilocarpine.

One of the most striking aspects of the pharmacologic actions of physostigmine is its effect on transmission at the neuromuscular junction. When administered systemically, physostigmine produces fasciculations and, with large doses, paralysis of striated muscle. As stated earlier, these responses are due to the inhibition of acetylcholinesterase and the resulting accumulation of acetylcholine in the neuromuscular junction. It is by this mechanism that physostigmine antagonizes the blockade of neuromuscular transmission produced by tubocurarine and other competitive neuromuscular blockers. Since tubocurarine blocks transmission by competing with acetylcholine for nicotinic receptor sites on the skeletal muscle end plate, the accumulation of acetylcholine which occurs following the inhibition of acetylcholinesterase shifts the competition in favor of the neurotransmitter and mediates the anticurare action of physostigmine. This is a useful tool for anesthesiologists. However, the use of physostigmine for this purpose has largely been replaced by pyridostigmine, neostigmine, and edrophonium since they have no central nervous system effects.

Because of the ability of physostigmine to penetrate into the central nervous system, the drug is useful to antagonize toxic concentrations of agents with anticholinergic properties, such as atropine, antihistamines, phenothiazines, and tricyclic antidepressants. For emergency treatment, the drug must be given in-travenously. Physostigmine has also been used, with limited success, in the treatment of Alzheimer's disease, which is characterized, in part, by serious reduction in acetylcholine levels in cerebral cortex and hippocampus.

The severity of adverse reactions associated with the drug depends on the route of administration. Topically in the eye, physostigmine often causes hyperemia of the conjunctiva and iris. Systemically, adverse reactions are the result of overstimulation of cholinergic effectors. Physostigmine can exacerbate peptic ulceration and bronchial asthma. It can also produce a reduction in heart rate and even bradyarrhythmias. Since it crosses the blood-brain barrier, physostigmine can worsen the symptoms of parkinsonism by further disrupting the balance of acetylcholine and dopamine.

Neostigmine Neostigmine is a synthetic cholinesterase inhibitor which differs from physostigmine in that it contains a quaternary nitrogen (Fig. 9-4). As a consequence, neostigmine has a limited pattern of distribution in the organism. Neostigmine is poorly and irregularly absorbed from the gastrointestinal tract although it is used by the oral route. In addition, it poorly penetrates other lipoidal barriers and membranes. Thus, it is difficult to regulate plasma levels of neostigmine when the drug is given orally. On the other hand, the poor penetration by the drug of the blood-brain barrier tends to minimize any occurrence of toxicity due to the inhibition of cholinesterases of the brain.

The presence of a quaternary nitrogen in the molecule introduces another important difference between physostigmine and neostigmine. The latter compound, in addition to inhibiting the cholinesterases, also has a direct stimulatory action on cholinergic receptors. Apart from these important differences, the general actions of neostigmine are like those of physostigmine and comparable to hyperactivity of cholinergic nerves.

Like other reversible cholinesterase inhibitors, neostigmine possesses a powerful anticurare action. This probably occurs by a combination of two mechanisms: (1) preservation of released acetylcholine by inhibiting acetylcholinesterase and (2) a direct stimulation of nicotinic II receptors on the skeletal muscle end plate. Use of this effect of neostigmine is made in anesthesiology to overcome the paralysis of skeletal muscles produced by curareform drugs.

The neuromuscular actions of neostigmine, more than those of physostigmine, have also been beneficial in the management of myasthenia gravis. For many years neostigmine was the drug of choice for this disorder. Although it is still used at present for this purpose, it has been displaced to some extent by newer cholinesterase inhibitors, such as pyridostigmine, which are better tolerated because of less intense side effects at therapeutic doses and have a longer duration of action.

There are some difficulties attending the use of neostigmine (and other cholinesterase inhibitors) for the treatment of myasthenia gravis. First, the dosage of neostigmine is difficult to regulate. With an overdose, the accumulation of acetylcholine at the end plate may be excessive and paralysis of transmission may occur. This situation due to excessive drug administration is termed *cholinergic crisis*. In the absence of prior knowledge of drug administration, it then becomes necessary to distinguish between the muscle weakness of the undertreated patient, i.e., *myasthenic crisis*, and the paralysis caused by an overdose of the anticholinesterase agent. The differential diagnosis is aided by the use of an ultra-short-acting anticholinesterase agent, edrophonium, which is described below. A second difficulty with neostigmine is the maintenance of a stable level of strength. Since neostigmine is a reversible cholinesterase inhibitor, its actions are relatively short-lived (mean half-life less than 1 h). Accordingly, muscle strength waxes and wanes as the drug effect takes place and then diminishes. This necessitates repeated administration of the drug and incurs the risk of cumulation. For some patients, it may also be necessary to interrupt their sleep for drug administration. The third problem is the ever-present one of side effects. For the cholinesterase inhibitors, these include excessive salivation, perspiration, abdominal distress, nausea, and vomiting. The side effects can be controlled by giving the drug in conjunction with atropine. However, these effects are the indicators of cumulation and overdose of the anticholinesterase agent, and their blockade by atropine may mask an impending cholinergic crisis.

In addition to its use in myasthenia, neostigmine has also been used for the treatment of postoperative abdominal distension and urinary retention.

Pyridostigmine Qualitatively, the pharmacologic properties of pyridostigmine are the same as those of neostigmine. Pyridostigmine, although useful by the oral route, is poorly absorbed from the gastrointestinal tract. Pyridostigmine is also slowly inactivated by plasma cholinesterases; the parent compound and metabolite are primarily excreted in the urine. The drug directly stimulates both muscarinic and nicotinic cholinergic receptors, in addition to its inhibition of cholinesterase. Pyridostigmine, however, is less potent than neostigmine.

Pyridostigmine is principally used for its nicotinic effects. It is the drug of choice for the treatment of myasthenia gravis. The improvement of muscle strength is more sustained than that produced by neostigmine. Accordingly, less frequent administration is required. Other advantages of pyridostigmine, compared to neostigmine, are (1) less danger of overdosage and (2) reduced frequency and severity of muscarinic side effects. Pyridostigmine is also used by anesthesiologists, to reverse the skeletal muscle blockade produced by curare-like drugs.

Adverse reactions associated with pyridostigmine include muscarinic (nausea, vomiting, diarrhea, miosis, increased bronchial secretions) and nicotinic (muscle cramps, fasciculation, and weakness) manifestations. Atropine may be used to reduce muscarinic side effects, but as mentioned can inadvertently mask *cholinergic crisis*.

Edrophonium Edrophonium is similar structurally to neostigmine, with two exceptions: (1) edrophonium has an ethyl group on the nitrogen and (2) it lacks an ester functional group (Fig. 9-4).

The pharmacologic properties of the compound qualitatively resemble those of neostigmine. However, the structural changes give edrophonium more selective direct receptor activity. In addition to inhibiting cholinesterases, edrophonium stimulates nicotinic receptors at the neuromuscular junction at lower doses than that which stimulate other cholinergic receptors. Therefore, edrophonium will enhance neuromuscular transmission at doses that do not stimulate the heart, smooth muscle cells, and glands. Two additional features distinguish the actions of edrophonium from those of neostigmine and pyridostigmine: (1) its onset of action is more rapid than either drug, and (2) its duration of action is considerably shorter, 10 to 15 min, compared with 0.5 to 2 h for neostigmine and 4 to 6 h for pyridostigmine. These characteristics are more consistent with a direct acting agent than with one that exerts its effect only by inhibiting an enzyme.

The brief duration of action of edrophonium compared with the longer-acting anticholinesterase agents is, for some purposes, a distinct advantage. It minimizes the problem of managing overdosage and reduces the possibility of cumulation of the drug.

Edrophonium plays a prominent role in establishing the diagnosis of myasthenia gravis and in making a differential diagnosis between myasthenic weakness and cholinergic crisis. In these situations, use is made of the transient actions of the drug. For the diagnosis of myasthenia, edrophonium is injected intravenously in divided doses. The brief duration of its effect requires that measurements of muscle strength be made quickly. The improvement in strength, if it occurs, will last for less than 5 min. The test can be repeated several times on the same day. For the differentiation between myasthenic and cholinergic crises, edrophonium is also given intravenously. If the crises is due to inadequate anticholinesterase therapy, edrophonium will result in an improvement of muscle strength. Conversely, edrophonium will further decrease muscle strength if the weakness if due to an overdose of the anticholinesterase agent. In the case of cholinergic crisis, the short-lived actions of edrophonium will not substantially prolong the crisis, and other measures, such as maintenance of airways and artificial ventilation, can be instituted.

A second important therapeutic use of edrophonium is based on its ability to antagonize curareform drugs. It is unlikely that the anticurare action is due to the inhibition of acetylcholinesterase, since doses of edrophonium which effectively antagonize the blockade of neuromuscular transmission have no effect on the sensitivity of end plate to injected acetylcholine.

Ambenonium Chloride   Ambenonium chloride is a cholinesterase inhibitor with pharmacologic properties similar to those of neostigmine and pyridostigmine (see Fig. 9-4 for structure). The pharmacologic actions of ambenonium are brought about primarily through the reversible inactivation of the cholinesterases.

The principal therapeutic use of ambenonium is in the management of myasthenia gravis. It is however considered a secondary agent to pyridostigmine. Though ambenonium appears to have a slightly more sustained action, it has a higher incidence of muscarinic side effects.

Demecarium   Demecarium is a bisymmetric compound containing two quaternary ammonium and two carbamate functional groups (Fig. 9-4). The compound is a reversible cholinesterase inhibitor, but with a duration of action longer than that of other reversible inhibitors. Demecarium has higher affinity for acetylcholinesterase than for plasma cholinesterase.

Demecarium is used in the management of glaucoma; when instilled topically into the eye, it lowers intraocular pressure. A single instillation into the conjunctival sac of normal subjects produces miosis, which is apparent within 1 h, attains a maximum within 4 h, and persists for 3 to 10 days. The miosis is accompanied by spasm of the intraocular muscles of accommodation.

Adverse reactions include local burning and itching. Systemic signs of cholinesterase inhibition can occur from prolonged administration.

Irreversible Cholinesterase Inhibitors

The second class of cholinesterase inhibitors is a group of organophosphorous compounds. They all have the same general formula:

$$\begin{array}{c} R_1O \diagdown \quad \diagup O \text{ (or S)} \\ P \\ R_2O \diagup \quad \diagdown X \end{array}$$

where R_1 and R_2 are alkyl functional groups and the X is a halogen or other functional group. Structures of individual compounds are shown in Fig. 9-4.

The organophosphates act by complexing to the serine hydroxyl group at the esteratic site of the cholinesterase enzymes; the phosphorous atom covalently bonds with this site. A schematic representation of the phosphorylated enzyme is illustrated in Fig. 9-5. In contrast with the rapid hydrolysis of acetylcholine

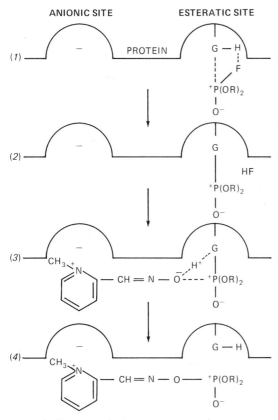

FIGURE 9-5 Steps in the inactivation of AChE by DFP and its regeneration by pralidoxime (2-PAM): (1) Attachment of DFP to the esteratic site. (2) Formation of a phosphoryl enzyme which, in contrast to the acetyl-AChE, is hydrolyzed extremely slowly, making the enzyme unavailable for hydrolysis of ACh. (3) Attachment of 2-PAM to the anionic site of the enzyme and to the phosphorylated esteratic site by virtue of the pronounced acidity of the oxime: the anionic (nucleophilic) O⁻ is attracted to the positively charged P atom, and the proton of the oxime to site G. (4) The complex formed in the preceding step breaks up into phosphorylated 2-PAM and regenerated AChE.

from the enzyme and slower hydrolysis of carbamates, the phosphorylated enzyme reacts very slowly with water, leading to essentially irreversible inhibition. For most of the organophosphorus compounds, de novo synthesis of the enzyme must take place for the cholinesterase activity of tissue to return. For others, a limited amount of spontaneous reactivation of the enzyme occurs. Although this type of inhibition is generally regarded as irreversible, chemical agents such as oximes can reactivate the enzyme. However, the phosphorylated enzyme can undergo a process called *aging*, in which the organophosphate loses an alkyl group, forming a tighter irreversible bond to the enzyme; this renders the enzyme insensitive to reactivation by oximes.

The signs and symptoms of acute toxicity which occur following the administration of an organophosphorus anticholinesterase agent can be readily predicted and are attributable to hyperactivity of the parasympathetic nervous system, neuromuscular junction, autonomic ganglia, and cholinergic nerves of the CNS. These signs and symptoms are listed in Table 9-2. Death is due primarily to depression of respiration caused by depression of the CNS, paralysis of the diaphragm and intercostal muscles, bronchospasm, and the accumulation of bronchosecretions. Each is due to the accumulation of excessive amounts of acetylcholine.

Some organophosphates are useful therapeutically, others are used as insecticides and potential chemical warfare agents based on their extreme toxicity. The pharmacology of representative individual agents is discussed below.

Isoflurophate (Di-isopropyl Fluorophosphate, DFP) The primary difference between isoflurophate and agents such as physostigmine lies in the persistency of action. By the mechanism described above for the organophosphorus cholinesterase inhibitors isoflurophate produces an irreversible inactivation of the cholinesterases. Both acetylcholinesterase and "nonspecific" plasma cholinesterase are inactivated by isoflurophate; however, isoflurophate has a greater affinity for the latter enzyme.

Isoflurophate is used in the treatment of certain types of glaucoma, when short-acting miotics are inadequate. The compound has also been used in certain types of strabismus. Maximal reduction in intraocular pressure occurs within 1 day of a single dose. Effects can persist for several days. The intensity and duration of action are much greater for isoflurophate than for pilocarpine or physostigmine and approximately the same as demecarium. Since isoflurophate is highly lipid-soluble, it must be administered in peanut oil, which is very irritating to the eye.

Echothiophate Iodide   Echothiophate is a phosphorylthiocholine (see Fig. 9-4 for structure). It is a long-acting cholinesterase inhibitor with pharmacologic actions on the peripheral nervous system similar to those of isoflurophate. Spontaneous regeneration of the phosphorylated enzyme occurs more rapidly with echothiophate than with isoflurophate.

Echothiophate is used in opthalmology for the treatment of glaucoma and other disorders of the eye amenable to therapy with cholinesterase inhibitors. In this regard, the water-soluble property of echothiophate affords one practical advantage over the lipid-soluble irreversible inhibitor. Lacrimation evoked by the irritation produced by solvents such as peanut oil may result in the removal of the anticholinesterase agent from the conjunctiva. Usually this does not occur with echothiophate. The use of echothiophate for ocular diseases is governed by the same precautions and limitations as are the other long-acting anticholinesterase agents. Long-term administration is limited due to the development of cataracts.

Other Organosphosphorous Cholinesterase Inhibitors   Several organophosphate compounds are available for use as household and agricultural insecticides. Most are highly lipid-soluble compounds, which are rapidly and completely absorbed by practically all routes, including the skin and the respiratory and gastrointestinal tracts. Some commonly used compounds include malathion and parathion.

Most organophosphates are biotransformed by hydrolysis of the carboxyl-ester linkage and are excreted in the urine. Malathion, widely used in the home and garden, has low toxicity in humans because it is readily detoxified by hydrolysis. This rapid inactivation does not occur in insects. Other organophosphates such as parathion and chlorpyrifos are not readily detoxified and are responsible for many cases of accidental toxicity every year.

Still other organophosphates, first synthesized in Germany during World War II, are some of the most toxic compounds known and are potential chemical warfare agents. These include soman, sarin, and tabun. What makes these compounds so toxic is the fact that they induce very rapid "aging" of the enzyme, making the enzyme insensitive to reactivation by oximes. Hence there is no adequate therapy for intoxication with these compounds.

Management of Organophosphate Poisoning

Treatment of organophosphate intoxication includes (1) artificial respiration; (2) atropine sulfate, a muscarinic receptor antagonist; and (3) pralidoxime, a cholinesterase reactivator. The pharmacology of atropine is covered in Chap. 10. The properties of pralidoxime are discussed below.

Pralidoxime Chloride   Studies of the reactivity of organophosphorus compounds and of the mechanism by which they inhibit the activity of acetylcholinesterase and other cholinesterases has resulted in the discovery of agents which are capable of reactivating the inhibited enzymes. These reactivators also possess considerable antidotal effect. The present compound of choice in this country is pralidoxime chloride (2-pyridine aldoxime methylchloride or 2-PAM chloride).

This drug is used as an adjunct to atropine in the treatment of organophosphate pesticide intoxication. It is not effective against carbamate cholinesterase inhibitors. Standard treatment of toxicity by soman and related compounds with atropine and pralidoxime (or other oximes) is not of practical value due to the rapid aging of these compounds to the enzyme.

Pralidoxime is a strong nucleophilic compound. It reactivates the phosphorylated enzyme in a two-step reaction (Fig. 9-5). First a complex forms between the oximate ion and the phosphorylated enzyme; this is followed by liberation of the phosphorylated oxime and regeneration of enzyme activity.

The high reactivating potency of pralidoxime has been attributed to its ability to combine with a negatively charged group on the enzyme surface and to a high degree of molecular fit between oxime and phosphorylated cholinesterase. The rate of the reactivation is very much dependent on the type of the phosphorylated enzyme and on other factors in addition to oxime concentration.

In summary, it appears that the oximes may, both in

vitro and in vivo, (1) react directly with the inhibitor, converting it to a harmless compound and (2) reactivate the inhibited enzyme, both in blood and tissues. At high concentrations, the oximes can act as mild cholinesterase inhibitors, a factor which does not appear to be of other than academic importance.

Pralidoxime is given by intravenous administration for severe organophosphate poisoning or by the oral route for mild poisoning. Being a quaternary compound, pralidoxime does not cross the blood-brain barrier and, therefore, will not reverse the central nervous system toxicities of organophosphates. Pralidoxime is largely metabolized in the liver, with its products excreted in the urine.

Pralidoxime may produce several adverse reactions including headache, dizziness, drowsiness, nausea, tachycardia, increased blood pressure, and muscle weakness when administered parenterally. There are no significant toxic effects following oral administration.

PREPARATIONS

Acetylcholine chloride (Miochol) is available in a combi-vial, one compartment containing 20 mg of acetylcholine chloride and 60 mg mannitol, the other containing 2 mL sterile water for the preparation of a 1:100 solution.

Methacholine chloride (Provocholine) is available as a powder for reconstitution into a 100 mg/5 mL solution.

Carbachol (Miostat, Isopto Carbachol) is available as sterile solutions (in concentrations of 0.01 to 3 percent) for intraocular use.

Bethanechol chloride (Urecholine) is available as tablets (5, 10, 25, 50 mg) for oral administration and in solution (5 mg/mL) for subcutaneous administration.

Pilocarpine hydrochloride (Pilocar, Isopto Carpine) and Pilocarine nitrate (P.V. Carpine) are available for topical administration as solutions (0.25 to 10 percent). The Pilocarpine Ocular Therapeutic System (Ocusert Pilo-20, Ocusert Pilo-40) delivers 20 to 40 μg/h of drug for up to 1 week.

Nicotine polacrilex (Nicorette) is available as a chewing gum containing 2 mg per square.

Lobeline sulfate (Bantron) is available as 2-mg tablets for oral administration.

Physostigmine salicylate (Isopto Eserine) is available as 0.25 and 0.5 percent solutions for topical use in the eye. It is also available as a 1-mg/mL solution for intravenous treatment of anticholinergic intoxication (Antilirium). Physostigmine sulfate (Eserine Sulfate) is available as a 0.25 percent ophthalmic ointment.

Neostigmine (Prostigmin) is available as the bromide in 15-mg tablets for oral administration and as the methylsulfate in sterile solution (0.25 to 1.0 mg/mL) for injection.

Pyridostigmine bromide (Mestinon) is available as a sterile solution in 2-mL ampuls (5 mg/mL) for injection; in 60-mg tablets, 180-mg sustained release tablets, and a syrup (60 mg/5 mL) for oral administration.

Edrophonium chloride (Tensilon) is available for injection in multiple-dose vials and ampuls containing 10 mg/mL.

Ambenonium chloride (Mytelase) is available in 10-mg tablets for oral administration.

Demecarium (Humorsol) is available as sterile solutions (0.125 and 0.25 percent) for topical administration into the conjunctival sac.

Isoflurophate (Floropryl) is available for topical administration in the eye as a sterile ointment (0.025 percent) in polyethylene-mineral oil gel.

Echothiophate iodide (Phospholine Iodide) is available for topical administration in the eye as a lyophilized powder (1.5, 3.0, 6.25, 12.5 mg) with 5-mL diluent to make 0.03, 0.06, 0.125, and 0.25 percent solutions, respectively.

Pralidoxime chloride (Protopam Chloride) is available as 500 mg tablets for oral administration and as a sterile powder (1 g in a 20-mL container) for intravenous administration.

BIBLIOGRAPHY

Abou-Donia, M. B.: "Organophosphorus Ester-induced Delayed Neurotoxicity," *Annu. Rev. Pharmacol. Toxicol.*, **21**:511–548 (1981).

Brown, J. H., G. T. Wetzel, and J. Dunlap: "Activation and Blockade of Cardiac Muscarinic Receptors by Endogenous Acetylcholine and Cholinesterase Inhibitors," *J. Pharmacol. Exp. Ther.*, **223**:20–24 (1982).

Dowdall, M. (ed.): *Cellular and Molecular Basis of Cholinergic Function*, Plenum, New York, 1988.

Drachman, D. H.: "Myasthenia Gravis," *N. Engl. J. Med.*, **298**:136–142, 186–193 (1978).

Hanin, I. (ed.): *Dynamics of Cholinergic Function*, Plenum, New York, 1986, vol. IV.

Hanin, I., and A. M. Goldberg: *Progress in Cholinergic Biology: Model Cholinergic Synapses*, Raven, New York, 1982.

Havener, W. H.: *Ocular Pharmacology*, 5th ed., Mosby, St. Louis, 1983, pp. 261–417.

Hirschowitz, B. I., R. Hammer, A. Giachetti, J. J. Kerns, and R. R. Levine (eds.): "Subtypes of Muscarinic Receptors," *Trends Pharmacol. Sci.*, (**Suppl**):1 (1984).

Johnson, M. K.: "The Target for Initiation of Delayed Neurotoxicity by Organophosphorus Esters," in E. Hodgson, E. Band, and R. M. Philpot (eds.), *Reviews in Biochemical Toxicology*, Elsevier, New York, 1982, vol. 4, pp. 141–272.

Karczmar, A. G.: "Pharmacologic, Toxicologic, and Therapeutic Properties of Anticholinesterase Agents," in W. S. Root and F. G. Hofman (eds.), *Physiological Pharmacology, Vol 3, The Nervous System-Part C: Autonomic Nervous System Drugs*, Academic, New York, 1967, pp. 163–322.

Kaufman, P. L., T. Weidman, and J. R. Robinson: "Cholinergics," in M. L. Sears (ed.) *Pharmacology of the Eye. Handbook of Experimental Pharmacology*, Springer-Verlag, Berlin, 1984, vol. 69, pp. 149–192.

Thai, L. J., P. A. Fuld, D. M. Masur, and N. S. Sharpless: "Oral Physostigmine and Lecithin Improve Memory in Alzheimer's Disease," *Ann. Neurol.*, **13**:491–496 (1983).

Wieland T.: "Poisonous Principles of Mushrooms of the Genus *Amanita*," *Science*, **159**:946–952 (1968).

———"Parasympathetic Neuroeffector Mechanisms in the Heart" (Symposium), *Fed. Proc.*, **43**:2597–2623 (1984).

Antimuscarinic Drugs and Ganglionic Blocking Agents

George B. Koelle

As discussed in previous chapters, there are three major types of cholinergic receptors: muscarinic (M), nicotinic I (N I), and nicotinic II (N II). Cholinergic receptor antagonists are classified based on their ability to selectively block one of these receptor types. *Antimuscarinic drugs* (muscarinic receptor blocking drugs) act at the muscarinic receptors of smooth muscle, cardiac tissues, and exocrine glands by blocking the actions of acetylcholine (ACh) liberated from cholinergic postganglionic autonomic nerve endings and administered cholinomimetic drugs. They also block M receptors in the central nervous system (CNS). *Ganglionic blocking agents* selectively interfere with transmission in autonomic ganglia mediated through N I receptors. *Neuromuscular blocking drugs* act at N II receptors of the skeletal muscle end plate.

The general pharmacology of the antimuscarinic drugs and some features of the ganglionic blocking agents are discussed in this chapter. Information concerning neuromuscular blocking drugs is presented with the pharmacology of the skeletal muscle relaxants (Chap. 11).

ANTIMUSCARINIC DRUGS

The oldest drugs of the group are the various galenical preparations of belladonna, hyoscyamus, and stramonium. All these are derived from plants of the potato family, the Solanaceae. The species used as drugs include *Atropa belladonna*, one of several plants known colloquially as "deadly nightshade"; *Hyoscyamus ni-*

ger (black henbane); and *Datura stramonium* (Jimson weed, Jamestown weed, or thorn apple). The active principles in all these plants consist mostly of *l*-hyoscyamine, with smaller and variable amounts of *l*-scopolamine (hyoscine). *l*-Hyoscyamine is much more active as a muscarinic receptor blocking drug than *d*-hyoscyamine, both peripherally and on the CNS, but the racemic mixture *dl*-hyoscyamine, better known as *atropine*, is preferred for most medicinal purposes because it is more stable chemically and therefore more dependable for action.

Atropine and its congener scopolamine are two of the most important antimuscarinic drugs, and as prototypes of the entire group, they will be discussed in more detail than some other derivatives or synthetic substitutes that have specialized uses.

Chemistry

Atropine is *dl*-tropyltropine, and scopolamine is *l*-tropyl-*d*-scopine (Fig. 10-1). They are, in fact, esters of tropic acid with the organic bases tropanol (tropine) and scopine, respectively. Scopine differs from tropine only by the oxygen bridge between C-6 and C-7.

Mechanism of Action

In recent years, subtypes of muscarinic receptors (M_1 and M_2) have been described, which are selectivity activated or blocked by various agents. However, both

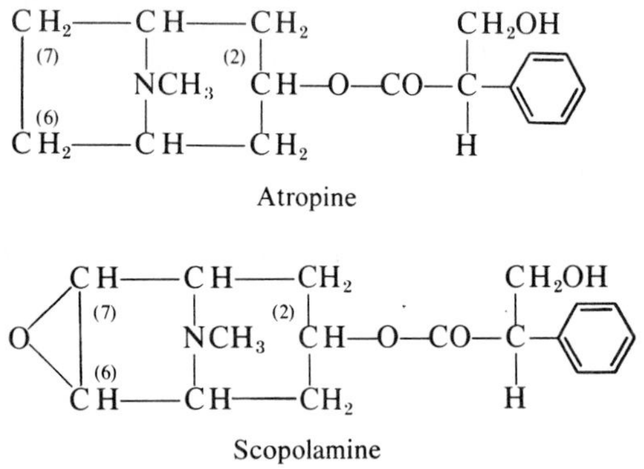

FIGURE 10-1   Structures of atropine and scopolamine.

types of muscarinic receptors are activated by the endogenous neurotransmitter ACh and blocked by atropine or scopolamine. Although atropine and scopolamine are competitive, reversible ACh-blocking agents, their dissociation constants with M receptors are several magnitudes lower than that of ACh. Accordingly their actions, such as mydriasis following intraconjunctival instillation, may persist for several days.

It has been observed repeatedly that atropine is more effective in blocking the effects of exogenously administered ACh and other parasympathomimetic agents than in blocking the effects following stimulation of parasympathetic, cholinergic nerve fibers. There are two likely reasons for this: (1) ACh is released by nerve impulses in close proximity to the M receptors of the effector cells; hence it competes more effectively with atropine arriving via the circulation than do parasympathomimetic agents arriving via the same route. (2) In certain organs, such as the urinary bladder, postganglionic parasympathetic fibers may release other neurotransmitters (e.g., ATP), in addition to ACh, which are not blocked by atropine.

These drugs have multiple actions. In addition to their M-receptor blocking action, atropine and scopolamine act at other sites and exhibit other effects. These drugs can block nicotinic cholinergic receptors at autonomic ganglion cells and the motor end plate of skeletal muscle, but only in doses far in excess of those employed clinically. The cutaneous flush that follows high doses of atropine is due to direct depression of arteriolar smooth muscle. Atropine is also a fairly potent local anesthetic and a histamine (H_1) receptor blocker in high doses.

Effects on Organ Systems

Atropine is somewhat more potent than scopolamine in its M-receptor blocking actions on the heart, gastrointestinal tract, and bronchial muscle; the reverse is true for the iris sphincter, ciliary muscle, and exocrine glands. In the following accounts, atropine is used as the prototype drug.

Heart   When atropine sulfate is administered by mouth or by subcutaneous, intramuscular, or intravenous injection, the heart rate first shows a temporary and moderate decrease, which is followed by a more marked acceleration. The tachycardia is accompanied by an increase in cardiac output. The P-R interval is shortened by all doses of atropine. The initial bradycardia is more prolonged following small doses, and it is attributed to atropine stimulating the cardioinhibitory center of the medulla in the presence of incomplete peripheral blockade. The subsequent cardiac acceleration is due to atropine blocking the tonic vagal impulses to the heart. The acceleration of the heart rate occurs earlier, is more marked, and is more prolonged as the dose of atropine is increased.

Atropine will also prevent or reverse the decrease in the refractory period, the lengthened P-R interval, the slowing of conduction, and the decrease in cardiac output and the cardiac oxygen consumption produced by vagal stimulation or cholinomimetic agents. The potassium liberation from and the sodium penetration into isolated atria produced by ACh are also reversed by atropine, and it will return the atrial fibrillation induced and maintained in animals by ACh or vagal stimulation to normal sinus rhythm.

Peripheral Circulation   Normal doses of atropine, given by mouth or parenterally, have little effect on blood pressure. Larger doses (2 mg or more), although causing a marked increase in heart rate, usually decrease the systolic blood pressure by a few millimeters of mercury. This fall in blood pressure is more marked in warm environments and may be caused by decreased cardiac filling due to excessive heart rate.

When atropine sulfate is injected intravenously, into either conscious volunteers or anesthetized patients, the heart rate increases and the cardiac output rises, but the stroke volume, central venous pressure, and total peripheral resistance decrease. The rise in the cardiac output is dependent on the degree of increase in the heart rate and is accompanied by a rise in the arterial blood pressure; in anesthetized patients, the extent of these changes varies with the anesthetic used.

Atropine abolishes the depressor response and the vasodilatation produced by ACh. On its own, it has a direct vasodilator effect on small blood vessels; this is not an anticholinergic phenomenon. Hence, a slight flushing of the skin may occur with small doses, and a pronounced reddening is a characteristic effect of toxic doses.

Central Nervous System   On the CNS, atropine first causes stimulation and then depression, whereas scopolamine generally has a purely depressant effect. With the usual dose of atropine sulfate, effects on the CNS are not striking, except for the slowing of the heart, mentioned above. Ordinary doses of scopolamine, given subcutaneously, have a profound soporific effect lasting 1 or 2 h. A similar dose given orally has very little soporific action, a fact that makes scopolamine given orally an effective treatment for motion sickness. Large doses of atropine produce drowsiness, hallucinations, disorientation, and eventually coma. Similar toxic effects are produced by relatively smaller doses of scopolamine. In occasional patients, particularly in the presence of severe pain, scopolamine may be excitatory. For this reason patients given scopolamine preoperatively should be kept under constant surveillance until taken to the operating room.

Medulla   A normal clinical dose of atropine has neither significant stimulatory nor depressant action on respiration. Atropine is not considered effective in counteracting respiratory depression in poisoning by barbiturates or opioids. However, it is a specific antidote for the central respiratory depression (and peripheral bronchoconstriction and increased tracheobronchial secretion) occurring in poisoning with anticholinesterase agents.

Higher Centers   Atropine decreases the muscle tremor and reduces the stiffness in parkinsonism. Scopolamine and many centrally active synthetic anticholinergic drugs have a similar action. This is probably due to their restoring the cholinergic-adrenergic (or dopaminergic) balance in the basal ganglia, since the primary deficit in parkinsonism has been shown to be a deficiency of dopamine. This is discussed further in Chap. 21.

Secretions   The exocrine sweat glands of the human skin are supplied by cholinergic fibers present in sympathetic nerves. Accordingly, sweating is diminished or abolished by small doses of atropine. This reduction or abolition of sweating may be responsible for the rise in rectal temperature that sometimes follows moderate doses of atropine and is a regular consequence of toxic doses.

One of the most obvious effects of ordinary doses of atropine and scopolamine is dryness of the mouth. The copious watery flow of saliva induced by parasympathetic nerve stimulation is essentially abolished by atropine. The secretions of the nose, pharynx, and bronchi are greatly reduced by ordinary doses of atropine and scopolamine.

Gastric secretion is under the influence of a large number of nervous, hormonal, and local factors. Atropine does block increased gastric secretion induced by vagal stimulation. This finds some clinical use, but much more effective block of gastric secretion is obtained by surgical vagotomy and more practically by histamine H_2-receptor blockers (see Chap. 12).

Atropine blocks the secretion of pancreatic juice caused by vagal stimulation or parasympathomimetic drugs, and this may be due to a blocking of the extrusion of zymogen granules. It has no effect on the secretion stimulated by secretin or pancreozymin.

Smooth Muscle

Alimentary Tract   In general, anticholinergic drugs reduce the tone and decrease the amplitude and frequency of peristaltic contractions of the stomach, small intestine, and, to a lesser extent, the colon. The inhibitory effect of atropine on gastrointestinal motility is more pronounced and less variable than on gastric secretion. Normal motility is not appreciably altered by therapeutic doses of atropine, but hypermotility associated with peptic ulcer and certain other gastrointestinal disorders is usually reduced markedly.

Bronchi   The smooth muscles of the bronchioles are slightly relaxed by atropine blocking the constrictor effects of the vagus nerves. The result is a freer airway, which is useful in anesthesia. Scopolamine has a longer bronchodilator action than does atropine. When these drugs or their congeners (e.g., ipratropium) are given by inhalation, side effects on other systems are minimized.

Biliary Tract Atropine has little effect on the secretion of bile, but it is thought to have some relaxant effect on the smooth muscle of the biliary tract, thus increasing bile flow through the duct. Consequently, even though its effect is slight, it is given with morphine for the relief of biliary colic.

Urinary Bladder Atropine decreases, but even in large doses does not abolish, the motor effect of the sacral cholinergic nerves supplying the bladder. Therapeutic doses are thought to diminish the tone of the fundus of the bladder and to increase the tone of the vesical sphincter. As a consequence, atropine may contribute to the retention of urine, which is often troublesome after surgical operations.

The Eye The circular smooth muscle of the iris, which constricts the pupil, is innervated by cholinergic fibers from the third cranial (oculomotor) nerve. Fibers from the same nerve cause contraction of the ciliary muscles, thus slackening the suspensory ligament of the lens and allowing the lens to become more convex. In addition, this action may result in opening of the canal of Schlemm, improving drainage of aqueous humor from the anterior chamber and thereby decreasing intraocular pressure. Atropine and scopolamine block the neurohumoral mediator at the smooth muscle of the iris, causing *mydriasis* (dilation of the pupil) and, at the ciliary muscle, causing *cycloplegia* (paralysis of accommodation). Relaxation of the ciliary muscle tends to occlude the angle of attachment of the iris to the cornea, and dilatation of the pupil causes the iris to crowd the angular space and thus obstruct the access of fluid to the venous sinus. The result is aggravation of the increased ocular pressure of glaucoma, a disease characterized by increased intraocular pressure. Therefore, atropine and other cycloplegics and mydriatics *should not* be used in the eyes of patients with glaucoma.

Pharmacokinetics

Atropine and scopolamine are almost completely absorbed in the intestinal tract and from the conjunctiva. Scopolamine can be absorbed across the skin (via

transdermal administration). The peak serum concentration occurs about 1 h after oral administration of atropine and 15 to 20 min after intramuscular injection. Measurement of the apparent volume of distribution shows values of about 2 to 4 L/kg with protein binding of about 50 percent. The half-life ($t_{1/2}$) is 13 to 38 h with a distribution phase of 6 h.

There is little hydrolysis of the ester bond. Rather, atropine is partially N-demethylated. About 33 to 50 percent appears in the urine as the intact molecule, the rest as metabolites.

Adverse Reactions

Excessive dosage with atropine, one of the galenical preparations of the belladonna group, or one of the many drugs (e.g., H_1 antihistamines, tricyclic antidepressants, and phenothiazines) that have anticholinergic properties, gives rise to distinctive signs, which include rapid pulse, dilated pupils, and dry, flushed skin. Patients may complain of thirst and difficulty in focusing their eyes, or may be restless, garrulous, excited, disoriented, or even delirious.

The classic description of atropine poisoning is: *red as a beet* (cutaneous vasodilatation), *dry as a bone* (blockade of salivary secretion), *hot as a hare* (blockade of sweat secretion), and *mad as a hatter* (cortical stimulation). While these and the accompanying symptoms (tachycardia, mydriasis, blurred vision) can be frightening, they are rarely fatal, except in children. Although there is individual variation and sensitivity to atropine and its congeners, there is a wide margin of safety between therapeutic and lethal doses. If recovery ensues, there may be no recollection of the distressing episode. If the outcome is fatal, it usually follows a period of coma in which the respirations become rapid and shallow and finally cease. The toxic effects of scopolamine are similar to those of atropine except that stupor and delirium are more prominent and excitement is less so.

If the poisonous dose was taken orally and the patient receives attention early, the stomach should be emptied as quickly as possible and washed out thoroughly. No specific antidote is very useful, but activated charcoal should be given to adsorb or inactivate the portion of the poison remaining in the alimentary tract. Physostigmine has been shown, however, to be beneficial in the treatment of scopolamine-induced delirium. Respiratory failure is a common feature in many of the reported deaths from atropine so that artificial respiration should also be administered. Hyperpyrexia can be alleviated by keeping the skin wet with water until spontaneous sweating occurs.

Therapeutic Uses

Atropine is given frequently in preparation for surgical anesthesia. The main purpose is to minimize bronchial, nasal, and salivary secretions, which may accumulate and obstruct the respiratory passages. Scopolamine is preferred if additional sedative action is desired.

Oral administration of atropine sulfate is often useful to dry the nasal secretions for the temporary relief of common colds or hay fever. Belladonna extract may be a common ingredient of over-the-counter cold remedies.

Atropine is useful in treating acutely ill patients when bradycardia is associated with a low cardiac output or ventricular irritability. The syndrome of bradycardia and falling arterial blood pressure is occasionally seen in patients with acute myocardial infarction. In such cases, atropine increases the heart rate and may restore the blood pressure to a normal range.

Atropine can allay the urgency and frequency of micturition, which often accompany cystitis, and may be useful as an adjunct in the treatment of enuresis in children, although substances such as propantheline may be more effective because they have in addition a ganglionic blocking action.

Scopolamine hydrobromide is used as a remedy for motion sickness. For this purpose it can be used orally, or it can be administered topically by application of an adhesive unit (Transderm Scop) behind the ear. It is also employed in obstetrics to promote drowsiness with amnesia, or "twilight sleep." It is given with a sedative analgesic agent such as morphine or meperidine.

Atropine, in conjunction with other measures, is recommended for the treatment of poisoning with anticholinesterase agents such as the organophosphorus insecticides and the nerve gases (see Chap. 9). In these cases atropine will block or reverse many of the toxic actions owing to this abnormal concentration of ACh. If a neuromuscular blockade is present, it will not be affected by the atropine. It is important to remember that large doses of atropine may be necessary for the adequate treatment of these cases of poisoning. An oxime, such as pralidoxime, should be given as an adjunct to atropine therapy.

In parkinsonism oral administration of atropine, with increasing doses until the limit of tolerance is reached, is often effective in relieving the muscular rigidity which impairs the speech, writing, and locomotion of patients with this disease. However, newer drugs (see below) are more commonly employed.

SYNTHETIC SUBSTITUTES

Gastrointestinal Antispasmodics

During the past few decades, a great number of synthetic atropine-like drugs with greater musculotropic spasmolytic action but less anticholinergic action have been introduced for clinical use in the hope that they (1) would be more effective than atropine in the treatment of peptic ulcer, pylorospasm, hyperperistalsis, spastic colon, and similar conditions, and (2) would have fewer side effects like dryness of the mouth or interference with accommodation. Most of these drugs act by three mechanisms: muscarinic blockade, direct depression of smooth muscle, and nicotinic blockade of parasympathetic ganglia. None of these newer drugs has been demonstrated conclusively to produce selectively the desired effect; all, like atropine, show undesirable side effects at other cholinergically innervated sites. The list of drugs includes a number of quaternary ammonium derivatives (e.g., propantheline, methscopolamine, tridihexethyl, anisotropine, mepenzolate, isopropamide, glycopyrrolate, clidinium and hexocyclium) and a tertiary amine (dicyclomine). A short discussion of propantheline will serve to describe the pharmacologic characteristics of the aforementioned drugs.

Propantheline Bromide The pharmacologic actions of this compound are qualitatively identical with those of atropine. The quaternary nitrogen (Fig. 10-2) makes the compound more polar, and thus it has less action on the CNS than atropine. In contrast to atro-

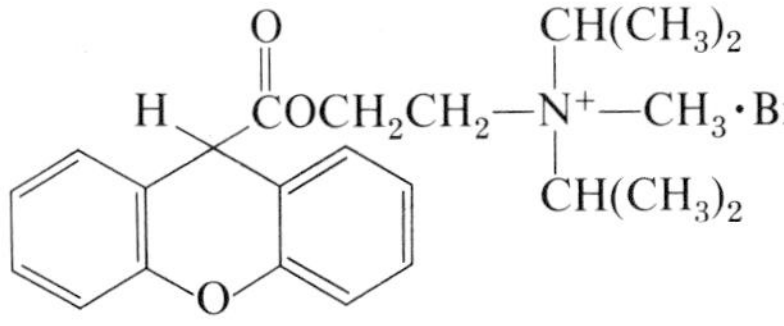

Propantheline bromide

FIGURE 10-2 Structure of propantheline bromide.

pine, propantheline has a high ratio of ganglionic blocking to antimuscarinic activity. Moreover, an unusual toxicity with overdosage is the production of neuromuscular blockade resembling a curare-like action. These actions may be attributed to the quaternary nitrogen and rather bulky rings and side chain.

Biotransformation is by hydrolysis, which begins even in the intestinal tract. After a single oral dose of 15 to 30 mg, peak serum concentrations occur in about 1 h. Plasma half-life is about 2 h. Only 5 percent is excreted in the urine as intact propantheline.

Overdosage produces toxicities similar to atropine. Additive effects are seen when combined with tricyclic antidepressants, antiparkinsonism drugs, quinidine, phenothiazines, antihistamines, and procainamide, all of which have antimuscarinic activity. Therapy of severe poisoning requires the use of intravenous physostigmine, sodium thiopental or diazepam to combat CNS agitation, and artificial respiration if progression of the curare-like respiratory muscle paralysis occurs.

Compounds Used in Ophthalmology

In the refraction of children, a potent cycloplegic is generally employed: atropine sulfate (1%) or scopolamine hydrobromide (0.5%). These drugs are also used in the treatment of acute iritis and other conditions where a potent, long-acting mydriatic is required.

Adults under the age of 40, in whom tension on the suspensory ligament of the lens is diminished, are generally refracted with shorter-acting, less potent cycloplegics such as homatropine hydrobromide (1%). After the age of 40, the use of cycloplegics for routine refraction is generally omitted. The ciliary muscle then exerts relatively little tone, and the danger of precipitating an attack of glaucoma by application of an antimuscarinic is present.

Less potent analogs that produce mydriasis of brief duration with relatively little cycloplegia are useful in performing ophthalmoscopic examinations (Table 10-1). The list includes cyclopentolate and tropicamide. Sympathomimetic agents such as epinephrine and phenylephrine can also be used as adjuncts to produce mydriasis (see Chap. 7).

Antiparkinsonian Agents

Atropine was the first effective drug introduced for the symptomatic treatment of parkinsonism. In contrast with the gastrointestinal antispasmodics, several synthetic compounds which cross the blood-brain barrier have proved to be much more effective. The list includes trihexyphenidyl, ethopropazine, benztropine, procyclidine, orphenadrine, and biperiden.

While levodopa is now generally considered to be the drug of choice in the treatment of parkinsonism (see Chap. 21), clinical experience in recent years has revealed its limitations. Among these is its restricted duration of efficacy. Consequently it is often preferable to initiate therapy with an anticholinergic agent and continue with such until more effective therapy is required. In addition, the drugs in the foregoing list are effective in controlling the parkinsonian side effects that frequently occur during therapy with antipsychotic drugs (phenothiazines, haloperidol). The pharmacology of the antimuscarinic drugs used in parkinsonism is discussed in Chap. 21.

TABLE 10-1   **Summary of peak and duration of mydriasis and cycloplegia with topical antimuscarinic drugs**

	Mydriasis		Cycloplegia	
Drug	Peak, min	Recovery, days	Peak, min	Recovery, days
Atropine (1%)	30–40	7–12	60–180	6–12
Homatropine (1%)	40–60	1–3	30–60	1–3
Scopolamine (0.5%)	20–30	3–7	30–60	3–7
Cyclopentolate (0.5–1%)	30–60	1	25–75	0.25–1
Tropicamide	20–40	0.25	20–35	0.25

GANGLIONIC BLOCKING DRUGS

During the 1950s and early 1960s, the ganglionic blocking agents were practically the only drugs available for the treatment of essential hypertension. They have now been almost totally superseded by more satisfactory agents (Chap. 31), and their clinical uses are few. However, they illustrate a number of important pharmacologic principles.

Mechanism of Action

The primary event in sympathetic and parasympathetic ganglionic transmission is the release of acetylcholine by the presynaptic nerve terminals. The neurotransmitter combines with nicotinic I receptors at the immediate subsynaptic site and, after a latent period of approximately 1 ms, results in the initial excitatory postsynaptic potential (EPSP); this in turn gives rise to action potentials in the postganglionic nerve fibers. However, subsequent events probably modify this process. These events include (1) the inhibitory postsynaptic potential (IPSP), which occurs after a latency of approximately 35 ms and involves both muscarinic (M) receptors probably found on small intraganglionic neurons that release norepinephrine or dopamine and stimulate α-adrenergic receptors on the postganglionic neuronal membrane; (2) the late EPSP, which occurs at about 300 ms and results from activation of postganglionic M receptors; and (3) the late slow EPSP, which occurs considerably later and persists for several minutes. The late slow EPSP is produced by various peptides released along with acetylcholine from the presynaptic terminals. While the physiologic significance of these modulatory influences is still obscure, it is clear that ganglion cells contain M and N I receptors, which accounts for cellular activation by muscarinic as well as by nicotinic agonists.

Ganglionic blocking agents can effectively block ganglionic transmission in both divisions of the autonomic nervous system by interacting with N I receptors on the postsynaptic membrane. These drugs can be classified into two groups: (1) *depolarizing ganglionic blocking drugs* and (2) *antidepolarizing blocking drugs*.

Depolarizing blocking drugs complex with and activate nicotinic I receptors of the ganglia, producing depolarization of the postganglionic neuronal membrane, as does acetylcholine, and then block transmission by persistent depolarization. Thus, these drugs have both a ganglionic stimulant and blocking action. Examples of drugs in this class are nicotine and lobeline. Since both of these are used therapeutically for their agonistic properties, the pharmacology of nicotine and lobeline is discussed in Chap. 9. The synthetic compounds, tetramethylammonium (TMA) and dimethylphenyl piperazinium (DMPP), also stimulate autonomic ganglia by activating nicotinic I receptors in the same manner as nicotine. However, they have a considerably wider range between the stimulant and depressant doses. They are used only as laboratory tools.

Antidepolarizing blocking drugs act as competitive antagonists of acetylcholine at the nicotinic ganglionic receptors. These agents possess a high affinity for the receptor site but lack intrinsic activity and therefore prevent the development of the initial EPSP; in this way they can produce total ganglionic blockade. Examples of drugs in this class include mecamylamine and trimethaphan. *d*-Tubocurarine acts similarly at both ganglionic synapses and the motor end plate of skeletal muscles.

Effects on Organ Systems

Theoretically, ganglionic blocking agents can abolish all autonomic activity. The effects that follow their administration reflect the predominance of sympathetic (adrenergic) or parasympathetic (cholinergic) tone before they were given. At the arteries and veins, adrenergic tone normally predominates. Accordingly, these drugs cause arteriolar vasodilatation with decreased peripheral resistance; venous dilatation leads to pooling of blood, diminished return to the heart, and decreased cardiac output. Both these effects result in hypotension with relatively little compromise of peripheral blood flow, the desired therapeutic effect. At the same time they cause orthostatic hypotension, an undesirable side effect.

At all other autonomic effectors, parasympathetic cholinergic tone normally predominates. These, and the consequences of their blockade, are the other side effects of the ganglionic blocking agents. They include the heart (tachycardia), iris (mydriasis), ciliary muscle (cycloplegia), gastrointestinal tract (reduced motility, constipation), urinary bladder (retention), salivary glands (xerostomia), and sweat glands (anhydrosis).

In addition to the foregoing side effects, the other limitations of the ganglionic blocking agents are their poor and irregular absorption from the gastrointestinal tract and the development of tolerance to their therapeutic effect in most patients.

The most surprising feature of the hemodynamic studies following the use of a ganglionic blocking drug is the improvement in allocation or distribution of cardiac output in favor of the heart and brain. Observations in humans indicate that after the autonomic nervous system is blocked the local regulatory mechanisms (such as the metabolic control of cerebral and coronary vessels) and the local unidentified vascular (autoregulatory) factors in the kidney and splanchnic bed come into play. These mechanisms, which are independent of the autonomic nervous system, are active in normotensive and hypertensive individuals and account for the relative safety of the use of autonomic blocking agents in antihypertensive therapy. Without these nonautonomic mechanisms, cerebral and coronary insufficiency, manifested by fainting and cardiac arrhythmias, would be more frequently encountered.

Mecamylamine   A secondary amine, mecamylamine, was introduced to overcome the problem of absorption following oral administration, common with most older quaternary amine ganglionic blocking drugs; it is absorbed practically completely. However, its structure also allows it to penetrate the blood-brain barrier so that it occasionally produces the additional side effects of malaise, choreiform movements, mania, and convulsions in some patients.

Mecamylamine is excreted slowly in the urine in an unmetabolized form. The drug has a long duration of action and generally can be taken two or three times daily.

At the present time, mecamylamine is the only ganglionic blocking agent administered orally for the treatment of essential hypertension. However, because of the development of tolerance and with the introduction of many other antihypertensive drugs (see Chap. 31), the routine use of mecamylamine in severe hypertension is no longer necessary.

Trimethaphan Camsylate   This differs from the foregoing drug in its extremely brief duration of action due probably to its rapid metabolism. In addition to blocking nicotinic I receptors, trimethaphan also exerts a direct peripheral vasodilator effect and liberates histamine from mast cells. By inducing vasodilation it causes blood to pool in the dependent periphery and the splanchnic system and reduces blood pressure. Trimethaphan is used for the production of controlled hypotension in surgery when a bloodless operative field is required. It is also used in the emergency treatment of pulmonary edema from acute left ventricular failure, for reducing blood pressure in acute dissecting aortic aneuryism, and in hypertensive crises. Since it is a charged compound it is not effective by the oral route and will not elicit significant CNS effects. Trimethaphan is administered by the intravenous infusion of a 0.1% solution in 5% dextrose at a rate of approximately 1.0 mL/min, with continuous monitoring of blood pressure; shortly after termination of the infusion, its effect wears off.

BIBLIOGRAPHY

Eger, E. L., II: "Atropine, Scopolamine, and Related Substances," *Anesthesiology*, **23**:365–383 (1962).

Hirschowitz, E. I., et al. (eds.): "Subtypes of Muscarinic Receptors," *Trends in Pharmacol. Sci.*, Suppl., 1–103 (1984).

Jan, Y. N., C. W. Bowers, D. Branton, L. Evans, and L. Y. Jan: "Peptides in Neuronal Function: Studies Using Frog Autonomic Ganglia," *Cold Spring Harbor Symp. Quant. Biol.*, **43**:363–374 (1983).

Paton, W. D. M., and E. J. Zaimis: "The Methonium Compounds," *Pharmacol. Rev.*, **4**:219–253 (1952).

Volle, R. L.: "Nicotinic Ganglion-Stimulating Agents," in D. A. Kharkevich (ed.), *Pharmacology of Ganglionic Transmission*, Springer-Verlag, Berlin, 1980, pp. 281–312.

Skeletal-Muscle Relaxants

Edward J. Barbieri

The skeletal-muscle relaxants are a diverse group of chemical compounds that share the capacity to interfere with the contraction of voluntary muscles. Some of these drugs are able to completely paralyze skeletal muscle; these compounds are used predominantly as adjuncts to anesthesia during surgical and orthopedic procedures in the controlled confines of the hospital environment. Other drugs in this broad category elicit a more modulatory effect on muscle contraction and do not completely block the activity of the skeletal musculature. These agents are useful in reducing muscle spasms and/or spasticity associated with myopathies and are commonly used in ambulatory patients.

Although the above separation of compounds is an appropriate therapeutic classification, the drugs discussed here are divided pharmacologically based on the site and mechanism of action. Three categories of drugs will be presented: (1) *neuromuscular blocking agents:* peripherally acting muscle relaxants that act at the myoneural junction and impair the transmission of impulses from somatic neurons to skeletal-muscle membranes; (2) a *direct-acting muscle relaxant:* one compound that acts directly on the muscle fiber by blocking the contractile process; and (3) *centrally acting drugs:* agents which depress the transmission of motor impulses at synapses within the central nervous system.

NEUROMUSCULAR BLOCKING AGENTS

These compounds block transmission from the motor nerve ending to skeletal-muscle fibers. Under the influence of these drugs, nerve conduction is not impaired and the muscle is capable of contraction following direct stimulation. The effect of the neuromuscular blocking agents is usually transitory, and recovery is complete upon cessation of drug administration.

Chemistry

Originally, neuromuscular blocking agents were extracted from *curare,* a generic term used to describe various resinous mixtures of paralyzing arrow poisons used by South American natives. Today synthetic neuromuscular blocking agents, including tubocurarine, an active alkaloid from curare, are used exclusively, and these are known as *curariform drugs.* The structural formulas of representative neuromuscular blocking agents are shown in Fig. 11-1. Tubocurarine and most other synthetic curariform agents contain two or more quaternary nitrogen groups (approximately 1.0 ± 0.1 nm apart), which appear to be important to the ability of the drugs to bind to nicotinic II receptors.

Mechanism of Action

By electron microscopy it has been estimated that the nicotinic II receptor density at the skeletal-muscle end plate is $10,000/\mu m^2$. Each nicotinic cholinergic receptor of the neuromuscular junction is envisioned to be an asymmetric complex of five proteins. This 250,000-dalton pentamer extends completely through the mus-

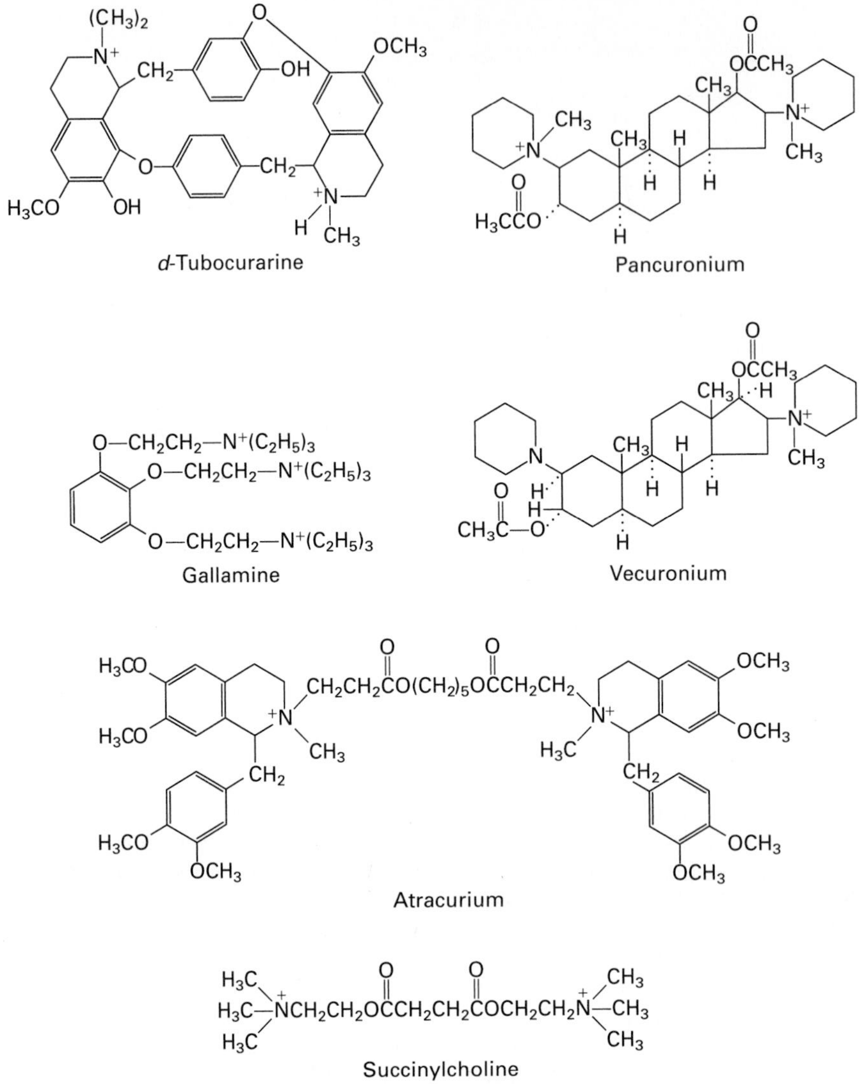

FIGURE 11-1   Structures of some neuromuscular blocking agents.

cle membrane and is composed of four subunits (two alpha, one each beta, gamma, and delta) arranged around a single Na^+-K^+ ion channel as shown in Fig. 11-2. The alpha subunits contain the primary recognition sites for the endogenous neurotransmitter, acetylcholine, and these proteins are also the sites for binding of the antagonists that act as neuromuscular blocking agents.

Following acetylcholine release from storage vesi-

cles of activated motor neurons, the neurotransmitter diffuses across the synaptic cleft and binds to the alpha subunits of the nicotinic II receptors. When one acetylcholine molecule binds to each alpha subunit, a conformational change occurs in the protein complex, opening the central ion channel (for about 1 ms) and making the muscle membrane permeable to the influx of Na^+ and the efflux of K^+. The ion flow induces a postjunctional end-plate potential, which gives rise to

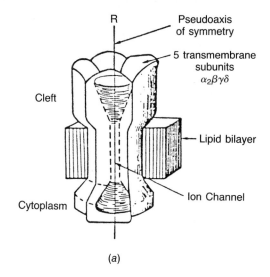

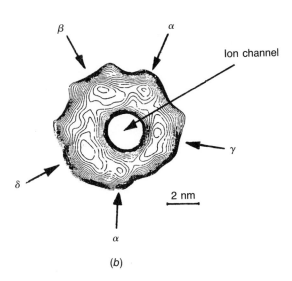

FIGURE 11-2 Morphology of the nicotinic II receptor. (*a*) Schematic model of the side view of the pentamer complex of the nicotinic receptor within the membrane of the neuromuscular junction. (*b*) Cross-sectional view of the asymmetric protein receptor complex showing the proposed positions of the alpha (α), beta (β), delta (δ), and gamma (γ) subunits relative to the central ion channel. [From J. -P. Changeux, A. Devillers-Thiery, and P. Chemouilli, *Science*, **225**:1335–1345 (1984).]

a propagated muscle action potential. The muscle action potential spreads throughout the myofibril conduction system and the muscle contracts.

When the muscle relaxes, it is refractory to another stimulus until repolarization of the muscle end plate is complete. This requires dissociation of acetylcholine from the nicotinic II receptor, reestablishment of the Na^+ and K^+ gradients across the membrane, and hydrolysis of acetylcholine by acetylcholinesterase located in the synaptic cleft. Neuromuscular blocking agents can depress skeletal-muscle contraction either by (1) preventing acetylcholine-induced depolarization of the muscle end plate, i.e., the *nondepolarizing drugs*, or (2) blocking repolarization of the muscle end plate, i.e., the *depolarizing neuromuscular blocking agents*.

Nondepolarizing Drugs Compounds in this group, which are also referred to as *antidepolarizing* or *competitive blocking agents*, include tubocurarine, metocurine, gallamine, pancuronium, vecuronium, and atracurium. The mechanism of action is competition by the blocking agent for the postsynaptic nicotinic II receptors. These drugs have affinity for, but no intrinsic activity on, the acetylcholine-binding sites on the alpha subunit of the nicotinic II receptor complex. Since two molecules of an agonist are required to open the ionic channel, binding of one molecule of antagonist to the receptor will cause it to be nonfunctional. If a sufficient number of receptors are occupied by the antagonist, the number activated by acetylcholine will be too small to lead to the production of an end-plate potential large enough to reach threshold for activation of the adjacent electrically excitable membrane. Thus transmission fails.

Depolarizing Drugs Succinylcholine is the only therapeutically useful neuromuscular blocker that acts as a *depolarizing agent* which blocks muscle repolarization. In contrast to the nondepolarizing agents, succinylcholine is not a competitive antagonist but rather a more stable agonist than acetylcholine: that is, as far as its action is concerned, succinylcholine differs from the transmitter acetylcholine only in duration of action. Both agents act at the same receptor, and with both, channel opening and depolarization of the end-plate regions result. Succinylcholine is inactivated more slowly than acetylcholine and, since it lasts longer in the synapse, differs only from the neurotransmitter in that it produces a persistent depolarization.

The persistent depolarization of the end plate leads, by local circuit action, to a persistent depolarization of the adjacent electrically excitable membrane of the muscle. This brief period of repetitive excitation appears as an initial muscle fasciculation on administration of succinylcholine. Since succinylcholine remains in the synaptic cleft for a relatively long period of time (in comparison to acetylcholine), the repolarization process is blocked and a flaccid paralysis results. This is *phase i* of the action of succinylcholine. Although stable depolarizing blocking agents can produce a depolarization which is quite prolonged compared with that produced by acetylcholine, they do not produce a depolarization of indefinite duration. Despite continued exposure to the depolarizing agent, the end plate does not stay depolarized to a constant extent and loses its reponsiveness to the depolarizing agent, i.e., it becomes desensitized. Since the action of the neurotransmitter is identical to that of the more stable depolarizing agent, the neurotransmitter loses its effectiveness as well. A situation is reached, therefore, where the depolarizing drug may no longer be present but the neuromuscular block persists. This is called a *phase ii block*, a *nondepolarization block*, or *desensitization block*.

Pharmacologic Actions

Neuromuscular Blockade   When a neuromuscular blocking agent is administered, a flaccid paralysis of the voluntary musculature develops. The muscles which produce fine movements (for example, the extraocular muscles and muscles of the head, face, and neck) are most sensitive to these drugs and are blocked first. Muscles of the trunk, abdomen, and extremities are affected next; respiratory muscles are the most resistant to blockade with paralysis affecting the intercostals prior to the diaphragm. Recovery of the musculature occurs in the reverse order following the cessation of drug administration.

When a depolarizing neuromuscular blocking agent (e.g., succinylcholine) is administered, the block is preceded by fasciculation, especially if the drug is given rapidly. Soon the fasciculation ceases, and the muscles become quiescent and superficially indistinguishable from those blocked by a competitive blocking agent.

The skeletal-muscle relaxant activity of the competitive neuromuscular blocking agents is enhanced by certain inhalational general anesthetics, e.g., halothane, enflurane, and isoflurane; these drugs appear to stabilize the neuromuscular membrane. Aminoglycoside antibiotics, such as streptomycin, neomycin, kanamycin, gentamicin, and tobramycin, inhibit acetylcholine release from cholinergic neurons and thus enhance neuromuscular blockade. Tetracyclines, clindamycin, polymyxin B, and colistin also increase the effect of curariform drugs by undetermined mechanisms. Enhanced neuromuscular blockade has occurred in antiarrhythmic therapy with quinidine and lidocaine. Fluid and electrolyte imbalances, such as acidosis, dehydration, and hypokalemia (produced by certain diuretics), will also enhance neuromuscular blockade. Postoperative respiratory depression due to neuromuscular blockade enhancement by quinine, magnesium, and lithium carbonate can occur. Patients with myasthenia gravis are extremely sensitive to nondepolarizing neuromuscular blocking agents.

The antagonism of neuromuscular blockade induced by the nondepolarizing blocking drugs is approached by the administration of a cholinesterase antagonist so that acetylcholine released from the motor neurons will reach the end plate in higher concentrations and therefore will compete more effectively for the nicotinic receptor. Drugs such as neostigmine, pyridostigmine, and edrophonium are useful in this regard (see Chap. 9). The choice of dose is not too critical, the antagonism is clear-cut, and the effect is well maintained. It seems that the action of these drugs is the result of a presynaptic action, an action to block cholinesterase, or a combination of both. There may also be a contribution from a direct depolarizing action on the nicotinic receptor.

Cholinesterase inhibitors should not be used in an attempt to reverse the action of the depolarizing blocker succinylcholine. Since succinylcholine is biotransformed via acetylcholinesterase at the neuromuscular junction, the use of a cholinesterase inhibitor would prolong the skeletal-muscle relaxant effect of this drug.

Ganglionic Blockade   Tubocurarine and metocurine are capable of producing ganglionic blockade at high therapeutic doses, which is, in part, responsible for the hypotension and tachycardia that may occur.

However, because the potency of these drugs is still greater at the neuromuscular junction than at autonomic ganglia, in most cases a prominant effect on the ganglia during clinical use is rarely observed. None of the other drugs shows any significant ganglionic blocking activity.

Histamine Resease Tubocurarine is a potent liberator of histamine from mast cells, which can account quantitatively for an episode of hypotension during anesthesia. Histamine release can also produce bronchospasm or an increase in respiratory tract secretion and is occasionally seen following the administration of tubocurarine or metocurine. Although other peripherally acting neuromuscular blocking agents possess the general structural properties for this action, they do not act as potent histamine releasers. However, histamine release can be problematic with these drugs at high therapeutic doses.

Pharmacokinetics

Since all clinically employed neuromuscular blocking agents are charged, independent of pH, absorption from the gastrointestinal tract is very poor; therefore, all these drugs are administered intravenously. For the same reason these drugs are largely distributed to the extracellular space only. The apparent volume of distribution for these drugs is low (0.15 to 0.45 L/kg); plasma protein binding is variable, with pancuronium being the highest of the group at about 87 percent and metocurine one of the lowest at 35 percent. Elimination is predominantly via the urine and, to a lesser extent, through the bile. Since the molecular charge will prevent reabsorption across the tubular membrane in the kidney, all the drugs that cross the glomerular membrane will be excreted. The major differences with respect to the pharmacokinetics of these drugs is in their biotransformation and elimination half-lives.

A negligible fraction of tubocurarine is metabolized. This drug, as well as its methyl derivative metocurine, contains few unstable bonds, and the only reactive groups (the charged quaternary heads) are not susceptible to conjugation, oxidation, or reduction. The elimination half-life of tubocurarine is between 2 and 3 h; that of metocurine is about 3.5 h. Both drugs appear to be eliminated primarily via the kidney. Gallamine is also reasonably inert. Its ether linkages are

stable, and so, like the aforementioned drugs, it is removed primarily by glomerular filtration. Such agents exert a prolonged action in patients with anuria.

Pancuronium and vecuronium are eliminated primarily unaltered by the kidneys, although up to 25 percent of these drugs may be deacetylated, mainly to a 3-hydroxy derivative but also to 17-hydroxy and 3,17-dihydroxy derivatives. 3-Hydroxypancuronium and 3-hydroxyvecuronium are about 50 percent as active as their parent compounds as neuromuscular blocking agents; the other metabolites are essentially inactive. Some of the unchanged pancuronium may undergo biliary excretion; up to 50 percent of vecuronium may be eliminated by this route. The elimination $t_{1/2}$ of pancuronium is 1.5 to 2.5 h, whereas that of vecuronium is only about 1 h.

As shown in Fig. 11-1, atracurium is a complex molecule with two ester groups joined by a 5-carbon chain. The drug is inactivated in plasma by two nonoxidation pathways: (1) ester hydrolysis, catalyzed by nonspecific esterases, and (2) a spontaneous chemical reaction at physiologic pH in which the carbon bridge is split from the quaternary nitrogens (known as Hofmann elimination). The metabolites and any remaining atracurium are eliminated through both the urine and the bile. The elimination $t_{1/2}$ of this drug is only 20 min.

Of all the neuromuscular blocking agents, succinylcholine is biotransformed most rapidly. It contains two ester bonds and is an excellent substrate for plasma pseudocholinesterase. The product of the hydrolysis is succinylmonocholine (an active product), which is also broken down by pseudocholinesterase to succinic acid and choline. Since the second stage is about 6 times slower than the first, appreciable quantities of the monocholine ester can accumulate, particularly during prolonged administration. The potency of the monocholine ester (about $\frac{1}{20}$ that of the dicholine ester) is great enough to contribute to the neuromuscular blockade.

The rapid destruction of succinylcholine not only makes the action brief ($t_{1/2}$ about 5 min) but also facilitates rapid onset. A larger dose can be given so that the effective concentration at the muscle end plate will be reached sooner, without prolonging unduly the overall duration of action. This feature has made succinylcholine popular for facilitation of endotracheal intubation during general anesthesia.

About one person in 3000 has atypical plasma cholinesterase which destroys succinylcholine less rapidly. If such a patient is given the usual dose of succinylcholine, an overdose will result, and this will bring on prolonged apnea. The problem should be regarded as a form of overdosing as well as a situation in which the terminal phase of drug elimination is slowed.

Succinylcholine also breaks down spontaneously by alkaline hydrolysis at a slow rate but fast enough to contribute to the biotransformation of the drug.

Since the neuromuscular blocking agents are charged ions, no marked transfer across the placenta would be expected. Some evidence of transfer has been reported for gallamine and tubocurarine, but it is negligible.

Effects on Organ Systems

Cardiovascular System Cardioacceleration, increased cardiac output, and mild hypertension may be seen with gallamine. These effects seem to be the result of both an atropine-like antimuscarinic action and a tyramine-like effect of the drug, whereby norepinephrine is released from the sympathetic nerve endings supplying the pacemaker region of the heart and the vasculature. Pancuronium also causes increases in heart rate, cardiac output, and blood pressure. These changes are moderate and have been attributed to four distinct actions: (1) blockade of the negative chronotropic and inotropic actions of acetylcholine, (2) release of norepinephrine from postganglionic adrenergic fibers, (3) blockade of the re-uptake of catecholamines into adrenergic terminals, and (4) a direct sympathomimetic effect. Although both tachycardia and bradycardia have been observed with the other neuromuscular blocking agents, these are not significant effects clinically.

Central Nervous System The charge on all these compounds makes permeation of the blood-brain barrier negligible, so that central nervous system effects are not observed in clinical practice.

Potassium Levels Depolarizing neuromuscular blocking agents liberate potassium from skeletal muscles. The continuous action of a depolarizing agent can lead to an elevation of the plasma potassium concentration. This should be borne in mind when patients are encountered who will need prolonged administra-

tion of a neuromuscular blocking agent and whose electrolyte concentrations are already disturbed.

Eye Succinylcholine can cause a slight increase in intraocular pressure immediately after its injection and during the fasciculation phase. This is usually attributed to a sustained contraction of the extraocular muscles. This effect is transient, and the drug is not contraindicated in patients with glaucoma.

Therapeutic Uses

Anesthesia The purpose of anesthesia is not only to render the patient insensible to pain but also, where possible, to facilitate surgery. Normally the motor nerves carry a constant low level of traffic to the skeletal muscles. These signals induce a contraction of only a small fraction of the muscle fibers at any time, but the activity of these fibers place a slight tension on the muscle which prepares it for more intense activity at a moment's notice. This background state of light contraction is called *muscle tone*. It can be a nuisance during anesthesia when the surgeon must struggle against it to reduce a fracture or when the tone in the flat muscles of the abdomen tends to expel the abdominal contents through an abdominal incision. Before the advent of neuromuscular blocking agents, larger doses of the anesthetic than were required simply to produce unconsciousness had to be administered in order to stop the tonic outflow at the source. General anesthetics, however, have a rather low margin of safety; the concentrations required for muscle relaxation are too close to stage IV of anesthesia. It is therefore desirable to use a second agent to abolish muscle tone so that lower concentrations of the general anesthetic can be used. The neuromuscular blocking agents have proved to be a satisfactory group of agents for this role. They have subsequently found even wider use during induction of anesthesia when they are given to relax the laryngeal muscles and thereby facilitate endotracheal intubation.

Electroshock Therapy When electroshock therapy is used in the treatment of psychiatric disorders, muscular contraction can be intense enough to cause fractures. Since the therapeutic effect of the convulsion does not depend on the muscular response, prior administration of a neuromuscular blocking agent can be used to abolish the muscular component. The chief hazard that may be encountered is a synergism between the drug and a postictal depression of respiration. Preparations should be made to maintain the airway and assist respiration if necessary. Succinylcholine is the most popular agent for this purpose; its short duration of action apparently outweighs its propensity to produce fasciculations and the ensuing discomfort.

Controlled Respiration   When a patient is unable to ventilate well enough to maintain a normal arterial P_{O2} and P_{CO2} or is becoming exhausted in the attempts to do so, it is advantageous to assist or control respiration by means of a mechanical ventilator. Controlled respiration is often ineffective because the patient's attempts to breathe are not synchronous with the cycle of the respirator. Frequently sedation and depression of the respiratory center with opioids will improve the situation, but occasionally it is necessary to block all respiratory effort. Intravenous competitive blocking agents are most satisfactory. Often repeated administration is not needed, since the return of arterial blood-gas tensions to normal with the improved ventilation reduces the stimulus to increased respiration, and the patient no longer "fights" the respirator. Alert patients should be sedated while paralyzed.

Myasthenia Gravis   Patients with myasthenia gravis are especially sensitive to the competitive neuromuscular blocking agents. Diagnosis of this disease can be facilitated in a borderline case by the use of a test dose of tubocurarine. However, tubocurarine is not used unless the more conventional tests with neostigmine or edrophonium have shown equivocal results.

Adverse Reactions

The most important adverse reaction to the neuromuscular blocking agents is apnea, which may extend into the postoperative period and may require artificial respiration over long periods. This may result following overdosage or, in the case of succinylcholine, may be due to the patient's inability to adequately biotransform the drug. The nondepolarizing blockers, such as tubocurarine and pancuronium, can be antagonized by cholinesterase inhibitors.

Other mild and infrequent adverse reactions that have occurred with the nondepolarizing drugs include bradycardia, tachycardia, hypotension, hypertension, bronchospasm, excessive salivation, and rash. In addition to those reactions listed above, succinylcholine may cause hyperkalemia, postoperative muscle pain, and malignant hyperthermia.

DIRECT-ACTING SKELETAL-MUSCLE RELAXANT

Dantrolene

Dantrolene is a substituted hydantoin that relieves spasticity by an action on muscle. Unlike all other skeletal-muscle relaxants, this agent acts directly on the contractile mechanism of skeletal-muscle by interfering with the release of calcium from the sarcoplasmic reticulum. This results in uncoupling the excitation-contraction mechanism of skeletal muscles and is more pronounced in fast muscle fibers than in slow ones. Dantrolene will depress the CNS; however, its skeletal-muscle relaxant effects do not appear to be mediated by actions on neurons.

Gastrointestinal absorption of dantrolene is incomplete and slow but consistent. The mean biologic half-life is approximately 9 h after oral dosing and 4 to 8 h following IV administration. Dantrolene is slowly biotransformed to inactive hydroxy and acetamino derivatives, which, along with the parent drug, are excreted in the urine.

Dantrolene is used orally for controlling the manifestations of clinical spasticity resulting from serious chronic disorders such as injury, stroke, cerebral palsy, and multiple sclerosis. It is not recommended for the treatment for skeletal-muscle spasms resulting from rheumatic disorders.

Because dantrolene interferes with the release of calcium from the sarcoplasmic reticulum to the myoplasma, it is also used in the therapy of life-threatening malignant hyperthermia caused by many inhalational general anesthetics and succinylcholine. For this purpose the drug is administered either orally or intravenously as soon as the malignant hyperthermia reaction is recognized. It can also be given preoperatively to prevent the development of this syndrome in patients who are judged to be susceptible to malignant hyperthermia.

The most frequent adverse effects of dantrolene are diarrhea, weakness, drowsiness, fatigue, dizziness, and general malaise. These are generally transient and disappear with continued drug use. The most serious adverse reaction is potentially fatal hepatocellular disease.

CENTRALLY ACTING SKELETAL-MUSCLE RELAXANTS

Unfortunately, skeletal-muscle paralysis achieved by curare-like drugs is not clinically useful in the large variety of common clinical spasticity states accompanying central nervous system lesions and local injury and inflammation. Neuromuscular block can relieve the spasm, but it also results in loss of voluntary control. The aim in conditions of muscle spasticity is to find an agent that relieves the painful muscle spasm without loss of voluntary muscle function and without impairment of cerebral function.

Many CNS depressants cause muscular relaxation. Notable among these are the alcohols and the barbiturates, but these are ordinarily of no use since they also produce marked sedation and other untoward effects.

The search for selective central nervous system agents capable of achieving muscular relaxation has produced a number of interesting compounds, none of which has been completely successful. Nevertheless, centrally acting skeletal-muscle relaxants are widely used in the treatment of sprains, arthritis, bursitis, and similar musculoskeletal disorders. This use is based on the assumption that spasms originating through spinal cord reflexes can be depressed by these muscle relaxants.

A number of heterogenous chemical compounds act within the spinal cord and depress monosynaptic and polysynaptic reflexes. Some of these are baclofen, cyclobenzaprine, carisoprodol, methocarbamol, chlorphenesin, chlorzoxazone, orphenadrine, and diazepam. The pharmacology of diazepam is presented in detail in Chap. 16. Baclofen and cyclobenzaprine are briefly discussed here as representative centrally acting skeletal-muscle relaxants.

Baclofen

$$H_2NCH_2CHCH_2COH$$

An analog of the inhibitory neurotransmitter gamma aminobutyric acid (GABA), baclofen reduces transmission at monosynaptic extensor and polysynaptic flexor reflex pathways in the spinal cord; actions at supraspinal sites may also contribute to the effect of the drug. In the spinal cord the action of baclofen appears to occur presynaptically and involves the interaction with, and activation of, specific $GABA_B$ receptors, which leads to the inhibition of release of excitatory neurotransmitters.

Baclofen is well absorbed following oral administration. Peak blood concentration is reached in 2 to 3 h. Plasma protein binding is only about 30 percent. Little of the compound is biotransformed; 70 to 85 percent of a dose is excreted unchanged by the kidney. The half-life of the drug is 3 to 4 h.

Baclofen is indicated for alleviating the signs and symptoms of muscle spasticity due to muscular sclerosis, clonus, and muscular rigidity. The drug may also be effective in patients with muscle spasms resulting from spinal cord injuries and other spinal diseases.

Drowsiness, dizziness, weakness, fatigue, confusion, headache, and insomnia are the most common adverse reactions observed with baclofen. These are often transient and will disappear with continued therapy. Gastrointestinal complaints including nausea, anorexia, and constipation may occur; hypotension and increased urinary frequency have also been reported.

Cyclobenzaprine

A compound which is structurally and pharmacologically related to the tricyclic antidepressants, cyclobenzaprine relieves muscle spasm associated with a variety of musculoskeletal conditions without interfering with skeletal-muscle function. The drug acts primarily at the level of the brain stem, although it has some activity at spinal motor neurons, which may contribute to its overall skeletal-muscle relaxant effects. The net response to cyclobenzaprine administration is a reduction in tonic somatic motor activity, influencing both descending alpha motor neurons and gamma motor neurons.

Cyclobenzaprine is generally well absorbed orally; however a significant first-pass effect occurs in some patients. Extensive hepatic biotransformation, primarily to inactive glucuronide conjugates, and renal excretion occur quite slowly and result in a half-life of 1 to 3 days. Because of the high plasma protein binding (93 percent) of the drug, cyclobenzaprine is not long-acting, and administration three times daily is recommended for most patients.

The most frequent adverse reactions to this drug are drowsiness, xerostomia, and dizziness. Other adverse effects are similar in nature and incidence to those which are to be expected from a tricyclic compound (see Chap. 20).

PREPARATIONS

Tubocurarine chloride is available as a solution for intravenous injection (3 mg/mL).

Metocurine iodide (Metubine) is available as a 2-mg/mL solution for intravenous injection.

Gallamine triethiodide (Flaxedil) is available as a 20-mg/mL solution for intravenous injection.

Pancuronium bromide (Pavulon) is available as 1- and 2-mg/mL solutions for intravenous injection.

Vecuronium bromide (Norcuron) is available as a lyophilized powder for intravenous injection (10 mg in 5- or 10-mL vials with diluent).

Atracurium besylate (Tracrium) is available as a solution (10 mg/mL) for intravenous injection.

Succinylcholine chloride (Anectine, Quelicin) is available as 20-, 50-, and 100-mg/mL solutions for intravenous or intramuscular injection and 100-, 500-, and 1000-mg vials of powder for injection.

Dantrolene sodium (Dantrium) is available as 25-, 50-, and 100-mg capsules. The drug is also available for intravenous administration as a powder in 20-mg vials.

Baclofen (Lioresal) is available as 10- and 20-mg tablets.

Cyclobenzaprine (Flexeril) is available as 10-mg tablets.

BIBLIOGRAPHY

Argov, Z., and F. L. Mastaglia: "Disorders of Neuromuscular Transmission Caused by Drugs," *N. Engl. J. Med.*, **301**:409–413 (1979).

Burke, D., C. J. Andrews, and L. Knowles: "The Action of a GABA Derivative in Human Spasticity," *J. Neurolog. Sci.*, **14**:199–208 (1971).

Changeux, J. -P., A. Devillers-Thiery, and P. Chemouilli: "Acetylcholine Receptor: An Allosteric Protein," *Science*, **225**:1335–1345 (1984).

Colquhoun, D.: "Mechanisms of Drug Action at the Voluntary Muscle Endplate," *Annu. Rev. Pharmacol.*, **15**:307–326 (1975).

Elenbaas, J. K.: "Centrally Acting Oral Skeletal Muscle Relaxants," *Am. J. Hosp. Pharm.*, **37**:1313–1323 (1980).

Ellis, K. D.: "Mechanisms of Control of Skeletal Muscle Contraction by Dantrolene Sodium," *Arch. Phys. Med. Rehabil.*, **55**:362–369 (1974).

Feldman, S.: "Neuromuscular Blocking Drugs," in H. C. Churchill-Davidson and W. D. Wylie (eds.), *A Practice of Anaesthesia*, 5th ed., Year Book Medical, Chicago, 1984, pp. 722–734.

Hubbard, J. I., and D. M. J. Quastel: "Micropharmacology of Vertebrate Neuromuscular Transmission," *Annu. Rev. Pharmacol.*, **13**:199–216 (1973).

Hughes, R., and D. J. Chapple: "The Pharmacology of Atracurium: A New Competitive Neuromuscular Blocking Agent," *Br. J. Anaesth.*, **53**:31–44 (1981).

Lambert, J. J., N. N. Durant, and E. G. Henderson: "Drug-Induced Modification of Ionic Conductance at the Neuromuscular Junction," *Annu. Rev. Pharmacol. Toxicol.*, **23**:505–539 (1983).

Reilly, C. S., and W. S. Nimmo: "New Intravenous Anaesthetics and Neuromuscular Blocking Drugs," *Drugs*, **34**:98–135 (1987).

Roizen, M. D., and T. W. Feeley: "Pancuronium Bromide," *Ann. Intern. Med.*, **88:**64–68 (1978).

Share, N. N., and C. S. McFarlane: "Cyclobenzaprine: A Novel Centrally Acting Skeletal Muscle Relaxant," *Neuropharmacology*, **14:**675–684 (1975).

Ward, A., M. O. Chaffman, and E. M. Sorkin: "Dantrolene," *Drugs*, **32:**130–168 (1986).

Young, R. R., and P. J. Delwaide: "Drug Therapy: Spasticity," *N. Engl. J. Med.*, **304:**28–33, 96–99 (1981).

PART III

Local Control Substances

SECTION EDITOR

Edward J. Barbieri

Histamine and Histamine Antagonists

Martin A. Wasserman and Leonard S. Jacob

HISTAMINE

The discovery and synthesis of histamine more than 80 years ago was a landmark achievement in pharmacology, immunology, and medicine. This naturally occurring and potent biogenic amine is widely distributed in tissues and is implicated in a variety of physiologic and pathophysiologic processes, although some uncertainty remains. The profound pharmacologic activity of histamine was first demonstrated in the early part of this century by investigations which established that similarities existed between pathophysiologic responses to histamine and to anaphylaxis. Both are characterized by smooth-muscle constriction (e.g., bronchioles, uterus, ileum), signs of inflammation (redness, swelling, edema), vasodepression, and shock-like symptoms. Presently it is known that histamine plays a central role in immediate hypersensitivity (allergic) reactions and is intimately involved in inflammatory responses.

Synthesis, Distribution, Localization, and Binding

Histamine is synthesized in many tissues by the decarboxylation of the amino acid L-histidine catalyzed by the pyridoxal phosphate-dependent enzyme, L-histidine decarboxylase (Fig. 12-1). Unlike its less specific counterpart, aromatic L-amino acid decarboxylase, this enzyme is specific for L-histidine. Histamine may also be ingested from food or formed by bacteria in the gastrointestinal tract; however, these sources do not contribute significantly to the body's store of histamine, since absorbed amounts are catabolized readily in the intestinal mucosa or liver and eliminated in the urine.

Following its synthesis, histamine is distributed and stored. The primary histologic site is the mast cell (especially in perivascular tissues of most organs) in which preformed histamine is stored in localized secretory cytoplasmic granules as a heparin-protease matrix (histamine constitutes approximately 10 percent of the weight of these granules). In the circulation the predominant site of storage is the basophil (the cytologic counterpart of the tissue mast cell), in which histamine is bound to chondroitin sulfate. Generally, histamine becomes pharmacologically active only when released from storage sites. There is scarcely a tissue or organ which does not contain some histamine. Those especially rich in histamine include gastrointestinal tract, lungs, and skin. Smaller amounts are found in the heart, liver, neural tissue, and reproductive mucosa. Furthermore, histamine has also been detected in bodily fluids, e.g., gastric juice, blood, urine, blister fluid, nasal washings, and pus.

Metabolism and Fate

There are two major enzymatic pathways for the metabolism of histamine (Fig. 12-1). Whereas only 2 to 3 percent of histamine is excreted unchanged in the urine, deamination with diamine oxidase (histaminase) and methylation via histamine *N*-methyltrans-

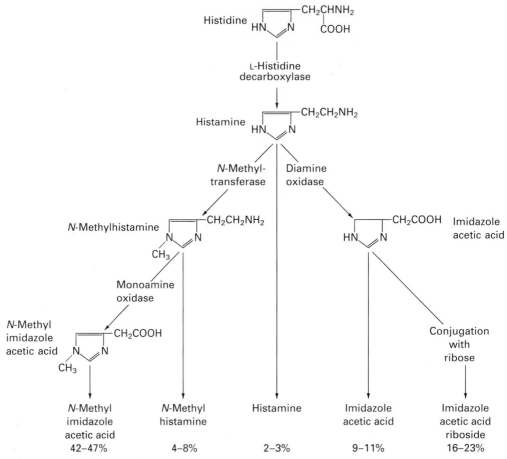

FIGURE 12-1 Pathways of histamine synthesis and catabolism. Major urinary metabolites are listed at the bottom.

ferase account for the bulk of histamine biotransformation. Ring *N*-methylation transfers a methyl group from *S*-adenosylmethionine to histamine in the presence of *N*-methyltransferase (small intestine, liver, kidney, and monocytes). *N*-methylhistamine is either excreted in small amounts (4 to 8 percent) or is deaminated subsequently by monamine oxidase to form *N*-methylimidazole acetic acid, which is the principal urinary metabolite of histamine in humans (42 to 47 percent). The other major catabolic pathway involves oxidative deamination of histamine by diamine oxidase (small intestinal mucosa, liver, skin, kidney, thymus, and leukocytes) to produce imidazole acetic acid,

which is either excreted (9 to 11 percent) or conjugated with ribose and excreted in the urine as imidazole acetic acid riboside (16 to 23 percent). It is interesting that histamine is the only known compound to be metabolized by conjugation with ribose, although the relative importance of this step is unclear.

Release and Inhibitors of Release

Although the liberation of endogenous histamine and other locally acting substances (autocoids) can be stimulated by a wide variety of conditions, perhaps the most important mechanism for induction of mast cell and basophil granule extrusion (exocytosis) and subsequent histamine release is immunologic, i.e., during anaphylaxis and allergy, wherein the specific interaction of immunoglobulin E antibody with antigen on the surface of mast cells and basophils triggers a cascade of biochemical events leading to mediator release without cell membrane disruption (Table 12-1). This "histamine hypothesis" of mediating immediate hypersensitivity reactions has achieved wide acceptance. The secretory behavior of histamine-containing cells is similar to that of exocrine and endocrine gland cells in which an increase in the concentration of intracellular calcium initiates stimulus-secretion coupling.

Individual sensitivity to this immunologic stimulus varies from species to species and person to person. In sensitized individuals, histamine will be produced along with a number of other key mediators of allergy and inflammation, e.g., leukotrienes C_4, D_4, E_4 (constituents of slow-reacting substance of anaphylaxis, "SRS-A"), prostaglandin D_2, thromboxane A_2, bradykinin, and platelet-activating factor. These mediators contribute directly or indirectly to the signs and symptoms of allergic disease.

There are many diverse classes of compounds which can liberate histamine without prior sensitization by affecting the integrity of the mast cell membrane so that the cell loses histamine from its granules. These

include: enzymes and venoms (phospholipase A_2, chymotrypsin, cobra venom), organic bases (morphine, d-tubocurarine), and macromolecular polymers (dextran). Clinically, the actions of some of the above substances may account for unexpected anaphylactoid reactions. In addition, tissue injury (trauma, burns, stress) may release histamine from storage sites possibly via released endogenous polypeptides, e.g., bradykinin.

Histamine release is blocked by various esterase inhibitors (isoflurophate), inhibitors of enzymes involved in energy production (fluoride), and other interfering agents (nicotinamide is a chymotrypsin inhibitor).

Cromolyn sodium is a drug which is presently employed as adjunct therapy in the management of allergic bronchial asthma. It is purported to behave as an inhibitor of mast cell degranulation, perhaps by mast cell membrane stabilization and, thus, is used prophylactically to prevent histamine release during allergic provocations; however, its clinical efficacy must also depend on other, as yet unknown, pharmacologic activities since a number of more effective and more potent mast cell stabilizers have failed clinically. The pharmacology of cromolyn is discussed in depth in Chap. 32.

H_1 and H_2 Receptors

The actions of histamine have been shown pharmacologically to be mediated through two separate and distinct membrane binding sites designated as H_1 and H_2 receptors (Table 12-2). The presence of more than one receptor was first suggested by the observation that the antihistamine mepyramine (pyrilamine) could block histamine-induced contractions of the guinea pig ileum but not affect gastric acid secretions; subsequently the presence of H_2 receptors was confirmed, and the first H_2 antihistamines were discovered. Whereas activation of H_1 receptors produces smooth-muscle contraction and increases in microvascular permeability, which are blocked by "classic" antihistamines, e.g., pyrilamine, diphenhydramine, and chlorpheniramine, stimulation of H_2 receptors mediates an increase in gastric acid secretion which is refractory to H_1 antihistamines but is sensitive to H_2 antihistamines as exemplified by cimetidine, ranitidine, famotidine, and nizatidine. There are some effects of histamine which are mediated by combined H_1 and H_2 stimula-

---

TABLE 12-1 Important biochemical events triggered by antigen-antibody interactions on mast cells and basophils

Activation of proteases

Influx of extracellular calcium via specific membrane channels

Phospholipase A_2 activation and arachidonate metabolism

Phospholipid methylation

Altered levels of cyclic nucleotides

Phosphorylation of a specific protein

Release of histamine and other mediators from the cells

TABLE 12-2   Differentiation of histamine receptor classes

Receptor	Actions	Agonists[a]	Antagonists
H_1	Contraction of bronchial and intestinal smooth muscle Vasodilation Increased capillary permeability Pruritis	2-Methylhistamine 2-Thiazolylethylamine 2-Pyridylethylamine	Chlorpheniramine Diphenhydramine Pyrilamine
H_2	Gastric acid secretion Vasodilation Inhibition of neutrophil activation Inhibition of T-cell cytotoxicity	4-Methylhistamine Dimaprit Impromidine	Cimetidine Ranitidine Famotidine Nizatidine

[a] All experimental compounds.

tion, including vasodilation, flushing, tachycardia, and headache. There are also species differences in the distribution of receptors, e.g., histamine contracts the uterus in most species (through H_1 receptors) but relaxes the uterus in the rat (an H_2-receptor effect). In addition, whereas the mouse and rat are highly resistant to the effects of histamine, the guinea pig and humans are extraordinarily sensitive.

The availability and applicability of highly selective H_1 and H_2 receptor agonists and antagonists have provided the necessary tools to unravel the complex physiology and pathophysiology of histamine and to provide new pharmacotherapy.

Pharmacodynamics

The most important pharmacologic actions of histamine are manifested principally on the cardiovascular system, extravascular smooth muscle, exocrine glands (especially the acid-secreting cells of the gastric musoca), and neural processes.

Cardiovascular System   The most prominent cardiovascular effects of histamine include an immediate fall in systemic blood pressure, flushing, and a lowering of peripheral resistance as a result of vasodilation of microcirculatory vessels (arterioles and capillaries). Histamine ranks among the most potent capillary vasodilators. This effect involves both H_1- and H_2-receptor activation and occurs diffusely throughout most vascular beds. H_1 receptors respond to low histamine concentrations in a rapid, short-lived fashion, whereas H_2-receptor activation leads to a slowly developing, yet more sustained, vasodilation. Thus, capillary vasodilator effects of histamine are completely blocked only by a combination of H_1- and H_2-receptor antagonists. Vasodilatation is most prominent in the skin and upper body as it produces heat, itching, and flushing ("blushing"). When cranial blood vessels dilate to histamine, abrupt and severe "cluster" headaches (also called *histamine headache* or *histamine cephalgia*) occur which are unilateral and involve the eye, temple, neck, and face.

Histamine also produces an increase in capillary permeability. Transudation of plasma and plasma macromolecules from vascular compartments to extracellular spaces in response to histamine occurs at postcapillary venules and is due to alterations in permeability manifested as increased hydrostatic pressure (venoconstriction) and enlarged endothelial intercellular spaces or gaps. This passage of fluid and proteins causes edema formation, a major component of the "triple response." This characteristic triad of reactions to intradermal histamine was described over 60 years ago and is composed of sequential localized vascular effects: (1) rapid reddening around the site of histamine injection ("erythema") resulting from direct local microcirculatory vasodilation, (2) bright red, diffusely shaped areas of hyperemia ("flare") around the initial erythema resulting from localized axonal reflex-induced arteriolar vasodilation, and (3) localized edema ("wheal") due to increased microvascular permeability. The triple response can also be induced by intradermal antigen in sensitized individuals, physical trauma, cold or thermal injury, or the injection of histamine liberators.

On the heart, histamine produces mechanical (positive inotropic and chronotropic) and electrophysiologic (slowed AV conduction) changes which are mediated by H_2 and H_1 receptors, respectively. Thus, cardiac pathophysiology due to either histamine or immediate hypersensitivity reactions should be effectively controlled by a combination of H_1- and H_2-receptor antagonists.

Smooth Muscle   Nonvascular smooth-muscle tone is generally stimulated in response to histamine (an H_1-mediated effect); however, depending on the species and the tissue studied, responses may vary greatly. Bronchial smooth muscle of humans is especially sensitive; indeed, even small amounts of histamine will provoke a marked bronchoconstriction in asthmatics and in patients with other hyperreactive airway diseases. Although airway constriction involves direct H_1-receptor activation, histamine is also capable of triggering a localized reflex cholinergic discharge by stimulating afferent vagal nerve endings.

With regard to other smooth muscles, the human uterus responds poorly to histamine; smooth muscle of the urinary bladder, gallbladder, intestine, and iris are inconsistently and weakly stimulated by histamine.

Exocrine Glands   Histamine is a potent stimulant of gastric acid and pepsin secretion, but a weak and relatively unimportant secretagogue for other exocrine glands, including salivary, bronchial, pancreatic, lacrimal, and intestinal mucosal glands. Its principal effect on gastric acid secretion results from a direct effect on parietal cell H_2 receptors. This can have important physiologic and pathophysiologic ramifications. As little as 0.025 mg injected subcutaneously will produce copious increases in acid secretion without evoking other histamine responses. Excessive production of acid induced by histamine (as in ulcers) is effectively reduced with H_2-receptor antagonists, e.g., cimetidine, which is discussed later in this chapter.

Peripheral Nerve Endings   Histamine stimulates various sensory and autonomic nerve endings. The stimulation of sensory nerve endings is most conspicuous in the epidermis and dermis where itching and pain result. Together with its effect on capillaries (dilation and increased permeability), histamine-induced sensory nerve stimulation is responsible for the triple response (described previously) and for some indirect effects on the heart and lungs.

Stimulation of autonomic nerve endings in the adrenal medulla is probably responsible for histamine-induced release of the catecholamines epinephrine and norepinephrine into the bloodstream. Whereas this sympathoadrenal discharge is insufficient to block the direct vasodepressor response to intravenous histamine in normal individuals, patients with functional pheochromocytoma respond with a rise in blood pressure following even a modest dose of histamine.

Central Nervous System   Little is known about the actual physiologic role of histamine in the central nervous system even though the brain does contain histamine, L-histidine decarboxylase, and diamine oxidase. Histamine does not penetrate the blood-brain barrier very well; however, when injected directly into the cerebral ventricles, histamine seems to stimulate both H_1 and H_2 receptors leading to a variety of effects, including changes in heart rate, blood pressure, body temperature, and state of arousal. Thus, there may be central histaminergic activities, but much remains to be elucidated before any definitive regulatory or pathologic role can be ascribed.

Tissue Growth and Repair   Tissues which are undergoing rapid growth or repair, e.g., embryonic tissue, malignant growths, bone marrow, and wound and granulation tissue, have an extraordinarily high histamine-forming capacity to enhance growth. Newly formed ("nascent") histamine appears to function in a facilitative fashion in the anabolic processes to accelerate reparative growth, but its precise role is still unknown.

Immunoreactivity   Histamine has the ability to bind to T cells by specific receptor interactions, especially the H_2 receptor. As a result, intracellular levels of cyclic AMP are elevated and T cell-mediated cytotoxicity is blocked. In addition, H_2-receptor activation suppresses lymphocyte proliferation and release of cytokines, inhibits E rosette formation, and stimulates T cells to release suppressor factors. Histamine also binds to H_1 receptors on T lymphocytes to inhibit suppressor cell function. With regard to other immunologic cells, histamine can reduce mast cell and basophil secretory capacity by increasing intracellular levels of cyclic AMP via H_2-receptor activation.

Molecular Mechanisms of Action   Molecular mechanisms underlying the actions of histamine on target cell responses have recently been the subject of intensive study. Altered ionic fluxes subsequent to an increase in cell membrane permeability can account for some stimulatory effects of histamine. For example, facilitation of calcium entry down its electrochemical gradient or release (mobilization) of intracellular calcium stores could provide the ionic link to histamine-induced smooth and cardiac muscle contraction. The positive inotropic effects in mammalian hearts, gastric acid secretion, and inhibition of basophil secretion are attributable to calcium influx and elevation of intracellular cyclic AMP, effects which are blocked by H_2 antihistamines. Thus, intracellular levels of free calcium are a key to the regulation of contraction and secretion. Relaxation of smooth muscle is also associated with H_2-receptor activation and a rise in cyclic AMP, while contraction involves H_1 receptors and a rise in cyclic GMP.

Stimulation of H_1 receptors also provokes a rapid turnover of inositol phospholipids (hydrolysis of phosphatidylinositides and formation of phosphorylated inositol derivatives) in concert with intracellular calcium mobilization. Additionally, H_1-receptor stimulation may activate phospholipase A_2 and trigger the arachidonic acid cascade leading to prostaglandin production. Since different prostaglandins have variable effects on cyclic nucleotide accumulation, this complicates the measurement of any direct effect of histamine. In bidirectional control systems found in a number of tissues, the signal transduction process that promotes a turnover of inositol phopholipids activates cellular functions, whereas the signal that raises cyclic AMP usually antagonizes such activation. Thus electrolyte, biochemical, and mechanical events are all linked in a complex process during stimulus-response coupling.

Diagnostic Uses

Currently, there are no therapeutic uses for histamine. It can be used in small doses (0.0275 mg/kg as the phosphate salt) for diagnosis, e.g., in the stimulation of gastric glands to test for their ability to produce hydrochloric acid; however, it is not frequently used anymore. Rather, more selective H_2-receptor agonists, e.g., impromidine (available in Canada and the United Kingdom), may be used instead, and also pentagastrin is now more commonly used to test for achlorhydria. Another application of histamine would be as a provocative test for pheochromocytoma, but it is indicated only for the occasional patient with paroxysmal signs of excessive catecholamine secretion.

Symptoms of Histamine Toxicity

The symptoms of histamine toxicity can be easily predicted on the basis of its pharmacologic activities. The primary finding is a precipitous fall in blood pressure accompanied by generalized vasodilation with a rise in skin temperature, headache, and visual disturbances. In addition, smooth-muscle stimulation leads to bronchoconstriction, dyspnea, and diarrhea. Further effects noted are vomiting and a metallic taste. In severe cases, shock may supervene, and appropriate measures must be taken to treat this serious complication. In general, nonshock cases can best be treated with epinephrine. Antihistamines do not provide adequate therapy in cases of severe histamine toxicity because their effect develops too slowly to cope with life-threatening toxicity and also because many histamine actions, e.g., bronchoconstriction, are complicated by concomitant effects of other endogenous substances which are released at the same time and are not antagonized by antihistamines.

H₁ ANTIHISTAMINES

Antihistamines were initially discovered in the late 1930s by investigators who reported that some amines with a phenolic ether substitution (1) afforded striking protection to guinea pigs from lethal doses of histamine, and (2) lessened the symptoms of experimental anaphylactic shock. Although the original antihistamines were too toxic for clinical use, these compounds led to future successes with more acceptable derivatives, which were competitive and reversible antagonists, e.g., pyrilamine. Shortly thereafter, some highly effective histamine antagonists, tripelennamine and diphenhydramine, were discovered, and by the 1950s there was a proliferation of these kinds of drugs.

Chemistry

Most conventional H_1 antihistamines resemble histamine structurally by sharing a substituted ethylamine side chain; however, they also have two aromatic moieties and are represented by the general formula shown in Table 12-3, where Ar_1 and Ar_2 (the "nucleus") are carbocyclic or heterocyclic aromatic rings, one or both of which may be separated from X by a carbon atom, where X is oxygen, carbon, or nitrogen connecting the aminoethyl side chain to the nucleus. R_1 and R_2 represent alkyl substitutions, usually methyl groups. As an example, the structure of chlorpheniramine, one of the most widely used antihistamines, is shown in Fig. 12-2.

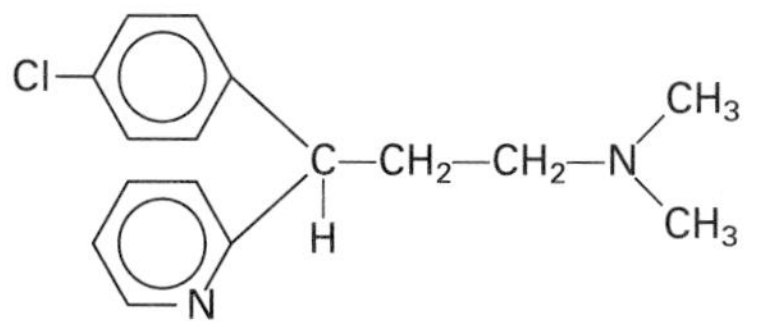

Chlorpheniramine

FIGURE 12-2   Structure of chlorpheniramine.

Mechanism of Action

All these compounds are competitive, reversible antagonists of histamine at H_1 receptors; they have no significant activity on H_2 receptors. Furthermore, these antihistamines only reduce or block the effects, not the synthesis, release, or metabolism of histamine.

All the H_1-receptor antagonists block to varying degrees most effects of histamine on different organs and systems of the body and can afford protection against allergic and anaphylactic reactions. By themselves these agents exert little, if any, significant direct effects, but rather by virtue of their affinity to H_1 receptors, they are therapeutically beneficial in antagonizing responses to histamine. Thus, antihistaminic effects are noted only in the presence of increased histamine activity. Although there are clearly differences in the relative potencies of these drugs when examined under different conditions, they do have comparable pharmacodynamic properties and therapeutic utility when considered as a group.

Pharmacodynamics

Smooth Muscle   Most smooth-muscle responses to histamine are blocked (or reduced) by H_1-receptor antagonists. For example, H_1 antihistamines can strikingly inhibit histamine-induced constriction of intestinal and respiratory smooth muscle. The therapeutic utility of these classic antihistamines against anaphylactic bronchospasm in human asthma remains controversial. A variety of mediators (including histamine) are implicated in asthma, e.g., leukotrienes, platelet-activating factor, acetylcholine, thromboxane. To date, H_1 antihistamines have been remarkably ineffective or only of limited value in these more severe respiratory diseases.

With regard to vascular smooth muscle, the vasoconstrictor effects of histamine (H_1-mediated) can be blocked with H_1 antihistamines, whereas a combination of H_1 and H_2 antagonists are required for complete suppression of histamine-mediated vasodilation and hypotension.

Vasopermeability   The ability of systemic or local histamine, allergic cutaneous reactions, or anaphylaxis to produce vasodilation and increased capillary permeability, resulting in edema and wheal formation at the tissue site, can be prevented or antagonized by H_1 antihistamines. Also, localized edema produced by vari-

TABLE 12-3   **Structural classes and representative examples of H_1 antihistamines**

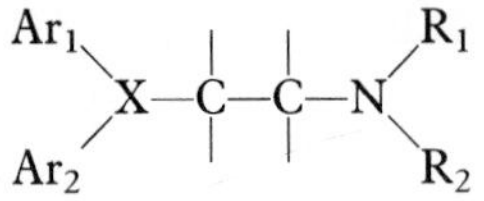

$$\begin{array}{c}
Ar_1 \\
\diagdown \\
\end{array}
X-\underset{|}{\overset{|}{C}}-\underset{|}{\overset{|}{C}}-N\diagup\overset{\displaystyle R_1}{}\diagdown_{\displaystyle R_2}$$

Structural classes	"X"	Examples
Ethylenediamines	$\diagup N-$	Pyrilamine (mepyramine) Tripelennamine
Aminoalkyl ethers	$-O-$	Diphenhydramine Dimenhydrinate
Alkylamines	$\diagup CH-$	Chlorpheniramine Dexchlorpheniramine Brompheniramine
Piperazines	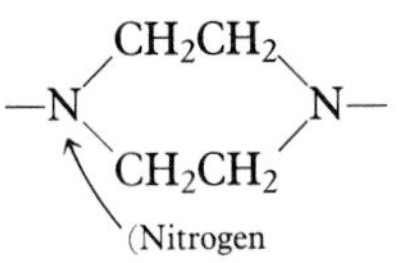 $-N\diagup\overset{\displaystyle CH_2CH_2}{\underset{\displaystyle CH_2CH_2}{}}\diagdown N-$ (Nitrogen in conjunction with a piperazine ring)	Meclizine Cyclizine Hydroxyzine
Phenothiazines	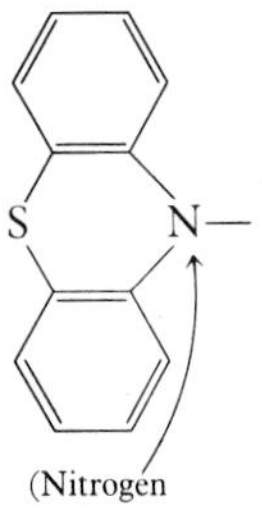 S $N-$ (Nitrogen in conjunction with a phenothiazine nucleus)	Promethazine Trimeprazine
Other		Cyproheptadine Terfenadine Aztemizole Loratadine

ous mechanical or chemical means and by inflammation can be reduced or blocked by antihistamines, which may be acting directly on vascular and sensory nerve ending H_1 receptors or by actions against other mediators, e.g., acetylcholine and serotonin, or by a local anesthetic effect. For example, some compounds of the phenothiazine class (promethazine) as well as a three-ringed nucleus derivative (cyproheptadine) possess both antihistamine and antiserotonin activities, which may afford clinical advantages in the treatment of cutaneous allergies with itching.

Immediate Hypersensitivity   Type I immediate hypersensitivity reactions, which include allergy and anaphylaxis, involve a number of autocoids, but the role of histamine as a primary mediator is universally accepted. Activated tissue-based mast cells and circulating basophils are the predominant cell sources which release histamine during type I immediate hypersensitivity reactions in quantities more than sufficient to account for much of the symptomatology of allergy and anaphylaxis. The relative importance of histamine vis-a-vis other mediators can vary with the tissue and species examined, and therefore, the therapeutic benefit of H_1 antihistamines may also be variable. Whereas these drugs are valuable in treating edema formation, itching, rhinorrhea, and lacrimation, they are less effective in controlling hypotension and allergic bronchoconstriction.

Central Nervous System   The effects of H_1 antihistamines on the central nervous system (CNS) are complex and dose-related. Depression of the CNS by therapeutic doses of most antihistamines will lead to varying degrees of diminished alertness, slowed reaction time, muscle weakness, mild sedation, and even somnolence. Some antagonists are more prone to produce these CNS manifestations than others, and patients seem to vary in susceptibility and responsiveness. The aminoalkyl ethers are especially liable to produce sedation; for example, diphenhydramine can produce drowsiness in 20 to 50 percent of the patients. In some circumstances, physicians may actually take advantage of this sedative effect and prescribe the drug for allergy patients who are also having problems sleeping. Some over-the-counter (OTC) preparations also include sedative antihistamines (including Sleep-Eze, Sominex, and Nytol), all of which contain diphenhydramine. However, there are always dangers inherent in this type of self-medication in that the patient may neglect to seek a proper medical diagnosis.

Paradoxically, H_1 antihistamines may occasionally produce CNS stimulation even within a therapeutic dose range, although stimulation occurs less frequently than sedation. This is manifested as restlessness, nervousness, hyperexcitability, and insomnia. Very small doses may provoke activation of the EEG, agitation, delirium, tremors, and epileptic seizures in some patients with focal CNS lesions. Infants may present with sensory and motor disturbances (convulsions) after H_1-antihistamine poisoning, which is followed by depression or paralysis of the medullary-pontine cardiovascular and respiratory centers.

The specific mechanism by which H_1 antihistamines produce CNS depression and excitation is unclear at present. They might be blocking responses to endogenously released histamine in the CNS, since these antagonists have been shown to be capable of high binding affinity to H_1 receptors in the brain. Alternatively, some compounds may replace α rhythms in the EEG with slow wave activity in the 3- to 4-s^{-1} range. Regardless, since these drugs are not all at risk of central liabilities, there does not appear to be a correlation between peripheral antihistaminic effectiveness and CNS activity.

The most important and exciting clinical advance in this field in some time has been the development of so-called new generation nonsedating antihistamines, which either do not enter the CNS or cross the blood-brain barrier only with great difficulty. Three of these newer antihistamines with reduced or minimal sedative liability are terfenadine, aztemizole, and loratadine.

Terfenadine was the first of this new class of pharmacologically distinct, specific, peripherally acting H_1 antihistamines. It has no significant effect on α- or β-adrenergic receptors and is relatively free of serotonergic, cholinergic, and local anesthetic activity. Whereas antihistaminic activity is comparable to chlorpheniramine, terfenadine reportedly produces little, if any, characteristic depression of the EEG, behavioral effects, or impairment of motor function seen frequently with older H_1 antagonists. Although terfenadine may have equal affinity for peripheral and central H_1 receptors, it is thought to poorly penetrate the blood-brain barrier at effective therapeutic doses and, hence, produces a low incidence of CNS effects. Aztemizole also has a high degree of H_1-receptor specificity, with little muscarinic, adrenergic, or other receptor activity. Loratadine may be less sedating because of either reduced ability to cross the blood-brain barrier or selective binding to peripheral rather than central H_1 receptors.

Another potentially useful CNS effect of some H_1 antihistamines is the ability to block emesis and motion sickness (car, sea, or air sickness). This activity is especially prominent with dimenhydrinate, diphenhydramine (the active moiety of dimenhydrinate), and meclizine. These drugs are helpful in alleviating most symptoms of disturbed equilibrium with minimal side effects. Perhaps promethazine owes its anti-motion sickness activity to the fact that it shows greater blockade of cholinergic muscarinic receptors than other H_1 antihistamines. After all, the anticholinergic scopolamine is considered to be the most effective drug for the prophylaxis and treatment of motion sickness and other labyrinthine disturbances, such as Ménière's disease.

Anticholinergic Many H_1 antihistamines have some capacity to inhibit responses to cholinergic muscarinic and serotonin receptor activation, but these ancillary effects do not appear to be related to antihistamine activity or potency. The atropine-like actions are prominent enough to be useful clinically, such as in drying of excessive secretions in allergic rhinitis patients. Among the classic H_1 antihistamines, diphenhydramine and promethazine have high anticholinergic activity; the one least liable to be anticholinergic is pyrilamine, and therefore it is more specific for histamine.

Local Anesthesia Most of the known H_1-receptor antagonists exert some degree of local anesthetic action. Numerous clinical studies have been performed using ointments or solutions containing diphenhydramine, tripelennamine, promethazine, or pyrilamine; however, much higher concentrations are required for local anesthesia than for antagonizing responses to histamine. In fact, some of these drugs have been shown to be more potent than procaine in comparative tests but are limited for use in minor surgical procedures by the incidence of mild-to-moderate irritation or the potential for local sensitization. They can be used locally for relief of itching and discomfort where the anesthetic component complements the antiallergic and antipruritic actions.

Pharmacokinetics

As a class, H_1 antagonists are well absorbed from the gastrointestinal tract following oral administration. With most, effects begin within 30 min, peak within 1 to 2 h and last approximately 3 to 6 h. Extensive pharmacokinetic data are available on only a few of these

drugs. For example, blood levels of diphenhydramine reach a maximum approximately 2 h after an oral dose and decrease exponentially with a plasma elimination half-life of 4 h. The drug is widely distributed through bodily tissues (including the CNS) and is biotransformed in the liver to inactive products, and these are excreted via the kidney within 24 h. Tripelennamine and other classical H_1 antihistamines have similar pharmacokinetic properties and are usually prescribed in doses which must be repeated every 4 h. These drugs are also capable of inducing liver microsomal enzymes which may facilitate their own metabolism.

Owing to a high degree of plasma protein binding (97 percent), terfenadine is longer lasting than most other antihistamines (elimination half-life of approximately 20 h) and is usually administered twice daily. Following biotransformation, 60 percent of terfenadine metabolites are eliminated in the feces, while 40 percent are excreted via the urine.

In contrast to all other H_1 blockers currently available for clinical use, loratadine is biotransformed to an active product, descarboethoxyloratadine. The plasma half-life of loratadine and its metabolite are 12 to 15 h and drug elimination occurs approximately equally through the feces and urine. This drug is used orally once a day.

Adverse Effects

The predominant central action of most H_1 antihistamines is sedation, but in children and some adults, agitation, nervousness, delirium, tremors, incoordination, hallucinations, and convulsions may occur. Sedation usually occurs within the therapeutic dose range for antihistaminic action and varies from diminished alertness and impaired ability to concentrate to muscle weakness and pronounced drowsiness. This effect interferes with daytime activities; patients are usually advised not to drive motor vehicles, operate heavy equipment and machinery, or imbibe alcohol or CNS depressants, which would be additive or, perhaps, synergistic.

Lesser side effects may manifest as digestive-tract-related, i.e., anorexia, nausea, vomiting, diarrhea or constipation, and epigastric distress. These are reduced if the drug is given with meals. Other untoward effects include: dryness of the mouth, throat and airways; cardiac palpitation; hypotension; urinary retention; headache; faintness; tightness in the chest; and visual disturbances. (Many of these may be accounted for by atropine-like effects.) Because they can also release histamine or induce hypersensitivity of the skin, topical antihistamines can produce drug allergy (urticaria, dermatitis, photosensitization).

Laboratory animal teratogenesis has been observed with some piperazine derivatives (cyclizine, meclizine). Even though this has not been demonstrated in humans, administration of antihistamines to pregnant women is discouraged.

In general, antihistamines possess a high therapeutic index such that it is rare to observe serious acute toxicity from their use. However, widespread use as self-medication or accidental overdose by children can lead to serious events as described earlier. Acute toxicity can culminate in coma, cardiorespiratory collapse, marked hyperthermia, and death within 2 to 15 h. Treatment is symptomatic and consists of supportive therapy with artificial ventilation.

Therapeutic Uses

Allergic diseases represent a complex series of disorders with acute and chronic manifestations which may vary from mild urticaria or rhinitis to severe and possibly fatal anaphylaxis. It is estimated that approximately 10 percent of the population may suffer from some form of allergy. Therapy directed toward removal or avoidance of the offending allergen from the environment and specific patient desensitization is not always practical or successful. In a number of allergies, the causative allergen cannot be demonstrated; also, associated chronic infection and inflammation often complicate therapy. Therefore, symptomatic management with a variety of drugs has been exceptionally beneficial. H_1 antihistamines have earned their deserved, time-proven place, acceptance, and value in treating immediate hypersensitivity reactions, especially seasonal hay fever, allergic rhinitis, dermatoses, and conjunctivitis.

Dermatoses Both acute and chronic urticaria respond well to H_1 antihistamines, although the effect is more striking in acute disorders. The pruritus (itching) and wheals are usually resolved rapidly in a high percentage of patients. Angioedema (angioneurotic edema) also responds favorably, but when the larynx is involved, epinephrine must also be used as a life-sparing measure. In patients with atopic dermatitis, con-

tact dermatitis, insect bites, stings, and poison ivy, these drugs are particularly useful in treating the itch (local anesthetic properties may also be operative here), while topical corticosteroids treat the inflammation. The sedative-tranquilizing effect of oral H_1 antagonists may reduce the urge to scratch by decreasing the associated anxiety. Urticarial and edematous lesions of serum sickness also respond well to H_1 antihistamines, but joint involvement and fever may require additional therapy. Caution should be exercised with individuals who may have a tendency to develop sensitization (allergic dermatitis) to topical application of these drugs.

Allergic Rhinitis H_1 antihistamines are especially effective in ameliorating the sneezing, rhinorrhea, and itching of the eyes, nose, and throat in most patients with seasonal allergic rhinitis and conjunctivitis (hay fever and pollinosis). They can be also used in combination with decongestants, e.g., phenylephrine or pseudoephedrine, and/or desensitization procedures. When exposure to the sensitizing allergen is prolonged or when nasal congestion is very prominent, these drugs become less effective. Similarly, they may only be of limited benefit in vasomotor rhinitis.

Bronchial Asthma Although normal daily doses of classic H_1 antihistamines have been ineffective in treating bronchial asthma, higher doses may have been effective but could not be used because of limiting adverse side effects, such as sedation. This issue may finally be nearing resolution with the advent of new, highly potent, long-lasting, "nonsedating" H_1 antihistamines, e.g., terfenadine, aztemizole, and loratadine. Their effectiveness (or lack of same) in asthma is presently undergoing intensive worldwide clinical investigations to determine just how important histamine really is as a mediator of bronchial asthma. Until this issue is resolved, the utility of these compounds in asthma remains unproven.

Common Cold H_1 antihistamines are generally considered as simple palliative therapy in treating the common cold. They will not "cure" the cold which is of viral origin but will affect any concomitant allergic component (such as nasal discharge and sneezing). When combined with other traditional agents, antihistamines will provide some degree of symptomatic relief against the common cold, while producing only mild, if any, side effects.

Motion Sickness and Emesis Antihistamines have been used extensively in the prophylaxis of motion sickness to prevent nausea and vomiting. This action cannot be correlated with antihistamine potency and is probably due to a nonspecific central effect. The most effective antihistamines used in motion sickness include dimenhydrinate, cyclizine, meclizine, and promethazine. Their effectiveness as general antiemetics is less than that of chlorpromazine and other phenothiazine tranquilizers, yet they are useful in vestibular disturbances such as Ménière's disease.

Miscellaneous Uses Several other uses of H_1 antihistamines include

1. *Insomnia* as mild hypnotics in OTC sleep-inducing medications, e.g., diphenhydramine
2. *Parkinson's disease* as an anticholinergic adjunct to modestly reduce tremors and muscular rigidity, e.g., diphenhydramine
3. *Anxiolytic* sedative and mild antianxiety effects, e.g., hydroxyzine
4. *Adverse reactions* to IV x-ray contrast media

Preparations and Doses

Many physicians familiar with the advantages and disadvantages of each of the H_1 antihistamines prefer to have a working pool for selection and variation as indicated by individual patient needs in terms of efficacy and side effects. Few other classes of drugs possess such depth in type and number for choice by the physician and acceptance by the patient.

Representative drugs for the various classes of H_1 antihistamines are presented in Table 12-4 along with usual single adult doses, available routes of administration, and frequency of use.

H_2-RECEPTOR ANTAGONISTS

While conventional ("classic") antihistamines block many histamine-induced effects that occur via H_1 receptors, they fail to antagonize H_2-receptor-mediated events, e.g., gastric acid secretion. In 1977, cimetidine was introduced in the United States as the first approved H_2-receptor antagonist and revolutionized the management of peptic ulcer disease. Several years

later, ranitidine, a chemically different H_2-receptor antagonist, was developed and marketed. Because of the significant benefits associated with these agents, other H_2-receptor antagonists, with minor pharmacologic differences, entered clinical development; famotidine and nizatidine are examples and have been recently approved for therapeutic use.

Chemistry

The structure of cimetidine (Fig. 12-3) is made up of a methylimidazole ring and a long side chain containing a sulfur atom and a small cyanoguanidine group. It was thought that the imidazole moiety, as found in histamine, was required for H_2-blocking activity; however, this proved untrue since ranitidine possesses a substituted furan ring and famotidine and nizatidine are thiazole derivatives and all are highly effective

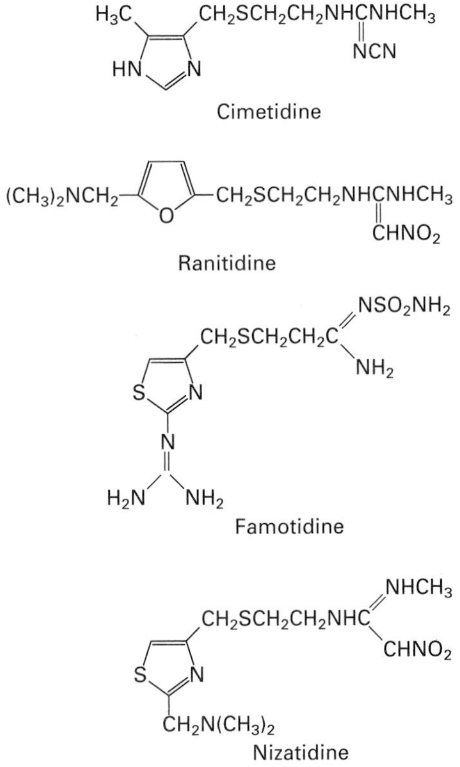

FIGURE 12-3   Structures of H_2-receptor antagonists.

TABLE 12-4   Doses and preparations of some representative H_1 antihistamines

Structural class and examples[a]	Usual adult dose (preparations)[b]	Frequency used
Ethylenediamines		
Pyrilamine	25–50 mg (O)	Every 4–6 h
Tripelennamine (PBZ)	25–50 mg (O, T)	Every 4–6 h
	37.5–75 mg (L)	Every 4–6 h
Aminoalkyl ethers		
Diphenhydramine (Benadryl)	25–50 mg(O, L, T)	3–4 times daily
	10–50 mg (I)	Every 3–4 h
Dimenhydrinate (Dramamine)	50–100 mg (O, L)	Every 4 h
	100 mg (S)	Twice daily
	50 mg (I)	Every 4 h
Alkylamines		
Chlorpheniramine (Chlor-	2–4 mg (O, L)	Every 4–8 h
Trimeton, Teldrin)	5–20 mg (I)	3–4 times daily
Dexchlorpheniramine	2 mg (O, L)	3–4 times daily
(Polaramine)		
Brompheniramine (Dimetane)	4–8 mg (O, L)	Every 6–12 h
	5–20 mg (I)	
Piperazines		
Meclizine (Antivert)	25–50 mg (O)	Once daily
Cyclizine (Marezine)	50 mg (O, I)	Every 4–6 h
Hydroxyzine (Atarax,	25–100 mg (O, L)	3–4 times daily
Vistaril)	25–100 mg (I)	Every 4–6 h
Phenothiazines		
Promethazine (Phenergan)	12.5–25 mg (O, L)	Twice daily
Trimeprazine (Temaril)	2.5 mg (O, L)	4 times daily
Other		
Cyproheptadine (Periactin)	4 mg (O, L)	3–4 times daily
Terfenadine (Seldane)	60 mg (O)	Twice daily
Aztemizole (Hismanal)	10 mg (O)	Once daily
Loratidine (Claritin)	10 mg (O)	Once daily

[a] Generic names with common trade names in parenthesis.
[b] Preparations available include oral solid (O), oral liquid (L), topical (T), injection (I), and rectal suppository (S).

H_2-receptor antagonists. All four compounds have a substituted methyl thioethyl side chain ($-CH_2SCH_2CH_2-$), which may be important for potent H_2-receptor blockade.

Mechanism of Action

The H_2-receptor antagonists reversibly and competitively inhibit the actions of histamine on H_2 receptors; they are pure antagonists, i.e., they have no agonistic activity. Numerous studies have lead to the conclusion that these drugs have no significant action at H_1 receptors, β-adrenoreceptors, or muscarinic receptors. Furthermore, neither the synthesis, release, or biotransformation of histamine is affected to any great extent by these compounds.

Pharmacodynamics

Although these drugs will block all H_2-receptor-mediated effects, the most important pharmacologic effect of the H_2-receptor antagonists is their ability to inhibit gastric acid secretion. All the drugs markedly reduce both daytime and nocturnal basal gastric secretory volume and acid output; gastric acid secretion induced by food, histamine, pentagastrin, insulin, and caffeine is also blocked. These drugs do not appear to affect gastric motility or gastric emptying time, and alterations in gastric mucous secretion have not been observed. Clinical data support the lack of pharmacodynamic differences between nizatidine 300 mg, cimetidine 800 mg, rantidine 300 mg, and famotidine 40 mg (all administered orally at bedtime) in the acute therapy of peptic ulcer disease. On a weight basis, famotidine is more potent than the other drugs, but their efficacy in peptic ulcer disorders appears to be similar.

Pharmacokinetics

Table 12-5 summarizes some of the pharmacokinetic characteristics of nizatidine, cimetidine, ranitidine, and famotidine. Cimetidine and nizatidine are well absorbed from the gastrointestinal tract following oral administration; the oral absorption of ranitidine and famotidine are incomplete. Cimetidine undergoes extensive first-pass biotransformation, while this is minimal with the other three compounds. Therefore the oral bioavailability of nizatidine is greater than that of cimetidine, famotidine, and ranitidine. All drugs have a relatively low plasma protein binding, and their apparent volumes of distribution range from 1.0 to 1.8 L/kg. The elimination half-lives of currently available H_2-receptor antagonists are relatively short (from 1.6 h for nizatidine to 3 h for famotidine).

The major biotransformation products of these drugs recovered in the urine are listed in Table 12-5. Approximately 50 percent of cimetidine is biotransformed (the sulfoxide is the major product); only a small percentage of the other drugs is metabolized. The only known active metabolite is monodesmethyl nizatidine (which represents 8 percent of the total nizatidine dose); it is 60 percent as active as the parent drug as an H_2-receptor antagonist.

For all these drugs the principal route of excretion is the urine. Renal elimination involves both glomerular

TABLE 12-5   Pharmacokinetic data for H_2-receptor antagonists

Drug	Oral bioavailability, %	Protein binding, %	Half-life, h	Major metabolites	Renal clearance, mL/min
Nizatidine	90	35	1.6	N^2-monodesmethyl N^2-oxide S-oxide	850
Cimetidine	60	20	2	Sulfoxide Hydroxymethyl	550
Ranitidine	50	15	2	N^2-oxide N-desmethyl S-oxide	600
Famotidine	45	20	3	S-oxide	350

filtration and tubular secretion. Precaution should be exercised when these H_2-receptor antagonists are administered to patients with renal insufficiency.

Adverse Reactions

In general, the H_2-receptor antagonists are remarkably safe agents, and side effects are usually moderate and reversible. These drugs infrequently produce headache, dizziness, constipation, diarrhea, skin rashes, and alterations of hepatic function. Various CNS disturbances, including somnolence, confusion, and hallucinations, have been reported. Small elevations of plasma creatinine have occurred with cimetidine, and dosage adjustment for patients with impaired renal function is necessary.

Cimetidine and ranitidine may elevate serum prolactin concentrations, while famotidine and nizatidine have not shown this effect. Cimetidine binds to androgen receptors, an action which may be responsible for the sexual dysfunction (reduced libido and impotence) and gynecomastia which has been reported for this drug. These effects are only rarely, if ever, observed with the other drugs. The frequency of these events appear greatest when cimetidine is administered in very high doses for the treatment of Zollinger-Ellison syndrome.

Drug Interactions

Cimetidine reversibly inhibits the cytochrome P-450 system of the liver in either a competitive or noncompetitive manner depending on the substrate and therefore reduces phase I biotransformation reactions. This appears to be explained by the imidazole binding to the heme portion of the enzyme, which is influenced by the lipophilicity of the molecule. Cimetidine does not inhibit phase II glucuronidation reactions. In contrast, ranitidine, famotidine, and nizatidine appear to have lower binding affinities to cytochrome P-450 and thus are only very weak inhibitors of drug metabolism. Therefore, cimetidine can interact with many drugs, thereby delaying their hepatic metabolism; for example, accumulation of the following drugs can occur: warfarin, phenytoin, theophylline, propranolol, diazepam, and phenobarbital. In contrast, none of the other three H_2-receptor antagonists affect P-450 drug metabolism to any significant extent.

By reducing gastric acid secretion, the absorption of drugs such as ketoconazole and clorazepate (enhanced at low stomach pH) is reduced by H_2-receptor blockers. In addition antacids will reduce the bioavailability of cimetidine by 20 to 30 percent, and the administration of antacids and oral cimetidine should be separated by a 1-h interval. Antacids may be given concomitantly with ranitidine, famotidine, and nizatidine.

Therapeutic Uses

H_2-receptor antagonists are effective in the treatment of peptic acid disorders. They have proven to be invaluable in the treatment of duodenal ulcer disease because of their ability to lower basal and nocturnal gastric acid secretion. In general, these agents also have proven to be effective therapy for the treatment of gastric ulcer and Zollinger-Ellison syndrome. All have been moderately effective in the prevention of duodenal ulcer recurrence. Ranitidine is the only H_2-receptor antagonist that is currently approved in the United States for the treatment of gastroesophageal reflux disease.

Preparations and Doses

Cimetidine (Tagamet) is available in tablets (200, 300, 400, and 800 mg), oral liquid (300 mg/5 mL), and for IM or IV injection (300 mg/2 mL). The recommended doses for active duodenal ulcer are 300 mg four times daily with meals and at bedtime, 400 mg twice daily, or 800 mg at bedtime. In those patients requiring maintenance therapy for duodenal ulcer, the recommended adult oral dose is 400 mg at bedtime. The oral dosage for short-term treatment of active benign gastric ulcer is 300 mg four times a day with meals and at bedtime. A similar dosing regimen is recommended for pathologic hypersecretory conditions. Higher doses may be necessary but should not exceed 2400 mg/day.

Ranitidine (Zantac) is available in tablets (150 and 300 mg) and injection (25 mg/mL). The recommended doses for active duodenal ulcer are 150 mg bid or 300 mg once daily at bedtime. In those patients requiring maintenance therapy for duodenal ulcer, the adult oral dose is 150 mg at bedtime. The oral dosage for short-term treatment of benign gastric ulcer is 150 mg twice a day. A similar dosing regimen is recommended for pathologic hypersecretory conditions;

however, higher doses may be required. The current recommended dose for gastroesophageal disease is 150 mg twice daily.

Famotidine (Pepcid) is marketed in tablets (20 and 40 mg), a powder for oral suspension (40 mg/5 mL when reconstituted), and an injectable solution (10 mg/mL). The recommended dosage of famotidine for oral treatment of active duodenal ulcer is 40 mg once daily at bedtime; 20 mg at bedtime is recommended for maintenance therapy. The intravenous dosage is 20 mg administered every 12 h. For hypersecretory conditions, 20 mg every 6 h is recommended, but doses up to 160 mg every 6 h have been used in patients with severe Zollinger-Ellison syndrome.

Nizatidine (Axid), the newest H_2-receptor antagonist, is available in capsules (150 and 300 mg) and is approved for the oral treatment of active duodenal ulcer at a recommened dose of 300 mg once daily at bedtime; 150 mg at bedtime is recommended for maintenance therapy.

BIBLIOGRAPHY

Ash, A. S. F. and H. O. Schild: "Receptors Mediating Some Actions of Histamine," *Br. J. Pharmacol.*, **27**:427–439 (1966).

Black, J. W., W. A. M. Duncan, C. J. Durant, C. R. Ganellin, and E. M. Parsons: "Definition and Antagonism of Histamine H_2-Receptors," *Nature*, **236**:385–390 (1972).

Bovet, D., and A. Staub: "Action Protectrice des Ethers Phenoliques au Cours de L'intoxication Histiminique," *Compt. Rent. Soc. Biol. (Paris)*, **124**:547–549 (1937).

Callaghan, R. F., et al.: "A Pharmacokinetatic Profile of Nizatidine in Man," *Scand. J. Gastroenterol.*, **22** (**Suppl. 136**):9–17 (1987).

Dale, H. H., and P. P. Laidlaw: "The Physiological Action of β-Imidazolylethylamine," *J. Physiol. (London)*, **41**:318–344 (1910).

Dale, H. H., and P. P. Laidlaw: "Histamine Shock," *J. Physiol. (London)*, **52**:355–390 (1919).

Dammann, H. G., et al.: "The 24-Hour Acid Suppression Profile of Nizatidine," *Scand. J. Gastroenterol.*, **22** (**Suppl. 136**):56–60 (1987).

"Famotidine (Pepcid)," *The Medical Letter*, **29** (**Issue 733**):17–18 (1987).

Ganellin, C. R., and M. E. Parsons: *Pharmacology of Histamine Receptors*, Wright-PSG, Bristol, England, 1982.

Jansen, R. T., et al.: "Cimetidine-Induced Impotence and Breast Changes in Patients with Gastric Hypersecretory States," *N. Engl. J. Med.*, **308**:883–888 (1983).

Klotz, V., et al.: "Comparative Effects of H_2 Receptor Antagonists on Drug Metabolism in Vitro and in Vivo," *Pharmac. Ther.*, **33**:157–161 (1987).

Lewis, T.: "The Blood Vessels of the Human Skin and Their Responses," Shaw & Sons, London, (1927).

Powell, J. R., and K. H. Donn: "The Pharmacokinetic Basis for H_2-Antagonist Drug Interactions: Concepts and Implications," *J. Clin. Gastroenterol.*, **5** (**Suppl. 1**):95–113 (1983).

Rohner, H. G., and R. Gugler: "Treatment of Active Duodenal Ulcers with Famotidine," *Am. J. Med.*, **81** (**Suppl. 4B**):13–16 (1986).

Van Hecken, A. M., et al.: "Ranitidine: Single Dose Pharmacokinetics and Absolute Bioavailability in Man," *Br. J. Clin. Pharmacol.*, **14**:195–200 (1982).

C H A P T E R **13**

Prostaglandins and Related Eicosanoids

J. Bryan Smith

The prostaglandins and related eicosanoids are a family of acidic lipids produced from cell membranes that are implicated in a great many biologic systems. The discovery of prostaglandins followed early studies of biologically active substances present in prostate glands and semen of various species. In 1934, smooth-muscle-stimulating material that was both acidic and lipid in nature was isolated from human semen and was given the name *prostaglandin*, owing to the mistaken belief that it came from the prostate gland. The isolation and identification of a family of prostaglandins from sheep seminal vesicles and from human semen was accomplished by the mid-1960s. Subsequently, other prostaglandins, such as *prostacyclin*, and related eicosanoids, such as *thromboxanes* and *leukotrienes*, were discovered.

It is now known that almost all cells in the body are capable of producing eicosanoids. The cells can do this because they contain both the appropriate fatty acid precursors, as esters in their membrane phospholipids, as well as the enzymes that are involved in the oxygenative transformation of these fatty acids once they are released from ester linkage. In part because of this almost ubiquitous biosynthetic potential of cells and in part because of their diversity of effects, the eicosanoids probably are involved in a great number of physiologic and pathologic processes including reproduction, blood pressure regulation, bronchoconstriction, inflammation, nerve transmission, gastric secretion, urine formation, and platelet aggregation. The participation of the eicosanoids in each of these areas is briefly discussed in this chapter.

The prostaglandins and related compounds can be used as drugs themselves to mimic the effects of endogenously produced eicosanoids. However, the use of prostaglandins as drugs has not become widespread because of the multiplicity of side effects due to the fact that prostaglandins act on so many systems. Alternatively, other drugs (most notably nonsteroidal anti-inflammatory drugs) can act by inhibiting the biosynthesis of the endogenous eicosanoids. An increasing number of experimental agents which inhibit the effects of endogenous eicosanoids at the receptor level are being synthesized.

CHEMISTRY

Biosynthesis of Eicosanoids

The fatty acid precursors of the eicosanoids are not freely available in cells, but they are abundant in ester linkage in phospholipids in the membranes of many cell types. The initiation of the biosynthesis of prostaglandins and related eicosanoids therefore depends on the release of the fatty acid precursors by enzymatic hydrolysis of the phospholipids. In general, it appears that this hydrolysis is catalyzed by phospholipase A_2, an enzyme that acts on most phospholipids and whose activity is enhanced by an increase in intracellular free calcium ions as occurs during cellular stimulation. In addition, there is some evidence that small amounts of the precursor fatty acids also may be released from one particular phospholipid, phosphatidylinositol, by the combined actions of phospholipase C (which produces diacylglycerol) and diacylglycerol lipase. Examples of stimuli which cause eicosanoid synthesis in cells include mechanical distortion of cell membranes, changes in ion fluxes, ischemia, hormones, enzymes such as thrombin, and antigens. It is important to remember that the prostaglandins and related eicosanoids (1) are not stored for later release like the catecholamines but are biosynthesized within seconds of the activation of phospholipase A_2 and (2) act as autocoids because they are rapidly metabolized.

The fatty acid precursors of the prostaglandins and related eicosanoids all contain 20 carbon atoms, which is signified by *eicosa*. In addition, these precursors contain three, four, or five double bonds; hence the names 8,11,14-eicosatrienoic acid, 5,8,11,14-eicosatetraenoic acid (arachidonic acid) and 5,8,11,14,17-eicosapentaenoic acid (EPA), where the numbers 5, 8, 11, 14, and 17 refer to the position of the double bonds with the carbon atom of the carboxyl group being numbered as 1 (Fig. 13-1). Of these three eicosanoid precursors, human cells and tissues contain almost exclusively arachidonic acid esterified to phospholipids with the major exception of human seminal vesicles, which contain equal amounts of 8,11,14-eicosatrienoic acid and arachidonic acid and lesser amounts of EPA in their phospholipid membranes. The first two eicosanoid precursor fatty acids either are derived from dietary linoleic acid, an essential fatty acid which cannot be biosynthesized by humans, or are ingested as constituents of meat. The third, EPA, is almost entirely assimilated by the ingestion of cold-water fish.

Once released, eicosanoid precursors (usually arachidonic acid) are rapidly transformed into oxygenated products by one or both of two distinct pathways involving either prostaglandin endoperoxide synthase or lipoxygenases (Fig. 13-2).

Prostaglandins and Thromboxanes All prostaglandins (PGs) are analogs of the hypothetical compound *prostanoic acid*, a 20-carbon fatty acid which contains a five-membered ring consisting of carbons 8, 9, 10, 11, and 12 (Fig. 13-3). The different prostaglandins are divided into several types or classes (A through I) according to the substituents present in the cyclopentane ring. They are further divided by a subscript (1, 2, or 3) which indicates the number of double bonds in the side chains. Prostaglandins D, E, F, and I are considered to be the compounds of primary interest since they are released from the activated cells.

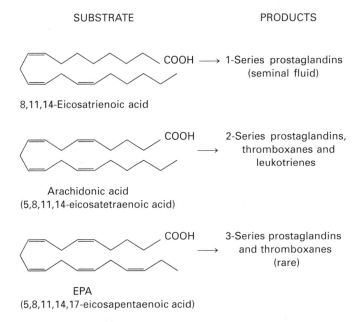

SUBSTRATE   PRODUCTS

COOH $\longrightarrow$ 1-Series prostaglandins
(seminal fluid)

8,11,14-Eicosatrienoic acid

COOH $\longrightarrow$ 2-Series prostaglandins,
thromboxanes and
leukotrienes

Arachidonic acid
(5,8,11,14-eicosatetraenoic acid)

COOH $\longrightarrow$ 3-Series prostaglandins
and thromboxanes
(rare)

EPA
(5,8,11,14,17-eicosapentaenoic acid)

FIGURE 13-1 Precursor substrates of the eicosanoids.

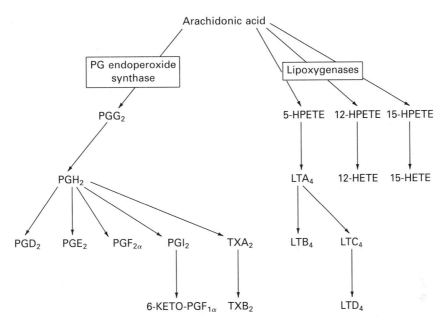

FIGURE 13-2 Overall schematic for the biosynthesis of prostaglandins and related eicosanoids.   PG = prostaglandin;   TX = thromboxane;   HPETE = hydroperoxyeicosatetraenoic acid; HETE = hydroxyeicosatetraenoic acid; and LT = leukotriene.

Prostaglandins A, B, and C can be derived chemically from prostaglandin E (PGE), but probably none of them occurs biologically. Prostaglandins G and H are intermediate cyclic endoperoxide derivatives that occur during prostaglandin biosynthesis as discussed below.

Prostaglandin endoperoxide synthase is a membrane-associated enzyme present in almost all cells. It consists of two protein subunits of 72,000 daltons and possesses both cyclooxygenase and peroxidase activities. Cyclooxygenase inserts two molecules of oxygen into arachidonic acid and causes an intramolecular rearrangement to yield an intermediate, PGG_2. The peroxidase then reduces PGG_2 to another chemically unstable ($t_{1/2}$ = 5 min at 37°C and pH 7.5) intermediate, PGH_2. PGH_2 is the precursor of all other known prostaglandins and thromboxanes containing two side-chain double bonds (see below). Prostaglandin endoperoxide synthase also will convert 8,11,14-eicosatrienoic acid into PGH_1 and 5,8,11, 14,17-eicosapentaenoic acid into PGH_3, and these endoperoxides can likewise be converted into other prostaglandins containing either one or three double bonds in their side chains, respectively.

The prostaglandin endoperoxides are isomerized enzymatically to a number of different products (Fig. 13-3). These products include PGD, PGE, PGF, PGI, and thromboxanes, and their formation depends on the presence of the appropriate isomerase or synthase within the cell. Brain tissue and mast cells contain a *PGH-PGD isomerase*, which can convert PGH_2 into PGD_2. Seminal vesicles contain *PGH-PGE isomerase* explaining the occurrence of large amounts of PGE_1 and PGE_2 in human semen. The precise mechanism of formation of $PGF_{2\alpha}$, by the uterus, for example, is still unclear. $PGF_{2\alpha}$ can be formed by the action of a reductase on PGH_2, PGD_2, or PGE_2. Endothelial cells contain *prostacyclin synthase* and convert PGH_2 primarily to prostacyclin (PGI_2). PGI_2 is unstable ($t_{1/2}$ = 3 min) and breaks down nonenzymatically to 6-keto-$PGF_{1\alpha}$. Blood platelets (thrombocytes) contain primarily *thromboxane synthase* and convert PGH_2 almost exclusively into thromboxane A2 (TXA_2). TXA_2 has a very short half-life ($t_{1/2}$ = 30 s) and converts nonenzymati-

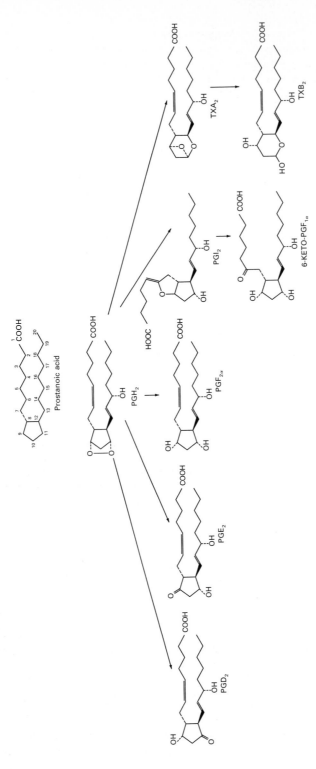

FIGURE 13-3 Structures of the hypothetical compound prostanoic acid and of prostaglandins and thromboxanes derived from arachidonic acid.

cally to TXB_2. Both prostacyclin and thromboxane synthases are cytochrome P-450 enzymes. Although thromboxanes are derived from prostaglandin endoperoxides, they are not prostaglandins because they contain a six-membered oxane ring rather than the cyclopentane ring of prostanoic acid.

Leukotrienes In contrast to prostaglandin endoperoxide synthase, which is present in the membranes of almost all cells, the *lipoxygenases* appear to be cytoplasmic and are almost entirely restricted to circulating or resident white blood cells. Three major mammalian lipoxygenases have been discovered so far, namely, those that catalyze the incorporation of a molecule of oxygen into the 5-, 12-, or 15-positions of arachidonic acid with the formation of the corresponding 5-, 12-, and 15-hydroperoxyeicosatetraenoic acids (HPETEs). Platelets contain *12-lipoxygenase* and produce 12-HPETE and its reduction product 12-hydroxyeicosatetraenoic acid (12-HETE). The function of these compounds is unknown. On the other hand, polymorphonuclear leukocytes, macrophages, basophils, and mast cells contain 5- and *15-lipoxygenases* and produce potent biologically active substances as a result of this activity. These substances include the *leukotrienes*.

The term *slow-reacting substance* (SRS) was first introduced in 1938 to describe a factor appearing in the perfusate of guinea pig lung following treatment with cobra venom. The factor produced a slow, prolonged contraction of a smooth-muscle preparation, in contrast to the rapid and transient action of histamine. A chemically and biologically similar material was subsequently found in the perfusate of sensitized guinea pig lungs following challenge with antigen. This immunologically released SRS was designated as *slow-reacting substance of anaphylaxis* (SRS-A) and was considered to be released together with other mediators (e.g., histamine and chemotactic factors) from mast cells after interaction between antigens, such as pollens, with IgE molecules bound to membrane receptors.

Studies of the transformation of arachidonic acid by polymorphonuclear leukocytes obtained from the peritoneal cavity of rabbits led initially to the identification of the major product as 5-hydroxyeicosatetraenoic acid (5-HETE). Further studies showed, however, that additional products also were formed; the major one was identified as 5,12-dihydroxyeicosatetraenoic acid and it was given the name leukotriene B_4 (LTB$_4$). It appears that arachidonic acid is transformed by a 5-lipoxygenase into 5-HPETE, which then is con-

verted into an intermediate, leukotriene A_4 (LTA$_4$). This compound is converted into LTB$_4$ by enzymatic hydrolysis (see Fig. 13-2). The name *leukotriene* was chosen to denote the cellular origin of these products (leukocytes) as well as the fact that they contained a conjugated double bond (triene) structure.

Physicochemical data on LTB$_4$ and SRS-A were similar and led to the hypothesis that there was some link between the two. After intensive study it was determined that the initial step in the biosynthesis of SRS-A is the formation of LTA$_4$. However, this LTA$_4$, instead of being converted into LTB$_4$ by hydrolysis, as in polymorphonuclear leukocytes, is transformed in mast cells by the addition of glutathione to produce the peptide-leukotriene LTC$_4$. Removal of glutamate from LTC$_4$ by a peptidase generates LTD$_4$, a peptide-leukotriene containing cysteinyl-glycine. It now appears that SRS-A is a mixture of LTC$_4$ and LTD$_4$ (Fig. 13-4).

Inhibition of Eicosanoid Biosynthesis

There is some indication that corticosteroids can inhibit prostaglandin, thromboxane, and leukotriene biosynthesis in polymorphonuclear leukocytes and certain other cell types by preventing the release of precursor arachidonic acid from membrane phospholipids. They do this by inducing the synthesis of a protein inhibitor of phospholipase A_2 called *macrocortin* (or *lipomodulin*). As described in greater detail in Chap. 39, corticosteroids induce the synthesis of many proteins, and it seems likely that the synthesis of macrocortin is at best only partly responsible for their anti-inflammatory action. On the other hand, the action of the nonsteroidal anti-inflammatory drugs (NSAIDs) such as aspirin, indomethacin, naproxen, and ibuprofen, depends to a great extent on their ability to selectively inhibit prostaglandin endoperoxide synthase and therefore block the synthesis of both prostaglandins and thromboxanes (see Fig. 13-2). It is known that aspirin acts by acetylating a hydroxyl group of a serine located in the active center of cyclooxygenase. The other agents act by complex mechanisms which seem to involve, in part, competition with arachidonic acid for access to the active site of the enzyme. Interestingly, salicylate, although closely related in structure to aspirin, has no acetylating capacity and is almost inactive as an inhibitor of cyclooxygenase. It is important to note that NSAIDs inhibit prostaglandin endoperoxide synthase but not lipoxy-

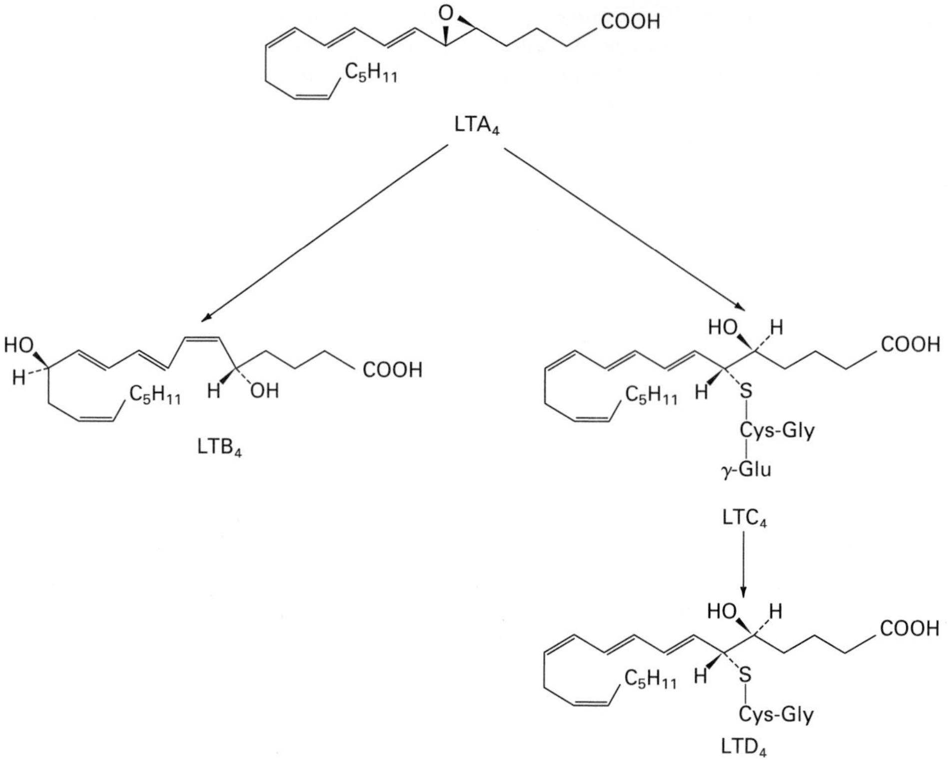

FIGURE 13-4   Structures of the leukotrienes.

genases. Therefore, it is possible that under certain conditions (for example, in mast cells which contain both prostaglandin endoperoxide synthase and 5-lipoxygenase activities) NSAIDs can actually increase the production of leukotrienes by diverting arachidonic acid to the 5-lipoxygenase pathway.

MECHANISM OF ACTION OF EICOSANOIDS

Prostaglandins, thromboxanes, and leukotrienes produce their effects on smooth muscle and other cells via interaction with membrane-bound receptors, which not only are specific for eicosanoids, as opposed to other hormones, but they also differentiate between the individual eicosanoids. Different cells contain specific receptors for many eicosanoids including PGE_1, PGE_2, $PGF_{2\alpha}$, LTB_4, and LTD_4, for example. The overall effect elicited by the eicosanoid-receptor inter-

action frequently appears to be mediated intracellularly by (1) an increase in cyclic AMP, (2) an increase in cyclic GMP, or (3) an increase in the level of free intracellular calcium ions. For example, PGE_1, PGD_2, and PGI_2 inhibit platelet aggregation by increasing the intracellular concentration of cyclic AMP, whereas PGG_2, PGH_2, and TXA_2 induce platelet aggregation by increasing the level of intracellular ionized calcium. Other eicosanoids such as PGE_2, $PGF_{2\alpha}$, 6-keto-$PGF_{1\alpha}$, TXB_2, LTB_4, and LTD_4 have little or no effect on platelets, although some of these eicosanoids have important effects on other cells.

PHARMACOKINETICS

As was previously mentioned, prostaglandins and other eicosanoids are not stored; rather they are formed quickly after the activation of phospholipase A_2 and are rapidly metabolized to inactive products after they enter the circulation. The lungs remove PGE_2 and $PGF_{2\alpha}$ from the circulation by an active uptake mechanism and subject them to enzymatic deactivation by *15-hydroxy-prostaglandin dehydrogenase* and *prostaglandin reductase*. The first enzymatic product, i.e., 15-keto-PGE_2, is less biologically active than its precursor, and the second metabolite, i.e., 15-keto-13,14-dihydro-PGE_2, is almost totally inactive. It has been estimated that 95 percent of E-type prostaglandins and 80 percent of F-type prostaglandins are inactivated in one single passage through the lungs. The prostaglandins are also biotransformed in the liver and elsewhere by beta and omega oxidation, and many of the metabolites of prostaglandins that appear in urine are dicarboxylic acids. The major metabolite of

LTC_4 and LTD_4 which appears in human urine is LTE_4, a relatively biologically inactive peptide-leukotriene containing cysteine.

PHYSIOLOGIC AND PHARMACOLOGIC EFFECTS

The physiologic and pharmacologic effects of prostaglandins and other eicosanoids are summarized briefly in Table 13-1 and are discussed in greater detail below.

The Reproductive System

The fact that there are large (microgram) amounts of PGE_1, PGE_2, $PGF_{1\alpha}$, and $PGF_{2\alpha}$ present in human semen has led to the "joint effort" hypothesis. This

TABLE 13-1 Physiologic and pharmacologic effects of prostaglandins and related eicosanoids

Biologic process	Eicosanoid	Effect
Reproduction	PGE_2	Contract pregnant uterus
	$PGF_{2\alpha}$	Destruct corpus luteum
		Contract pregnant uterus
Blood pressure regulation	PGE_1, PGE_2, PGI_2	Dilate blood vessels
	$PGF_{2\alpha}$	Constrict veins
	TXA_2	Constrict arteries
Gastric secretion	PGE_1, PGE_2	Contract longitudinal smooth muscle, stimulate bicarbonate secretion
	$PGF_{2\alpha}$, LTC_4, LTD_4	Contract smooth muscle
Inflammation	PGE_1, PGE_2, PGI_2	Increase local blood flow, increase vascular permeability
	LTB_4	Chemotactic for leukocytes
	LTC_4, LTD_4	Increase vascular permeability
Bronchoconstriction	PGD_2, $PGF_{2\alpha}$, TXA_2, LTC_4, LTD_4	Cause bronchoconstriction
	PGE_1, PGE_2, PGI_2	Cause bronchodilation
Platelet aggregation	PGE_1, PGD_2, PGI_2	Inhibit platelet aggregation
	PGG_2, PGH_2, TXA_2	Induce platelet aggregation

theory states that in males the prostaglandins stimulate the smooth-muscle contraction necessary for ejaculation, whereas in females the prostaglandins are absorbed by the vagina and contract the myometrium and oviducts. It should be pointed out, however, that, while there does seem to be some correlation between the levels of prostaglandins in semen and male fertility, the requirement for the prostaglandins does not seem to be absolute and their precise role remains to be determined.

In many subprimate species, luteolysis (destruction of the corpus luteum in the ovary) is undoubtedly caused by $PGF_{2\alpha}$. This prostaglandin is released in a pulsatile manner from the uterus at term and passes by local vascular transfer from the utero-ovarian vein into the closely positioned ovarian artery whereby it reenters the ovary. The parenteral injection of $PGF_{2\alpha}$ is associated with decreased output of progesterone by the corpus luteum and interrupts early pregnancy, which is dependent on luteal rather than placental progesterone. The luteolytic activity of prostaglandins of the F type has been put to veterinary use in synchronizing estrus in farm animals such as sheep, cattle, and pigs, which has simplified the breeding of the animals. The prostaglandins also can be used to provide safe, early abortions before the animals are put to market.

PGE_2 and $PGF_{2\alpha}$ can cause contraction of uterine smooth muscle of primates including that of the human uterus. It is thought that the increased synthesis of one or both of these prostaglandins may modulate menstruation in the human female. In keeping with this concept, NSAIDs (e.g., ibuprofen) are now prescribed for relieving menstrual cramps (dysmenorrhea).

Increased concentrations of prostaglandins have been found in the circulating blood of females during labor or spontaneous abortion. Thus, it is thought that increased intrauterine synthesis of prostaglandins initiates and maintains uterine contractions during labor. Labor may actually be induced by PGE_2 given orally (0.5 mg/h); if labor is not established by 12 h, an intravenous infusion of oxytocin is substituted. However, since this practice is accompanied by increased risk of uterine hypertonus and fetal bradycardia, the primary use of prostaglandins in gynecologic practice has been as abortifacients (see "Therapeutic Uses").

Inflammatory and Immune Responses

Prostaglandins of the E type are inflammatory, i.e., they can cause erythema, pain, and hyperalgesia (increased tenderness). They are produced locally in response to many different types of stimuli such as heat, foreign particles, and bacteria, and, by sensitizing nerve endings and increasing local blood flow, enhance the pain and increased vascular permeability induced by other agents such as complement, bradykinin, serotonin, and histamine. PGE_1 and PGE_2 have been shown to elicit pain and induce a wheal and flare responses when injected into human skin in nanogram amounts and to directly increase vascular permeability when injected subcutaneously in animals. PGI_2 also is likely to be generated during inflammation and it, too, can cause erythema and increase local blood flow, but other prostaglandins such as PGD_2 (the major prostaglandin from mast cells) and $PGF_{2\alpha}$ have not been implicated to any great extent in the inflammatory response. In contrast to the short-lived effects of other inflammatory mediators, E-type prostaglandins produce long-lasting effects (up to 10 h) upon subcutaneous blood vessels after intradermal injection. The release of prostaglandins during the inflammatory process thus produces both a direct response as well as a mechanism for the amplification of the effects of other inflammatory mediators.

The leukotrienes may also be involved in inflammation; LTB_4 is an extremely potent chemotactic agent for polymorphonuclear leukocytes, and LTC_4 and LTD_4 have the capacity to increase vascular permeability. It is known that, early in the inflammatory process, leukocytes migrate into the injured area and phagocytize the bacteria, antigen-antibody particles, or other noxious agents that may be present. During this process, the leukocytes release lytic enzymes from their lysosomes and synthesize and release LTB_4. The lysosomal enzymes then cause damage to surrounding tissue, while the LTB_4 recruits more leukocytes to the scene. Furthermore, there is evidence that the peptide-leukotrienes, LTC_4 and LTD_4 not only are formed in response to the combination of antigen with the IgE bound to the membranes of mast cells but also can be produced in increased amounts following mechanical trauma such as in surgery.

The fact that NSAIDs inhibit the formation of prostaglandins but not the formation of leukotrienes specifically implicates the prostaglandins as contributing to the symptoms of inflammation. Furthermore, NSAIDs have little or no effect on the release or activity of histamine, serotonin, or lysosomal enzymes and, similarly, potent antagonists of serotonin or histamine have little or no therapeutic effect in inflammation. Consequently, the contribution of these latter mediators in inflammation is of doubtful importance. However, this does not exclude the leukotrienes as making a contribution to the inflammatory response. It is possible that the steroidal anti-inflammatory drugs may act by inhibiting the production of both prostaglandins and leukotrienes by inducing the synthesis of the inhibitor of phospholipase A_2, macrocortin.

Human blood monocytes have the capacity to produce PGE_2. This prostaglandin has been implicated in the control of the immunologic response as it elevates cyclic AMP in the T lymphocyte and thereby inhibits mitogenesis. The production of interleukin 2 (T-cell growth factor) is inhibited indirectly via PGE_2-induced activation of an $OKT8^+$ (T-suppressor) population of lymphocytes.

Platelet Aggregation

Platelets respond to vessel injury by adhering to exposed connective tissue and clumping together to form a hemostatic plug to stem blood loss. A very similar series of events seems to occur in arterial thrombosis, with the formation of a thrombus that can lead to stroke or myocardial infarction. During the adhesion of platelets to collagen, they synthesize and release TXA_2, which can induce platelet aggregation and constrict brain and coronary arteries. The coagulation protein thrombin also is a powerful stimulus for platelet TXA_2 formation. The TXA_2 acts together with adenosine diphosphate, another aggregating agent released from the platelets, to recruit passing platelets to build up the thrombus.

A single tablet of aspirin (325 mg) totally inhibits platelet thromboxane production and hence considerably reduces the aggregation induced by collagen. The effect of aspirin on platelet aggregation lasts for 3 to 4 days because platelets (unlike most other cells) have little or no capacity for the synthesis of new protein. The return of cyclooxygenase activity, and the associated thromboxane formation, must await the entry of fresh platelets (with cyclooxygenase that has not been acetylated) from the bone marrow. It has been shown in clinical trials that aspirin reduces the incidence of transient ischemic attacks in the brain as well as myocardial infarctions in men with unstable angina. These benefits presumably result from the ability of aspirin to inhibit collagen-induced platelet aggregation.

Prostacyclin (PGI_2) is much more potent than aspirin as an inhibitor of platelet aggregation and also dilates coronary arteries. PGD_2 and PGE_1 also inhibit platelet aggregation but are less potent and seem to be less important. Endothelial cells and smooth-muscle cells can synthesize PGI_2 in response to certain stimuli such as bradykinin, but the circulating levels are too low to produce systemic effects. PGI_2 has been used clinically to prevent platelet loss during extracorporeal circulation of blood during dialysis, cardiopulmonary bypass, and hemoperfusion through charcoal. However, PGI_2 has to be infused continuously because of its rapid metabolism, and its use is complicated by a profound hypotensive effect.

Substitution of EPA (fish oil) for arachidonic acid in the diet seems to reduce plasma triglycerides and cholesterol and inhibits platelet aggregation. This, coupled with the knowledge that Eskimos who eat a lot of fish have a reduced incidence of atherosclerosis, has led to the hypothesis that the formation of more derivatives of PGH_3 and fewer derivatives of PGH_2 is beneficial. However, the evidence obtained to support this hypothesis is presently inconclusive.

The Gastrointestinal Tract

Longitudinal smooth muscle from stomach to colon contracts in response to prostaglandins of the E and F type. Circular smooth muscle contracts in response to $PGF_{2\alpha}$ but is relaxed by PGE_2. Leukotrienes C_4 and D_4 are very potent in contracting gastrointestinal smooth muscle. Prostaglandins are also involved in normal and abnormal gastrointestinal motility. Administration of PGE_2 or $PGF_{2\alpha}$ orally or intravenously often causes diarrhea, and endogenously produced prostaglandins are implicated in diarrhea associated with medullary carcinoma of the thyroid and with cholera. In contrast to PGE_2 and $PGF_{2\alpha}$, PGI_2 does not cause diarrhea.

Prostaglandins E_1, E_2, and I_2 inhibit acid output and the volume of gastric acid secretions. They stimulate bicarbonate secretion in the stomach and duodenum and increase the production of the protective mucin in the stomach. Analogs are being developed to take advantage of these protective properties; one such analog, misoprostol (15-deoxy-16-hydroxy-16-methyl-PGE_1) is approved and marketed in over 20 countries for the treatment of ulcers.

The use of NSAIDs increases fecal blood loss and is sometimes associated with gastrointestinal disturbances. This may be due in part to their ability to inhibit the formation of prostaglandins by the stomach.

Blood-Flow Regulation

PGE_1, PGE_2, and PGI_2 are potent dilators of almost all blood vessels. Intravenous infusion of PGE_2 and PGI_2 in humans induces facial flushing, vasodilatation in the systemic and pulmonary vascular beds, and hypotension. Endogenously produced PGE_2 and PGI_2 may be local regulators of blood flow in many vascular beds. For example, PGE_2 is synthesized by the kidney medulla and can regulate blood flow to the inner and outer cortex. Renal synthesis of PGE_2, a vasodilator, increases in response to angiotensin II, a vasoconstrictor, thereby causing negative feedback. Inhibition of prostaglandin synthesis by NSAIDs reduces blood flow to the inner cortex and increases flow to the outer cortex.

It is thought that renal prostaglandins are involved in Bartter's syndrome. In this rare condition there are increased levels of renin and aldosterone in blood and increased amounts of potassium and prostaglandins (PGE_2 and PGI_2) in urine. However, the patients are normotensive. If the patients are given indomethacin chronically, the urinary excretion of prostaglandins is inhibited and aldosterone returns to normal.

$PGF_{2\alpha}$ constricts superficial veins of the hand, and TXA_2 constricts cerebral and coronary arteries; their metabolites, 6-keto-$PGF_{1\alpha}$ and TXB_2, respectively, are inactive on the cardiovascular system. It is possible that Prinzmetal's angina, a vasoconstrictive problem in coronary arteries, may in part be due to the TXA_2 release from platelets. The peptide-leukotrienes C_4 and D_4 also have been shown to have the ability to constrict coronary arteries.

Bronchoconstriction

Not only can lungs remove prostaglandins from the circulation and inactivate them as noted above, but they can also produce $PGF_{2\alpha}$, PGE_2, PGI_2, TXA_2,

LTC_4, and LTD_4. The source of PGD_2 and the leukotrienes is most likely the mast cells which line the respiratory passages. Overproduction of PGD_2 or the leukotrienes will result in bronchoconstriction, and both are thought to be potential mediators of asthma. $PGF_{2\alpha}$ and TXA_2 also are potent constrictors of bronchial and tracheal muscle. On the other hand, PGE_1, PGE_2, and PGI_2 are potent bronchodilators, with PGE_2 being much more active than PGI_2. Unfortunately prostaglandins are irritant to the airways and cause coughing when inhaled, which has precluded their use as antiasthmatic drugs.

Nerve Transmission

PGE_1 and PGE_2, but not PGI_2, have been found to be potent inhibitors of norepinephrine output from nerve endings and to depress the responses of the innervated tissues. However, these effects vary greatly depending on the species, tissue, and experimental conditions used for the studies. Many stimulant and depressant effects of prostaglandins on the central nervous system also have been reported. In general, these effects have been elicited with rather high concentrations of prostaglandins, and they require further study to shed light on their relevance to physiologic or pathologic conditions.

THERAPEUTIC USES

Abortifacients

Since they stimulate the uterus to contract, certain prostaglandins, specifically $PGF_{2\alpha}$ (generic name dinoprost), PGE_2 (dinoprostone), and 15-methyl $PGF_{2\alpha}$ (carboprost), are available for use as abortifacients.

In contrast to oxytocin, prostaglandins will induce contractions of human uterus at all stages of pregnancy. However, the state of contractile responsiveness of the uterus to the prostaglandins is at its greatest at term and at its lowest early in pregnancy. Thus, larger doses of PGE_2 or $PGF_{2\alpha}$ are needed to induce early, second trimester abortion, as compared with producing labor. The drugs are given locally either by intravaginal or intra-amniotic administration to reduce the metabolism of the prostaglandins and systemic side effects.

Dinoprost (Prostin F2 alpha) is indicated for use during the 16th to 20th gestational weeks and is administered by intra-amniotic injection. The mean response time is 20 h following a single dose. After 24 h a second dose may be given, which may take up to an additional 24 h to elicit a response.

Dinoprostone (Prostin E2) is indicated for use between the 12th and 20th gestational weeks. It is also used to evacuate the uterus in intrauterine fetal death up to 28 gestational weeks. This drug is administered by vaginal suppository (20 mg) given every 3 to 5 h until abortion occurs. Continuous administration for more than 48 h is not recommended.

Carboprost (Hemabate) is available only for intramuscular administration and is recommended for use during the 13th to 20th gestational weeks. An additional indication includes second trimester abortions following the failure of other methods to expel the fetus. Typically the drug (250 μg) is given every 1.5 to 3 h based on the uterine response. This drug is also used for refractory postpartum bleeding of uterine atony.

Regardless of which drug is used, the response that occurs takes the form of a sharp rise in tonus with superimposed rhythmic contractions. This abortifacient action of prostaglandins in early human pregnancy is not associated with a decreased output of progesterone, and luteolysis does not seem to be a significant factor.

None of these drugs are specific for the gravid uterus and will elicit all the effects associated with the prostaglandins throughout the body. A high incidence of gastrointestinal upset (nausea, vomiting, and diarrhea) has been observed with all these drugs.

Ductus Arteriosus

Especially in premature deliveries, sometimes the ductus arteriosus of the newborn will remain patent (open) such that 90 percent of the cardiac output is shunted away from the lungs. The delayed spontaneous closure of the ductus is almost certainly due to the continued high production of prostaglandins (probably PGI_2) after delivery. Indomethacin inhibits prostaglandin formation and closes the patent ductus arteriosus, and it is approved by the FDA for this use.

Conversely, certain neonates with congenital heart defects including pulmonary atresia or stenosis, tricuspid atresia, tetralogy of Fallot, interruption of the aortic arch, coarctation of the aorta or transposition of the great vessels, depend on an open ductus for survival.

The smooth muscles of the ductus are especially sensitive to PGE_1, and the compound causes dilatation to occur.

Prostaglandin E_1 (generic name alprostadil) is useful therapeutically to temporarily maintain the patency of the ductus arteriosus until corrective surgery is performed. Alprostadil (Prostin VR Pediatric) is administered by continuous intravenous infusion or by catheter through the umbilical artery and should only be used in pediatric intensive care facilities. Commonly 0.05 to 0.1 μg/kg/min is used; this dose may be reduced as the therapeutic response is achieved. The more common adverse reactions to this drug include fever, flushing, bradycardia or tachycardia, hypotension, and apnea.

Prevention of Gastric Ulcers

Endogenous prostaglandins secreted by the gastric mucosa, i.e., PGE_1, PGE_2, and PGI_2, inhibit gastric acid output and the volume of gastric acid secretions. In addition, they stimulate the secretion of bicarbonate and mucin from the stomach and, therefore, protect the mucosa from the ulcerogenic effects of acid. The most common adverse effect of NSAIDs is gastric irritation, which may lead to gastric ulceration and bleeding. These effects result from the ability of NSAIDs to inhibit prostaglandin formation in the gastrointestinal tract.

Misoprostol is a synthetic analog of PGE_1. In the United States it is indicated for the prevention of gastric ulcers in patients taking NSAIDs; in other countries the drug is approved and marketed for the treatment of idiopathic peptic ulcers unrelated to NSAIDs.

Misoprostol (Cytotec) is available as tablets (200 μg) and is administered orally in a dose of 100 to 200 μg 4 times daily. It is rapidly absorbed in the intestine and is biotransformed to its free acid, which is the product responsible for the drug's activity. The $t_{1/2}$ of the compound is only 20 to 40 min; excretion is mainly via the urinary tract and partly through the feces.

The most common adverse effects of this drug are diarrhea and abdominal pain, which are usually transient. Gynecological disturbances, e.g., spotting, cramps, and dysmenorrhea, have also been reported. Rarely do the adverse effects of misoprostol require cessation of therapy.

BIBLIOGRAPHY

Bergstrom, S.: "Prostaglandins: Members of a New Hormonal System," *Science*, **157**:382–391 (1967).

Caldwell, B., and H. R. Behrman: "Prostaglandins in Reproductive Processes," *Med. Clin. North. Am.*, **65**:927–936 (1981).

DiPalma, J. R.: Misoprostol: Prostaglandin for Peptic Ulcer, *Am. Fam. Physician*, **40**:217–219 (1989).

Dunn, M. J., and V. L. Hood: "Prostaglandins in the Kidney," *Am. J. Physiol.*, **233**:F169–F184 (1977).

Flower, R. J.: "Drugs Which Inhibit Prostaglandin Biosynthesis," *Pharmacol. Rev.*, **26**:33–67 (1974).

Horton, E. W., and N. L. Poyser: "Uterine Luteolytic Hormone. A Physiologic Role for Prostaglandin $F_{2\alpha}$," *Physiol. Rev.*, **56**:595–651 (1976).

Piper, P. J.: "Formation and Actions of Leukotrienes," *Physiol. Rev.*, **64**: 744–761 (1984).

Samuelsson, B. et al.: "Prostaglandins and Thromboxanes," *Annu. Rev. Biochem.*, **47**:997–1029 (1978).

Smith, J. B.: "The Prostanoids in Hemostasis and Thrombosis," *Am. J. Pathol.*, **99**:742–804 (1980).

PART IV

Central Nervous System Drugs

SECTION EDITOR

G. John DiGregorio

General Anesthetics

Jan C. Horrow and Ruby M. Padolina

Anesthesia, literally, denotes a loss of sensibility. In current practice, surgical anethesia is a controlled degree of central nervous system depression with the following components: analgesia (lack of pain), amnesia (lack of memory), inhibition from reflexes such as bradycardia and laryngospasm, and skeletal muscle relaxation. Although frequently called sleep, anesthesia is an altered state of consciousness quite different from sleep. The general anesthetics depress or block neurologic impulses throughout the central nervous system. An ideal anesthetic would possess all the above properties, including a wide margin of safety without serious adverse effects. Presently, there are two types of general anesthetics. They are the inhaled or gaseous agents and the intravenous anesthetics.

This chapter includes a discussion of the inhaled anesthetic agents (halothane, enflurane, isoflurane, methoxyflurane, and nitrous oxide) and the intravenous anesthetic agents (barbiturates, ketamine, and etomidate). Included also are the adjuncts to anesthesia such as sufentanil, diazepam, lorazepam, midazolam, propofol, althesin, and propanidid. This chapter also contains discussion of the following three major principles underlying the use of general anesthetics:

1. *Minimum alveolar concentration (MAC)* This concept is utilized to explain or quantitate the pharmacodynamic properties of general anesthetics.
2. *Uptake and distribution* These topics are presented to quantitate the pharmacokinetics of these agents.
3. *Mechanism of action* A general mechanism of action is presented to explain why these agents are capable of producing a sequential depression of the central nervous system.

MINIMAL ALVEOLAR CONCENTRATION

The effects of any oral or parenteral drug are characterized by a dose-response curve relating serum concentration to a measured organ response. However, with inhalational anethetics, the end organ of interest is the brain, and its desired response is unconsciousness to a noxious stimulus such as surgical incision.

Drugs administered as gases are unusual in that most of the drug inspired is immediately exhaled with only a fraction being absorbed and retained. The dose administered is measured not by weight but by that percent of an atmosphere containing the drug. Since gases in the alveoli are equilibrated with blood, the dose of anesthetic is measured by its alveolar concentrations. Furthermore, end-tidal gas concentrations reflect alveolar gas concentrations. Thus anesthetic dose (alveolar concentration) is conveniently measured by analyzing exhaled gas.

The anesthetic potency is characterized by the minimal alveolar concentration (MAC) of a drug that abolishes motion in response to a noxious stimulus in 50 percent of people. The more potent an anesthetic, the lower its value for MAC. The dose-response curve is steep: 99 percent of people remain immobile when given 1.3 times the MAC of an anesthetic.

Why is MAC important? Just as uptake and distribution (see the next section) describe the pharmacokinetics of inhaled anesthetics, MAC describes their pharmacodynamics. The analog of MAC for noninhalational drugs is the steady-state plasma concentration at 50 percent effect, or $Cpss_{(50)}$. Inhaled anesthetics have very low therapeutic indices, ranging around 2 to 4. Safe use thus requires accuracy in choosing and administering a dose. MAC allows safe selection of an initial dose (concentration) of drug. The MACs for currently used agents are listed in Table 14-1. Note that the MAC of nitrous oxide is very different from the MACs of volatile anesthetics.

MAC is highest in infants and steadily decreases with age to a value in the elderly of about one-half that of the infant. MAC is less during pregnancy. It also declines as body temperature drops. There is no synergism or antagonism among inhalational anesthetics when they are administered concurrently: MAC is additive. Thus 1.3 MAC may be provided by adding 0.7 MAC of nitrous oxide to 0.6 MAC of halothane. MAC is increased in the presence of increased sympathetic neurotransmitter activity in the central nervous system. Thus agents that increase the concentration and release of catecholamines centrally, such as cocaine and amphetamines used acutely, will elevate MAC. MAC is decreased by agents depleting CNS catechols, such as alpha-methyldopa, clonidine, and chronic amphetamine use. Concurrent administration of intravenous anesthetics, sedatives, or opioids will lower the MAC of inhaled agents. Acute ethanol intoxication decreases MAC (with ethanol providing the balance of CNS depression in additive fashion), while tolerance to alcohol elevates MAC.

UPTAKE AND DISTRIBUTION OF INHALED AGENTS

The effect of a given concentration of an anesthetic agent on humans is dependent on its anesthetic potency (MAC) and the manner in which it is handled by the transport mechanisms and storage depots of the body. The process governing uptake of inhalational anesthesia can be divided into several sections (Fig. 14-1).

Since uptake and distribution depend on the tension or pressure of the dissolved gas in blood and tissues, these aspects of inhalation anesthesia are presented in terms of the partial pressure of anesthetics rather than their concentrations. The partial pressure of inhaled anesthetic depends on the vapor pressure and the volume of oxygen in which the anesthetic is mixed.

TABLE 14-1 Properties of modern inhalational anesthetics

	MAC, % atm	Vapor pressure at 20°C, mmHg	Blood-gas solubility coefficient
Nitrous oxide	110.	—	0.43
Halothane	0.77	243	2.4
Enflurane	1.68	175	1.9
Isoflurane	1.15	238	1.4
Methoxyflurane	0.16	23	12.

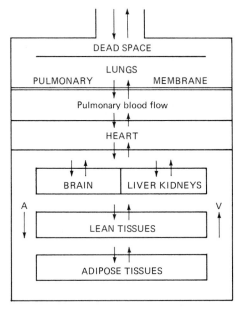

FIGURE 14-1 Diagram illustrating some of the physiologic and physical factors underlying the uptake of inhalation anesthetics by the body.

After volatization and mixing in the anesthesia machine, gases are delivered via a breathing circuit. The patient inhales anesthetic agent producing an alveolar partial pressure with which each tissue equilibrates. The tissue in which an anesthetizing partial pressure must develop is the brain. In order to increase the fraction of anesthetic in the alveolus (F_A), the anesthesiologist must deliver a suitable inspired fraction of anesthetic agent (F_I) and the patient must breathe. Ventilation delivers anesthetic to the alveoli, while uptake removes anesthetic from the alveoli. The alveolar concentration results as a balance between these two forces.

Uptake into blood is a product of three factors: anesthetic solubility, cardiac output, and the difference of anesthetic partial pressure between alveolar gas and venous blood. An increase in any of these causes a proportional increase in uptake, presuming the other two factors remain constant. If any of these approaches zero, uptake approaches zero and F_A rapidly approaches F_I.

Anesthetic solubility is a specific type of partition coefficient. If the affinity of gas anesthetic for phase A is twice the affinity for phase B, then we say that gas anesthetic has an A/B partition coefficient of 2. Partition coefficients are measured by determining the relative concentration of gas anesthetic in phases A and B when the partial pressure of gas anesthetic is the same in both phases. Tables 14-1 and 14-2 give representation values for the blood-gas partition coefficient, for the tissue-blood partition coefficients for two tissues, brain and fat, and for the oil-gas partition coefficient.

On the first inspiration of an anesthetic, the blood coming to the alveolus via the pulmonary capillaries is suddenly exposed to the tension of the anesthetic present in the alveolus. If the anesthetic is totally insoluble in blood (i.e., blood-gas partition coefficient = 0), then none of it will be taken up by the circulation and alveolar concentration rises rapidly as permitted by ventilation.

Anesthetics with high blood solubility produce high uptake but slow induction, since alveolar partial pressure rises slowly. With anesthetics of low blood solubility only a small quantity is dissolved in blood, so the alveolar concentration rises rapidly. This process is somewhat analogous to a drug administered intravenously that is highly bound to plasma proteins: more drug must be given to saturate binding sites so that enough unbound, free drug remains to exert its effect.

An increase in cardiac output presents more blood to the anesthetic within the alveolus, leading to an increase in uptake, a slower rise of alveolar partial pressure, and prolonged induction.

The uptake of an anesthetic agent by the tissue depends on the same factors as described for the blood—the tension gradient between the circulation and the tissue, the solubility of the agent in a particular organ, and finally the blood flow. A high tissue solubility (a high tissue-blood partition coefficient), a high tissue volume relative to blood flow, and a high arterial to tissue anesthetic partial pressure difference all increase uptake.

Subsequent distribution throughout the body is shown by the directional arrows of Fig. 14-1. On the arterial side (A), the tension of anesthetic reaching tissues is the same. The volume of blood flow to the brain, heart, and kidneys is high compared with their mass. Diffusion of anesthetic gas into and out of tissues occurs according to the prevailing partial pressure gradient on the venous side (V) of the circulation. The tension of anesthetic returning to the right heart and lungs represents the flow-weighted average of tensions of anesthetic returned from the various tissues.

In Fig. 14-2, curves demonstrate the rate of the increase in arterial partial pressure of several anesthetics expected to occur during administration of anesthetics. The curves show how arterial anesthetic gas tensions approach a constant inhaled tension of the gas or vapor which would be expected to produce anesthesia. Because of the excellent blood supply of the brain and the rapid exchange of dissolved gas between brain and blood, the curves also indicate the partial pressures reached in the brain, leading to the induction of the

TABLE 14-2   Partition coefficients at 37°C

Anesthetic	Brain-blood	Fat-blood	Oil-gas
Nitrous oxide	1.06	2.3	1.4
Isoflurane	2.6	45	98
Enflurane	1.45	36.2	98
Halothane	2.3	60	224
Methoxyflurane	2.0	49	970

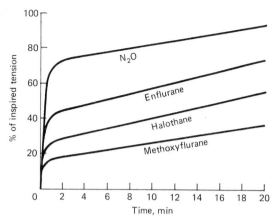

FIGURE 14-2 Exchange of gas at lungs and tissues. Graphic representation of how the tension of anesthetic gas in arterial blood approaches inspired tension during the course of inhalational anesthesia (values calculated from a formula derived by Kety). With the inspired tension of anesthesia gas shown as 100 percent, the tension of anesthetic in arterial blood is read from the ordinate as a percentage of the inspired tension. Time in minutes is shown on the abscissa.

anesthetic state. It is assumed that the minute volume of respiration, the size of the lung compartments, and the cardiac output are average normal values for adults. The general shape and direction of the curves in Fig. 14-2 are similar for each anesthetic, indicating the constancy of the physiologic conductions. The variations are explained by differences in the physical properties of the anesthetics. Initially, within 2 to 3 min, there is a sharp rise in the arterial curve and a leveling off at the knee of the curve, with a different height for each anesthetic. The heights reached indicate that nitrous oxide approaches the inhaled tension most rapidly. This is again a manifestation of the relative solubilities in blood, those anesthetics with the lesser solubilities maintaining an alveolar pressure close to the inhaled tension. Thus the height of the knee for each anesthetic inversely corresponds to its solubility in the blood, so that nitrous oxide may be expected to induce anesthesia quickly, methoxyflurane more slowly.

It appears from Fig. 14-2 that anesthesia is never reached with the anesthetics most soluble. Practically, however, the anesthesiologist does not maintain a constant inhaled partial pressure of anesthetic, as the diagram suggests, but increases the partial pressure for rapid induction and subsequently varies the level according to the patient's reactions and the surgical needs. When saturation of tissues is approached, the arterial anesthetic tension approximates that of the inhaled tension. The process of desaturation and emergence from anesthesia can be followed graphically by inverting the curves shown in Fig. 14-2, but this is true only if equilibration was reached; otherwise, redistribution among tissues could still be most rapid with the agents that are least soluble in blood, e.g., nitrous oxide. At the same time, rapid diffusion into the alveoli lowers the blood level quickly, and within the period of lung washout there should be an approach to recovery of consciousness. Even in this case, however, a residual concentration is present in blood as long as the tissues retain the anesthetic, this again being a function of circulation and distribution between blood and tissues.

The actual sequence of anesthesia induction provides insight into the choice of modern anesthetic agents. The anesthetist employs a precision calibrated vaporizer to increase gradually the inspired concentration of volatile anesthetic in oxygen. Corrugated tubing delivers this gas mixture to a mask placed snugly over the patient's mouth and nose. Anesthetic concentration is increased by about 0.5 percent every other breath. The patient passes through several "stages" of anesthesia. In the first stage, the stage of analgesia, sensation to pain is blunted while consciousness remains intact. During stage 2, the stage of excitability, inhibitory reflexes are depressed, and the patient is unable to follow commands. Respirations become irregular, heart rate increases, and cardiac dysrhythmias may appear. The patient may attempt to sit up and leave the room, or may pull out intravenous catheters and disengage monitoring devices. Vomiting and regurgitation may occur; inhibition of the appropriate reflex laryngeal closure to entry of this foreign material may result in pulmonary aspiration of gastric secretions, an event associated with high mortality. For these many reasons, the intensity and duration of stage 2 should be kept to a minimum.

As delivery of anesthetic to the brain progresses,

stage 2 ends and the stage of surgical anesthesia begins. Anesthetics refer to the planes, or levels, of this stage as being light or deep, with deep indicating greater depression. Finally, if administration of large doses of anesthetic is continued, stage 4 is achieved. At this stage, depressant effects result in cardiovascular collapse and death.

Mechanism of Action

From 1899 to 1901, Meyer and Overton proposed a theory regarding "the action of the anesthetic agents." They correlated the potency of anesthetics with their degree of solubility in olive oil, the more fat-soluble anesthetic agents being more potent. Others related anesthetic potency to surface-tension-reducing properties or to the ease of formation of "icebergs" within the cell. Anesthetics most likely act by changing the physical properties of the phospholipid matrix of the biologic membrane, resulting in altered function of receptors and ion channels.

General anesthetics have neurophysiologic effects on the neurons of the central nervous system. These compounds decrease the firing rate of nerve cells by decreasing the rise of the action potential. The proposed molecular mechanism is based on the effects of these agents on sodium movement across the membrane. The general anesthetics apparently attach to the sodium channels by interacting with the lipid and hydrophilic areas of the channel causing a distortion of this structure. The resulting distortion of the channel causes an interference in sodium conductance across the membrane.

INHALED ANESTHETIC AGENTS

Halothane

The ongoing research for a potent inhalation agent that was neither explosive nor highly toxic led to the development of halothane, a halogenated hydrocarbon. Halothane was one of the most significant advances in general anesthesia since the introduction of ether 110 years earlier.

Chemistry Halothane is similar to the pioneering anesthetic chloroform, a substituted alkane. In contrast to halothane are the substituted methyl-ether ethers, enflurane and isoflurane.

$$\begin{array}{ccc} F & Br \\ | & | \\ F-C-C-H \\ | & | \\ F & Cl \end{array}$$

Halothane

At room temperature, halothane exists as a volatile liquid with a vapor pressure of 243 mmHg, about one-third of an atmosphere at sea level. Since low concentrations of inspired halothane provide surgical anesthesia, the mixture of inspired gases containing halothane must be controlled accurately. A precision, calibrated vaporizer provides this control with correction for changes of vapor pressure with temperature. Halothane is administered only by inhalation of vaporized liquid, never intravenously.

Halothane corrodes many metals and some plastics. Addition of thymol to liquid halothane prevents degradation during storage. Halothane has a sweet, pleasant odor and is not irritating to respiratory mucosa.

Pharmacokinetics Halothane undergoes significant metabolism in humans, with about 20 percent of the absorbed dose recovered as metabolites. Both oxidative and reductive metabolism occur, but oxidative metabolism predominates.

The major metabolite of oxidative metabolism is trifluoroacetic acid, which is excreted in the urine. Other oxidative metabolites that appear in the urine are chloride and bromide. Trifluoroacetic acid has no known adverse effects. However, serum bromide concentration will increase approximately 0.5 meq/L per MAC per hour of halothane administration. Signs of bromide toxicity (somnolence, mental confusion) occur when the serum bromide concentration exceeds 6 meq/L.

Reductive metabolism of halothane is more likely to occur in the presence of inadequate oxygen delivery to hepatocytes and stimulation of hepatic microsomal enzyme activity by drugs (phenobarbital) or chemicals (polychlorobiphenyls). This results in the formation of reactive intermediary metabolites and fluoride. The reactive intermediaries may produce liver damage either directly or via an immune-mediated hypersensitivity.

Pharmacodynamics

Central Nervous System Inhalation of increasing concentrations of halothane results in progressive obtundation leading to the state of surgical anesthesia and, if continued, on to cardiovascular collapse and death. Halothane is analgesic in sub-MAC concentrations. Amnesia occurs as well. The EEG reflects these CNS events. The baseline EEG consisting of a fast, low-voltage signal becomes a slow, higher-voltage signal with clinical doses of halothane. Cerebral blood flow increases even though the cerebral metabolic rate of oxygen use declines: this disparity defines a state of impaired cerebral autoregulation. Halothane increases CSF pressure.

Cardiovascular System Halothane induces a dose-dependent decrease in systemic blood pressure: mean arterial pressure is inhaled at 2 MAC. Cardiac output is decreased while systemic vascular resistance changes little. Myocardial blood flow and extraction of oxygen and lactate decrease proportionally, indicating preservation of coronary vascular autoregulation. Heart rate decreases during halothane inhalation secondary to diminished sympathetic tone. Obtundation of the baroreceptor reflex permits heart rate to remain constant or decrease despite a fall in systemic blood pressure. Adrenergic stimulation during halothane inhalation induces ventricular dysrhythmias. The source of this stimulation may be extrinsic, as from a surgical incision or administration of epinephrine, or intrinsic, as occurs with hypercarbia and light planes of anesthesia. Although overall systemic vascular resistance remains unchanged, splanchnic beds constrict while skin and muscle beds dilate.

Respiratory System Halothane decreases tidal volume and increases respiratory rate in humans, yielding a net decrease in minute ventilation. As a consequence, the arterial P_{CO_2} rises to almost 50 mmHg at 1 MAC. The normal ventilatory response to carbon dioxide is attenuated: the curve is shifted to the right (decreased minute ventilation for a given P_{CO_2}), and its slope is less steep (smaller increase in ventilation per mmHg increase in P_{CO_2}). These alterations are centrally mediated and not secondary to an effect on peripheral chemoreceptors. The ventilatory response to hypoxia is also obtunded by halothane. Only 1.1 MAC obliterates the normal hyperventilatory response

to hypoxia. Unlike halothane's attenuation of the effects of hypercarbia, halothane depresses hypoxic respiratory drive by directly affecting peripheral chemoreceptors.

Halothane dilates a bronchoconstricted airway via a direct action on bronchial smooth muscle as well as via depression of local reflex arcs: its effect is not dependent on obtaining blood concentrations of drug. A resting, unstimulated airway with normal bronchial tone is not further dilated by halothane. Mucociliary function is depressed during halothane inhalation.

Neuromuscular Junction By itself, halothane provides inadequate muscle relaxation for surgery, although it does potentiate the action of nondepolarizing muscle relaxants. A 1 MAC halothane, the dose of neuromuscular blocking drug may be reduced by about one-third to one-half. The site of action appears to be the muscle membrane.

Other Effects Renal blood flow and glomerular filtration rate both decrease during halothane inhalation. Renovascular autoregulation is not disturbed. The rate of urine production decreases by more than half. Hepatic blood flow and hepatic enzymatic activity decreases. Halothane relaxes the uterus: it is used clinically to treat tetany during labor.

Adverse Reactions

Halothane Hepatotoxicity Soon after the discovery of halothane, reports of postoperative jaundice and hepatic necrosis appeared with findings similar to those caused by chloroform. Repeated administration of halothane has been associated with liver damage in rare instances. Prolonged exposure to halothane, even following enzyme induction with phenobarbital, has failed to produce liver damage. However, both pretreatment and hypoxia produce centrilobular necrosis following exposure to halothane.

Multiple exposures to halothane in short intervals may increase the risk of liver damage, possibly via an immune response mechanism. Other proposed but unsubstantiated mechanisms include enhanced biotransformation of halothane and reductive halothane metabolism. The U.S. National Halothane Study reviewed 85,000 anesthetics. It concluded that the incidence of massive hepatic necrosis associated with halothane is 1 in 10,000 and recommended that unexplained fever and jaundice following halothane might reasonably be considered a contraindication to subsequent use.

Dysrhythmias   Aminophylline, like epinephrine and other sympathomimetic agents, may cause ventricular tachycardia or fibrillation during halothane anesthesia. The use of alternative inhalation agents with a bronchodilator effect, such as enflurane or isoflurane, is recommended for asthmatic patients who must receive aminophylline before or during surgery. Patients who are being treated for depression with the tricyclic compound amitriptyline may suffer life-threatening ventricular dysrhythmias when given halothane and pancuronium, probably related to the blocking effect of tricyclic compounds on reuptake of the neurotransmitter norepinephrine.

Malignant Hyperthermia   A rare patient (one in 10,000 to 20,000) experiences rapid temperature elevation upon exposure to volatile anesthetics or depolarizing muscle relaxants. This syndrome, which occurs only in genetically susceptible individuals, arises from a primary disorder of muscle involving poor control of intracellular calcium sequestration during muscle contraction. Although malignant hyperthermia is of little consequence when a susceptible individual is not anesthetized, when it occurs untreated under anesthesia, death is likely. Metabolic acidemia, cardiac dysrhythmias, and hyperkalemia accompany episodes of malignant hyperthermia. Prophylaxis for susceptible patients and treatment of ongoing episodes utilize dantrolene, a drug which interferes with the release of calcium from the sarcoplasmic reticulum (see Chap. 11).

Therapeutic Use   Halothane induces analgesia, amnesia, loss of consciousness, and obtundation of noxious reflexes such as bradycardia and laryngospasm. These properties define a complete anesthetic. Halothane may serve as the sole agent in providing anesthesia in suitable patients for procedures not requiring muscular relaxation although, for reasons already discussed, a single drug is rarely used to provide anesthesia. Despite the attraction of a certain simplicity in providing anesthesia with a single drug, one agent, such as halothane, is rarely administered by itself. More commonly, other anesthetic agents and adjuvants combine with halothane to provide a smoother

and safer passage from consciousness to stage 3. A rapid-acting intravenous agent such as thiopental will bypass stages 1 and 2 altogether; the term *induction agent* is suitably applied. Addition of nitrous oxide to a halothane-oxygen gas mixture utilizes the additive properties of MAC and the more favorable blood-gas partition coefficient of nitrous oxide to accelerate anesthetic delivery to brain and shorten stage 2. Following induction of anesthesia, controlled ventilation, as opposed to spontaneous breathing, prevents the adverse consequences of hypercarbia attendant with inhalation of volatile anesthetic (see below).

The factors determining choice of volatile anesthetic agent are varied and complex. The patient's pathophysiologic derangements related to concurrent disease states provide the primary motivations to select or avoid particular drugs. For example, severe asthmatics who require general anesthetics often do best with a volatile agent, which dilates constricted bronchi. Patients with congestive heart failure, on the other hand, may develop worsening failure with the volatile anesthetics owing to myocardial contractile depression. Some clinicians avoid halothane in patients with a history of abnormal liver function, so that in the event of postoperative worsening of hepatic function, the differential diagnosis is not complicated by the specter of halothane hepatitis.

During a mask induction of anesthesia using halothane and oxygen, with or without nitrous oxide, large concentrations of halothane, up to 5 percent or even higher, will be administered transiently. The purpose of this "overpressuring" is to establish as quickly as possible a brain partial pressure of anesthetic that is consistent with stage 3 anesthesia. Following induction, inspired concentrations are decreased to match the level of surgical stimulation. For example, during placement of surgical drapes, stimulation is minimal; the anesthetic requirement may be less than 1 MAC, say 0.5 percent. In contrast, the deeper plane of anesthesia needed for manipulation of the peritoneum often demands concentrations around 1.5 percent, or about 2 MAC.

Enflurane

Following synthesis of halothane, a substituted ethane, the search continued for a halogenated anesthetic similar in structure to diethyl ether. A series of substituted ethers emerged, including fluroxene, methoxyflurane, enflurane, and isoflurane. Of these enflurane and isoflurane remain in common use today.

Chemistry Enflurane is a substituted methyl ethyl ether. The other linkage combined with increased fluorine substitution yields greater molecular stability compared with halothane. Enflurane is less volatile and less potent than halothane. Its room temperature vapor pressure of 175 mmHg is about one quarter of an atmosphere at sea level. MAC for enflurane is 1.68 percent, more than twice that of halothane. Like halothane, enflurane has a sweet odor, although enflurane inhalation is slightly less pleasant and more irritating to respiratory mucosa.

$$\begin{array}{ccc} F & F & F \\ | & | & | \\ HCOC & & CH \\ | & | & | \\ F & F & Cl \end{array}$$

Pharmacokinetics The lower blood-gas partition coefficient for enflurane allows for more rapid onset and offset of anesthesia compared with halothane. A lower solubility in fat results in more rapid excretion and less time for metabolism to occur. Small amounts of enflurane are defluorinated in the liver yielding several metabolic products including fluoride ion. While excessive fluoride is nephrotoxic, peak fluoride levels rarely exceed even half the threshold for toxicity.

Pharmacodynamics The cerebral blood flow increase during enflurane inhalation is less than that during halothane. Enflurane profoundly depresses the oxygen and glucose needs of the brain. Like halothane, enflurane increases intracranial pressure. Large doses of enflurane result in seizure-like activity, especially in the presence of hypercarbia. Both abnormal muscular contraction and spike-and-dome complexes on the EEG can occur. Enflurane-induced seizure activity markedly elevates the cerebral metabolic rate.

Blood pressure decreases during enflurane administration secondary to decreases in both cardiac output and systemic vascular resistance. Heart rate remains unchanged. Junctional rhythm occurs on occasion, while ventricular ectopy is rare even during sympathetic stimulation.

Tidal volume and respiratory rate both decrease, producing profound ventilatory depression and arterial P_{CO_2} values greater than 60 mmHg at 1 MAC. Like

halothane, enflurane dilates a bronchoconstricted airway and obtunds the ventilatory responses to hypercarbia and hypoxia. Potentiation of nondepolarizing muscle relaxants is greater with enflurane than with halothane, thus reducing the dose of relaxant by two-thirds. Enflurane and halothane have similar effects on the kidney, liver, and uterus.

Isoflurane

Chemistry Isoflurane is an isomer of enflurane. The MAC of isoflurane is about 1.15 percent, which is lower than the MAC of its isomer enflurane (1.68 percent). The blood-gas and oil-gas partition coefficients are 1.4 and 99, respectively. Isoflurane is more pungent than both halothane and enflurane.

$$\begin{array}{ccc} F & & \\ | & & \\ HC & \!\!-O-\!\! & CHCF_3 \\ | & & | \\ F & & Cl \end{array}$$
Isoflurane

Pharmacokinetics Isoflurane causes direct coronary vascular dilatation leading to redistribution of coronary blood flow away from diseased vessels that are unable to dilate to healthy vessels capable of dilation, thereby worsening ischemia. However, the existence of this syndrome has not been proven in humans, and its effect on the outcome in humans undergoing anesthesia with isoflurane is not clear.

The amount of isoflurane metabolized in the body is insignificant. As a result, the amounts of fluoride ion and trifluoroacetic acid released by metabolism are negligible. Though enzyme induction by phenobarbital, ethanol, and isoniazid increases metabolism if isoflurane, the amount of fluoride released is of no clinical significance. Liver damage caused by isoflurane has not been reported.

Pharmacodynamics Isoflurane increases cerebral blood flow and decreases cerebral metabolic rate for oxygen (CMR_{O_2}). At 1.5 to 2 MAC, isoflurane decreases CMR_{O_2} by 50 percent and produces an isoelectric EEG. Further increases do not produce deeper metabolic depression. Isoflurane's effect on the EEG is dose-dependent: fast activity with low amplitude occurs at 0.5 MAC, progressing with increasing dose through slow waves and burst suppression to an isoelectric tracing at 2 MAC. Isoflurane promotes muscle relaxation and enhances the effects of muscle relaxants on neuromuscular junction to the same extent as enflurane. This characteristic is attributed to the increase in the effects on the central nervous system and neuromuscular junction. Mean arterial pressure decreases with the administration of isoflurane in a dose-dependent fashion, due mostly to a decrease in systemic vascular resistance.

Methoxyflurane

Another substituted methyl ethyl ether, methoxyflurane, has a characteristic fruity odor.

$$\begin{array}{c} Cl \quad F \\ | \quad | \\ HC{-}COCH_3 \\ | \quad | \\ Cl \quad F \end{array}$$

Methoxyflurane

With a MAC of 0.16 percent, it is the most potent anesthetic available. Its high blood-gas solubility coefficient of about 12 makes for a prolonged induction and emergency from anesthesia. Methoxyflurane use is exceedingly rare, owing to the drug's potential for nephrotoxicity. Biotransformation liberates a significant amount of fluoride ion leading to high output renal failure.

Nitrous Oxide

Chemistry Nitrous oxide, N_2O, the only inorganic gas used to produce anesthesia in humans, has a molecular weight of 44 and specific gravity of 1.527 (air = 1). It is neither inflammable nor explosive but will support combustion of other agents, even in the absence of oxygen, owing to its decomposition to N_2 and O_2 at temperatures about 450°C. The oil-water solubility ratio is 3.2. The blood-gas solubility coefficient is 0.47.

Pharmacokinetics Despite the relative insolubility of N_2O in blood, a large amount is rapidly taken up because high concentrations are given. Within 20 min of administration, as much as 30 L may be absorbed via the lungs and distributed to body tissue. At the termination of anesthesia, if the patient is abruptly permitted to breathe room air, a correspondingly large volume of nitrous oxide diffuses outward, thus lowering $P_{A_{O_2}}$ and temporarily causing hypoxemia (diffusion hypoxia). At the same time, $P_{A_{CO_2}}$ is lowered, causing respiratory depression. This undesirable sequence is avoided by administration of pure oxygen for a few minutes before permitting inhalation of room air.

Pharmacodynamics Nitrous oxide is a weak anesthetic agent. Clinical doses are limited to 80 percent, an amount not sufficient to progress beyond stage 2 in most patients. With a MAC of 101 percent, it cannot be used as the sole anesthetic agent. However, when combined with another agent, nitrous oxide provides additive anesthetic action: 30 percent N_2O (0.3 MAC) reduces the amount of enflurane needed by 0.3 MAC, from 1.68 to 1.17 percent. Likewise, 70 percent N_2O reduces enflurane requirement to 0.5 percent, which is 0.7 of its MAC. Seventy percent N_2O also reduces halothane or isoflurane MAC by six-tenths of its usual value.

Adverse Reactions

Hematologic Effects There is evidence of interference with production of both leukocytes and red blood cells by the bone marrow, following very prolonged administration of nitrous oxide. Nitrous oxide can oxidize the cobalt atom in vitamin B_{12} and, thereby, cause megaloblastic changes in the bone marrow and a neuropathy in experimental animals.

Teratogenic Effects Many epidemiologic surveys have investigated the possible adverse reproductive effects of working in operating or dental suites. The most consistent finding is a higher than expected incidence of spontaneous abortion among female personnel directly exposed to waste anesthetic gases. Spontaneous abortion may be 25 percent more frequent among exposed women. Spontaneous abortion rates for chairside assistants of dentists increase with increasing duration of exposure to nitrous oxide, reaching a maximum of 2 times the control rate. The data from studies on congenital abnormalities are less consistent. Malformations may be slightly more frequent in the offspring of exposed women.

Diffusion into Air-Containing Spaces The blood-gas partition coefficient of nitrous oxide (0.47) is 34 times greater than that of nitrogen (0.014). This differential solubility means nitrous oxide can leave the blood to enter an air (79% nitrogen)-filled cavity 34 times more rapidly than nitrogen can leave the cavity to enter the blood. Hence, the volume of or pressure within the cavity increases. Air-filled cavities surrounded by a complaint wall (intestinal gas, pneumothorax, lung distal to a pulmonary embolus, pulmonary vascular air embolism) will expand; for those cavities surrounded by a noncomplaint wall (middle ear, cerebral ventricles, supratentorial subdural space), intracavity pressure will increase.

Therapeutic Uses

Analgesia At a concentration of 6 to 25 percent of nitrous oxide, analgesia (stage 1) is achieved, but patients remain in full contact with their surroundings. As a sole agent, nitrous oxide may thus be used intermittently to provide analgesia for dental procedures and during the first stage of parturition. The drug is used in some countries in this manner to produce postoperative analgesia.

Surgical Anesthesia Since nitrous oxide is an incomplete anesthetic, it must be administered with adjuvant drugs. Commonly, volatile anesthetics are used, but not infrequently large doses of a short-acting opioid such as fentanyl are given in order to produce an anesthetic state.

Abuse Potential Recreational inhalation of nitrous oxide, which began with the early experiments of Humphrey Davy, has gained popularity in recent years owing to the extensive use of nitrous oxide analgesia in dentistry. Nitrous oxide possesses a (false) reputation as a harmless, chemically inert substance.

In a recent survey of medical and dental students at a university via an anonymous questionnaire, up to 20 percent of medical and dental students has used nitrous oxide to produce euphoria. Nitrous oxide had been obtained from a variety of sources, most often from cylinders used in the production of whipped cream. Health professionals with easy access to the agent are especially vulnerable to this practice. Some of the 524 students who responded to the questionnaire reported nausea, diarrhea, cyanosis, and syncope. Hypoxia and asphyxia leading to malignant arrhythmias and death may occur during inhalation of nitrous oxide when adequate concentrations of inspired oxygen are not given.

INTRAVENOUS ANESTHETICS

The first attempt at producing insensibility by means of intravenous injection occurred in 1656, when Percival Christopher Wren, with the encouragement of Dr. Robert Boyle, injected tincture of opium into the vein of a dog. Since then, many drugs have been tried with varying degrees of success. But it was not until the introduction of thiopental, a sulfur derivative of pentobarbital, independently by Lundy and Waters in 1934, that the intravenous method began to achieve popularity. The simplicity of the intravenous induction technique, combined with its ready acceptance by patients, has created widespread popularity among clinicians. However, its utility is limited by side effects and a lack of rapid reversibility.

These agents are discussed here briefly, highlighting their uses in the practice of anesthesia. Full presentations for several drugs appear in other chapters (see Chaps. 16 and 22).

Short-Acting Barbiturates

The short-acting barbiturates are highly lipid-soluble. Therefore, they are suitable for induction of anesthesia. The two most commonly used are thiopental and methohexital. The uptake by brain is very rapid and reaches a maximum within 30 s. Anesthesia lasts for 5 min. This short duration of action is due to rapid redistribution of the drug from brain to muscle and skin. Redistribution to fatty tissue is much slower owing to minimal perfusion of this tissue group.

Thiopental has a profound, direct, and dose-dependent depression effect on the myocardium. An induction dose decreases stroke volume and cardiac output, resulting in hypotension. Thiopental decreases venous tone, thus decreasing venous return to the heart. This effect is mediated through depression of the central nervous system and, to a lesser degree, through direct relaxation of venous smooth muscle.

Barbiturates decrease cerebral blood flow (CBF) and the metabolic rate for oxygen (CMR_{O_2}) in a dose-dependent fashion. Both components are reduced by 30 percent with an induction dose of thiopental. Larger doses of thiopental decrease these parameters by 50 percent and produce an isoelectric EEG. Doses greater than those which provide an isoelectric EEG do not further decrease CBF and CMR_{O_2}. Cerebral blood flow autoregulation and its response to carbon dioxide remain intact at a mean arterial pressure above

60 mmHg. The depressant effect of barbiturates on CBF makes these drugs ideal for induction of anesthesia and management of patients within increased intracranial pressure. The salutary effects of barbiturates on CBF, CMR_{O_2}, and intracranial pressure suggest that patients predisposed to cerebral ischemia, such as those with carotid occlusive disease, may benefit from their use. This approach remains controversial. Limited protection can be achieved with barbiturates in incomplete ischemia, while in complete ischemia the brain does not benefit from the effect of barbiturates.

The termination of action of thiobarbiturates depends on redistribution of the drug away from the brain (see Fig. 14-3). Accumulation of the drug in other tissue depots accrues, however, which may lead to continued low levels of drug entering the bloodstream. Thus, if given in sufficiently high doses, ultra-short-acting hypnotics may have a long duration of action.

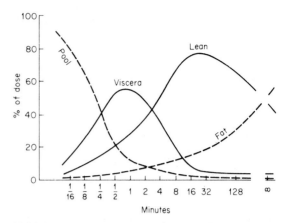

FIGURE 14-3   Distribution of thiopental in different body tissues at various times after intravenous injection. Time scale (in minutes) progresses geometrically. Final values are at infinity.

Ketamine

Cl

O

$\overset{+}{N}H_2CH_3$ Cl^-

Ketamine

Phencyclidine and ketamine produce a state called *dissociative anesthesia,* which provides amnesia and analgesia while preserving respiratory drive and muscle tone and augmenting sympathetic nervous system tone. Phencyclidine has been abandoned owing to the high frequency of its side effects: hallucinations, unpleasant dreams, and excitement. These dysphoric sequelae occur less frequently with ketamine, which is still used for sedation and anesthesia. Induction is complete within 30 s and lasts for 15 min. Analgesia is profound and lasts about 40 min. The amnestic effect may linger for 1 to 2 h.

Premedication with morphine and scopolamine, benzodiazepines, or butyrophenones reduces the dysphoric effects of ketamine. Young adults and children have a lower incidence of these side effects than adult patients. Ketamine is a valuable induction agent for critically ill and pediatric patients and as an analgesic during parturition. It enjoys an expanding role in outpatient procedures.

Etomidate

Etomidate is an imidazole-containing molecule not structurally similar to other anesthetics.

H_3C

$H-C-$ (phenyl)

O

CH_3CH_2OC- N

N

Etomidate

Since intravenous bolus doses provide rapid loss of consciousness, etomidate is classified as a sedative-hypnotic agent. Owing to poor solubility in water above pH 3, clinical preparations employ a propylene glycol solvent, which often engenders pain on injection.

The speed of onset and offset of unconsciousness is slightly less rapid than that of the thiobarbiturates. Rapid redistribution from brain to other tissues provides the rapid offset, as with the thiobarbiturates. Both hepatic microsomal enzymes and plasma esterases participate in metabolism of etomidate. The cerebral effects of etomidate and thiopental are similar: cerebral blood flow, cerebral metabolic rate, and intracranial pressure all decrease; both drugs are anticonvulsant; neither drug is analgesic. Unlike thiopental, etomidate occasionally causes transient myoclonic activity, which is not accompanied by seizure activity on the EEG.

Heart rate remains unchanged while systemic vascular resistance and blood pressure decrease slightly. There is a high incidence of nausea and vomiting postoperatively. Steroid production in the adrenal gland is inhibited for several hours following induction doses of etomidate. Inhibition of steroid genesis can lead to Addisonian crisis in patients maintained on continuous infusion of etomidate for long-term sedation in intensive-care units.

Etomidate is useful for rapid induction of anesthesia in patients with cardiovascular instability, particularly in patients with elevated intracranial pressure. Pain on injection and postoperative nausea and vomiting limit its widespread use.

Potent Opioids

Use as Adjuvants Opioids are used widely in the practice of anesthesia as adjuvant drugs. Since opioid analgesics are essential for relief of pain after operation, patients often receive an opioid prior to the termination of anesthesia. Clinical doses of opioids permit use of smaller doses of anesthetic agents. Patients frequently receive an opioid prior to surgery as part of their premedication. The usual choice in this regard is intramuscular morphine. Recent clinical trials have shown sufentanil-impregnated lollipops to be equally successful in small children.

Use in Balanced Anesthesia Opioid analgesics form an essential part of the "balanced" anesthetic technique, in which about 0.7-MAC nitrous oxide, muscle relaxant, and opioid are administered together. Other components of balanced anesthesia are thiobarbiturate, hyperventilation, and a potent sedative-amnestic such as scopolamine. Balanced anesthesia provides selected patients with rapid awakening to a lucid, intensely analgesic state. Two analgesics that are currently used to anesthesia are morphine and fentanyl. Morphine is usually employed in long procedures. However, fentanyl is the drug of choice for shorter surgical procedures.

Fentanyl is a synthetic opioid with the following structure:

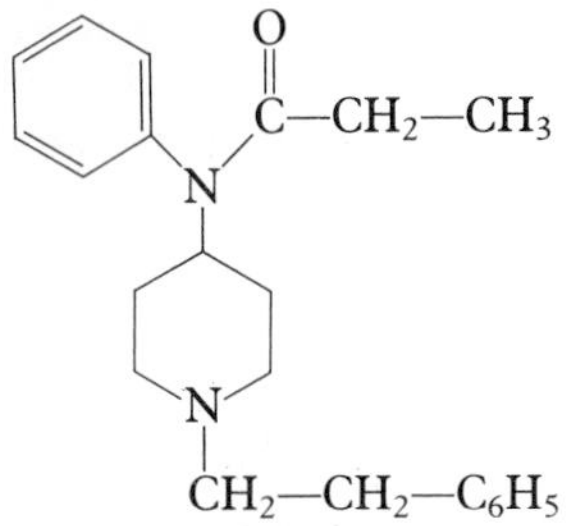

Fentanyl

It is usually administered intravenously. It binds to plasma proteins by 80 percent with a volume of distribution of 40 L/kg and an elimination half-life of 3 to 4 h. Redistribution of fentanyl from brain to other tissues accounts for its shorter duration of action.

Morphine, 1 to 2 mg/kg, was the first opioid to gain widespread use as the sole opioid anesthetic for patients with cardiovascular compromise. The rapidity of injection is limited severely by histamine release and need for fluid administration. Compared with morphine, fentanyl is more lipophilic and 80 times more potent; it does not release histamine. Intravenous induction doses of fentanyl vary from 20 to 100 μg/kg. With these large doses, duration of action is no longer determined by redistribution but rather by elimination half-life. Compared with fentanyl, sufentanil is more lipophilic and 10 times more potent. Induction is more rapid, and histamine release is likewise absent. Alfentanil is less potent than fentanyl (1:4 ratio) but much more lipophilic; its short duration of action makes it inappropriate for procedures lasting many hours. Partial agonist-antagonist agents do not provide satisfactory oxygen-opioid anesthesia owing to their limited efficacy. More comprehensive information on opioids is found in Chap. 22.

Use as Sole Anesthetic Agent High doses of potent opioids produce profound analgesia and anesthesia in most patients. The opioid is given intravenously while the patient inhales pure oxygen. As with balanced anesthesia, an amnestic agent is frequently employed. Opioids given rapidly act in the central nervous system to cause bradycardia and muscular rigidity, the latter most notably affecting the chest wall, thus impairing ventilation. Cardiovascular stability is prominent with all opioids except meperidine. Respiratory depression is profound and long-lasting, necessitating controlled ventilation for as long as 24 h.

An occasional patient is not completely anesthetized with this technique and exhibits a hyperdynamic circulatory state characterized by tachycardia, hypertension, and high cardiac output. Sub-MAC doses of volatile anesthetics usually control these undesirable hemodynamics.

Miscellaneous Agents

Benzodiazepines Many benzodiazepines are available in the United States. Their primary use lies in the treatment of anxiety. The CNS effects of all the benzodiazepines include anxiolysis, sedation, anticonvulsant action, amnesia, and muscle relaxation. Three compounds in the group are of particular interest to anesthesiologists: diazepam, lorazepam, and midazolam. These drugs are utilized in various surgical procedures as preanesthetic medications for their calming effect. All these agents potentiate the action of gamma-aminobutyric acid (GABA), an inhibitory neurotransmitter in the cerebrum, substantia nigra, hippocampus, cerebellum, and spinal cord.

Diazepam (Valium) Diazepam is used widely as a premedicant, an adjunct to regional anesthesia, and an induction agent for minor procedures including endoscopy. Owing to poor solubility in water, the parenteral form is a glycol-alcohol solution that causes pain and venous irritation upon intravenous administration as well as unpredictable absorption when given intramuscularly. Diazepam has a high volume of distribution and a low clearance rate, resulting in an elimination half-life of 20 to 40 h. Oxidative metabolism in the liver yields active metabolites. Elderly patients exhibit prolonged excretion owing to changes in tissue distribution and protein binding.

Diazepam has minimal circulatory effects. It produces less depression of ventilation than barbiturates. However, in combination with narcotics and anesthetics, significant respiratory depression will occur. It is highly effective as an anticonvulsant and useful to control the muscle rigidity and spasm in patients with tetanus or cerebral palsy.

Lorazepam (Ativan) Lorazepam is slow in onset of action (10 to 20 min). Its chief use has been as a premedicant (0.05 mg/kg intramuscularly) and as an adjuvant to regional anesthesia (0.04 mg/kg intravenously) owing to its profound anxiolytic, amnesic, and tranquilizing effects. Pharmacologic actions are similar to those of diazepam. Although its elimination half-life (16 h) is shorter than that of diazepam, its clinical duration of action is longer than the action of diazepam. The less-lipid-soluble lorazepam terminates more by elimination than redistribution.

Midazolam (Versed) Midazolam is a water-soluble benzodiazepine. Pain on injection and postinjection phlebitis are rare. Despite a large volume of distribution, elimination half-life is 2 to 4 h owing to rapid hepatic clearance. Midazolam has little effect on the cardiovascular system. Ventilation is usually preserved, although intravenous administration demands the presence of equipment to control ventilation in case apnea ensues. Midazolam is approximately 1.5 to 2 times more potent than diazepam. For premedication, 70 to 80 μg/kg intramuscularly is given; for conscious sedation, 0.1 to 0/15 μg/kg intravenously is usually adequate.

Propofol Propofol is a newer hypnotic agent used for anesthetic induction maintenance. A dose of 1.5 to 3 mg/kg causes unconsciousness within seconds. High lipid solubility permits ready penetration of the blood-brain barrier, resulting in rapid induction. Recovery occurs in about 5 min at a plasma concentration of about 1 mg/mL. Propofol is 96 percent protein-bound, with a distribution half-life of 2.2 min and elimination half-life of 70 min. Its brief action after a single injection results from redistribution and hepatic metabolism. Active metabolites are not known.

Propofol is a respiratory depressant and may produce brief periods of apnea. Systemic blood pressure, stroke volume, and systemic vascular resistance decrease minimally. Cardiac output remains unchanged. The drug has no known adverse effects in the liver or kidneys.

Althesin Althesin is a mixture of two steroids, alphaxalone 9 mg/mL and alphadolone 3 mg/mL. It is not used in the United States. It causes rapid unconsciousness, a short period of anesthesia, and rapid recovery with little hangover. Althesin finds particular application in poor risk patients, in asthmatics, and in patients having intraocular and outpatient surgery. The induction dose is 0.05 to 0.08 mL/kg. Repeated doses can be given but may need to be accompanied by an analgesic.

Althesin has minimal effect on blood pressure and cardiac output. Heart rate increases slightly. Althesin produces transient depression of ventilation. It has bronchodilating properties. Elimination is hepatic, but liver damage does not greatly prolong its effects. Very little postoperative nausea and vomiting follows the use of althesin. It has a low incidence of thrombophlebitis. A high frequency of anaphylactic reactions severely limits its use.

Propanidid Propanidid is a phenoxyacetic amine which is a eugenol derivative with the chemical composition propyl 4-N,N'-diethylcarbamoylmethoxy-3-methoxy-phenylacetate. It is prepared as a 5% solution in oxyphenylated castor oil. This solution is viscous but can be diluted with distilled water or normal saline. The drug binds to plasma proteins.

Propanidid is useful for short operations, e.g., in dental patients and outpatients. The dose is 5 to 10 mg/kg intravenously. Propanidid causes hyperpnea following intravenous injection, usually followed by a short period of apnea. It may cause tremors and muscular movements. Histamine release may result in severe hypotension. Cardiovascular depression or even cardiac arrest may occur. Propanidid is not hepatoxic in clinical doses. It is not approved for use in the United States.

BIBLIOGRAPHY

Buffington, C. W., J. L. Romson, A. Levine, N. C. Futtlinger, and A. M. Muang: "Isoflurane Induces Coronary Steel in a Canine Model of Chronic Coronary Occlusion," *Anesthesiology*, **66**:280 (1987).

Edwards, R. E., R. K. Miller, and M. F. Roizen: "Cardiac Effects of Imipramine and Pancuronium During Halothane and Enflurane Anesthesia," *Anesthesiology*, **50**:421 (1979).

Newburg, L. A., J. H. Milde, and J. D. Michenfelder: "The Cerebral Metabolic Effects of Isoflurane at and above Concentrations That Suppress Atrial Electrical Activity," *Anesthesiology*, **59**:23 (1983).

Nussmeier, N. A., C. Arlund, S. Slogoff: "Neuropsychiatric Complication after Cardiopulmonary Bypass: Cerebral Protection by a Barbiturate," *Anesthesiology*, **64**:165 (1986).

Roizen, M. F., and V. C. Stevens: "Multiform Ventricular Tachycardia due to Interaction of Aminophylline and Halothane," *Anesth. Analg.*, **57**:738 (1978).

Rsenberg, H., F. K. Orkin, and J. Springstead: "Abuse of Nitrous Oxide," *Anesth. Analg.*, **58**:104–106 (1979).

White, P. F., W. L. Wary, and A. J. Trevor: "Ketamine: Its Pharmacology and Therapeutic Uses," *Anesthesiology*, **56**:119 (1982).

Wood, M., M. L. Berman, and R. D. Harbison: "Halothane-Induced Hepatic Necrosis in Triiodothyronine-Pretreated Rats," *Anesthesiology*, **52**:470 (1980).

Sedatives and Hypnotics

Andrew P. Ferko

The sedative-hypnotic agents are classified into the barbiturates, the benzodiazepine hypnotics, and a miscellaneous group. These drugs, which possess sedative and hypnotic properties, are frequently used as adjuncts in the treatment of organic and emotional disorders to provide a calming effect and induce sleep. The majority of drugs in this chapter are indicated in the treatment of insomnia. With some exceptions the same drugs can be utilized for sedation and hypnosis. The differences in effects are dependent on the dose. Sedation is a mild degree of central nervous system depression, while hypnosis is a degree of central nervous system depression that resembles natural sleep.

BARBITURATES

The barbiturates are derivatives of barbituric acid, which is a condensation of malonic acid ($HOOC—CH_2—COOH$) with urea ($NH_2—CO—NH_2$). Barbiturates are weaks acids, and salts of the compounds are formed at position 2. The formulas of some barbiturates, as well as the classifications to which they belong, are shown in Table 15-1.

In order for derivatives of barbituric acid to have central depressant activity they must possess two substitutions at the 5 position. Barbital, which is a 5,5-diethyl derivative, is a weak hypnotic, while barbiturates with an ethyl group and a longer chain are more potent than barbital. Compounds with a branched chain at position 5 usually have greater hypnotic activity than the corresponding drug with a straight chain.

Barbiturates containing a phenyl group in the 5 position are less potent hypnotics than their aliphatic or alicyclic analogs, but they have enhanced anticonvulsant and antiepileptic activity. N-methylation of the barbituric acid nucleus increases lipid solubility and decreases duration of action. It also may confer antiepileptic activity, while alkylation of both nitrogens yields derivatives that show convulsant activity. Replacement of the oxygen in the 2 position by sulfur (thiobarbiturates) causes a marked increase in the lipid-to-water partition coefficients of 5,5-disubstituted barbiturates (Table 15-2). The resulting drugs have greater hypnotic potency than their oxygen analogs when given intravenously, but their low water solutility and their localization in depot fat make them unsuitable for oral administration as hypnotics. Their greatest usefulness is as intravenous anesthetics (ultrashort-acting barbiturates).

Mechanism of Action

Actions on the central nervous system of barbiturates are expressed in many ways, ranging from subtle changes in mood to more profound effects such as sedation, sleep, or anesthesia, depending on the dose administered. The pharmacologic basis of such central nervous system depression appears to be complex in its nature. Although a detailed mechanism of action for the barbiturates is not fully delineated at the present time, it appears that gamma aminobutyric acid (GABA) receptor-mediated chloride ion fluxes have a

TABLE 15-1   Classification and formulas of some clinically useful barbiturates

$$\text{Barbituric acid}$$

Barbituric acid

Barbiturate	R_1	R_2	R_3
Ultrashort-acting			
Methohexital	Allyl	1-Methyl-2-pentynyl	CH_3
Thiopental[a]	Ethyl	1-Methylbutyl	H
Short to intermediate-acting			
Amobarbital	Ethyl	Isopentyl	H
Butabarbital	Ethyl	sec-Butyl	H
Pentobarbital	Ethyl	1-Methylbutyl	H
Secobarbital	Allyl	1-Methylbutyl	H
Long-acting			
Mephobarbital	Ethyl	Phenyl	CH_3
Metharbital	Ethyl	Ethyl	CH_3
Phenobarbital	Ethyl	Phenyl	H

[a] Sulfur present at position 2 instead of 0.

role in the central depressant properties of these drugs. The barbiturates potentiate $GABA_A$-induced chloride influxes into neuronal tissue.

GABA is an inhibitory neurotransmitter in the central nervous system. It binds to both $GABA_A$ and $GABA_B$ receptors. $GABA_A$ receptors are associated with the chloride ionophore, which is a macromolecular complex that also contains receptor sites for barbiturates and benzodiazepine (Fig. 15-1). Four subunits of proteins, two alpha and two beta subunits, are pres-

TABLE 15-2   Barbiturates: pharmacokinetic data

Barbiturate	Half-life[a]	Partition coefficient[b]	Plasma protein binding[c]
Amobarbital	16–24	—	—
Butarbital	62–138	—	—
Pentobarbital	21–48	39	35
Phenobarbital	72–96	3	20
Secobarbital	20–28	52	44
Thiopental	—	580	65

[a] Plasma half-life in hours in adult humans.
[b] Concentration in methylene chloride/concentration in water.
[c] Percent binding to bovine serum albumin.

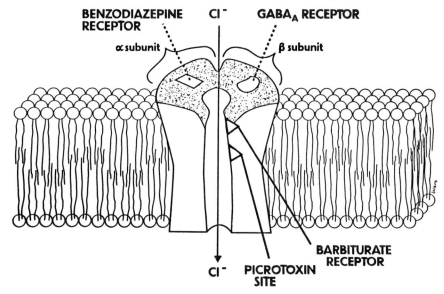

FIGURE 15-1 Diagrammatic representation of a hemi section of the chloride ionophore showing the location of the receptor sites for GABA, barbiturates, benzodiazines, and picrotoxin.

ent in the chloride ionophore. The benzodiazepine receptor sites are located on the alpha subunits. The GABA recognition sites, the barbiturate receptors, and the binding sites for picrotoxin are carried on the beta subunits. The $GABA_B$ receptor is a smaller molecular structure and appears to be involved with potassium ion and possible calcium ion conductances. Activation of $GABA_B$ receptor occurs with GABA and the drug baclofen.

When GABA binds to the $GABA_A$ receptor site in the postsynaptic chloride ionophore, there results an influx of chloride ions into neuronal tissue, which results in hyperpolarization of the membrane. Barbiturates and benzodiazepine derivatives, such as the benzodiazepine hypnotics discussed in this chapter, potentiate $GABA_A$ receptor-mediated chloride influx by binding to their specific receptor sites on the chloride ionophore. In the presence of GABA, barbiturates prolong the duration of the $GABA_A$-activated chloride ion influx. In addition barbiturates can enhance the affinity of GABA for its receptor site on the chloride ionophore. The benzodiazepines potentiate the activity of GABA on chloride influx by increasing the frequency of the openings of the $GABA_A$ receptor-mediated chloride channels.

Another effect of the barbiturate in the central ner-

vous system that is also possibly related to their mechanism of action is the ability of barbiturates to increase membrane fluidity when they are administered acutely. The drug molecules appear to position themselves into the lipid components of the membrane and reduce the rigidity of the structural arrangement. By increasing neuronal membrane fluidity, the barbiturates may alter (1) the conformation of enzymes, (2) ion fluxes, and (3) neurotransmitter release. Other drugs such as ethanol and the general anesthetics are also reported to produce their pharmacologic effects by increasing neuronal membrane fluidity. These drugs alter membrane fluidity not by a receptor mechanism but by their physical presence in the membrane.

Therefore, it appears that potentiation of $GABA_A$ receptor-mediated chloride fluxes by the barbiturates and the effect of these drugs to increase membrane fluidity play a role in the central depressant properties of the barbiturates.

Pharmacodynamics

Central Nervous System The central depressant actions of the barbiturates resemble those of the general anesthetics, alcohol, and most of the hypnotic drugs discussed in subsequent sections of this chapter.

Barbiturates are uniformly distributed within the central nervous system, and the reticular activating system appears to be the most sensitive area to the depressant effects. Depending on the dose administered, all the clinically useful drugs produce a broad range of effects extending from mild sedation to deep coma or anesthesia. The effects of the sedative-hypnotic barbiturates depend on the nature of the subject and the situation in which the drug is administered.

Sedation and Hypnosis   Although the doses employed for hypnosis are larger than those for sedation, the therapeutic goal is the same: to reduce awareness of external stimuli and, in appropriate circumstances, to promote sleep. The barbiturates most favored for daytime sedation are those which have a long or intermediate duration of action, for example, phenobarbital or butabarbital, respectively.

In general, barbiturates with a short to intermediate duration of action, such as secobarbital or amobarbital, are employed as hypnotic agents. The hypnotic action is sometimes apparent as early as 15 min after ingestion of the drug, but usually 30 to 60 min is needed. Sleep is usually maintained uninterrupted for 5 to 6 h. The incidence of rapid eye movement (REM) sleep and dreams is reduced. In REM sleep, also called *paradoxical* sleep, periods of rapid eye movements under closed eyelids alternate with periods of quiescence during physiologic sleep. Episodes of rapid eye movement have been correlated and associated with dreaming. Prolonged deprivation of REM sleep will generally result in reversible gross behavioral effects. The barbiturates reduce REM sleep somewhat but do not obliterate it totally and therefore do not generally alter the personality behavior of the individual.

Anesthesia   In sufficiently large doses, all the barbiturate hypnotics are capable of producing surgical anesthesia. However, only ultrashort-acting barbiturates are useful anesthetics. The ultrashort action of useful intravenous anesthetics, such as thiopental and methohexital, depends on redistribution of the drugs from the brain (which is entered rapidly) to the other tissues (which are entered more slowly). Pentobarbital does not enter the brain as rapidly as thiopental or methohexital, and redistribution plays a relatively small role compared with biotransformation in determining its duration of effects.

Anticonvulsant Effects   All the sedative-hypnotic barbiturates are effective antidotes to convulsant drugs, and in anesthetic doses they suppress the convulsions of tetanus and status epilepticus. Phenobarbital, however, differs from other barbiturates in that it has a more satisfactory action, which is utilized to prevent epileptic seizures, particularly of the generalized tonic-clonic seizure type. Apart from phenobarbital, the only barbiturates which have proved useful in the treatment of epilepsy are metharbital (*N*-methylbarbital) and mephobarbital (*N*-methylphenobarbital). The pharmacology of antiepileptic drugs is discussed in Chap. 21.

Analgesia   The barbiturates differ from opioids and nonnarcotic analgesics in lacking significant ability to obtund pain in doses not impairing consciousness. The remarkable effectiveness of the ordinary analgesic drugs precludes using barbiturates routinely for relief of pain. However, increased comfort is often achieved by combining barbiturates with aspirin or small doses of narcotics.

Respiratory System   Sleep induced by hypnotic doses of barbiturates involves no more depression of the respiratory system than occurs in normal sleep. Larger doses cause progressive reduction of the minute volume; the rate may be increased or decreased. The respiratory-stimulating action of 5 to 10% carbon dioxide becomes weaker and weaker and finally disappears. Death from acute barbiturate poisoning is usually attributed to respiratory failure. With toxic doses the mechanism appears to be a direct paralysis of the medullary respiratory center as a result of the loss of the response to the carbon dioxide drive. However, in general, in overdoses with barbiturates in abusers, pulmonary edema or hypostatic pneumonia often plays a role in decreasing the respiration. Laryngospasm appears to be a rare complication of ordinary barbiturate poisoning but is of considerably importance in connection with the intravenous administration of the ultrashort-acting thiobarbiturates.

Circulatory System   The circulation is not significantly affected by sedative or hypnotic doses of barbiturates. Greater effects on the blood pressure are observed in hypertensive patients; the decreases in both systolic and diastolic pressure are attributable to inhibition of the central neurogenic component of the hypertension. Doses large enough to cause coma or anesthesia generally produce a sustained decrease in the mean arterial pressure and pulse pressure.

Liver   Hypnotic doses do not alter the results of any of the usual clinical tests of hepatic function. Even in patients with severe liver disease the tests reveal no changes suggestive of deleterious effects of the drugs.

Barbiturates in the liver may cause a striking enhancement of the activity of enzymes involved in the biotransformation of a variety of drugs and certain normal body constituents. The mechanism of this effect is not fully understood but appears to involve increased synthesis of enzymes in the cytoplasmic reticulum. Barbiturates have a definite effect on the drug-metabolizing microsomal system, which may be of clinical significance (see Chap. 3). For example, a few therapeutic doses of phenobarbital may increase the rate of biotransformation of the coumarin anticoagulants sufficiently to necessitate increased doses to achieve the desired reductions in clotting time. Moreover, withdrawal of the barbiturates without an adjustment in the dose of the anticoagulant may result in hemorrhage. The barbiturates may also competitively interfere with the biotransformation of a number of substrates of cytochrome P-450. They also increase the activity of glucuronyl transferase and increase delta-aminolevulinic acid synthetase.

Pharmacokinetics

The barbiturates are readily absorbed from the stomach, small intestine, rectum, and intramuscular sites. The mechanism of absorption from the gastrointestinal tract is simple passive diffusion. Following absorption, the drugs are present in all tissues and fluids of the body. Furthermore, barbiturates cross the placental barrier and become widely distributed in the fetal tissues. The drugs differ considerably in their binding to plasma protein (Table 15-2). Binding to tissue proteins parallels the binding to plasma proteins. Therefore, the drugs are rather uniformly distributed throughout the body. Ultrashort-acting barbiturates attain much higher concentrations in depot fat than in other tissues of the body. One of the highly lipid-soluble barbiturates is thiopental.

Barbiturate hypnotics are biotransformed primarily in the liver by oxidation of the substituents in the 5 position. Ethyl groups are quite resistant to oxidation. Therefore, barbital, which contains two ethyl groups, is excreted almost completely unchanged. Longer alkyl chains are oxidized to form secondary alcohols, ketones, or carboxylic acid derivatives; the latter are sometimes subjected to beta oxidation to form carboxylic acids with two fewer carbon atoms. The phenyl group in phenobarbital is hydroxylated in the para position. N-dealkylation and desulfuration may occur when the appropriate substituents are present. Phenolic as well as alcoholic biotransformation products are conjugated with glucuronic acid to varying extents. The allyl ($CH_2 = CHCH_2$) group present in a number of barbiturates usually escapes biotransformation, but in secobarbital it is converted in part to a 2,3-dihydroxypropyl ($CH_2OHCHOHCH_2$) group. Hydrolysis of the barbituric acid ring is generally only a minor reaction.

The barbiturates and their biotransformation products are eliminated primarily by renal excretion. Alkalinization of the urine does little to expedite the elimination of most barbiturate hypnotics but does have an effect on the excretion of phenobarbital. The basis for this difference is that phenobarbital has a lower pK_a (7.2) than do the other barbiturates. Therefore, increasing pH in the physiologic range converts a greater fraction of phenobarbital to the anionic form, to which tubules are impermeable.

Barbiturates are administered orally, rectally, intramuscularly, or intravenously. The oral route should be employed whenever possible. In infants or in patients who are vomiting, the drugs may be given rectally in the form of a suppository or retention enema. When rapid onset of action is needed, as in patients with convulsions, the drugs may be injected intramuscularly or intravenously.

Adverse Reaction

Acute Poisoning   The wide use of the barbiturate hypnotics provides ample opportunities for accidental intoxication and suicide attempts. Most cases of barbiturate poisoning stem from attempted suicide, but some are accidental, and a few may result from what has been called *automatism*. This is a state of drug-induced confusion in which the patient forgets having taken the medication and ingests more of it. The fairly wide difference between the usual hypnotic dose and toxic dose of barbiturates casts doubt on the plausibility of automatism as a common source of serious poisoning in nondependent persons. Nevertheless, many clinicians are persuaded that automatism is a genuine phenomenon of considerable importance.

The diagnosis of barbiturate intoxication is based on the history, physical examination, and detection or determination of drugs in the blood, urine, or gastric contents. Poisoning by barbiturates seldom can be distinguished on purely clinical grounds from that caused by other hypnotic drugs. The cardinal signs are stupor or coma and respiratory depression. The respiration is affected early in the course of intoxication. The minute respiratory volume is decreased, sometimes sufficiently to cause cyanosis. The rhythm may be slow or rapid or may have a Cheyne-Stokes pattern. Ordinarily the blood pressure falls appreciably only in the presence of marked respiratory depression. Undoubtedly, hypoxia plays an important role in causing the hypotension, since merely providing adequate ventilation often restores blood pressure to normal. However, severely poisoned patients may develop circulatory shock.

The treatment of barbiturate poisoning includes removing any unabsorbed drug from the stomach, supporting the respiration and circulation, performing hemodialysis, and preventing complications. It should always be kept in mind that acute intoxication may be superimposed upon chronic intoxication. After emerging from coma, every patient poisoned by barbiturates should be questioned about chronic use of the drugs and treated accordingly.

Chronic Toxicity   The clinical picture of chronic barbiturate intoxication resembles that of mild acute barbiturate or alcohol intoxication. Barbiturate abusers differ from alcoholics in that they usually maintain a good state of nutrition. The signs and symptoms vary considerably in different individuals and in the same subject at different times. The effects are greatest when the drug is taken on an empty stomach. They are least marked upon arising and increase during the day as successive doses are consumed. The mental changes include impairment of intellectual ability, defective judgment, loss of emotional control, and accentuation of pathologic features of the personality. Most abusers prefer shorter acting barbiturates such as pentobarbital, secobarbital, or amobarbital to phenobarbital. The

drugs are usually taken by mouth, although some abusers inject them intravenously.

The severity of the abstinence syndrome depends on the individual patient as well as on the daily dose and the duration of the intoxication. Abrupt withdrawal of barbiturates from chronically intoxicated individuals is absolutely contraindicated. The patient should be hospitalized and stabilized on the smallest amount of the drug which maintains a continuous state of mild intoxication. A period of 2 to 3 weeks is usually required to withdraw barbiturates safely. Rehabilitation and psychotherapeutic treatment of recovered barbiturate abusers is the same as that for alcoholics or opioid abusers.

Idiosyncrasy   Abnormal reactions to the barbiturates may be encountered in certain patients who have not had prior experience with the drugs (natural idiosyncrasy). In some individuals hypnotic doses of the barbiturates consistently produce excitement and inebriation. Others respond with headache, nausea, and vomiting or diarrhea. Occasionally the drugs appear to be responsible for myalgia, neuralgia, or arthralgia, which may persist for several days after discontinuation of medication.

Hypersensitivity   Hypersensitivity reactions to the barbiturates most commonly involve the skin, although the blood and blood-forming organs may also be affected. Phenobarbital occasionally causes exfoliative dermatitis, which may be accompanied by parenchymatous hepatitis. A few cases of agranulocytosis and thrombocytopenic purpura have also been attributed to the drug.

Drug Interactions   When a barbiturate is administered to an individual who has received opioids, other sedatives or hypnotics, general anesthetics, neuromuscular blocking agents, alcohol, or antianxiety agents, an additive respiratory depressant effect may occur. When barbiturates are used by chronic alcohol abusers, in the absence of ethanol, there is a decreased sedative effect from the barbiturate due to its increased biotransformation by the microsomal system, which is induced by the chronic use of ethanol; acute intoxication by concomitant use of ethanol and barbiturates results in increased central nervous system depression due to an additive effect of two CNS depressants plus decreased biotransformation of the barbiturate. Acute ethanol administration can inhibit the metabolism of barbiturates. Rifampin will decrease the effect of barbiturates because of induction of the drug-metabolizing microsomal system. Barbiturates may also diminish the response to coumarin anticoagulants, resulting in less suppression of prothrombin. This effect is due primarily to the increased activity of the drug-metabolizing microsomal system caused by the barbiturates. There is thus an increase in the biotransformation of the coumarin anticoagulant, making less coumarin anticoagulant available for therapeutic action. Withdrawal of the barbiturate without a dose alteration of the anticoagulant may result in hemorrhage. Other drugs biotransformed by the drug-metabolizing microsomal system may similarly have their therapeutic activity adversely affected by barbiturates; these include tricyclic antidepressants, corticosteroids, digitoxin, phenothiazines, quinidine, and tetracyclines.

Contraindications   The barbiturates are definitely contraindicated in patients who have become sensitized to them. Severe pulmonary insufficiency constitutes a contraindication, since patients with disorders such as chronic emphysema are often extremely sensitive to the respiratory-depressant action of ordinary hypnotic doses. Barbiturates are contraindicated in patients with intermittent porphyria. This is because individuals with this condition have a defect in the regulation of delta-aminolevulinic acid synthetase, and the administration of a barbiturate which increases this enzyme may cause a dangerous and precipitous increase in the level of porphyrins, which may result in paralysis and death.

Barbiturates should be used with caution in patients with decreased liver function or renal insufficiency because these conditions will alter, respectively, the biotransformation and excretion of the barbiturate. Great caution must be exercised in prescribing barbiturates for the individual with a suicidal tendency or a predilection to abuse them.

Clinical Uses

Sedation and Hypnosis   Barbiturates are effective sedatives and hypnotics; however, they are used on a limited basis in therapy due to the availability of the benzodiazepine derivatives. The barbiturates have a greater potential to cause dangerous adverse reactions, dependence, and abuse than the benzodiazepines.

When the barbiturates are used to treat ordinary insomnia, they should not be regarded as a substitute for a concerted effort to discover and treat the basic causes of the disorder. Patients should be urged to provide an environment maximally conducive to sleep and to seek methods of relaxing at bedtime. In recommending drugs to be administered during the night, it is advisable that the dose to be taken be isolated from the main supply to guard against accidental ingestion of an excessive amount. Continuous use of barbiturates in recommended doses may result in tolerance and dependence. The patient should be told that the first night after discontinuing the drug may be less restful than usual. Sleep laboratory research on most hypnotics has found them to lose their sleep-promoting properties within 3 to 14 days of continuous use. Physicians should look for and treat underlying disorders causing insomnia and restrict even further the prescribing of hypnotics.

Anticonvulsant and Antiepileptic Uses   The barbiturates may be used in the treatment of acute convulsions arising from various disease processes or from the ingestion of poisons. Thus they have been employed in the therapy of status epilepticus, eclampsia, and cerebral hemorrhage. The therapeutic use of phenobarbital, metharbital, and mephobarbital in the treatment of epilepsy is discussed in Chap. 21.

Preanesthetic Medication   Pentobarbital, amobarbital, and secobarbital are employed as preanesthetic medication. In the absence of pain, they provide the serenity desired before anesthesia.

Hyperbilirubinemia and Kernicterus   In the neonate these conditions have been successfully treated with phenobarbital because it increases the activity of glucuronyl transferase and consequently decreases elevated levels of bilirubin.

Preparations and Doses

Amobarbital (Amytal) is available in capsules containing 65 or 200 mg; in tablets containing 15, 30, 50, or 100 mg; as an elixir containing 44 mg in 5 mL; and in vials containing 125, 250, or 500 mg. The usual adult oral hypnotic dose is 100 to 200 mg.

Butabarbital (Butisol) is available in tablets and capsules containing 15, 30, or 100 mg and as an elixir containing 30 mg in 5 mL. The usual adult oral hypnotic dose is 50 to 100 mg.

Pentobarbital (Nembutal) is available in capsules containing 30, 50, or 100 mg; in timed-release tablets containing 100 mg; as an elixir containing 20 mg in 5 mL; in suppositories containing 30, 60, 120, or 200 mg; in ampuls and multiple-dose vials containing 50 mg/mL; and in vials containing 130 and 325 mg/mL. The usual adult oral hypnotic dose is 100 mg.

Phenobarbital (Luminal) is available in tablets containing 16, 32, 65, or 100 mg; as an elixir containing 20 mg in 5 mL; in vials containing 65, 130, or 162 mg/mL; and as suppositories ranging from 8 to 125 mg. The usual adult oral hypnotic dose is 100 to 200 mg.

Secobarbital (Seconal) is available in capsules containing 30, 50, or 100 mg; as an elixir containing 22 mg in 5 mL; and in suppositories containing 30, 60, 120, or 200 mg. The usual adult oral hypnotic dose is 100 mg.

BENZODIAZEPINES

Flurazepam, Temazepam, and Triazolam

These benzodiazepine derivatives are effective pharmacologic agents used exclusively for their hypnotic effect in the treatment of sleep disorders. Other benzodiazepines that are used primarily for their antianxiety effect are discussed in Chap. 16. All benzodiazepine compounds possess the same basic structural nucleus as is illustrated by flurazepam.

Flurazepam

Mechanism of Action At the present time evidence in the literature suggests that these hypnotic agents are involved in an interaction with the inhibitory neurotransmitter, GABA. Flurazepam, temazepam, and triazolam appear to increase the inhibitory effect of GABA in the central nervous system. The site of this interaction between GABA and the benzodiazepines is the chloride ionophore, a macromolecular complex, that contains specific receptors of GABA, benzodiazepines, and barbiturates (Fig. 15-1).

Flurazepam and the other drugs bind to the benzodiazepine receptor and enhance the GABA-mediated chloride influx which results in hyperpolarization of neuronal membranes. Details about the GABA-benzodiazepine-barbiturate relationship are presented earlier in this chapter.

Pharmacokinetics

These benzodiazepine hypnotics are well absorbed from the gastrointestinal tract after oral administration and exhibit very good bioavailability. They are biotransformed in the liver by the drug-metabolizing microsomal system. Flurazepam undergoes an *N*-dealkylation reaction to yield *N*-desalkylflurazepam, which is the major active product and has an elimination $t_{1/2}$ of 76 to 160 h. For temazepam and triazolam the parent compound is the active hypnotic, and the elimination half-lives are 8 to 38 h and 1.6 to 5.4 h, respectively. These three drugs and their metabolites are eliminated from the body primarily by renal excretion.

Adverse Reactions

Drowsiness, dizziness, lethargy, and ataxia may occur particularly in elderly and debilitated patients. Confusion, dry mouth, headache, and gastrointestinal disturbances have been observed. Idiosyncratic excitement, stimulation, hyperactivity, and hallucinations have been reported.

Tolerance to the hypnotic effect has not been observed following one or two months of continuous nightly usage. Dependence does not appear to develop in individuals taking therapeutic doses of these drugs. However, as with any CNS depressant, there is always the possibility that dependence may occur. In cases of overdosage, ataxia, hypotension, respiratory depression, and coma have been reported. The benzodiazepine hypnotics have an additive depressant effect with other central nervous system depressants. During pregnancy the benzodiazepines should be avoided.

Clinical Use

Flurazepam, temazepam, and triazolam are used for the treatment of insomnia. They are of value in treating persons who have difficulty in falling asleep, frequent nocturnal awakenings, or early morning awakening. When the drugs are taken at bedtime, the least preferred hypnotic to use in patients who have difficulty in falling asleep is temazepam. In order for temazepam to influence a patient's sleep latency the compound should be taken 1 to 2 h before bedtime.

These benzodiazepines decrease time to onset of sleep and number of awakenings and increase total sleep time. At ordinary therapeutic doses flurazepam and the other benzodiazepine drugs neither suppress REM sleep nor cause a rebound after withdrawal; however, the percentage of REM sleep is decreased because there is an increase in total sleep time. Stages 3 and 4 of sleep are reduced but stage 2 is lengthened. In addition little or no rebound insomnia occurs when the drug is discontinued. The usual adult doses for flurazepam, temazepam, and triazolam are 30, 30, and 0.25 mg, respectively. In some patients as little as one-half of the recommended dose may be effective.

Preparations

Flurazepam (Dalmane) is available in capsules containing 15 or 30 mg.

Temazepam (Restoril) is available in capsules containing 15 or 30 mg.

Triazolam (Halcion) is available in tablets containing 0.125 or 0.25 mg.

MISCELLANEOUS GROUP

Chloral Hydrate

Chloral hydrate [$CCl_3CH(OH)_2$] is an aldehyde hydrate which has a pungent odor and somewhat caustic taste. Chloral hydrate is usually taken by mouth but is sometimes given rectally. Its irritant action precludes subcutaneous or intramuscular injection.

The sedative-hypnotic action of chloral hydrate can be attributed almost entirely to trichloroethanol formed by the chemical reduction of the drug in tissues. Although the exact mechanism of action of chloral hydrate is unknown, the drug probably acts in a manner similar to ethanol in the central nervous system to increase the fluidity of membranes, which results in sedation or sleep (Chap. 17).

Pharmacokinetics Very little chloral hydrate is available to the central and systemic circulations because of a large first-pass effect in the liver that transforms it to trichloroethanol by the enzyme alcohol dehydrogenase. The drug and its products of biotransformation appear to be widely distributed throughout the body. Chloral hydrate is partly oxidized to trichloroacetic acid and partly reduced to trichloroethanol. Trichloroethanol, with a half-life of 4 to 8 h, is responsible for most of the hypnotic effect of chloral hydrate, while trichloroacetic acid is devoid of hypnotic action. Chloral hydrate and trichloroethanol are biotransformed by the liver to trichloroacetic acid and urochloralic acid, both of which are excreted by the kidney.

Pharmacodynamics The central depressant actions of chloral hydrate resemble those of alcohol, the barbiturates, and the general anesthetics. In small doses the principal effect is sedation. Somewhat larger doses taken under appropriate circumstances induce sleep. In ambulatory individuals, the drug may produce the signs and symptoms of drunkenness. Larger doses lead to coma or anesthesia. However, the drug is not used for anesthesia because the margin of safety is too narrow.

Controlled clinical studies have proved the effectiveness of the usual hypnotic dose (0.5 to 1 g) of chloral hydrate in inducing and maintaining sleep. In most individuals sleep occurs within 1 h after swallowing the drug and continues for 5 h or longer. At any time during the hypnotic response, the patient can be readily aroused. The duration of action of chloral hydrate is short enough so that the incidence of aftereffects (hangover) is insignificant.

Chloral hydrate has minimal effects on the various stages of normal sleep, including REM sleep, when given in therapeutic doses. At high doses REM sleep may be suppressed.

Doses of chloral hydrate larger than the therapeutic dose cause deeper and longer sleep and increase the incidence of hangover. Pain is obtunded, and the body temperature may fall. Loss of all reflexes and depression of the medullary respiratory and vasomotor centers occur after doses in the lethal range.

Therapeutic doses of chloral hydrate ordinarily cause no changes in the respiration, blood pressure, or heart rate beyond those occurring in normal sleep. However, extremely large doses may cause myocardial depression or arrhythmias, in which central vagal stimulation appears to be involved. Chloral hydrate has an irritant action on the gastric mucosa and therefore should be taken well diluted; otherwise it may cause nausea and vomiting.

Adverse Reactions and Precautions   Undesirable reactions occurring in individuals taking chloral hydrate include hangover, drowsiness, headache, nausea, vomiting, flatulence, staggering gait, and ataxia. Idiosyncratic excitement and delirium may also occur.

Chloral hydrate has additive CNS-depressant effects with other drugs such as alcohol, barbiturates, and antianxiety agents. It may also alter the therapeutic response of any drug which is biotransformed by the drug-metabolizing microsomal system.

Acute Poisoning   The signs of poisoning by chloral hydrate resemble those from alcohol or the barbiturates. The usual features are coma, depressed respiration, hypotension, and hypothermia. The ingestion of large doses may cause death almost immediately. If the patient survives for several hours, the prognosis is generally good, although transient jaundice or albuminuria may be present during recovery. The average *lethal* dose has been estimated to be about 10 g. In the past many cases of poisoning occurred from chloral hydrate added illicitly to alcohol beverages ("knockout drops," "Mickey Finn"); however, the belief that the activity of chloral hydrate is enhanced by a chemical reaction with alcohol is erroneous. The metabolism of ethanol is not appreciably altered by chloral hydrate. However, blood trichloroethanol reaches earlier and higher peak levels when chloral hydrate is administered with ethanol, an effect attributed to decreased oxidation of the halogenated drug to trichloroacetic acid.

Treatment of acute poisoning consists of gastric lavage, support of respiration and circulation, and maintenance of normal body temperature.

Chronic Poisoning   Chloral hydrate is very similar to alcohol, the barbiturates, and other hypnotics in respect to tolerance and psychological and physical dependence. Dependence on chloral hydrate is uncommon, and protocols for treatment have not been formulated in detail, although experience with barbiturate dependence suggests that gradual reduction of the daily dose would be preferable to abrupt withdrawal of the drug. Delirium, mania, or convulsions occurring during withdrawal should receive the same treatment as that given for alcohol or barbiturate abstinence.

Precautions   The drug should be used cautiously in the presence of severe hepatic, renal, or cardiac disease. Oral administration is wisely avoided in patients with esophagitis, gastritis, or gastric or duodenal ulcers. Continued administration of chloral hydrate may increase the activity of the drug-metabolizing microsomal system. This effect is of particular importance in patients receiving coumarin anticoagulants because withdrawal of the hypnotic may decrease the rate of biotransformation of the anticoagulant and thereby increase bleeding tendency.

Trichloroacetic acid binds strongly to plasma proteins. Therefore it may interact with other drugs or natural substances which bind to plasma proteins by displacing them, resulting in a sharp rise in blood level of the free drug or natural substance.

Clinical Use   Chloral hydrate is used in adults and children for the short-term treatment of insomnia. Its rapid onset of action and short duration of effect make it suitable for individuals whose main difficulty is falling asleep. In certain patients chloral hydrate may be considered as an alternative to the benzodiazepine hypnotics. The drug is also indicated as a sedative in children and adults.

Preparations and Dose   *Chloral hydrate* (Noctac) is available in capsules of 250 and 500 mg; as a syrup containing 250 or 500 mg per 5 mL; and as suppositories containing 500 mg. The usual adult oral hypnotic dose is 0.5 to 1.0 g.

Paraldehyde

Paraldehyde, a trimer of acetaldehyde, has the following structure:

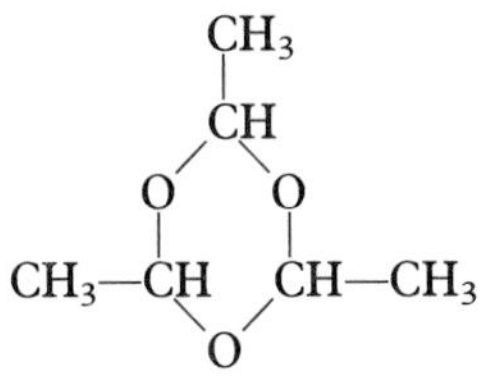

$$CH_3$$
$$CH$$
$$O \qquad O$$
$$CH_3-CH \qquad CH-CH_3$$
$$O$$

Paraldehyde

It is a colorless liquid with a characteristic penetrating odor and a disagreeable burning taste.

Most studies on the mechanism of action of hypnotics have involved the benzodiazepines and barbiturates rather than paraldehyde. The exact mechanism of action for paraldehyde is unknown. It appears likely that the central depressant actions of paraldehyde can be attributed to the drug rather than one of its biotransformation products.

Paraldehyde is absorbed rapidly from the gastrointestinal tract including the rectum. The drug is extensively metabolized in the body; 11 to 28 percent is excreted unchanged through the lungs and 0.1 to 2.5 percent through the kidneys. The fate of the remaining drug appears to involve conversion to acetaldehyde and subsequent oxidation via the tricarboxylic acid cycle to carbon dioxide and water.

The liver seems to be the principal organ involved in the metabolism of paraldehyde. In some patients with severe hepatic disease, the drug is detoxified at an abnormally slow rate, and the hypnotic effects are prolonged. The abstinence syndrome resembles delirium tremens.

Paraldehyde is quite similar to chloral hydrate, alcohol, and the barbiturates in regard to tolerance and dependence. The usual features of acute poisoning are coma, depressed respiration, and hypotension. After intravenous administration, signs of pulmonary edema, right-sided heart failure, and severe coughing may also be present. The use of decomposed paraldehyde, which contains acetic acid, has been responsible for several cases of serious corrosion of the stomach and rectum.

The treatment of acute poisoning by paraldehyde consists of gastric or rectal lavage to remove unabsorbed drug, maintenance of body temperature, and support of respiration and circulation. The patient may remain in coma for many hours, since the rate of biotransformation of paraldehyde is low.

Because of its irritant action, oral administration of paraldehyde is contraindicated in esophagitis, gastritis, or gastric or duodenal ulcers, and rectal administration should be avoided in the presence of inflammatory conditions of the anus or lower bowel. Some physicians consider the drug contraindicated in patients with asthma or other bronchopulmonary diseases. Paraldehyde is also contraindicated in patients taking disulfiram, a drug that inhibits acetaldehyde biotransformation.

The odor it imparts to the breath restricts the use of paraldehyde for most ambulatory patients, thus the drug has found limited use as a sedative and hypnotic. Paraldehyde may be considered as an alternative drug in the treatment of status epilepticus when other drugs do not control this life-threatening condition.

Preparation and Dose *Paraldehyde* (Paral) is available as a liquid in bottles containing 30 mL. The usual adult oral hypnotic dose is 5 to 10 mL.

Ethchlorvynol

The sedative-hypnotic ethchlorvynol has approximately the same potency and toxicities as phenobarbital, but its hypnotic effects are achieved more rapidly (within 30 min) and disappear more quickly (5 h). Its effect on REM sleep has not been assessed.

After oral administration ethchlorvynol is rapidly absorbed from the gastrointestinal tract. It is highly localized in body lipids, biotransformed primarily by the liver, and slowly excreted by the kidney. The compound can induce the liver drug-metabolizing microsomal system.

Acute toxicities of ethchlorvynol produce an array of signs and symptoms indistinguishable from those caused by other hypnotics, and chronic intoxication resembles chronic poisoning by alcohol or the barbiturates. Patients may exhibit ataxia, confusion, disorientation, and occasionally visual or auditory hallucinations. A daily dose of 2 g appears sufficient to cause physical dependence. Withdrawal of the drug may result in generalized tonic-clonic seizures or psychotic behavior.

Due to the availability of other hypnotics such as the benzodiazepine derivatives, ethchlorvynol is seldom used in the treatment of insomnia.

Ethinamate

Ethinamate is a hypnotic agent whose effects resemble those of pentobarbital or secobarbital. The drug is rapidly absorbed from the gastrointestinal tract. In the liver it is biotransformed by hydroxylation and glucuronide conjugation. The metabolites are excreted in the urine. The drug has an elimination half-life of 2.5 h.

Acute overdosage with ethinamate has been reported, but fatalities have been relatively few, and these have often involved complicating factors. Death is usually attributed to respiratory failure, although circulatory collapse has also been observed. Treatment of ethinamate poisoning consists of maintaining body temperature and supporting the respiration and circulation; gastric lavage is useful if the patient is seen shortly after taking the drug. Extracorporeal hemodialysis is effective in eliminating the drug but is probably less useful for this purpose than for the treatment of poisoning from hypnotics with a longer duration of action.

Dependence on ethinamate has been reported. The clinical picture resembles that of chronic barbiturate intoxication.

Although ethinamate is an effective hypnotic agent, it is infrequently used over a benzodiazepine in the short-term management of insomnia.

Glutethimide

Glutethimide possesses hypnotic and sedative properties. The hypnotic effect is about the same as that of pentobarbital. Its abuse can lead to psychological and physical dependence and acute poisoning.

After oral absorption the drug is widely distributed and reaches somewhat higher concentrations in fat than in other tissues because of its lipid solubility. Glutethimide is almost completely biotransformed by hydroxylation. It has a half-life of 45 h.

Glutethimide was originally indicated for the treatment of insomnia in individuals who could no tolerate barbiturates. However, the drug offers no therapeutic advantages over the benzodiazepine hypnotics and is rarely used.

Methyprylon

Methyprylon is a hypnotic agent whose pharmacologic effects closely resemble those of pentobarbital and secobarbital. Large doses of the drug cause coma, which may be accompanied by respiratory depression or hypotension or both. Chronic abuse of methyprylon results in the development of tolerance and physical dependence.

As with glutethimide this drug is rarely used in the treatment of insomnia since the introduction of the benzodiazepine hypnotics.

Preparations and Doses   *Ethchlorvynol* (Placidyl) is available in capsules containing 100, 200, 500, or 750 mg. The usual adult oral hypnotic dose is 500 mg.

Ethinamate (Valmid) is available in capsules containing 500 mg. The usual adult oral hypnotic dose is 0.5 to 1.0 g.

Glutethimide (Doriden) is available as tablets containing 250 or 500 mg; and as capsules containing 500 mg. The usual adult oral hypnotic dose is 500 mg.

Methyprylon (Noludar) is available as tablets containing 50 or 200 mg; and as capsules containing 300 mg. The usual adult oral dose is 200 to 400 mg.

Nonprescription Sleep Medication

There are several over-the-counter (OTC) products that can be obtained by individuals to aid in the induction of sleep at bedtime. The active ingredient in these preparations is diphenhydramine or doxylamine. They are antihistamines (H_1 blockers). Both antihistamines can cause a sufficient degree of sedation. It is this sedative property of the antihistamine that decreases the latency to sleep when the medication is taken at bedtime.

The sedative effect of antihistamines is enhanced by the concurrent administration of other central nervous system depressants and ethanol. In addition, it is possible that the use of OTC sleep aids may interfere with prescription drugs that the individual is taking. If satisfactory results are not obtained by the use of an OTC sleep medication, the individual should seek medical treatment for the insomnia. For more information about these antihistamines see Chap. 12.

BIBLIOGRAPHY

Bliwise, D., W. Seidel, I. Karacan, M. Mitler, T. Roth, F. Zovick, and W. Dement: "Daytime Sleepiness as a Criterion in Hypnotic Medication Trials: Comparison of Triazolam and Flurazepam," *Sleep*, **6**:156–163 (1983).

Eldefrawi, A. T., and M. E. Eldefrawi: "Receptors for γ-Aminobutyric Acid and Voltage-Dependent Chloride Channels as Targets for Drugs and Toxicants," *FASEB J.* **1**:262–271 (1987).

Lader, M., and H. Petursson: "Long-Term Effects of Benzodiazepines," *Neuropharmacol.*, **22**:527–533 (1983).

Owen, R. T., and P. Tyrer: "Benzodiazepine Dependence: Review of the Evidence," *Drugs*, **25**:385–398 (1983).

Richter, J. A., and J. R. Holman "Barbiturates: Their *in vivo* Effects and Potential Biochemical Mechanisms," *Prog. Neurobiol.*, **18**:275–319 (1982).

Rickels, K.: "Clinical Trials of Hypnotics," *J. Clin. Psychopharmacol.*, **3**:133–139 (1983).

Sellers, E. M., and U. Basto: "Benzodiazepines and Ethanol: Assessment of Effects and Consequences of Psychotropic Drug Interaction," *J. Clin. Psychopharmacol.*, **2**:249–262 (1982).

Shiromani, P. J., J. C. Gillin, and S. J. Henriksen: "Acetylcholine and the Regulation of REM Sleep: Basic Mechanisms and Clinical Implications for Affective Illness and Narcolepsy," *Annu. Rev. Pharmacol. Toxicol.*, **27**:137–156 (1987).

Smith, A. G., and F. DeMatteis: "Drugs and Hepatic Porphyria," *Clin. Haematol.*, **9**:399–424 (1980).

Snyder, S. H.: "Drug and Neurotransmitter Receptors in the Brain," *Science*, **224**:22–31 (1984).

Stephenson, F. A.: "Understanding the GABA$_A$ Receptor: A Chemically Gated Ion Channel," *Biochem. J.*, **249**:21–32 (1988).

Trifiletti, R. R., A. M. Snownan, and S. H. Snyder: "Barbiturate Recognition Site on the GABA/Benzodiazepine Receptor Complex Is Distinct from the Picrotoxin/TBPS Recognition Site," *Eur. J. Pharmacol.*, **106**:441–447 (1985).

C H A P T E R   **16**

Antianxiety Drugs

G. John DiGregorio

Anxiety is a diffuse, unpleasant feeling associated with various medical conditions. By far, the most common situation is anxiety neurosis. The syndrome is characterized by diffuse symptoms, such as helplessness, apprehension, faintness, and headaches, but it is also characterized by somatic symptoms such as pain, sweating, tachypnea, tachycardia, nausea, palpitations, and dry mouth. These symptoms can be mild and require little or no treatment but at times may be severe and cause patients to have considerable distress. Various studies have shown that benzodiazepines are very effective in the treatment of neurotic anxiety. Benzodiazepines have also found a place in the treatment of anxiety associated with organic disease such as coronary heart disease, cancer, hypertension, and gastrointestinal tract disorders. The drugs commonly used for the treatment of anxiety are referred to as *antianxiety*, or *anxiolytic*, drugs.

BENZODIAZEPINES

Prior to the discovery of the benzodiazepines, the major drugs used for the treatment of anxiety were primarily sedatives and hypnotics. These drugs, which included secobarbital, phenobarbital, glutethimide, and even alcohol, were used extensively in various situations. Unfortunately, because of their widespread use and their pharmocologic properties, the drugs caused a number of therapeutic problems including (1) high incidence of drug overdose and death due to their

potent depressive effect on the respiratory system and (2) high incidence of drug dependency. The benzodiazepines are considered to be specific antianxiety drugs, which possess less depression of the respiratory system and potentially less dependency. For these reasons, the benzodiazepines are the drugs of choice for the treatment of anxiety.

The primary application for benzodiazepine drug therapy is in patients who experience anxiety so debilitating that their life-styles, work, and interpersonal relationships are severely hampered. However, the absolute necessity for concurrent psychologic support and counseling cannot be overemphasized.

The benzodiazephines are a group of many compounds, the first of which was synthesized in the 1930s. The first useful drug of this group was chlordiazepoxide, which was developed in the late 1950s. Since that time a dozen or so benzodiazepines with useful pharmacologic properties have been successfully introduced into clinical medicine. The agents discussed in this chapter include alprazolam, chlordiazepoxide, clorazepate, diazepam, halazepam, lorazepam, oxazepam, and prazepam. All possess similar efficacy, differing quantitatively (i.e., in degree and duration of effect) rather than qualitatively. There are a number of other benzodiazepines on the market used therapeutically for conditions other than anxiety. These agents are discussed in detail in other chapters. They are carbamazepine (anticonvulsant, see Chap. 21) and flurazepam, triazolam, and temazepam (hypnotics, see Chap. 15).

Chemistry

The benzodiazepines are divided into two major categories: 1,4-benzodiazepines (e.g., chlordiazepoxide, diazepam, lorazepam) and heterocyclic 1,4-benzodiazepines (e.g., alprazolam). The electronegative group at the C-7 position and the halogen (C-7) or nitro group (N_4) are necessary for optimal antianxiety activity. Substitution at the C-5 position with a phenyl ring and/or halogen will also increase pharmacologic activity (Fig. 16-1).

Mechanism of Action Evidence now suggests that the mechanism of action for benzodiazepines involves the gamma aminobutyric acid (GABA) receptor. The benzodiazepines as a class potentiate the activity of GABA, an inhibitory neurotransmitter, at receptors within the CNS, particularly in the limbic system. The benzodiazepines do not directly interact with "GABA receptors" nor do they prevent re-uptake of GABA into presynaptic storage vesicles. They bind to a specific receptor on the chloride ionophore. This benzodiazepine-receptor interaction appears to increase the inhibitory activity of GABA by inducing an allosteric change in the GABA receptor, which results in an increased influx of chloride ions through GABA-activated chloride ion channels (see Chap. 15). In summary, they increase the frequency of the chloride channel openings in conjunction with GABA. Review Chap. 15 for a complete discussion of the GABA receptor.

Pharmacokinetics

A great deal of information has accumulated concerning the pharmacokinetics of the benzodiazepines. This information has been utilized as a means of classifying the drugs as short-acting versus long-acting benzodiazepines. To fully understand the kinetics of these drugs, one must discuss this topic in terms of single-dose versus steady-state kinetics (see Table 16-1).

In single dose kinetics, the onset of action of the benzodiazepines is based on the absorption and distribution of the particular drugs. The duration of action after single-dose therapy depends largely on the lipid solubility of the drugs as well as their elimination processes. However, after steady state has been established (approximately 5 times elimination half-life), the duration of action depends mainly on biotransfor-

mation and elimination. It is this later concept on which the classification of the benzodiazepines is based. For example, oxazepam, lorazepam, halazepam, and alprazolam are classified as short-acting (half-life between 3 and 20 h) due to their rapid elimination; chlordiazepoxide, diazepam, clorazepate, and prazepam (half-life of 20 h or more) are long-acting, slowly eliminated benzodiazepines.

Three benzodiazepines are available for administration by injection: diazepam, chlordiazepoxide, and lorazepam. Absorption of diazepam and chlordiazepoxide is faster and more predictable after oral dosing than following intramuscular injection, which may produce low and inconsistent plasma levels if the site of administration is the gluteal muscle. Therefore, if diazepam is to be given by the intramuscular route, it should be injected into the deltoid muscle where absorption is complete and predictable. Lorazepam is well absorbed by both the oral and intramuscular routes and consistently develops peak plasma levels more rapidly after IM injection [60 to 90 min, compared to oral dosing (2 h)]. The remaining benzodiazepines—alprazolam, clorazepate, halazepam, oxazepam, and prazepam—are administered by the oral route. Clorazepate is the only benzodiazepine that is converted to an active product, *N*-desmethyldiazepam, by the acid in the stomach. The rate of conversion of clorazepate is inversely proportional to gastric pH.

In general, benzodiazepines are highly bound to human serum albumin. Plasma protein binding is greatest for diazepam (98 to 99 percent). Binding for the remaining agents varies from 88 to 97 percent with the exception of alprazolam which exhibits an in vitro plasma protein binding of 67 to 73 percent. The distribution of diazepam and some other benzodiazepines is complicated somewhat by a considerable degree of biliary excretion, which occurs early in the distribution of these agents. This enterohepatic recirculation occurs with biotransformation products as well as parent compounds and may be clinically important for agents and metabolites with a long elimination half-life. The presence of food in the upper bowel delays reabsorption and contributes to the late resurgence of plasma drug levels and activity.

The benzodiazepines exhibit a rather complex interrelationship of biotransformation reactions and products, which contributes in most cases to a prolongation of pharmacologic activity. The major biotransforma-

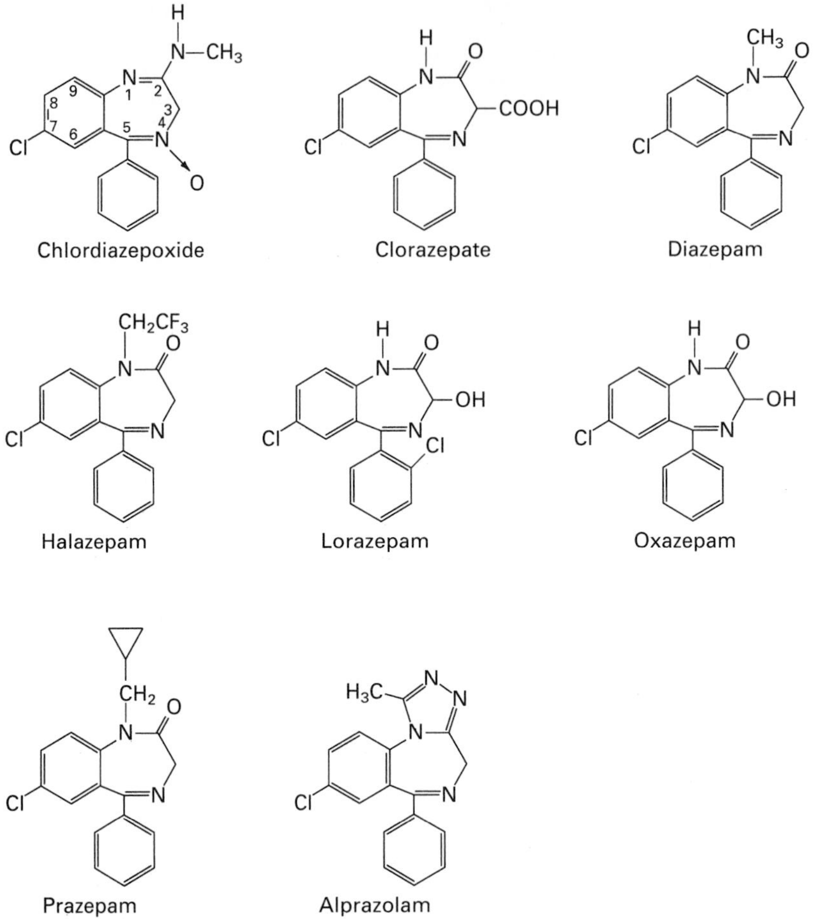

FIGURE 16-1   Chemical structures of various benzodiazepines.

tion reactions associated with benzodiazepines are oxidation and conjugation. Most biotransformation reactions occur in the liver via the drug-metabolizing microsomal system (DMMS), and in many cases the benzodiazepines are biotransformated to active products such as N-desmethyldiazepam (nordazepam). Lorazepam and oxazepam are metabolized only to inactive metabolites.

Although the benzodiazepines are biotransformed via the DMMS, they do not significantly induce the activity of the DMMS and, consequently, do not accelerate the biotransformation of other agents metabolized via the microsomal system. Biotransformation of certain benzodiazepines can be influenced by cimeti-

dine. Cimetidine, an H_2 antagonist which is a P-450 inhibitor, can increase the blood concentrations of benzodiazepines by inhibiting their oxidation, whereas the biotransformation of other benzodiazepines that go by a metabolic route other than oxidation is not altered (Fig. 16-2).

In order to illustrate the complexities of benzodiazepine biotransformation, the reactions are summarized in Fig. 16-2. It should be noted that since hepatic biotransformation is important to the termination of pharmacologic activity of all the benzodiazepines discussed, the duration of action of these agents may be significantly prolonged in patients with hepatic dysfunction or failure.

TABLE 16-1 Pharmacokinetic characteristics of selected antianxiety drugs

Drug name — Generic	Drug name — Trade	Classification (duration of action)	Route(s) of administration	Parent compound — Time, h By mouth dose of peak plasma levels	Parent compound — Plasma protein binding	Parent compound — Elimination half-life, h	Biotransformation — Reaction	Biotransformation — Product	Biotransformation — Active	Biotransformation — Elimination half-life, h
Alprazolam	Xanax	Benzodiazepine (short)	PO	1.0–2.5	67–73	7–15	Hydroxylation, N-demethylation	α-Hydroxyalprazolam, N-desmethyldiazepam	Yes Yes	12–15 30–200
Chlordiazepoxide	Librium	Benzodiazepine (long)	PO IM, IV	1.0–2.5	94–97	5–30	N-Demethylation 3-hydroxylation	N-Desmethyldiazepam, oxazepam	Yes Yes	30–200 3–21
Clorazepate	Tranxene	Benzodiazepine (long)	PO	0.5–1.5[a]	[b]		N-Demethylation, 3-hydroxylation	N-Desmethyldiazepam[a] oxazepam	Yes Yes	30–200 3–21
Diazepam	Valium	Benzodiazepine (long)	PO IM, IV	0.5–1.5	98–99	20–70	N-Demethylation, 3-hydroxylation, N-demethylation	N-Desmethyldiazepam, 3-hydroxydiazepam, oxazepam	Yes Yes Yes	30–200 8–25 3–21
Halazepam	Paxipam	Benzodiazepine (short)	PO			5–15	N-Demethylation	N-Desmethyldiazepam	Yes	30–200
Lorazepam	Ativan	Benzodiazepine (short)	PO IM, IV	1.0–2.5	88–92	8–25	Conjugation	Glucuronide	No	
Oxazepam	Serax	Benzodiazepine (short)	PO	1.5–3.0	94–97	5–15	Conjugation	Glucuronide	No	
Prazepam	Centrax	Benzodiazepine (long)	PO	1.0–8.0	[b]		N-Demethylation, 3-hydroxylation, N-demethylation	N-Desmethyldiazepam, 3-hydroxyprazepam, oxazepam	Yes Yes Yes	30–200 3–21
Meprobamate	Equanil, Meprospan, Miltown, Meprobamate, USP	Propanediol Parbamate (short)	PO	2–3		6–17	Hydroxylation and conjugation	None		

[a] N-Desmethyldiazepam, the active principle, is formed from clorazepate in the stomach; the rate of conversion of clorazepate to N-desmethyldiazepam is inversely proportional to gastric pH. [b] Clorazepate and prazepam are "prodrugs," i.e., they never achieve effective levels in the plasma compartment. *Note:* Modified and reproduced with permission from: G. J. DiGregorio, S. J. Smith, and T. E. Sudol, *Clinical Pharmacology: A Teaching Resource,* Roche, 1984.

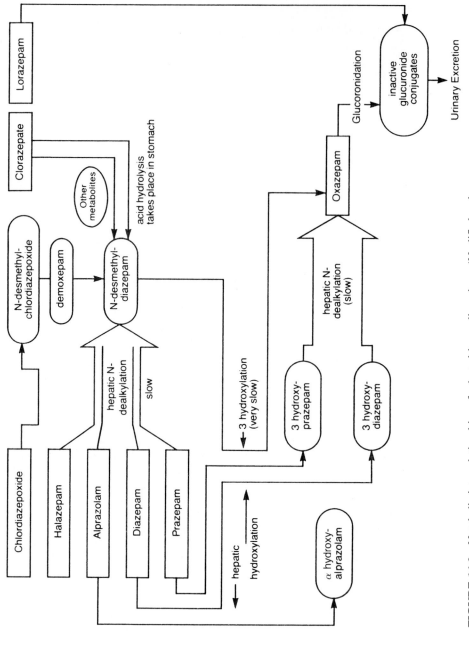

FIGURE 16-2   Metabolic interrelationships of selected benzodiazepines. (Modified and reproduced with permission from: G. J. DiGregorio, S. J. Smith, and T. E. Sudol, *Clinical Pharmacology: A Teaching Resource*, Roche, 1984.)

Pharmacodynamics

Central Nervous System   As a class, the benzodiazepines produce five main effects within the CNS: antianxiety, sedation, skeletal muscle relaxation, anticonvulsant activity, and hypnosis. The *antianxiety effect* of the benzodiazepines appears to be related to a specific activity within the limbic system. This is one effect that makes these drugs unique and separate from the sedatives and hypnotics. Although the benzodiazepines qualitatively posses the same effect, they differ, quantitatively. On a weight basis the antianxiety potency of the benzodiazepines discussed here is (in decreasing order) alprazolam, lorazepam, diazepam, clorazepate, chlordiazepoxide, prazepam, halazepam, and oxazepam.

At therapeutic doses, *sedation/drowsiness* occurs as an effect of these drugs on the central nervous system. It is interesting to note that patients tend to become tolerant to this particular effect but do not become increasingly tolerant to the antianxiety effects. Those benzodiazepines employed as hypnotic agents have less of an effect on the sleep cycle pattern than barbiturates and other nonbarbiturate sedative hypnotics. The benzodiazepines appear to have an effect on the cycle of reducing stages 3 and 4 of the sleep cycle but have less effect on REM sleep than the sedative hypnotics. The clinical significance is not understood.

The benzodiazepines produce *skeletal muscle relaxation* by a combination of central effects related to their actions on polysynaptic nerve tracts modulated by GABA in the spinal cord and the brain stem. Their antianxiety effects may be a significant contributing factor here. Specifically, it has been demonstrated that benzodiazepines (more precisely, diazepam) can depress monosynaptic reflex pathways in the spinal cord. This is accomplished by enhancing the presynaptic inhibition provided by GABA. The physiologic significance of presynaptic inhibition is that it produces an intense negative feedback which converts afferent impulses that normally perpetuate spastic contraction into inhibitory impulses which block or reduce subsequent contraction. This is the major site of muscle relaxant action. Diazepam appears to be the most potent of all the benzodiazepines as a muscle relaxant.

The ability of the benzodiazepines to increase the *convulsive seizure threshold* is well documented. The major sites of anticonvulsant activity appear to be the limbic system and the mesencephalic reticular forma-

tion. The anticonvulsant activity of benzodiazepines is associated with an increase of fast beta EEG activity and enhancement of subcortical inhibitory mechanisms which suppress epileptiform activity. This may be the result of benzodiazepine (specifically, diazepam) enhancement of the inhibitory effects of GABA in abnormal neuronal populations, especially in the Purkinje cells of the cerebellum.

Adverse Effects

Acute   The adverse reactions most frequently encountered during benzodiazepine therapy are sedation, lightheadedness, ataxia, and lethargy. The mild sedative actions of these drugs vary quantitatively from benzodiazepine to benzodiazepine. For example, the short-acting lorazepam, although it clears the body rapidly, possesses a prolonged sedative action compared to the other benzodiazepines. Usually these mild reactions occur early in therapy and disappear after a few days of treatment. Occasional reactions with hypnotic doses are impaired mental and psychomotor function, confusion, euphoria, delayed reaction time, uncoordinated motor function, dysarthria, headache, and xerostomia. Rare reactions may include syncope, hypotension, blurred vision, altered libido, skin rashes, nausea, menstrual irregularities, agranulocytosis, lupus-like syndrome, edema, and constipation. The effect of the benzodiazepines on respiration has been extensively investigated. Unlike the barbiturates, the benzodiazepines have only a mild effect on respiration when given by the oral route, even in toxic doses. There are very few documented cases where high oral doses of benzodiazepines are responsible for respiratory failure. However, when given parenterally or in conjunction with other depressants like alcohol, all the benzodiazepines have the potential of causing significant respiratory depression. Individuals, particularly the elderly and debilitated, should be warned of the potential danger of these drugs to respiratory system in these situations. Some benzodiazepines, in therapeutic doses, also can cause anterograde amnesia. This amnesia, which is described by patients as a "blank feeling," has beneficial as well as adverse effects. Clinical advantage of this particular effect can be taken by using the benzodiazepines, administered parenterally, for various presurgical or diagnostic procedures such as "endoscopy." However, given orally, most benzodiazepines do not cause this effect. Patients should be warned of this effect, especially if the patient is being treated as an outpatient.

Adverse reactions associated with intravenous use of some injectable benzodiazepines include pain during injection, thrombophlebitis, hypothermia, restlessness, cardiac arrhythmias, coughing, apnea, vomiting, and a mild anthicholinergic effect.

Deaths from overdose of benzodiazepines alone rarely occur. Patients have taken as much as 50 times the therapeutic doses of these drugs without causing mortality. This particular property of these drugs is another example of how they differ from the potent respiratory depressant sedatives and hypnotics.

Overdose of benzodiazepines, when taken in combination with other drugs, such as heavy doses of alcohol, have been reported to cause death.

Chronic Benzodiazepines present a major problem when administered over long periods of time. This problem has been described as *benzodiazepine dependence*. The dependence associated with the benzodiazepines should not be compared with the situation one observes with alcohol, narcotic, or barbiturate dependencies. If taken at therapeutic doses for short periods of time (4 to 6 weeks), the benzodiazepines usually can be stopped abruptly without causing significant symptoms. However, if the drugs are taken in higher than recommended doses and/or for longer periods of time and given to patients with histories of drug or alcohol abuse, the incidence of developing symptoms when the drug is discontinued increases significantly. Apparently, the onset of the withdrawal symptoms is based on the elimination half-life of the benzodiazepines. The onset of withdrawal symptoms will occur sooner with the shorter-acting drugs due to rapid elimination.

With the longer-acting benzodiazepines, the onset is much slower due to their longer half-lives and slower disappearance from the plasma. The benzodiazepine withdrawal symptoms produced should be characterized into three stages. The first, or initial, symptoms occur usually immediately after the drug is stopped; the patient may experience an acute, mild anxiety reaction due to the realization that the benzodiazepines will no longer be available. After a period of time (2 to 3 days for shorter-acting benzodiazepines, 5 to 14 days for longer-acting benzodiazepines) withdrawal symptoms associated with dependence are usually mild and consist of nervousness, insomnia, headache, and fa-

tigue. However, in rare instances, severe reactions, which are characterized by hypotension and convulsions, may develop. Only a few reports have been published concerning the severe withdrawal reactions of these drugs. The third reaction, which may occur after the withdrawal reactions have subsided, is the reintroduction of the original anxiety symptoms. These symptoms tend to be very similar to the symptoms experienced before the benzodiazepines were started.

Drug Interactions Benzodiazepines produce additive CNS depression when administered with other depressant agents, including (especially) ethanol, antihistamines, and sedative-hypnotic agents, as well as psychotropic agents including phenothiazines, MAO inhibitors, and narcotic analgesics.

Owing to the availability of ethanol, this interaction with benzodiazepines is commonly seen. Generally the interaction is described as an increase in CNS depressant effects. Individuals may experience episodes of mild to severe ataxia and "drunkenness" which will severely retard their performance level. No one benzodiazepine is considered safer than another in combination with ethanol. Therefore, physicians should indicate to their patients this potential interaction and tell patients *not* to drink alcoholic beverages while taking the benzodiazepine, especially if a patient is relatively new to the benzodiazepine. For individuals who have been taking alcohol or benzodiazepines for long periods of time, when they take them together they experience this interaction, but to a milder degree.

Another drug-drug interaction involving the benzodiazepines is that with the H_2 blocker, cimetidine. Cimetidine will decrease the biotransformation of the long-acting benzodiazepines by inhibiting the P-450 enzyme system necessary for oxidation of these drugs. This interaction does not involve the short-acting benzodiazepines such as oxazepam or lorazepam since these drugs undergo only glucuronidation in the liver. Clinically the interaction probably has been overemphasized. Although blood levels increase, clinical symptoms have not increased significantly. The interaction will have to be reinvestigated to determine the clinical significance.

Contraindications As with any drug or class of drugs, the benzodiazepines should be avoided in patients with a known hypersensitivity to these agents. Alprazolam, clorazepate, diazepam, halazepam, lorazepam, and prazepam are contraindicated in individuals with acute narrow-angle glaucoma presumably due to their anticholinergic side effects.

Owing to the considerable lipid solubility of most benzodiazepines, these agents cross the placenta and are secreted in mother's milk. Consequently, they should be avoided in pregnant and nursing women.

Precautions The dose of benzodiazepines in elderly and debilitated patients should be limited to the smallest effective amount initially. This can be increased gradually as needed and tolerated.

As with other psychotropic medications, the usual precautions with respect to administration of the drug and size of the prescription are indicated for severely depressed patients or those in whom there is reason to expect concealed suicidal ideation or plans.

Therapeutic Uses The primary use of the benzodiazepines is in the management of anxiety such as anxiety neurosis and/or the short-term relief of the symptoms of anxiety, which may manifest themselves in other psychoneuroses or as a result of an organic disease. Other uses of selected benzodiazepines include the following: (1) treatment of acute alcohol withdrawal symptoms (chlordiazepoxide, clorazepate, diazepam, and oxazepam); (2) relief of skeletal muscle spasms, spasticity, and athetosis (diazepam); (3) treatment of severe recurrent convulsive seizures (status epilepticus) (diazepam); (4) as a preanesthetic medication to reduce the apprehension and anxiety which a patient may experience prior to surgery (diazepam or lorazepam); (5) treatment of partial seizures or as an adjunct in the management of convulsive disorders (clorazepate or diazepam); (6) as a premedication prior to endoscopic procedures or cardioversion to reduce the anxiety stress and tension associated with these procedures and to diminish the patient's recollection of the procedure (diazepam and lorazepam); and (7) as hypnotic agents used in the treatment of insomnia (see Chap. 15).

PROPRANEDIOLS

Meprobamate

Introduction Meprobamate is the prototype for a group of antianxiety agents (the propanediol carbamates) which have been used in the treatment of anxi-

ety and for daytime sedation. In light of recent developments and the advent of the benzodiazepines these agents are now less commonly used.

$$H_2NCOCH_2\overset{\overset{\displaystyle O}{\|}}{C}CH_2OCNH_2$$
$$\underset{CH_2CH_2CH_3}{\overset{\displaystyle CH_3}{|}}$$

Meprobamate

Mechanism of Action The effects of meprobamate are somewhat similar to those of the barbiturate phenobarbital, although shorter in duration. The precise mechanism(s) by which meprobamate produces these effects is unknown. Meprobamate produces a widespread but uneven depression of the central nervous system; polysynaptic reflexes are depressed, while monosynaptic reflexes are undisturbed. Little skeletal muscle relaxation is produced at therapeutic doses. This agent possesses no analgesic effect of its own but has been reported to enhance the analgesia produced by other agents when used in combination for musculoskeletal pain. Meprobamate promotes sleep in patients with insomnia; however, in a fashion similar to the barbiturates, it depresses the stage of rapid-eye-movement (REM) sleep which is associated with dreaming and the resolution of psychological conflicts.

Pharmacokinetics Peak blood levels of meprobamate occur 2 to 3 h after oral administration. This agent is not significantly bound by plasma proteins and is extensively biotransformed by hydroxylation and subsequent conjugation in the liver's drug metabolizing microsomal system (DMMS).

Meprobamate's major biotransformation product, 2-methyl-2(betahydroxy-propyl)-1,3-propanediol dicarbamate, is inactive. Meprobamate induces the DMMS and may thereby speed its own biotransformation. About 10 to 20 percent of the parent compound is excreted unchanged in the urine. The availability of meprobamate in timed-release dosage forms has been reported to provide more consistent bioavailability but offers no marked benefit compared to ordinary preparations with regard to duration of action or dosing interval for most patients.

Adverse Reactions The untoward effects most commonly associated with meprobamate are drowsiness and ataxia. Anaphylaxis, allergic reactions, hypotension, and syncope have also been reported. Other adverse reactions reported rarely include thrombocytopenia, leukopenia, dermatitis, urticaria, purpura, leukemia, and aplastic anemia. Reports indicate that prolonged use of meprobamate in daily doses does not produce withdrawal symptoms. However, long-term, high-dose use has been shown to cause psychological and physical dependence. Abrupt discontinuation of this agent after such a course of therapy may produce withdrawal symptoms. Typical withdrawal symptoms include anorexia, anxiety, ataxia, insomnia, muscle spasms, tremors, nausea, and vomiting.

Uses   Meprobamate is somewhat useful in the management of anxiety but is less effective than the benzodiazepine in this application, and is potentially more sedative and causes greater dependency.

Warnings   Patients should be warned that this drug may impair the mental and/or physical abilities required for the performance of potentially hazardous tasks such as driving a motor vehicle or operating machinery.

Precautions   The lowest effective dose should be administered, particularly to elderly and debilitated patients in order to preclude oversedation.

The possibility of suicide attempts should be considered, and the least amount of drug feasible should be dispensed at any one time.

Meprobamate occasionally may precipitate seizures in epileptic patients.

AZASPIRODECANEDIONE

Buspirone

Buspirone is a member of a new series of antianxiety drugs. Buspirone is chemically unrelated to the benzodiazepines or the barbiturates.

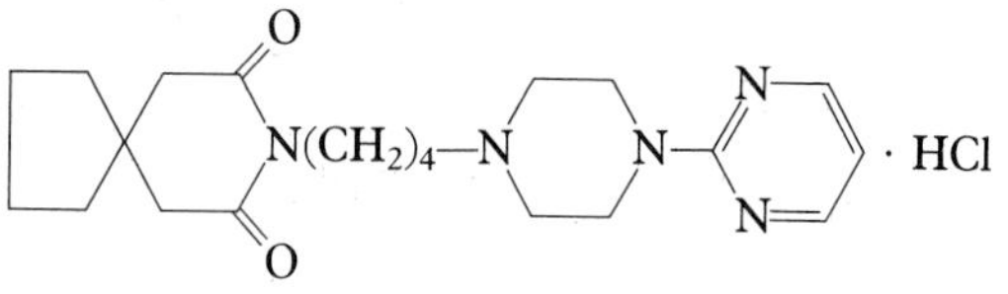

Buspirone

Mechanism of action of buspirone is unknown. It does not affect or alter the GABA receptors but appears to have a high affinity for certain serotonin (5-HT) receptors and also moderate affinity for brain D_2-dopamine receptors.

Buspirone is effective as an antianxiety drug but lacks the anticonvulsant and muscle relaxant effects of the benzodiazepines. It also has minimal sedative effects as compared to other antianxiety drugs. Buspirone is rapidly absorbed and goes through a first pass effect. Approximately 95 percent of the drug is bound to plasma proteins. It is metabolized by oxidation to an active metabolite, 1-pyrimidinyl piperazine. The elimination half-life is about 2 to 3 h less. Less than 50 percent of the drug is excreted in the urine unchanged.

Some adverse reactions of buspirone includes dizziness, drowsiness, dry mouth, headaches, nervousness, fatigue, insomnia, weakness, lightheadedness, rash, and infrequent urinary frequency.

Buspirone is indicated for the management of anxiety states, both chronic and acute. The drug used chronically appears to cause less tolerance and potential for abuse when compared to other anxiolytic drugs.

HETEROGENOUS CHEMICALS

Hydroxyzine

Hydroxyzine possesses antihistaminic, antiemetic, and sedative activities.

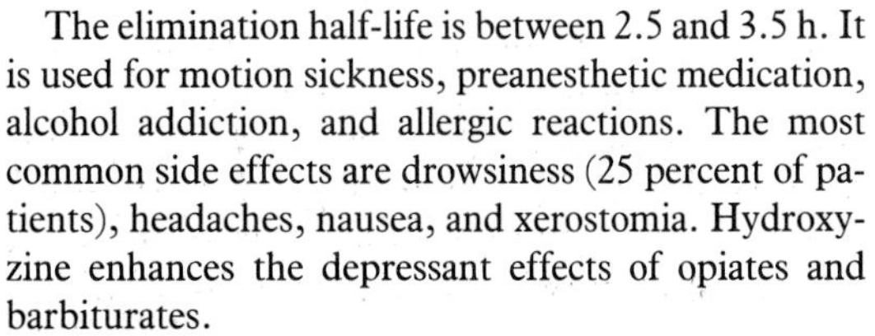

Hydroxyzine

The elimination half-life is between 2.5 and 3.5 h. It is used for motion sickness, preanesthetic medication, alcohol addiction, and allergic reactions. The most common side effects are drowsiness (25 percent of patients), headaches, nausea, and xerostomia. Hydroxyzine enhances the depressant effects of opiates and barbiturates.

PREPARATION

Buspirone (BUSPAR) is available in 5- and 10-mg tablets.

Diazepam (Valium) is available in the following preparations: scored tablets containing 2, 5, and 10 mg; 2-mL ampuls and vials containing 5 mg/mL of IM or IV injection; and slow-release capsules containing 15 mg.

Halazepam (Paxipam) is available in the following preparations: scored tablets containing 20 to 40 mg.

Lorazepam (Ativan) is available in the following preparations: 0.5-mg. tablets; 1.0- and 2.0-mg scored tablets; as a liquid for injection in sterile cartridge needles; and multiple dose vials in concentration of 2 and 4 mg//mL.

Oxazepam (Serax) is available in the following preparations: capsules containing 10, 15, and 30 mg and tablets containing 15 mg.

Prazepam (Centrax) is available in the following preparations: capsules containing 5 and 10 mg and scored tablets containing 10 mg.

Meprobamate (Equanil, Meprospan, Miltown, Me-probamate U.S.P.) is available in the following preparations: timed-release capsules containing 200 and 400 mg; tablets containing 200, 400, and 600 mg; and as an oral suspension containing 40 mg/mL.

BIBLIOGRAPHY

Abernethy, D. R., D. J. Greenblatt, and R. I. Shader: "Benzodiazepine Hypnotic Metabolism: Drug Interactions and Clinical Implications," *Acta Psychiatr. Scand.*, **74**:32–38 (1986).

Burrows, G. D., T. R. Norman, B. Davis: "Antianxiety Agents," vol. 2, *Drugs in Psychiatry*, Elsevier, Amsterdam, 1984.

File, S. E., and S. Pellow: "Behavioral Pharmacology of Minor Tranquilizers," *Pharmacol. Ther.*, **35**:265–290 (1987).

Morse, D. R., and M. L. Furst: "The Antianxiety Agents," *Intern. J. Psychosomatics*, **34**:8–14 (1987).

Rosenbaum, J. F.: "The Drug Treatment of Anxiety," *N. Engl. J. Med.*, **306**:401 (1982).

Skolnick, P., and S. M. Paul: "The Mechanism of Action of Benzodiazepines," *Med. Res. Rev.*, **1**:3 (1981).

Ethanol and Related Alcohols

Andrew P. Ferko

Ethanol is a central nervous system depressant that possesses important pharmacologic and toxicologic properties. In addition it has become one of the most widely abused drugs in our society. The basic concepts of the effects of ethanol in the body are presented in this chapter. Furthermore, several other alcohols are discussed from the standpoint of their toxicology. They are methanol, ethylene glycol, and isopropyl alcohol.

ETHANOL

Ethanol is one of the oldest drugs used by humans in the course of civilization. The drug is employed for both medicinal and social uses. Although ethanol has several therapeutic indications, its primary medical interest today is related to the fact that ethanol is commonly used as a drug of abuse. Ethanol produces central nervous system euphoria and depression. Although ethanol is a simple compound, its pharmacology is complex and diverse. On repeated administration over a period of time, tolerance and physical dependence can develop. Prolonged ingestion of ethanol can lead to pathologic changes in body organs, e.g., cirrhosis of the liver. Ethanol consumption can seriously affect the lives of alcoholics and their families. Alcoholics have 15 times the suicide rate of the general population. Ethanol is significantly involved in many cases of wife and child abuse. In addition, the drinking of ethanol is associated with about 50 percent of all deaths that occur in automobile accidents. Al-

though ethanol has many social implications in its use, the intent of this chapter is to be an introduction to the basic pharmacology of ethanol.

Chemistry and Source

Ethanol is a water-soluble aliphatic alcohol (CH_3—CH_2—OH); it is also referred to as *ethyl alcohol*, or *alcohol*. Ethanol is manufactured by the process of fermentation. In the presence of yeast, sugar is converted to ethanol. If the starting product is a cereal which contains starch, the starch is first malted so that the starch is converted to the sugar maltose.

The ethanol content of alcoholic beverages such as wines and distilled liquors are listed as the percentage of alcohol expressed by volume or as a number followed by the word *proof*. In the United States the proof number is twice the percentage of alcohol by volume. The term *proof* originated in an old English custom of testing the alcohol content of whisky. The whisky was poured over gunpowder and a flame applied to it. If the gunpowder exploded, the whisky was said to be of "proof strength." For whisky to ignite, it must contain at least 50% ethanol by volume.

Mechanism of Action

Ethanol is a central nervous system depressant. Depending on the dose, there may occur sedation, ataxia, hypnosis, anesthesia, or even death due to respiratory paralysis. At the present time, the exact mechanism of action for ethanol in the central nervous system is not fully delineated, however, it is proposed that the site of action for ethanol is the cellular membrane. It is suggested that acute ethanol administration acts in a physical manner to cause the disordering of membranes and thereby increase membrane fluidity. The ethanol molecules dissolve into cell membranes and cause the lipid bilayer of the membrane to become less rigid in its structural arrangement. The enhanced fluidity of neuronal membranes produced by ethanol may alter such events as (1) ion fluxes across the membrane, (2) conformational changes in enzymes, or (3) neurotransmitter mechanisms.

It is reported that some behavioral effects of ethanol are attributed to an enhancement of chloride ion influx, resulting in hyperpolarization of membranes. In neuronal membranes this stimulated influx of chloride ions occurs through the chloride ionophore, a macromolecular complex that contains receptors for gamma aminobutyric acid (GABA), benzodiazepines, and barbiturates. It appears that ethanol modifies the microenvironment of the postsynaptic $GABA_A$ receptor-mediated chloride ion channel to augment the influx of chloride ions. Although chloride ions have been implicated in some of the behavioral actions of ethanol, this chloride ion proposal does not explain fully the pharmacologic effects of ethanol. Ethanol also alters the fluxes of other ions such as sodium and calcium. In addition, a variety of neurotransmitters such as norepinephrine, dopamine, and GABA are affected by the administration of ethanol.

When ethanol is administered in repeated doses over a period of time, it has been shown that the drug induces less alteration of membrane fluidity as compared with single-dose administration of it. This adaptation of the components of membranes to repeated exposure of ethanol may play a role in the phenomena of tolerance and physical dependence that are associated with ethanol.

The various actions of ethanol occur in a complex manner, and further research is required before a more definitive statement can be made about a detailed mechanism for the action of ethanol.

Pharmacokinetics

Upon oral administration ethanol is initially absorbed in the stomach, but the major portion of the drug is absorbed in the small intestine. This neutral, low-molecular-weight compound is transported across membranes by simple diffusion. The absence of food in the stomach and increasing the concentration of ethanol up to 40% enhance the rate of ethanol absorption. High concentration of ethanol (40% or greater) can produce gastric irritation, pylorospasm, and gastric mucous secretion, which tend to impede the absorption of ethanol from the gastrointestinal tract.

Ethanol is widely distributed in the body according to the water content of tissues. The rate of ethanol accumulation in the various tissues depends on the blood supply to them. As blood level of ethanol increases, ethanol tissue concentrations build up quite readily in the brain but more slowly in skeletal muscle and adipose tissue. At equilibrium the exhaled air from the lungs contains 0.05% of the ethanol concentration that is present in the blood. Therefore, the analysis of expired air serves as a method for the determination of the concentration of ethanol in the blood.

Over 90 percent of ethanol is biotransformed, primarily in the liver. The remainder is eliminated unchanged in the urine, exhaled air, sweat, and saliva. For humans the average rate at which this occurs is 100 (mg/kg/h) and is reflected as a corresponding fall in blood ethanol in the body. In other words, a 150-lb person can eliminate 7 g (9 mL) of absolute ethanol or about 2/3 oz of 100-proof whisky every hour. For each gram of ethanol biotransformed, 7 kcal is made available to the body.

The biotransformation of ethanol may be divided into three stages, which take place concurrently (Fig. 17-1).

Stage I During this stage, ethanol is oxidized to acetaldehyde by alcohol dehydrogenase, with nicotinamide adenine dinucleotide (NAD^+) acting as the immediate hydrogen acceptor. Alcohol dehydrogenase, a zinc-containing enzyme, is present in the liver to a large extent, and smaller concentrations are found in the gastrointestinal tract and kidney. Stage I occurs almost exclusively in the liver. The rate at which alcohol is changed to acetaldehyde is constant, and it essentially follows zero-order kinetics. It appears that the velocity of the reaction and therefore the ethanol elimination rate are primarily dependent on the concentration of NADH and the total enzyme activity of alcohol dehydrogenase.

Stage I $CH_3—CH_2OH + NAD^+ \xrightarrow[\text{dehydrogenase}]{\text{alcohol}}$

$CH_3—CHO + NADH + H^-$

Stage II $CH_3CHO + H_2O \xrightarrow[\text{dehydrogenase}]{\text{aldehyde}} CH_3—COOH + (2H)$

Stage III $CH_3—COOH + 4(O) \longrightarrow 2CO_2 + 2H_2O$

FIGURE 17-1   Biotransformation of ethanol by the alcohol dehydrogenase pathway.

Stage II   In this step the acetaldehyde is oxidized to acetic acid and the latter buffered to form acetate. The enzyme responsible for the oxidation of acetaldehyde to acetate is a mitochondrial aldehyde dehydrogenase, and the hydrogen acceptor is NAD^+. Stage II is a very rapid reaction, so that only small traces of acetaldehyde appear in the blood, even after excessive consumption of alcohol.

Stage III   The acetate formed in stage II increases the body's pool of acetate, which is finally oxidized to CO_2 and H_2O. The actual reaction is much more complicated, and most of the acetate probably goes through the Krebs cycle. The CO_2 formed then enters the body's pool of bicarbonate, almost all of which finally exists as pulmonary CO_2.

Two other biotransformation systems have been implicated in the oxidation of ethanol to acetaldehyde (Fig. 17-2). They are the hepatic microsomal ethanol oxidizing system (MEOS) and the catalase system. The MEOS requires NADPH-cytochrome P-450 reductase, cytochrome P-450, molecular oxygen, and phospholipids. The catalase system, which is also present in the liver, requires the availability of hydrogen peroxide. Although the major pathway for oxidation of ethanol to acetaldehyde is by alcohol dehydrogenase, under normal conditions the MEOS seems to participate in the oxidation of ethanol when high blood levels are present in the body and during chronic consumption of ethanol. The increased rate of ethanol biotransformation that is observed during chronic use of ethanol is believed to be due to enhanced activity of the MEOS. The catalase system probably has little or no significant role in the biotransformation of ethanol in the body.

Pharmacodynamics

The main effect of ethanol is depression of the central nervous system. This depressant effect begins with the higher functions and later extends to the lower centers of the brain as the concentration of ethanol in the central nervous system increases. The reticular activating system is most sensitive to the depressant action of ethanol. The common misconception that ethanol is a stimulant is due to its effect to lessen inhibitory influences in other areas of the brain, particularly the cor-

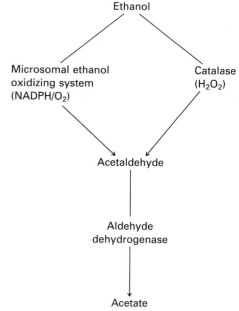

FIGURE 17-2   Alternate pathways for the oxidation of ethanol to acetaldehyde.

tex, by suppression of the integration function of the reticular activating system. Some important effects of ethanol on the central nervous system are as follows:

1. *Euphoria*   Drinkers see the world and themselves through rose-colored glasses. The desire to secure this effect is the chief reason for the popularity of alcoholic beverages, except for those who use these beverages sparingly as a condiment. Euphoria usually begins at levels of blood ethanol below those causing definite muscular incoordination.

2. *Removal of inhibitions*   Ethanol, even in rather small amounts, causes loss of inhibitions, and the individual responds to many impulses which are ordinarily repressed. The resultant behavior may consist of silly speech and harmless antics, but sometimes becomes vicious and antisocial.

3. *Impairment of vision*   Ethanol reduces visual acuity. The ethanol in two or three cocktails may cause a reduction in visual acuity of more than 50 percent. Diplopia may occur if the blood ethanol concentration reaches 200 to 300 mg per 100 mL.

4. *Muscular incoordination*   Small doses of ethanol impair the ability of the brain to coordinate muscular activity. With high concentrations of ethanol in the body, the manifestations of muscular incoordination are slurred speech and staggering gait, the complete loss of the power of speech and locomotion, and finally coma and general anesthesia.

5. *Lengthened reaction time*   The mean normal reaction time is around 0.29 s to light and 0.19 s to sound. Blood ethanol concentrations below 100 mg per 100 mL have very little effect on reaction time. Levels between 100 and 200 mg per 100 mL usually lengthen the reaction time from 10 to 50 percent.

In the posterior pituitary, ethanol produces depression, and this results in a reduction in the release of antidiuretic hormone. As a consequence of the suppression of antidiuretic hormone, less water is reabsorbed from the collecting duct of the nephron of the kidney and diuresis ensues. This diuretic effect occurs primarily as blood ethanol concentrations are increasing. Another area of the brain that is affected by ethanol is the hypothalamus. Higher concentration of ethanol (greater than 1 g/kg) can induce hypothermia, and this effect is enhanced when the environmental temperature is low. In addition, when blood ethanol concentrations are increasing, depression of the vasomo-

tor center and the respiratory center leads to a decrease in blood pressure and a suppression of respiration. The lethal effect of ethanol is attributed to respiratory depression.

Ethanol exerts effects on the gastrointestinal tract and liver. In the gastrointestinal tract ethanol increases in gastric acid secretion; however, when concentrations of ethanol are greater than 20%, there is a reduction in gastric acid and pepsin secretion. Ethanol also enhances salivary secretion. In the liver, following ethanol ingestion, high concentrations of ethanol reach the liver via the portal vein, and since the liver bears the brunt of oxidizing ethanol to acetaldehyde, it is apparent that ethanol may eventually produce hepatic dysfunction. In the chronic abuse of ethanol, the hepatic cirrhosis that can develop is due to prolonged high intake of ethanol rather than to the associated dietary deficiencies, and therefore ethanol has a direct hepatotoxic action.

Adverse Reactions

Acute   There is a direct correlation between the concentration of ethanol in the blood and pharmacologic effects leading to impairment. One type of impairment, frank intoxication, exhibits the common signs of drunkenness, including slurred speech, difficulty of locomotion, and obvious loss of inhibitions. The results of several studies have been summarized as follows: For six zones of blood ethanol concentration (expressed in milligrams per 100 mL), the average percentage of subjects judged to be intoxicated were 0 to 50, 10 percent; 51 to 100, 34 percent; 101 to 150, 64 percent; 151 to 200, 86 percent; 201 to 250, 96 percent; and 251 to 300, 99 percent. These studies agree that almost all subjects with blood alcohol levels above 200 mg per 100 mL were definitely drunk. The blood ethanol level to be considered intoxicated for operating a motor vehicle from a legal standpoint is 100 mg per 100 mL.

The symptoms of severe, acute toxicity are much like those of an overdose of any general CNS-depressant drug, with shallow respiration and some impairment of circulation. The face and body surface are pale, and the extremities are cold. Depression of the respiratory and vasomotor centers is observed at 350 mg per 100 mL of ethanol. Although deaths have been reported at this blood ethanol concentration, it is uncommon. Greater suppression of the respiratory, cardiac, and vasomotor centers occurs when the blood ethanol concentration increases to 550 mg per 100 mL. Acidosis, hypoglycemia, and elevated intracranial pressure are noted. The patient may be in a stupor or coma at this point, and if not treated, death can occur. Death is due to respiratory failure. Chief postmortem findings are hyperemia of the stomach mucosa and edema at the base of the brain.

No specific treatment for severe acute intoxication has been found. Treatment is symptomatic, such as the administration of pressor amines, glucose, or mannitol, and the correction of metabolic acidosis by sodium bicarbonate. If the patient can be kept alive and hypoxia avoided, he or she will usually recover as the absorbed ethanol is biotransformed.

The consumption of ethanol in a very cold environment, which can induce hypothermia, is dangerous under certain circumstances. Ingestion of moderate quantities causes dilation of skin blood vessels, with flushing of the face, neck, and upper trunk area. This effect prevents normal cutaneous vasoconstriction on exposure to cold, so that intoxication hastens the fatal outcome in "freezing to death." Central vasomotor depression probably plays a role in the production of this vasodilatation.

Chronic   Alcoholism presents a serious medical, social, and economic problem. At present there is no scientific explanation for the fact that some persons continue excessive drinking to the point where their lives become "utterly unmanageable," to quote a phrase from Alcoholics Anonymous.

The alcoholic cannot refrain from excessive drinking and is distressed and upset without the euphoria produced by alcohol in his or her system. Some chronic alcoholics often do not drink to the point of marked intoxication; others are quite drunk most of the time. The outstanding symptom is an intense craving for alcohol, the desire to drink being about the only interest in life. There are, of course, varying gradations of the affliction.

Chronic consumption of ethanol produces tolerance and physical dependence. The degree and severity of the withdrawal syndrome that occurs upon abrupt discontinuation of ethanol drinking depends on the amount of ethanol ingested and the duration of time that the ethanol was used. On termination of ethanol consumption, the individual can have *acute alcoholic*

hallucinosis. These hallucinations can be auditory, visual, tactile, or olfactory in their manifestation. In most severe cases of physical dependence, *delirium tremens* occurs. Delirium tremens usually occurs as a sequel to heavy, excessive drinking over a period of 2 to 6 weeks. The initial symptoms are restlessness, insomnia, tremor, fear, perspiration, and headache. This is followed by the second stage, which is characterized by hallucinations and delirium. The hallucinations are predominantly visual but may be tactile and auditory; they generally involve great fear. Alcoholics call the first stage the "shakes" and the second stage the "horrors." Convulsions sometimes occur. The delirium usually lasts 3 or 4 days. The reported mortality in delirium tremens varies from 10 to 15 percent. Management of delirium tremens may involve the use of benzodiazepines such as diazepam and chlordiazepoxide.

Other chronic effects from ethanol abuse include morning nausea and vomiting, gastritis, ulceration of the gastrointestinal tract, pancreatitis, cardiomeglia, alcoholic hepatitis, and cirrhosis of the liver. Ethanol may alter male fertility by reducing serum testosterone levels and decreasing sperm motility. *Alcoholic polyneuropathy*, which is associated with numbness, pain, and muscle wasting in the legs, may be produced. *Wernicke encephalopathy* is the result of excessive ethanol use and a deficiency of thiamine. This disorder is characterized by ocular abnormalities, e.g., nystagmus, ataxia, and mental confusion.

Korsakoff's syndrome appears in a few alcoholics, the incidence of this disorder being about one-tenth that of delirium tremens. The chief signs of Korsakoff's syndrome are impairment of memory of recent events, lessened learning ability, disorientation in space and time, and polyneuritis involving pain in the extremities and partial or total paralysis of the arms and legs. The polyneuritis appears to be due to a marked deficiency of vitamin B_1 (thiamine).

The daily consumption of ethanol during pregnancy increases the risk of birth defects. As little as 1 oz of ethanol (two drinks), but definitely 3 oz (six drinks) or more a day is associated with a significant incidence of congenital anomalies which are referred to as the *fetal alcohol syndrome* (FAS). The neonate may exhibit such signs as growth deficiency, developmental delay or mental retardation, craniofacial abnormalities, and structural anomalies of the heart and genitals. Complete safety from the threat of FAS can be assured only by abstinence from ethanol during the entire pregnancy.

Some cases of chronic alcoholism, both psychotic and nonpsychotic, terminate fatally in a few months or years. However, many chronic alcoholics have a fairly normal life expectancy, aside from being bad safety risks. Chronic alcoholics have a serious illness and should be treated as such.

Drug Interactions

Since ethanol causes central nervous system depression and can influence the drug-metabolizing microsomal system (DMMS), various drugs, when taken in combination with ethanol, may produce altered therapeutic responses or adverse reactions in the patient. Acute ethanol administration increases the central depressant properties of barbiturates, benzodiazepines, H_1-antihistamines with sedative effects, and narcotic analgesics. This effect is due to the fact that these drugs and ethanol depress the central nervous system and their combined effect is additive. Ethanol can have an additive effect on the adverse reaction of sedation that is associated with phenothiazines and tricyclic antidepressants, particularly those antidepressants with significant sedative properties, e.g., amitriptyline and doxepin. Also acute ethanol consumption may inhibit the microsomal biotransformation of these drugs listed above and thus enhance their effects, particularly on the central nervous system. Chronic ethanol administration, however, induces the microsomal system and may accelerate drug metabolism, thereby possibly attenuating their pharmacologic action.

Chronic ingestion of ethanol can enhance the hepatotoxic effect of acetaminophen, particularly when acetaminophen is taken in large doses or in an overdose situation. It appears that ethanol increases the formation of metabolites that are toxic to the liver, e.g., N-acetyl-p-benzoquinone. Aspirin and related drugs (NSAID) may exhibit a greater tendency to cause gastrointestinal bleeding in the presence of ethanol. These analgesics and ethanol can adversely affect the gastric mucosal barrier. Ethanol can also enhance bleeding time. Cimetidine may increase the intoxication of ethanol by inhibiting ethanol's biotransformation and possibly enhancing its absorption from the gastrointestinal tract. The greater degree of central nervous system depression that is noted with chloral

hydrate and ethanol appears to be related to a reduction in the biotransformation of ethanol and an increased rate of metabolism of chloral hydrate to trichloroethanol, which is the active component of chloral hydrate. Ethanol can increase or decrease the prothrombin time of a patient who is receiving anticoagulants. Other drug interactions with ethanol are listed in Table 17-1.

Several drugs appear to interfere with the oxidation of ethanol and increase the blood levels of acetaldehyde which produces a disulfiram-like reaction in the patient (see Disulfiram). This reaction is associated with such symptoms as sweating, vomiting, weakness, and tachycardia. Some drugs that may produce a disulfiram-like reaction, are listed in Table 17-2. Since the drugs that are capable of interaction with ethanol are so numerous, it is reasonable to suggest that when patients are on any medication they should refrain from the consumption of ethanol.

Clinical Uses

Ethanol is used as an antiseptic in solutions of 50 to 95%. A 70% solution is generally considered the optimum concentration for penetration and denaturation of bacterial protein. Ethanol evaporates readily from

TABLE 17-1 Some drug interaction with ethanol

Drug	Reaction
Chlorpropamide	Facial flushing
Cyclobenzapine	Enhanced CNS depression
Glutethimide	Increased blood ethanol levels
Nitrates	Enhanced hypotensive effect
Nitrtates (IV preparations)	Ethanol content may cause CNS and cardiac depression
Phenytoin	Decreased phenytoin serum levels
Oral hypoglycemic agents (sulfonylureas)	Risk of hypoglycemia

TABLE 17-2   Drugs which cause a disulfiram-like reaction in the presence of ethanol

Acetohexamide	Chlorampheicol	Phentolamine
Cefoperazine	Griseofulvin	Procarbazine
Cephamandole	Metronidazole	Tolazamide
Cetriaxone	Moxalactam	Tolbutamide

the skin, producing a cooling effect. It lowers surface tension and is also a good solvent for many substances on the skin. Sponge baths with ethanol or isopropyl alcohol are sometimes useful for cleansing and as an aid in reducing fevers.

The use of alcohol to dilate coronary vessels and for treating peripheral vascular diseases is unreliable. However, alcoholic drinks may be of benefit to patients with cardiac disease in that the mild sedation permits rest and relaxation.

Ethanol is used as an antidote in methanol and ethylene glycol poisoning. These uses of ethanol are discussed later in the chapter.

Ethanol and hydroalcoholic solutions are excellent solvents and preservatives for many drugs.

DISULFIRAM

Many physicians refer their alcoholic patients to Alcoholics Anonymous. However, sometimes disulfiram (Antabuse) is employed to bolster sobriety by the production of unpleasant symptoms.

$$C_2H_5 \quad\quad\quad\quad\quad\quad C_2H_5$$
$$N-C-S-S-C-N$$
$$\quad\quad \underset{S}{\|} \quad\quad \underset{S}{\|}$$
$$C_2H_5 \quad\quad\quad\quad\quad\quad C_2H_5$$
Disulfiram

When taken by itself in small doses, disulfiram produces no apparent pharmacologic effects. If, however, after several days of such medication, small amounts of alcohol are imbibed, a toxic reaction follows, which persists as long as the alcohol is being metabolized. Roughly in order of their appearance, the symptoms

and signs are a cutaneous sensation of heat, flushing, vasodilatation, hypotension, palpitation, increased heart rate, dizziness, vomiting, unconsciousness, and collapse. The magnitude of these symptoms is subject to individual variation and is proportional to the dosage of both disulfiram and alcohol. In some patients only discomfort has been observed; in a few instances death has occurred.

The mechanism by which disulfiram produces this unpleasant reaction or the "acetaldehyde syndrome," as it is sometimes called, is due to interference with the oxidation of ethanol. Disulfiram irreversibly inhibits the enzyme aldehyde dehydrogenase by binding to sulfhydryl groups of the enzyme and also chelating zinc, which is present in the enzyme. In addition disulfiram is biotransformed to diethyldithiocarbamic acid, which also inhibits aldehyde dehydrogenase. As a result of the inhibition of aldehyde dehydrogenase, the blood acetaldehyde level can be 5 to 10 times higher than with the consumption of ethanol in the absence of disulfiram.

The drug is adequately absorbed (80 percent) from the gastrointestinal tract and achieves a peak plasma concentration within 1 to 2 h. The drug is widely distributed in the body because of its lipid solubility; however, only small concentrations of the drug are present in the brain. Disulfiram is reduced in the body to diethyldithiocarbamic acid. In addition, this metabolite undergoes several other reactions such as methylation, oxidation, and conjugation with glucuronic acid.

Disulfiram is contraindicated in patients with a history of severe myocardial disease or coronary occlusion, psychosis, or hypersensitivity reaction to disulfiram. This drug should be used only in selected patients to bolster their determination not to drink and should be accompanied by good psychiatric and medical treatment. Disulfiram (Antabuse) is available as tablets which contain either 250 or 500 mg.

METHANOL

Methanol is a simple compound with the following chemical structure: CH_3—OH. This aliphatic alcohol is also known as methyl alcohol, wood spirit, and wood alcohol. It is used mainly as an industrial solvent and is found also in such products as paint thinner, solid canned heat, gasoline (as an additive), and paint remover. Methanol poisoning can result from industrial exposure and accidental or intentional ingestion of products containing it.

After oral ingestion of methanol, the compound is readily absorbed from the gastrointestinal tract and distributed in the body. Methanol is oxidized by the alcohol dehydrogenase system, the same pathway that biotransforms ethanol. The oxidation of methanol follows zero-order kinetics, but the rate of disappearance of methanol from the blood occurs at a much slower rate than that of ethanol elimination (about one-seventh). Methanol is biotransformed to formaldehyde and formic acid. The metabolite, formic acid, appears to be responsible for the blindness that is associated with methanol ingestion. The possibility of blindness is enhanced in the presence of acidosis. It has been suggested that some of the methanol may be metabolized by the catalase system. If the catalase system does play a role in the oxidation of methanol, it is probably a minor component when compared with the alcohol dehydrogenase system.

The symptoms of methanol poisoning include initial visual disturbances, which may lead to partial or complete blindness due to damage of retinal cells and degeneration of the optic nerve by the metabolites of methanol. Central nervous system depression occurs along with nausea, vomiting, slowed respiration, bradycardia, and coma.

Therapeutic measures that are taken to treat methanol toxicities can include (1) correction of acidosis, (2) maintenance of respiration, (3) monitoring of electrolytes and providing nutrition, and (4) administration of ethanol. Ethanol is given to the patient to reduce the rate of methanol metabolism. Ethanol competes with methanol for alcohol dehydrogenase and, therefore, decreases the formation of formaldehyde and formic acid. In serious methanol poisoning, hemodialysis is also employed. Another antidote that has been proposed for the treatment of methanol poisoning is 4-methylpyrazole. This compound is an inhibitor of alcohol dehydrogenase and prevents the formation of the toxic metabolite of methanol.

ETHYLENE GLYCOL

Ethylene glycol (CH_2—OH—CH_2—OH) is a dihydroxyalcohol. This agent is found in antifreeze solutions and as an industrial solvent for plastics and paints. Ethylene glycol is discussed in this chapter because of the toxicities that can occur upon accidental or intentional ingestion.

In the body ethylene glycol is first oxidized by alcohol dehydrogenase and then further metabolized to oxalic acid and other products (glycolic and formic acids). Calcium oxalate crystals that are formed, deposit in a variety of tissues, particularly the kidney, where they are nephrotoxic. Oxalate crystals also appear in the urine.

The symptoms of ethylene glycol poisoning may be central nervous system depression, convulsions, acidosis, renal damage, and respiratory failure. Management of ethylene glycol intoxication can include (1) gastric lavage, (2) maintenance of airway, (3) maintenance of body temperature (4) vigorous diuresis, (5) correction of acidosis, (6) hemodialysis, and (7) administration of ethanol. Ethanol will slow the biotransformation of ethylene glycol and reduce the formation of toxic metabolites. Another compound that has been suggested for the treatment of ethylene glycol intoxication is 4-methylpyrazole. This antidote reduces the biotransformation of ethylene glycol into oxalate by inhibition of the enzyme alcohol dehydrogenase, which is the first step in its biotransformation.

ISOPROPYL ALCOHOL

Isopropyl alcohol (isopropanol, 2-propanol) is widely available as a rubbing alcohol (a 70% solution), an antiseptic, and a topical agent to reduce fever. It readily evaporates from the skin and lowers elevated body temperature. This alcohol, however, is probably a better antibacterial agent than ethanol.

Isopropyl alcohol is about twice as potent as a central nervous system depressant when compared with ethanol. It is slowly biotransformed in body, possibly by alcohol dehydrogenase to acetone, which also possesses depressant properties. The half-life of isopropyl alcohol is 2.5 to 3 h.

Isopropyl alcohol produces toxicities when it is intentionally or accidentally ingested or inhaled. Toxicities of isopropyl alcohol can include nausea, vomiting, dizziness, central nervous system depression, coma, and respiratory depression. Treatment of isopropyl alcohol poisoning consists of supportive measures to maintain vital functions and hemodialysis.

BIBLIOGRAPHY

Becker, C. E.: "Methanol Poisoning," *J. Emerg. Med.*, **2**:47–49 (1983).

Bloom, F. E., and G. R. Siggins: "Electrophysiological Action of Ethanol at the Cellular Level," *Alcohol*, **4**:331–337 (1987).

Chin, J. H., and D. B. Goldstein: "Effects of Low Concentrations of Ethanol on the Fluidity of Spin-Labeled Erythrocytes and Brain Membranes," *Mol. Pharmacol.*, **13**:435–441 (1977).

Chin, J. H., and D. B. Goldstein: "Membrane-Disordering Action of Ethanol," *Mol. Pharmacol.*, **19**:425–431 (1981).

Crabb, D. W., W. F., Bosron, and T. K. Li: "Ethanol Metabolism," *Pharmacol. Ther.*, **34**:59–73 (1987).

Berglund, M.: "Alcoholics Committed to Treatment: A Prospective Long-Term Study of Behavioral Characteristics, Mortality, and Social Adjustment," *Alcohol Clin. Exp. Res.*, **12**:19–24 (1988).

deWit, H., E. H. Whlenhuth, J. Pierri, and C. E. Johanson: "Individual Differences in Behavioral and Subjective Responses to Alcohol," *Alcohol Clin. Exp. Res.*, **11**:52–59 (1987).

Ferko, A. P.: "Present Status of Disulfiran," *Am. Family Physician*, **28**:183–185 (1983).

Hartung, G. H., J. P. Foreyt, R. E. Metchell, J. E. Mitchell, R. S. Reeves, and A. B. Gotto: "Effect of Alcohol Intake on High-Density Lipoproteins in Runners and Inactive Men, *J.A.M.A.*, **24**:747–750 (1983).

Mattucci-Schiavone, L., and A. P. Ferko "Effect of Muscimol on Ethanol-Induced Central Nervous System Depression," *Pharmacol. Biochem. Behav.*, **27**:745–748 (1987).

Suzdak, P. D., and S. M. Paul: "Ethanol Stimulated GABA Receptor-Mediated Cl^- Ion Flux *in vitro:* "Possible Relationship to Anxiolytic and Intoxicating Actions of Alcohol," *Psychopharmacol. Bull.*, **23**:445–451 (1987).

Sullivan, J. T., and E. M. Sellers: Treating Alcohol, Barbiturate and Benzodiazepine Withdrawal," *Rational Drug Ther.*, **20**:1–4, (1986).

Psychotomimetic Drugs

Henry W. Hitner

The nonmedical use of psychoactive substances has increased significantly in recent years. Psychotomimetic drugs possess the ability to induce psychic and behavioral patterns which are characteristic of psychosis. At one time, lysergic acid diethylamide (LSD) and other psychotomimetic drugs were investigated for the treatment of alcoholism, drug addiction, and mental illness. Currently, these drugs have no therapeutic indications and are classified as schedule 1 drugs under the Controlled Substance Act. Psychotomimetic drugs are also referred to as *hallucinogens* and are abused "recreationally." The novel sensory and hallucinogenic effects produced by these drugs are claimed to provide "mind expansion" where universal understanding and creativity are enhanced. Use of LSD-type hallucinogens has decreased; however, abuse of other psychoactive drugs such as phencyclidine, amphetamine, cocaine, and marijuana are causing significant health and social problems.

CLASSIFICATION OF PSYCHOTOMIMETIC SUBSTANCES

The psychotomimetic drugs do not form a distinct drug class. Current classification is based on psychopharmacologic drug profiles and the ability of some drugs to display cross-tolerance.

Psychotomimetic drugs can be divided into three general groups. Cross-tolerance exists between the drugs usually identified as hallucinogenic: LSD, psilocybin, *N,N*-dimethyltryptamine (DMT), mescaline,

and 2,5-dimethoxy-4-methylamphetamine (DOM). Results of receptor binding studies confirm that these drugs act on a specific serotonin receptor subtype. Consequently, they appear to share a common mechanism of action and constitute one group, the *LSD-type hallucinogens*. The second group is composed of centrally acting *anticholinergic drugs* such as atropine and scopolamine. The *miscellaneous psychotomimetics* are a diverse group of drugs, which include phencyclidine, the psychomotor stimulants (amphetamine, cocaine), and marijuana. These drugs do not share cross-tolerance with the LSD-type drugs and produce psychic effects qualitatively different from each other and from the other two groups.

LSD-TYPE HALLUCINOGENS

The grouping of these drugs is based on common pharmacologic properties, which include mechanism of action, psychotomimetic effects, and development of tolerance and cross-tolerance. The prototype of this group is LSD; therefore, it is discussed in detail, and the others will be described in relation to it. Structurally, LSD, psilocybin, and DMT all possess a tryptamine nucleus, which is also found in the centrally acting neurotransmitter serotonin (5-hydroxy-tryptamine or 5-HT). The structure of LSD is shown in Fig. 18-1, the broken line indicating the tryptamine structure within the LSD molecule.

Although mescaline and DOM do not possess the tryptamine structure and are derivatives of the β-

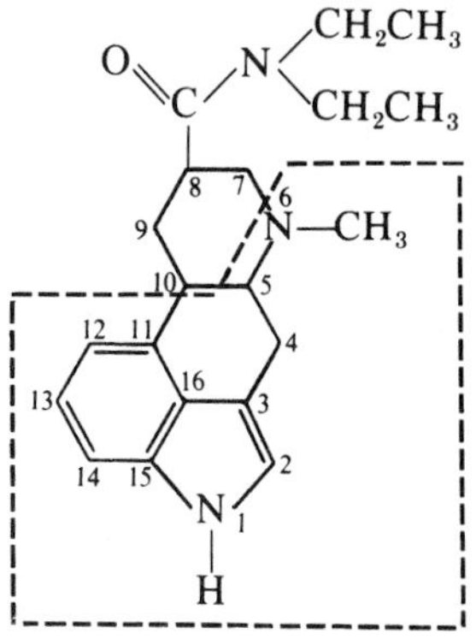

LSD

FIGURE 18-1   Lysergic acid diethylamide (LSD).

phenethylamines (catechol structure), this does not appear to produce significant differences in the psychotomimetic actions of these drugs.

Mechanism of Action

How LSD produces its effects is not exactly known. Early theories emphasized the CNS interactions of LSD with catecholamines and serotonin (5-HT) neurotransmitters. Structural similarities of LSD to 5-HT and the finding that LSD was a potent antagonist of the peripheral actions of 5-HT suggested that the psychic effects of LSD might be related to antagonism of 5-HT within the CNS. Subsequent investigations revealed that the peripheral and central interactions of LSD with 5-HT differed. In the CNS, LSD suppressed the activity of serotonergic neurons—a presynaptic effect. Additional experiments showed, however, that the effects of LSD persisted and were even enhanced after destruction of serotonergic neurons. This suggested that the site of action of LSD for psychotomimetic effects was postsynaptic.

Recent receptor binding studies show that LSD displays high-affinity binding to a specific subtype of serotonin receptor found in the brain, the 5-HT$_2$ receptor, where LSD acts as an *agonist* on both excitatory and inhibitory receptors.

The psychic effects of LSD have been shown to be decreased after prolonged pretreatment with monoamine oxidase inhibitors (MAOIs increase 5-HT levels). Pretreatment with MAOIs reduces the number of postsynaptic serotonin receptors ("down regulation"

due to elevated 5-HT levels) and, consequently, the availability of the proposed site of action of LSD—the 5-HT$_2$ receptor. This finding adds support to the hypothesis that LSD is acting on postsynaptic serotonin receptors.

Numerous serotonergic pathways originate in the brain stem and project to all major areas of the brain. The agonist actions of LSD on 5-HT$_2$ receptors are thought to trigger a series of neuronal actions involving other neurotransmitter systems (especially noradrenergic and dopaminergic), which then by some yet unexplained mechanism contribute to the psychotomimetic syndrome. The other drugs of this group—psilocybin, DMT, mescaline, and DOM—have also been shown to bind to 5-HT$_2$ receptors.

Psychotomimetic Syndrome

Following administration of LSD and similar hallucinogens, a common sequence of dose-related effects occur. They have been divided into three phases: (1) the *somatic phase* occurs initially after absorption and consists of CNS stimulation and autonomic changes which are predominantly sympathomimetic in nature; (2) the *sensory phase* is characterized by sensory distortions and pseudohallucinations, which are the effects desired by the drug user; and (3) the *psychic phase* signals a maximum drug effect where disruption of thought processes, depersonalization, true hallucinations, and psychotic episodes may occur. Experiencing the latter phase would be considered a "bad trip."

Pharmacokinetics of LSD

After oral administration, LSD is readily absorbed from the gastrointestinal tract and widely distributed throughout the body. The average hallucinogenic dosage ranges from 50 to 100 μg with only about 0.01 percent reaching the brain. Since we assume the significant actions of LSD take place within the brain, this makes its potency all the more impressive. The psychic effects of LSD usually last about 12 h, with peak effects occurring 1 to 2 h after oral administration. The half-life of LSD is approximately 3 h.

LSD is metabolized in the liver by hydroxylation, with subsequent conjugation to glucuronide. Excretion is primarily through the biliary tract into the intestinal tract (80 to 90 percent), with the remainder eliminated by urinary excretion.

Pharmacodynamics of LSD

LSD is a very potent stimulant of the central nervous system; individuals remain sleepless for many hours after ingesting it. The earliest and longest-lasting effect, occurring even with very small doses, is pupillary dilation. Pupillary inequality (anisocoria) is common, as is hippus, a rhythmic dilation and contraction of the pupils, often synchronous with respiration. Hyperreflexia, also occurring uniformly, is another evidence of overstimulation of the nervous system. This may progress to spontaneous clonus of the antigravity muscles, especially the quadriceps group. Masseter hyperreflexia causes feelings of tightness of the jaw which, however, does not progress to actual trismus. Waves of piloerection often occur. The pupillary and hyperreflexic effects are inversely correlated with age, being greater in young adults and lesser in older subjects. Increases in body temperature are sometimes encountered but are not very great. Even without fever, the subjects feel hot and look flushed.

Sialorrhea, nausea, and vomiting are common gastrointestinal effects. Subjects may feel unusually hungry but be unable to eat much. Hypermotility of the gastrointestinal tract is frequently present.

Cardiovascular effects include tachycardia and a moderate increase in blood pressure. These may be secondary to the general state of excitement rather than direct effects of the compound. LSD does not affect cerebral circulation significantly.

LSD is believed to have the potential to cause both mutagenic and teratogenic effects. Reports of chromosomal damage and birth defects involving limb deformities and spina bifida have yet to be adequately investigated.

Sensory and Subjective Effects of LSD

Along with the overexcitation and hyperreflexia described above, sensory distortions occur regularly. A sense of variation in lighting progresses to vivid visual illusions, pseudohallucinations, and, after sufficiently large doses, true hallucinations. Typically, the visual images are of vividly colored geometric patterns, often moving kaleidoscopically, or of halos or rainbows around lights. Often, any moving object seems to be followed by a stream of color. True auditory hallucinations are extremely rare, although illusions, distortions, and synesthesias occur. Bizarre paresthesias and

distorted proprioception are frequent, ranging from formications to sensations of walking on a pebbly or hot surface.

Distortions in perceptions of size and distance and other spacial distortions are very common and are often associated with distortions of body image. Feelings of separation of part of the body, or loss of a part, or failure to recognize a part as one's own are also common. Sometimes a subject may feel quite small, and cower in the middle of a bed, terrified of falling off and being killed. In others, perceptions of other people may be altered so that they look horrid and threatening.

LSD possesses a unique pharmacologic property known as flashbacks. This phenomenon, which can occur at any time (months to years) after single or multiple exposures to LSD, is characterized by many of the sensory and subjective effects of LSD without readministration of the drug. Flashbacks often occur after the use of other psychoactive drugs, which may somehow trigger the flashback episode.

Tolerance and Physical Dependence

Tolerance develops rapidly to the psychotomimetic effects of LSD, usually within 3 or 4 days of daily use. Also, cross-tolerance exists between LSD and the other drugs of this group so that subsequent doses of one drug taken shortly after another drug will produce decreased effects. The tolerance is not accompanied by physical dependence, and abrupt discontinuance after chronic use does not precipitate withdrawal symptoms.

Intoxication and Treatment

The signs and symptoms of LSD intoxication include elevated body temperature and blood pressure, tachycardia, hyperreflexia, dilated pupils, anxiety, hallucinations, and psychotic behavior. LSD has a high therapeutic index and virtually no known cases of death have been related to overdose toxicity by LSD alone. Consequently, treatment is aimed at protecting the patient from accidental injury until drug effects subside. The individual should be placed in a quiet, nonthreatening environment and given reassurance that everything will be all right. Benzodiazepine antianxiety agents or barbiturates can be used for their sedative effects. Phenothiazine antipsychotic drugs are pharmacologic antagonists of LSD but may cause additional undesirable effects and are generally avoided. These drugs are indicated when individuals are uncontrollable. This approach to treatment is considered standard therapy for most hallucinogenic drug intoxication.

Other LSD-Type Hallucinogens

Tryptamine Derivatives Psilocybin and *N,N*-dimethyltriptamine are obtained from natural sources. Psilocybin is found in a variety of *Psilocybe* mushroom species, which have been eaten ceremonially by primitive cultures for centuries. Psilocybin is converted to an active metabolite, psilocin, which is believed to be responsible for the majority of psychotomimetic effects. The hallucinogenic dose of psilocybin is approximately 25 mg, which produces effects lasting 3 to 6 h.

DMT occurs in many plants and has been used as a snuff by various Indian cultures. It is ineffective when taken orally and must be inhaled or administered parenterally. The usual hallucinogenic dose given by injection is 1 mg/kg of body weight, which produces psychotomimetic effects lasting approximately 1 h.

β-Phenethylamine Derivatives Mescaline and 2,5-dimethoxy-4-methylamphetamine are phenethylamine derivatives similar in structure to norepinephrine and amphetamine. CNS stimulation and sympathomimetic effects are prominent features of both drugs. Mescaline, found in the peyote cactus, is among the least potent of the hallucinogenic drugs. It

is readily absorbed from the gastrointestinal tract and produces effects which last about 6 h. Humans excrete about 58 percent of mescaline unchanged. The remainder is mostly oxidized to 3,4,5-trimethoxyphenylacetic acid, which is inactive.

DOM or STP (serenity, tranquility, peace) is a synthetic compound. The usual hallucinogenic dose is 3 to 5 mg, which produces effects lasting 6 to 8 h. The chemical structures of mescaline and DOM are compared to norepinephrine and amphetamine in Fig. 18-2.

ANTICHOLINERGIC PSYCHOTOMIMETIC DRUGS

The prototypes of this group are atropine and scopolamine. Their basic pharmacology is given in Chap. 10. At present, the most plausible explanation for the actions of these compounds is that by blocking cholinergic mechanisms in the brain, they allow predominance of other neurotransmitter systems, most likely adrenergic, dopaminergic, and serotonergic. The anticholinergic drugs are not widely abused, and psychic effects can occur when these drugs are used therapeutically.

The peripheral effects of anticholinergic psychotomimetics resemble those of the parent compound atropine and include dilated pupils; dry, hot, flushed skin; dry mouth; and tachycardia. Blood pressure changes are those of postural hypotension and are usually unimpressive except in severe toxicity when hypotension occurs because of ganglionic blockage.

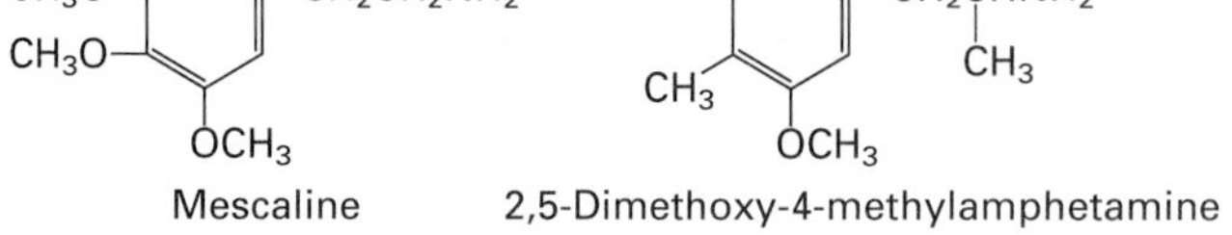

FIGURE 18-2 Comparison of the chemical structures of norepinephrine, amphetamine, mescaline, and DOM (2,5-dimethoxy-4-methylamphetamine).

Psychotomimetic effects are similar to those of a toxic psychosis. The most marked effects are delirium, mental confusion, and disorientation. Attention span is reduced along with loss of memory for recent events. Auditory and visual hallucinations occur regularly. Restlessness and overactivity may continue for many hours. Exhaustion with dehydration and electrolyte depletion can result from sustained activity and refusal of food and drink.

In advanced toxicity, CNS depression, respiratory failure, cardiovascular collapse, and hyperpyrexia are contributing factors in fatalities due to these compounds. Treatment of anticholinergic poisoning includes: gastrointestinal tract decontamination via emesis, lavage, and saline cathartics; cardiopulmonary support; and administration of physostigmine, a reversible cholinesterase inhibitor with CNS activity. The administration and actions of physostigmine should be monitored by ECG.

MISCELLANEOUS PSYCHOTOMIMETIC DRUGS

Phencyclidine

Phencyclidine (PCP) was investigated for use as a general anesthetic in humans. However, because of the high incidence of emergence delirium, it was dropped from further consideration for this purpose. PCP is still used in veterinary practice to immobilize primates. Because of its psychotomimetic effect, the drug has gained wide popularity as a drug of abuse, especially for replacing LSD as a hallucinogen. Street names for phencyclidine include angel dust, elephant or horse tranquilizer, killer weed, and *peace pill*.

Phencyclidine [*N*-(1-phenylcyclohexyl)piperidine] (Fig. 18-3) is a white, stable solid. It is readily soluble in water, alcohol, and lipids.

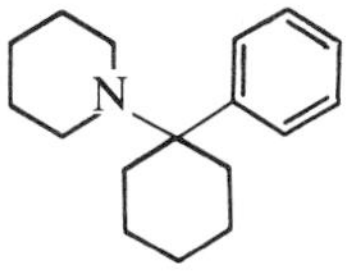

Phencyclidine

FIGURE 18-3 Phencyclidine.

Mechanism of Action The pharmacology of phencyclidine is very complex. PCP produces multiple pharmacologic actions including CNS stimulation, CNS depression, peripheral autonomic effects, analgesia, and anticonvulsant activity. The psychotomimetic effect which occurs at nonanesthetic doses is varied and the result of mixed CNS stimulant and depressant actions exerted at multiple brain sites. PCP interacts with several neurotransmitters including dopamine, norepinephrine, acetylcholine, serotonin, and the excitatory amino acids glutamate and aspartate. These interactions have been used to account for many of the actions of PCP. In addition, a specific receptor has been identified which is believed to mediate some of the psychotomimetic effects caused by PCP and PCP-like drugs.

PCP has been claimed to produce psychic disturbances which more closely mimic those of schizophrenia than any other drug. Since antipsychotic drugs affect dopamine activity, an interaction between PCP and dopamine was suggested to explain the psychotomimetic effects of PCP. Some of the effects of PCP such as increased motor activity, suppression of appetite, stereotyped behavior, and suppression of prolactin are common to dopamine agonist, like the amphetamines. Antipsychotic drugs, which block dopamine receptors, have been shown to antagonize the dopamine-related actions which both PCP and amphetamine produce. This indicates that some of the effects of PCP are mediated by a dopaminergic action. Additionally, PCP has been demonstrated to block the reuptake of dopamine, norepinephrine, and serotonin; enhance the release of dopamine, norepinephrine, and probably serotonin; and antagonize the excitatory actions of glutamate and aspartate.

Structure activity relationships among PCP and several PCP-like drugs (ketamine and PCP derivatives) and the ability of various animal species to discriminate between these drugs has contributed to the hypothesis that a specific receptor may mediate some aspects of the behavioral actions of PCP. The proposed receptor is currently referred to as the PCP σ receptor. Further research will be needed to elucidate the role of this receptor with the psychotomimetic actions of PCP.

Pharmacokinetics PCP can be administered by various routes including inhalation (smoking), oral, insufflation (snorting), and intravenous. Like other anesthetics, PCP is lipid-soluble and widely distributed to peripheral tissues where it accumulates and persists in fat. PCP is also secreted into gastric acid and then reabsorbed in the intestine. This recycling when combined with PCPs persistence in fat tissue contributed to a prolonged half-life (48 to 72 h) and protracted systemic effects. PCP is readily metabolized by the liver to various hydroxylated derivatives, which are then conjugated with glucuronic acid and excreted in the urine.

Pharmacologic Effects   The effects of PCP vary significantly with increasing dosage. At low doses there is CNS stimulation, euphoria, and sympathetic stimulation similar to the effects produced by amphetamines. With increasing dosage, thought processes become disoriented and speech is slurred. This is followed by paresthesias, slowed reflexes, and ataxia. Disorders of body image are common, with both elongation and shrinkage of extremities. This state may last 4 to 6 h, after which a depressive state occurs with a paranoid behavior pattern. It may take several days before the affected individual returns to normal. In acute toxicity, the individual will exhibit marked anxiety, agitation, hallucinations, and occasionally violent behavior. This may progress to dysphoria, catatonia, muscle rigidity, convulsions, nystagmus, hypertensive crisis, coma, and death.

Treatment of Intoxication   Initial treatment is similar to that with LSD-type hallucinogens: a nonstimulating environment and reassurance. Propranolol to control excess sympathetic stimulation and diazepam for sedation may be administered when deemed necessary. Acidification of the urine to pH 5.5 will increase excretion of PCP and shorten the half-life. Continuous gastric suction will increase elimination of PCP by interfering with intestinal reabsorption after gastric secretion. Seizures can be treated with phenytoin or diazepam.

Tolerance and Dependence   Tolerance develops fairly rapidly to the behavioral and toxic effects of PCP during chronic use. PCP has been demonstrated to be a positive reinforcer of behavior in some animal species. This indicates the development of some degree of dependency. The drug dependence appears to be predominantly psychological rather than physical. Withdrawal symptoms, when present, include a craving for the drug, increased anxiety, and mental depression.

Psychomotor Stimulants

Amphetamine and cocaine are potent CNS stimulants which are widely abused. At higher doses these drugs produce prominent psychotomimetic effects. The basic pharmacology of amphetamines and cocaine related to their therapeutic uses is given in Chaps. 7 and 24, respectively, and only the stimulant and psychotomimetic properties will be presented here. The central actions of these drugs are very similar, and many experienced drug users have difficulty discriminating between them following intravenous administration.

Mechanism of Action   The major actions of amphetamine and cocaine occur within the brain. Both drugs increase the amounts of norepinephrine (NE) and dopamine (DA) that are available for stimulation of adrenergic and dopaminergic receptors. Amphetamine enhances the release of NE and DA from presynaptic nerve terminals and, in addition, blocks the neuronal reuptake of both neurotransmitters. The stimulant actions of cocaine are related to its ability to block the neuronal reuptake of NE and DA. There is also evidence that both drugs affect the levels of serotonin. The increased levels of NE produce prominent peripheral and central sympathomimetic effects. The higher levels of DA influence behavioral activity, particularly that involving the limbic system. The behavioral actions account for the ability of these drugs to act as potent reinforcers of behavior. In animal studies, this is defined by the rapidity of acquisition of self-administration. Cocaine has been shown to be one of the most potent drug reinforcers of behavior yet studied. Supporting this action of dopamine is the finding that dopamine antagonists will eliminate the reinforcing properties of both amphetamine and cocaine while specific adrenergic antagonists of NE do not.

Amphetamines

A number of drugs are referred to as the "amphetamines." This includes amphetamine itself (racemic form), dextroamphetamine (dextrorotary isomer of amphetamine), methamphetamine, and a few related drugs. The amphetamines are basically sympathomimetic amines with chemical structures very similar to NE and DA. There are however, some important pharmacokinetic differences between the drugs and the neurotransmitters.

Pharmacokinetics In comparison to NE and DA, the amphetamines are lipid-soluble and not affected by the enzymes and inactivation mechanisms, which quickly terminate the effects of the neurotransmitters. Consequently, the amphetamines are well absorbed orally, readily pass into the brain, and produce effects lasting several hours. Intravenous injection of amphetamines, especially methamphetamine ("speed"), has become a significant problem. Large amounts are often injected over several days. It is during these sustained high-dosage bouts that the psychotomimetic effects of the drug frequently occur.

Biotransformation of the amphetamines occurs in the liver with formation of several active metabolites which produce pharmacologic actions similar to the parent compounds. One of these is *p*-hydroxyamphetamine, which is subsequently converted to another active metabolite, *p*-hydroxynorephedrine. The latter metabolite has a prolonged half-life, undergoes reuptake like NE, and functions as a "false transmitter." Following deamination and conjugation, the metabolites are excreted primarily in the urine along with 20 to 40 percent of the unmetabolized parent compound.

Pharmacologic Effects Abuse of amphetamines is based on the action of these drugs to influence physical performance and psychological mood. After oral administration, people feel more confident, alert, talkative, and are generally hyperactive. Amphetamines increase endurance and reduce feelings of fatigue. Following intravenous administration, the user experiences an initial "rush" which has been described as orgasmic. The euphoria and excitement produced by amphetamines are important for the reinforcing properties on behavior. This compulsive behavior drives the user to repeat the drug again and again in order to maintain the good feelings, "the reward."

Initially, the hyperactivity may stimulate the user to be more industrious and diligent, but eventually performance deteriorates. Activity may continue for hours but may also become compulsive and highly stereotyped. The user gets "hung up" doing one thing over and over again. As amphetamine usage increases and the dosages become larger, the psychotomimetic effects become apparent and can lead to psychotic behavior.

The amphetamine psychosis is paranoid in character and similar to paranoid schizophrenia. Although the users may feel elated, they appear glum, depressed, and withdrawn. Suspicion, hostility, and ag-gressive behavior may lead to violent acts. Sensory illusions, auditory and visual hallucinations, and distortions of body image may occur. The psychosis can occur after only a few doses but usually occurs after chronic use of high doses.

After discontinuance of the drug, profound sleep usually occurs. Upon awakening, the user experiences disagreeable depressed feelings ("crash") and wants to resume drug taking immediately.

Tolerance and Dependence Tolerance to the amphetamines, especially after prolonged IV administration, develops rapidly, and larger amounts are usually administered with continuous use. The peripheral sympathomimetic effects show greater tolerance than the central effects. Tolerance does develop to some of the central effects such as the euphoria and appetite suppression. Other CNS effects, however, do not appear to develop tolerance and may demonstrate sensitization (reverse tolerance). The development of tolerance to amphetamines is not completely understood.

Abrupt discontinuance of amphetamines after chronic use results in only mild physical withdrawal symptoms. Withdrawal effects appear to be predominantly psychological in nature and include extreme fatigue, mental depression, and a strong desire for the drug.

Intoxication and Treatment There are a number of adverse effects and potential complications caused by overstimulation of the sympathetic and central nervous systems. The psychotomimetic effects of the paranoid psychosis have already been described. Sympathetic stimulation produces hyperthermia and profuse sweating, respiratory difficulties, tremors, and various cardiovascular effects. Intense cardiovascular stimulation results in tachycardia, arrythmias, and hypertension, which may contribute to intracranial hemorrhaging, necrotizing angiitis, and sudden death. After prolonged IV use, severe fatigue and exhaustion may be followed by convulsions, coma, and death. Chronic intoxication can produce all these effects, and, in addition, there may be extreme weight loss due to the anorexic effect.

Treatment of amphetamine intoxication is aimed at supporting vital functions and providing symptomatic therapy. Acidification of the urine increases excretion. Adrenergic blockers and vasodilators can be administered to control excessive sympathetic and cardiovascular stimulation. Diazepam is generally preferred to control seizures and can also be used for sedation when necessary. Highly agitated individuals can be given antipsychotic drugs, which reduce psychotic symptoms by antagonizing the actions of DA and NE.

Cocaine

Cocaine was isolated from the leaves of *Erythroxylon coca* in 1855. Native Indians of South America have chewed coca leaves for centuries to ward off fatigue and hunger. In the late nineteenth century cocaine was considered a "wonder drug" and advocated for numerous medical conditions, including the treatment of morphine and alcohol addiction. After recognizing the potential dangers of cocaine abuse, the government enacted legislation in 1914 which restricted and controlled the use of cocaine. Cocaine was "rediscovered" in the 1970s as the phenomenon of recreational drug use dramatically increased. Presently, cocaine is considered the "illicit drug of choice," and widespread abuse has generated major social and medical problems.

The pharmacologic effects of cocaine are similar to those of the amphetamines. However, cocaine possesses a number of features which make it more popular with drug users. Cocaine is prepared in different forms, which can be administered by a variety of methods. The intensity and duration of drug effects are highly dependent on the preparation used and the route of administration. The structure of cocaine is shown in Fig. 18-4.

Preparations of Cocaine   Cocaine base (benzoylmethylecgonine) is extracted from coca leaves and converted to the water-soluble hydrochloride salt. It is in this form that cocaine is exported and adulterated with other substances such as sugars and local anesthetics. Cocaine hydrochloride can be administered orally, intranasally, and intravenously. It is, however, destroyed by the high temperatures generated during smoking. Several methods exist for conversion of cocaine hydrochloride back into the free-base form. Free-base cocaine possesses greater lipid solubility and a lower melting point. Consequently, it can be smoked, which allows almost instantaneous delivery of cocaine to the brain in a concentrated bolus. The intensity of effect is greatly increased. One form of free base cocaine, "crack," is prepared by an alkalinization-water process, which forms a crystalline rocklike substance that makes a cracking sound when it is smoked.

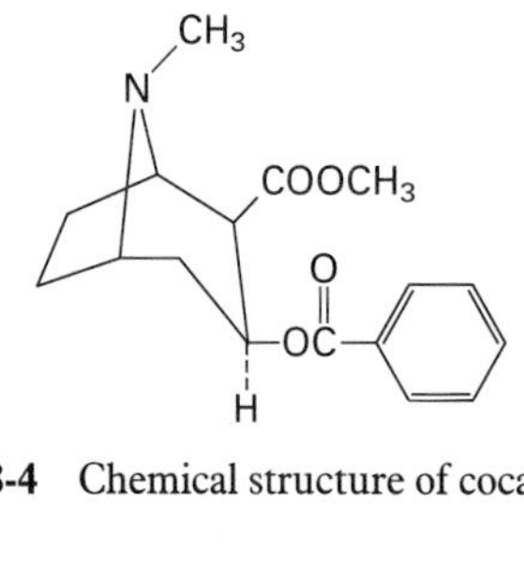

Pharmacokinetics   Cocaine is absorbed from the intestinal tract and from all mucous membranes. Pharmacologic effects are delayed (30 to 60 min) and less intense after oral administration compared to other routes. Drug effects are detectable 3 to 5 min after intranasal administration, peak in 20 to 30 min, and last 60 to 90 min. Plasma levels measured an hour or more after oral or intranasal administration are comparable; however, it is the concentration of cocaine in the brain that is important. Intranasal administration provides higher drug levels in the brain within a shorter period of time; therefore, effects are more intense. Intravenous injection and smoking both provide immediate effects of high intensity but of shorter duration. Peak effects by these routes occur in minutes and last about 20 min. Smoking cocaine is the most popular route of administration; it is more convenient than making injections, and there is less nasal irritation and septal perforation than when taken intranasally.

The plasma half-life of cocaine is approximately 40 to 60 min; however, there is considerable variability. Cocaine is metabolized primarily by serum and liver cholinesterases. Serum cholinesterase or pseudocholinesterase is genetically influenced, and variations in enzyme activity may account for individual sensitivities to cocaine. The major metabolites which are excreted in the urine are benzoylecgonine and ecgonine methyl ester, which can be further metabolized to ecgonine, benzoic acid, and methanol. Demethylation also occurs in the liver, and one metabolite, norcocaine, possesses some ability to inhibit re-uptake mechanisms.

Pharmacologic Effects   Cocaine is a powerful CNS stimulant producing marked euphoria, self-confidence, and heightened feelings of physical and mental

FIGURE 18-4   Chemical structure of cocaine.

ability. These ego reinforcing effects can lead to delusions of grandeur, which have been referred to as *cocainomania*. These positive psychological effects are followed by dysphoria, anxiety, and feelings of depression as the drug effect wears off. This creates a desire in the user to repeat the drug again, which often leads to prolonged binges where cocaine use becomes compulsive. This is similar to the situation which develops with amphetamines. However, the duration of action after smoking or injecting cocaine is only 20 to 30 min, compared to several hours for amphetamines. Consequently, cocaine must be administered much more frequently in order to maintain the "good feelings." This contributes to the reinforcing properties of cocaine on behavior and leads to drug dependency.

As dosages of cocaine are increased, CNS stimulation becomes excessive. Tremors and myoclonic jerks develop and may progress to clonic-tonic convulsions. Peripheral sympathomimetic effects increase, and cardiovascular stimulation resulting in hypertension, tachycardia, and arrthymias may progress to serious complications and sudden death. A toxic psychosis, similar to that caused by amphetamines, can develop after high dosages or prolonged use. Symptoms include hostility, social withdrawal, paranoid ideation, hallucinations, delusions, and violent behavior.

Tolerance and Dependence   The question of tolerance to cocaine is not entirely clear. Acute tolerance does develop to sympathomimetic and psychological effects when cocaine is used frequently within short periods of time. The tolerance does not appear to involve any changes in metabolism or distributional disposition. Users often purposefully increase dosage in an attempt to supercede the "high" of the previous dose. There is also evidence that reverse tolerance or "kindling" may develop to some of the effects of cocaine after chronic use. The development of paranoid psychosis has been suggested to involve a kindling phenomenon.

Before widespread abuse in the 1970s, cocaine was considered a relatively safe drug which did not cause physical dependency. However, with the technique of free-basing where higher doses are administered frequently on a daily basis, the evidence suggests that cocaine does produce some degree of physical dependence. There is a mistaken perception by many that substances which only cause psychological dependence are generally safe. Cocaine is one of the most psy-

chologically habituating drugs known, and those who become dependent on it suffer fates similar to those individuals addicted to alcohol, narcotics, and other physically addicting drugs. It would not be expected that the withdrawal symptoms from depressant drugs such as alcohol and narcotics would be identical to withdrawal symptoms from stimulant drugs such as amphetamine and cocaine. The symptoms of withdrawal from cocaine include a craving for the drug, dysphoria, irritability, anxiety, depression, tremors, eating and sleeping disturbances, and suicidal ideation.

Intoxication and Treatment   Depending on the dosage and time since administration, the user may be euphoric and excited or dysphoric, anxious, and depressed. After prolonged binges of cocaine use, extreme fatigue, exhaustion, hyperthermia, seizures, and coma may occur. The most serious effects of acute cocaine poisoning are on the CNS and cardiovascular system, leading to convulsions and cardiac complications. Tachycardia and arrthymias may precipitate ventricular fibrillation and sudden death. CNS stimulation is followed by severe depression resulting in respiratory failure and cardiovascular collapse. Individuals with underlying cardiovascular disease are at greater risk of complication and sudden death. The psychotic reactions which usually occur after prolonged use are similar to those observed with amphetamines.

Treatment of cocaine intoxication is similar to that of amphetamine poisoning, supportive and symptomatic. Diazepam is useful to control seizures and for sedation. Since the half-life of cocaine is short, the greatest danger in acute intoxication occurs within the first few hours. Antipsychotic drugs, such as chlorpromazine and haloperidol, are useful because of their multiple effects to antagonize DA and NE.

Treatment of cocaine dependence usually involves education of the individual to the dangers of continued use and behavioral modification to control impulsive desires for the drug. A newer approach to control cocaine dependence is the use of tricyclic antidepressants (TCAs). Treatment with TCAs has been reported to lessen the euphoric effects of cocaine and reduce cravings for continued use of the drug.

Identification of Cocaine in Body Fluids   Under certain legal and medical circumstances, determination of cocaine levels in plasma and urine may be important. Since cocaine has a relatively short half-life (40 to 60 min), it will be present in plasma for only a few hours. However, the metabolites of cocaine: benzylecgonine, ecgonine methyl ester, and norcocaine can be identified in plasma and urine for approximately 24 h. High pressure liquid chromatography (HPLC) and electron capture-mass spectrometry (ES-MS) methods are used for identification and quantitation.

Marijuana

The source of marijuana is a species of hemp plant, *Cannabis sativa*. The marijuana plant is dioecious; the flowering tops of the female plant are particularly rich in a sticky resin in which the active psychotropic principles are found in highest concentrations. The resin can be extracted from the plant and is known as *hashish*. Marijuana generally refers to the dried, chopped plant (seeds, flowers, twigs, leaves) which is smoked like tobacco. The psychoactive effects of the marijuana plant have been known for many centuries and in many cultures. This is reflected in the many names given to different preparations by different countries: bhang (India), ganja (Jamaica), kif (North Africa), kabak (Turkey), and grass or pot (United States).

Various preparations from the marijuana plant have been tried medicinally over the centuries for anesthesia, analgesia, hypnosis, bronchodilation, and anti-emetic effects. Tinctures and extracts of cannabis were used officially in the United States until 1937, when the Marijuana Tax Act eliminated further widespread use. Presently, there are efforts to develop synthetic derivatives of the active principles of the marijuana plant that retain useful pharmacologic actions but do not produce psychotropic effects. Currently, marijuana has the distinction of being the most frequently used illicit drug.

Chemistry The pharmacologically active substances in marijuana are nitrogen-free tricyclic compounds referred to as *cannabinoids*. Two systems of nomenclature are used to describe these compounds: the formal or dibenzopyran system and the monoterpene system. The dibenzopyran system is used in this chapter. Cannabinoids of major interest that are found naturally in the marijuana plant are shown in Fig. 18-5. The major active cannabinoid present in the plant is l-Δ^9-*trans*-tetrahydrocannabinol (Δ^9THC), hereafter referred to as THC. Another isomer, Δ^8THC, is similar in potency to THC but is found in very small quantities. Cannabinol (CBN) possesses about one tenth the potency of THC, while cannabidiol (CBD) is devoid of psychoactive activity.

Marijuana cigarettes supplied by the National Institute of Drug Abuse for research purposes weigh about 900 mg and contain 1.0 to 1.5 percent of THC, which is average for most varieties of marijuana. The resin,

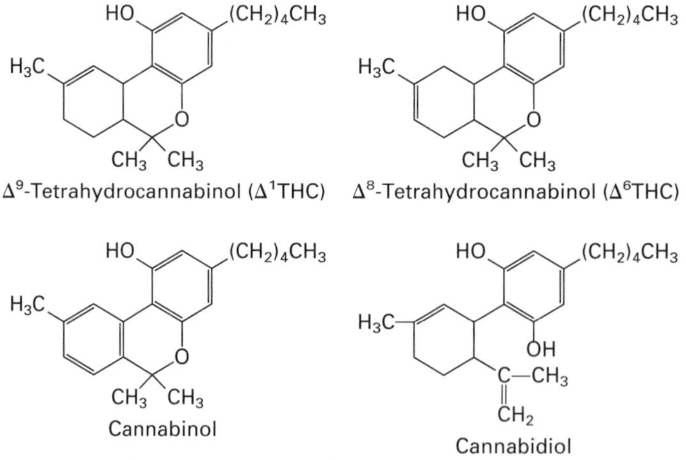

FIGURE 18-5 Natural cannabinoids of *Cannabis sativa*. The monoterpine numbering system is shown in parentheses for Δ^9THC and Δ^8THC.

hashish, usually contains about 10 percent of THC. It should be noted that there are hundreds of chemical compounds in the marijuana plant, with more than 60 identified as cannabinoids. During the pyrolysis of smoking, many chemical conversions occur, including conversion of the inactive monocarboxylic acid of THC to the active THC. Also, about 30 percent of THC is estimated to be destroyed during the smoking process.

Pharmacokinetics The cannabinoids are highly lipid-soluble compounds. Bioavailability after oral administration averages only 6 percent. Effects begin within 30 to 60 min, peak in 1 to 2 h and last about 4 to 6 h. The most common rate of administration of marijuana is smoking, which provides bioavailability of 10 to 25 percent, depending on the efficiency of smoking technique. Effects after smoking begin within 5 to 15 min, peak in 30 to 90 min, and generally last 3 to 4 h.

THC is widely distributed throughout the body; however, the initial volume of distribution (V_d) is small because of high plasma protein binding (97 to 99 percent). With continued use, the V_d increases as the highly lipid-soluble THC is taken up by peripheral body compartments and sequestered in adipose tissue. The initial plasma level of THC decreases rapidly after absorption as distribution to peripheral tissues occurs.

Biotransformation of THC occurs predominantly in the liver by the microsomal enzyme system. Metabolic degradation is complex, with approximately 80 different metabolites already identified. The primary metabolite of THC is 11-hydroxy-Δ^9THC (11-OH-THC), which is active and equipotent with THC. This compound is subsequently biotransformed to a number of inactive metabolites, which are then excreted. Figure 18-6 illustrates the principal metabolites of THC.

Approximately 60 to 70 percent of THC metabolites are slowly eliminated, via the bile, into the feces with the remainder excreted in the urine. THC is readily metabolized when it is in the plasma. However, rapid redistribution from the plasma to peripheral tissue compartments removes approximately 70 percent of the THC administered. Because of its high lipid solubility THC is released slowly back to the plasma, biotransformed by the liver, and excreted in the feces and urine. After 72 h, approximately 50 percent of an original dose is still present in the tissues and organs. The

elimination half-life of THC ranges from 20 to 36 h, and THC can persist to some extent in adipose tissue for 2 weeks or more.

Pharmacologic Effects

Acute Effects Conjunctival reddening and increases in heart rate have been the most consistently reported effects of marijuana. Heart rate increases of 20 to 50 beats per minute may occur and are dose-related. Tolerance develops to this effect with chronic use. After one marijuana cigarette, there is usually physical and mental relaxation, feelings of euphoria, and increased sociability. These feelings come and go as if in waves. Conversation and ideas tend to concentrate on the "here and now" and not on past or future circumstances. There is a sense that time is passing slowly. With moderate intoxication, there is drowsiness, lapses of attention, and impairment of short-term memory. At high levels of intoxication, reflexes are slowed, muscle coordination decreases, ataxia is evident, and speech and the ability to concentrate become more difficult. Performance of a variety of tasks deteriorates. The more complex the task, the greater the degree of disruption produced. Dreamlike states with alterations of auditory and visual perceptions reflect the psychotomimetic actions of marijuana. Psychic effects may also include dysphoria, acute panic-anxiety reactions and psychotic episodes. Marijuana psychosis may, in part, be caused by an unmasking of latent psychiatric disorders by the drug. It appears to occur under conditions of unusually heavy drug use. Symptoms are characterized by delirium, disorientation, and schizophrenic-like behavior.

Chronic Effects Chronic use of marijuana in the young has frequently been related to the development of an "amotivational syndrome." This is a highly controversial issue. Many studies have concluded that the lack of interest and motivation demonstrated by many heavy users of marijuana was present before drug use and that amotivation is not a specific effect of marijuana. However, students who frequently use marijuana during school and study time are certainly shortchanging their academic and future potential.

At low doses, marijuana produces a slight bronchodilatation. However, marijuana smoke contains higher concentrations of tar and some carcinogens than tobacco smoke. Chronic use can produce hoarseness,

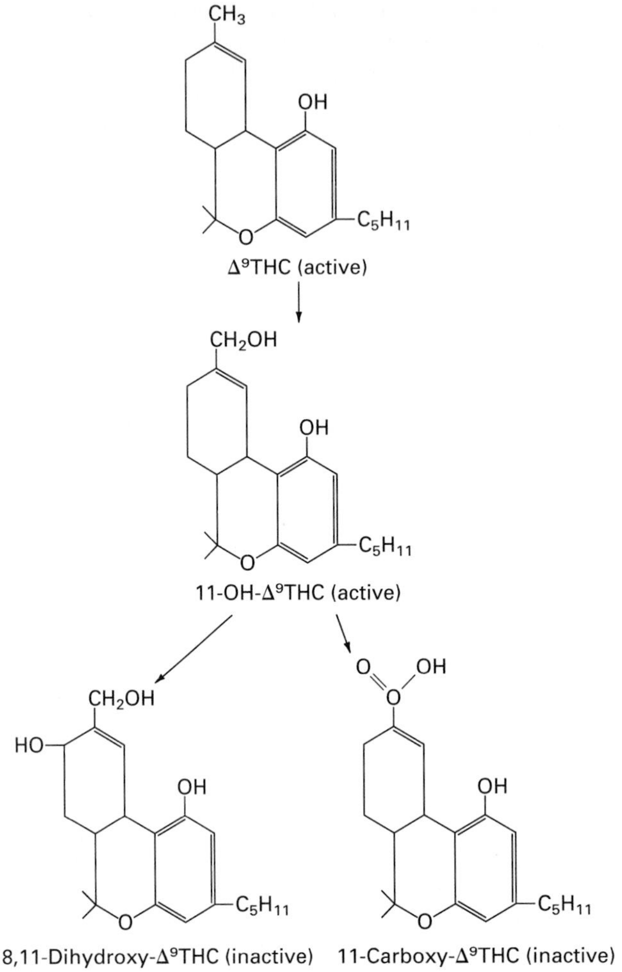

FIGURE 18-6   Principal metabolites of Δ^9THC.

cough, and bronchitis. Heavy use results in increased airway resistance and has been associated with precancerous changes in the respiratory epithelium.

Marijuana alters the plasma levels of some reproductive hormones. In males, lower testosterone levels decrease the sperm count and motility. In females, levels of LH and prolactin are suppressed resulting in sporadic ovulation and irregular menstrual cycles. THC readily crosses the placenta, and teratogenic effects have been demonstrated in animal studies. Specific birth defects have not been observed in humans, but lower birth weights have been recorded in mothers who smoked marijuana during pregnancy. Marijuana appears to have some teratogenic potential, and use during pregnancy should be strongly discouraged.

Experimental studies have shown marijuana to cause a mild, transitory immunosuppressant effect. Decreased levels of T lymphocytes have been observed in some chronic users. The clinical significance of this effect has not been determined.

Tolerance and Dependence   Tolerance to marijuana, i. e., diminished response to a given dose when repeated, has been demonstrated. However, the development of tolerance usually occurs only after prolonged use of higher amounts of marijuana. The tolerance is variable and develops to a greater degree for some effects such as tachycardia, CNS depression, and euphoria. Tolerance is rapidly reversed after cessation of marijuana use. Some of the tolerance may be metabolic in origin and caused by induction of microsomal enzymes. As with chronic tobacco smoking, tars and residues in marijuana smoke stimulate the drug microsomal enzyme system. However, this effect on metabolism does not explain all the tolerance which develops. Cross-tolerance with other psychoactive drugs has not been demonstrated.

Abrupt cessation of marijuana after prolonged use has been associated with the development of some dependency. The dependence appears to be more psychological than physical and of considerably less intensity than observed with cocaine and amphetamines. Withdrawal symptoms are mild and not unlike those observed on individuals who quit the tobacco habit. Symptoms include dysphoria, anxiety, tremors, eating and sleeping disturbances, and increased sweating which usually lasts for only a few days. Since most use of marijuana is social, development of tolerance and dependency is not a major problem.

Intoxication and Treatment   The most common intoxication reaction requiring treatment is the acute panic-anxiety reaction where the users appear to lose control and feel as if they were losing their minds. This reaction occurs most frequently with inexperienced users who are unfamiliar with the effects of marijuana. The effects rarely last more than a few hours. Diazepam may be administered to individuals who are particularly agitated. Psychotic reactions, which were previously discussed, occur after high doses or prolonged use and may require hospitalization and treatment with antipsychotic drugs.

Identification in Plasma and Urine   Determination of marijuana use by analysis of body fluids is more difficult than with other drugs. Separation of THC from endogenous lipids requires various "clean-up" methods. Although some assays for measurement of THC and 11-OH-THC in plasma have been devel-

oped, the most common method is identification of the urinary metabolites of THC. One of the metabolites frequently measured is 11-carboxy-Δ^9THC using gas chromatography-mass spectrometry. The metabolites can be identified in the urine and feces for more than a week.

Therapeutic Potential of THC   THC and various derivatives are currently undergoing clinical investigation in the treatment of glaucoma and as an antiemetic for cancer patients who are receiving chemotherapy. Dronabinol (Marinol) is a drug formulation of THC for use in cancer patients. Other properties of THC including analgesia, bronchodilation, and anticonvulsant effects are also under investigation at the present time.

BIBLIOGRAPHY

Agurell, S., M. Halldin, J. E. Lindgren, et al: "Pharmacokinetics and Metabolism of Δ'-Tetrahydrocannabinol and Other Cannabinoids with Emphasis on Man," *Pharm. Rev.*, **38(1)**:21 (1986).

Anderson, P. O., and G. G. McGuire: "Delta-9-Tetrahydrocannabinol as an Antiemetic," *Am. J. Hosp. Pharm.*, **38**:639 (1981).

Brawley, P., and J. C. Duffield: "The Pharmacology of Hallucinogens," *Pharm. Rev.* **24(1)**:31 (1972).

Clonet, D. H. (ed.): *Phencyclidine: An Update*, Research Monograph 64, NIDA, Washington D.C. 1986.

Grabowski, J. (ed.): *Cocaine: Pharmacology, Effects and Treatment of Abuse*, Research Monograph 50, NIDA, Washington D.C. 1984.

Hollister, L. E.: "Health Aspects of Cannabis," *Pharm. Rev.*, **38(1)**:1 (1986).

Jacobs, B. L.: "How Hallucinogenic Drugs Work," *Am. Sci.*, **75**:386 (1987).

Meltzer, H. Y. (ed.): *Psychopharmacology: The Third Generation of Progress*, Raven, New York, 1987.

Ray, O. (ed.): *Drugs, Society and Human Behavior*, Mosby, St. Louis, 1978.

Schultes, R. E., and A. Hofmann: *The Botany and Chemistry of Hallucinogens*, Charles C Thomas, Springfield, Ill., 1980.

C H A P T E R 19

Antipsychotic Drugs and Lithium

G. John DiGregorio

Antipsychotic drugs are agents which produce tranquilization or "peace of mind" and have been primarily used for the treatment of psychotic or schizophrenic patients. The drugs produce emotional calmness and mental relaxation and are, therefore, highly effective in controlling the symptoms of acutely and chronically disturbed patients. Many of these drugs are also used in treatment of nonpsychotic conditions including the control of nausea, emesis, hiccups, itching, and potentiation of the action of other drugs. In Europe, these drugs are called *neuroleptics* because they have diffuse activities throughout the central nervous system, including suppression of spontaneous movement and complex behavior.

The term *major tranquilizer* for antipsychotic drugs has been used in the past to differentiate these agents from the "minor tranquilizers" (antianxiety drugs).

CLASSIFICATION

The antipsychotic drugs are subdivided into five groups based on their chemical structure. These are the phenothiazines, butyrophenones, thioxanthenes, dihydroindolones, dibenzoxazepines and diphenylbutylpiperidines.

PHENOTHIAZINE DERIVATIVES

The phenothiazines have a complex pharmacology with effects on both central and peripheral nervous systems, in addition to important metabolic and endocrine effects. Each compound differs quantitatively and qualitatively in the extent to which it produces each of these pharmacologic effects. All of them act on the central nervous system to produce (1) mild sedation; (2) antiemetic effects, (3) alteration of temperature regulation, which may result in either hypothermia or hyperthermia, depending on environmental temperature; (4) alteration of skeletal-muscle tone; (5) endocrine alterations; and (6) potentiation of analgesics. They also act on the autonomic nervous system to produce (1) alpha-adrenergic receptor blockade, (2) inhibition of biogenic amine uptake and adrenergic potentiation, and (3) cholinergic blocking effects at both nicotinic and muscarinic receptor sites. They also block serotonin and histamine receptors.

Chemistry

The basic chemical nucleus of the phenothiazines and various substitutions are illustrated in Table 19-1. Depending on the substitution on the nitrogen at position 10, the phenothiazines are subdivided into three subgroups, namely, the open-chain, piperazine, and piperidine derivatives.

Sites and Mechanism of Action

The specific etiology of psychotic disorders is presently unknown. However, an imbalance of dopaminergic function in the central nervous system has been suspected as one of the primary causes of psychotic behavior. Most investigators believe that increasing

TABLE 19-1 Some therapeutically useful phenothiazines

Name	R_1	R_2
Open chain		
Promazine	$CH_2—CH_2—CH_2—N(CH_3)_2$	H
Chlorpromazine	$CH_2—CH_2—CH_2—N(CH_3)_2$	Cl
Triflupromazine	$CH_2—CH_2—CH_2—N(CH_3)_2$	CF_3
Promethazine	$CH_2—CH—N(CH_3)_2$ with CH_3	H
Piperazine		
Prochlorperazine	$CH_2—CH_2—CH_2—N$ (piperazine) $N—CH_3$	Cl
Trifluoperazine	$CH_2—CH_2—CH_2—N$ (piperazine) $N—CH_3$	CF_3
Fluphenazine	$CH_2—CH_2—CH_2—N$ (piperazine) $N—CH_2—CH_2OH$	CF_3
Piperidine		
Thioridazine	$(CH_2)_2—$ (piperidine with $N—CH_3$)	SCH_3

dopamine activity in specific areas of the CNS is responsible for this abnormal behavior pattern. The site of antipsychotic activity for phenothiazines is the mesolimbic and hippocampal areas of the central nervous system. These compounds appear to block the activity of dopamine on dopaminergic receptor sites, thus decreasing psychotic activity.

The central dopamine receptors are divided into D_1 and D_2 receptors. Both receptors have a high affinity for dopamine but differ in their sensitivity to antipsychotic drugs. The D_1 receptor site is excitatory and activates directly the adenylate cyclase system. The D_2 receptor is also related to the adenylate cyclase system and may be inhibitory in some brain tissues. Phenothiazines are nonselective, competitive D_1 and D_2 antagonists. Butyrophenone antipsychotics such as halo-

peridol are known to selectively antagonize at D_2 receptors. This suggests that the antipsychotic activity of these drugs is primarily related to the blockade of the D_2 receptors.

The mechanism responsible for its action is also responsible for at least some of its side effects. For example, by blocking the action of dopamine in the nigrostriatal pathway, it causes a parkinsonism-like syndrome.

Blockade of other dopamine receptors in the tuberoinfundibular dopamine pathway by these drugs releases prolactin, resulting in hyperprolactinemia.

The antipsychotic drugs also possess antiserotonin, antihistamine, and α-adrenergic blocking activities. Some researchers believe that these activities also contribute to the therapeutic effectiveness of these drugs.

For example, the antihistamine effect may be related to the sedative activity of these drugs. The α-adrenergic blocking activity may be related to the decrease in central nervous system stimulation as well as the cause for the orthostatic hypotension. Still it remains to be established whether these mechanisms play a major role in the antipsychotic activity.

Effects on Organ Systems

Central Nervous System The administration of chlorpromazine and related phenothiazines depresses the central nervous system. The open-chain phenothi-azines and the piperidines tend to be more sedative than the piperazine derivatives (Table 19-2). Depression resulting in anesthesia, however, is seldom produced even with large doses. After receiving phenothiazines, psychotic patients appear less severely disturbed and have fewer hallucinations and delusions. However, the antipsychotic effect is not seen until several weeks or months after initiation of therapy. Administration of these agents for acute conditions produces a quieting effect in grossly agitated and disturbed patients. After long-term administration of phenothiazines, tolerance develops to their sedative effect with no reduction in antipsychotic activity.

TABLE 19-2 Comparison of some pharmacodynamic properties of antipsychotics

	Equivalent doses, mg, (antipsychotic activity)	Sedation	EPR[a]	Anti cholinergic activity	α-Adrenergic blocking (orthostatic hypotension)
Aliphatics					
Chlorpromazine	50	High	Moderate	Moderate	High
Promazine	100	Moderate	Moderate	High	Moderate
Piperidine					
Thioridazine	50	High	Low	High	High
Mesoridazine	25	High	Low	Moderate	Moderate
Piperazine					
Prochlorperazine	8	Moderate	High	Low	Low
Fluphenazine	1	Low	High	Low	Low
Trifluoperazine	2.5	Low	High	Low	Low
Butyrophenones					
Haloperidol	1	Low	High	Low	Low
Thioxanthenes					
Chlorprothixene	50	High	Moderate	Moderate	Moderate
Thiothixene	2	Low	High	Low	Low
Dihydroindolone					
Molindone	5	Low	High	Low	Low
Dibenzoxazepine					
Loxapine	5	Moderate	High	Low	Moderate

[a]EPR = extrapyramidal reactions (excluding tardive dyskinesia).

The piperazine phenothiazines (for example, prochloroperazine) possess the greatest antipsychotic potency when compared on a weight basis with the open-chain or piperidine derivatives.

Antiemetic Actions There is a bilateral area on the floor of the fourth ventricle known as the area postrema which, when stimulated by chemical agents such as apomorphine, will cause emesis. This area is referred to as the *chemoreceptor trigger zone*. The phenothiazines act as antiemetics by suppression of the chemoreceptor trigger zone. They cannot prevent vomiting induced by gastrointestinal irritants such as copper sulfate or vomiting induced by vestibular dysfunction.

Alteration of Temperature Regulation The phenothiazines depress hypothalamic temperature-regulating mechanisms. They may produce hypothermia or hyperthermia, depending on the environmental temperature. In climates where the temperature is high, patients on phenothiazine medication may suffer a hyperthermic episode because of failure to lose body heat. Normally, phenothiazines have a hypothermic effect.

Endocrine Actions The endocrine effects of the phenothiazines are due primarily to their action on the brain, at the hypothalamus, and pituitary. Dopamine normally inhibits prolactin release. The phenothiazines, which are dopamine receptor antagonists block this action of dopamine. They may as a result of this activity, increase prolactin levels and lactation. The phenothiazines will increase lactation when used chronically.

The effects of the phenothiazines on ovulation and menstruation depend on the dose and duration of treatment. Therapeutic doses delay ovulation, as judged by biopsy, basal body temperature, and menstruation. It has been shown that some phenothiazines, especially in high doses, produce amenorrhea by decreasing gonadotropin liberation.

False-positive human chorionic gonadotropin pregnancy tests may result with phenothiazine use. This may be due to the stimulation of hypothalamic release of pituitary hormones. Phenothiazines also interfere with the release of corticotropin from the pituitary.

Dopamine also inhibits the release of melanocyte-stimulating hormone (MSH). The phenothiazines therefore stimulate the release of melanocyte-stimulating hormone from the pituitary, which results in abnormal pigmentation. There is a direct correlation between the effectiveness of various phenothiazines in releasing melanocyte-stimulating hormone and their antipsychotic potency.

Peripheral Nervous System The phenothiazines have multiple actions on the peripheral nervous system. These compounds produce α-adrenergic receptor blocking, depending on the dose and duration of therapy. With a single small dose, especially with chlorpromazine, the α-adrenergic blockade is more consistent. Owing to the blockade of these receptor sites, orthostatic hypotension will occur in a significant number of patients (Table 19-2). Although most of the phenothiazines produce α-adrenergic receptor blockade, their actions are considered to be much less specific compared with a classic α-adrenergic blocking agent such as phenoxybenzamine. The phenothiazines also block cholinergic receptor, primarily muscarinic (Table 19-2). These actions are weak and are seen primarily as side effects. However, some phenothiazines such as thioridazine are effective anticholinergics. The phenothiazines also vary widely in antihistaminic actions. Those phenothiazines having an ethyldiethylamino group, e.g., promethazine, generally have higher antihistaminic action and are used mainly for that purpose.

Skeletal Muscle It is believed that phenothiazines have skeletal-muscle relaxant properties. This activity is probably mediated centrally through the basal ganglia but may also block nicotinic skeletal-muscle receptors. Shivering, which is a protective action against cold weather, may be diminished. This may contribute to the hypothermia of patients taking phenothiazines in cold weather.

Pharmacokinetics

Many of the phenothiazines can be given intravenously, subcutaneously, intramuscularly, rectally, and orally. They must be given very slowly intravenously because of local irritation and possible severe hypotension due to central vasomotor depression and alpha-adrenergic blockade.

Ordinarily, the oral absorption of phenothiazines is slow and incomplete; peak plasma levels are reached within 2 to 4 h. The effect of intramuscular and/or intravenous injection is immediate and may persist for 4 h. Fluphenazine is available in depot form, which has a duration of 1 to 4 weeks.

The biotransformation of chlorpromazine and similar phenothiazines is accomplished by the drug-metabolizing microsomal system in the liver. The most common pathway is ring hydroxylation and subsequent conjugation with glucuronic acid. The second most common pathway is the formation of sulfoxides. In addition, demethylation and side-chain oxidation can occur. The half-life of chlorpromazine is between 16 and 30 h, and its plasma protein binding is more than 90 percent. About 1 percent of chlorpromazine appears in the urine unchanged. However, at least five biotransformation products of chlorpromazine are found: chlorpromazine sulfoxide, desdimethyl-chlorpromazine sulfoxide, glucuronides, hydroxyl derivatives, and promazine (via dechlorination). There are more than 150 proposed metabolites of chlorpromazine.

Thioridazine undergoes sulfoxidation to a sulfoxide and sulfone metabolites. Mesoridazine and sulforidazine are active metabolites. The metabolism of the piperazine phenothiazine is similar to that of chlorpromazine. There are apparently no active metabolites from this group.

Although the elimination of chlorpromazine and related phenothiazines may take many weeks, the duration of action of these drugs is relatively short, especially on single-dose administration. Compounds such as chlorpromazine have a duration of action after oral administration of 6 h; it is necessary to medicate 3 to 4 times a day to maintain an adequate blood level. In the case of some phenothiazines, such as trifluoperazine, drug administration twice a day is sufficient.

Correlations of plasma concentrations of phenothiazines and efficacy are difficult to establish. Chlorpromazine causes an improvement in clinical situations with plasma levels in wide range of 50 to 300 ng/ml. Higher concentration may not increase efficacy.

Therapeutic Uses

The phenothiazines have a number of therapeutic uses. The phenothiazines are used widely as antipsychotics. Although these agents are not curative, they do reduce psychiatric symptoms sufficiently to allow mentally disturbed patients to have better contact with reality and to be discharged to a home and family environment. Therapeutic use of these drugs has made community psychiatric treatment a reasonable possibility. When used as an antipsychotic, the dose of the drug should be increased gradually. Once maximum therapeutic efficacy is obtained, the dose should be gradually reduced to the lowest effective maintenance level.

Occasionally phenothiazines are used to relieve very severe anxiety and especially panic reactions induced by abuse of amphetamines and lysergic acid diethylamide. Children having serious behavioral problems which cannot be controlled by psychotherapy or other nonneuroleptic drugs may be given antipsychotics. The drugs are also useful as preanesthetics because of the following reasons: (1) they reduce anxiety and apprehension; (2) they control nausea and vomiting, which are very common in surgical patients; (3) they cause muscle relaxation during surgery. Phenothiazines administered intramuscularly, rectally as a suppository, or orally are useful antiemetics if the patient can retain the drug. The antiemetic effect of the drug may suppress vomiting from illnesses such as intestinal obstruction and brain tumors and thus obscure their signs and symptoms. This fact must be borne in mind when they are prescribed. Other uses include the treatment of intractable hiccup, tetanus, and acute intermittent porphyria and as antihistaminics.

Adverse Reactions

The phenothiazines produce various undesirable side effects such as CNS disturbances including extrapyramidal symptoms, endocrine disorders, autonomic nervous system disturbances, hematologic abnormalities, jaundice, and skin pigmentation. The potency of the substituted phenothiazines as antipsychotics correlates inversely with sedation, undesirable autonomic effects, seizures, dermatitis, jaundice, and agranulocytosis. It follows that the autonomic nervous system effects are most prevalent with less potent antipsychotic drugs such as promazine and that autonomic side effects are less frequent with the potent agents such as trifluoperazine and fluphenazine.

Allergic reactions to the phenothiazines usually occur in the first few months of treatment. These include various forms of dermatitis, urticaria, photosensitivity, asthma, laryngeal edema, angioneurotic edema, and anaphylaxis.

Most blood dyscrasias occur within the first few weeks of therapy. Agranulocytosis, although rare, is more prevalent with chlorpromazine and promazine than with the other more potent phenothiazines. If this is recognized and the drug is stopped, the patient will recover completely. Eosinophilia, leukopenia, aplastic anemia, and thrombocytopenia have also been reported.

Phenothiazines can produce a wide range of metabolic and endocrine effects. Weight gain, one major adverse effect, may be due to increased appetite. Galactorrhea is observed in chronically treated women and is due to increased levels of prolactin. Amenorrhea is also produced owing to variable concentrations of luteinizing hormone (LH). In males, there is gynocomastia and a decrease in libido. Impotence and sterility may occur. These effects are probably associated with hyperprolactinemia.

Usually following chronic, but occasionally after acute, administration of some phenothiazines, extrapyramidal side effects may develop. The phenothiazines produce their extrapyramidal symptoms presumably by blocking dopamine receptors in the basal ganglia. The extrapyramidal reactions are divided into three areas: (1) parkinsonism, (2) akathisia, and (3) dystonic reactions. The phenothiazines with the greatest antipsychotic activity produce the highest incidence of extrapyramidal reactions. The reduction in dopaminergic activity produced by the phenothiazines results in a relative increase in cholinergic activity in the basal ganglia. Therefore, anticholinergic therapy can control these symptoms. Those substituted phenothiazines with the highest anticholinergic activity (e.g., thioridazine) produce the lowest incidence of parkinsonian-like symptoms (Table 19-2). Extrapyramidal symptoms induced by the phenothiazines are frequently dramatic. In one study akathisia (motor restlessness) occurred in approximately 21 percent, tremors 15 percent, and dystonic reactions in 2 percent of cases. A correlation has been found between the percentage of occurrence of such reactions and the milligram potency of the drugs. Some interesting sex differences have been observed. Akathisia and tremors occur twice as often in women as in men. In men, dyskinesia occurred earliest (90 percent within $4\frac{1}{2}$ days), akathisia next, and tremors last. Dystonic reactions include bizarre neuromuscular manifestations which could be mistaken for seizures, tetanus, meningitis, encephalitis, and poliomyelitis. These extrapyramidal symptoms are completely reversible upon discontinuation of the drug or by reduction of dose.

A life-threatening syndrome known as *neuroleptic malignant syndrome* has been reported. This syndrome is characterized by muscular rigidity, hyperthermia, altered consciousness, and autonomic dysfunction. It develops suddenly over a 24- to 72-h time period and can occur within hours to months after initial drug therapy. Mortality has been 20 percent in reported cases. No specific therapy is available. Management consists of immediate discontinuance of the antipsychotic agent and supportive medical care. Usually, the symptoms improve within 5 to 10 days of stopping the drug.

Tardive dyskinesia is a syndrome associated with administration of large chronic doses of phenothiazines. It appears to be caused by an imbalance of acetylcholine and dopamine in which there is an increase in dopaminergic activity and a relative decrease in cholinergic activity. However, there is no direct relationship between the potency of the phenothiazines and their ability to produce this syndrome. This phenomenon appears to be a consequence of a decrease in dosage or increase in tolerance to the phenothiazine effects possibly due to supersensitivity of dopamine receptors. Anticholinergics have been found to intensify the symptoms of tardive dyskinesia while the administration of higher doses of the phenothiazines or a cholinergic drug has been found to be useful in decreasing the symptoms of this syndrome. This syndrome usually occurs in older patients and more commonly in women after administration of large doses of phenothiazines for long periods. The onset is insidious, and the movements are rhythmic and coordinated rather than spasmodic. The tongue, lips, face, and jaw are most commonly involved. The late dyskinesia is not only irreversible, but it is usually intensified when the phenothiazine is withdrawn. This state may be suppressed with high doses of phenothiazines. This reaction is difficult to reverse. There is no effective therapy of tardive dyskinesia. Present treatment consists of slowly reducing the dose of the phenothiazine and removing or stopping all anticholinergic agents.

Large doses of most antipsychotic drugs are capable of causing convulsions. However, this is rarely seen clinically. Epileptics are more susceptible because of the ability of the phenothiazines to decrease the seizure threshold.

Thioridazine appears to produce significantly fewer untoward side effects such as extrapyramidal symptoms, lethargy, drowsiness, orthostatic hypotension, convulsions, and photosensitivity, compared with other phenothiazines. However, this compound has its own side effects including atropine-like actions, and when given in massive doses, pigmentary retinopathy and lens opacities may occur. Temporary failure of ejaculation has also been described following this medication.

Three types of pathologic liver conditions are associated with phenothiazine medication. The most frequent type is a diffuse inflammatory change associated with biliary stasis. The clinical picture is that of obstructive jaundice with a moderate elevation of alkaline phosphatase level. The next type of liver-induced ailment resembles acute hepatitis with evidence of parenchymal liver damage. In the third and least common type of reaction, early cirrhosis is observed.

Autonomic nervous system disturbances can be either anticholinergic, antiadrenergic (alpha-blocking), or both depending on the drug administered. Antiadrenergic symptoms include nasal stuffiness, dry mouth, hypotension, ejaculatory disorders, and miosis. Anticholinergic side effects can be obstipation, constipation, impotence, urinary retention, and mydriasis.

Exposed portions of the skin may develop pigmentation. Eye complications consisting of corneal and lenticular deposits, epithelial keratopathy, and pigmentary retinopathy may also occur.

The most common adverse effects in children are extrapyramidal reactions, which may be confused with encephalitis or other neurologic syndromes. The less common complications of phenothiazine therapy in children include jaundice, granulocytopenia, cutaneous eruptions, and hyperpyrexia.

Patients who take an excessive amount of phenothiazines present with two different clinical pictures. The first is related to extreme somnolence: with prodding, the patient can be aroused but promptly falls back into a deep sleep. The second is hypotension. There may be a mild to moderate drop in blood pressure; the patient may or may not be conscious. The skin may be markedly gray but warm and dry. The nail beds are usually still pink, and the pulse is strong but more rapid than normal. Respiration usually is slow and regular. Hypotension may be severe, in which case the patient may present symptoms of shock, including weakness, cyanosis, perspiration, and a rapid, thready pulse.

Drug Interactions

By induction of liver microsomal enzymes, chlorpromazine can accelerate its own biotransformation. Similarly, potent enzyme inducers such as phenobarbital and other barbiturates will increase the biotransformation of chlorpromazine and possibly lead to a reduced antipsychotic effect. There is also evidence that phenothiazines and haloperidol can inhibit the biotransformation of tricyclic antidepressants and vice versa. CNS depressants such as barbiturate narcotics and anesthetics and anticholinergics such as atropine should not be used or be used very cautiously in patients taking neuroleptics because of additive effects. Chlorpromazine has been shown to depress the level of alcohol dehydrogenase, causing increasing blood levels of ethanol.

The concurrent administration of antidiarrheal mixtures or a colloidal antacid such as aluminum hydroxide gel with chlorpromazine could decrease the absorption of chlorpromazine and lead to reduced plasma levels. Similarly, the combination of a potent anticholinergic agent and chlorpromazine could decrease chlorpromazine plasma levels by decreasing gastric motility and allowing more chlorpromazine to be biotransformed in the gastrointestinal tract before it is absorbed. By an unknown mechanism, caffeine can diminish the antipsychotic effect of the drugs, so drinks containing caffeine should not be taken. Phenothiazines can block the therapeutic response to levodopa in patients with parkinsonism by blocking dopamine receptors at the target sites. These drugs can also interact with guanethidine and negate its antihypertensive action. The combination of methyldopa with phenothiazines can lead to a decreased antihypertensive effect. When epinephrine is used with phenothiazines there is predominant activity of beta receptors because alpha receptors are blocked by the later drug. This can be dangerous, and so epinephrine should be avoided. Propranolol and phenothiazine together increase plasma levels of both drugs by an unknown mechanism. Cardiac depression caused by quinidine can be enhanced by phenothiazines. Encephalopathy has been reported in a few patients receiving both haloperidol and lithium carbonate. When the phenothiazines are administered along with lithium, the phenothiazine blood level decreases. Phenytoin toxicity may be increased by phenothiazines via altered hepatic metabolism.

Contraindications

Phenothiazine antipsychotics are contraindicated in individuals with previous hypersensitivity reactions to these agents. The possibility of cross-sensitivity among various phenothiazines exists. All antipsychotic compounds are contraindicated in comatose patients or those with CNS depression due to alcohol or other centrally acting depressants. The presence of liver disease or bone marrow depression is a relative contraindication to the use of these agents. The more potent agents should not be used in patients with Parkinson's disease of an extreme degree. Thioridazine should be avoided in patients with severe heart disease. The drugs should be avoided in children suspected to have Reye's syndrome since confusion may arise between the disease and the extrapyramidal symptoms produced by the drug.

The safety of all antipsychotic compounds for use during pregnancy has not been established. Therefore, these drugs should be given to pregnant patients only when, in the judgment of the physician, the expected benefits from treatment exceed the possible risks to mother and fetus.

THIOXANTHENE DERIVATIVES

Structurally, the thioxanthenes differ from phenothiazines only in that they have a carbon in place of a nitrogen in the center ring. Chlorprothixene, the first clinically successful thioxanthene, and thiothixene are very similar pharmacologically to their corresponding phenothiazine analogs. They have the same mechanism of action and similar effects on the central and peripheral nervous systems. They differ quantitatively. Chlorprothixene is as potent as chlorpromazine as an antipsychotic drug. Compared to chlorpromazine, chlorprothixene produces the same degree of sedation, extrapyramidal symptoms, anticholinergic effects, and orthostatic hypotension. Thiothixene is more potent an antipsychotic than chlorprothixene. It causes less sedation but has more extrapyramidal effects. Thiothixene also causes fewer anticholinergic and orthostatic hypotensive effects.

Thiothixene is rapidly absorbed, and peak plasma levels are obtained in 1 to 2 h. The drug has a half-life of 34 h.

BUTYROPHENONE DERIVATIVES

Although the butyrophenone dervatives have pharmacologic properties which are very similar to those of the phenothiazines and thioxanthenes, they are chemically quite different. Haloperidol, a potent butyrophenone antipsychotic agent, has the following structure:

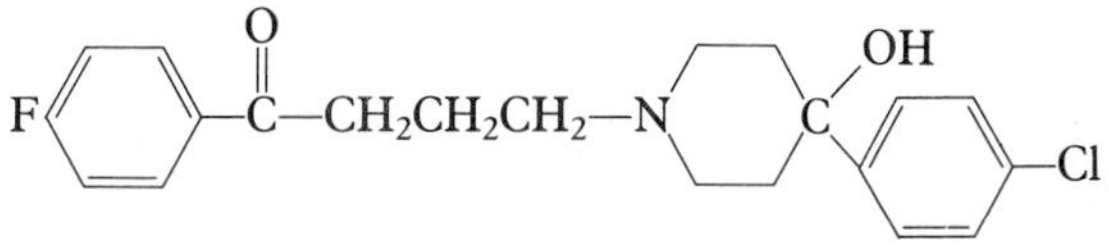

Haloperidol has a mechanism of action that is identical with that of the phenothiazines, that is, blockade of dopaminergic receptors. However, it is more selective for D_2 receptors. Haloperidol has good oral absorption with peak plasma levels in 3 to 6 h. It has an

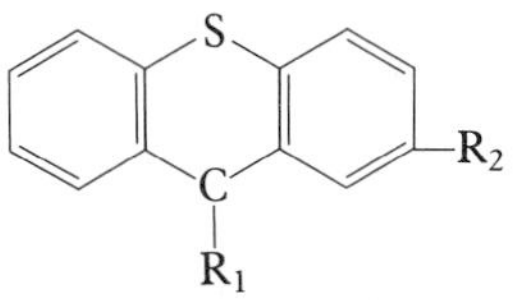

Generic name	R_1	R_2
Chlorprothixene	$=CH—CH_2—CH_2—N(CH_2)_2$	Cl
Thiothixene	$=CH—CH_2—CH_2—N$⬠$N—CH_3$	$\begin{array}{c} O \\ \uparrow \\ S—N(CH_3)_2 \\ \downarrow \\ O \end{array}$

elimination half-life of 12 to 20 h. The major metabolites are inactive. Approximately 40 percent of the drug is eliminated in the urine unchanged. Correlation of haloperidol blood levels and therapeutic effect is poor.

Haloperidol has similar pharmacodynamic properties to chlorpromazine (see Table 19-2). It is more potent as an antipsychotic drug than chlorpromazine. It produces weaker sedative, anticholinergic effects and orthostatic hypotension than chlorpromazine. Haloperidol, however, produces greater incidence of extrapyramidol reactions. Haloperidol is indicated for the treatment of psychosis associated with schizophrenia or acute delirium. It is also used as an adjunct in the therapy of the manic phase of manic depression. It is also useful in suppressing the symptoms (tics and vocal utterances) of Gilles de la Tourette's syndrome. The drug can be used in hyperactive children showing excessive motor activity with conduct disorder. Neuroleptics should be used in children only after failure of psychotherapy and other medications. It has also been used as an adjunct to narcotics in the therapy of chronic pain.

DIHYDROINDOLONE DERIVATIVE

Molindone is a dihydroindolone drug whose structure is unrelated to the phenothiazines, the butyrophenones, or the thioxanthenes.

It has a mechanism of action which is similar to that of the phenothiazines. Molindone is more potent as an antipyschotic drug when compared with chlorpromazine (see Table 19-2). It produces less sedation, anticholinergic effects, and orthostatic hypotention but possesses greater extrapyramidal activity than chlorpromazine. It is well absorbed orally with peak levels reached in 30 to 60 min. It is believed to be metabolized in the liver and has 36 recognizable metabolites. The metabolites are excreted in the urine. Less than 3 percent of the parent drug is excreted in the

urine. Elimination by hemodialysis or peripheral dialysis is insignificant.

The adverse reactions and therapeutic uses are similar to the phenothiazines.

DIBENZOXAZEPINE

Loxapine is a dibenzoxazepine compound which represents a tricyclic antipsychotic agent similar to the phenothiazines.

The mechanism of action is identical with that of the phenothiazines. Loxapine is more potent as an antipsychotic drug than chlorpromazine. It induces less sedation, anticholinergic effects, and orthostatic hypotension but has greater extrapyramidal activity than chlorpromazine. The drug is completely absorbed orally, and after absorption it is rapidly distributed to tissues. The drug has a half-life of 6 to 8 h. It is metabolized in the liver and has conjugated and unconjugated metabolites. The conjugated metabolites are excreted in the urine, while unconjugated metabolites are excreted in the feces.

The adverse reactions and uses of loxapine are identical with those of the phenothiazines.

DIPHENYLBUTYLPIPERIDINES

Pimozide is a diphenylbutylpiperidine, which is used for patients having uncontrolled Tourette's syndrome.

The drug has a number of side effects, many of which are similar to the phenothiazines. In addition to the extrapyramidal symptoms, neuroleptic malignant syndrome, tardive dyskinesia, and allergies, it can cause prolongation of ST, flattening or inversion of T wave, nausea, vomiting, dizziness, blurred vision, chest pain, periorbital edema, and urinary frequency. The mechanism of action, although largely unknown, is believed to be by its blocking action on dopaminergic activity. The use of the drug is contraindicated in patients having hypersensitivity, CNS depression, prolonged QT or cardiac arrhythmias, in patients taking drugs known to cause motor tics, and in patients having tics from disorders other than Tourette's syndrome.

Preparations and Doses

Phenothiazine Derivatives *Chlorpromazine* (Thorazine) is available in tablets, 10, 25, 50, 100, and 200 mg; suppositories, 25 and 100 mg; sustained-release capsules, 30, 75, 150, 200, and 300 mg; solutions (oral use), 30 mg/mL: injection, 25 mg/mL, 50 mg in 2 mL, and 250 mg in 10 mL; syrup, 2 mg/mL.

Fluphenazine (Permitil, Proloxin) is available in tablets, 0.25, 1, 2.5, 5, and 10 mg; extended-action tablets, 1 mg; elixir, 0.5 mg/mL; solution (injection), 25 mg in 10 mL. Fluphenazine decanoate and enanthate are also available in 1- and 5-mL vials at 25 mg/mL.

Prochlorperazine (Compazine) is available in tablets, 5, 10, and 25 mg; solution (injection), 10 mg in 2 mL, and 50 mg in 10 mL; syrup, 1 mg/mL; suppositories, 2.5, 5, and 25 mg; sustained-release capsules, 10, 15, 30, and 75 mg.

Promazine (Sparine) is available in tablets, 10, 25, 50, 100, and 200 mg; solution (injection), 50 mg in 1, 2, and 10 mL, and 250 and 500 mg in 10 mL; syrup, 2 mg/mL.

Thioridazine (Mellaril) is available in tablets, 10, 15, 25, 50, 100, 150, and 200 mg; solution (oral), 30 and 100 mg/mL.

Trifluoperazine (Stelazine) is available in tablets, 1, 2, 5, and 10 mg; solution (injection), 20 mg in 10 mL, and 10 mg/mL; dosage.

Triflupromazine (Vesprin) is available in tablets, 10, 25, and 50 mg; solution (injection), 10 and 20 mg in 1 mL.

Chlorprothixene (Taractan) is available in capsules, 1, 2, 5, 10, and 20 mg; solution (injection) 5 mg/mL and 4 mg in 2 mL.

Haloperidol (Haldol) is available in tablets, 0.5, 1, 2,

5, and 10 mg; oral concentrate 2 mg/mL; solution (injection), 5 mg/mL and 50 mg in 10 mL.

Molindone (Moban, Lidone) is available in tablets, 5, 10, and 25 mg.

Loxapine (Daxolin, Loxitane) is available in capsules, 5, 10, 25, and 50 mg; solution, 25 mg/mL.

Pimozide (Orap) is available as 2-mg tablets.

LITHIUM CARBONATE

Bipolar affective disorder is a mental disorder which combines episodes of mania and depression. The mania is characterized by elation of mood, grandiosity, and hyperactivity. It may either precede or follow a period of normal mood or a depressed phase. Lithium is indicated for the control of the manic episodes of manic-depressive illness. The drug is also used as a maintenance treatment for bipolar disorders in order to reduce frequency and intensity of the mania episodes. This is the only FDA approved use of this agent.

Lithium is a monovalent cation that belongs chemically to the same family as sodium and potassium. It has similarities to calcium and magnesium.

Mechanism of Action

In normal situations, therapeutic levels of lithium have no sedative, depressant, or euphoric effects on the central nervous system.

Lithium is absorbed and apparently exerts its effects as the lithium ion. Lithium as an ion increases neuronal re-uptake of norepinephrine and serotonin. Electrolytes may play a key role in maintaining the synthesis, storage release and inactivation of neurotransmitters. Lithium could induce changes in these electrolytes, which may induce changes of neurotransmitters such as mentioned previously with norepinephrine and serotonin.

Pharmacokinetics

Absorption, Distribution, and Elimination Absorption of lithium carbonate is virtually 100 percent. Food does not impair this absorptive process. Peak serum levels are reached in 2 to 4 h with complete absorption in 8 h. Average serum half-life is approximately 24 h; steady state is reached within 5 to 7 days.

Lithium is not bound to plasma proteins or metabolized but is freely filtered through the glomerular membrane. The volume of distribution is equal to that of total body water. When steady state is reached, the concentration in the cerebrospinal fluid is about 40 to 50 percent of the concentration in plasma. The therapeutic serum level ranges from 0.4 to 1.0 meq/L. Adverse and toxic reactions usually occur when serum lithium levels exceed 2 meq/L. Approximately 95 percent of a single dose of lithium is eliminated in the urine. About 80 percent of filtered lithium is reabsorbed by the renal tubules; lithium clearance by the kidney is about 20 percent of that for creatinine, ranging between 15 and 30 mL per minute. This is lower in elderly persons and in patients with renal impairment.

Adverse Effects

Adverse reactions are seldom seen when lithium levels are below 2 meq/L but can be observed in patients sensitive to the drug. Blood samples for serum lithium levels should be drawn prior to the next dose. Levels should be determined daily until serum levels are stabilized. The following reactions have been reported to be related to serum lithium levels, including therapeutic levels:

Neuromuscular/central nervous system   tremor, muscle hyperirritability (fasciculations, twitching, clonic movements of whole limbs), ataxia, choreoathetotic movements, hyperactive deep tendon reflex, extrapyramidal symptoms, blackout spells, epileptiform seizures, slurred speech, dizziness, vertigo, incontinence of urine or feces, somnolence, psychomotor retardation, restlessness, confusion, stupor, coma, tongue movements, tics, tinnitus, hallucinations, poor memory, slowed intellectual functioning, startled response.

Cardiovascular   Cardiac arrhythmia, hypotension, peripheral circulatory collapse, bradycardia.

Gastrointestinal   Anorexia, nausea, vomiting, diarrhea, gastritis, salivary gland swelling, abdominal pain, excessive salivation, flatulence, indigestion.

Genitourinary   Albuminuria, oliguria, polyuria, glycosuria, decreased creatinine clearance.

Dermatologic   Drying and thinning of hair, alopecia, anesthesia of skin, chronic folliculitis, xerosis cutis, psoriasis or its exacerbation, itching, angioedema.

Autonomic   Blurred vision, dry mouth.

Thyroid abnormalities   Euthyroid goiter and/or hypothyroidism (including myxedema) accompanied by lower T_3 and T_4. ^{131}I uptake may be elevated. Paradoxically, rare cases of hyperthyroidism have been reported as diffuse nontoxic goiter with or without hypothyroidism.

EEG changes   Diffuse slowing, widening of the frequency spectrum, potentiation and disorganization of background rhythm.

EKG changes   Reversible flattening, isoelectricity, or inversion of T-waves.

Miscellaneous   Fatigue, lethargy, dehydration, weight loss, tendency to sleep, leukocytosis, headache, transient hyperglycemia, generalized pruritus with or without rash, cutaneous ulcers, albuminuria, worsening of organic brain syndrome, excessive weight gain, edematous swelling of ankles or wrists, thirst or polyuria, sometimes resembling diabetes insipidus, metallic taste, impaired or distorted taste, salty taste, swollen lips, tightness in chest, impotence/sexual dysfunction, swollen and/or painful joints, fever, polyarthralgia, dental caries.

A few reports have been received of the development of painful discoloration of fingers and toes and coldness of the extremities within one day of the starting of treatment with lithium. The mechanism through which these symptoms (resembling Raynaud's syndrome) developed is not known. Recovery followed discontinuance.

Lithium should generally not be given to patients with significant renal or cardiovascular disease, severe debilitation or dehydration, or sodium depletion, and to patients receiving diuretics, since the risk of lithium toxicity is very high in such patients. If the psychiatric indication is life-threatening, and if such a patient fails to respond to other measures, lithium treatment may be undertaken with extreme caution, including daily serum lithium determinations and adjustment to the usually low dose ordinarily tolerated by these individuals. In such instances, hospitalization is a necessity.

Chronic lithium therapy may be associated with diminution of renal concentration ability, occasionally presenting as nephrogenic diabetes insipidus, with polyuria and polydipsia. Such patients should be carefully managed to avoid dehydration with resulting lithium retention and toxicity. This condition is usually reversible when lithium is discontinued.

Morphologic changes with glomerular and interstitial fibrosis and nephron atrophy have been reported in patients on chronic lithium therapy. Morphologic changes have also been seen in manic depressive patients never exposed to lithium. The relationship between renal function and morphologic changes and their association with lithium therapy have not been established.

In humans, lithium carbonate may cause fetal harm when administered to a pregnant woman. Data from lithium birth registries suggest an increase in cardiac and other anomalies, especially Ebstein's anomaly. If this drug is used during pregnancy, or if a patient becomes pregnant while taking this drug, the patient should be apprised of the potential hazard to the fetus.

Drug Interactions

Acetazolamide, aminophylline, mannitol, sodium bicarbonate, and urea can substantially increase renal clearance of lithium.

Lithium excretion decreases with sodium depletion and increases when large doses of sodium chloride are given.

Long-term therapy with ethacrynic acid, furosemide, or thiazide diuretics has been shown to decrease renal clearance of lithium. Reduced urine output, paradoxical fluid retention, and a rise in serum lithium levels to toxic concentrations may occur during concomitant therapy. Dosage modification may be necessary. Spironolactone and triamterene appear to have little or no effect on lithium clearance.

Lithium may prolong the effects of neuromuscular blocking agents. Therefore neuromuscular blocking agents should be given with caution to patients receiving lithium.

Management of Intoxication

The best therapy is prophylactic avoidance of toxicity. Periodic serum lithium measurements are mandatory along with dosage adjustments. Ordinarily 6 days are required to stabilize the serum level after a change in dose.

Water and sodium intake must not be restricted at any time. Excessive sweating such as during exercise in hot weather may lead to lithium intoxication because of sodium and water loss.

Severe lithium intoxication is a medical emergency and requires hospitalization. Lithium and diuretics are to be discontinued immediately. The condition is treacherous and despite corrective measures may worsen. The primary aim of therapy is to restore water and sodium balance. This can be cautiously accomplished by mild diuresis and sodium infusion. Experience has shown that caution is to be exercised, and sometimes half-normal saline is a wiser choice.

In extreme cases hemodialysis is the preferred therapy. If this is not available peritoneal dialysis is a good substitute. Complete recovery may be prolonged, and some instability of water balance and renal and neurologic function may persist for weeks or months.

Doses and Preparations

Lithium carbonate is available as 300-mg tablets and 150-, 300-, and 600-mg capsules. It is also available as a syrup having 8 meq of lithium per 5 mL or 16 meq/mL.

BIBLIOGRAPHY

Carlton, P. L., and P. Manowitz: "Dopamine and Schizophrenia: An Analysis of the Theory," *Neurosci. Biobehav. Rev.*, **8**:137 (1984).

Delini-Stula, A.: "Neuroanatomical, Neuropharmacological and Neurobiochemical Target Systems for Antipsychotic Activity of Neuroleptics," *Pharmacopsychiat.* **19**:134 (1986).

DiPalma, J. R.: "Lithium Toxicity," *Am. Family Physician*, **36**:225–228 (1987).

Hashimoto, F., C. B. Sherma, and W. H. Jeffrey: "Neuroleptic Malignant Syndrome and Dopaminergic Blockade," *Arch. Intern. Med.*, **144**:629 (1984).

Hetmar, O., L. Clemmesen, J. Ladefaged, and O. J. Rafaelsen: "Lithium, Long-Term Effects on the Kidney III. Prospective Study," *Psychiat. Scand.*, **75**:251–258 (1987).

Hollister, L. E.: "Drug Treatment of Schizophrenia," *Psychiatric Clin. North Am.*, **7**:435 (1984).

Kishimoto, A.: "Longterm Prophylactic Effects of Carbamazepine in Affective Disorder," *Br. J. Psychiatry*, **143**:327 (1983).

Antidepressant Drugs

Alan Frazer and David J. Brunswick

Affective disorders, or disorders of mood, are a very common occurrence. At some time, almost everyone has felt "blue" or "down in the dumps." In most people, this mood state is quite transient (hours to several days) and can clearly be identified with some precipitating event. Therefore, it deserves emphasis that major affective disorder, which is the state of clinical depression for which antidepressant drugs should be prescribed, is a distinct psychiatric diagnosis which is not made on the basis of a transient dysphoric mood. Rather, the mood disturbance should be prominent and persistent and be accompanied by other symptoms like sleep disturbance, change in appetite, psychomotor disturbances, pervasive loss of interest of pleasure, feelings of worthlessness or guilt and even thoughts of death or suicide. The use of an antidepressant drug should be limited to patients with major affective disorder and not to those experiencing relatively transient feelings of sadness. The magnitude of importance can be realized by the fact that about 15 percent of adults in the United States may suffer from significant depressive symptomatology in any given year, and about 40 to 80 percent of suicides are by individuals who have a major affective disorder.

CLASSIFICATION

There are three classes of antidepressant drugs. They are the tricyclic antidepressants (TCAs), monoamine oxidase inhibitors (MAOIs), and a group of newly developed drugs which are heterogenous in structure and pharmacologic properties. This group of drugs is termed *second-generation*, or *atypical*, antidepressants (Fig. 20-1).

TRICYCLIC ANTIDEPRESSANTS

Chemistry

These drugs are the most commonly prescribed antidepressants and are tricyclic due to their similar three joined-ring structures as shown in Fig. 20-1. Their structures consist of two benzene rings attached to a central seven-membered ring. An amine-containing side chain is attached to the central ring. Based on the substituents on the terminal nitrogen, there are two classes of tricyclic antidepressants: the tertiary amines and the secondary amines. Examples of tertiary amines are imipramine, amitriptyline, trimipramine, and doxepin. Desipramine (also called desmethyl-imipramine), nortriptyline, and protryptyline are examples of secondary amines. The tricyclic antidepressants are closely related chemically to the phenothiazines, which are used widely as antipsychotic agents.

Mechanism of Action

The tricyclic compounds that are presented in this chapter are effective agents in the treatment of endogenous depression. Initially it was thought that depression may be a consequence of a reduction in biogenic amines such as norepinephrine and serotonin in the

I. TRICYCLIC ANTIDEPRESSANTS

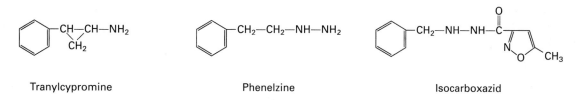

Imipramine

Amitriptyline

Trimipramine

Doxepin

Desipramine

Nortriptyline

Protriptyline

II. MONOAMINE OXIDASE INHIBITORS

Tranylcypromine

Phenelzine

Isocarboxazid

III. SECOND GENERATION ANTIDEPRESSANTS

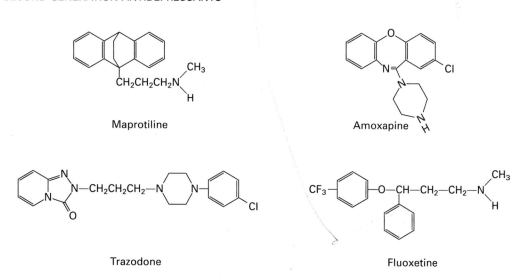

Maprotiline

Amoxapine

Trazodone

Fluoxetine

FIGURE 20-1 Chemistry of representative antidepressant drugs.

TABLE 20-1   Antidepressant drugs

Generic name	Trade name	Usual daily dose,[a] mg	Maximal daily dose, mg	Plasma elimination half-life
Tricyclics				
Amitriptyline	Amitril, Elavil, Endep, Enovil	75–150	300	10–25 h
Desipramine	Norpramin, Pertofrane	75–150	300	7–60 h
Doxepin	Adapin, Sinequan	50–150	300	8–25 h
Imipramine	Janimine, Tofranil	50–200	300	4–18 h
Nortriptyline	Aventyl, Pamelor	75–100	150	13–90 h
Protriptyline	Vivactil	15–40	60	2–5 days
Trimipramine	Surmontil	50–150	300	Similar to imipramine?
MAOIs				
Isocarboxazid	Marplan	10–30	40	?
Phenelzine	Nardil	45–60	90	1.5–4 h
Tranylcypromine	Parnate	20–30	60	1.5–3 h
Second generation				
Amoxapine	Asendin	200–300	600	Approx 8 h
Fluoxetine	Prozac	20–40	80	1–3 days
Maprotiline	Ludiomil	75–150	225	1.5–4.5 days
Trazodone	Desyrel	150–400	600	2–11 h

TABLE 20-1 (*continued*)   **Antidepressant drugs**

Active metabolite	Active metabolite plasma elimination half-life	Sedative or stimulant	Anticholinergic effect	Cardiovascular effects	
				Potential for ortho-static hypotension	Potential for condu-tion dis-turbance[b]
Nortriptyline	17–108 h	Sedating	Marked	High	High
—	—	Stimulant	Moderate	High	High
Desmethyl-doxepin	33–80 h	Sedating	Marked	High	High
Despiramine	13–62 h	Sedating	Marked	High	High
—	—	Neither	Marked	Low	High
—	—	Stimulant	Marked	High	High
Desmethyl-trimipramine	—	Sedating	Marked	High	High
—	—	Neither	None	High	None
—	—	Neither	None	High	None
—	—	Stimulant	None	High	None
8-OH-Amoxapine	Approx 30 h	Sedating	Moderate	Moderate to high	Moderate to high
Norfluoxetine	3–15 days	Stimulant	None	Low	None
—	—	Sedating	Moderate	Moderate to high	Moderate to high
m-Chlorophenyl-piperazine	—	Sedating	None	None	None

[a] Usual dosage range for depressed patients without other serious medical diseases. Adolescent, brain-injured, or elderly patients generally require lower doses.
[b] At usual therapeutic doses, drug-induced conduction disturbances are unlikely to be clinically significant in patients without preexisting cardiac disease. The entries in the table indicate the likelihood that a given drug will produce clinically significant disturbances in either high dosages or in patients with preexisting cardiac disease.

central nervous system. This assumption was based on the fact that certain drugs such as reserpine, which decreased biogenic amines in the brain, produced depression in patients as an adverse reaction. Studies showed that tricyclic antidepressants blocked the reuptake of norepinephrine and/or serotonin (Table 20-1) into the presynaptic nerve terminal, and this pharmacologic effect of tricyclic antidepressants, therefore, added support to the biogenic amine hypothesis that depression may be associated with a deficiency of norepinephrine and serotonin.

In order for the tricyclic antidepressants to start to alleviate depression in a patient, these drugs must be administered for 2 to 3 weeks; however, their ability to block the re-uptake of biogenic amines occurs immediately. It appears that some other biochemical events, although related to the increased presence of amines in the synapse, may be responsible for the antidepressant activity of these agents. Recent evidence indicates that chronic administration of tricyclic antidepressants blocks the re-uptake of biogenic amines and as a consequence of this blockade produces a down-regulation of beta-adrenergic and serotonin receptors that are present in the postsynaptic membrane. This down-regulation of biogenic amine receptors, which can cause a modification of cellular responses, is suggested as a mechanism of action of these antidepressants.

Another effect of the tricyclic antidepressants that may be involved in their therapeutic effect is their action on alpha$_2$-adrenergic receptor sites. These drugs may antagonize the effect of norepinephrine at the presynaptic alpha$_2$-adrenergic receptor and cause an enhanced release of norepinephrine from the adrenergic nerve terminal. This increased release of norepinephrine can possibly produce an eventual down-regulation of beta-adrenergic receptors.

It also should be mentioned that the antimuscarinic effect of some tricyclic antidepressants may contribute to their mechanism of action. By blocking the parasympathetic nervous system, there can be an increase in the activity of the sympathetic nervous system in the central nervous system. Some investigators have suggested that this antimuscarinic effect, if it occurs, plays a minor role in the overall antidepressant effect and is probably more so related to the adverse reactions produced by these drugs.

The mechanism of action of the tricyclic antidepressants is not completely known; it appears that the anti-depressant effect of these drugs is complex in nature and that at the present time no one hypothesis can fully explain their antidepressant effect.

Pharmacologic Effects

Antidepressant Effects   The antidepressant effects of the tricyclic drugs are not akin to the acute stimulant or mood-elevating effects produced by drugs such as amphetamine or methylphenidate in normal subjects. TCAs do not cause mood-elevating effects in nondepressed persons. The acute effect of the TCAs in normal subjects is sedation often accompanied by unpleasant anticholinergic effects. Repeated administration of these drugs to nondepressed subjects usually accentuates these symptoms and can lead to difficulty in concentrating. By contrast, repeated administration of the same drugs to depressed patients results in an elevation of mood. Thus, in contrast to stimulant drugs, the mood-elevating properties of antidepressants are dependent on the initial behavioral state. In general, this seems true for MAOIs as well, although tranylcypramine may have some stimulant properties, probably owing to its structural similarity to amphetamine. Further distinguishing antidepressants from stimulants is the fact that drugs such as amphetamine, cocaine, and methylphenidate are not effective antidepressants.

It is widely believed that the beneficial therapeutic effect of all types of chemical antidepressants takes 2 to 3 weeks before becoming evident. This lag period has been interpreted as indicating that there is a time delay in the onset of action of antidepressants. Although claims have been made that some of the newer second-generation compounds have a faster onset of action, there is no conclusive evidence that this is so. However, what most clinical trials also show is that there is clinical improvement in patients on an antidepressant drug within the first couple of weeks of treatment, but that the response to the antidepressant is no better than the response to placebo. From such data, it is difficult to determine when the *onset* of drug-induced antidepressant effects occurs. In reality, the lag period really seems to pertain to maximal therapeutic benefit with antidepressants in that all studies show that this takes 4 weeks or longer to occur. We still have no drug that rapidly produces maximal amelioration of depressive symptomatology.

Not all depressed patients respond equally well to the TCAs. Melancholic patients with symptoms such as loss of appetite and weight loss, early morning awakening, psychomotor retardation or agitation and lack of reactivity tend to respond well to TCAs. By contrast, depressions that are accompanied by delusions or hallucinations (i.e., psychotic depressions) tend to respond poorly to TCAs.

One final point about the clinical use of antidepressants is noteworthy. At least one-half of the individuals with an initial episode of major depression have at least one recurrence during their lifetime. There is an accumulating body of data that TCAs are effective in preventing or attenuating new episodes and are beginning to be used as preventative treatments. Also, patients are being continued on TCAs longer than they were previously to try to maintain control of an acute episode after the initial symptomatology has subsided. Such continuation treatment may often occur for up to 16 to 20 weeks. Because of this longer duration of treatment with TCAs, it is likely that all types of physicians will encounter patients being treated with these drugs in their clinical practices.

Anticholinergic Effects   Apart from antidepressant effects, the TCAs have anticholinergic effects such as dry mouth, constipation, mydriasis, blurred vision, and retention of urine. The degree of anticholinergic effect varies with the choice of drug (see Table 20-2).

Cardiovascular Effects   The most important and troublesome action is to produce orthostatic hypotension by blocking alpha$_1$-adrenergic receptors (Table 20-2). Although TCAs can cause severe arrhythmias in overdosage, they actually have strong antiarrhythmic activity at usual plasma concentrations. These effects are best documented for imipramine and nortriptyline but may pertain to the other TCAs as well. The antiarrhythmic activity seems mainly to be due to a direct action on the heart in that these drugs produce changes in the electrophysiologic profile like type 1 antiarrhythmic drugs such as quinidine. On the electrocardiogram these drugs can increase the PR interval and produce AV block and flattening or inversion of the T wave.

Pharmacokinetics

Following oral administration, the tricyclic antidepressants are absorbed relatively rapidly with peak plasma levels generally occurring within 2 to 4 h. Although absorption of tricyclic antidepressants from the gastrointestinal tract is complete, these drugs are not 100 percent bioavailable because the amount of drug is reduced by the hepatic "first-pass" effect. There is considerable intersubject and interdrug variability in the magnitude of the first-pass effect owing mainly to differences in the activity of the hepatic microsomal metabolizing enzymes. This appears to be of major importance in determining the steady-state concentration of drug for an individual. The tricyclic antidepressants are highly lipid-soluble drugs and are, therefore, widely distributed in the body. They are strongly bound to plasma proteins and to constituents of tissue. Blood levels are low (generally in the 20 to 300-ng/mL range), leading to large apparent volumes of distribution, typically 10 to 50 L/kg.

Tricyclic antidepressants are metabolized extensively by hepatic microsomal enzymes. Only small quantities of the tricyclics are excreted intact. A major pathway for the tertiary amine tricyclics is demethylation to the corresponding secondary amine; e.g., imipramine is demethylated to desipramine, amitriptyline to nortriptyline, and doxepin to desmethyldoxepin (see Table 20-1). Thus patients treated with tertiary amine tricyclics will be exposed, in addition, to the corresponding secondary amine metabolites, which themselves have antidepressant activity. (Desmethyldoxepin has antidepressant activity although it is not marketed as a separate drug, in contrast to desipramine and nortriptyline.) In some subjects, the extent of demethylation is so great that the predominant pharmacologically active compound present in the body in patients taking a tertiary amine tricyclic is the secondary amine metabolite. Since the demethylation reaction is not reversible, patients treated with a secondary amine tricyclic are exposed only to the parent compound and not to the corresponding tertiary amine. Thus patients treated with desipramine or nortriptyline are not exposed to imipramine or amitriptyline.

Hydroxylation on the ring structure is another important metabolic pathway for these drugs. The hydroxylated metabolites are excreted in urine, mainly in

TABLE 20-2   Potency of TCAs and second-generation antidepressants to block either monamine uptake or receptors

Drug	Monoamine uptake NE[a]	5-HT[b]	Histamine$_1$ receptors	Muscarinic receptors	Alpha$_1$ receptors	Serotonin$_2$ receptors
TCAs						
Amitriptyline	Low	Moderate	High	Moderate	Moderate	Moderate
Desipramine	High	Low	Moderate	Low	Low	Low
Doxepin	Low	Very low	Very high	Moderate	Moderate	Moderate
Imipramine	Moderate	Moderate	High	Moderate	Moderate	Moderate
Nortriptyline	High	Low	High	Low	Moderate	Moderate
Protriptyline	High	Low	Moderate	Moderate	Low	Moderate
Trimipramine	Very low	Very low	Very high	Moderate	Moderate	Moderate
2nd-Generation antidepressants						
Amoxapine	Moderate	Low	Moderate	Very low	Moderate	High
Fluoxetine	Low	Moderate	Very low	Very low	Very low	Low
Maprotiline	Moderate	Very low	High	Low	Moderate	Low
Trazodone	Very low	Low	Low	Very low	Moderate	High

[a] NE: norepinephrine.
[b] 5-HT: serotonin.

the form of their glucuronides. Other more relatively minor metabolic pathways for the tricyclics include loss of the side chain, oxidation of the amine group to form N oxides and demethylation of the secondary amine to form primary amines. With the possible exception of the N oxides, these pathways lead to inactive metabolites.

The half-lives of the different tricyclics vary widely, not only among themselves but also among individuals. Some estimates of these half-lives are shown in Table 20-1. In general, the half-lives of the secondary amine tricyclics are longer than those of the tertiary amine drugs. For the tertiary tricyclics, it is, however, important to consider not only the half-life of the parent compound but also the secondary amine metabolite. The rate of metabolism of tricyclic antidepressants varies widely among individuals. Differences in plasma levels of threefold and greater have been found among groups of patients treated with the same dose of tricyclic drug, and variations of five- to tenfold are relatively common. This variability arises primarily from genetic differences in the activity of the hepatic microsomal metabolizing enzymes. Interindividual differences in volume of distribution of drug also contribute to these variations. Additional factors may involve concurrent administration of other drugs and possibly smoking.

Adverse Effects

These drugs do produce prominent side effects. Most common are their antimuscarinic effects, which may be evident in over 50 percent of treated patients. Clinically, the antimuscarinic effects may manifest as dry mouth, blurred vision (due to loss of accommodation), constipation, tachycardia or palpitations, dizziness, and/or urinary retention. Such side effects may be nothing more than bothersome in young, depressed adults who are otherwise healthy but can be intolerable in the elderly. The anticholinergic properties of the TCAs can precipitate an acute confusional state in the elderly. Also, constipation can lead to fecal impaction, or acute glaucoma may be precipitated in the presence of a narrow-angle glaucoma. As depression is one of the most common psychiatric disorders in the elderly, with prevalence rates of from 2 to 18 percent, antidepressants with minimal anticholinergic effects may be of particular use in this patient population (see Table 20-2).

In addition to antimuscarinic effects, the TCAs can cause cardiovascular side effects. In otherwise healthy individuals, perhaps the most clinically significant cardiovascular effect is orthostatic hypotension, due, at least partly, to the alpha$_1$-adrenergic blocking properties of the TCAs (see Table 20-1). There is some evidence that nortriptyline may cause less orthostatic hypotension than imipramine. Changes in myocardial conduction are caused also by the TCAs. At "therapeutic" plasma concentrations, these drugs usually do not cause changes in the electrocardiogram (EKG). However, at plasma concentrations only moderately higher than the usual "therapeutic" ones, these drugs will increase the PR interval because of an increase in intraventricular conduction time (i.e., the HV interval). These drugs also cause an inversion or flattening of the T wave. In depressed patients with normal cardiac conduction, the changes in cardiac conduction caused by the TCAs are, in the main, not clinically significant. However, there is an increased tendency for patients with preexisting cardiac conduction disease to develop AV block when treated with a TCA.

The direct cardiac effects of the TCAs are important in overdosage, as death from these agents can result from heart block and/or arrhythmias. Unfortunately, overdosage is not an uncommon event, since these drugs are prescribed for depressed patients, some of whom may be suicidal. The third most common cause of drug-related death is alcohol-drug combinations and heroin. Symptoms of TCA overdosage include slurred speech, confusion, coma, tachycardia, hypotension, respiratory distress, conduction delays, and seizures. Such symptoms may persist for days, given the relatively long half-lives of the TCAs. Treatment should be directed at removal of the drug from the stomach and support of vital functions.

There are a number of central side effects produced by the TCAs that are clinically significant. These drugs lower the seizure threshold and can increase the risk of tonic-clonic seizures. Other CNS effects may include confusion or delirium, and a fine tremor may be produced in some patients, especially the elderly. Many of the TCAs are sedative, presumably because of either their strong antihistaminic and/or alpha$_1$-adrenergic antagonist properties (see Table 20-2). In depressives with the diagnosis of bipolar illness, TCAs can precipitate the transition from depression into mania or hypomania, the so-called switch process. Because of this, caution should be exercised in prescribing TCAs to bipolar patients not taking lithium carbonate or to first-time depressives with a strong family history of mania or hypomania. Although not a side effect, it should be noted that the TCAs cause changes in the characteristic stages of sleep, in particular an increase in stage 4 sleep and a very marked decrease in time spent in paradoxical, or rapid-eye-movement (REM), sleep.

Finally, the safety of these drugs during pregnancy or in the treatment of young children is not well established. Although there are no convincing data linking TCAs with teratogenic effects, it is advisable when possible to avoid the use of TCAs in the first trimester of pregnancy.

Drug Interactions

A number of drug interactions involving the tricyclic antidepressants are of potential importance. Tricyclic antidepressants block the antihypertensive effects of guanethidine and similarly acting agents by blocking their uptake into adrenergic neurons. They also block the centrally mediated antihypertensive effect of cloni-dine. The tricyclic antidepressants potentiate the ef-fects of sympathomimetic agents such as norepineph-rine and epinephrine, which are normally inactivated by neuronal uptake; these effects can be severe. In contrast, they block the effects of indirectly acting sympathomimetic agents, such as tyramine, which must be taken up into neurons to cause release of nor-epinephrine. Tricyclic antidepressants may potentiate the effects of CNS depressants such as alcohol, seda-tives, or hypnotics. Barbiturates stimulate the metabo-lism of the tricyclic antidepressants and hence reduce plasma levels. The clinical importance of this effect has not been demonstrated. Benzodiazepines do not appear to affect the metabolism of the tricyclic antide-pressants. Concurrent administration of amitriptyline and ethychlorvynol has been reported to produce tran-sient delirium. Although monoamine oxidase inhibi-tors and tricyclic antidepressants can be administered together safely in the majority of patients, these drugs, when coadministered, have been occasionally reported to produce severe CNS toxicity, including hyperpy-rexia, convulsions, and coma. It is generally recom-mended that these drugs not be given together and that at least 2 weeks separate the initiation of the ad-ministration of tricyclic antidepressants following ter-mination of monamine oxidase therapy. Conversely, it is generally recommended that monoamine oxidase inhibitors not be administered until 7 to 10 days fol-lowing tricyclic antidepressant therapy. The anticho-linergic effects of the tricyclic antidepressants may delay gastric emptying; this can result in substantial inactivation in the stomach of drugs such as levodopa and phenylbutazone, which are absorbed from the in-testine. A number of drugs increase plasma levels of the tricyclic antidepressants by inhibiting the activity of the hepatic microsomal metabolizing enzymes. Most neuroleptics increase tricyclic plasma levels, and this has occasionally been associated with ECG changes (AV block or changes associated with myocar-dial ischemia). Other drugs which have been demon-strated to increase tricyclic plasma levels are methyl-phenidate and cimetidine. Whereas the clinical significance of these effects has not been demonstrated conclusively, it would be expected that drugs that in-hibit the metabolism of tricyclics would decrease the dose of tricyclic necessary for beneficial therapeutic effect.

MONOAMINE OXIDASE INHIBITORS

These drugs appear to act by combining irreversibly with the enzyme monoamine oxidase, thereby inacti-vating it. Phenelzine, isocarboxazide, and tranylcy-promine are the only three monoamine oxidase inhibi-tors available in the United States.

Chemistry

Phenelzine is the hydrazine analog of phenyleth-ylamine. Isocarboxazide is a hydrazide derivative which appears to act as a prodrug for the correspond-ing hydrazine derivative. Tranylcypromine is *trans*-2-phenylcyclopropylamine, a cyclopropyl analog of phenethylamine and amphetamine; it consists of a ra-cemic mixture (see Fig. 20-1).

Mechanism of Action

The monoamine oxidase inhibitors used in clinical practice—phenelzine, isocarboxazid, and tranylcy-promine—inhibit monoamine oxidase by forming covalent bonds at the active site of the enzyme. Phen-elzine inactivates MAO by reacting with the flavin prosthetic group of the enzyme. Isocarboxazid appears to act in a similar manner following its initial conver-sion to an active hydrazine intermediate. Inactivation of MAO by tranylcypromine appears to involve reac-tion of an activated intermediate with a group (proba-bly a sulfhydryl group) in the active site of the enzyme itself.

The MAOIs increase the availability of endogenous amines such as norepinephrine and serotonin in the central nervous system by inhibiting intracellular de-amination of these amines, and their antidepressant effect might result from this inhibitory action. Al-though these antidepressants inactivate MAO almost immediately and their maximum effect on the enzyme occurs within 24 to 48 h, the therapeutic effect from administration of these drugs is not observed for about 2 to 3 weeks. Like the tricyclic antidepressants, one hypothesis for the mechanism of action of the MAOI antidepressants suggests that chronic administration of these drugs increases the concentration of biogenic amines in the synapse and causes eventually a downregulation of the beta-adrenergic and serotonin receptors in the postsynaptic membrane. Although downregulation of biogenic amine receptors might play a role in the antidepressant effect of MAOI, it appears that their mechanism of action is complex and not completely understood at the present time.

The MAOI tranylcypromine possesses two modes of action. The first is due to its potent inhibition of MAO, and the second is the result on amphetamine-like action. The latter effect has been attributed to the release of norepinephrine from central neurons.

The more rapid onset of action of tranylcypromine may be a consequence of its amphetamine-like action, and its sustained antidepressant effects are related to the biochemical events produced by the inhibition of MAO. This nonhydrazide derivative has sometimes been referred to as a bimodal antidepressant.

Pharmacokinetics

Surprisingly little is known about the metabolism and pharmacokinetics of the monoamine oxidase inhibitors due, in part, to the fact that these drugs received FDA approval before 1962, a time when such detailed studies were not required. Despite extensive clinical use for over 20 years, the metabolism of phenelzine is poorly understood. Although the effects of phenelzine on monoamine oxidase are long-term, the drug itself is rapidly absorbed following dosing orally and is rapidly cleared from plasma (half-life, 1.5 to 4 h) (see Table 20-1). Until recently, it had been thought that acetylation represented the major pathway for drug inactivation. However, more recent studies have failed to find the acetylated derivative in plasma or urine, and it appears now that oxidation rather than acetylation is the major metabolic pathway for this drug. The major metabolic products are phenylacetic acid and *para*-hydroxyphenylacetic acid. The drug may inhibit somewhat its own metabolism, since steady-state plasma concentrations gradually increase over the initial 5 to 8 weeks of chronic treatment.

Tranylcypromine is absorbed rapidly with peak levels occurring 40 min to 3.5 h after each dose. Elimination is also rapid with a half-life of from 1.5 to 3 h. Essentially little or no information is available on the pharmacokinetics of isocarboxazid.

Adverse Effects

Some of the side effects caused by MAOIs are similar to those produced by the TCAs. For example, orthostatic hypotension is produced by MAOIs. The hypo-

tensive effect has been attributed to either (1) heightened stimulation of central alpha$_2$-adrenoceptors due to the buildup of NE in brain, which can lead to a reduction in sympathetic outflow from the CNS or (2) the accumulation of the "false transmitter" octopamine in sympathetic nerve terminals, with the displacement of NE from the same terminals. Octopamine has much less of an effect at alpha$_1$-adrenoceptors than does NE, and consequently sympathetic tone is diminished. In addition, the MAOIs may also precipitate hypomanic or manic episodes in bipolar depressives. Again similar to the TCAs, inhibitors of MAO produce very marked reductions in the time spent in REM sleep.

Other clinically significant side effects caused by these drugs include excessive weight gain, sexual dysfunction, insomnia, and bipedal edema. As opposed to TCAs, inhibitors of MAO do not seem to have any important direct cardiac effects or prominent anticholinergic effects. Because of this, their use is increasing in the treatment of the elderly depressive.

MAOIs can elicit a hypertensive crisis, and this has, perhaps unduly, led practitioners to avoid their use. Oftentimes, the high blood pressure elicits a headache which may be associated with sweating, pallor, nausea, and vomiting. These painful, frightening attacks usually end in several hours. However, more serious and even fatal syndromes can develop, such as intracranial hemorrhage. The MAOI-induced hypertensive crises result from the ingestion of foodstuffs containing agents that can cause the release of stored NE, i.e., indirectly acting sympathomimetic amines such as tyramine, a substance containing tyramine increase. This substance is normally metabolized by MAO in the gastrointestinal tract and does not enter into the circulation in appreciable amounts. However, when MAO is inhibited, tyramine enters the circulation to release greater than normal amounts of NE stored in sympathetic nerve terminals and the adrenal medulla. Foodstuffs such as aged and overripe cheeses, certain prepared meats such as chicken liver pâté, smoked meats such as sausages, preserved foods such as pickled herring, broad bean pods, and certain yeast products contain a variety of indirectly acting sympathomimetic amines. For this reason, patients treated with MAOIs are placed on diets which either eliminate entirely or reduce substantially such foodstuffs. Perhaps even more problematic for patients on MAOIs are sympathomimetic drugs contained in over-the-counter medications (see "Drug Interactions," below).

Documented deaths due to overdosage with MAOIs have been infrequent. However, overdosage with these drugs can cause a toxic syndrome characterized by altered mental status, hyperpyrexia, and hyperreflexia, which may progress to metabolic acidosis, seizures, and cardiovascular collapse. Treatment of this state is primarily supportive in nature and should include procedures to reduce or retard further drug absorption.

Drug Interactions

The hypertensive effects of sympathomimetic agents during monoamine oxidase inhibitor therapy can be potentiated. This effect is greater with indirectly acting amines than with directly acting amines. Significant interactions have been observed with both centrally acting sympathomimetics or peripherally acting agents including nonprescription or prescription cold remedies that contain pressor agents. Parenteral administration of guanethidine with a MAOI may cause a severe pressor response as a result of a sudden release of accumulated catecholamines. It is generally recommended that MAOIs not be administered concurrently with levodopa, since agitation and hypertension can result. It is also recommended that CNS depressants be administered cautiously to patients receiving MAOIs to avoid excessive sedation and acute hypotension. The hypotensive and CNS depressant effects of general and local anesthetics may also be enhanced in patients taking MAOIs. Meperidine should not be given to patients on MAOIs, since a rapid hyperpyrexic reaction, which appears to be mediated via serotonin release, can occur. Finally, a period of at least 2 weeks is recommended when switching from one MAOI to another.

SECOND GENERATION ANTIDEPRESSANTS

A number of compounds which are neither tricyclic antidepressants nor monoamine oxidase inhibitors have been demonstrated to be effective antidepressants. These compounds are termed *second-generation*, or *atypical*, antidepressants. Four such drugs—

amoxapine, fluoxetine, maprotiline, and trazodone—are currently approved for use as antidepressants in the United States (see Fig. 20-1).

Chemistry

Amoxapine is sometimes included in the category of tricyclic antidepressants. However, its structure is somewhat different from that of the tricyclics. Amoxapine is a dibenzoxazepine derivative with a side chain that contains a piperidine group. Fluoxetine is a phenylpropylamine derivative, and trazodone is a triazolopyridine derivative. Fluoxetine and trazodone are chemically unrelated to other antidepressants. Fluoxetine is a secondary amine, whereas trazodone is a tertiary amine. Maprotiline is a secondary amine that is also closely related in structure to the tricyclic antidepressants; it has a four-ring "bridged" structure rather than the three-ring structure of the tricyclics.

Mechanism of Action

Among the second-generation antidepressants, maprotiline and amoxapine are selective inhibitors of the uptake of NE. Trazodone is a rather weak inhibitor of the uptake of 5-HT and actually is more potent as an antagonist at receptors for 5-HT (see Table 20-2). Fluoxetine, marketed as an antidepressant in the United States in 1988, is a potent selective inhibitor of the uptake of 5-HT. If these monoamine uptake inhibiting effects are related to the clinical efficacy of these drugs, it is noteworthy that primary actions on either NE or 5-HT uptake can result in an antidepressant effect.

Pharmacokinetics

Amoxapine is a lipophilic compound which is rapidly absorbed and reaches peak blood levels 1 to 2 h following oral administration. The elimination half-life of amoxapine is approximately 8 h. Amoxapine is metabolized by hydroxylation mainly at the 8-position ring structure with hydroxylation at the 7-position minor pathway. These hydroxy metabolites do possess pharmacologic activity and appear able to penetrate the brain to some extent. The 8-hydroxy metabolite has an elimination half-life of approximately 30 h. The relationship between amoxapine blood levels and clinical effect has not been established.

Fluoxetine is absorbed almost completely following oral administration although the rate of absorption is relatively show with maximal blood levels generally not seen until 4 to 8 h after dosing. Bioavailability is close to 100 percent, since the first-pass effect is small. Fluoxetine is a lipophilic compound which, like the tricyclics, is highly bound to plasma proteins and has a large apparent volume of distribution (averaging approximately 30 L/kg). Fluoxetine is demethylated hepatically to a pharmacologically active compound, norfluoxetine. The half-lives of fluoxetine and its normetabolite are long, with values reported in the range of 1 to 3 days for fluoxetine and 3 to 15 days for norfluoxetine. There is also some preliminary evidence that the half-life of fluoxetine increases on repeated administration of drug although the half-life of the metabolite does not appear to be affected. The long half-lives of fluoxetine and norfluoxetine are consistent with the clinical practice of prescribing this drug on a once-a-day dosing schedule. Only small amounts of fluoxetine and its normetabolite are excreted intact. Most of the compound is excreted in the form of conjugated metabolites whose identities have not yet been determined. Plasma levels of fluoxetine and its nonmetabolite vary widely between individuals, but it is not known whether these levels correlate with clinical response.

Maprotiline, like fluoxetine, is absorbed completely but relatively slowly. Maximal blood levels are not observed until 8 to 24 h after dosing. Also, like fluoxetine, the first-past effect is small for this drug, and plasma half-lives are relatively long, being in the range of 36 to 105 h. As in the tricyclics, steady-state levels of this drug vary widely among individuals. No consistent relationship has been demonstrated between plasma levels of the drug and clinical response.

Trazodone is absorbed relatively rapidly and almost completely. Maximal blood levels are generally found 30 min to 4 h after dosing. It is extensively bound to plasma proteins. Trazodone is metabolized extensively, mainly by oxidation and hydroxylation with a half-life of 2 to 11 h. Very little trazodone is excreted unchanged. The steady-state plasma levels of trazodone are somewhat higher than those found for the tricyclic antidepressants. Levels have been found to vary approximately eightfold among patients on the same dose but have not been demonstrated to differ between responders and nonresponders to the drug. Levels up to 5000 ng/mL have been well tolerated,

even in an elderly population. The principal metabolite in humans appears to be *meta*-clorophenyl-piperazine. It is not known if this or any other metabolite contributed to clinical activity.

Adverse Effects

The hopes for these drugs were that they would act quickly on a greater percentage of patients than the earlier-developed antidepressants, have fewer side effects, be safer in overdosage, and not have serious side effects. Although the second-generation antidepressants do not seem to be superior to TCAs or MAOIs with regard to clinical efficacy, some of these drugs do have a different profile of side effects than do the earlier antidepressants, which may make them particularly useful in certain patients.

None of these drugs are inhibitors of MAO, so they do not have the risk of precipitating a hypertensive crisis following the ingestion of certain foodstuffs. Although amoxapine and maprotiline have anticholinergic properties, trazodone and fluoxetine have little affinity for muscarinic receptors. When administered clinically, these latter two drugs produce the same incidence of anticholinergic side effects as seen upon administration of placebo. Also, neither trazodone nor fluoxetine seems to have any effect on the conduction system of the heart. Maprotiline seems to cause similar cardiac effects as TCAs do, whereas the effects of amoxapine may be slightly less but not as insignificant as those with trazodone or fluoxetine. Whereas maprotiline, amoxapine, and trazodone are sedating, similar to the more sedative TCAs like doxepin or amitriptyline, fluoxetine does not seem to have sedative properties (see Table 20-1). Rather, fluoxetine may produce nervousness and insomnia and have somewhat of a stimulant rather than a sedative profile.

These second-generation antidepressants do have some specific adverse effects that are either qualitatively or quantitatively unique in nature. For example, about 25 percent of patients taking fluoxetine experience nausea, and about 10 percent have diarrhea; weight loss with this drug may also occur. There does seem to be an increased risk for seizure development in patients treated with maprotiline, and certainly there is a greater incidence of seizures after overdosage with maprotiline than with other antidepressants. The incidence of seizures after overdosage with amoxapine is also relatively high. By contrast, the incidence of seizure development with either trazodone or fluoxetine is quite low, perhaps even lower than with the TCAs.

Among antidepressants, amoxapine is unique in having neuroleptic activity in vivo, presumably because of its structural relationship to the antipsychotic drug loxapine. Consequently, with the exception of trimipramine, this drug is more potent than other antidepressants in blocking D_2 dopamine receptors. Treatment with amoxapine can produce many of the movement disorders, e.g., dystonia, akathesia, akinesia, and parkinsonism, that can be associated with neuroleptic treatment. Amoxapine raises plasma concentrations of prolactin, which can lead to galactorrhea. It is interesting that trimipramine does not cause these effects even though it is as potent an antagonist of D_2 dopamine receptors as amoxapine. In comparison with amoxapine, trimipramine has greater affinity for muscarinic cholinergic receptors (see Table 20-2), and this might contribute to its lack of causing extrapyramidal effects.

Of serious concern with trazodone is that it can cause priapism (protracted and painful penile erection), a number of cases of which have required corrective surgery or caused permanent loss of erectile function.

The symptoms of overdosage with either trazodone or fluoxetine are somewhat more benign than with other antidepressants, and no deaths have been reported in cases when the patient took just trazodone or fluoxetine alone. By contrast, overdose with either maprotiline or amoxapine produces as serious sequelae as those seen upon overdosage with TCAs. Particularly troublesome with maprotiline is the high incidence of seizures (35 percent) and prolonged coma (72 h), which it causes in some patients. Overdosage with amoxapine can have acute renal failure as an associated complication.

Drug Interaction

Current data indicate that there are relatively few drug interactions involving fluoxetine. L-Tryptophan coadministration has been associated with increased agitation and restlessness. Fluoxetine is a potent inhibitor of the metabolism of many drugs in animals, but similar effects have not been observed in humans. Concurrent administration of alcohol and fluoxetine has not produced any evidence of potentiation.

Trazadone appears to potentiate, somewhat, the action of CNS depressants. Otherwise, significant drug interactions have not been demonstrated. It is not known whether interactions between trazodone and MAOIs can occur, although such an interaction appears unlikely.

AMOXAPINE AND MAPROTILINE

In general, amoxapine and maprotiline drugs have similar drug interaction profiles to the tricyclic antidepressants.

Therapeutic Uses

Antidepressant As stated previously, the use of these drugs should be restricted to patients having a psychiatric diagnosis of depression rather than a transient dysphoric mood.

The physician is faced with a choice from a number of drugs. The choice between MAOI and TCA would weigh in favor of the TCAs because of the risk of hypertensive crises with MAOI. However, many trials indicate that MAOI may be more effective in patients presenting with "atypical" depression.

While starting treatment with TCA, it is better to start with a lower dose and gradually to increase the dose until good clinical results are obtained in the absence of serious side effects. The TCAs have a sedative effect, so the dose is generally given at bedtime. Some drugs of the second generation are claimed to be faster-acting. Trazodone is relatively less toxic, except for some cases of priapism. For this purpose patients should be told to report immediately if they have a persistent, nonsexual excretion.

BIBLIOGRAPHY

Blackwell, B.: "Newer Antidepressant Drugs," in H. Y. Meltzer (ed.), *Psychopharmacology. The Third Generation of Progress*, Raven, New York, 1987, pp. 1041–1049.

Blier, P., C. de Montigny, and Y. Chaput: "Modifications of the Serotonin System by Antidepressant Treatments: Implications for the Therapeutic Response in Major Depression," *J. Clin Psychopharmacol.*, 7:24S–25S (1987).

Brotman, A. W., W. E. Falk, and Gelenberg A. J.: "Pharmacologic Treatment of Acute Depressive Subtypes," in

H. Y. Meltzer (ed.), *Psychopharmacology. The Third Generation of Progress*, Raven, New York, 1987, pp. 1031–1040.

Glassman, A. H., S. P. Roose, E.-G. V. Giardina, and J. T. Bigger, Jr.: "Cardiovascular Effects of Tricyclic Antidepressants," in H. Y. Meltzer (ed.), *Psychopharmacology. The Third Generation of Progress*, Raven, New York, 1987, pp. 1437–1442.

Heninger, G. R., and D. S. Charney: "Mechanism of Action of Antidepressant Treatments: Implications for the Etiology and Treatment of Depressive Disorders," in H. Y. Meltzer (ed.), *Psychopharmacology. The Third Generation of Progress*, Raven, New York, 1987, pp. 535–544.

Katz, M. M., S. H. Koslow, J. W. Maas, A. Frazer, C. L. Bowden, R. Casper, J. Croughan, J. Kocsis, and E. Redmond, Jr.: "The Timing, Specificity and Clinical Prediction of Tricyclic Drug Effects in Depression," *Psychol. Med.*, **17**:297–309 (1987).

Murphy, D. L., C. S. Aulakh, N. A. Garrick, and T. Sunderland: "Monamine Oxidase Inhibitors as Antidepressants: Implications for the Mechanism of Action of Antidepressants and the Psychobiology of the Affective Disorders and Some Related Disorders," in H. Y. Meltzer (ed.), *Psychopharmacology. The Third Generation of Progress*, Raven, New York, 1987, pp. 545–552.

Plotkin, D. A., C. Gerson, and L. F. Jarvik: Antidepressant Drug Treatment in the Elderly," in H. Y. Meltzer (ed.), *Psychopharmacology. The Third Generation of Progress*, Raven, New York, 1987, pp. 1149–1158.

Wander, T. J., A. Nelson, H. Okazaki, and E. Richelson: "Antagonism by Antidepressants of Serotonin S_1 and S_2 Receptors of Normal Human Brain in Vitro," *Eur. J. Pharmacol.*, **132**:115–121 (1986).

Antiepileptic and Antiparkinsonian Drugs

Neil M. Sussman

Epilepsy is a syndrome characterized by recurrent seizures, which can be described as paroxysmal alterations in behavior associated with abnormalities in the brain's electrical activity. Seizures are brief events lasting from seconds to several minutes. Epilepsy was described in ancient times and is a common illness affecting 0.5 to 1 percent of the population. Approximately 80 percent of patients with epilepsy can have their seizure frequency dramatically reduced by drug therapy. In those cases not adequately controlled by medication, surgical therapy may be an option.

With the large number of seizure types that can occur, an overview of the international classification of seizures helps in the communication among health care workers and between health care workers and patients. The classification which follows is a simplified version suitable for a rational approach to drug therapy.

I. Partial, or focal, seizures
   A. Simple partial seizures—motor or sensory (Jacksonian)
   B. Complex partial seizures
   C. Partial seizures (secondarily generalized)
II. Generalized seizures
   A. Tonic-clonic seizures—grand mal
   B. Absence seizures—petit mal
   C. Tonic seizures
   D. Atonic seizures

PARTIAL, OR FOCAL, SEIZURES

Focal seizures arise from one area of the brain. Occasionally they can arise from more than one particular focus. Wherever in the brain the seizures begin, the initial symptomatology is related to that area. For instance, if seizures start near the motor strip, clonic movements of the opposite limb, face, or tongue occur initially. The abnormal electrical discharges can then spread to involve the entire brain, producing a generalized seizure. According to the classification, this is a simple partial seizure evolving to a generalized tonic-clonic seizure (formerly called *Jacksonian epilepsy*). If the focus of the seizure is in the posterior temporal or occipital lobe, then visual hallucinations may occur. A seizure focus in the temporal lobe in the region of the hippocampus or amygdala (mesial surface) or frontal lobe can produce complex partial seizures. The term *complex* means that there is loss of awareness. A person in a complex partial seizure can wander about in a dazed state, picking at clothing, lip smacking, or having other stereotyped behaviors. After the seizure occurs, neurons are exhausted, and as a result the person may sleep or be confused.

GENERALIZED SEIZURES

Tonic-Clonic Seizures

Tonic-clonic seizures, or convulsions, have two phases. The tonic phase is related to rapid spikes on the EEG, and the person becomes stiff with stretched out arms and legs, not taking breaths, and unconscious, and the jaw is tightly closed. Tongue biting occurs with the initial jaw closure. Urinary or fecal incontinence may occur at this time as well. The person may fall and injure himself or herself. This phase lasts 20 to 40 s, and then the person enters the clonic phase, which is alternating relaxation with stiffening of the skeletal muscles. The EEG shows spike and slow wave complexes. The clonic phase lasts 20 to 40 s. Confusion or sleep follows the seizure.

Absence Seizures

Absence seizures are primarily encountered in childhood and have their onset in the first decade of life but may persist into adulthood and occasionally may begin after the age of 20. The attacks are characterized by sudden, brief lapses in consciousness which may be accompanied by clonic movements of the eyes, head, or extremities. Falling rarely occurs, but there may be staggering and drooping of the head or picking movements of the hands. The attack is brief, lasting 5 to 30 s. Afterward the patient is immediately alert and able to resume normal activity. These seizures can be induced in some cases by 3 to 5 min of hyperventila-

tion. Absence seizures can occur with great frequency many times per day. The EEG is normal between attacks and shows the generalized 3 per second spike and wave abnormality during the attack.

ANTIEPILEPTIC DRUGS

The antiepileptic drugs fall into basically two categories (Table 21-1)—those that are effective against absence seizures and those effective against tonic-clonic seizures.

Those antiepileptic drugs effective against the tonic-clonic and focal seizures include phenytoin, mephenytoin, ethotoin, carbamazepine, phenobarbital, and primidone. In the treatment of absence seizures, the following drugs are useful: ethosuximide, valproic acid, clonazepam, acetazolamide, trimethadione, and

TABLE 21-1 Selected antiepilepsy drugs

Name of drug	Usual dosages, mg/kg	Usual plasma levels, μg/mL	Half-life, h	Doses/day
Absence seizures				
Ethosuximide	10–20	40–120	60 ± 6	2
Valproic acid[a]	15–60	50–150	12 ± 6	3–4
Clonazepam	0.03–0.3	15–70	27 ± 5	2
Acetazolamide	10–15	10–15	1.5, 48	3
Trimethadione	20–40	10–40	16	2
Tonic-clonic and focal seizures				
Phenytoin	15–25	6–12	24 ± 6	3–4
Carbamazepine	4–6	10–25	14 ± 6	2
Phenobarbital 15, 30, 60 or 100 mg	2–4	15–40	96 ± 12	1
Primidone	1–20	5–12	6 ± 4	3–4

[a] Secondary drug for focal and tonic-clonic seizures.

par, paramethadione. In addition, valproic acid is considered to be a secondary drug for focal and tonic-clonic seizures. Only occasionally are drugs helpful in both categories.

Hydantoin Derivatives

The chemical structures of two hydantoins are shown in Table 21-2. It will be noted that they have five-membered rings, in contrast to the six-membered ring of the barbiturates (Table 21-3), which will be discussed later. Another point of difference lies in the absence of a C=O group in the ring structure. All the hydantoins are highly fat-soluble and essentially insoluble in water.

Phenytoin   In its overall effect on the central nervous system this drug comes close to being an ideal antiepileptic drug, since in full antiepileptic doses it has only minor sedative effects. Even in large doses it does not cause hypnosis.

Mechanism of Action   Certain aspects of the mechanism by which phenytoin causes a suppression of seizure spread have now been clarified to some extent. One current theory concerns the function of the PTP (posttetanic potential) in the spread of excitation throughout the cerebral cortex. At a focal point in the

TABLE 21-2   Hydantoin derivatives mainly effective in tonic-clonic seizures

Drug	R_1	R_2	R_3
Phenytoin (diphenylhydantoin)	(phenyl)	(phenyl)	—H
Mephenytoin	(phenyl)	—C_2H_5	—CH_3

cerebral cortex, where there is a rapid negative firing and rapid discharge of impulses (as in an epileptic focus), the spread of such excitation requires the formation of the PTP, which results in an enhancement of synaptic transmission. The PTP is an important mechanism in developing high-frequency trains of impulses for excitatory feedback circuits and in spreading impulses to other areas of the cortex. It is believed that phenytoin reduces the influx of sodium and calcium ions into neuronal fibers during depolarization of the action potential. In addition, phenytoin decreases the efflux of potassium ions during repolarization. The alteration in these ionic fluxes appears to inhibit the formation of the PTP, and consequently phenytoin retards significant spread of excitation throughout the brain.

Phenytoin may also have an influence on the gamma aminobutyric acid (GABA)-mediated transmission within the central nervous system. It is believed that the drug can interfere with GABA uptake and increase the sensitivity of the GABA receptor by inducing an increase in the number of GABA receptors. These actions result in an increase of GABAergic inhibition.

Pharmacokinetics   Phenytoin is readily absorbed from the gastrointestinal tract, reaching highest concentrations in the liver and central nervous system. Protein binding is approximately 90 percent. Mean plasma half-life is 24 ± 6 h. The half-life of phenytoin in the blood increases to 72 h if phenytoin levels go above 30 $\mu g/mL$, based on saturation kinetics. The steady-state level of phenytoin in plasma can be obtained in 5 days. Phenytoin is biotransformed by hydroxylation in the microsomal system in the liver. Biotransformation can be increased by drugs such as phenobarbital, which induces increased activity of hepatic microsomal enzymes. Drugs which appear to decrease phenytoin biotransformation include dicumarol and isoniazid.

One of the major metabolic pathways for disposition of phenytoin is parahydroxylation of one of the phenol groups, with subsequent glucuronic acid formation and excretion. The urinary output of this compound may account for 50 to 70 percent of the total amount of drug given, with the unchanged drug accounting for less than 5 percent. Some patients have been subject to adverse events on ordinary doses of the drug as a result of a defect in parahydroxylation or because of drug interactions mentioned above. Also side effects may occur at standard or conventional blood levels when the albumin is reduced considerably such as in kidney disease. The free or unbounded phenytoin would increase in relation to total phenytoin measured in the blood. When this occurs, measurement of unbound phenytoin as well as total phenytoin is helpful. Unbound phenytoin usually constitutes 10 percent of the total phenytoin.

Therapeutic Uses   The major clinical use of phenytoin is in the treatment of tonic-clonic epilepsy. Clinical response determines the dosage of antiepileptic medication. However, drug blood level measurements are helpful in the management of some patients, particularly those who do not respond to average or maximal doses and who manifest signs or symptoms of toxicity while receiving small or conventional doses of anticonvulsant agents. The usual therapeutic blood serum level of phenytoin is 10 to 20 μg/mL. Minor clinical usefulness of phenytoin is in cardiac arrhythmias and paroxysmal pain syndromes such as tic douloureux, phantom limb, or peripheral nerve damage.

Adverse Reaction   Side effects can occur in a paient at plasma levels of phenytoin greater than 20 μg/mL when it is used as the only agent. Patients experience ataxia, lack of coordination, diplopia, drowsiness, and nystagmus. Drowsiness can cause behavioral irritability. A skin rash is fairly common in as much as 5 percent of the patients. The drug should be stopped if a rash occurs, and another medication should be prescribed. Long continued use of phenytoin can lead to hyperplasia of the gums, especially in children and adolescents. The connective tissue and capillaries of the gums proliferate with no evidence of pain or inflammation. Often the subject is unaware that gum hyperplasia is occurring. The mechanism of action is unknown. There may be no improvement upon withdrawal of the drug. Hirsutism is another troubling symptom which is seen occasionally with this drug. Fortunately, phenytoin has rarely caused serious blood dyscrasias.

   A rare complication of phenytoin therapy is lymphadenopathy. The distribution of the lymphoid enlargement may closely resemble malignant lymphoma and is termed *pseudolymphoma*. All signs disappear with cessation of therapy. Other rare adverse reactions are megaloblastic anemia due to interference with the absorption of folic acid from the gastrointestinal tract. Folic acid supplementation corrects this anemia. Induction of antinuclear antibodies with a lupuslike syndrome and erythema multiforme exudativum occasionally occurs. Both may represent hypersensitivity reactions. Teratogenicity has been reported with phenytoin, but this remains controversial and the amount of teratogenicity may be related to the number of antiepilepsy drugs used rather than any particular one, except for trimethadione or paramethadione, which are clearly teratogenic. Neuropsychological tests for concentration, memory, and cognitive abilities show mild impairment with phenytoin use.

Mephenytoin

As seen in Table 21-2, mephenytoin differs in two respects from phenytoin. At position 5 an ethyl group is substituted for one of the phenyl rings; at position 3 a methyl group is added. These changes, while retaining the fundamental characteristics of phenytoin, make mephenytoin better tolerated than phenytoin but occasionally produce fatal blood dyscrasias.

   Depression of the bone marrow occurs occasionally. Patients on mephenytoin must have frequent blood counts. The half-life of the mephenytoin metabolite is 7 days. Once blood dyscrasias are found, in spite of stopping the drug, the metabolite remains in the system for several weeks.

Ethotoin

The third antiepileptic hydantoin derivative is ethotoin. It is less potent than phenytoin and also less toxic. It is a poor substitute for mephenytoin but is used when the person is allergic to phenytoin. Because the half-life is 4 h, it must be given 6 to 7 times a day.

Carbamazepine

Carbamazepine is an iminostilbene carboximide. This drug is emerging as the treatment of choice for focal epilepsy in the pediatric age group. Either carbamazepine or phenytoin is the treatment of choice for focal epilepsy in adults. It is the best tolerated of the antiepileptic drugs for focal and major motor seizures and has the least cognitive impairments as measured by

CONH$_2$

Carbamazepine

neuropsychologic tests. Carbamazepine is also used for paroxysmal pain disorders such as tic douloureux and may have some use in bipolar manic-type disorders.

Pharmacokinetics Carbamazepine is readily absorbed upon oral administration. Peak absorption is usually 6 to 8 h after administration. Its half-life in a chronically treated epileptic population is 14 ± 6 h. Volume of distribution of the drug is 1 L per kilogram of body weight. It is bound 70 percent to plasma proteins. After several months of use, the serum levels of carbamazepine decline slowly because it induces its own metabolism in the liver. The first metabolic product of carbamazepine is 10,11-dihydro derivative, which also possesses antiepileptic activity. This compound is inactivated by conjugation.

Adverse Reaction In high doses carbamazepine causes a reduction of granulocytes, almost invariably to blood levels of approximately 1000 granulocytes per cubic millimeter. The granulocytes rarely go below that level, and it is a dose-dependent phenomenon. Aplastic anemia has also been reported with carbamazepine, but the number of cases is so small that it may not be greater than the expected occurrence of aplastic anemia in a population not taking the drug. Other adverse reactions are urinary retention, impotence, and elevated blood pressure. Dose-related side effects are disequilibrium, drowsiness, blurred vision, and disturbances of coordination. Skin allergies to carbamazepine occur but are less frequent than with phenytoin.

Barbiturates

Phenobarbital Phenobarbital is the prototype barbiturate antiepileptic (Table 21-3). This drug is useful in the treatment of tonic-clonic seizures and simple partial seizures. Generally phenobarbital is given in combination with some other antiepileptic compound such a phenytoin. Recent evidence suggests that phe-

TABLE 21-3 Barbiturates and related compounds effective in tonic-clonic seizures

Compound	R$_1$	R$_2$	R$_3$
Phenobarbital	(phenyl)	—C$_2$H$_5$	—H
Mephobarbital	(phenyl)	—C$_2$H$_5$	—CH$_3$
Metharbital	—C$_2$H$_5$	—C$_2$H$_5$	—CH$_3$
Primidone[a]	(phenyl)	—C$_2$H$_5$	—H

[a] Not a barbiturate; replacement of C=O at position 2 by CH$_2$ changes ring to pyrimidine.

nobarbital is no longer the treatment of choice for any seizure-type, particularly in children, because the major problems with barbiturate use are sedation and cognitive impairment as measured by neuropsychologic tests.

The efficacy of phenobarbital as an antiepileptic agent may be related to its effects on GABAergic transmission in the central nervous system, in which it enhances the inhibitory action of GABA. In addition, this drug may reduce the effects of the excitatory amino acid glutamate. Which of these mechanisms is more important for antiepileptic activity has not been determined. In the treatment of epilepsy the dosage of phenobarbital is approximately 2 to 3 mg/kg with a usual therapeutic blood level of between 15 and 40 μg/mL. The half-life of the drug is 96 h in adults and 80 h in children. Plasma protein binding is in the range of 40 to 60 percent.

Adverse Reaction The toxicity of phenobarbital when used in epilepsy is the same as that when it is given as a general sedative and hypnotic. However, in epilepsy the drug is used for long periods of time (months and years); thus certain adverse effects are more likely to develop. Skin rashes may eventually occur even after the drug has been used for years. This requires withdrawal of the drug, for there is always the possibility of exfoliative dermatitis.

Sudden withdrawal of the drug from epileptic patients may precipitate seizures and occasionally leads to status epilepticus (repeated seizures without rest periods). For this reason barbiturates should be withdrawn slowly and replaced by other drugs to prevent this complication. Rarely do the usual doses employed in epileptic therapy lead to dependence or barbiturate "inebriation." Further information on phenobarbital is presented in Chap. 15.

Mephobarbital Mephobarbital (Table 21-3) is the 3-methyl derivative of phenobarbital. This structural change makes the compound more fat-soluble and less water-soluble, a characteristic of many antiepileptic drugs.

The potency of mephobarbital is somewhat less than that of phenobarbital, and its actions on the central nervous system are quite similar to those of phenobarbital.

Gastrointestinal absorption of mephobarbital is less complete than that of phenobarbital. In the liver, demethylation occurs. About 75 percent of a given oral dose is converted to phenobarbital within 24 h. Chronic administration of the drug leads to accumulation of phenobarbital, rather than mephobarbital, in the plasma. Thus it is difficult to establish whether mephobarbital or its product of biotransformation, phenobarbital, is the primary active component in long-term use.

Metharbital Metharbital is the 3-methyl derivative of barbital (Table 21-3). It bears the same structural relationship to barbital that mephobarbital bears to phenobarbital. Like the former drug, it is demethylated in the liver to barbital, although the process of conversion is slower than that of mephobarbital.

Primidone The chemical structure if primidone is shown in Table 21-3. It has a close resemblance to the barbiturates: the only difference lies in the replacement of the C=O group in position 2 by CH_2. Primidone is oxidized in the liver to phenobarbital. It

is also biotransformed to phenylethylmalonamide, which possesses anticonvulsant activity.

Primidone is useful in the treatment of tonic-clonic seizures and simple and complex partial seizures. Side effects such as ataxia and sedation are quite marked, even in minimal anticonvulsant doses. Because of the high incidence of drowsiness, it can seldom be used alone. The somnolence tends to decrease as the drug is continued. Other side reactions common to barbiturates, such as skin rashes, also occur. Rare instances of megaloblastic anemia have been reported. The elimination half-life is 6 ± 4 h, and the therapeutic blood level is 5 to 12 μg/mL.

Succinimides

A group of five-membered-ring structures effective in absence seizures are the succinimides. The most important drug in this category is ethosuximide.

Ethosuximide Ethosuximide, or 2-ethyl-2-methyl-succinimide, has the following structure:

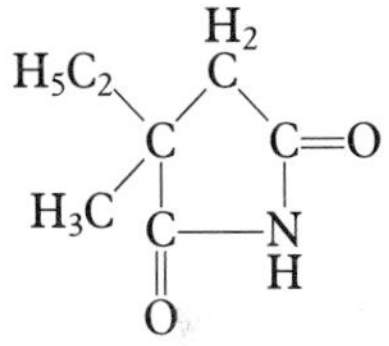

Ethosuximide

The compound is absorbed well from the gastrointestinal tract. Peak blood levels occur between 3 and 7 h after oral administration. The volume of distribution is 0.7 L/kg. Ethosuximide is almost completely metabolized by hydroxylation in the liver, which is then followed by conjugation. The elimination half-life is approximately 30 ± 6 h in children and may be as long as 60 h in adults. The therapeutic blood level is 40 to 120 μg/mL. Ethosuximide is the treatment of choice for uncomplicated absence seizures. If a particular patient has both absence seizures and tonic-clonic seizures, then the addition of either carbamazepine or phenytoin is required because ethosuximide will not prevent tonic-clonic seizures.

Adverse Reactions The succinimides cause sedation and drowsiness, particularly when they are given in large doses. Ethosuximide causes the least sedation in this group of antiepileptic drugs. Minor side effects are headaches, nausea, vomiting, and disequilibrium. Severe blood dyscrasias have been reported with ethosuximide but are quite rare. There are other reports of hepatic and renal dysfunction associated with this drug.

Phensuximide and Methsuximide Two other drugs in this category are phensuximide and methsuximide, but they are less well tolerated than ethosuximide and probably less effective as well. There are reports in the literature that methsuximide may also be effective in complex partial seizures.

Valproic acid

Valproic acid (VPA) is a simple eight-carbon branched-chain fatty acid.

$$CH_3-CH_2-CH_2$$
$$CH-COOH$$
$$CH_3-CH_2-CH_2$$

Valproic acid

Valproic acid is very effective in absence seizures and has a wider range of clinical effectiveness than the succinimides. It is also effective for myoclonic epilepsy and somewhat effective for atypical absence seizures. This drug is reported by some investigators to be helpful as adjunctive therapy with complex partial seizures.

Valproic acid has been shown to increase brain levels of gamma aminobutyric acid by competitive inhibition of GABA transaminase and succinic semialdehyde dehydrogenase. This effect of valproic acid to inhibit the biotransformation of GABA has been suggested as a possible explanation for its antiepileptic action in the central nervous system.

Valproic acid is well absorbed by the oral route, and peak plasma concentrations of valproic acid are reached in 0.5 to 4 h. Its volume of distribution is 0.15 to 0.40 L per kilogram of body weight, indicating that the drug is distributed chiefly in the intramuscular and fatty tissues and in exchangeable extracellular fluid. Circulating valproic acid is 80 to 95 percent bound to serum protein. The major biotransformation pathways are beta and omega oxidations followed by conjugation. The elimination half-life is 12 ± 6 h, and the therapeutic plasma level is at least 50 μg/mL and can be as high as 150 μg/mL.

Adverse Reactions Anorexia, nausea, and vomiting occur in 20 percent of patient receiving valproic acid, but these effects occur much less frequently with patients who are administered the coated tablet divalproex. When valproic acid is given in combination with phenobarbital, it raises the phenobarbital levels by 25 percent because of the decreased rate in the biotransformation of phenobarbital. Valproic acid increases the appetite, and there can be up to a 50-lb increase in weight. It occasionally causes some sedation and produces alopecia. In high doses, valproic acid can cause delirium and hallucinations. A common side effect is an action tremor of the hands, which can be severe enough to alter handwriting and make drinking from a cup almost impossible. This is a dose-related phenomenon.

There are dose-related effects of valproic acid which produce (1) an increase in liver enzymes to 2 to 3 times the baseline level, (2) a decrease in platelet count to as low as 13,000, and (3) a decrease of fibrinogen with an associated increased bleeding time. Reduction in dosage of the drug improves these side effects. An idiosyncratic hepatic failure can occur, which usually improves upon stopping the drug. Rarely does pancreatitis occur. However, there have been reported deaths from hepatic failure and pancreatitis with the use of valproic acid. This may present as Reye's syndrome. Carnitine is reported to be beneficial in counteracting this valproic acid toxicity.

Benzodiazepines

These drugs, represented by chlordiazepoxide and diazepam, are used mainly as antianxiety agents. They have mild sedative effects along with anticonvulsant and muscle-relaxing properties. The pharmacology of these agents is presented in Chap. 16. Diazepam is also used in the treatment of status epilepticus. This drug is very effective in controlling the state of continuous convulsions when it is administered intravenously. Diazepam may also have some value as a secondary drug in myoclonic spasms and atonic seizures. Another benzodiazepine derivative reported to be effective in status epilepticus is lorazepam. A third benzodiazepine derivative is clonazepam, which is described below.

Clonazepam Clonazepam is a chlorinated benzodiazepine that is not used as an antianxiety drug but in the treatment of absence seizures, myoclonic seizures, and atonic seizures.

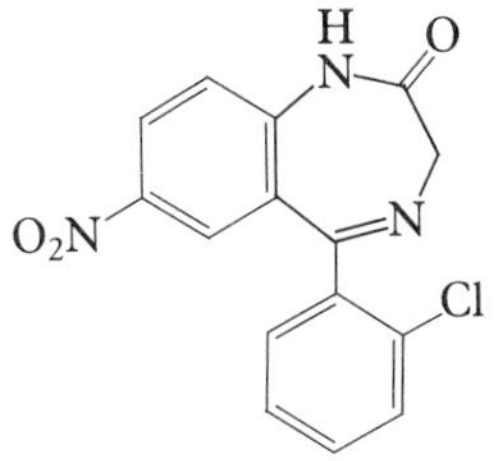

Clonazepam

Pharmacokinetics Between 80 and 100 percent of clonazepam is absorbed via the oral route. Biotransformation involves reduction, acetylation, and hydroxylation with the formation of inactive metabolites. Protein binding is approximately 50 percent, and the elimination half-life is approximately 27 ± 5 h. The therapeutic plasma level is 15 to 70 μg/mL. Because of its extreme sedation, the medication should be started at a very low dosage such as 0.5 mg/day and increased slowly.

Adverse Reactions Ataxia, drowsiness, and dysarthria are commonly seen. Exacerbation of preexisting or new seizures has been reported in 2 to 10 percent of patients. Excessive salivation and bronchial secretion, elevated liver enzymes, and blood dyscrasias are rare toxic effects.

Acetazolamide

The carbonic anhydrase inhibitor, acetazolamide, has been found clinically useful in absence seizures. It is best used in conjunction with other antiepilepsy drugs. The adverse reactions are drowsiness, anorexia, and paresthesias of the hands and feet. Skin rashes and blood dyscrasias have been rarely reported. Further information on the pharmacology of acetazolamide is presented in Chap. 30.

Phenacemide

Phenacemide, or phenurone, is structurally similar to hydantoin with an open hydantoin ring at positions 1 and 5.

The drug is very well absorbed from the gastrointestinal tract. It is biotransformed in the liver, and its

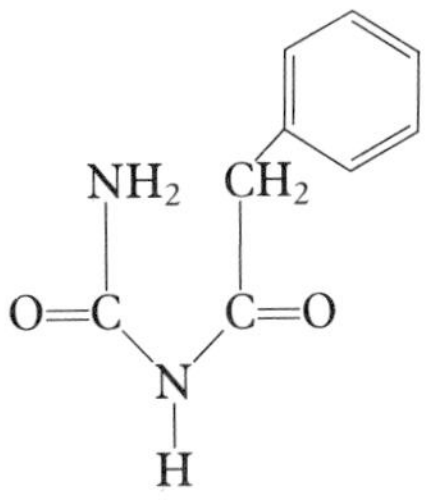

Phenacemide

metabolites are excreted in the urine. Phenacemide is probably as efficacious as carbamazepine or phenytoin as an antiepileptic drug but is very toxic. It should be used only in the most severe forms of complex partial (psychomotor) seizures refractory to other agents. The major side effects are hepatotoxicity and bone marrow depression, and in approximately one-third of the patients taking this medication a toxic psychosis occurs, appearing as a major depression.

Oxazolidines

In this group there are two drugs which are closely related, trimethadione and paramethadione. They are used exclusively in absence seizures. Paramethadione has no advantage over trimethadione. Trimethadione is a five-membered ring structure similar to the hydantoins except that oxygen replaces the nitrogen in the 1 position.

Pharmacokinetics Absorption from the gastrointestinal tract is efficient and rapid for trimethadione. The methyl group on the nitrogen atom is removed by the liver. The demethylated product dimethadione is excreted slowly by the kidney. It has an elimination half-life of 16 h. This metabolic product also has antiepilepsy properties.

Adverse Reaction Large doses are required for the antiepileptic effect of trimethadione, and its therapeutic index is small; hence frequent side effects occur such as ataxia and sedation. The most common complaints are minor skin allergies, photosensitivity, and gastric irritation. About a fourth of the patients complain of a visual disturbance, called *hemeralopia*, in which there is a visual aberration with diminished visual acuity and objects appearing whitish and at times dazzling as if seeing objects through snow. No optic nerve damage has been documented, but it is an intolerable side effect. Liver, kidney, and bone marrow damage have been reported.

Preparations and doses

Acetazolamide (Diamox) is available in 125- and 25-mg tablets and 500-mg vials. The usual adult dose is 0.5 to 1.0 g daily.

Carbamazepine (Tegretol) is 200 mg twice a day, which is then gradually increased. The minimum effective dose is 800 to 1200 mg daily. Available in 100- and 200-mg tablets and suspensions.

Phenytoin (Dilantin) is available in capsules of 30, 50, 100 mg; tablets of 50-mg oral suspension of 30 mg and 125 mg per 5 mL; and injection of 50 mg/mL.

Ethosuximide (Zarontin) is available in capsules of 250 mg and a syrup containing 250 mg per 5 mL.

Ethotoin (Peganone) is available in 250-mg tablets.

Mephenytoin (Mesantoin) is available in 0.1-g tablets.

Mephobarbital (Mebaral) is available in tablets of 32, 50, 100, and 200 mg.

Metharbital (Gemonil) is available in tablets containing 0.1 g.

Methsuximide (Celontin) is available in capsules of 0.3 g and 0.15 g.

Phensuximide (Milontin) is available in capsules of 0.5 g in a suspension of 62.5 mg/mL.

Primidone (Mysoline) is available in 50- and 250-mg tablets and a 5% suspension for children.

Trimethadione (Tridione) is available in capsules containing 0.3 g in tablets of 0.15 g and as a solution containing 40 mg/mL.

Valproic acid dosage for infants and children is 20 to 60 mg/kg/day, and adult dosages range from 750 to 400 mg daily. The drug is available as 250-mg capsules and in a liquid preparation of 250 mg per 5 mL.

Divalproex is a coated tablet in dosages of 125, 250, and 500 mg.

Phenacemide (Phenurone) is available as 0.5-g tablets.

PARKINSONISM

Parkinsonism is a movement disorder with pathology in the substantia nigra and diverse etiologies. The chief manifestations are rigidity, akinesia, resting tremor, and a characteristic flexed posture and shuffling gait. Iatrogenic parkinsonism due to antipsychotic drugs also accounts for a large number of cases, seen mostly in psychiatric practice. Parkinsonian features may be among the symptoms of cerebral vascular disease and other degenerations of the central nervous system.

Antiparkinsonian Agents

For more than a century, the treatment of parkinsonism has rested primarily on the use of centrally active anticholinergic agents. Initially, various preparations of the belladonna alkaloids were used, including stramonium, atropine, and hyoscine. Recognition of the role of acetylcholine in nervous function, and particularly its probable role in the central nervous system, led to the suggestion that the clinical efficacy of atropine and scopolamine in parkinsonism might be due to their antagonism of acetylcholine.

An appreciable body of evidence has accumulated to show parkinsonism as a pathophysiologic state resulting from disease or dysfunction of a dopaminergic neuronal system arising in the midbrain, chiefly in the substantia nigra, and projecting to the corpus striatum. Physiologic studies indicate that dopamine exerts an inhibitory influence on the striatum. Thus in parkinsonism, the striatum would appear to be released from an inhibitory dopaminergic influence. The observation that centrally active cholinergic agents such as physostigmine exacerbate the parkinsonian state, whereas centrally active anticholinergic agents reduce its intensity, suggests that the symptomatology reflects the disinhibited activity of striatal cholinergic systems. According to this hypothesis, a beneficial action could be exerted in parkinsonism either by blocking the excessive stimulation of the cholinergic system or restoring the normal function of the inhibitory dopaminergic system by restoration of its deficient neurohumor.

Levodopa   Of the several methods attempted to correct dopamine deficiency in parkinsonism, administration of the immediate precursor of dopamine, levodopa, is the logical therapy because dopamine does not cross the blood-brain barrier but levodopa does. It is believed that the therapeutic effect of levodopa reflects the restoration of striatal dopamine toward normal (Fig 21-1).

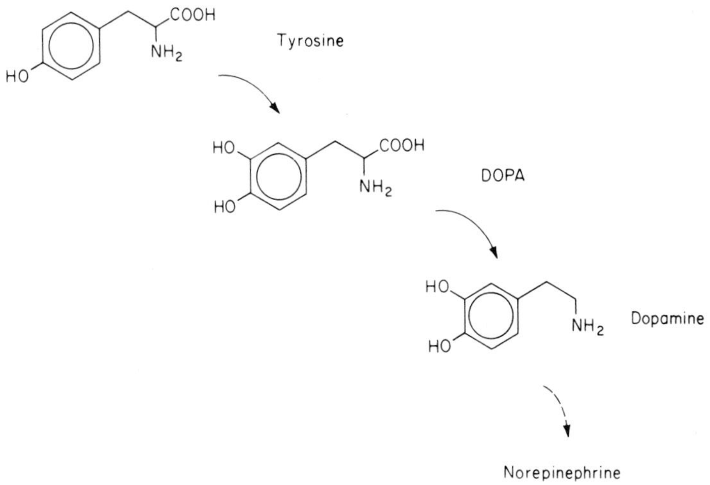

FIGURE 21-1 Synthesis of dopamine from tyrosine. Schematic pathway of synthesis of dopamine from tyrosine in dopaminergic neurons. Presumably, increasing the supply of dioxyphenylalanine (dopa) would increase the production of dopamine.

Pharmacokinetics

Levodopa is administered orally. Peak plasma levels occur within 0.5 to 2 h. Food may delay the absorption. Enzymes of the gastric mucosa can delay absorption by degradation. Levodopa is extensively metabolized in the gastrointestinal tract and the liver. Less than 1 percent of the unmetabolized drug passes to the central nervous system. Elimination half-life is approximately 1 to 3 h. The major urinary metabolites are dihydroxyphenylacetic acid and homovanillic acid.

Adverse Reaction Anorexia, nausea, and vomiting are the chief dose-limiting side effects in the initial period of treatment. Others include tachycardia, palpitations, orthostatic hypotension, insomnia, agitation, and occasionally more severe mental disturbances with delusions and hallucinations. Cardiac arrhythmias can be quite severe. These effects diminish with lowering the daily dosage or increasing the frequency of dosing while maintaining effective total daily dose. Choreiform involuntary movements may develop in patients receiving long-term treatment. Chorea is a side effect of high dose *l*-dopa. If the movements are severe and interfere with function, the dose should be decreased until a satisfactory compromise is achieved.

Drug Interactions The dosage requirement of levodopa can be reduced without altering clinical effectiveness by combining it with the decarboxylase inhibitor carbidopa. This compound does not penetrate the blood-brain barrier to inhibit central decarboxylase. As a result levodopa is not degradated in the peripheral blood and more levodopa can enter the brain, thus permitting the dosage to be reduced without reducing the striatal dopamine effect. A combination of carbidopa and levodopa is the drug product of choice in the United States. It is well tolerated by 96 percent of patients. Many patients benefit from the combination of levodopa with one of the anticholinergic agents.

Pyridoxine markedly reduces or completely annuls the beneficial effect of levodopa administration. Pyridoxine appears to accelerate the biotransformation of the drug in extracerebral tissues by increasing the effects of decarboxylation, thereby preventing it from gaining access to the central nervous system. Phenothiazines such as chlorpromazine antagonize the effect of levodopa and are best avoided. The therapeutic effect of levodopa is reduced by methyldopa and reserpine and enhanced by tricyclic antidepressants. Concurrent administration of levodopa and a monoamine oxidase inhibitor will result in a hypertensive crisis. Levodopa is contraindicated in narrow-angle glaucoma and malignant melanoma.

Anticholinergic Agents

Today the belladonna alkaloids have been replaced in the treatment of parkinsonism by the synthetic anticholinergic antiparkinsonian agents listed in Table 21-4. Although less potent than the natural alkaloids, these synthetic agents possess similar pharmacologic properties and are strongly anticholinergic. The wide distribution of cholinergic neurons in the central nervous system makes it difficult to identify the specific structure involved in the beneficial effect of the anticholinergic drugs.

Clinical Use   There is little reason for preferring one of the anticholinergic antiparkinsonian drugs over another. In general, treatment is begun with small doses which may be increased gradually until further increases yield no benefit or side effects are encountered. The benefits obtained are limited to a partial and often unsatisfactory reduction in the intensity of the parkinsonian state. A decrease in muscular resistance to passive movement, i.e., rigidity, is the most striking effect observed. There is also a general improvement in motor function and posture. Tremor may be reduced but is rarely abolished and is generally the least responsive feature of the parkinsonian syndrome.

Adverse Reactions   Side effects attributable to the anticholinergic activity of these drugs are encountered in nearly all patients, and usually some compromise must be made in adjusting the dosage between levels that produce therapeutic effects and those that induce the side effects common to all anticholinergic drugs.

Amantadine

The antiviral agent amantadine was accidentally discovered to relive parkinsonism when used prophylactically against A_2 influenza viral infection in patients suffering with parkinsonism. The antiparkinsonian action of amantadine has been associated with release of dopamine from storage sites and increases in the concentration of gamma aminobutyric acid in the striatum and substantia nigra.

Amantadine

Amantadine has a peculiar chemical structure consisting of four fused cyclohexane rings substituted with a single amine group. It is well absorbed from the gastrointestinal tract. Among the numerous reactions are hyperexcitability, tremors, ataxia, slurred speech, psychic depression, insomnia, lethargy, and, in high doses, convulsions. Other side effects are dry mouth, gastrointestinal symptoms, skin eruptions, polyuria, and nocturia.

TABLE 21-4   Preparations and doses of anticholinergic antiparkinsonian agents

Drug	Availability	Usual Daily Dosage, mg
Trihexyphenidyl	Tablets, 2 and 5 mg	
Procyclidine	Tablets, 2 and 5 mg	1–15
Biperiden	Tablets, 2 mg Ampuls, 5 mg	
Benztropine	Tablets, 0.5, 1, and 2 mg Ampuls, 2 mg	1–6
Diphenhydramine	Capules, 25 and 50 mg	
Orphenadrine	Tablets, 100 mg Ampuls, 60 mg	50–200

The treatment of parkinsonism by combining levodopa, anticholinergic agents, and amantadine has produced better results than are seen with any of these drugs alone. This combined therapeutic program is of particular importance in those individuals who cannot tolerate higher doses of levodopa because of toxicity. Amantadine may be used as initial therapy for parkinsonism.

Miscellaneous Agents

Bromocriptine   The dopamine receptor agonists such as bromocriptine are used for Parkinson's disease (Fig. 21-2). Bromocriptine mimics the action of dopamine in the brain. It apparently causes fewer abnormal involuntary movements than levodopa but more mental aberrations, including hallucinations, possibly because of chemical similarity to lysergic acid diethylamide (LSD). Since, unlike levodopa, bromocriptine does not require enzymatic transformation in the brain to have a therapeutic effort, it is useful for patients not responding to levodopa.

About 28 percent of the oral dose of bromocriptine is absorbed from the gastrointestinal tract. The drug is 90 to 96 percent bound to serum albumin. Bromocriptine undergoes complete biotransformation, and the major route of excretion is biliary. Approximately 85 percent of the administered dose is excreted in the feces in 120 h. It is also indicated for short-term treatment of amenorrhea and galactorrhea associated with excessive secretion of prolactin. Also it helps to reduce in size prolactin-secreting pituitary tumors.

The major adverse effects of bromocriptine are nausea, nasal congestion, and orthostatic hypotension. Other less common side effects include constipation, headaches, fatigue, and hallucinations. Bromocriptine is useful in the treatment of prolactinomas, acromegaly, and Parkinson's disease.

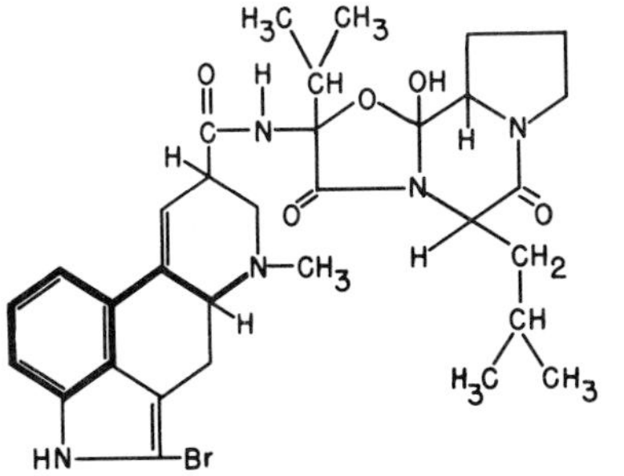

Preparations and Doses

Levodopa is available as tablets and capsules containing 100, 250, and 500 mg.

Carbidopa (Lodosyn) is available in tablets of 25 mg.

Carbidopa and *levodopa* (Sinemet) is available in tablets of 10/100 (10 mg of carbidopa and 100 mg of levodopa), 25/100 (25 mg of carbidopa and 100 mg of levodopa), and 25/250 (25 mg of carbidopa and 250 mg of levodopa).

Amantadine (Symmetrel) is available in capsules of 100 mg and syrup containing 50 mg per 5 mL. The usual daily dose is 100 mg twice a day.

Trihexyphenidyl (Artane) is available in tablets containing 2 and 5 mg and 5-mg sustained-release capsules. The usual daily dosage is 1 to 15 mg.

Procyclidine (Kemadrin) is available in tablets containing 2 and 5 mg. The usual daily dose is 1 to 15 mg.

Biperiden (Akineton) is available in tablets containing 2 mg and ampuls containing 5 mg. The usual daily dose is 1 to 15 mg.

Benztropine (Cogentin) is available in tablets containing 0.5, 1, and 2 mg. The usual daily dose is 1 to 6 mg.

Diphenhydramine (Benadryl) is available in capsules containing 25 and 50 mg. The usual daily dosage is 50 to 200 mg.

Orphenadrine (Dispal) is available in tablets containing 50 and 100 mg and ampuls containing 60 mg. The usual daily dosage is 50 to 200 mg.

Bromocriptine (Parlodel) is available as tablets containing 2.5 or 5 mg. Usual dosage is 2.5–7.5 mg/day.

FIGURE 21-2   Chemical structure of bromocriptine (heavy lines represent dopamine moiety).

BIBLIOGRAPHY

Bergmann, K. J., M. R. Mendoza, M. D. Yahr: "Parkinson's Disease and Long Term Levodopa Therapy," in K. J. Bergmann and M. D. Yahr (eds.), *Parkinson's Disease, Advances in Neurology*, Raven, New York, **45**:463–468 (1987).

Borowski, G. D., and L. I. Rose: "Bromocriptine Update," *Am. Fam. Physician*, **30**:218 (1984).

Commission on Classification and Terminology of the International League Against Epilepsy: "Proposal for Revised Clinical and Electroencephalorgraphic Classification of Epileptic Seizures," *Epilepsia*, **22**:489–501 (1981).

Delorenzo, R. J.: "Mechanisms of Action of Anticonvulsant Drugs," *Epilepsia*, **29**:535–547 (1988)

Guelen, P. J. M., and E. Vanderklein: "Practical Pharmacokinetics" in D. M. Woodbury, J. K. Penry, and C. E. Pippenger (eds.), *Antiepileptic Drugs*, Raven, New York, 1982, pp. 57–72.

Marsden, C. D., and S. Fahn: "Problems in Parkinson's Disease and Other Akinetic Rigid Syndromes," in C. D. Marsden and S. Fahn (eds.), *Movement Disorders II*, Butterworth, Boston 1987, pp. 65–72.

Treiman, D. M.: "Efficacy and Safety of Antiepileptic Drugs: A Review of Controlled Trials," *Epilepsia* **28**:51–58 (1987).

Wotten, G. F.: "Progress in Understanding the Pathophysiology of Treatment Related Fluctuations in Parkinson's Disease," *Ann. Neurology* **24**:263–365 (1988).

Narcotic Analgesics

Martin W. Adler

The *narcotic analgesics* are a group of drugs which obtund pain without producing loss of consciousness. In large doses, the drugs can depress the central nervous system and may produce sleep or narcosis—hence the term *narcotic analgesics*. Even though the term *opiate* is sometimes applied to this group of drugs, it is correctly applied only to those alkaloids (i.e., morphine and codeine) obtained from the poppy plant, opium. In this chapter, the term *opioid* will be used to define drugs, naturally occurring and synthetic, which have properties similar to morphine, the oldest known opium derivative.

These agents are the most effective drugs for the relief of pain. An understanding of the mechanisms involved in opioid action, especially the interplay between drug and receptor, is essential for the rational use of these drugs.

MOLECULAR BASIS OF ACTION

Endogenous Opioid Peptides

In 1975, the structures of two pentapeptides, Met- and Leu-enkephalin, were identified. Since that time a number of other endogenous opioid peptides have been identified, the most prominent of which are beta-endorphin and dynorphin.

Like many other peptides present in the nervous system, the endogenous opioid peptides are not synthesized individually. Instead, a single gene encodes a large inactive polypeptide that contains within its structure the sequences of several small active molecules that are subsequently split from the precursor. As with virtually all other neuropeptides, the active peptides have pairs of basic amino acids on both sides. A trypsin-like enzyme splits the larger peptide at the C-terminal side, leaving the active peptide. A carboxypeptidase beta-like enzyme removes the basic amino acid at the N-terminus. Furthermore, the sites where the molecule is split may vary from tissue to tissue, making possible the generation of different combinations of peptides from a single gene. There are three families of endogenous opioid peptides, and they arise from precursor or prohormone molecules: pro-opiomelanocortin (POMC), proenkephalin, and prodynorphin (Fig. 22-1). These precursors and their products have different distributions in the nervous system.

POMC was the first of the precursors to be identified. This polypeptide is produced in the anterior and intermediate lobes of the pituitary gland, in the hypothalamus, and in other areas of the brain. It is also made in several peripheral tissues, including the placenta, gastrointestinal tract, and lungs. Beta-endorphin is the 61-91 amino acid chain in beta-lipotropin. POMC also gives rise to nonopioid peptides of great importance, including ACTH and alpha-melanocyte stimulating hormone (alpha-MSH).

Although the 61-65 amino acid sequence of beta-endorphin is Met-enkephalin, we now know that this compound is not the source of Met-enkephalin in the brain. The source of Met-enkephalin is proenkephalin. In addition, proenkephalin cleavage leads to the formation of several other peptides (e.g., Leu-enkeph-

A. POMC

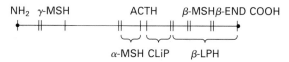

B. Proenkephalin

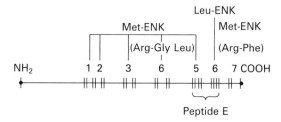

C. Prodynorphin

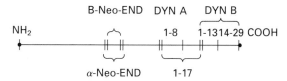

FIGURE 22-1 Schematic representation of the protein precursor structures of the three opioid peptide families. POMC = Proopiomelanocortin [Duplicated with permission from H. Akil et al., "Endogenous Opioids," *Ann. Rev. Neurosci. 7:223–255 (1984).*]

alin, Met-enkephalin-Arg-Phe, Met-enkephalin-Arg-Leu, peptide E). Prodynorphin, the last of the precursors to be identified, is the source of dynorphin A, dynorphin B, Leu-enkephalin, and other dynorphins. The endogenous opioid peptides are widely but not equally distributed to the CNS; they are found in discrete locations.

Of particular relevance to this chapter is that some of the endogenous opioid peptides, especially beta-endorphin, produce morphine-like analgesia. The most sensitive sites seem to be located in the periaqueductal grey (PAG) and other medial thalamic sites. Beta-endorphin also produces analgesia by an effect at the level of the spinal cord. The enkephalins in contrast to beta-endorphins have a very fleeting action due to their rapid degradation. The analgesic action of dynorphin is more selective and appears to be effective only against certain types of pain (e.g., mechanical, cold) working primarily by actions on the spinal cord.

In addition to analgesia, the endogenous opioid peptides produce a variety of other effects, including an increased electrical activity, respiratory depression,

antidiarrheal activity, release of prolactin and growth hormone, alteration of body temperature, modifications of learning and memory, changes in the immune system responsiveness and, with repeated administration, tolerance and physical dependence. Of the endogenous opioid peptides, only β-endorphins have been administered intravenously to patients; effects on mood, cognitive function, and autonomic responses have been noted. In some depressed patients, an antidepressant effect was reported. The effects of the endogenous opioid peptides are remarkably similar to those seen following the administration of morphine and other narcotic analgesics.

Opioid Receptors

It is currently believed that a substantial proportion of opioid binding sites are receptors. There are several types of opioid receptors: mu, kappa, sigma, and delta. The delta receptor and part of the mu receptor were recently cloned and sequenced. Some types of opioid receptors may even have subtypes, just as we find in several other systems (e.g., adrenergic). Mu receptors were named after morphine; thus the agonist actions associated with the interaction of a ligand and the mu receptor are those typically seen with morphine. Beta-endorphin is the endogenous ligand that appears to interact primarily with this receptor type. The kappa receptor appears to be involved with certain types of analgesia, diuresis, and thermoregulation; dynorphin appears to be the endogenous ligand. The enkephalins have their primary effects on the delta receptor. The functions of the delta receptor are unknown, but learning, memory, gastrointestinal motility, and analgesia may be involved. The sigma receptor has been implicated in the dysphoria and other undesirable psychic effects associated with some of the agonists and mixed agonist-antagonists, and a subtype of the sigma receptor may be identical to the so-called PCP (phencyclidine) receptor.

Opioid receptors seem to be localized in membrane fragments of synaptosomal fractions, and they are probably glycoproteins. They undergo conformational changes under certain conditions, which affects affinity for the binding of agonists or antagonists. For example, sodium increases antagonist and decreases agonist binding. As would be expected from studies of other neurotransmitter systems, receptors for the endogenous opioid peptides are generally located in the same areas as the ligands themselves. The brain site with the highest concentration of mu receptors is the PAG.

It now appears quite certain that the physiologic role of the endogenous opioid system is not restricted to pain and analgesia. This system seems to be important in terms of endocrines, behavior, thermoregulation, the gastrointestinal tract, and immune competence. It is likely that the endogenous opioids may influence other systems as well as several other neurotransmitter systems (e.g., cholinergic and adrenergic) and other neuropeptide systems. Opioid receptors are also involved in the development of tolerance to and dependence on narcotic analgesics.

Classification

The opioids are classified into three major subgroups according to their activities at the opioid receptors: (1) agonists, (2) mixed agonist-antagonists, and (3) antagonists. Table 22-1 lists the various narcotic drugs according to their classification.

The opioid *agonist* drugs have both affinity and efficacy for the opioid receptors, therefore mimicking the activity of the endogenous opioid peptides. The *mixed agonist-antagonists* are semisynthetic derivatives of morphine which have agonistic activity at some opioid receptors but antagonistic activity at others. The *antagonists* bind to receptor sites throughout the body but fail to activate them. These compounds are not used for analgesia: rather the therapeutic utility of these drugs lies in their ability to reverse the adverse effects associated with acute overdose or addiction to an agonist opioid. Table 22-2 shows representative narcotic agonists, agonist-antagonists, antagonists, and the receptors to which they bind.

AGONISTS

The opioid agonists act primarily at mu receptors to produce analgesia but have varying activity at the kappa and sigma receptors. In general, analgesic activity resides in the *levo* isomer of the drugs. The analgesic activity of opium is due largely to the alkaloid morphine. Morphine, the oldest narcotic analgesic, is the best understood and remains the standard against which all other analgesics are compared.

Morphine

Source and Chemistry Morphine is obtained from opium, which is the dried sap of the unripe fruit capsules of the poppy plant (*Papaver somniferum*), and its analgesic efficacy has been known for more than 3000 years. A number of alkaloids are present in the plant, and they fall into two categories, phenanthrenes and benzylisoquinolines. The former is the important one from the perspective of analgesia. The phenanthrenes in opium include morphine (about 10 percent) and codeine (about 0.5 to 1 percent). The benzylisoquinolines include papaverine, an alkaloid with vasodilator and antispasmodic properties but lacking analgesic properties. The structure of morphine is shown below:

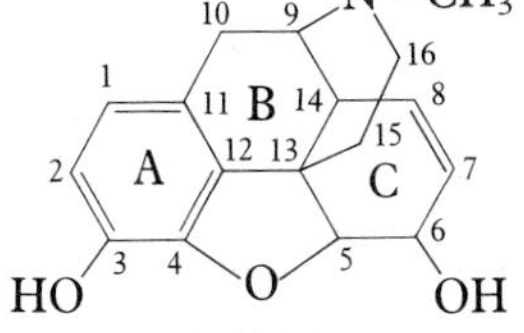

Morphine

TABLE 22-1   Selected narcotic compounds

Classification	Generic name	Common trade name
Agonists		
Phenanthrene derivatives		
	Morphine	
	Codeine	
	Hydromorphone	DILAUDID
	Oxymorphone	NUMORPHAN
	Oxycodone	
Morphinan derivative		
	Levorphanol	LEVO-DROMORAN
Phenylpiperidine derivatives		
	Meperidine	DEMEROL
	Propoxyphene	DARVON
Antagonists		
	Naloxone	NARCAN
	Naltrexone	TREXAN
Mixed agonist-antagonists		
	Buprenorphine	BUPRENEX
	Butorphanol	STADOL
	Nalbuphine	NUBAIN
	Pentazocine	TALWIN

Source: Modified and reproduced with permission from G. J. DiGregorio, E. Barbieri, and G. Sterling (eds.), *Handbook of Pain Management*, Medical Surveillance Inc., Philadelphia, 1989.

Relatively simple modifications of the morphine molecule result in a number of compounds varying with analgesic potency. *Codeine* is formed from the substitution of methoxy for the 3-hydroxy group of the phenol ring. *Heroin* (3,6-diacetylmorphine) is made by acetylation of the two hydroxyl groups. Methylation of the two hydroxyls and addition of a double bond to one of them results in the formation of *thebaine*, a precursor of the narcotic antagonist naloxone, and buprenorphine, the mixed agonist-antagonist. Many other agonists can also be formed by such alterations of the morphine molecule. A number of other opioids with analgesic activity, however, are derived from chemical structures unrelated to morphine. These compounds include the agonist meperidine. The benzomorphans, compounds that have mixed agonist-antagonist properties, have only a partial chemical relationship to morphine.

Pharmacokinetics   Morphine can be administered either by the oral, intramuscular, or subcutaneous routes. The oral bioavailability of morphine is relatively poor (10 to 20 percent), due to a high first-pass biotransformation effect. Morphine is metabolized in the liver to an inactive glucuronide metabolite, which is then excreted in the urine.

The onset of action of morphine after intramuscular injection is approximately 30 min (see Table 22-3). The peak effects occur between 30 and 90 min, with a 3- to 7-h duration of action. The elimination half-life is

TABLE 22-2   Opioid receptor binding of representative narcotic agonists, antagonists, and agonist-antagonists

Drug	Opioid receptor types		
	μ (mu)	κ (kappa)	σ (sigma)
Morphine[a]	Agonist	Agonist	—[b]
Naloxone[c]	Antagonist	Antagonist	Antagonist
Pentazocine	Antagonist	Agonist	Agonist
Nalbuphine	Antagonist	Partial agonist	Agonist
Buprenorphine	Partial agonist	—	—
Butorphanol	—[d]	Agonist	Agonist

[a] All the narcotics of the agonist type listed in this table bind to and stimulate μ and κ receptors similar to morphine.
[b] Indicates that no significant activity has been observed.
[c] Both naloxone and naltrexone bind to and block these opioid receptors.
[d] Although experimental data suggest that there is little binding at μ receptors, some authorities consider butorphanol to possess weak antagonistic activity at this site.
Source: Modified and reproduced with permission from G. J. DiGregorio, E. Barbieri, and G. Sterling (eds.), *Handbook of Pain Management*, Medical Surveillance Inc., Philadelphia, 1989.

TABLE 22-3   Pharmacokinetic data of narcotic analgesics

Drug	Onset of effect,[a] min	Peak effect,[a] min	Duration of effect, h	Plasma half-life, h
Narcotic agonists				
Morphine	30	30–90	3–7	2–3
Codeine	30	45–90	4–6	3–4
Fentanyl	10	20–30	1–2	3–4
Hydromorphone	30	30–90	4–5	2–4
Levorphanol	30	60–90	4–8	10–12
Meperidine	15	30–60	2–4	3–4
Methadone	15	60–120	4–6	21–25
Oxycodone	—	—	4–5	—
Oxymorphone	10	30–90	3–6	—
Propoxyphene[b]	30	60–90	4–6	6–12
Narcotic agonist-antagonists				
Buprenorphine	15	45–60	4–6	2–3
Butorphanol	10	30–60	3–4	2–4
Nalbuphine	15	45–60	3–6	4–6
Pentazocine	15	30–60	2–3	2–3

[a] Based on intramuscular administration.
[b] Based on oral administration.
Source: Modified and reproduced with permission from G. J. DiGregorio, E. Barbieri, and G. Sterling (eds.), *Handbook of Pain Management*, Medical Surveillance Inc., Philadelphia, 1989.

relatively short, 2 to 3 h. Heroin and codeine can be metabolized to morphine to some extent before inactivation by glucuronide conjugates.

Effects on Organ Systems

Central Nervous System In its analgesic action, morphine does not interfere with pain sensation either at nerve endings or in the conduction of pain impulses to the brain. Rather, it depresses the cortical processes which would interpret the afferent signal as pain. Differences in potency to induce analgesia among the compounds varies greatly (see Table 22-4). Otherwise, morphine has both stimulant and depressant effects on the central nervous system, and there are great variations in the degree to which either of these is more prominent.

The usual effect of morphine on humans is sedation. However, some humans are made excited, even maniacal, by morphine. Typically, a level of sedation is produced which is not so deep as that of a hypnotic agent such as a barbiturate: the patient may doze but can be readily aroused. Morphine is often described as producing a sense of euphoria. This is not always true. Some persons are made euphoric by morphine; others, dysphoric. The feeling of dissociation is regarded as pleasant by some persons and unpleasant by others. Accompanying the sedation and mood effect, morphine produces feelings of dizziness, warmth, itching, and frequently nausea. The nausea produced by morphine is probably due to a combination of two factors: (1) morphine stimulates the chemoreceptor trigger zone of the medulla oblongata and (2) morphine can

TABLE 22-4   Potency comparisons of selected narcotic analgesics[a]

Drug	Equianalgesic doses, mg		Parenteral/oral dose ratio
	IM	PO	
Narcotic agonists			
Morphine	10	60	1.17[b]
Codeine	120	200	0.60
Fentanyl	0.1	—[c]	—
Hydromorphone	1.5	7.5	0.20
Levorphanol	2	4	0.50
Meperidine	75	300	0.25
Methadone	10	20	0.50
Oxycodone	15	30	0.50
Oxymorphone	1	6	0.17
Propoxyphene	—[c]	130	—
Narcotic agonist-antagonists			
Buprenorphine	0.3	—[c]	—
Butorphanol	2	—[c]	—
Nalbuphine	10	—[c]	—
Pentazocine	30	150	0.20

[a] The data in this Table are based on morphine, 10 mg, administered intramuscularly, and represent the medical consensus. Variability will occur among patients; therefore, these values should be used only as a guide for comparison.
[b] These data were calculated as the ratio of the IM: PO equianalgesic doses of the compounds. The equianalgesic doses were estimated from dose-response curves and are based on the analgesic efficacy of the drugs. These data are not reflective of bioavailability, which is based on plasma concentrations of the drugs.
[c] Not used by this route.
Source: Modified and reproduced with permission from G. J. DiGregorio, E. Barbieri, and G. Sterling (eds.), *Handbook of Pain Management,* Mĕdical Surveillance Inc., Philadelphia, 1989.

cause some degree of orthostatic hypotension. Therefore, subjects given morphine who sit up or walk about are more prone to nausea than are those who lie quietly in bed. The chemoreceptor trigger zone activates the nearby emetic center of the medulla. Antagonistic to the effect of stimulating the trigger zone, in larger doses, morphine depresses the emetic center. Morphine also possesses antitussive activity. The effects of morphine on spinal cord reflexes are very complex. Spinal cord stimulation is always present but is often masked by central nervous system depression.

Morphine causes marked constriction of the pupil in those species in which the drug is sedative. This effect is apparently accomplished by an excitatory action on the visceral nuclei of the oculomotor nuclear complex. The effect can be blocked by atropine. Tolerance does not develop to this miosis, and the effect is so uniform that it has been used for evaluating analgesic drugs.

Respiratory System Morphine is a powerful respiratory depressant, acting by medullary depression, which in turn reduces carbon dioxide drive. Alveolar and serum P_{CO_2} both increase after morphine administration, and this may occur before any reduction in respiratory rate or tidal volume is noted.

Cardiovascular System Morphine causes orthostatic hypotension in some patients because of depression of the vasomotor center of the medulla or possibly because of histamine release. Sufficiently large doses of morphine can cause hypotension, even in the horizontal position; very large doses cause bradycardia.

Gastrointestinal System The emesis following oral morphine administration is caused by a direct effect on the upper portion of the gastrointestinal tract, which produces vigorous contractions and spasms of the smooth muscles of gut walls and sphincters. This results in hypertonic delay of peristalsis, with delayed gastric emptying time, and in constipation, which can become very severe, alternating with waves of overactivity. Tolerance does not develop to this effect of opiates, the mechanism of which remains unknown.

Hepatic System The drug has no significant effect on the liver, even in large chronic doses. The action of morphine on the gallbladder, bile ducts, and sphincters is the same as that on the gut; as a result, morphine produces greatly increased cholecystic and choledochal pressures.

Skin Morphine occasionally causes urticaria, and some cases of contact dermatitis have been reported. Morphine causes an increase in sweating as well as histamine release, which in turn accounts for the reddened eyes and itching skin.

Genitourinary System Morphine decreases the volume of urine, probably because of release of antidiuretic hormone from the neurohypophysis. As in the gut, morphine causes spasm of the smooth muscles of the urinary tract, so that the detrusor and sphincter are spastic. The result of all these effects is oliguria, which may become clinically significant. Morphine also depresses sexual activity. Chronic dosage in humans causes absence of libido; addicts are reportedly able to maintain erection, but ejaculation is delayed or absent. In women, chronic morphinism causes oligomenorrhea or amenorrhea. Involution of the female genitals may eventuate. These effects are due to suppression by morphine of hypophyseal gonadotropins. Despite these profound effects, sterility does not necessarily ensue. Morphine has no significant direct effect on contractions of the uterus in labor, but it mitigates the concomitant, involuntary ("bearing down") contractions of the abdominal musculature and thus can delay labor.

Miscellaneous System Morphine inhibits thyroid hormone release, probably by interfering with the central (hypothalamic) pathways which permit release of thyroid-stimulating hormone from the adenohypophysis. Morphine stimulates the postsynaptic elements of the adrenal medulla, causing release of epinephrine and norepinephrine and partial depletion of adrenal medullary catecholamine stores. The release of catecholamines causes hyperglycemia, which can be blocked by adrenergic blockade.

Adverse Reactions and Acute Poisoning Most adverse reactions are the result of the pharmacologic actions noted above. These include nausea, vomiting, dizziness, pruritis, constipation, and CNS depression. Urticaria and other allergic phenomena may occasionally occur.

When death occurs from opioid overdosage, the cause is almost always respiratory depression. Although individual variability is great, serious toxicity and even death may occur from morphine. Respiratory depression is always a potential problem associated with the use of opioids, as mentioned earlier, and opioids should be used with extreme caution in patients with decreased respiratory reserve. Opioids, as a group, are CNS depressants, and synergism or potentiation with other CNS depressants may occur. In the fetus, respiratory depression may pose an even greater risk, since the relative absence of a blood-brain barrier allows larger amounts of drugs such as morphine to enter the brain.

The triad of coma, pinpoint pupils, and markedly depressed respiration is strongly suggestive of opioid poisoning. The treatment of choice is the administration of small doses (e.g., 0.4 mg) of naloxone intravenously, repeated every few minutes as needed. In the absence of an opioid antagonist, adequate ventilation must be maintained. When naloxone is used, it should be remembered that its duration of action is much shorter than that of the agonist, so the patient must not be left unattended when respiration recovers as a result of the antagonist administration. Use of the antagonist in an opioid addict may precipitate a severe abstinence syndrome, so particular care should be exercised in such patients.

The use of naloxone is particularly beneficial when the cause of poisoning is unknown or when a mixture of drugs is involved. Naloxone will antagonize all the opioids, including the mixed agonist-antagonist group. Since naloxone has no agonist properties, however, it will not make the patient's condition worse if the offending drug is something other than an opioid.

Tolerance and Physical Dependence When the narcotic agonists are administered over long periods of time (chronically), both tolerance and physical dependence may be observed. Tolerance occurs when the dose of a drug causes a decreased effect following repeated administration or when high doses are required to obtain the initial effect caused by the initial dose of the drug. Physical dependence is an addictive state that refers to a continued administration of the drug, which leads to a pattern of use that causes alterations in the biochemical and psychologic state of individuals. One of the cardinal signs of physical dependence is the characteristic withdrawal symptom which occurs when the drug is stopped abruptly.

Tolerance occurs to some of the effects of morphine. Most commonly, patients become tolerant to central nervous system effects such as analgesia, sedation, respiratory depression, nausea and vomiting, euphoria, and cough suppression. Minimal tolerance occurs to

the constipating or the pinpoint-pupil effects of morphine. Tolerance to and dependence on morphine are both dose- and time-dependent. Large doses of morphine in a short time interval will cause faster tolerance and higher degree of dependence than will small doses administered further apart. Tolerance to morphine does not become important until after 2 or 3 weeks of continued administration of morphine. The time required to produce physical dependence following long-term use may be as short as 1 to 2 weeks if large quantities of the drug are used. Cross-dependency within the opioid group is common.

Therapeutic Uses. The most important use of the *narcotic analgesics* is to relieve pain. The differences among the various agonists relate primarily to oral efficacy, duration of action, and specific side effects. These potent agents, with their liabilities of respiratory depression and physical dependence, should never be used when less potent measures will suffice. Where the lesser measures do not produce satisfactory pain relief, however, opioids may be necessary. No patient should be denied the use of opioids where other forms of pain relief are inadequate. This is particularly true in chronic pain states such as cancer. When given for chronic pain, opioids are generally administered at irregular intervals. Currently, use of "on demand" doses is on the increase, and there is accumulating evidence that patients may require less drug this way. Use of oral administration for chronic pain treatment is becoming more common, and there are reports that there is less tolerance when the drug is administered by this route. Additional studies, however, are needed to confirm these early impressions. Intrathecal administration of opioids is also on the increase, and this route appears to be very useful in certain pain states. Recent findings indicate that the epidural administration of small volumes of morphine can produce spinal analgesia with little in the way of side effects associated with supraspinal actions of the drug. As tolerance develops to the opioids, irrespective of the route of administration, dosage should be advanced only to the point of pain relief. These measures will delay the progress of tolerance. Since the drugs used today act on the mu opioid receptor, cross-tolerance exists among all the agonists and switching drugs is of no help in avoiding or delaying tolerance.

With regard to other uses, opioids have proven to be beneficial in the relief of some forms of *diarrhea*. In myocardial infarction, when not only pain but apprehensiveness is often intense, morphine relieves the pain, calms the patient, and may decrease oxygen consumption and cardiac work. Morphine is valuable in treating *acute pulmonary edema*. Another very common use of opioids is as part of *premedication for surgery*. The drugs can reduce the apprehension of the patient before induction of general anesthesia, as well as reduce the amount of anesthetic drug necessary. Some agonists can be used by themselves or combined with a neuroleptic (neuroleptanalgesia) to produce a state in which surgery can be performed. Some opioids, especially codeine, are useful as *antitussives*, although morphine is not employed for this purpose.

Codeine

Like morphine, codeine is a naturally occurring alkaloid from the poppy plant. Structurally, it differs from morphine only in that a methoxy group is substituted for the 3-hydroxyl group on the aromatic ring.

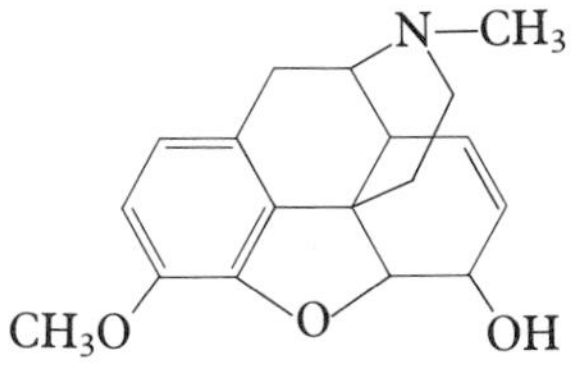

Codeine

About 10 percent of orally administered codeine is converted to morphine; some is demethylated to norcodeine, and the rest is largely conjugated by the liver. Although its pharmacodynamic actions are similar to those of morphine, there are some significant differences. Codeine is more effective orally and has wide use as an analgesic for the treatment of mild to moderate degrees of pain and as an antitussive agent. Although morphine is at least 10 times more potent than codeine on a weight basis, codeine can produce very effective analgesia if given in proper dosage (Table 22-4). The maximum oral dose commonly used for analgesia is 60 mg, while the antitussive dose is usually about 15 mg. The antitussive activity of codeine has been postulated to result from interactions with a set of receptors that differ from the opioid receptors discussed earlier. As with morphine, tolerance and dependence can develop to codeine, but the dependence is not seen as frequently as with morphine. Codeine

has more central stimulatory and less sedative properties than morphine. Toxic doses can produce seizures, especially in children.

Heroin

Heroin, or diacetylmorphine, is a synthetic opioid.

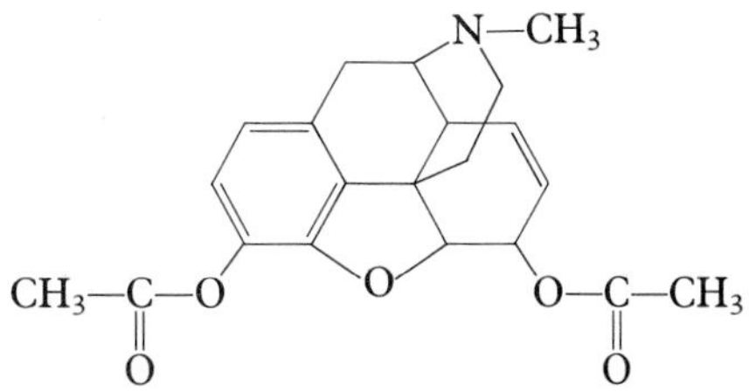

Heroin

Despite repeated claims by some that heroin possesses special properties, controlled clinical studies have shown that it serves no therapeutic purpose that cannot be achieved by other drugs. Possession and use of heroin is illegal in the United States and elsewhere. The greater lipid solubility of heroin, compared with that of morphine, accounts for its rapid passage through the blood-brain barrier but its actions are those of morphine, the compound to which heroin is biotransformed in the brain.

Methadone

Methadone is a synthetic opioid with activity primarily on the mu receptor and with properties very similar to those of morphine.

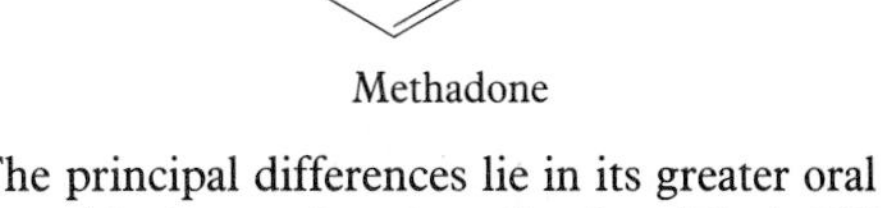

Methadone

The principal differences lie in its greater oral efficacy and its longer duration of action. The half-life of methadone is on the order of 24 to 36 h. That, coupled with its accumulation in the tissues after repeated administration and its slow release from receptors, accounts for the milder but protracted abstinence syndrome associated with methadone. In addition to its usefulness as an analgesic, methadone is used to treat opioid abstinence (it can substitute for other mu agonists) and to treat heroin users (so-called methadone maintenance). Its use during pregnancy in heroin-addicted mothers is discussed in the chapter on drug abuse (see Chap. 25).

Methadone hydrochloride is available for oral or parenteral administration. The usual oral dose range for analgesia is 2.5 to 10 mg. The usual intramuscular or subcutaneous dose is 7.5 mg; this may be repeated after 4 h. There is a broad range of doses used for oral maintenance to treat narcotic addiction, but 40 mg daily is often a stabilizing dose level. Reduction of dosage can begin after 2 or 3 days.

Meperidine and Other Phenylpiperidines

Meperidine is a phenylpiperidine that differs markedly from morphine and many other agonists in chemical structure. Fentanyl, loperamide, and diphenoxylate are chemically related.

Meperidine

The effects of meperidine on the CNS are similar to those of morphine, and many of its actions are on the mu receptor. Toxic doses cause CNS excitation due to the formation of normeperidine. Equianalgesic doses (meperidine is only about one-tenth as potent as morphine) depress respiration and induce sedation as much as does morphine (Table 22-4). It is less constipating than morphine, has less effect on the pupil, and is not an effective antitussive. The pharmacology of meperidine shows both opioid and atropine-like (anticholinergic) characteristics. Like morphine, meperidine causes both histamine release and spasm of smooth muscle and, therefore, bronchoconstriction and biliary spasm. Meperidine is shorter-acting than morphine (about 2 to 3 h) and, contrary to popular belief, is not particularly useful when administered orally. Approximately 4 times the parenteral dose is needed for equivalent oral efficacy.

The dependence liability of meperidine is similar to that of morphine, although signs of abstinence differ somewhat. Adverse reactions to meperidine resemble those of atropine: mydriasis, dry mouth, tachycardia, and excitement that progresses to delirium with disorientation and hallucinations. The acute toxic effects of meperidine are not so completely counteracted by naloxone as are the effects of morphine because naloxone antagonizes only opioid but not atropine-like actions. Administration of meperidine to a patient being treated with a monoamine oxidase inhibitor may result in excitation, delirium, and convulsions as a result of increased formation of normeperidine.

Fentanyl is a chemical relative of meperidine that is nearly 100 times more potent than morphine.

Fentanyl

It is rarely used as an analgesic by itself; its most frequent use is in anesthesiology, either alone or in combination with droperidol, an antipsychotic butyrophenone, for a procedure called *neuroleptanalgesia*, in which the indifference to painful stimuli induced by the antipsychotic, combined with the abolition of the perception of pain by the opioid, makes certain surgical procedures possible without actually anesthetizing the patient. Newer congeners are sufentanil and alfentanil, both of which have a shorter half-life and are more potent than fentanyl. Fentanyl citrate (Sublimaze) is available in ampuls containing 50 μg/mL. Dosage should be individualized depending on use, age, and general state of the individual. In combination with droperidol, it is marketed as Innovar in ampuls containing 50 μg/mL fentanyl base and 2.5 mg/mL droperidol.

Loperamide and *diphenoxylate* are poorly absorbed from the gastrointestinal tract and exert their antidiarrheal actions there.

Addiction liability, especially with loperamide, is extremely low. Diphenoxylate hydrochloride is available in tablets of 2.5 mg, containing also 0.025 mg of atropine sulfate; also in a liquid containing the same

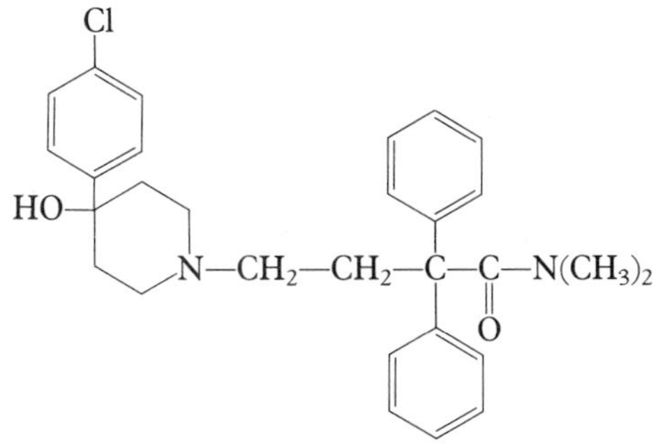

Loperamide

Diphenoxylate

amounts in 5 mL. Initial dosage is two tablets or 10 mL, four times daily until control is achieved, then gradual reduction of dosage. Loperamide hydrochloride is available in 2-mg capsules of a liquid containing 1 mg per 5 mL. Initial dose is 4 mg, followed by 2 mg after each unformed stool. Maximum daily dosage: 16 mg.

Hydromorphone and Oxymorphone

These agents are congeners of morphine. Hydromorphone is approximately 8 times more potent than morphine (Table 22-4). Its absorption following oral administration is better than that of morphine; its onset of action is faster, while the duration of action is briefer. Hydromorphone is more sedative and less euphoriant than morphine.

Oxymorphone is about 10 times as potent as morphine and causes more euphoria and more nausea and vomiting than do otherwise equivalent doses of morphine. The time-action curve of oxymorphone is about the same as that of morphine.

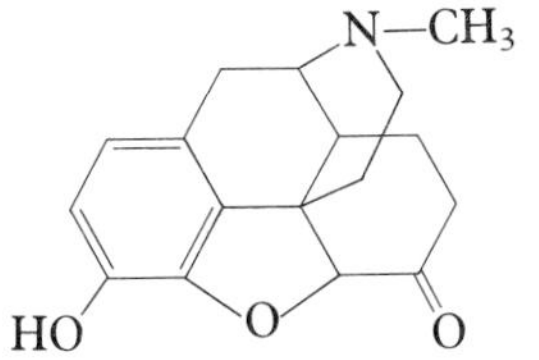

Hydromorphone

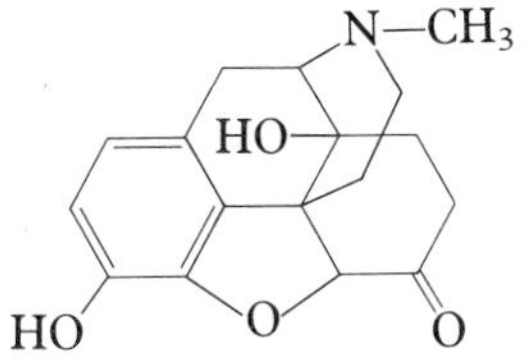

Oxymorphone

Hydrocodone and Oxycodone

These two drugs are chemically related to codeine and morphine. Both are absorbed quite well from the gastrointestinal tract, both are analgesics and good antitussives. The latter is the only clinical use of hydro-

codone, while oxycodone is also used as an analgesic in combination with either acetylsalicylic acid or acetaminophen. Both can produce tolerance and dependence.

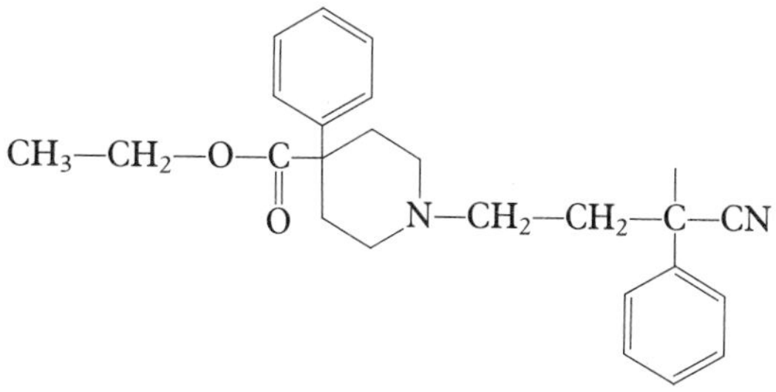

Propoxyphene

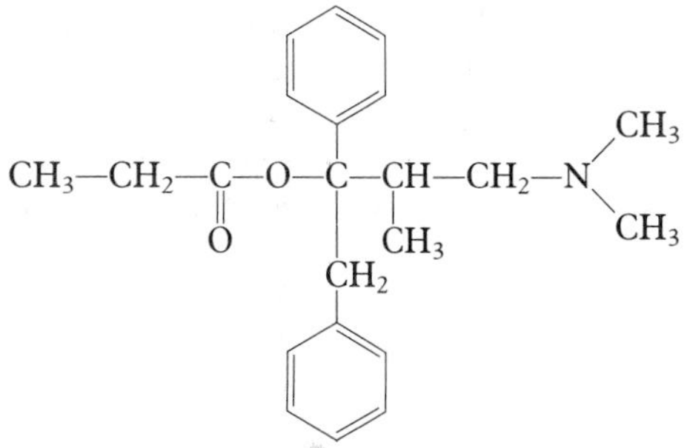

Propoxyphene

Propoxyphene has some structural similarity to methadone. Although still quite widely used, its analgesic potency is less than that of codeine and, perhaps, no more effective than aspirin. In large doses, propoxyphene can produce respiratory and CNS depression, and sometimes convulsions. Propoxyphene can produce dependence.

Levorphanol

The pharmacologic effects of levorphanol are similar to those of morphine except that the incidence of nausea, vomiting, and constipation are reported to be less than with the prototype agent. By injection the compound is approximately 5 times more potent than morphine, and like codeine has a high parenteral/oral dose ratio (Table 22-4). The onset and peak analgesic effects are comparable to those of morphine; however, the duration of the analgesia is somewhat longer, since levorphanol is biotransformed less rapidly, resulting in a longer elimination half-life (see Table 22-3).

Levorphanol

Methorphan

The levorotatory isomer levomethorphan produces intense opiate-like effects; it can be substituted for morphine, and it is fully addictive. The dextro isomer, dextromethorphan, is not analgesic, will not substitute for morphine, and is not addicting. However, it has useful antitussive activity.

MIXED AGONIST-ANTAGONIST

Drugs in this group possess both agonist and antagonist activity. Generally speaking, the antagonist actions are primarily at the mu receptor, with the agonist activity at other opioid receptors, especially kappa and sigma. Although their use can result in the production of analgesia, respiratory depression, and other agonist effects associated with drugs such as morphine, they can also block and reverse the effects of the agonists and may precipitate an abstinence syndrome if administered to individuals who are dependent on the opioid agonists. Tolerance develops to the agonist actions of this group of drugs, but no tolerance develops to the antagonist properties. Although dependence liability to this group of drugs is relatively low, dependence can result from their continued use. The abstinence syndrome that may result differs considerably from that associated with dependence to the mu agonists such as morphine or heroin. The principal use of this group of agents is for analgesia, and they are quite effective against moderate and even fairly severe forms of pain. Despite a few studies to the contrary, it is generally held that these agents are somewhat less effective than morphine in treating severe pain. The mixed agonist-antagonists can antagonize the respiratory depression associated with overdosage from the agonists. How-

ever, if the respiratory depression is due to agents other than opioids (e.g., sedative-hypnotics such as barbiturates), the patient may be made worse, since the drugs in this group cause respiratory depression as part of their agonist profile.

Nalorphine, or *N*-allylnormorphine, is an effective analgesic when administered parenterally but often produces dysphoria, confusion, and visual hallucinations. Although no longer used clinically in the United States, it was the first agent found to be efficacious in the treatment of heroin overdose. Nalorphine has a much shorter duration of action than morphine, and in the treatment of severe narcotic-induced respiratory depression the patient must be carefully monitored and repeated doses of nalorphine administered as required.

Pentazocine

Pentazocine is a weak antagonist of morphine, much weaker than nalorphine or levallorphan, but with a strong analgesic effect. Its agonistic effects, including analgesia, are largely on the kappa receptor.

Pentazocine

Structurally, pentazocine is a benzomorphan derivative. It can precipitate an abstinence syndrome in an opioid-dependent individual, but it will not antagonize morphine-induced respiratory depression. It cannot suppress withdrawal symptoms associated with abstinence from morphine or other mu agonists, an indication that its agonist actions are not on mu receptors. It should be recalled that agonists acting on the same receptors (e.g., mu receptors) can suppress abstinence signs associated with other agonists acting on that receptor. Pentazocine is about one-third to one-fourth as active orally as parenterally, and its use as an analgesic is primarily by the oral route, although subcutaneous and intramuscular administration can provide more effective analgesia (Table 22-4). When administered orally, its analgesic potency is about equal to that of codeine. The half-life in plasma is 2 to 3 h. It is metabolized in the liver, primarily by oxidation and conjugation to glucuronides. Untoward effects that are fairly common are dizziness, sweating, nausea, and vomiting. Respiratory depression has a ceiling, is not of the usual dose-related type, and can be antagonized with naloxone. Effects on the gastrointestinal tract are similar to those of the opioid agonists. Large doses can produce tachycardia, elevated blood pressure, and dysphoria. The last action is probably due to interactions with the sigma receptor.

Tolerance develops to the actions of pentazocine but may be slower and less complete than that seen with morphine. Although originally touted as a compound essentially devoid of abuse liability, psychologic and physical dependence on pentazocine has been reported after parenteral self-administration. The increasing incidence of such abuse a few years ago, especially in combination with tripelennamine (an antihistamine), led to placement of the drug in schedule IV of the Federal Controlled Substances Act (see Chap. 25). It also led to the inclusion of small amounts of the antagonist naloxone in an oral preparation of pentazocine as a means of preventing misuse of tablets by injections.

Despite problems associated with the use of pentazocine, the drug remains an important and useful analgesic, especially because of its oral efficacy. The risk of drug dependence is lower than that associated with the use of full agonists such as morphine.

Nalbuphine

Nalbuphine is equipotent to morphine as an analgesic.

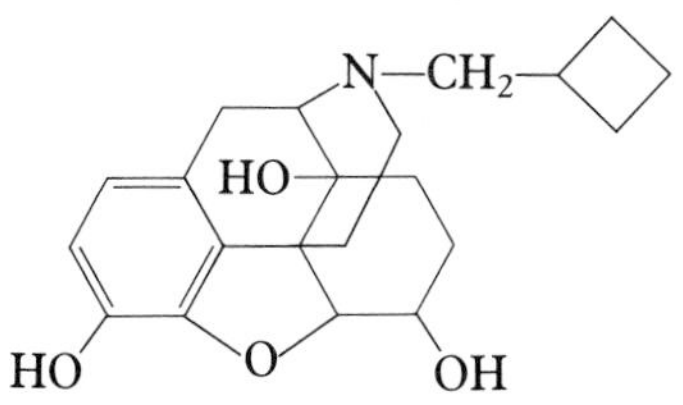

Nalbuphine

It is reported to cause less vomiting and to have less potential for drug abuse. Although qualitatively similar to pentazocine, it is a more potent mu antagonist (Table 22-4). It is somewhat effective orally but is markedly only for injection, with a duration of action of 3 to 6 h. Although nalbuphine can produce respiratory depression comparable to that seen with low to moderate doses (10 to 30 mg) of morphine, there is a ceiling effect, and the respiratory depression with higher doses is much less than that associated with morphine. All effects can be antagonized by naloxone. Higher doses (70 mg) can produce dysphoria and other side effects as does nalorphine. Abuse potential, although lower than for morphine, probably exists and is similar to that seen with pentazocine.

Butorphanol

This drug is similar, in most ways, to nalbuphine. However, like pentazocine, it can increase cardiac work.

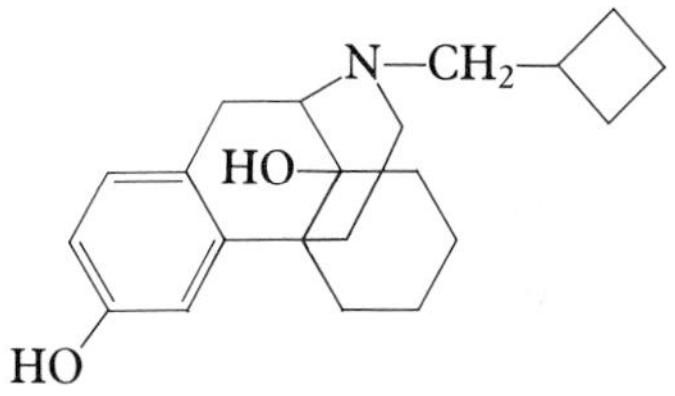

Butorphanol

It does not seem to precipitate abstinence as readily as nalbuphine in individuals dependent on mu agonists, and its potential for abuse appears to be low. It is available only for parenteral use.

Buprenorphine

Buprenorphine, like nalbuphine and butorphanol, is a derivative of thebaine, a compound closely related chemically to morphine. The chemical modification that leads to buprenorphine, however, markedly changes the pharmacologic profile.

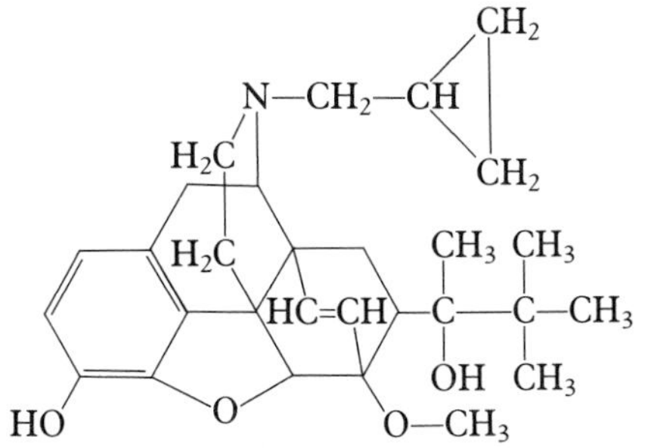

Buprenorphine

Buprenorphine has recently become available in the United States, but only in injectable form. Buprenorphine is 25 to 50 times more potent than morphine as an analgesic and has 10 times the potency of nalorphine as an antagonist (Table 22-4). Its duration of action (about 6 h) is considerably longer than that seen with the other drugs of this group, and naloxone may fail to antagonize the associated respiratory depression, probably an indication of buprenorphine's high affinity for and slow dissociation from opioid receptors. This drug is sometimes referred to as a partial agonist, rather than a mixed agonist-antagonist. Side effects are similar to those seen with morphine. Although some of the drug is excreted unchanged in the feces, some is metabolized in the liver.

Unlike the other mixed agonist-antagonists, the abstinence syndrome associated with its use bears many similarities to that seen with morphine, it can suppress morphine withdrawal, and it can precipitate abstinence. However, buprenorphine abstinence is of much longer duration than that seen after morphine withdrawal, and the symptoms are milder. Some reports indicate that abrupt withdrawal produces no symptoms, and it appears that a final evaluation awaits more experience with the drug.

OPIOID ANTAGONISTS

These agents have marked antagonist activity but, unlike the mixed agonist-antagonists, possess no agonist activity. The effectiveness and the potency of the opioid antagonist activity vary with the type of opioid receptor. In general, the order is mu, delta, kappa, sigma. Questions have arisen as to whether these so-called pure narcotic antagonists are totally devoid of any agonist activity. What seems apparent is that any effects associated with low to moderate doses of the drugs are most likely due to the antagonism of the toxic effects of endogenous opioid peptides. Very high doses of the antagonists can produce other effects, but these may or may not be related to activity at the opioid receptors. For all practical purposes, these effects can be ignored in terms of clinical medicine. Tolerance and physical dependence do not occur, since the antagonists have no intrinsic activity. They are capable, however, of precipitating the abstinence syndrome, and they can also antagonize the actions of the agonists and the mixed agonist-antagonists.

Naloxone

Chemically, naloxone is *N*-allylnoroxymorphone. In general, *N*-allyl substitution leads to antagonist properties.

$$N-CH_2-CH=CH_2$$

HO

HO　　O　　O

Naloxone

Naloxone is several times more potent as an antagonist than nalorphine, the exact ratio depending on the effect being studied and the agonist or mixed agonist-antagonist it is antagonizing. Its role as the drug of choice for the treatment of opioid overdosage has been discussed above.

The half-life of naloxone is on the order of 20 to 40 min, and the duration of action is about 1 to 2 h. Onset of action following intravenous administration is within 1 to 2 min. The drug is metabolized in the liver by glucuronide conjugation. For the treatment of overdoses of mu agonists, intramuscular, subcutaneous, or intravenous doses of 0.4 to 0.8 mg are generally administered and the dose is repeated at 2- to 3-min intervals until a response is seen. If no response is noted after a total of 10 mg has been administered, the offending agent is probably not an opioid. For respiratory depression of the newborn as a result of opiates given to the mother, the usual dose is 0.01 mg per kilogram of body weight given intravenously, intramuscularly, or subcutaneously.

Special care must be exercised in the administration of naloxone to an individual dependent on opioids, since an abstinence syndrome may be precipitated. Similarly, care should be exercised in treating newborns of mothers suspected of opioid addiction.

Naltrexone

Naltrexone is a cyclopropylmethyl derivative of oxymorphone. It is essentially identical to naloxone in its actions, but it differs in two important ways: it is effective orally and it has a long duration of action, on the order of 24 h. It is subject to "first-pass" metabolism in the liver, but one of its metabolic products, 6-β-naltrexol, is also a potent opioid antagonist.

Naltrexone

The principal use of naltrexone is as an adjunct in the treatment of detoxified opioid users. If used in an individual still taking opioids, an abstinence syndrome can be precipitated. However, once the person has been taken off opioids, the use of naltrexone will prevent the effects associated with the subsequent use of agonists. This may be very beneficial in a certain subpopulation of former addicts. The therapeutic range associated with the use of naltrexone is potentially hepatotoxic. Patients being treated with the drug should be carefully monitored for hepatic function.

Drug Interactions

Opioid drug interactions occur with

1. *Sedative–hypnotics* which increase respiratory depression as well as other central nervous system depressant effects
2. *MAO inhibitors* which produce a high incidence of hyperpyrexia leading to coma

Contraindications

The opioid drugs are contraindicated in various clinical situations as follow:

1. Avoid use of agonist with mixed agonist-antagonist drugs because of the possibility of inhibiting the analgesic activity. In addition, the possibility may exist of producing a state of withdrawal.
2. Avoid use in patients with poor liver function, since the major metabolic pathways of the opioids is via the liver.
3. Avoid use in patients with poor respiratory func-

tion because of the respiratory depressant effects of the opioid analgesics.
4. Avoid chronic use in pregnant women, which may cause addiction in utero and produce withdrawal symptoms in the newborn after birth.

Preparations

Morphine sulfate is available in tablets of 5, 8, 10, 15, and 30 mg. These can be given orally or dissolved in water for parenteral use.

Hydromorphone hydrochloride is available as follows: ampuls for injection containing 1 to 4 mg/mL; rectal suppositories containing 3 mg; and tablets containing 1 to 4 mg. Multiple-dose vials are also marketed, containing 10 to 20 mL, with 2 mg/mL.

Oxymorphone hydrochloride is available as follows: solutions for injection containing 1 mg/mL; tablets of 10 mg for oral use; and suppositories of 2 or 5 mg.

Codeine phosphate is available in 15-, 30-, and 60-mg tablets for oral or hypodermic use.

Oxycodone hydrochloride is available in tablets or capsules of 5 mg, containing also 325 mg of acetaminophen, a nonnarcotic analgesic.

Meperidine hydrochloride is available in the following solutions for injection: 25, 50, 75, or 100 mg/mL. Meperidine is also available in tablets of 50 or 100 mg and in elixir containing 10 mg/mL.

Diphenoxylate hydrochloride is available in tablets of 2.5 mg, containing also 0.025 mg of atropine sulfate; also in a liquid containing the same amounts in 5 mL.

Loperamide hydrochloride is available in capsules of 2 mg. Initial dose is 4 mg, followed by 2 mg after each unformed stool.

Fentanyl citrate is available in solution containing 0.05 mg of fentanyl and 2.5 mg of droperidol per milliliter.

Methadone hydrochloride is available in solutions of 10 mg/mL. It is also available in tablets of 2.5, 5, 7.5, and 10 mL and a syrup of 0.33 mg/mL.

Propoxyphene hydrochloride is available in capsules of 32 and 65 mg for oral use.

Propoxyphene napsylate is available as 100-mg tablets and as a suspension containing 50 mg per 5 mL.

Levorphan tartrate is available in solutions containing 2 mg/mL. Tablets containing 2 mg are also available.

Pentazocine hydrochloride is available as 50-mg tablets.

Pentazocine lactate is available in solutions containing 30 mg of base per milliliter.

Nalorphine hydrochloride is available in ampuls for injection containing 0.2 mg/mL, 5 mg/mL, and a multiple-dose vial containing 50 mg per 10 mL.

Naloxone hydrochloride is available in ampuls for injection containing 0.4 mg/mL.

Levallorphan tartrate is available in solution of 1 mg/mL.

BIBLIOGRAPHY

Beumont, A., and J. Hughes: "Biology of Opioid Peptides," *Annu. Rev. Pharmacol.*, **19**:203–244 (1979).

Brady, J. V. and S. Lukas (eds.): Testing Drugs for Physical Dependence Potential and Abuse Liability, NIDA Research Monograph 52, U.S. Government Printing Office, Washington, D.C., 1984.

Braude, M. C., E. L. Harris, J. P. May, J. P. Smith, and J. E. Villareal (eds.): "Narcotic Antagonists," in *Advances in Biochemistry and Psychopharmacology*, vol. 8, Raven, New York, 1973.

Delitala, G., M. Motta, and M. Serio (eds.): *Opioid Modulation of Endocrine Function*, Raven, New York, 1984.

DiGregorio, G. J., E. Barbieri, G. Sterling, R. Fruncillo, and S. Kozen: *Handbook of Pain Management*, Medical Surveillance Inc., Philadelphia, 1986.

Hughes, J., H. O. J. Collier, M. J. Rance, and M. B. Tyers (eds.): *Opioids—Past, Present, and Future*, Taylor and Francis, London, 1984.

Kosterlitz, H. W. (ed.): *Opiates and Endogenous Opioid Peptides*, North-Holland, Amsterdam, 1976.

Pasternak, G.: *The Opiate Receptors*, Humana Press, Clifton, New Jersey, 1988.

Simon, E. J., and J. M. Hiller: "The Opiate Receptors," in H. W. Kosterlitz (ed.), *Opiates and Endogenous Opioid Peptides*, North-Holland, Amsterdam, 1976, pp. 371–394.

Terenius, L.: "Endogenous Peptides and Analgesia," *Annu. Rev. Pharmacol.*, **18**:189–204 (1978).

Wiler, A.: *Opioid Dependence—Mechanisms and Treatment*, Plenum, New York, 1980.

Nonnarcotic Analgesics

James M. Ross and Raphael J. DeHoratius

Analgesic drugs which are not related to opiates have a different spectrum of activity than do the narcotic analgesics dealt with in the preceding chapter. Most of these drugs are also antipyretic, and some also have anti-inflammatory properties. Nonsteroidal anti-inflammatory drugs (NSAIDs) are one class of agents which have anti-inflammatory, antipyretic, and analgesic effects. In general these agents are most effective in pain associated with inflammation such as arthritis. Still another category of agents such as colchicine and probenecid is useful in the therapy of gouty arthritis.

NONSTEROIDAL ANTI-INFLAMMATORY DRUGS

Aspirin and Salicylates

Aspirin, the acetyl derivative of salicylic acid, is today probably used more widely and in larger quantity than any other therapeutic agent. The first pharmacologic data on aspirin appeared in 1899. Aspirin and a number of other drugs possess analgesic, antipyretic, and anti-inflammatory actions. Aspirin is the prototypic NSAID. NSAIDs are prescribed for a wide variety of clinical uses such as rheumatic conditions, analgesia, and dysmenorrhea. In addition to aspirin, there are several NSAIDs available in the United States (Table 23-1) which are commonly prescribed. Aspirin is the standard by which all other NSAIDs are compared, and no other NSAID has been proven to be more effective than aspirin in the treatment of several rheumatic conditions. Aspirin is a very effective cyclooxygenase inhibitor, compared with some of the newer nonacetylated salicylates which are only weak inhibitors.

Chemistry Aspirin and other salicylates are derivatives of salicylic acid; all are prepared synthetically.

Salicylic acid   Acetylsalicylic acid

Methyl salicylate

Mechanism of Action According to present concepts, the mechanism of action by which aspirin and the other NSAIDs are analgesic, antipyretic, and anti-inflammatory results from their ability to inhibit prostaglandin formation. A simplified scheme for the production of prostaglandins (PG) is given in Fig. 23-1. Arachidonic acid bound to phospholipids is present in cell membranes. In response to various stimuli, the arachidonic acid is hydrolyzed from the phospholipids by phospholipase A_2, then rapidly oxygenated by a cyclooxygenase (prostaglandin synthetase-enzyme complex) to form the cyclic endoperoxides PGG_2 and PGH_2. These cyclic endoperoxides, which produce pain and vasoconstriction, may be further metabolized by different enzymes in the prostaglandin synthetase

TABLE 23-1 **Classification and half-lives of some nonsteroidal anti-inflammatory drugs**

Nonsteroidal anti-inflammatory drugs	Half-life, h
Salicylates	
Aspirin (acetyl salicylic acid)	2–15
Choline magnesium trisalicylate	2–15
Diflunisal	11–14
Magnesium salicylate	2–15
Salsalate	2–15
Proprionic acids	
Fenoprofen	2
Ibuprofen	2
Ketoprofen	2
Naproxen, naproxen sodium	12–15
Acetic acids	
Indomethacin	4–8
Sulindac	16
Tolmetin	4–6
Diclofenac	2
Oxicams	
Piroxicam	50
Pyrazoles	
Phenylbutazone	43–83
Fenamates	
Meclofenamate	2–3
Mefenamic acid	2

complex to form other prostaglandins (e. g., PGE_2 and $PGF_{2\alpha}$), thromboxanes, or prostacyclin. These end products are not stored in the body; they are produced as required, exert their various physiologic or pathologic effects, and are quickly metabolized to inactive products. By a similar pathway PGE_1 is produced from linoleic acid. In addition, arachidonic acid can be converted to leukotrienes by the lipoxygenase pathway. Aspirin has been shown to inhibit conversion of arachidonic acid to cyclic endoperoxides by irreversible acetylation of cyclooxygenase. This irreversible inhibition results in reduction of levels of prostaglandins and thromboxane A_2. Other NSAIDs, in contrast, are reversible inhibitors of cyclooxygenase.

Other mechanisms of action of the NSAIDs have been suggested, but the effect on cyclooxygenase appears the best explanation for the action of these drugs. Further information on prostaglandins is presented in Chap. 13.

Anti-Inflammatory Effect The release of prostaglandins, especially PGE_2, during an inflammatory reaction causes edema, erythema, pain, and heat. These effects are inhibited by the NSAIDs. Clinically the drugs are useful in the treatment of inflammatory arthritis, such as rheumatoid arthritis. Unfortunately, they do not affect the proliferation of synovium in rheumatoid arthritis and therefore do not prevent progression of the disease. NSAIDs are highly protein-bound and, since sites of inflammation allow extravasation of serum proteins, NSAIDs may reach greater concentrations in areas of inflammation.

Analgesic Effect Local prostaglandin formation intensifies the pain-producing properties of bradykinin, lowering the threshold to pain and producing a hyperalgesic state. Thus the role of prostaglandins in production of pain seems to be in combination with other mediators and can be described as a modulator of pain production. Aspirin and the other NSAIDs act as analgesics by decreasing the synthesis of prostaglandins and also by affecting release or action of bradykinin. Clinically the NSAIDs are much more effective in relieving pain associated with inflammation; thus their mechanism is quite different than that of the centrally acting analgesics such as morphine.

Antipyretic Effect One of the prostaglandins (PGE_1) is the most potent physiologic pyrogen (fever-producing agent) known and has been found to be generated in the brain during fever. Following intravenous injection of pyrogens, PGE_1 has been found in the cerebrospinal fluid. The NSAIDs effectively inhibit generation of prostaglandins in the brain during conditions producing fever. Aspirin and the other NSAIDs are effective drugs when used to lower elevated body temperature, but they have no effect on normal body temperature.

Effect on Organ Systems

Central Nervous System It has been suggested that aspirin has a slight calming action and may be synergistic with the hypnotic effect of barbiturates. Central

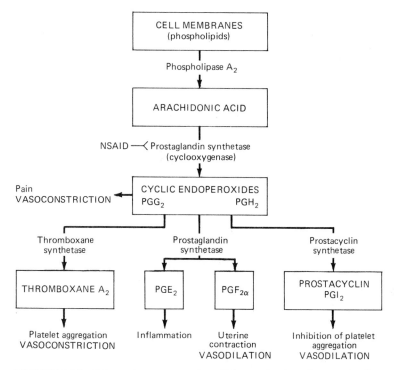

FIGURE 23-1 Schematic representation of the production of prostaglandins. [Adapted from Nickander, McMahon, and Ridolfo, *Annu. Rev. Pharmacol. Toxicol.*, **19**:469 (1979).]

nervous system disturbances such as delirium and occasionally psychoses may develop in patients after high doses of aspirin. These symptoms in their mild form are so common that the term *salicylism* is generally applied to them (see "Adverse Reactions," below). Other NSAIDs can cause confusion, delirium, dizziness, drowsiness, depression, and headaches, and these effects are especially prominent in the elderly.

Gastrointestinal Tract Nausea, vomiting and gastric irritation are common. Prostaglandin E_2 plays a significant role in gastric mucus production and maintains the integrity of the gastric mucosal barrier. Aspirin and the other NSAIDs reduce gastric prostaglandin E_2 resulting in diminished gastric cytoprotection. Therefore NSAID therapy is associated with a variety of gastrointestinal disorders, including gastritis, peptic ulcer disease, and upper gastrointestinal bleeding. This effect is independent of the route of administration. Nausea and vomiting are produced partially by central stimulation. In rheumatic fever patients in

whom high plasma levels of aspirin are maintained, nausea is common as a side effect. Hepatotoxicity manifested by hepatitis or mild elevation of liver enzymes has occurred with all NSAIDs.

Respiratory System The average analgesic dose of aspirin (325 mg) does not affect respiration; however, respiration is increased in both rate and depth after large doses of aspirin or other salicylates. This is largely the result of a direct stimulation of the medulla. It has also been suggested that peripheral metabolic stimulation and overproduction of carbon dioxide may contribute to this effect.

Acid-Base Balance Acid-base balance changes and disturbances in electrolyte pattern are related to both respiratory stimulation and metabolic alterations. The respiratory stimulation tends to lead to respiratory alkalosis. As more aspirin is absorbed, more acidic intermediary metabolites are formed (see "Salicylate Overdose," below). These, as well as the acidity of the drug itself, lead to metabolic acidosis.

Blood In susceptible individuals large doses of aspirin produce a degree of hypoprothrombinemia, probably by antagonizing vitamin K and thereby decreasing the synthesis of certain blood coagulation factors in the liver. Changes in sedimentation rate are common after aspirin ingestion and occur by an unknown mechanism. Sedimentation rates are inversely related to the fibrinogen concentration in both normal subjects and patients with rheumatic fever or rheumatoid arthritis.

Platelets Thromboxane A_2 synthesized in platelets causes aggregation of platelets and vasoconstriction. Prostaglandin I_2 (prostacyclin) released by endothelial cells inhibits platelet aggregation. When tissue injury occurs, platelets are exposed to thromboplastin and aggregation occurs. In atherosclerosis, PGI_2 production is believed to decrease, thus increasing the chances for thrombosis. Aspirin and other NSAIDs inhibit the production of thromboxane A_2 and prostacyclin by platelets and the endothelial cells, respectively. Inhibition of platelet thromboxane production predominates, since platelets are unable to synthesize new cyclooxygenase after it is irreversibly acetylated by aspirin. Trials with low-dose aspirin have demonstrated antithrombotic effects, which can be explained by this reduction in thromboxane production. Aspirin in doses of 324 to 1300 mg/day has been shown to be effective in preventing myocardial infarction, transient ischemic attacks, and occlusion of coronary grafts.

Kidney There are several clinical renal syndromes associated with NSAID use, including papillary necrosis, acute interstitial nephritis, nephrotic syndrome, hyperkalemia, and acute renal failure. Intrarenal prostaglandins maintain renal blood flow and glomerular filtration rate (GFR) when there is diminished effective intravascular volume or a preexisting renal condition. When NSAID therapy is instituted in these conditions, the subsequent decrease in renal prostaglandins may result in diminished GFR and acute renal failure. Risk factors for NSAID-induced renal failure include cirrhosis, chronic renal disease, congestive heart failure, use of diuretics, and possibly advanced age. If NSAIDs are used in these conditions, it is necessary to follow renal function, since acute renal failure is reversible if recognized early. NSAIDs may also cause sodium and water retention, and certain NSAIDs have been shown to interfere with antihypertensive drug therapy.

Uric Acid Excretion Drugs which tend to enhance the excretion of uric acid are termed *uricosuric agents*. There seems to be no doubt that aspirin can lower the renal threshold for uric acid and the urate level in the blood; however, it has long been recognized that aspirin may produce an opposite effect, depending on the dose administered. At doses in the range of 5 g/day, aspirin increases urate excretion by 40 percent, and when given with sodium bicarbonate, excretion increases up to 80 percent. However, at low doses, such as 1 g/day, it will decrease urate excretion by 20 percent. Furthermore, even at high doses it will antagonize the uricosuric effect of probenecid, phenylbutazone, and sulfinpyrazone.

Skin Free salicylic acid and methyl salicylate irritate the skin. Topical application of salicylic acid produces a slow and painless destruction of the epithelium (keratolytic effect), which is useful for the removal of corns and warts. While it may have some direct action against certain fungi, it is more likely that its effectiveness in this area is due chiefly to its keratolytic action.

Uterus Prostaglandins, especially $PGF_{2\alpha}$, are potent stimulants of uterine contraction. Prostaglandin $F_{2\alpha}$ is used clinically to induce abortions. The NSAIDs have been shown to relax uterine spasm occurring during menstrual cramps and are used in treating dysmenorrhea. Their value in preventing spontaneous abortion has not been shown.

Ductus Arteriosus Prostaglandins are important agents during neonatal life where they act to keep the ductus arteriosus patent. In the neonatal period, if the ductus arteriosus does not close, the NSAIDs, notably indomethacin, may induce closure. Formerly the condition was treatable only by surgery. Conversely, infusion of PGE_1 has been used in infants with congenital cardiac anomalies where potency of the ductus arteriosus is essential for survival until surgery can be performed.

Pharmacokinetics Aspirin is well absorbed after oral administration, reaching a peak blood level in 1 to 2 h. The presence of food or antacid delays its absorption. Aspirin is 50 to 80 percent protein-bound and will compete with other highly protein-bound drugs. Aspirin is rapidly hydrolyzed in the plasma and liver to the pharmacologically active salicylic acid. The metabolism of aspirin follows first-order and zero-order kinetics. At low doses, increments result in proportional increases in serum levels. At higher doses the metabolic pathway becomes saturated and a small dose will result in a relatively large increase in serum levels. The half-life of aspirin is 15 to 20 min, but that of salicylic acid is 3 h after administration of 300 mg of aspirin. The half-life of salicylic acid after administration of 1000 mg of aspirin is 5 to 6 h, after a toxic dose of 20 g is 20 h.

Salicylic acid is biotransformed in the liver. The major product is the glycine conjugate, salicyluric acid. Other products are gentisic acid, salicyl acyl glucuronide, and salicyl phenolic glucuronide. These biotransformation products as well as free drug are excreted by the kidney. Administration of soluble antacid such as sodium bicarbonate markedly promotes the excretion of unchanged aspirin by the kidney by increasing ionization and reducing reabsorption. At pH 4, 10 percent of aspirin is excreted unchanged, whereas at pH 8, 80 percent is excreted.

Therapeutic Uses Analgesia constitutes the major use of aspirin. The general public employs aspirin mainly in the treatment of simple headache or neuralgic pain in doses of 325 to 650 mg. Aspirin is especially useful in pain of low intensity associated with inflammation.

An important application of aspirin is in the treatment of rheumatic arthritis. In order to achieve an anti-inflammatory effect it must be administered in doses greater than 4 g/day. At this dose objective changes such as decrease of joint size, increase in grip strength, reduction of erythrocyte sedimentation rate, and decrease in morning stiffness are seen in addition to relief of pain. It is important to stress that for the anti-inflammatory effect to be optimum, aspirin must be administered at a dose higher than that used for simple analgesia. Preferably, therapy should be monitored. With salicylate blood levels, a level of 20 to 25 mg per 100 mL is considered the therapeutic range.

Acute rheumatic fever, an inflammatory disease following infection with β-hemolytic streptococci, manifests itself in arthritis, carditis, chorea, and skin rash. Large doses of aspirin are of value in the symptomatic therapy of the disease. Aspirin, however, is of no value in preventing later attacks of rheumatic fever. Aspirin has long been recognized as an antipyretic and is commonly employed for this purpose, i. e., to reduce or prevent fever and to relieve the discomfort associated with fever.

NSAID Therapy in the Elderly Many patients taking NSAIDs are elderly, since this population has an increased prevalence of arthritic conditions. The elderly also frequently have coexisting medical problems or are receiving concurrent medical therapy which may predispose to adverse effects of NSAID therapy. Renal, gastrointestinal, and central nervous system toxicity is particularly a concern in the elderly. Therefore these patients should be monitored closely while on NSAIDs. Use of nonacetylated salicylates is preferred, since these agents are weak cyclooxygenase inhibitors and therefore should hold less risk for adverse effects.

Adverse Reactions Gastric irritation, which may lead to gastric ulceration and bleeding, is the principal adverse reaction seen with aspirin and all the other NSAIDs. The mechanism responsible for gastric irritation and ulcerations is described above.

Salicylism is a series of reactions frequently recurring when the therapeutic dose of aspirin is high, such as used in rheumatic fever and rheumatoid arthritis. These symptoms, which may be manifest at plasma levels in excess of 25 mg per 100 mL, consist of nausea and vomiting, tinnitus, deafness, severe headache, mental dullness and confusion, quickened pulse, and increased respiration. The condition resembles cinchonism and may be quite troublesome, but it disappears completely on stopping or reducing the drug.

Hypersensitivity manifested by bronchoconstriction, urticaria, angioneurotic edema, or anaphylactic shock may develop from the administration of relatively small doses of aspirin. The cause of hypersensitivity is unknown but is commonly seen in asthmatics with nasal polyps and may be due to an airway response to a decrease in prostaglandins. Another hypothesis is that inhibition of cyclooxygenase results in shunting of arachidonic acid metabolism to the lipoxygenase pathway, increasing certain mediators of allergic response (see Fig. 23-1). In very sensitive patients the reaction may be fatal. Cross-sensitivity with all the other NSAIDs occurs, and therefore all NSAIDs are contraindicated in patients with hypersensitivity to aspirin.

Aspirin may be involved in a number of interactions with other drugs, and since it is a nonprescription item widely used by the general public, patients receiving certain medications should be warned against the use of aspirin. Competition occurs with anticoagulant drugs such as warfarin, since both drugs are protein-bound. Aspirin may increase the hypoglycemic effect of insulin and oral hypoglycemic agents. Its action on uric acid clearance by the kidney causes it to interfere with the uricosuric action of probenecid and sulfinpyrazone.

There is evidence linking Reye's syndrome to aspirin intake during viral illnesses. Reye's syndrome is an illness which is directly related to viral epidemics and can result in hepatic failure, severe neurologic symptoms, and death. Most cases occur in children 4 to 12 years of age. Therefore, it is recommended that aspirin not be used in children and teenagers with viral illnesses.

Pregnancy During pregnancy salicylates may reach substantial levels in the fetus. Women who used aspirin habitually have been shown to have children with smaller birth weights, but birth defects are not more common. Aspirin taken at the term of pregnancy may delay onset of labor and is associated with bruising of the newborn child.

Salicylate Overdose Despite its relatively low toxicity, aspirin is responsible for many accidental poisonings as well as poisoning with suicidal intent. It also ranks very high as a cause of poisoning in children under 5 years of age. There is no clear-cut evidence of chronic toxicity, since arthritic patients taking up to 10 g a day for many years often develop no adverse reactions. Controversy exists as to the possible role of aspirin in analgesic-abuse nephritis. In higher doses, aspirin will produce serious toxicity and even death. Because of its pleasant odor, methyl salicylate is often ingested by children and causes salicylate intoxication. Fatalities have occurred after ingestion of 4 mL of oil of wintergreen (methyl salicylate). Fatalities result from salicylate ingestion with greater frequency in children than in adults, apparently because of the lesser ability of children to withstand acid-base changes and dehydration. Initially the effects of salicylate overdose are those of respiratory stimulation, both in depth and rate, with resultant hypocapnia and respiratory alkalosis. Accompanying these signs may be irritability, dizziness, tinnitus, hallucinations, fever, nausea, and vomiting. Therapeutic anti-inflammatory concentrations are in the range of 20 to 25 mg per 100 mL. Above 30 to 40 mg per 100 mL, signs of toxicity appear. Levels above 90 mg per 100 mL are frequently lethal. In early stages the pH of the blood is

usually high, ranging up to 7.6, but after several hours, particularly in children, both the serum carbon dioxide content and the pH are frequently distinctly decreased. A series of metabolic alterations caused by ingestion of aspirin are responsible for production of the acidosis and ketosis. There may be acidic intermediates such as ketone bodies and lactic acid, resulting from incomplete carbohydrate and lipid metabolism. Furthermore, the concentration of salicylate itself in plasma may be appreciable, namely 40 to 80 mg per 100 mL, representing several milliequivalents per liter of acid. Finally, unidentified anions may accumulate in the blood and may amount to 8 to 18 meq/L.

The net result of these effects is a disturbance which may be either respiratory alkalosis or metabolic acidosis or a combination of both. Blood pH is a better measure of the acid-base balance than urinary pH. Some of the interrelationships are illustrated in Fig. 23-2. The picture of hyperpnea, hyperglycemia, ketosis, acidosis, polyuria, and dehydration may be similar to that seen in diabetic acidosis. It can be distinguished by a

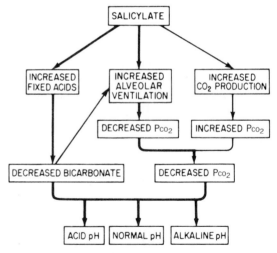

FIGURE 23-2 Summary of the pathogenesis of mixed disturbances of acid-base equilibrium in salicylate intoxication. From above downward are depicted the basic actions of salicylate, the separate effects of these actions on acid-base equilibrium, and the interaction of these effects in dictating the final pH. The line connecting "decreased bicarbonate" and "increased alveolar ventilation" is meant to imply that low blood pH may augment the primary effect of the drug upon respiration.

history of salicylate ingestion, the presence of tinnitus, muscle irritability, petechiae, and salicylate blood level.

Other disturbances associated with acute salicylate intoxication may be vomiting and diuresis occurring during the early phases of intoxication. Accompanying these are electrolyte disturbances, including hyponatremia and hypokalemia. Tetany and changes in the ECG have been reported. Delirium, coma, and oliguria may follow, and death may occur after 2 h to several days. Treatment of acute poisoning should be aimed at preventing absorption, at treating the acid-base and other electrolyte problems, and at promoting elimination of the drug. Activated charcoal may be of considerable value in reducing absorption. In severe cases hemodialysis may be used.

NONACETYLATED SALICYLATES

The nonacetylated salicylates available in the United States are diflunisal, magnesium choline trisalicylate, and salsalate (Table 23-1). These drugs have been shown to be effective in rheumatic conditions. In the body magnesium choline trisalicylate and salsalate are metabolized into salicylic acid. The serum salicylate levels that are achieved show a wide variability. Careful titration is required to produce therapeutic levels, since at or near therapeutic levels a small increment in dose may cause large increases in serum salicylate levels.

Diflunisal

Diflunisal is a derivative of salicylic acid but is not metabolized into salicylic acid. It is a reversible cyclooxygenase inhibitor and has an elimination half life of 11 to 14 h. Ninety percent is excreted in the urine as a soluble glucuronide conjugate. This drug has uricosuric activity and also has a dose-related effect on platelet function. Adverse reactions include nausea, vomiting, gastrointestinal toxicity, renal insufficiency, headache, and tinnitus.

Choline Magnesium Trisalicylate

Choline magnesium trisalicylate is a combination of choline salicylate and magnesium salicylate. These compounds are weak inhibitors of cyclooxygenase.

They are metabolized into salicylic acid and provide effective anti-inflammatory activity when salicylate levels are maintained in the therapeutic range. Glycine and glucuronide metabolites are excreted through the renal system. Adverse reactions include nausea, vomiting, uricosuric effects, salicylism and tinnitus. Choline magnesium trisalicylate does not affect platelet aggregation, and it produces minimal gastrointestinal and renal toxicity.

Salsalate

Salsalate is hydrolyzed in the small intestine into two molecules of salicylic acid. This drug is weak cyclooxygenase inhibitor and exhibits similar adverse effects to those seen with choline magnesium trisalicylate. During therapy salicylate levels should be monitored.

OTHER NONSTEROIDAL ANTI-INFLAMMATORY DRUGS

The mechanism of action of NSAIDs such as indomethacin, ibuprofen, and naproxen is the same as that of aspirin, namely, inhibition of cyclooxygenase. These drugs are used in the treatment of rheumatoid arthritis, osteoarthritis, acute attacks of gout or pseudogout, ankylosing spondylitis, and other seronegative spondyloarthropathies. However, the newer NSAIDs have not been shown to be more effective than aspirin in the treatment of rheumatoid arthritis although some adverse reactions may occur less frequently with these drugs than with aspirin. These agents are also used in the treatment of dysmenorrhea and mild to moderate pain. Also, there is considerable individual variation in response to these drugs, and there is no way to predict which NSAID will be most effective in an individual patient. All NSAIDs have a high degree of protein binding and therefore have a potential for displacement of highly bound drugs such as warfarin. NSAIDs are metabolized principally through hepatic mechanisms, and metabolites are primarily excreted by the kidney.

These drugs may be classified chemically as listed in Table 23-1. Specific characteristics of the agents are discussed under each chemical group. The structural formulas of some nonsteroidal anti-inflammatory drugs are shown in Fig. 23-3.

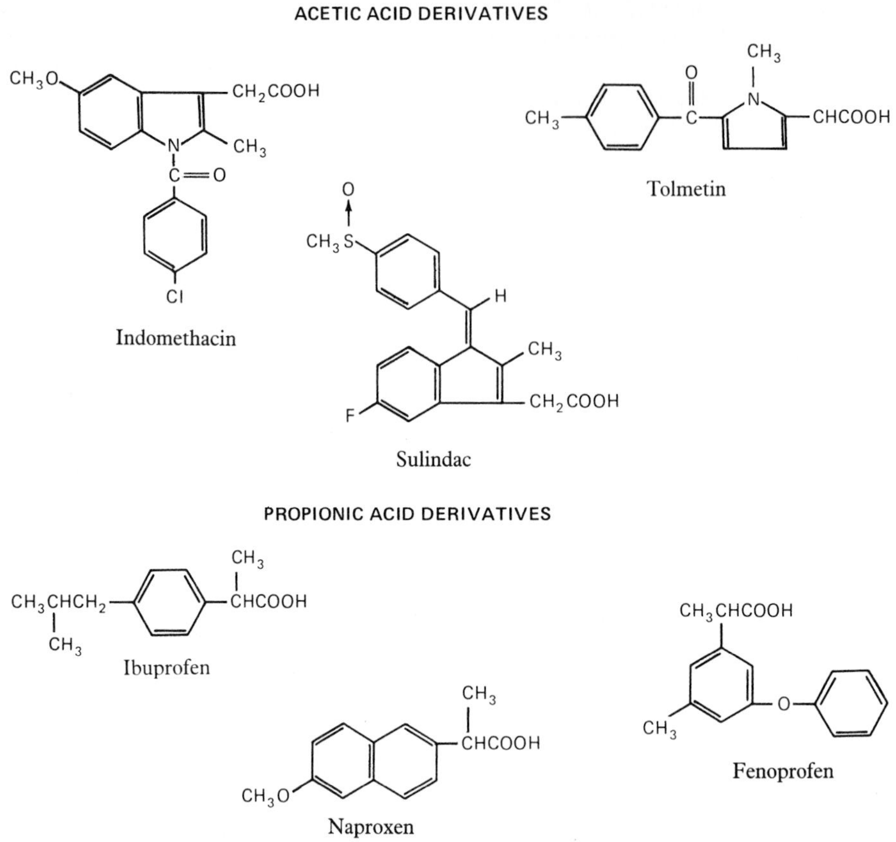

ACETIC ACID DERIVATIVES

Indomethacin

Tolmetin

Sulindac

PROPIONIC ACID DERIVATIVES

Ibuprofen

Naproxen

Fenoprofen

FIGURE 23-3   Structural formulas of some nonsteroidal anti-inflammatory agents.

Propionic Acid Derivatives

Ibuprofen   Ibuprofen was the first of the propionic acid derivatives to be released for clinical use for its anti-inflammatory effect and also is available without prescription. Like aspirin it possesses anti-inflammatory, analgesic, and antipyretic actions and has the same mechanism of action as that of aspirin. Ibuprofen is well absorbed orally; peak serum concentrations are attained in 1 to 2 h after oral administration. In the presence of food there is a decrease in the rate but not in the extent of absorption. Ibuprofen is rapidly biotransformed with a serum half-life of 1.8 to 2 h. The drug is completely eliminated 24 h after the last dose. The principal adverse reaction of ibuprofen is gastrointestinal irritation. Epigastric distress occurs in 14 to 16 percent of patients. Skin rashes, dizziness, tinnitus, renal failure, and edema may occur. Aseptic meningitis has been observed rarely and has occurred most commonly in individuals with systemic lupus erythematosus. Renal failure and aseptic meningitis have also been seen with over-the-counter preparations. Although some studies have failed to show interaction between ibuprofen and warfarin, because of its high protein binding, ibuprofen should be used with caution if at all in patients receiving oral anticoagulants. As mentioned above, patients with hypersensitivity to aspirin manifested by nasal polyps, angioneurotic edema, and bronchospasm will show hypersensitivity to ibuprofen as well as the other NSAIDs.

Naproxen Naproxen is completely absorbed from the gastrointestinal tract. Peak plasma levels are attained in 2 to 4 h. The mean biologic half-life is 13 h. Naproxen is 99 percent protein-bound. Approximately 95 percent is excreted in the urine as unchanged drug and desmethylnaproxen. As with ibuprofen, the principal toxicity is gastrointestinal irritation, which may lead to ulceration and hemorrhage. Rare cases of bone marrow depression have occurred. The drug is contraindicated in aspirin hypersensitivity. It is approved for treatment of juvenile rheumatoid arthritis and is available in suspension form. Naproxen sodium is also available and is more rapidly absorbed than naproxen. It provides pain relief within 1 h and is useful in the management of acute and chronic pain.

Fenoprofen Calcium A third propionic acid derivative, fenoprofen, is related chemically and pharmacologically to the other two compounds. Fenoprofen is rapidly absorbed from the fasting stomach, reaching peak plasma levels with 2 h. The plasma half-life is 3 h. Fenoprofen is 99 percent protein-bound; 90 percent of the drug is eliminated within 24 h as fenoprofen glucuronide and hydroxyfenoprofen glucuronide. The major adverse reaction is gastrointestinal irritation. Skin rashes, somnolence, palpitations, headache, and tinnitus have been reported.

Flurbiprofen Flurbiprofen is well absorbed from the gastrointestinal tract and produces peak plasma levels in approximately 1.5 h. The compound is extensively biotransformed by the liver with an elimination half-life of 5.7 h. Excretion of the drug occurs primarily through the kidney, and in the urine are found parent drug as well as conjugated and hydroxylated metabolites. Flurbiprofen exhibits a very high degree of protein binding (99 percent).

The mechanism of action for its anti-inflammatory, analgesic, and antipyretic properties appears to be related to the inhibition of prostaglandin synthesis. The drug is used in acute and chronic conditions of rheumatoid arthritis and osteoarthritis. The adverse reactions reported for flurbiprofen are similar to those of the other NSAIDs. Dyspepsia, gastrointestinal bleeding, abdominal pain, diarrhea, edema, and tinnitus are some reactions that can occur. In addition, flurbiprofen is contraindicated in patients who have hypersensitivity to it or the other NSAIDs.

Ketoprofen This compound is a proprionic acid derivative which is rapidly and completely absorbed from the gastrointestinal tract. Ketoprofen attains peak plasma levels in 0.5 to 2 h and has a mean plasma half-life of 2 h. Sixty percent of the glucuronide metabolite is excreted in the urine. Some adverse reactions reported for ketoprofen include renal and gastrointestinal toxicities, edema, fluid retention, and abnormalities in liver function test.

Acetic Acid Derivatives

Indomethacin This drug is an indole acetic acid derivative and is a very potent cyclooxygenase inhibitor. It also is an inhibitor of phosphodiesterase and therefore can increase intracellular concentrations of cyclic AMP. Indomethacin is rapidly and completely absorbed from the gastrointestinal tract, attaining peak plasma concentrations in 1 to 2 h. The half-life is about 4.5 h. Indomethacin is 90 percent protein-bound. The drug is biotransformed by demethylation and N deacylation. Both the parent drug and the biotransformation products undergo enterohepatic circulation. Thirty-three percent is eliminated in the feces and the remainder in the urine. Indomethacin has a significant amount of gastrointestinal toxicity. Other adverse reactions include headaches, dizziness, tinnitus, vertigo, and nephrotoxicity.

Tolmetin Sodium This drug is rapidly and almost completely absorbed from the gastrointestinal tract; peak plasma levels are reached within 30 to 60 min. Virtually all the drug is eliminated within 24 h in the urine as conjugated tolmetin and an inactive product of oxidative biotransformation. Tolmetin may also produce pseudoproteinuria. This drug is approved for the treatment of juvenile rheumatoid arthritis. The toxicities are similar to those of the other NSAIDs.

Sulindac This drug is an indene acetic acid derivative. It has the same pharmacology as the other members of the acetic acid group. Sulindac is well absorbed after oral administration, with peak plasma levels appearing in 1 h. Sulindac is biotransformed into its sulfide derivative. It is believed that sulindac sulfide is the active form of the drug and has a plasma half-life of 16.4 h. Both compounds as well as an inactive derivative, a sulfone, undergo extensive enterohepatic circulation, and this effect appears to account for the long duration of the drug. Both sulindac and its sulfide are highly protein-bound (95 percent).

About 25 percent of the drug and its biotransformation products are excreted in the feces and the remainder in the urine. As with other NSAIDs, gastrointestinal toxicity is the main effect of sulindac. Skin rash, tinnitus, dizziness, headaches, edema, and renal toxicity have been reported. Sulindac does not appear to interfere with antihypertensive drug therapy. As with all NSAIDs, sulindac is contraindicated in aspirin hypersensitivity.

Diclofenac Sodium Diclofenac sodium is a phenylacetic acid derivative. It is administered as an enteric coated tablet, which is completely absorbed from the GI tract. First-pass metabolism occurs, and only 50 percent of the dose is systemically available. Mean plasma half-life is 2 h. Adverse reactions include gastrointestinal, renal, and hepatic toxicity, edema, dizziness, and tinnitus. It is contraindicated in individuals with porphyria.

Pyrazolone Derivatives

Phenylbutazone Phenylbutazone is metabolized to oxyphenbutazone, which is the active form of this drug. Its mechanism of action and pharmacology are similar to those of other NSAIDs. Another pyrazolone derivative, sulfinpyrazone, is discussed in the treatment of gout, below. Phenylbutazone should not be administered for periods over 1 week except in highly selected cases of severe ankylosing spondylitis where less toxic NSAIDs such as indomethacin have not proven effective. The most serious adverse reaction seen with phenylbutazone is agranulocytosis. Two types of agranulocytosis are found. One is idiosyncratic and irreversible, while the other is dose-related and reversible with discontinuation of the drug. Agranulocytosis may appear at any time following administration and severely limits the use of these drugs.

Gastrointestinal toxicity leading to ulceration and bleeding may be caused by this drug as well as by other NSAIDs. Liver-function tests and histologic studies show evidence of toxic hepatitis in some patients and a cholangiolitic change in others. Jaundice and increased prothrombin time with purpura have been observed, and toxic cirrhosis has led to death. Kidney

damage has been caused by hematuria, anuria, and uremia, with severe destruction of the convoluted tubules. Sodium retention due to increased reabsorption of sodium has been observed regularly and is frequently associated with water and chloride retention and edema. Presumably the effect occurs without impairment of general renal function, and the mechanism can be due to inhibition of prostaglandin production as described above. Skin irritation in the form of a drug rash with an occasional fatal exfoliative dermatitis is not uncommon after administration of this drug.

Oxicam Derivatives

Piroxicam Piroxicam is the first oxicam derivative available in the United States. It has a similar mechanism of action and pharmacology when compared with other NSAIDs. Peak absorption is in 3 to 5 h, and piroxicam has a mean half-life of 50 h. It is metabolized by hydroxylation on the 5 position of the pyridyl side chain and then conjugated. The compound also undergoes hydrolysis of the amide ring. Sixty-six percent of piroxicam and its metabolites are excreted in the urine and 33 percent in the feces. Adverse reactions include gastrointestinal toxicity, renal insufficiency, papillary necrosis, edema, and abnormalities in liver function tests. Interactions with warfarin have been reported.

Fenamate Derivatives

Meclofenamate Sodium Meclofenamate sodium has a mechanism of action similar to that of the other NSAIDs. The mean plasma half-life is 2 h. Adverse reactions are also similar to those of the other NSAIDs, except that diarrhea is a frequent side effect. In addition, the effect of the oral anticoagulant warfarin is enhanced by meclofenamate.

Mefenamic Acid Mefenamic acid is indicated for use in dysmennorhea and moderate pain for no more than 1 week. The use of mefenamic acid for greater than 1 week is not recommended because of development of possible serious gastrointestinal toxicity, nephrotoxicity, hemolytic anemia, and bone marrow hypoplasia. Autoimmune hemolytic anemia is associated with continuous administration of the drug for more than 12 months.

Preparations and Doses

Aspirin is available in 325- and 500-mg tablets. A variety of buffered and enteric-coated preparations are available. The usual dosage for pain is 650 mg. As an anti-inflammatory, the starting dose is 975 mg four times a day.

Diflunisal (Dolobid) is available in 250- and 500-mg tablets. Usual dosage is 500 to 1000 mg divided in two doses.

Choline magnesium trisalicylate (Trilisate) is available in 500-, 750-, and 1000-mg tablets and is available in liquid form. Usual starting dose is 2000 to 3000 mg divided in two or three doses.

Salsalate (Disalcid) is available in 750-mg tablets. Usual starting dose is 2150 to 3000 mg divided in two or three doses.

Ibuprofen (Motrin, Rufen) is available in 300-, 400-, 600-, and 800-mg tablets. Over-the-counter preparations (Nuprin, Advil, Medeprin) are available in 200-mg tablets. Usual anti-inflammatory dose is 300 to 800 mg three to four times a day.

Naproxen (Naprosyn) is available in 250-, 375-, and 500-mg tablets. Usual dose is 250 to 500 mg twice a day. It is also available in suspension with 125 mg per 5 mL. Naproxen sodium is available in 275-mg tablets.

Fenoprofen (Nalfon) is available in 200-, 300-, and 600-mg tablets. Usual dosage is 300 or 600 mg three or four times a day.

Flurbiprofen (Ansaid) is available in 50- and 100-mg tablets. The recommended starting dose is 200 to 300 mg divided in two to four doses.

Ketoprofen (Orudis) is available in 50- and 75-mg tablets. Usual dosage is 150 to 300 mg divided in three or four doses.

Indomethacin (Indocin) is available in capsules of 25 and 50 mg and also 75-mg capsules (Indocin SR). Usual dosage is 75 to 200 mg daily in divided doses.

Tolmetin sodium (Tolectin) is available in 200-mg tablets and 400-mg capsules (Tolectin DS). Usual dosage is 400 mg three or four times a day.

Sulindac (Clinoril) is available in 150- and 200-mg tablets. Usual dosage is 150 to 200 mg twice a day.

Phenylbutazone (Butazolidin) is available in 100-mg tablets. The usual dose is 100 mg one to four times a day not to exceed 400 mg a day.

Piroxicam (Feldene) is available in 10- and 20-mg capsules. Usual dose is 20 mg once daily.

Meclofenamate sodium (Meclomen) is available in 50- and 100-mg tablets. Usual dose is 50 or 100 mg three or four times a day.

Diclofenac sodium (Voltaren) is available in 25-, 50-, and 75-mg enteric coated tablets. Usual dose is 100 to 200 mg daily divided in two doses.

OTHER ANALGESIC AND ANTIPYRETIC DRUGS

Acetaminophen

Acetaminophen is employed for its analgesic and antipyretic effects. Acetophenetidin (Phenacetin) is a similar agent which is no longer available in the United States. The primary use of acetaminophen is for relief of ordinary aches and pains and elevated body temperatures. In contrast to the NSAIDs, however, it is devoid of anti-inflammatory or antirheumatic properties and therefore is not classified as a nonsteroidal anti-inflammatory drug.

$$NH-CO-CH_3$$

OH
Acetaminophen

Mechanism of Action   Since it has been demonstrated that acetaminophen inhibits brain cyclooxygenase even more strongly than does aspirin, it is probable that both drugs are antipyretic by an effect on heat regulatory centers. On the other hand, the mechanism of the analgesic action of acetaminophen is uncertain because this drug is only a weak inhibitor of peripheral cyclooxygenase. Therefore, in contrast to aspirin, its analgesic action may be central.

Effect on Organ Systems   There is little effect on organ systems with short-term use of acetaminophen. The hepatotoxic effects of high doses of acetaminophen are described under "Adverse Reactions," below.

Pharmacokinetics   Acetaminophen is totally absorbed from the gastrointestinal tract, attaining a peak plasma level in 1 to $1\frac{1}{2}$ h. Acetaminophen is metabolized into a number of metabolites, and these, together with free drug, are excreted in the urine.

Therapeutic Use   Acetaminophen is widely used as an analgesic and antipyretic in the treatment of mild pain and fever. Acetophenetidin was available in the past and for many years was an ingredient of the popular "APC" tablet containing aspirin, acetophenetidin (Phenacetin), and caffeine. APC tablets are no longer available because of potential kidney toxicity on chronic administration.

Adverse Reactions

Liver   Because of the widespead use of acetaminophen as a substitute for aspirin in the treatment of mild pain and fever, there has been an increased incidence of toxicity due to overdose of drug with suicidal intent or by accident. Ingestion of over 7.5 g of drug at one time has been associated with severe hepatic toxicity. After ingestion, nausea, vomiting, and lethargy develop within 12 h. These symptoms resolve, and then liver damage occurs 48 h after ingestion, often resulting in death from hepatic failure if left untreated. The hepatotoxicity and hepatic damage may be due to an *N*-hydroxylated biotransformation product, *N*-acetyl-benzoquinoneimine. Treatment consists of gastric lavage followed by administration of *N*-acetylcysteine within 12 h of acetaminophen ingestion. Following recovery from overdose, there appears to be complete resolution of hepatic damage. Dialysis is not recommended in the treatment of acetaminophen overdose.

Gastrointestinal Tract   As mentioned above, acetaminophen does not cause gastrointestinal irritation as do the NSAIDs and may be used in patients exhibiting gastrointestinal toxicity from the other drugs. Acetaminophen may be used in patients with hypersensitivity to aspirin.

Preparations and Doses   Acetaminophen is available in 300-mg tablets and 500-mg capsules. It is also available in various elixirs. The usual dose is 300 to 1000 mg every 4 h.

DRUGS USED IN THE TREATMENT OF GOUT AND HYPERURICEMIA

Acute gout is caused by precipitation of sodium urate crystals in a synovial joint. It is a classic example of acute inflammation. Hyperuricemia (serum urate lev-els above 7 mg per 100 mL) may be caused by a variety of secondary etiologies or may be idiopathic. If idiopathic, it may be caused by overproduction of uric acid or underexcretion by an otherwise normal kidney. The defects causing idiopathic hyperuricemia are unknown. The disorder may be asymptomatic, requiring no treatment. When present for many years, it may cause acute gouty arthritis, tophi (precipitation of sodium urate crystals in interstitial tissues), or uric acid stones in the urinary system.

Drugs used in the treatment of gout may be divided into two groups. The first group includes drugs used to treat an acute attack of gouty arthritis occurring in a synovial joint. Most of the NSAIDs are effective for this purpose. Colchicine, as described below, is also effective in acute attacks of gout. The second group includes drugs to treat hyperuricemia if such treatment is indicated.

Colchicine

Chemistry   *Colchicine* is an alkaloid found in the meadow saffron (or autumn crocus). Aside from its use in the therapy of acute gouty arthritis for about 1500 years, colchicine is of considerable biologic interest because of its remarkable ability to arrest cell division in metaphase when given in larger doses.

Mechanism of Action   Colchicine has the ability to penetrate the cell and migrate into the microtubular system. By an unknown mechanism it stabilizes the intracellular membranes, and inflammatory cells lose their ability to respond to the inflammatory reaction caused by sodium urate crystals. Colchicine has no effect on the urinary excretion of uric acid or its biosynthesis and therefore is of no value in the treatment of hyperuricemia. There is little evidence that it acts primarily as an analgesic and is usually ineffective in arthritis other than that caused by sodium urate deposition. Colchicine does provide rapid relief of acute gouty pain and can also be used prophylactically to prevent recurrent exacerbations of gout.

Therapeutic Use   Administration of colchicine should begin at the earliest possible moment after the appearance of one or more symptoms suggestive of acute gouty arthritis, since it may be ineffective if administration is delayed for more than 24 h. Treatment of an acute attack of gout requires the ingestion of one tablet (0.6 mg) every hour until there is an unmistakable subsidence of articular symptoms or until the patient develops severe diarrhea. Usually the total amount of drug required is between 1.8 and 3 mg administered over several hours. The drug may also be given intravenously, and by this route 1 or 2 mg is administered as one dose, which may be repeated once in 2 to 4 h. In case of renal impairment, the dose of colchicine should be reduced and should not be used in presence of simultaneous hepatic and renal disease. Adverse reactions include nausea, diarrhea, and severe neutropenia, while an acute overdose of 7 mg may be fatal.

Preparation *Colchicine* is available in 0.5- and 0.6- mg tablets and as an intravenous solution.

Probenecid

Chemistry Probenecid is a sulfonamide with the following chemical structure:

Probenecid

Mechanism of Action Uric acid is derived chiefly from the catabolism of nucleic acids. In a person on a low purine diet, about 700 mg of uric acid is excreted daily, two-thirds of it via the kidney. Uric acid is filtered in the glomerulus, reabsorbed in the proximal tubule, and secreted in the distal tubule. There is some evidence that there may be further reabsorption in the distal tubule. Probenecid inhibits renal tubular secretion and reabsorption of a variety of organic acids, including uric acid.

Pharmacokinetics Probenecid is totally absorbed on oral administration, reaching a peak in 1 to 5 h. The drug is almost totally metabolized and is excreted by the kidney.

Therapeutic Use Probenecid produces a large negative balance of uric acid when first administered particularly at a time when the uric acid concentration in the plasma is high. Probenecid and other uricosuric agents are of no value in relieving the pain and inflammation in acute attacks of gout, since they are not anti-inflammatory. In fact by altering the serum uric acid level, acute attacks of gout may be precipitated. Pro-

benecid is used in the presence of underexcretion of uric acid with normal renal function. When probenecid does not lower the uric acid blood level sufficiently or in the presence of severely impaired renal function, allopurinol may be used.

Adverse Reactions Probenecid is well tolerated by most patients. Gastrointestinal irritation and hypersensitivity causing nausea and vomiting or skin rashes may occur.

Aspirin, even at uricosuric doses, should not be administered with probenecid, since the actions of the two drugs are antagonistic. If an analgesic agent is needed, acetaminophen may be used. Probenecid decreases the renal clearance of penicillin, indomethacin, certain cephalosporins, and thiazides. When administered in conjunction with these drugs, increased blood levels will occur, and if not corrected may cause toxicity. Probenecid, by altering the excretion of penicillin, may be used as a therapeutic modality to increase the blood level of penicillin.

Sulfinpyrazone

Sulfinpyrazone is a pyrazolone derivative closely related chemically to phenylbutazone. It has the following chemical structure:

Sulfinpyrazone

Sulfinpyrazone is a uricosuric agent which acts by inhibiting tubular secretion of uric acid as well as its reabsorption. This results in an increased uric acid excretion and decreased serum urate concentration. In addition, the drug inhibits platelet aggregation. Sulfinpyrazone is used as a uricosuric agent in the treatment of hyperuricemia. The toxicity of sulfinpyrazone is similar to that seen with phenylbutazone, namely, gastrointestinal irritation, which may lead to ulceration and bleeding. Agranulocytosis, however, is much less frequent than that reported with phenylbutazone. Because of its relation to sulfonamides, sulfinpyrazone may interact with the oral hypoglycemic agents and increase the hypoglycemic effect. The drug is completely absorbed from the gastrointestinal tract, obtaining a peak level in 1 h. It is highly protein-bound and is excreted 50 percent unchanged and 50 percent as the parahydroxy metabolite.

Salicylates at any dose will block the uricosuric effect of sulfinpyrazone. Probenecid will have a synergistic effect on the uricosuric action of sulfinpyrazone but will increase the plasma level of the drug.

Preparation and Dose   *Sulfinpyrazone* (Anturane) is available in tablets of 100 mg. The usual dose is 100 to 200 mg twice a day.

Allopurinol

Allopurinol has the following chemical structure:

Allopurinol

Like the uricosuric agents, allopurinol has no analgesic or anti-inflammatory effect and is therefore of no value in the treatment of acute gouty arthritis.

Mechanism of Action   Allopurinol is an antimetabolite of xanthine and hypoxanthine and inhibits xanthine oxidase; thus the conversion of hypoxanthine and xanthine to uric acid is reduced. Since the solubility of hypoxanthine and xanthine is considerably greater than that of uric acid, there is a net loss of urate from the total body pool.

Effect on Organ Systems   Despite the fact that allopurinol inhibits an enzyme and is an antimetabolite, it is relatively free of effect on organ systems except when it causes adverse reactions.

Pharmacokinetics   Allopurinol is about 80 percent bioavailable, reaching a maximum blood level in 2 to 6 h. It is oxidized by xanthine oxidase to alloxanthine (oxypurinol). Both allopurinol and alloxanthine in-

hibit xanthine oxidase. The half-life of allopurinol is 2 to 3 h and of alloxanthine is 18 to 30 h. Both drugs are excreted entirely in the urine.

Adverse Reactions   Mild reactions to allopurinol include fever, skin rash, headache, vertigo, and nausea. Severe reactions, frequently fatal, may occur in hypersensitive individuals. Severe skin involvement causing exfoliative dermatitis with Stephens-Johnson syndrome may be seen. Severe renal damage with eosinophilia, frequently associated with skin rash of a severe degree, has been recorded and is frequently fatal. Hepatitis may occur in mild form or may go on to hepatic insufficiency. Since allopurinol is a xanthine oxidase inhibitor, it will interfere with the biotransformation of azathioprine and 6-mercaptopurine. If allopurinol must be administered concurrently with these drugs, such as in the treatment of acute leukemia, the dose of the cytotoxic agent must be reduced by one-third to one-half. The dose should also be reduced in the presence of renal insufficiency.

Preparation and Dose   *Allopurinol* (Zyloprim) is available in tablets of 100 and 300 mg. The usual dose is 100 to 300 mg/day. The dose may be administered once a day.

BIBLIOGRAPHY

Baum, C., D. L. Kennedy, and M. B. Forbes: "Utilization of Nonsteroidal Anti-inflammatory Drugs," *Arthritis Rheum.*, **28**:686–692 (1985).

Clive, D. M., and J. S. Stoff: "Renal Syndromes Associated with Nonsteroidal Anti-inflammatory Drug," *N. Engl. J. Med.*, **310**:563–572 (1984).

Graham, G. G., R. O. Day, G. D. Champion, E. Lee, and K. Newton: "Aspects of the Clinical Pharmacology of Nonsteroidal Antiinflammatory Drugs," *Clin. Rheum. Dis.*, **10**:229–249 (1984).

Huskisson, E. C. (ed.): *Anti-rheumatic Drugs*, Praeger Publishers, New York, 1983.

LaMontage, J. R.: "Summary of a Workshop on Disease Mechanism and Prospects for Prevention of Reye's syndrome," *J. Infect. Dis.*, **148**:943–950 (1983).

Nikander, R., F. G. McMahon, and A. S. Ridolfo: "Nonsteroidal Anti-inflammatory Agents," *Annu. Rev. Pharmacol. Toxicol.*, **19**:469–490 (1979).

Oates, J. A., et al: "Clinical Implications of Prostaglandin and Thromboxane A_2 Formation," *N. Engl. J. Med.*, **319**:689–698, 761–767 (1988).

Roberts, W. N., M. H. Liang, and S. H. Stern: "Colchicine in Acute Gout—Reassessment of Risks and Benefits," *JAMA*, **257**:1920–1922 (1987).

Shirota, H., M. Goto, and K. Katayama: "Application of Adjuvant-Induced Local Hyperthermia for Evaluation of Anti-inflammatory Drugs," *J. Pharmacol. Exp. Ther.*, **247**:1158–1163 (1988).

Simon, L. S., and J. A. Mills: "Nonsteroidal Anti-inflammatory Drugs," *N. Engl. J. Med.*, **302**:1179–1185, 1237–1243 (1980).

Stevenson, D. D.: "Diagnosis, Prevention and Treatment of Adverse Reactions to Aspirin and Nonsteroidal Anti-inflammatory Drugs," *J. Allergy Clin. Immunology*, **74**:617–633 (1984).

C H A P T E R **24**

Local Anesthetics |

Lawrence Levit and Jerry D. Levitt |

Local anesthetics are drugs which in therapeutic concentrations reversibly block nerve conduction. Complete reversibility is basic to this definition because many substances (e.g., ethanol) and surgical procedures (e.g., neural damage) can block nerve conduction irreversibly and therefore are not useful as local anesthetics. As agents which block *conduction* in axons and dendrites, local anesthetics are distinguished from agents which block neural *transmission* at synapses. Although local anesthetics are also capable of blocking at synapses, usually they are applied along the course of axons and dendrites.

Cocaine, an alkaloid derived from the *Erythroxylon coca* plant, was first used clinically as a local anesthetic in 1884. It was found to block pain as a topical anesthetic in a patient undergoing an operation for glaucoma. Today its therapeutic usefulness is limited, but it is an important drug of abuse (see Chap. 18). Procaine, the first synthetic local anesthetic, was introduced into clinical practice in 1905. Since then hundreds of local anesthetics have been synthesized and evaluated. However, only a dozen or so compounds have properties which have kept them in current use. Other landmarks in the history of local anesthetics include the introduction in 1947 of lidocaine, the first amide-type local anesthetic, and in 1963 the introduction of bupivacaine, a long-acting amide-type local anesthetic.

CHEMISTRY AND STRUCTURE ACTIVITY RELATIONSHIPS

Most useful local anesthetics are composed of three parts: an aromatic ring (the lipophilic portion), an in-termediate chain, and an amino group (the hydrophilic portion) (see Fig. 24-1). Local anesthetics are classified as either *esters* or *amides* according to the structure of the intermediate chain. This classification is of more than academic interest, as the metabolism, allergic potential, stability, and to some extent the toxicities of the local anesthetics are determined by this intermediate chain. The longer known local anesthetics (e.g., cocaine, procaine) are esters, while most agents introduced more recently are amides (e.g., lidocaine, bupivacaine). Substitutions on the aromatic ring and on the amino group change the lipid solubility and the degree to which the local anesthetic molecule binds to protein. The lipid solubility and protein binding, in turn, determine the potency and duration of action of drugs such as etidocaine (see Table 24-1). The intrinsic vasodilator properties of the local anesthetic and its solubility in other tissues may limit the amount of drug at the nerve membrane. Clinically, then, these properties also determine potency and duration.

The structure-activity relationships are important in determining the usefulness of the agents. The structure and properties of mepivacaine and bupivacaine offer an instructive comparison. Bupivacaine differs from mepivacaine only in the substitution of a butyl group for the methyl group on the nitrogen of the amine end. This substitution increases the potency and duration of action. The toxicity of the drug is also increased.

The pK_a of a local anesthetic is another important chemical characteristic. Most local anesthetics are weak bases. The free base is poorly soluble in aqueous solutions, so the drug is usually supplied in a solution of low pH as the hydrochloride "salt." Because of the amino group, aqueous solutions consist of a mixture of the free (uncharged) base form and the protonated (cationic) form in equilibrium. The relative amount of each form is determined by the dissociation constant (pK_a) of the cationic form and pH of the solution.

Clearly, the higher the pK_a of a drug, the less will be in the free-base form at physiologic pH. The penetration of a local anesthetic to its site of action is largely dependent on its ability to cross lipid membranes. The free-base form has a high lipid-to-water partition coefficient and can therefore penetrate such membranes easily. Cationic forms, because of their charge, are unable to penetrate lipid membranes. In general, local anesthetics with lower pK_a's exhibit faster onset than drugs with higher pK_a's.

MECHANISM OF ACTION

In the resting state, the axoplasm is at about -90 mV with respect to the outside of the cell. This "resting potential" is maintained by the relative concentrations and permeabilities of sodium and potassium ions across the nerve membrane. In the resting state, the membrane is highly impermeable to sodium ions, but relatively more permeable to potassium ions through the potassium channels. When the nerve is stimulated, the transmembrane potential becomes less negative (depolarizes), some sodium channels in the region of the depolarization open, and sodium moves inward along its concentration gradient. At the peak of depolarization the axoplasm is +20 mV with respect to the exterior of the cell. Near this peak, potassium channels open, potassium ions leave the cell, and the cell repolarizes. The propagated sequence of depolarization and repolarization takes 1 to 2 ms and is called an *action potential*. Only a small proportion of the available sodium and potassium ions move during a single action potential. After repolarization, the sodium-potassium pump reestablishes the ion gradients.

Local anesthetics have been shown to (1) increase the threshold for electrical excitation in nerve, (2) slow propagation of the depolarization, (3) reduce the rate of rise of the action potential, and (4) eventually block conduction of the action potential. Local anesthetics have no effect on the resting membrane potential.

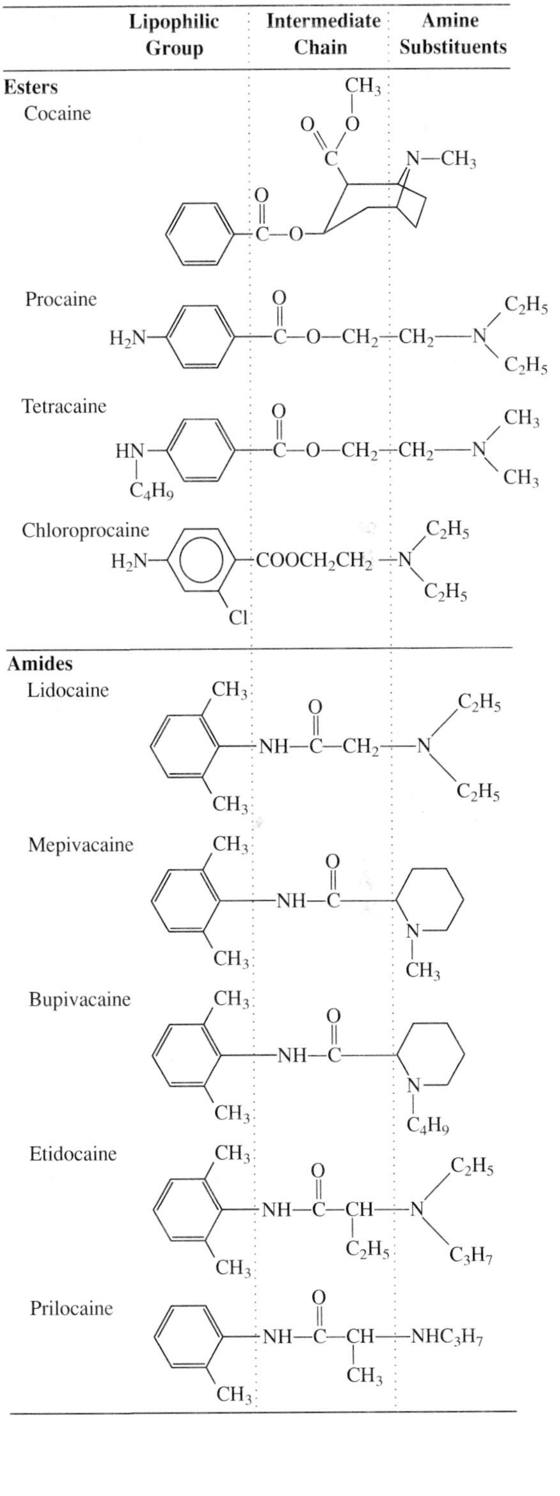

FIGURE 24-1 Chemical structures of some local anesthetics.

TABLE 24-1   Pharmacokinetic comparison of various local anesthetics[a]

Drug	Potency (procaine = 1)	Lipid solubility	Percent protein binding	Site of metabolism, min	Elimination half-life, min	Duration of action
Esters						
Procaine	1	Low	6	Plasma	—	Short
Chloroprocaine	4	—	—	Plasma	—	—
Tetracaine	16	Moderate	76	Plasma	—	Long
Amides						
Lidocaine	4	Low	70	Liver	96	Moderate
Mepivacaine	2	Low	77	Liver	114	Mod.–long
Bupivacaine	16	Moderate	95	Liver	210	Long
Etidocaine	16	High	94	Liver	156	Long
Prilocaine	3	Low	55	Liver & moderate, extrahepatic tissues	—	

[a] Surface anesthetics such as cyclomethycaine, benzocaine, and butamben are used for topical or surface anesthesia and are not significantly absorbed.

Experiments utilizing isolated "voltage-clamped" nerve fibers have demonstrated that local anesthetics cause a dose-related decrease in sodium conductance and that the block of sodium channels is sufficient to account for the action of these drugs.

The sodium channels pass through at least three states: closed, open, and inactivated. From the closed state depolarization opens the "gate," allowing sodium ions to enter the channel and local anesthetics also to enter. Upon entering the open sodium gate, the local anesthetics interfere with sodium influx and subsequently change the gate to become more refractory to depolarization. Local anesthetics block nerve fibers more strongly when the fiber is stimulated at higher frequency. This phenomenon, termed *use-dependent block,* may occur because the sodium channel is in the open state more when stimulated at higher frequencies and this may permit more access for the local anesthetic. In the inactive state the channel is refractory to depolarization. Local anesthetics may increase the time the sodium channel is in the inactive state (see Chap. 27 for a schema of the sodium channel and additional discussion).

In summary, the following is a likely sequence for the production of clinical local anesthesia. After injection, the uncharged (free-base) and cationic forms of the local anesthetic are in equilibrium in the extracellular space in a proportion determined by the pK_a of the local anesthetic and the pH of the tissue. The uncharged form passes through the connective tissue surrounding the nerve fiber and through the phospholipid of the plasma membrane to the axoplasm. In the axoplasm the free base ionizes to a degree determined by the intracellular pH. The cationic form attaches to the intracellular opening of the sodium channel, decreases sodium conductance, and blocks depolarization. The process is reversed by diffusion of the local anesthetic into the vasculature and redistribution.

Benzocaine is a local anesthetic which is permanently uncharged and has a mechanism somewhat different than other agents. It seems to work by dissolving in and expanding the phospholipid membrane. This expansion deforms the sodium channel to reduce sodium conductance. Membrane expansion has also been proposed as a mechanism of action of general anesthetics.

PHARMACOKINETICS

Table 24-1 represents some pharmacokinetic parameters of representative local anesthetics. Etidocaine possesses the highest lipid solubility. Protein binding is the highest for bupivacaine (95 percent) and etidocaine (94 percent).

Local anesthetics are administered normally at their anatomic site of action, that is, in close proximity to the nerves to be blocked. For most other drugs, initial uptake and distribution moves the drug from the site of administration to the target organ. In contrast, for local anesthetics, uptake into the blood and distribution will remove the drugs from their intended targets and carry them to sites where systemic toxicity is manifest and where biotransformation occurs. The blood level of a local anesthetic depends on (among other factors) the dose, the vascularity at the site of administration, and the clearance of the drug from the blood. If, by accident, the drug is injected directly into a vein, uptake is instantaneous and a relatively small dose may produce a toxic blood level.

Local anesthetics are absorbed from different sites at markedly different rates, so that for the same dose of a given local anesthetic the peak blood level is a function of what type of nerve block has been initiated. The relative rates of absorption, in decreasing order, for various nerve blocks are as follows: intercostal > caudal > epidural > brachial plexus > subcutaneous infiltration.

Vasoconstrictors, usually epinephrine and occasionally phenylephrine, may be added to local anesthetic solutions to slow absorption of the anesthetic from the site of injection. This prolongs the duration of the nerve block, reduces the peak blood concentration of the anesthetic, reduces surgical bleeding in local infiltration anesthesia, and may permit a larger dose of anesthetic to be injected without systemic toxicity. The effect of a vasoconstrictor is greater when used with local anesthetics which are intrinsically strong vasodilators and are not highly lipid-soluble such as procaine and lidocaine. When used in epidural anesthesia, epinephrine increases the duration of lidocaine by about 80 percent: in contrast, the duration of bupivacaine is increased by only 15 percent. Local anesthetics containing vasoconstrictors should not be used for infiltration of structures supplied by end arteries such as fingers, toes, and penis because of the possibility of causing ischemia. The vasoconstrictor itself may cause systemic toxicity if injected directly into a blood vessel or in an excessive dose.

The initial step in the metabolism of the *ester* local anesthetics is hydrolysis by cholinesterases, especially pseudocholinesterase in plasma (see Table 24-1). The ester linkage is cleaved by plasma cholinesterase, forming *para*-aminobenzoic acid and an amino alcohol. A small proportion of the population is allergic to *para*-aminobenzoic acid (the allergen also in sulfonamide hypersensitivity), and this is the basis of allergic reactions to the ester local anesthetics. The amides are degraded in the liver and are very rarely associated with allergic reactions. The amides are more stable in solution during storage and heat sterilization than are the esters. Conversely, some ester-type local anesthetics, notably procaine and chloroprocaine, are metabolized so rapidly by plasma cholinesterase that toxic reactions (as distinguished from allergic reactions) are rare. The rate of hydrolysis of chloroprocaine is extremely rapid, with the result that blood concentrations of this drug remain low and systemic adverse reactions seldom occur. Tetracaine, on the other hand, is slowly hydrolyzed. Therefore, tetracaine is used almost exclusively for spinal anesthesia, where the low dose and slow uptake of the drug result in very low blood levels. The rates of hydrolysis in increasing order are tetracaine, procaine, and chloroprocaine. Genetic variations in the activity of pseudocholinesterase may affect the rates of hydrolysis of these drugs.

The *amide* local anesthetics are not susceptible to hydrolysis by esterases. They are metabolized predominantly in the liver. Lidocaine is biotransformed by several pathways. The primary route involves the removal of one of the ethyl groups on the terminal tertiary nitrogen followed by hydrolysis of the amide linkage to form 2,6-xylidine and monoethylglycine. Oxidation occurs prior to sulfate conjugation. Both free and conjugated forms are excreted in the urine with less than 3 percent of the total administered dose excreted unchanged. The elimination half-life of lidocaine is 96 min. However, one of its metabolites, glycinexylide, has a half-life of 10 h. Several of the metabolites of lidocaine have local anesthetic, antiarrhythmic, and convulsant properties. These may contribute to the systemic toxicity of lidocaine administered by infusion or repeated doses, especially in patients with renal insufficiency.

The elimination half-lives of mepivacaine, bupivacaine, and etidocaine are considerably longer than the esters. Bupivacaine and etidocaine are considered to be long-acting local anesthetics.

PHARMACODYNAMICS

Clinically, small, nonmyelinated nerve fibers, which transmit pain and autonomic impulses, seem more susceptible to local anesthetic action than more myelinated larger fibers. In spinal anesthesia, the order of blockade by local anesthetics occurs initially with the sympathetic outflow followed by the sensations of pain, cold, warmth, touch, deep pressure, proprioception, and motor activity. Recovery usually proceeds in the reverse order. However, etidocaine does not seem to follow this pattern. Motor blockade may be more intense than sensory blockade with this drug. Local anesthetics influence all neurons, as well as all other excitable tissues. As a consequence, the "local" action of these agents is a function of dose, site, method of administration, anatomy of the neural structures, and the physical properties of the agent employed. Systemic absorption of these compounds may initiate undesirable pharmacologic actions.

ADVERSE EFFECTS

In addition to their local anesthetic actions, these drugs may produce several other manifestations. Systemic effects on susceptible organ systems, primarily the central nervous and cardiovascular systems, occur at high blood levels. Allergic and hypersensitivity reactions have been reported. Certain local anesthetics and their additives also caused damage to nerves and surrounding muscle tissue.

Blood levels of local anesthetic sufficient to cause systemic toxicity may result from accidental intravascular injection or absorption of a toxic dose of anesthetic from the site of injection. Factors which contribute to systemic toxicity of local anesthetics include vascularity of the site and the addition of vasoconstrictors to slow absorption.

Central Nervous System

Local anesthetic agents initially produce CNS excitation followed by generalized CNS depression. This seemingly biphasic effect is due to early selective blockade of inhibitory pathways in the cerebral cortex. Consequently, facilitatory neurons function unopposed, causing increased excitatory activity which can progress to seizure. Generalized central nervous system depression follows, as all neural conduction is blocked by local anesthetic. Only cocaine is a true central nervous system stimulant.

Subjective central nervous system symptoms of lightheadedness and dizziness followed by visual and auditory disturbances such as diplopia and tinnitus have been reported following intravenous infusions of local anesthetics. Additional symptoms may include drowsiness, circumoral paresthesia, and numbness of the tongue. Objective signs of central nervous system toxicity include muscular twitching, shivering, and tremors which can progress to a generalized tonic-clonic seizures. Large doses of local anesthetic reaching the central nervous system can cause brain-stem depression resulting in severe respiratory depression or apnea.

The central nervous system toxicity of local anesthetics is related primarily to the intrinsic anesthetic potencies. The speed at which blood levels are attained is another determinant of toxicity. Rapid infusion will produce toxicity at lower doses. Severe CNS toxic reactions have occurred while anesthetizing nerves of the neck after very small quantities of local anesthetic were injected directly into an artery supplying the brain (carotid or vertebral artery).

Cardiovascular System

Local anesthetic toxicity of the cardiovascular system is manifest by hypotension and arrhythmias secondary to depressed electrical conduction and cardiac contractility as well as vasodilatory effects on peripheral vasculature. As with CNS toxicity, there is a close relationship between intrinsic local anesthetic potency and the dose required to produce cardiovascular effects. However, the cardiovascular system is more resistant to toxicity than the CNS. The dose of local anesthetic required to produce cardiovascular collapse is 4 to 7 times greater than that which will cause seizure.

The electrophysiologic effects of local anesthetics on cardiac muscle are covered extensively in Chap. 27. These effects include decreased electrical excitability and conduction. High levels of local anesthetic can cause bradycardia progressing to sinus arrest as a result of sinoatrial pacemaker depression. Additionally, partial or complete atrioventricular dissociation may result from depressed atrioventricular node conduction.

High blood levels of local anesthetic will also impair mechanical activity of cardiac muscle in a dose-dependent manner. There is evidence that local anesthetics with greater potency, lipid solubility, and protein binding (specifically bupivacaine and to a lesser extent etidocaine) are relatively more cardiotoxic than other agents. Resuscitation from bupivacaine-induced cardiovascular collapse is much more difficult than that following other local anesthetics. In addition, severe cardiac arrhythmias including ventricular tachycardia and ventricular fibrillation occur after rapid infusion of bupivacaine but not after the administration of lidocaine or mepivacaine.

Hypersensitivity

True hypersensitivity or allergic-type reactions to local anesthetic agents are most likely to occur with the aminoesters than with amino-amides. These agents are chemically similar in structure to *para*-aminobenzoic acid, a sunscreen as well as a metabolite of procaine, which is a common allergen. Allergic-type reactions with amino-amide local anesthetics are extremely rare. The preservative methylparaben, whose structure is similar to *para*-aminobenzoic acid, can be found in multiple-dose containers of amino-amides and may be thought to be responsible for some hypersensitivity reactions.

A meticulous history can be helpful in distinguishing possible allergic reactions from other local anesthetic reactions. The effectiveness of skin testing is unclear, although it may be helpful in making such a diagnosis. However, it is important to perform these tests with agents free of preservatives or additives to avoid misleading results.

Local Tissue Reactions

Local-anesthetic-induced tissue toxicity is extremely rare when approved agents in appropriate concentrations are used. Local neurotoxicity is an especially feared complication. There are a number of mechanisms which may result in neurotoxicity. Direct trauma from the injection needle, intraneural injection, or neural ischemia produced by the pressure of injection may cause a neurologic deficit. Excessive concentration of local anesthetic or contamination of local anesthetic with foreign substances can also cause toxic neural injury.

Recently chloroprocaine has been suspected of being neurotoxic. Persistent and possibly permanent neurologic deficits were reported to follow the unintentional subarachnoid injection of large doses of chloroprocaine. Sodium bisulfite, an antioxidant used in chloroprocaine solutions, when buffered to a low pH, causes irreversible neural injury in the absence of chloroprocaine. Chloroprocaine itself does not appear to be neurotoxic.

CLINICAL APPLICATIONS OF LOCAL ANESTHETICS

Local anesthetics permit those skilled in their administration to render various regions of the body insensitive to pain. In contrast to general anesthetics, these agents cause loss of sensation without loss of consciousness. General anesthetics alter many centrally mediated controls of body function such as temperature regulation and medullary control of respiration and circulation. Barring systemic toxicity, the effect of local anesthetics is limited to that part of the body which is anesthetized.

Local anesthetics are used clinically in a variety of locations and applications. Neural blockade is established at terminal nerve endings and receptors (surface and infiltration anesthesia), at the peripheral nervous system (discrete nerve blocks and plexus blocks), and at the level of the central nervous system (spinal and epidural anesthesia). The following section reviews these techniques.

Surface Anesthesia

Topical application of local anesthetic agents to mucous membranes of the nose, mouth, throat, tracheobronchial tree, eyes, urinary tract, and gastrointestinal tract induces surface anesthesia. Following such application local anesthetics are absorbed rapidly into the circulation and carry the risk of systemic toxicity. Cocaine can be used as a topical anesthetic because of its vasoconstrictive properties, which will decrease its own absorption as well as improve surgical conditions through shrinkage of mucous membranes and decreasing local bleeding. Phenylephrine in dilute concentrations can be added to other local anesthetics to produce similar vasoconstrictive effects. Epinephrine is not effective in producing topical vasoconstriction.

Surface anesthetic agents include cyclomethycaine sulfate, hexylcaine hydrochloride, cocaine, lidocaine, and tetracaine. The following agents have primarily ophthalmologic application in the production of corneal anesthesia: benoxinate hydrochloride, and proparacaine hydrochloride.

Infiltration Anesthesia

The direct injection of local anesthetics into skin or deeper structures to facilitate surgery or painful procedures is called *infiltration anesthesia*. This technique is most commonly used for superficial procedures such as skin or breast biopsy and suture of wounds. However, in the absence of other anesthetic options infiltration anesthesia has been used to facilitate emergent procedures such as appendectomy or cesarean delivery. As previously mentioned, the addition of vasoconstrictors to local anesthetics for infiltration anesthesia has desirable features of decreased systemic absorption, decreased bleeding, and prolonged duration of anesthesia.

Field block anesthesia is a technique of infiltrating local anesthetics so as to produce a wall of anesthesia around an operative field. A clinical example of this would be field block anesthesia for inguinal herniorrhaphy. Local anesthetic agents commonly used for infiltration or field block anesthesia include lidocaine, mepivacaine, bupivacaine, etidocaine, and chloroprocaine.

Peripheral Nerve Block

Interruption of neural pathways of the peripheral nervous system is accomplished by depositing local anesthetics onto or about individual nerves or groups of nerves called *plexuses*. These techniques as well as spinal and epidural anesthesia are referred to as *regional anesthesia*. At appropriate local anesthetic concentrations they result in anesthesia of all nerve fibers and therefore block sensory, motor, and autonomic pathways.

Many surgical procedures are performed under regional anesthesia. Examples include brachial plexus blocks for arm and hand procedures, cervical plexus blocks for surgery of the neck, intercostal blocks for abdominal and thoracic wall procedures, and blocks of individual nerves at the wrist or ankle for hand and foot procedures.

The most commonly used local anesthetic agents for peripheral nerve blocks are lidocaine, mepivacaine, and bupivacaine.

Spinal Anesthesia

Spinal anesthesia, also called *intrathecal* or *subarachnoid block* is accomplished by the injection of local anesthetic into the cerebrospinal fluid (CSF) of the spinal subarachnoid space. Injections of anesthetics are made most commonly below the termination of the spinal cord, which correlates with the body of second lumbar vertebra. The development of spinal anesthesia, manifested by sympathetic block, loss of sensation, and muscular relaxation, is due primarily to the action of local anesthetics at the spinal nerve roots and in the dorsal root ganglia. The extent of neural blockade is determined by the distribution of local anesthetic in the CSF. Important factors governing local anesthetic spread include the density of the anesthetic solution relative to the density of the CSF, the position of the patient, and the dose and volume of the agent.

The ratio of anesthetic solution density (density equals mass in grams per milliliter of solution) to CSF density is known as *baricity*. Anesthetic solutions can be either hypo-, iso-, or hyperbaric. Hyperbaric solutions are the most commonly used in clinical practice. A hyperbaric solution spreads cephalad, causing a higher level of subarachnoid block, when patient positioning can control spread of the anesthetic agent to the desired level of neural contact within the subarachnoid space.

Onset of spinal anesthesia is very rapid, with detectable analgesia within 1 or 2 min and progression to desired levels of sensory and motor blockade in 5 to 10 min. Factors such as total dose of agent, baricity, use of vasoconstrictor, and lipid solubility determine the intensity and duration of spinal anesthesia.

Accompanying the blockade of motor and sensory modalities, spinal anesthesia will also cause profound physiologic alterations due to the interruption of the sympathetic nervous system. The preganglionic sympathetic fibers leave the spinal cord between T-1 and L-2 and travel in the corresponding anterior roots across the subarachnoid and epidural spaces. Because of the increased sensitivity of preganglionic autonomic (B) fibers, the level of sympathetic nervous system blockade will extend higher than sensory and motor blockade. Physiologic effects of this blockade include venous (capacitance vessels) and arterial (resistance vessels) dilatation, causing decreased cardiac output and blood pressure.

Preservative-free solutions of lidocaine, bupivacaine, and tetracaine are most frequently used agents for spinal anesthesia.

Epidural Anesthesia

Epidural or peridural anesthesia is produced by injection of local anesthetic into the space surrounding the dura mater, within the bony cavity of the spinal canal. Spinal nerves with their dural cuffs pass through the epidural space on their way to the intervertebral foramina. Following epidural injection, local anesthetics gain access to their site of action by diffusing through the dural cuffs, into the cerebrospinal fluid, and to the paravertebral area through the intervertebral foramina. Larger doses of local anesthetic (approximately 10-fold) are required for epidural anesthesia, compared with doses needed for spinal anesthesia, owing to the increased distance from neural tissue and dependence on diffusion to the site of action. As a consequence there is a greater potential for systemic local anesthetic toxicity with this technique. Another concern is the risk of injecting large doses of local anesthetic intended for epidural anesthesia into the subarachnoid space. A high, or "total," spinal can then occur, which may be accompanied by hypertension, bradycardia, and respiratory arrest secondary to intercostal and diaphragm muscle paralysis. Onset of epidural anesthesia is slower than spinal anesthesia.

Epidural anesthesia induced by administration of anesthetic solution into the sacral canal through the sacral hiatus is referred to as *caudal anesthesia*. It has applications in obstetric, perineal, and lower extremity procedures. Both epidural and spinal anesthesia may be administered and maintained via a catheter placed in the proper anatomic location. Anesthesia can then be maintained and closely titrated for indefinite periods of time. Agents used for epidural anesthesia include lidocaine, mepivacaine, bupivacaine, etidocaine, and chloroprocaine.

THERAPEUTIC USES OF LOCAL ANESTHETIC CONGENERS

Amino-Amide Agents

Lidocaine Lidocaine is the most versatile of all local anesthetic agents. It has excellent potency, rapid onset, a moderate duration of action and can be used for all the above-mentioned clinical applications.

Mepivacaine Mepivacaine has similar properties to lidocaine. Duration of its action is somewhat longer than that of lidocaine. This agent is not used in obstet-

ric anesthesia due to its prolonged metabolism in the fetus and neonate, leading to an increased possibility of toxicity.

Bupivacaine Bupivacaine is characterized by slow onset, long duration of action, and high quality anesthesia. Most notable is the separation of sensory analgesia and motor blockade. At lower concentrations bupivacaine can provide sensory analgesia with minimal motor block. As described, bupivacaine exhibits more serious cardiovascular toxicity owing probably to its high affinity for the sodium channels of myocardial conduction fibers.

Etidocaine Etidocaine is distinguished by the profound muscular relaxation it produces. It is similar in profile to bupivacaine with respect to duration of action and production of high-quality anesthesia; however, it has a more rapid onset.

Prilocaine Prilocaine is comparable to lidocaine in clinical profile, yet it has a lower potential for systemic toxic reactions. Because of the formation of methemoglobinemia at high doses, this drug is not commonly used.

Dibucaine Dibucaine is very potent and has a long duration of action. It is used primarily for spinal anesthesia and is similar to tetracaine in this clinical application.

Amino-Ester Agents

Procaine Procaine is an agent of low potency and short duration of action. Allergic reactions are more common with this agent due to its metabolism to *para*-aminobenzoic acid.

Chloroprocaine Chloroprocaine is notable for rapid onset of action and low systemic toxicity, which is due to rapid hydrolysis in plasma. It is popular in obstetric anesthesia because of its low fetal and maternal toxicity.

Tetracaine Tetracaine has a profile of high potency and long duration. In contrast to chloroprocaine, tetracaine undergoes slow plasma hydrolysis. Systemic toxicity at large doses has deterred its use in many regional anesthetic techniques. It is most commonly used for spinal anesthesia.

Cocaine Cocaine is used primarily as a surface anesthetic because of its vasoconstrictor properties. Its widespread abuse as a central nervous system stimulant warrants more extensive discussion (see Chaps. 18 and 25).

Surface Anesthetics

Many of the compounds described above possess the ability to produce good surface anesthesia when applied topically, as well as local anesthetic action upon injection. However, a number of compounds, because of poor solubility or other chemical properties which limit their diffusion capabilities, are not useful upon injection but demonstrate excellent therapeutic qualities when applied to the skin or mucous membranes. It should be noted that most of the compounds in this classification do not conform to the structure previously described for classic local anesthetics. The following drugs are representative of those utilized as surface anesthetics.

Cyclomethycaine Cyclomethycaine [3-(2-methylpiperidino)propyl-*p*-cyclohexyloxybenzoate] is used for topical application only. The compound induces sustained anesthesia when applied to the mucous membranes of the rectum, vagina, urethra, and urinary bladder, but it exhibits little effect on the mucous membranes of the bronchi, trachea, nose, and eyes. As with most poorly soluble local anesthetics, it can be applied to the skin whether abraded or intact. Cyclomethycaine is utilized for the relief of surface irritation and itching due to pruritus, insect bites, minor burns, and hemorrhoids, and it is also used for urethral instillation prior to urologic examination.

Benzocaine and Butamben Benzocaine (ethyl aminobenzoate) and its close relative butamben (butyl aminobenzoate) are esters of *para*-aminobenzoic acid, yet differ from the parent procaine-type esters in that they do not contain the terminal hydrophilic amine group.

$$H_2N-\text{⟨benzene ring⟩}-\overset{\overset{\displaystyle O}{\|}}{C}OCH_2CH_3$$

Benzocaine

Benzocaine is, therefore, very slightly soluble in water and is slowly absorbed, with a prolonged duration of action. Sensitization may occur with these compounds when in contact with susceptible patients, when applied over extensive areas, and when utilized repeatedly. Benzocaine produces a sustained and effective local anesthetic action when applied to abraded skin. These drugs are employed as topical anesthetics on intact or abraded skin, as antipruritics, and for various dermatologic conditions.

Ethyl Chloride Ethyl chloride is a highly flammable and volatile liquid which is used in the form of a spray on surface areas to obtain brief periods of local anesthesia. Its anesthetic action is based on the principle of rapid evaporation, which produces localized freezing of the tissue, promoting loss of peripheral sensory function. (Fluorocarbons, because of similar physical properties, also exhibit this action.) Ethyl chloride is useful for the temporary relief of pain in inflamed areas and for muscle spasms.

Preparations and Doses

Benzocaine (ethyl aminobenzoate) is available in 1 and 5% cream; 1, 2, 5, 9, and 20% ointment; 5, 13.6, and 20% aerosol; 0.75 and 10% spray; 6.37% liquid; and 0.5% lotion.

Butamben (butyl aminobenzoate, Butesin) is available in a 1% ointment for topical use on skin. It is also available in a 6.37, 10, and 22% liquid and a 7.5, 20, and 22% gel. All are for topical use on mucous membranes.

Cocaine is available in bulk powder for preparation of solutions for topical use on mucous membranes.

Cyclomethycaine (Surfacaine) is available in 0.5% cream and 1% ointment for topical use on the skin.

Dibucaine (Nupercaine) is available in 1:1500 to 1:500 solutions for injection; in 0.5% cream, 1% ointment, and 0.25% spray for topical use on skin.

Etidocaine (Duranest) is available in 0.5 to 1.5% solutions for injection.

Ethyl chloride is available in spray bottles.

Lidocaine (Xylocaine) is available in 0.5 to 5% solutions for injection; in 0.25 and 0.5% ointment for topical use on skin; in 2 and 4% solutions, 2% jelly, 3% cream, and 5% ointment for topical use on mucous membranes.

Mepivacaine (Carbocaine) is available in 1 to 3% solutions for injection.

Procaine (Novocain) is available in 0.25 to 10% solutions for injection.

Tetracaine (Pontocaine) is available in 0.2 to 2% solutions for injection; in 0.5% ophthalmic solution; in 0.5% ophthalmic ointment; in 0.5% ointment and 1% cream for topical use on skin; and in 2% solution for topical use on mucous membranes.

BIBLIOGRAPY

Adriani, J., and M. Naraghi: "The Pharmacologic Principles of Regional Pain Relief," *Annu. Rev. Pharmacol,* **17**:223–242 (1977).

Bingol, N.: "Teratogenicity of Cocaine in Humans," *J. Pediatrics,* **110**:93–96 (1987).

Campbell, A. H., J. A. Stasse, G. H. Lord, and J. E. Wilson: "In Vivo Evaluation of Local Anesthetics Applied Topically," *J. Pharm. Sci.,* **57**:2045–2048 (1968).

Covino, B. G.: "Pharmacology of Local Anaesthetic Agents," *Br. J. Anaesth.,* **58**(7):701–716 (1986).

Covino, B. G.: Clinical Pharmacology of Local Anesthetic Agents, in M. J. Cousins and P. O. Bridenbaugh (eds.), *Neural Blockade in Clinical Anesthesia and Management of Pain,* 2d ed., Philadelphia, J. B. Lippincott Company, 1988, Chap. 4.

Covino, B. G., and H. G. Vassalo: *Local Anesthetics, Mechanism of Action and Clinical Uses,* Grune & Stratton, New York, 1976.

Haddad, I. M.: "1978: Cocaine in Perspective," *J. Am. Coll. Emergency Physicians,* **8**:374–376 (1979).

Hodgkin, A. L.: *The Conduction of the Nerve Impulse,* Charles C Thomas, Springfield, Ill, 1964.

Ludena, F. P.: "Duration of Local Anesthesia," *Annu. Rev. Pharmacol.,* **9**:503–520 (1969).

Reiz, S., and S. Nath: "Cardiotoxicity of Local Anaesthetic Agents," *Br. J. Anaesth.,* **58**:736–746 (1986).

Reynolds, F.: "Adverse Effects of Local Anaesthetics," *Br. J. Anaesth.,* **59**:78–95 (1987).

Scott, D. B.: "Toxic Effects of Local Anaesthetic Agents on the Central Nervous System," *Br. J. Anaesth.,* **58**:732–735 (1986).

Seeman, P.: "The Membrane Actions of Anesthetics and Tranquilizers," *Pharmacol. Rev.,* **24**:583–655 (1972).

Stewart, D. M., W. P. Rogers, J. E. Mahaffey, S. Witherspoon, and E. F. Woods: "Effect of Local Anesthetics on the Cardiovascular System of the Dog," *Anesthesiology,* **24**:620–624 (1963).

Strichartz, G., T. Rando, G. K. Wang: "An Integrated View of the Molecular Toxinology of Sodium Channel Gating in Excitable Cells," *Ann. Rev. Neurosci.,* **10**:237–267 (1987).

Tucker, G. T.: "Pharmacokinetics of Local Anaesthetics," *Br. J. Anaesth.,* **58**(7):713–717 (1986).

Wildsmith, J. A. W.: "Peripheral Nerve and Local Anaesthetic Drugs," *Br. J. Anaesth.,* **58**:692–700 (1986).

C H A P T E R 25

Drug Dependence

Charles O'Brien

Drug dependence is a problem of continuously increasing medical and social importance, largely because of the spread of drug abuse: ingesting them not for legitimate medical needs but for real or imagined psychologic gratification. Many of these drugs can induce dependence, with the result that eventually users become addicted and continue taking the drug with increasing frequency. There has been mounting public concern about drug abuse, partly because of increased availability of drugs that act on the brain and may have potential abuse liability, and partly because no totally satisfactory and effective means has been developed to cope with abuse and addiction.

The situation has assumed crisis proportions in the 1980s because of the appearance of a new form of cocaine which is more highly addictive than any drug previously available and because of the association of intravenous drug abuse with the acquired immune deficiency syndrome (AIDS).

TERMS CONCERNED WITH DRUG DEPENDENCE AND ABUSE

The terminology of drug dependence essentially derives from the concept of drug enslavement and designates different degrees of enslavement or compulsion to seek and take drugs. *Psychologic dependence* generally means that the effect of the drug satisfies some psychologic need and is gratifying to the individual. Addiction refers to a pattern of repeated drug-taking behavior where the need or compulsion is much stronger than psychologic dependence. This definition of addiction has been formalized and extended to include, in addition to a strong compulsion, the tendency to increase the dose and the production of physical dependence (see below).

The term *drug abuse* is now frequently employed to designate the inappropriate as well as excessive use of drugs. Drug abuse also implies that harm is done to the individual user and/or to society in general. Society attempts to limit drug abuse and dependence by determining the abuse potential of drugs, both new and old, and subjecting the agents to appropriate controls according to their abuse potential. The Drug Enforcement Administration of the U.S. Department of Justice has classified such drugs into schedules according to their abuse potential and has issued stringent regulations on their possession and administration.

Schedule I

Drugs in this schedule have a high potential for abuse and no currently accepted medical use in the United States. Examples of such drugs include heroin, marijuana, peyote, mescaline, some tetrahydrocannabinols, and various opioid derivatives. Substances listed in this schedule are not for prescription use; they may be obtained for chemical analysis or research instruction by submitting an application and a protocol of the proposed use to the Drug Enforcement Administration.

Schedule II

The drugs in this schedule have a high abuse potential with severe psychologic or physical dependence liability. Schedule II substances consist of certain opioid drugs, preparations containing amphetamines or methamphetamines as the single active ingredient or in combination with each other, and certain sedatives. Examples of opioids included in this schedule are opium, morphine, codeine, hydromorphone, methadone, meperidine, cocaine, oxycodone, and oxymorphone. Also included are stimulants, e.g., dextroamphetamine, methamphetamine, methylphenidate, and depressants, e.g., amobarbital, pentobarbital, and secobarbital.

Schedule III

The drugs in this schedule have a potential for abuse that is less than that for those drugs in schedules I and II. The use of these drugs may lead to low or moderate physical dependence or high psychologic dependence. Included in this schedule, for example, are glutethimide, methyprylon, phendimetrazine, maxindol, and paregoric.

Schedule IV

The drugs in this category have the potential for limited physical or psychologic dependence and include barbital, phenobarbital, paraldehyde, chloral hydrate, ethchlorvynol, meprobamate, chlordiazepoxide, diazepam, clorazepate, flurazepam, oxazepam, clonazepam, prazepam, lorazepam, and propoxyphene.

Schedule V

Schedule V drugs have a potential for abuse that is less than that for those listed in schedule IV. These consist of preparations containing moderate quantities of certain opioids for use in pain (i.e., buprenorphine) or as antidiarrheals (e.g., diphenoxylate) or as antitussives (such as codeine-containing cough mixtures, e.g., Robitussin A-C). They may be dispensed without a prescription order, provided that specified dispensing criteria are met by the pharmacist. Physicians should be clearly aware of the abuse potential of drugs: (1) their capacity to induce compulsive drug-seeking behavior: (2) their toxicity; and (3) the social consequences of abusing drugs as well as the attitude of society toward drug abuse.

TOLERANCE

Tolerance is defined as decreased response to a subsequent dose of a previously administered drug—hence the need for an increased dose to obtain a given response. With some drugs the original effect cannot be completely reproduced once tolerance has developed, no matter how much the dose is increased. When tolerance develops very rapidly, following either a single dose or a few doses given over a short period of time, it is called *acute tolerance*, or *tachyphylaxis*. When the drug must be administered over a long period of time to induce tolerance, it is called *chronic tolerance. Cross-tolerance* exists when tolerance to one drug confers tolerance to another.

Mechanisms involved in tolerance may be classified in three categories: (1) *metabolic*, which involves more efficient disposition of the drug; (2) *pharmacodynamic*, which includes synaptic adaptations such as changes in numbers or sensitivity of receptors so as to counteract the effects of a drug at the synapse; and (3) *behavioral*, which involves learning to function in the presence of drug impairment of conditioned reflex changes which counteract the changes produced by the drug. With regular dosing, tolerance increases and a state of physical dependence follows.

PHYSICAL DEPENDENCE

Physical dependence is a state of drug-induced physiologic change which becomes manifest as an abstinence syndrome when the drug effect is diminished by either withdrawing the agent or by administering appropriate antagonists which displace it from its site of action. When physical dependence develops at a very rapid rate over a matter of hours, it is called *acute physical dependence*. When it is produced by prolonged treatment with a drug, it is called *chronic physical dependence*. The abstinence syndrome that results from termination of the drug is termed *withdrawal syndrome*. The withdrawal syndrome includes bodily changes that tend to be opposite to the effects of the drug which produced the dependence. Thus a drug that produces stimulation, such as cocaine, is followed by weakness and depression during withdrawal. A drug that produces sedation, such as diazepam, produces hyperreflexia, anxiety, and irritability during withdrawal.

The drugs of abuse are divided into four major categories: (1) *depressants*, including opioids, benzodiazepines, and alcohol; (2) *stimulants*, including cocaine and the amphetamines; (3) *hallucinogens*, including lysergic acid diethylamide (LSD) and phencyclidine (PCP); and (4) *miscellaneous*, including marijuana and nicotine.

DEPRESSANTS

Opioids Dependence

(See Chap. 22 for pharmacologic details.) There are two major clinical patterns of opioid abuse. The first occurs in individuals who receive prescription analgesic medication because of chronic pain. Tolerance to opioids begins with the first dose, and when patients receive these drugs chronically, tolerance and physical dependence are inevitable. This is why such drugs generally should not be used in the treatment of chronic pain unless the pain is associated with a terminal illness or unless the pain is so severe that the opioids must be used as a last resort. Problems such as chronic headaches, back pain, or neuritis should rarely be treated with opioids.

On the other hand, acute pain is often undertreated by physicians because of the fear of producing addiction. If pain is caused by a known source such as surgery or myocardial infarction, opioids can be prescribed on a short-term basis. It is important to be sure that the patient has adequate pain relief. There should be a clear distinction between the tolerance and physical dependence, which are expected occurrences when opioids are used repeatedly, and the opioid dependence syndrome, which involves drug-seeking behavior and the intention to use the drug in order to "get high" rather than simply to relieve pain.

The second type of opioid abuse pattern is that seen in street heroin addicts. These are most commonly young men who begin the use of heroin between 14 and 18 years of age and typically increase their dose over time so that within several years they are using the drug 3 to 6 times per day. The actual dose of heroin obtained in purchases on the streets of the United States is actually small. Perhaps 4 to 6 percent of the material in each heroin bag is actually heroin; the other 96 percent contains fillers such as quinine, maltose, bicarbonate, or worse. Thus even a person injecting as often as 6 times per day is not usually receiving a large amount of opiate.

The opioid dependence syndrome is associated with many medical problems, in addition to preoccupation with drug-seeking behavior. Street heroin addicts tend to have multiple infections because of contaminated substances injected into their veins. These produce abscesses, sclerosed veins, lung lesions (because of contaminants filtered in the pulmonary circulation), cardiac lesions (such as bacterial endocarditis), and hepatitis (as many as 70 percent of street heroin addicts have some type of hepatitis). Street addicts are also often malnourished and suffering from associated psychiatric disorders, especially depression and anxiety.

In recent years drug abuse has become a major risk factor for AIDS. Not only does the virus spread because of addicts' habit of sharing dirty needles, but it is also possible that some of the drugs used and the deteriorated condition of the addicts may make the drug abuser more susceptible to infection with HIV.

Tolerance and Dependence

Tolerance develops very rapidly to repeated use of opioids, but it develops in different systems at different rates. Thus a chronic user who no longer gets a "high" from a given dose may still continue to suffer from constipation and endocrine suppressant effects. Cross-tolerance refers to tolerance to all opioids produced by repeated dosing with a single opioid. The phenomenon of cross-tolerance forms the basis of the most widely used treatment for heroin dependence, methadone maintenance. Methadone is a long-acting opioid, given orally, which blocks opioid withdrawal and produces a level of tolerance such that the effects of the usual dose of street heroin can barely be perceived. Since there is little or no reward in taking heroin, properly maintained patients stop or at least greatly diminish their use of street opiates. They are required to come to a clinic daily or at least three times per week, and thus they are available for psychotherapy, counseling, and other treatment which might be indicated.

When a chronic user stops taking opioids, a withdrawal syndrome develops, which consists of signs opposite to the effects seen when opioids are administered. For example, opioids produce pupillary constriction, and during withdrawal there is pupillary dilatation. Opioids produce calming, and in withdrawal extreme anxiety is common. The severity of the withdrawal syndrome depends on the dose of the opioid. Most cases of opioid withdrawal require little medication, and some patients can stop on their own without assistance although relapse under those circumstances is almost universal. Short-acting drugs such as heroin have a brief severe withdrawal syndrome, which peaks at 36 to 48 h and lasts up to 7 to 10 days. Long-acting drugs such as methadone have significantly longer withdrawal syndromes, which are just beginning at 36 to 48 h. In addition to the acute withdrawal syndrome, all opioids produce a protracted withdrawal syndrome, which consists of subtle but measurable signs and symptoms for at least 6 months. Most of the signs and symptoms of opioid withdrawal are related to rebound hyperactivity of central adrenergic pathways. Clonidine, a drug used in the treatment of hypertension, will reduce most of the symptoms of opioid withdrawal. The major advantages in the use of clonidine over a drug such as methadone is that clonidine (1) is nonaddictive, (2) causes a removal of the withdrawal symptoms without itself producing a withdrawal symptom, and (3) can detoxify certain individuals in a relatively shorter period of time. It is believed that clonidine centrally stimulates certain depressor areas thereby decreasing the release of norepinephrine in the peripheral tissues. In addition, clonidine apparently attaches to the same opioid receptors as morphine and will relieve the symptoms of the narcotic withdrawal syndrome. Therefore, by decreasing sympathetic outflow and stimulating morphine receptors, clonidine in certain patients can be used successfully in the treatment of narcotic withdrawal symptoms.

Opioid antagonists

Because opioids act at specific receptor sites, their effects can be blocked by other drugs which can occupy those receptors. Naloxone is such an antagonist, and it represents perhaps the only true antidote in medicine. Persons suffering from an acute overdose of opioids will be immediately awakened by intravenous naloxone because it competes successfully with opioid molecules at receptor sites.

In addition to the treatment of overdose, there are two other uses of opioid antagonists in the treatment of dependence. Antagonists can be used to diagnose dependence because, when injected, they will displace opioids from receptors producing an acute withdrawal syndrome. The prevention of relapse is yet another use of opioid antagonists. When given to a drug-free formerly dependent person, the antagonist will occupy opiate receptors and prevent the user from experiencing opioid effects. For this relapse-prevention function, a long-acting antagonist, naltrexone, is used. The completeness of the blockade depends on the dose of naltrexone, the time since the last dose of naltrexone, and the dose of the opioid used in the attempt to override the blockade. Naltrexone is effective in antagonizing typical doses of street opioids for 48 to 72 h. In practice, most patients do not test the blockade, and the treatment is effective for well-motivated patients when combined with a comprehensive rehabilitation program.

SEDATIVE DEPENDENCE

(See Chaps. 16 and 17 for pharmacologic details.) The most important sedative is alcohol, which is covered in a separate chapter. However, it should be noted that alcohol, while it has sedating effects, also has general anesthetic effects and is often used in combination with other sedatives to be described here. The subjective effects of all sedatives are somewhat similar to alcohol. In low doses they cause a suppression of inhibition, which produces a feeling of relaxation, even euphoria, although not as intense as that produced by stimulants. At higher doses, the sedation is more intense and the subject goes to sleep. The balance between euphoria and sedation is a function of dose, speed of entry into the nervous system, and the prior experience of the user. Benzodiazepine dependence is the most common type of sedative dependence apart from alcoholism, and thus it will be discussed in more detail.

Benzodiazepine Abuse and Dependence

Benzodiazepines are used mainly in the treatment of anxiety disorders. The abuse liability of the benzodiazepines is a controversial subject because they are so widely prescribed and there is uncertainty over what level of usage constitutes abuse. About 15 percent of the population of the United States takes a benzodiazepine at least once during a given year. About a third of these users take the drug chronically. Most, if not all, chronic users develop some degree of physical dependence, and they will experience withdrawal symptoms when the drug is terminated. This does not necessarily mean, however, that these patients are abusing benzodiazepines, providing that they are taking them in accordance with a doctor's prescription.

Many cases can be cited of individuals who were unable to function because of chronic anxiety, but with the use of low and steady doses of benzodiazepines they are able to lead normal lives. When the drug is withdrawn, such long-term users experience typical withdrawal symptoms, and later they may experience symptoms of the return of the anxiety disorder which were present prior to the original prescription of the benzodiazepine. Such a patient would be physically dependent on benzodiazepines.

Iatrogenic or inadvertent dependence on benzodiazepines can still be a clinical problem when benzodiazepines are prescribed by a physician. Some patients tend to gradually increase their dose of benzodiazepines as their tolerance to the sedating effects of the drug increases. This may be more common with those benzodiazepines that have a relatively rapid onset of action such as alprazolam. It is also a problem with the very potent benzodiazepines such as alprazolam where doctors may be willing to prescribe doses of 5 to 10 mg/day because this seems like a low dose. However, when translated to diazepam equivalents, this is 50 to 100 mg/day.

There is also a significant problem with deliberate abuse of benzodiazepines. Benzodiazepines have a street value, and they are sold on the black market. Drug abusers use them to "get high" or to ameliorate the withdrawal symptoms from opiates, alcohol, or other sedatives. Because of the capacity to develop tolerance to the sedating effects of benzodiazepines, huge doses are sometimes taken by drug abusers.

Benzodiazepine Tolerance

Benzodiazepines exhibit an excellent illustration of the phenomenon of differential tolerance. That is, tolerance develops within different systems for different functions at different rates. It is very clear that a large degree of tolerance can develop for the sedating effects of benzodiazepines. However, it is equally clear that the memory impairment effects of benzodiazepines do not diminish with repeated use. Benzodiazepines have

significant disruptive effects on short-term memory as demonstrated by tests of recall and speech fluency. These effects are relatively greater than those caused by barbiturates or alcohol. Memory impairment after a benzodiazepine dose is found in subjects who have taken low or moderate doses of benzodiazepines consistently for 10 years.

A very important clinical question is whether tolerance develops to the antianxiety effects of benzodiazepines. This question is difficult to answer in clinical studies because benzodiazepine withdrawal resembles the symptoms of anxiety. Only one double-blind study has clearly addressed this issue, and it suggests that while tolerance develops to the sedating effects of the drugs, tolerance does not develop to the antianxiety effects, and thus it is rational to continue to medicate patients with chronic anxiety. Another argument in this direction by inference is the lack of tolerance to the memory disrupting effects. Since there is clearly lack of tolerance for these effects of benzodiazepines, there may also be lack of tolerance for the antianxiety effect.

Benzodiazepine Withdrawal

The benzodiazepine withdrawal syndrome depends on the dose, duration, and half-life of the benzodiazepine used. Those taking even a moderate dose of benzodiazepines may show withdrawal symptoms if the drug is abruptly discontinued after about 4 months of chronic use. The severity of the withdrawal syndrome and the time of onset depend on the above variables. The symptoms include irritability, tremors, dysphoria, sweating, headache, unpleasant dreams, insomnia, anorexia, dizziness, muscle twitches, and paresthesias. After higher doses, generalized seizures, panic, paranoia, and delirium have been observed. It should also be noted that mild but definite withdrawal symptoms have been documented after as little as 15 mg of diazepam per day.

Treatment

Benzodiazepine withdrawal should be suspected in all alcoholics and other sedative abusers at the time of detoxification. Symptoms may occur unexpectedly, especially in individuals taking long-acting benzodiazepines such as diazepam where the syndrome may occur 5 to 7 days after the patient is admitted to the hospital and the diazepam discontinued. The standard detoxification regimen consists of placing the patient on a long-acting benzodiazepine and gradually reducing the dose over 7 to 10 days, but sometimes a much longer treatment is required. The particular treatment circumstances may require an even longer term outpatient detoxification.

When deliberately abused, benzodiazepines are usually taken in combination with other drugs, and the dangers of accidental overdose are increased markedly. This is particularly true when benzodiazepines are combined with alcohol. After the acute detoxification, the treatment for prevention of relapse is aimed at the overall drug-dependence syndrome. This involves psychotherapy, possibly living in a therapeutic community, group therapy, and behavioral relapse prevention techniques. Benzodiazepines should rarely be prescribed for people with a history of alcoholism or other forms of drug abuse. If an antianxiety agent is found to be absolutely necessary, physicians should consider a benzodiazepine with a low abuse potential.

Barbiturate and Other Nonbenzodiazepine Sedative Abuse

Barbiturates tend to have a greater abuse potential than benzodiazepines, but they are prescribed less often since the benzodiazepine era. Slow-onset, long-acting barbiturates such as phenobarbital are very rarely abused despite widespread use in the treatment of seizure disorders. Accidental overdose is a danger with barbiturates and other nonbenzodiazepines because tolerance to the "high" effects occurs more rapidly and extensively than tolerance to the brain stem depressant effects. Sleeping pills such as glutethimide or methaqualone are notorious in this regard. The abuser who keeps increasing the dose to obtain a "high" may unexpectedly suffer cardiorespiratory arrest as the toxic range for the brain stem is reached. In general, barbiturates and other nonbenzodiazepine sedatives are far more dangerous than benzodiazepines from the perspective of abuse potential and overdose risk.

The withdrawal syndrome from sedative dependence is more dangerous than opiate or stimulant withdrawal. All patients being detoxified from sedative dependence require at least a medical evaluation to determine whether hospitalization and treatment with medication to assist the withdrawal is necessary.

STIMULANTS

Cocaine and Amphetamine Dependence

(See Chap. 18 for pharmacologic details.) Oral cocaine has been used for centuries by Indians of the Andes who chew coca leaves with an alkaline material which facilitates absorption of the alkaloid base through oral mucous membranes. This technique produces relatively mild stimulation which results in increased endurance but no known abuse. The hydrochloride salt can be produced from coca leaves and placed in the nose for absorption through the nasal mucous membranes ("snorting"). By this route the local vasoconstricting effects of the drug slow absorption and prolong the effect. The hydrochloride salt can also be taken intravenously, and this produces a much more rapid effect which is difficult to regulate and may result in seizures. The hydrochloride salt cannot be smoked because it will be volatilized only at temperatures which degrade it. However, the alkaloidal cocaine, called *freebase*, or crack, is readily volatilized undegraded at much lower temperatures. Simply heating crack enables a person to smoke it and absorb the cocaine through the lungs, where it is rapidly absorbed into the pulmonary circulation and carried to the left side of the heart. It then reaches the brain in seconds and produces an intense euphoric effect. The smoking of crack cocaine thus produces rapid and strong effects, and dependence can occur within days to weeks of initial use.

With the next use, perhaps one to several days later, the tolerance is no longer present and the original effects are again present. Under certain conditions, reverse tolerance or sensitization occurs. This phenomenon has not been studied systematically in humans, but it may be the explanation for some of the cases of seizures or cardiac arrhythmias which have been seen in people who have previously taken the same dose without significant toxicity.

Cocaine is an effective topical local anesthetic and vasoconstrictor of mucous membranes. Stimulants do reduce appetite, but significant tolerance to this effect develops. When stimulants are discontinued, a rebound increase in weight can leave the person heavier than before the drug was taken.

Amphetamine has a longer duration of action than cocaine, but many of the effects are similar. Amphetamine has been used by physicians for a variety of conditions, including weight reduction, narcolepsy, and attention-deficit disorder. Amphetamine has not been shown to be of value in weight reduction programs, and the prescription of stimulants has been curtailed by legal restrictions.

Methylphenidate has a much lower abuse potential than either cocaine or amphetamine. It has been useful in the treatment of attention deficit disorder in children and in narcolepsy.

Detoxification

The withdrawal syndrome from cocaine dependence consists of fatigue, lack of energy, and a depressed mood. There is also intense craving for the drug. The withdrawal syndrome is thought to represent a dopamine depletion syndrome because the blockage of dopamine re-uptake results in lack of dopamine conservation and eventual depletion of available dopamine stores. During acute intoxication, stimulants can also produce a paranoid syndrome which resembles an acute paranoid schizophrenic episode. After a binge, the withdrawal syndrome is often referred to as a *crash* because of the severe depression and desire for sleep.

Toxic Effects

The most likely complication of cocaine use is dependence. Another common consequence is the development of a psychiatric disorder such as paranoid symptoms or a depressive syndrome. While sexual drive and sexual appreciation may be increased during early cocaine use, subsequently there is often loss of interest in sex and difficulty with sexual performance.

There are also important toxic effects on the cardiovascular system. There is evidence that cocaine is capable of causing acute myocardial infarction even in patients with normal coronary arteries. There is also evidence that cases of sudden death may be due to cocaine-induced ventricular arrhythmia. The arrhythmia may be the result of the direct effect of cocaine on the cardiac conduction system or an indirect effect that is mediated via the effect of cocaine on the central nervous system. There is also evidence that cocaine can produce myocarditis.

Treatment

Cocaine withdrawal usually does not require pharmacologic intervention although some have advocated the use of dopamine receptor stimulants such as bromocriptine to ease the withdrawal syndrome. The major clinical problem is the prevention of relapse of compulsive cocaine use. There are reports that tricyclic antidepressants, especially desipramine, can reduce some of the effects of cocaine craving.

HALLUCINOGENS

Lysergic Acid Diethylamide (LSD) and Phencyclidine (PCP) Dependence

(See Chap. 18 for pharmacologic details.) There are many mechanisms for producing hallucinations, and drugs which act on the serotonergic, cholinergic, and adrenergic systems can produce such effects by various mechanisms. The drug which is currently the greatest problem is phencyclidine, which has pharmacologic effects similar to those of anesthetics, and it produces amphetamine-like stimulation. Phencyclidine is easily synthesized, however, and it is found in many street samples misrepresented as other drugs, for example as LSD or as THC.

LSD is effective at doses as low as 20 μg; however, the usual street dose is around 200 μg. The drug produces central sympathomimetic stimulation characterized by dilatation of the pupils, hyperthermia, rapid heartbeat, elevated blood pressure, pyloerection, and increased alertness. Nausea and vomiting occasionally occur. The psychologic effects of LSD depend on the expectations of the user, the setting, the dose and the previous experiences. Individuals with a preexisting psychiatric disorder often have a very frightening response to the hallucinations produced by LSD. Typical reactions include a feeling that insights are enhanced and that ordinary sights and sounds seem louder and clearer. Perceptual distortions commonly occur, causing an individual, for example, to see his or her hand suddenly grow large or the hairs on the hand look like snakes. Usually visual hallucinations occur, and they may occur in vivid colors. The reaction to LSD persists for about 10 h, but fatigue and tension may continue for an additional 24 h. Other hallucinogenic drugs such as mescaline and dimethyltryptamine are shorter in duration.

Phencyclidine produces a rapid stimulant effect similar to that seen with amphetamine, and it may produce a feeling of euphoria. Numbness, clumsiness, slurred speech, and nystagmus are common. Phencyclidine also produces frightening hallucinations, especially visual and tactile hallucinations. There may be assaultive and hostile behavior, and the person has amnesia for these actions. Occasionally individuals inadvertently take a large dose of phencyclidine which can produce catatonia and coma. Phencyclidine overdose should always be considered in a comatose patient with dilated pupils and elevated blood pressure.

Tolerance and Dependence

Tolerance develops to some of the effects of hallucinogens after several administrations. Thus experienced users may require a somewhat higher dose in order to get the effects that they are seeking. A withdrawal syndrome has not been described for these drugs in human subjects although signs of withdrawal in animal subjects after high chronic doses of phencyclidine have been reported.

Toxic Effects

Significant toxic problems can occur with the use of hallucinogens after only one administration. Individuals may have a "bad trip," which involves terror, anxiety, and a prolonged psychotic reaction. Occasionally individuals have harmed themselves or others when having a bad trip. Phencyclidine appears the most toxic of the hallucinogens, with severe reactions being more common than mild reactions. Several studies have indicated a high frequency of phencyclidine abuse in individuals admitted to psychiatric hospitals with a diagnosis of acute psychotic reaction and no diagnosis of drug abuse on admission. Phencyclidine appears to be capable of producing a psychosis which can be indistinguishable from an acute schizophrenic disorder. Patients being treated for chronic schizophrenic disorders in mental health clinics often give a history of hallucinogen abuse in the past, but it is not possible to determine whether the hallucinogen caused chronic schizophreniform disorder or whether hallucinogen abuse was merely associated with the onset of schizophrenia which would have occurred even in the absence of drug abuse.

Frequent hallucinogen users may report the occurrence of flashbacks after stopping hallucinogen use. These flashbacks consist of brief periods of hallucinations resembling the acute effects of the drug but occurring days, weeks, or months after last ingestion of the drug.

MISCELLANEOUS

Marijuana Dependence

(See Chap. 18 for pharmacologic details.) Cannabis is called *marijuana*, *hashish*, or *hemp*, depending on the part of the world and the part of the marijuana plant prepared. Actually, cannabis is not a single drug, but a complex preparation containing many biologically active chemicals. Studies have shown that delta 9-tetrahydrocannabinol (Δ^9THC), produces most of the pharmacologic effects of the complex. Throughout the 1970s the use of marijuana increased dramatically among young people so that in 1979 more than 60 percent of high school seniors reported trying it and 9 percent were using it daily. During this time period, the potency of marijuana also increased dramatically so that some cigarettes were found to contain up to 14% THC, which is more than has been found in potent forms such as hemp seen in other parts of the world.

In the United States, marijuana is usually taken by inhalation. This route is 3 to 4 times more potent than the oral route, and it permits users to more accurately titrate their dose. The effects of inhaled marijuana begin within minutes and subjectively persist for 2 to 3 h, depending on the dose and the experience of the user. However, psychomotor impairment has been demonstrated for up to 11 h after taking a single dose even though the subjects reported that they felt normal at the time of the testing.

Marijuana, of course, is taken for its psychoactive effects, and these include relaxation, giddiness, a feeling of enhanced perceptions, and a feeling that time is passing slowly. Attention and learning are impaired. Anxiety reactions are occasionally reported, and sometimes there is acute pain which causes the user to be brought to an emergency room. There are also increases in heart rate, conjunctival vascular injection ("red eyes"), decreases in intraocular pressure, peripheral vasodilatation, bronchodilatation, and increases in airway conductance. Ataxia, nystagmus, fine tremors, and dryness of the mouth may occur.

Cannabis has been found to be an effective antiemetic for some patients, and it has been taken by cancer patients receiving chemotherapy. The antinausea effect is not seen without the psychoactive changes which prevent normal daily functions. Thus, the antinausea effect has not been found to be useful for many patients who do not like the psychoactive side effects.

It is important to note that motor vehicle operation is definitely impaired by cannabis, and the impairment may persist for hours after the user feels normal and confident about driving ability.

Δ^9 THC and other cannabinols have unusually high lipid solubility, and thus they persist in brain tissue for long periods of time. In regular users who terminate their use, the metabolites remain detectable in the urine for several weeks. Of course the biologic significance of low levels is unknown. Cannabis metabolites can also be detected in the urine of individuals who have sat for several hours in a room filled with marijuana smoke but who have not smoked marijuana cigarettes themselves. Under ordinary circumstances, however, the levels produced by such passive inhalation do not reach the usual threshold for calling a test positive.

Tolerance and Dependence

Tolerance to the sedating and cardiovascular effects of marijuana has been observed in experimental subjects given marijuana at regular intervals on a research unit. When the drug was stopped, a definite withdrawal syndrome was noted. In clinical situations, however, most patients do not take marijuana in high enough doses and at regular intervals so as to produce clinically significant dependence and a noticeable syndrome. Also, when present, the withdrawal syndrome is usually mild and does not require treatment with medication. While compulsive marijuana use is seen in some patients, the marijuana-seeking behavior does not resemble the frantic drug-craving and drug-seeking behavior seen among cocaine addicts and heroin addicts.

Toxic Effects

Regular marijuana use by adolescents is associated with impairment of psychologic maturation and poor social and scholastic adjustment. There has been no experimental demonstration that marijuana is the cause of such deterioration in social behavior, but there is general agreement that the drug is at least a contributing factor. Young people who exhibit the so-called amotivational syndrome also have many other problems besides marijuana use. Successful treatment of this syndrome requires that the individual cease

marijuana use as well as become engaged in psychotherapy, often family psychotherapy.

Occasional users of marijuana have fewer problems, but even intermittent users report episodes of acute panic, paranoid reactions, and frightening distortions of body images at times. These reactions seem to occur more frequently with higher doses and in individuals who take large doses by the oral route, where the dose cannot be readily controlled, instead of smoking the drug. Certain individuals seem to be extremely sensitive to the toxic effects of marijuana, and these often include individuals who are recovering from a psychotic episode or who suffer from a chronic psychiatric disorder.

Since cannabis stimulates the cardiovascular system, it may pose a problem for individuals with heart disease. There is also clear evidence that marijuana cigarettes cause inflammatory changes in the bronchi and in the mucosa of the sinuses. In experimental tests cannabis products are found to produce carcinoma, but it is difficult to find cases of this phenomenon clinically because it is rare to find a marijuana smoker who does not also use tobacco cigarettes.

DESIGNER DRUGS

In an attempt to synthesize derivatives of meperidine, two derivatives were developed that have gained popularity as street drugs as new heroin compounds. These compounds are commonly known as "designer drugs." The two most popular ones are MPPP (1-methyl-4-phenyl-proprionoxy-piperidine) and MPTP (1-methyl-4-phenyl-1,2,5,6-tetrahydropyridine).

MPPP   MPTP

These compounds are administered by injection and produce a syndrome of muscle rigidity, weakness, and tremulousness which resembles idiopathic Parkinson's disease. A significant number of individuals who abused these chemicals have developed permanent damage to their central nervous system. Because of their severe toxic effects, the illicit use of these so-called designer drugs has decreased drastically, so they play only a small part in the overall dependence area.

NICOTINE DEPENDENCE

(See Chap. 10 for pharmacologic details.) Nicotine is the dependence-producing component of tobacco and as such it results in the most severe mortality of any drug of abuse. Nicotine in the typical smoker produces relaxation of skeletal muscle and a reduction in deep tendon reflexes. There is also an increase in hand tremor and a desynchronization of the electroencephalogram, a pattern associated with increased alertness. Subjects report a sense of alertness with relaxed muscles and a facilitation of memory and attention. There is also a reduction of appetite. The mechanisms by which nicotine produces these effects are multiple, and they include changes in the release of acetylcholine depending on the dose and facilitation of the release of dopamine and norepinephrine.

The net effect of these changes is to produce something which smokers describe as pleasant. Each puff on a cigarette produces a small bolus of nicotine which is absorbed by the lungs and delivered rapidly to the brain via the arterial circulation. Since each cigarette takes approximately 10 puffs, one-pack-a-day smokers deliver approximately 200 reinforcements to their brains each day. This establishes a very strong habit.

Tolerance and Dependence

With repeated use, the unpleasant side effects of cigarettes including nausea, vomiting, and dizziness no longer occur. The other effects of nicotine also show tolerance, but some of the tolerance is lost each morning, since cigarettes are not ordinarily used during the night. Thus the first cigarette in the morning seems to have a greater effect than cigarettes later in the day. Also, experienced smokers show tolerance to the effects of intravenous nicotine as compared with nonsmokers.

Sudden cessation of smoking usually produces a withdrawal syndrome. While this is not seen in all smokers, it can be very unpleasant, lasting for at least several days and in some cases for several weeks. The signs and symptoms of nicotine withdrawal consist of irritability, restlessness, anxiety, shortened attention span, drowsiness, increased appetite, insomnia, headaches, and upset stomach. The withdrawal symptoms respond to doses of nicotine, including nicotine chewing gum. There is also evidence that the antihypertensive drug clonidine, which reduces opioid withdrawal symptoms, is also effective in nicotine withdrawal. This suggests that many of the symptoms of nicotine withdrawal are related to sympathetic nervous system rebound hyperactivity.

Toxicity

The significant toxic effects of smoking are related to the tars found in tobacco. Carcinomas, emphysema, and other diseases have been related to carbon monoxide produced by burning tobacco. The cardiovascular effects of nicotine may be harmful to individuals with heart disease.

CONCLUDING COMMENTS

Drug abuse is a complicated disorder which results from the interaction of a number of variables. These include the availability of the drug, the characteristics of the user, and the setting in which the drug is used. Virtually any drug described in this book can be abused by some people at some time. However, certain drugs, because of their pharmacologic characteristics carry a much higher potential for abuse. While pharmacology is very important in understanding the phenomenon of drug abuse, the problem actually goes far beyond pharmacology; the problem is at the interface of behavior, pharmacology, sociology, psychology, and clinical medicine.

BIBLIOGRAPHY

Chiang, C. N., and R. S., Rapaka : "Pharmacokinetics and Disposition of Cannabinoids," *Natl. Inst. Drug Abuse Res. Mang. Ser.*, **79**:173–188 (1987).

DiGregorio, G. J., and M. A. Bukovinsky: "Clonidine for Narcotic Withdrawal," *Am. Family Physician*, **33**:203 (1981).

Gawin, F. H., and E. H. Ellinwood: "Cocaine and Other Stimulant Actions, Abuse and Treatment," *N. Engl. J. Med.*, **318**:1173–1182 (1988).

Schuster, C. R.: "The United States Drug Abuse Scene: An Overview," *Clin. Chem.* **33**:7B–12B (1987).

Semlitz, L. and M. S. Gold: " Diagnosis and Treatment of Adolescent Substance Abuse," *Psychiatric-Med*, **3**:321–323 (1985).

Tractenberg, M. C., and K. Blum: "Alcohol and Opioid Peptides," *Am. J. Drug Alcohol Abuse*, **13**:365 (1987).

Yahya, M. D., and R. R. Watson: "Immunomodulation by Morphine and Marijuana," *Life Sci.* **41**:2503–2510 (1987).

PART V

The Cardiovascular and Renal and Respiratory Systems

SECTION EDITOR
Joseph R. DiPalma

Congestive Heart Failure: Cardiac Glycosides and Other Inotropes and Vasodilator Therapy

Joseph R. DiPalma

Heart failure is a very common disorder. It may be defined simply as a failure of the heart to pump enough blood to supply the oxygen and nutritive demands of peripheral tissues. Heart failure may present clinically in two major forms: (1) forward failure, which is acute and represents a dramatic decrease in cardiac output and is manifest by the symptoms of circulatory failure, i. e., low blood pressure, fast pulse, cold clammy skin, and collapsed veins, and (2) congestive heart failure, which presents clinically as either with severe dyspnea (left-sided heart failure) or peripheral edema (right-sided heart failure). More often the two are combined and really represent a form of chronic failure of the heart as a pump that has been compensated for by a number of adjusting mechanisms. Consequently the output of the heart is not severely compromised. Indeed, it may be high as in high output failure, and shock does not result, but the individual is embarrassed by a number of distressing symptoms and the ability to do useful work is compromised. The treatment of this syndrome, commonly called *congestive heart failure (CHF)*, is the focus of this chapter.

CAUSES OF CONGESTIVE FAILURE

There are numerous disorders which can precipitate CHF, and these are shown in Table 26-1. By far the most common cause is ischemia of cardiac muscle caused by atherosclerotic disease of the coronaries. Other causes are less common. CHF secondary to other causes is best treated by alleviating the cause.

Beriberi heart failure is cured by thiamine and thyrotoxicosis by antithyroid drugs and surgery. Valvular disease is cured by surgery, and even ischemic heart disease is amenable to bypass coronary repair. The emphasis in this chapter is on those cases not amenable to therapy for the primary disease which need to have therapy for the CHF. Three groups of drugs have great utility in CHF. These are the diuretics (Chap. 30); the inotropic agents comprising mainly digitalis glycosides, sympathomimetic agents (Chap. 7), nonsympathomimetics, amrinone, and related compounds; and vasodilators such as nitrates, nitroprusside, angiotensin converting enzyme (ACE) inhibitors, and calcium-channel blockers (Chaps. 28 and 31).

To understand drug therapy for CHF, it is necessary to appreciate the mechanisms by which the body attempts to compensate for the heart with an inadequate output.

MECHANISMS OF COMPENSATION

As the heart fails to pump enough blood to answer the demands of peripheral tissues, certain neuronal and endocrine reflexes become activated. These are

1. *Neuronal* The afferent arcs are baroreceptors from the atrium and mediastinum, the great vessels in the mediastinum, and the carotid sinus. These terminate in the vasomotor center in the brain. Reinforcement of the afferent arc occurs from somatic sensations from skin and muscle and from the cortex as the individual experiences apprehension over

TABLE 26-1   Some common causes of congestive heart failure

Coronary artery disease (ischemia)

Metabolic muscle disease
  Lipodystrophy
  Amyloidosis
  Hemachromatosis
  Sarcoidosis
  Thyrotoxicosis
  Vitamin deficiency (beriberi)

Infectious
  Viral cardiomyopathy
  Subacute bacterial endocarditis

Elevated afterload
  Hypertension
  Aortic stenosis
  Hypertrophic cardiomyopathy

Elevated preload (increased venous pressure)
  Aortic insufficiency
  Mitral insufficiency
  Tricuspid insufficiency
  Congenital left to right
  AV fistula

his or her condition. The efferent arc is the sympathetic nervous system expressed as increased release of norepinephrine and other catecholamines. The result is an increase in heart rate and a moderate rise in blood pressure, but more significant is a redistribution of blood flow to the most vital organs. The brain and the heart do not vasoconstrict under sympathomimetic stimulation. The kidney does; consequently its ability to excrete and control water balance is compromised. Sodium and water are retained.

2. *Neuroendocrine*   The main reaction is stimulation of the renin-angiotensin aldosterone system. As a result of anoxemia, the kidneys secrete more renin, which is converted to angiotensin (see Chap. 31). Angiotensin is a powerful vasoconstrictor. Meanwhile more aldosterone is secreted by the adrenal cortex. The progression of these events is manifest

by a rise in blood pressure, redistribution of blood flow, and retention of sodium and water. Another seldom mentioned endocrine reflex is the stimulation of erythropoiesis. Anoxemia of the kidney leads to the increased production of erythropoietin (a peptide rather close in structure to angiotensin), which stimulates red blood cell production. The patient with chronic heart failure may have an increased blood volume not only because of fluid retention but also on account of an increased red blood cell volume.

3. *Autoregulatory*   The heart, particularly in the ventricles, is very rich in neuronal structures capable of secreting catecholamines. Thanks to this, there are apparently local reflexes, perhaps due to anoxemia, which cause self-stimulation of the heart—the so-called catecholamine heart drive. This self-stimulatory effect works well in the normal heart but is less effective in the heart with CHF, and, indeed, it is thought to wear out in the later stages.

An even more intriguing self-regulatory mechanism has been discovered recently. This concerns atrial natriuretic factor (ANF), or atriopeptin. As the name suggests, this is a peptide produced by the atrium, which has natriuretic and vasodilatory properties. The normal level of ANF is 10 to 70 ng/mL. It rises in response to volume expansion and atrial tachycardia, both factors in increasing atrial pressure. ANF acting on the kidneys causes natriuresis and diuresis. Furthermore, it suppresses vasopressin release and aldosterone secretion and has a direct action in the relaxation of blood vessels. Apparently ANF is the major hormone whose function is to modulate the compensatory mechanisms which lead to CHF.

4. *Mechanical factors*   The Frank-Starling law is often used to explain some of the features of CHF. It states that an increase in the length of ventricular muscle fibers is related to an increase in work output. In other words, an increase in filling pressures (increased atrial pressure) will cause an increase in cardiac output. This law works nicely in the isolated heart and the heart-lung preparation. In the intact human heart changes in heart rate, inotropy, and peripheral resistance complicate the picture. Nevertheless, the law is useful particularly in its extreme extent for there is a point beyond which increased filling pressure and overdistention of the

ventricular muscle result in decreased rather than increased cardiac output.

The increased filling pressure (increased preload) brought about by the mechanisms described above has more important consequences than the Frank-Starling law. The ventricles dilate, the diastolic size is larger; the heart does not empty itself as completely of blood (ejection fraction reduced), the ventricular wall is thinner, contraction is more isotonic than isometric, the velocity of ejection is reduced (*dv/dp* reduced), and, most important, at the price of an increased cardiac output, the efficiency of the heart as a pump is reduced. The heart in CHF uses more oxygen per unit of work than the normal heart. Moreover, because of the consequences of anoxemia, the heart depends on a less efficient carbohydrate rather than fat metabolism to produce the energy for muscle contraction.

In summary, the pathophysiology of CHF consists of a precipitating cause which results in a decrease in contractile capacity of the heart. This is followed by a complex series of compensatory measures, which include fluid volume, heart rate, blood pressure, and redistribution of blood flow to vital organs. Eventually the heart dilates and hypertrophies. In the beginning the compensatory measures allow the heart to function marginally, but gradually the compensatory measures become excessive and fluid collects in the lungs and periphery. Increases in heart rate and peripheral resistance can no longer cope with an inadequate pumping action.

The therapy of CHF, therefore, consists of correction and modulation of the compensatory responses of the body which have become excessive and self-destructive. By far the most important measure is the reduction of fluid volume by the induction of diuresis. The various diuretics are described in Chap. 30 and are not further discussed here. The aim is to approach the dry weight of the individual but not to cause hyponatremia. This measure reduces preload by diminishing venous filling pressure.

The second most important measure is to improve the pumping action of the heart. The ideal heart rate is about 60 beats per minute. If there is any arrhythmia such as atrial fibrillation or flutter with a rapid ventricular response, this may be corrected by agents which produce block at the AV node. Similarly bradycardia (less than 40 beats per minute) should be treated with chronotropic drugs or a pacemaker. Inotropic drugs

such as the digitalis glycosides, which do not exhaust the energy production of the heart, are ideal. In some instances inotropic drugs such as amrinone may be preferable.

Finally an attempt is made to adjust the peripheral circulation so that "preload" and "afterload" of the heart is at an ideal level. Preload refers to atrial filling pressure, which is determined by blood volume and venous tone. Afterload refers to the peripheral resistance. Obviously the ventricle performs less work when pumping a given volume of blood at a blood pressure of 120/70 than 150/90 mmHg. Preload and afterload are decreased by agents which decrease venous tone and arteriolar tone, respectively. Such therapy is collectively called, *vasodilation therapy* and is usually applied in the later stages of therapy but may be used initially in selected cases.

CARDIAC GLYCOSIDES

The drugs known collectively as *digitalis glycosides* exert a unique and valuable action on heart muscle. This action derives from active principles found in *Digitalis lanata* and *D. purpurea*, as well as from various other plant and animal sources.

Chemistry

These compounds are glycosides (sugar derivatives of alcohols). Their sugar components may be mono-, di-, tri-, or tetrasaccharides built from characteristic sugars, whereas the aglycones or genins (the nonsugar part of the glycosides) are steroids with certain typical structural features. The simplest cardiac genin is digitoxigenin, the aglycone of one of the principal gly-

Digitoxigenin

cosides of *D. lanata* (lanatoside A) as well as of *D. purpurea* (purpurea glycoside A). The sugar component, attached to the C-3 hydroxyl of the steroid structure, is in both cases a tetrasaccharide composed of one molecule of glucose and three molecules of *d*-digitoxose.

$$
\begin{array}{c}
CHO \\
| \\
CH_2 \\
| \\
HCOH \\
| \\
HCOH \\
| \\
HCOH \\
| \\
CH_3
\end{array}
$$

Digitoxose

Lanatoside A carries an acetyl group attached to one of the digitoxose units. This is the sole difference between lanatoside A and purpurea glycoside A. Schematically, therefore, the structure of lanatoside A is

O—C-3 of the steroid structure
|
digitoxose—digitoxose—digitoxose—glucose
|
acetyl

The structure of two further glycosides of *D. lanata*, lanatoside B and lanatoside C, is the same, except that lanatoside B also has a hydroxyl group attached to C-16 of its genin (gitoxigenin), whereas in the genin of lanatoside C (digoxigenin) the extra hydroxyl is attached to C-12. *D. purpurea* also contains a glycoside B, which differs from lanatoside B in the same way that purpurea glycoside A differs from lanatoside A, i. e., by the absence of an acetyl group from the sugar component of purpurea glycoside B. There is no glycoside in *D. purpurea* corresponding to lanatoside C,

i. e., with a hydroxyl group at C-12. Figure 26-1 illustrates the relationships among the glycosides derived from *D. lanata* and *D. purpurea*. The main function of the sugars appears to be to solubilize the genins.

Both species of *Digitalis* contain hydrolyzing enzymes which easily split off the acetyl group and the glucose. What is ordinarily extracted from both species of *Digitalis* are the partially hydrolyzed glycosides, digitoxin and gitoxin. Digoxin is obtained only from *D. lanata*.

All digitalis genins are steroids which have an unsaturated lactone ring attached to C-17 in beta orientation, a hydroxyl group at C-14, and, most interesting, a cis junction of rings C and D—features unique to digitalis compounds.

Today from a realistic point of view digoxin is the only glycoside widely used in the United States. Digitoxin and deslanoside (deacetyl lanatoside C) are only occasionally employed. By common usage the name *digitalis* generically relates to all glycosides.

Mechanism of Action: Inotropic Effect

Digitalis appears to affect the flux of calcium across the sarcolemmal membrane of the myocardial cell (Fig. 26-2). In the generation of myocardial contraction, the action potential at the surface membrane and at its related invaginations, the transverse, or T tubules, causes release of free calcium from the lateral cisternae into the cytoplasm. Recently, however, it has been suggested that the major source of contractile-dependent calcium is derived from the cell surface membrane rather than the lateral cisternae of the sar-

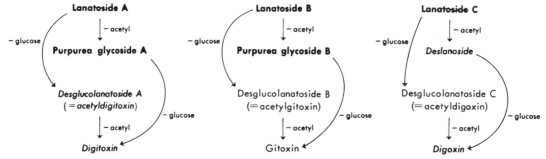

FIGURE 26-1 Schema showing structural relationships among some cardiac glycosides derived from *Digitalis lanata* and *D. purpurea* and their hydrolysis products. (Native glycosides are shown in heavy print; those medicinally used in italics.)

cotubular sacs. Whatever may prove eventually to be the major source of calcium which enters the cytoplasm, it is this free calcium that attaches to troponin on the actin filaments, and this action removes the barrier to actin-myosin interaction. (Normally, the troponin-tropomyosin complex inhibits actin-myosin interaction during diastole.) These events, in turn, initiate contraction, activating myosin ATPase (E_1 in Fig. 26-2) to provide energy from ATP (adenosine triphosphate). Following repolarization, reaccumulation of calcium by the sarcoplasmic reticulum or the cell surface sufficiently lowers the level of free cytoplasmic calcium to permit relaxation.

There is some evidence to suggest that cardiac glycosides, as well as numerous other positive or negative inotropic agents, act by altering calcium ion movement. Whereas some drugs, such as epinephrine, appear to affect calcium stores by stimulating the adenylate cyclase-cyclic AMP system (cyclic AMP increases tubular stores of calcium), it has been suggested that digitalis works through a separate mechanism to inhibit Na^+, K^+-sensitive ATPase (E_2) in the transverse tubular system and on the sarcolemma. Normally, following repolarization, Na^+, K^+-sensitive ATPase restores sodium ions to the outside and potassium ions to the inside of the cell. A secondary sodium-calcium exchange mechanism also functions to remove intracellular sodium. When digitalis inhibits Na^+, K^+-sensitive ATPase, the sodium-calcium exchange predominates, and the influx of calcium ions into the cardiac cells increases. Therefore, more calcium is available to the myofibrils and a positive inotropic effect is manifest during systole.

The electrical toxic effects of the digitalis glycosides on cardiac tissue may be due to their action on sarcolemmal membrane ATPase (E_2). Sarcolemmal membrane effects of digitalis are commonly interpreted as being due to a remarkably potent inhibition of Na^+- and K^+-activated ATPase, which normally provides energy for the extrusion process by which sodium is removed from the cell, and is followed by a reciprocal inflow of potassium. This inhibitory effect results in a loss of intracellular potassium ions and may produce dysrhythmias. Quite possibly, the positive effect of digitalis on contractility may in time be found to be due to a combination of actions on both the sarcotubular sacs and the surface membrane.

Exquisite proof that the action of digitalis is associated with a transient calcium increase has been ob-

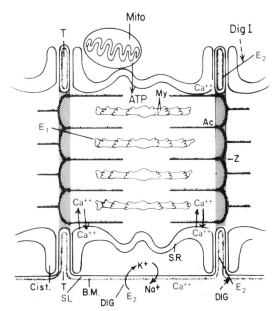

FIGURE 26-2 Schematic representation of proposed sites of action of digitalis in a cardiac muscle cell. SL = sarcolemma; B.M. = basement membrane; S.R. = sarcoplasmic reticulum or longitudinal tubular system; T = transverse tubular system (T tubules); My = myosin filaments; Ac = actin filaments; Z = Z line; Cist = terminal sisternae of S.R.; Mito = mitochondrion; E_1 = myosin ATPase; E_2 = sarcolemmal ATPase and T-tubular ATPase; DIG = proposed site of action of digitalis for inotropic effect and sites for toxic arrhythmic effects.

tained by using *aequorin*, a photoprotein which undergoes luminescence on exposure to calcium. Using direct recordings from a canine Purkinje fiber, a close coupling can be demonstrated between depolarization, free calcium level and contraction. Digoxin causes increase in calcium and increased muscle tension. At toxic levels of digoxin there is an abnormal calcium increase during diastole accompanied by a depolarization and muscle contraction.

In summary, it appears certain that digitalis has two distinct effects on the heart: (1) an effect on contractility mediated through intracellular changes in calcium stores and (2) an effect on the electrical behavior of cellular membranes mediated through changes in transport of sodium, potassium, and calcium evolving indirectly from the known inhibitory effects of digitalis on cell membrane ATPase.

Interactions between digitalis and ionic calcium and potassium at a membrane level have important clinical and toxicologic implications. There is a synergistic action between calcium ions and digitalis. Sudden increases in serum calcium may result in arrhythmias in the digitalized patient. On the other hand, digitalis and potassium ions are antagonistic. Hypokalemic patients have a decreased tolerance to digitalis. In patients with digitalis toxicity, raising the serum levels of potassium tends to alleviate the toxic effects.

In occasional cases magnesium seems to play an interactive role with digitalis which is similar to that of potassium. It must be recalled that vigorous diuresis results in depletion of magnesium as well as potassium.

Electrophysiologic Effects

The digitalis changes are best described by an analysis of the monophasic action potential of a Purkinje fiber (Fig. 26-3) (for a complete description of this recording, see Chap. 27). Moreover, comparison of the monophasic potential with the ECG allows a further analysis.

The intrinsic deflection of the R wave of an ECG coincides in time with phase 0, the S-T segment with phase 2, and the T wave with phase 3. In contrast to

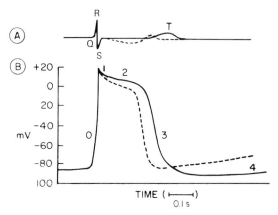

FIGURE 26-3 Representation of (*a*) electrocardiogram and (*b*) ventricular intracellular action potential before (solid line) and after (broken line) digitalis administration. Note depression of S-T segment of the ECG related to a more rapid decline of phase 2. In addition, the Q-T duration is shortened correlating with a shorter action potential duration.

this ventricular record, the transmembrane potential recorded from a pacemaker fiber (i. e., SA node, AV node, or His-Purkinje fibers) does not remain constant after repolarization but exhibits slow diastolic depolarization during phase 4. If this slow depolarization carries the membrane potential to the threshold potential, firing occurs. Many fibers develop this phase, but the one that first attains the threshold potential usually acts as the dominant pacemaker, and the others, with slower depolarization during phase 4, are latent pacemakers. Digitalis affects this slow diastolic depolarization of Purkinje fibers by increasing the rate of diastolic depolarization, i. e., it increases the slope of phase 4 and therefore ultimately enhances automaticity with resultant ventricular ectopic beats and ventricular tachycardia.

In the atrioventricular (AV) node the cardiac glycosides slow phase 0 (depolarization), thereby diminishing conduction velocity and possibly leading to various degrees of heart block. On the surface ECG this effect is manifest as a lengthening of the P-R interval. A direct effect of digitalis on repolarization of cardiac tissue is an alteration of phases 1, 2, and 3, resulting in a shortening of the duration of the intracellular action potential and a subsequent decrease in refractoriness. In the ECG this is seen as a shortening of the Q-T interval. Furthermore, the quickening of phases 1 and 2 of repolarization is reflected as an S-T segment depression of the ECG, sometimes referred to as the *boot heel depression*.

Effects on Organ Systems

Cardiac Effects At therapeutic dose levels, digitalis acts primarily by increasing the force of myocardial contraction. In the failing heart, this results in an increase in cardiac output and, usually, a decrease in heart size because of an increase in the ejection fraction. In the AV node and bundle of His, the refractory period is lengthened and conduction is slowed by heightened vagal activity and possibly by reduced adrenergic activity, as well as by direct effects. This increased refractoriness is particularly beneficial in atrial fibrillation, since the number and irregularity of ventricular contractions are reduced.

Digitalis directly increases contractility of the myocardium in both the failing heart and the normal heart. In the failing, dilated heart, digitalis has been shown to double the stroke volume or cardiac output. The heightened contractility causes more complete ejection with less residual systolic volume. In this manner, the glycosides correct the depressed contractility which is responsible for ventricular failure. It must be recalled that when digitalis is used alone, its most dramatic manifestation is diuresis. This diuresis is believed to be due to improved renal circulation, although when digoxin is injected directly into the renal artery it causes diuresis. At therapeutic doses administered systemically the direct diuretic effect is considered to be minimal.

The cardiac output in normal subjects who are given digitalis generally remains unchanged, although occasionally it decreases. Obviously normal subjects have a normal blood volume, and no diuresis occurs. Besides exerting a positive inotropic action on the normal (nonfailing) heart, the cardiac glycosides also produce a direct contraction of peripheral arterial and venous smooth muscle. This increased peripheral resistance, along with increased contractility, generally results in unchanged cardiac output. However, in congestive heart failure, there is already increased peripheral resistance, a compensatory mechanism. In the patient with CHF this results in an increased redistribution of blood flow, which favors the kidney and promotes diuresis. It is this rather than the increased contractility which causes a decrease in the diastolic size of the heart. These latter changes are not attributed to digitalis today because diuretics are administered first or simultaneously with digitalis.

The improved cardiac efficiency which occurs with digitalis suggests a relationship to some direct effect on energy production. However, extensive studies have demonstrated no direct action of this sort. Even the feature of increased energy utilization has been questioned, since oxygen consumption, which is considered an ultimate measure of this variable, reportedly does not change in proportion to cardiac work. This implies an increase in efficiency which could be attributed to some obscurely understood chemical phenomenon but is more acceptable if interpreted on the basis of the important mechanical advantage which comes from the decrease in heart size during diastole, typically caused by digitalis action.

Vagal Effects Vagal effects occur at early stages or with minimal therapeutic dose levels and increase with higher dose levels. Pacemaker activity is slowed at the SA and AV nodes, conduction rate is decreased, and refractory intervals of the conduction tissue are increased. Vagal effects decrease contractility in the atria but have no pronounced effects on the ventricles, and apparently the direct positive inotropic effects of digitalis overshadow these negative inotropic effects. The heightened vagal activity has been attributed to action on afferent nerves in the nodose ganglion and the parotid sinus, as well as to effects at peripheral sites and central vagal nuclei.

Early effects on conduction and refractoriness at the AV node and the bundle of His are now generally thought to be mediated almost entirely through the vagal action, except for a component of action which is antiadrenergic and which can be relatively more important under conditions of heightened sympathetic nervous system activity, as in heart failure.

Digitalis-induced vagal influences on automaticity are complicated by the marked difference in responsiveness of pacemaker or automatic cells, on the one hand, and muscle fibers of the atria and ventricles, on the other, which do not generate spontaneous action potentials. The pacemaker cells of the SA node (and possibly other specialized atrial cells) respond to vagal simulation by a decrease in the ascending slope of the diastolic phase (phase 4) and an increase in transmembrane negativity. These effects, acting to maintain the subthreshold state, result in a pronounced reduction in heart rate, and with more intense vagal stimulation, there may be arrest of automatic activity of these cells. Under these conditions, pacemaker activity of the bundle of His and the Purkinje system may assume dominance, since automaticity in these conduction systems is not as responsive to vagal activity. This type of "vagal escape" is enhanced by adrenergic influences and by decreased levels of intracellular potassium. Release from the control of higher pacemakers and increased automaticity correspond to the later stages of digitalis arrhythmias such as induced nodal rhythms, ventricular ectopic beats, and ventricular tachycardia.

The activity at the SA node has been demonstrated by injecting cardiac glycosides into its localized blood supply; the results are predominantly bradycardia but with some occurrence of tachycardia, the latter attributed to some local release of catecholamines. Effects appear to be peripheral to strict vagal control and may be related to intracellular potassium levels.

Peripheral Vascular Effects Rapid intravenous injection of cardiac glycosides in normal human subjects leads to increased arterial pressure and increased peripheral resistance, usually of moderate degree. When administered more slowly, as by oral ingestion, digitalis does not have important effects on arterial pressure, although venous constriction may be observed. In patients with heart failure the existing sympathetic influences are more pronounced and the relief of failure may act to reduce the sympathetic effects. This may be because the improved renal blood flow may reduce the renal production of renin and hence angiotensin, a potent vasoconstrictor.

Effects on Other Organs The frequent gastrointestinal effects of digitalis (nausea, vomiting) are attributable to direct effects as well as chemoreceptor trigger-zone stimulation. With the use of pure glycosides, as compared with that of crude preparations, these effects are minimal.

In the elderly, disorientation and hallucinations may occur. It is difficult to ascribe these changes to digitalis or to the rapid diuresis and sometimes dehydration. Yellow vision is a fairly frequent phenomenon which may not be noticed by some patients.

Gynecomastia and galactorrhea are rarely reported. These may be the result of a direct effect (recall steroid structure of digitalis) or more likely hypothalamic stimulation.

Pharmacokinetics

Digoxin and digitoxin are effective both orally and parenterally. Table 26-2 indicates some of the pharmacokinetic parameters determined on each drug. For digoxin the kidney is the chief route of elimination. The drug is excreted unchanged mainly by glomerular filtration, and some of it is eliminated by tubular secretion. Seriously depressed kidney function can result in accumulation of the drug. This is considered a major factor contributing to its toxicity. The time course of elimination is slower in elderly patients and individuals with decreased kidney function.

Digitoxin is biotransformed in the liver by the drug-metabolizing microsomal system, predominantly to inactive products; a small portion (8 percent) of digitoxin is hydroxylated to digoxin. Most biotransformed products are excreted in the urine, while approximately 25 percent of them appear in feces. Digitoxin exhibits a higher degree of protein binding, a longer half-life, and better oral absorption than digoxin (Table 26-2).

Following oral administration of digoxin or digitoxin, it is possible to determine serum concentrations of these drugs in the nanogram-per-milliliter (ng/mL) range by radioimmunoassay. Typical average plasma levels for digoxin and digitoxin are given in Table 26-2. Note the much larger serum half-life of digitoxin as compared to digoxin, which may be due to the more avid binding of digitoxin to plasma proteins (95 percent versus 25 percent).

Therapeutic Uses

Congestive Heart Failure The main indication for digitalis is CHF whatever the cause or mechanism. Though not so effective in high-output failure of the type seen in cor pulmonale and thyrotoxicosis, it may be used here together with other measures. The response to digitalis is less in conditions associated with mechanical obstruction or insufficiency, such as in valvular lesions or constrictive pericarditis, although a sufficient improvement warrants its use. In heart failure associated with acute rheumatic fever or myocarditis, digitalis should be used concomitantly with other drugs. Thus clinical improvement may be expected in congestive failure regardless of cause, level of cardiac output, or type of cardiac rhythm.

TABLE 26-2 Pharmacokinetic characteristics

Drug	Oral absorption, %	Protein binding, %	V_d, L/kg	Serum half-life $(t_{1/2})$	Therapeutic plasma concentration, ng/mL	Cardiac tissue concentration, ng/g
Digoxin	65–80	25	6–10	33–51 h	0.8–2	56–160
Digitoxin	90–100	96	0.5	4–6 days	15–25	105–175

Left-sided heart failure may develop quite precipitously as acute pulmonary edema with widely distributed rales and frothy sputum. In these cases, digitalis glycosides are given intravenously.

A practical view of the treatment of congestive heart failure is that diuretics provide the best management of congestive heart failure and edema and that digitalis is an auxiliary measure to be used only in certain cases, especially the arrhythmias.

Diuretics administered to a digitalized but still edematous patient often bring on copious diuresis but coincidentally bring on the typical arrhythmias of digitalis overdose. An acceptable explanation for this phenomenon is that the diuresis lowers intracellular potassium levels, which in turn increases sensitivity to digitalis-induced arrhythmias. For this reason some clinicians are wary of giving digitalis first or even simultaneously with the initial period of diuresis. The diuretics are so effective in relieving CHF that digitalis is considered unnecessary in the early stages of therapy. Once stabilized with respect to fluid and electrolyte balance, the patient is given digitalis for what added benefit it may contribute in improvement of exercise tolerance.

Arrhythmias

Atrial Fibrillation and Atrial Flutter In atrial fibrillation, digitalis reduces the ventricular rate by increasing the refractory period of the conduction tissue. The rapid, irregular atrial impulses showered on the AV node are extinguished in greater numbers as the refractory interval is increased by digitalis. The refractory interval of the atria, on the other hand, may be shortened; this favors perpetuation of atrial fibrillation and increased atrial rate. Similarly, atrial flutter may be altered to reach the state of atrial fibrillation. The vagal effect of digitalis is responsible for the early shortened refractory period of the atrium. General improvement in myocardial function, measured as increased contractile force, may have the later effect of converting the arrhythmias into normal sinus rhythm.

This has been a most satisfactory action of digitalis and effectively cures CHF that is due to this cause. With the advent of the calcium-channel blockers, namely, verapamil and diltiazem, the block between atrium and ventricle can be produced just as effectively and with less toxicity than with digitalis. Today for this purpose many clinicians will use calcium-

channels blockers alone or in combination with digitalis.

Similarly digitalis was often used to control paroxysmal atrial tachycardia (not caused by digitalis). Again the calcium-channel blockers have gained ascendancy for this purpose.

Myocardial Infarction with Failure Digitalis is one of the inotropic agents considered in myocardial infarction associated with heart failure, and here it has an advantage over adrenergic agents in that its effects are better sustained and are associated with less of an imposed load due to pressor effects.

Adverse Reactions

The prime danger with digitalis is the dose-related progressively severe arrhythmias terminating in ventricular fibrillation. The common predisposing influence is a decrease in intracellular potassium which may develop following the use of potassium-excreting diuretics or any condition causing vomiting or diarrhea. Other predisposing situations occur in the elderly with decreased kidney function and correspondingly decreased renal excretion of the drug; in premature infants deficient in the usual excretory and metabolic processes; in conditions such as hypothyroidism, with decreased biotransformation; in any condition of decreased kidney function; and during variabilities in absorption from the alimentary tract. Additionally, hyperthyroidism is associated with a faster rate of elimination of digitalis and hypothyroidism with a slower rate, as compared with the euthyroid state.

Digitalis toxicity is common and is increasing in incidence. Some estimates indicate that 10 percent of hospitalized patients receive digitalis and that 20 percent of these develop toxicity. Cardiac effects may include the various stages of AV block, premature systoles and tachycardia (especially when ventricular in origin), paroxysmal atrial tachycardia with AV block, AV dissociation with nonparoxysmal nodal tachycardia, and ventricular fibrillation. The most common arrhythmia produced in digitalis poisoning is paroxysmal tachycardia with AV block. A representative summary of the incidence of the signs and symptoms of digitalis poisoning is given in Table 26-3.

As a result of all the toxicities of digitalis, there has been more conservative use. Reliance on other agents

TABLE 26-3 Symptoms and signs in 44 cases of digitalis poisoning

Symptom or sign	No. of cases
Anorexia	21
Nausea	18
Vomiting	16
Diarrhea	5
Weakness and fatigue	4
Yellow vision	6
Scotoma	3
No symptoms but ECG irregularities	17
Paroxysmal tachycardia with AV block	20
S-T and T-wave depression	15
Premature contractions, irregular	6
Bigeminy	12
Trigeminy	1
Extreme bradycardia	2
AV block	7
SA block	1
Nodal rhythm	2
Atrial fibrillation, developing during observation	10
Atrial flutter, developing during observation	1
Death, presumably due to ventricular fibrillation	2

such as vasodilators, newer inotropic agents, calcium-channel blockers, and angiotensin converting enzyme inhibitors is increasing the scope of therapy of CHF.

Drug Interactions

Adverse interactions between digitalis glycosides and other drugs have been reported. Simultaneous administration of digoxin and oral antacids or kaolin-pectin products decreases the pharmacologic effect of digoxin by interfering with its absorption from the gastrointestinal tract. It has been known for some time that diuretics which produce hypokalemia may augment digitalis toxicities. Recently, spironolactone has been implicated in increasing the effect of digoxin. The probable mechanism of this interaction is a reduction in renal digoxin excretion caused by spironolactone. Also quinidine has been implicated in increasing serum digoxin concentration. The exact mechanism of this interaction is unknown, although it has been suggested that quinidine displaces digoxin from tissue-binding sites. The cardiac effects of digitoxin may be decreased by barbiturates or rifampin, both of which induce the microsomal enzymes. Cholestyramine, which can bind digitoxin and digoxin in the intestine, may reduce their effectiveness. In addition, when sympathomimetic amines are administered in the presence of digitalis compounds, there may be an increased predisposition to cardiac arrhythmias.

Contraindications

Digitalis may be harmful in subaortic hypertrophic stenosis in which hypertrophied ventricular myocardium obstructs the left ventricular outflow tract. Increasing the force of contraction of the outflow tract intensifies the resistance to ventricular ejection. Also, the drug is contraindicated in patients allergic to digitalis.

Treatment of Digitalis Toxicity

The use of potassium salts for treating digitalis-induced arrhythmias is based on considerable clinical experience. Potassium chloride may be administered orally or by intravenous infusion. Obviously, the antidotal regimen is pointless without discontinuing all forms of digitalis or diuretics, such as thiazides or furosemide, which remove potassium.

There is broad agreement that increased extracellular potassium decreases automaticity and suppresses the ectopic beats induced by digitalis by forcing potassium into the cell. Conversely, lowered potassium levels are associated with the appearance of arrhythmias in the presence of even small doses of cardiac glycosides, and this may occur with potassium-excreting diuretics or hemodialysis. Depressed conduction due to digitalis is further depressed by increasing potassium levels or, again, by rapidly rising potassium levels. Abnormally low potassium levels also may act to depress conduction.

Antiarrhythmic drugs, such as lidocaine or phenytoin, can be used to correct disturbances in cardiac rhythm caused by digitalis. If lidocaine or phenytoin is ineffective, propranolol and procainamide are used, but with caution, since these drugs may aggravate AV block produced by digitalis.

Direct-current shock may be indicated and used in certain arrhythmias such as ventricular tachycardia and fibrillation secondary to the cardiac glycosides. However, if cardioversion must be employed, an initial small energy of countershock should be used and the patient should be pretreated with lidocaine or phenytoin. Also electrical conversion of arrhythmias may require that digitalis be eliminated before the countershock is applied.

In accidental overdoses or suicidal attempts the above measures are usually unsuccessful. Such extreme toxicity is best treated with newly developed antibodies. These consist of immune Fab fragments of digoxin. The immune Fab fragments have a very high affinity for the glycoside binding it, thus reducing the concentration available to the heart. The Fab-digitalis combination is readily excreted in the urine.

Preparations

Digoxin (Lanoxin) is a crystalline glycoside isolated from the leaves of *D. lanata*, available as tablets of 0.125, 0.25, and 0.5 mg and as ampuls of 0.5 mg in 2 mL and 0.1 mg/mL.

Digoxin elixir contains 0.05 mg/mL.

Digitoxin (Crystodigin) is a crystalline glycoside from *D. purpurea* or *D. lanata* and is available in tablets of 0.05, 0.1, 0.15, and 0.2 mg and ampuls of 0.2 mg/mL.

Deslanoside (Cedilanid-D, desacetyl lanatoside C) is available in ampuls of 0.4 mg in 2 mL.

The most significant difference which could exist among the various digitalis preparations would be a difference between the ratio of doses producing therapeutic effects and those producing toxic effects. In cases of progressively deteriorating cardiac function, particularly in the aged, doses of digitalis preparations must be progressively increased into the toxic range. Any superior therapeutic index of any one of these preparations would mark it the drug of choice under these conditions. The bulk of evidence, however, demonstrates that the cardiac glycosides do not exhibit any significant difference in this vital ratio of safety.

The trial-and-error method must be used, and dosage should be individualized and largely empirical. Extensive clinical experience has produced some average dosages that can be used as rough guidelines (Table 26-4).

OTHER INOTROPIC AGENTS

There is no doubt that digitalis is the most satisfactory cardiac inotropic agent. However, there is a subset of patients who have a slow sinus rhythmn for whom digitalis seems to add no benefit and only toxicity. In all patients afflicted with CHF eventually there comes a time when digitalis and diuretics no longer are able to restore compensation. There is, therefore, a desire to find an inotropic agent which can rescue the heart in intractable heart failure.

In the past 20 years many agents have been tested. They fall into two categories: (1) sympathomimetic derivatives and (2) nonglycoside nonsympathomimetics. In Table 26-5 listed is a selection of agents, some old, some new. A natural inclination is to try sympathomimetic agents. A wide selection is available, which permits particular action on alpha, beta, and dopamine receptors. The alpha agonists cause mainly vasoconstriction, along with some cardiac inotropic action (because of latent beta activity of higher doses). The beta agonists stimulate the heart increasing output, but they also increase heart rate, which is disadvantageous. They do not cause vasoconstriction but do dilate some vascular beds, thus causing redistribution of blood flow. Levodopa, of course, is converted to dopamine in the body and is thus a convenient oral form of dopamine in the form of a prodrug. All these sympathomimetic agents have a usefulness in short-term (24 h or less) support of the heart. The de-

TABLE 26-4 Commonly used digitalis preparations

Preparation	Digitalizing-dose range		Daily maintenance dosage, oral
	Oral	IV	
Digitalis	1.2–2.0 g		0.1–0.2 g
Digitoxin	1.0–1.6 mg	1.0–1.6 mg	0.05–0.3 mg
Digoxin	0.75–1.5 mg	0.5–1.5 mg	0.125–0.5 mg
Deslanoside		1.0–1.6 mg	

TABLE 26-5　Cardiac inotropic agents

Class	Agent	Principal mechanism of action
Sympathomimetics	Norepinephrine Epinephrine	Alpha and beta agonists
	Isoproterenol Terbutaline Albuterol Pirbuterol	Beta$_2$-selective agonists
	Dopamine Dobutamine Prenalterol	Beta$_1$-selective agonists
	Propylbutyl- dopamine	Alpha agonist
	Levodopa	Dopamine receptor agonist
Nonsympathomimetic	Cyclic nucleotides Dibutyl-cAMP	Increases cardiac contractibility Peripheral vasodilation
	Theophylline Amrinone Milrinone	Inhibit phosphodiesterase

velopment of tolerance or unacceptable side effects such as arrhythmias further limits the usefulness of these agents. (See Chap. 7 for more detail about these agents.) The nonsympathomimetic agents all appear to function by augmenting or stimulating the action of cyclic AMP. The cyclic nucleotides substitute directly for cyclic AMP, and the rest augment it by inhibiting phosphodiesterase. Theophylline in the form of aminophyllin was extensively studied some 20 years ago as a cardiac inotropic agent but was found unsatisfactory for long-term use and expecially as an oral drug. Other methylxanthines have been synthesized but none has made the grade as a useful cardiac inotrope. On the other hand some related bipyridines have been successful.

Amrinone

This bipyridine has become the accepted inotropic agent to use in advanced CHF for short-term application when there has been an inadequate response to diuretics, digitalis, and vasodilators (Table 26-5). Its chemical structural formula along with that of milrinone is

Amrinone　　　　　Milrinone

Amrinone is unique because it also causes vasodilation by smooth-muscle relaxation and thus reduces both preload and afterload. Meanwhile, unlike theophylline, it does not easily produce arrhythmias or signs of myocardial ischemia.

The mechanism of action is not understood. It does inhibit phosphodiesterase (like theophylline), increasing cellular levels of cyclic AMP. Bipyridines also increase calcium flux favoring inward flow, and this effect is not caused by inhibition of Na^+, K^+-ATPase.

Oral absorption is good, but it is used only intravenously because unacceptable toxicity results by this route. These include dose-dependent reversible thrombocytopenia, liver dysfunction, fever, and gastrointestinal disturbances. In CHF patients after an IV loading dose, satisfactory plasma levels are maintained by continuous infusion. Amrinone is inactivated by conjugation and mainly excreted in the urine, although some is eliminated in the feces. The toxicity by the intravenous route is much less than that of the oral route but it is still wise to do platelet counts before and during therapy. Obviously, amrinone can be used only in a hospital setting where continuous monitoring is available.

Milrinone has better oral tolerance than amrinone and is actually more potent. It appears to be effective for oral long-term use but has not been approved by the FDA.

VASODILATOR DRUGS

In the past 10 years the vasodilators have established themselves as primary agents in the therapy of CHF. As shown in Table 26-6, many drugs are available. They may be selected with major effects on venous tone, such as the nitrates, thus reducing preload. Similarly hydralazine and minoxidil act almost entirely on arteriolar tone and thus primarily lessen afterload. Some drugs affect both arteriolar and venous tones and are suited for long-term therapy. These are the antihypertensive drugs prazosin, captopril, and enalapril. The latter are angiotensin converting enyzme inhibitors and are expecially suitable for CHF therapy where presumably the renin-angiotensin-aldersterone system is overactive and benefit is to be obtained by its modulation. The calcium-channel blockers such as nifedipine are also useful.

Tolerance development is a major source of difficulty with nitrates (see Chap. 26). For this reason abstinence from this therapy at night might help to avoid its development. Unfortunately, tolerance also develops in about 50 percent of patients on prazosin. The other drugs in Table 26-6 do not suffer from this problem.

At the present time, the angiotensin converting enyzme inhibitors appear to be the most satisfactory for long-term vasodilator therapy both from the viewpoint of efficacy and toxicity. Even with this therapy which certainly relieves symptoms and improves the quality of life, improvement in long-term survival in patients with heart failure has not been proven.

MANAGEMENT OF CHF

CHF may present as an acute event which is dramatic and life-threatening. Pulmonary edema and consequent anoxemia and dyspnea, along with signs of hypervolemia such as dilated veins, dominate the picture. Required are hospitalization and intravenous

TABLE 26-6 Vasodilators commonly employed in congestive heart failure

Drugs	Dilatation of vascular beds	
	Venous (reduction of preload)	Arteriolar (reduction of afterload)
Nitroglycerin, Isosorbide dinitrate	++++	++
Hydralazine	−	+++
Minoxidil	−	+++
Sodium nitroprusside	+++	+++
Prazosin	+++	++
Captopril	+++	++
Enalapril	+++	++
Nifedipine	+	++

TABLE 26-7   **Major steps in the management of CHF**

Principal	Theraphy
Reduce heart-work	Limit activity, bed rest, etc.
	Control hypertension as required
	Weight reduction
	Sedation (as needed)
Reduce blood volume	Diuretics
	Restrict sodium
	Restrict water (seldom needed)
Improve efficiency of heart	Digitalis
	Correct arrhythmias (verapamil, antiarrhythmics)
Fine-tune control of circulation	Vasodilators
	Nondigitalis inotropes

therapy, along with airway and oxygen support. However, the principles of therapy are the same as in chronic CHF and follow the same stepwise therapeutic modalities. In Table 26-7 these steps are outlined. All these steps may be applied at once or progressively as required. In chronic CHF it is wise to move slowly. For example, overenthusiastic use of diuretics may lead to hyponatremia, which may precipitate circulatory failure and renal shutdown.

BIBLIOGRAPHY

Abrams, J.: "Vasodilator Therapy for Chronic Congestive Heart Failure," *JAMA*, **254**:3070 (1985).

Awan, N. A., et al.: "Long Term Hemodynamic and Clinical Efficacy of Captopril Therapy in Ambulatory Management of Severe Chronic Congestive Heart Failure," *Am. Heart J.*, **103**:474–479 (1982).

Cody, R. J., D. W. Franklin, and J. H. Laragh: "Combined Vasodilator Therapy for Chronic Congestive Heart Failure," *Am. Heart J.*, **105**:575–580 (1983).

Cohn, J. N.: "Marriage of the Heart and the Peripheral Circulation," *Prog. Cardiovac. Dis.*, **24**:189–190 (1981).

Cohn, J. N., et al.: "Effect of Vasodilator Therapy on Mortality in Chronic Congestive Heart Failure: Results of a Veteran Administration Cooperative Study," *N. Eng. J. Med.*, **314**:1547 (1986).

DiPalma, J. R.: "The Digitalis Controversy," *Am. Fam. Physician*, **26**:217–218 (1982).

DiPalma, J. R.: "Vasodilator and Inotropic Therapy for Heart Failure," *Am. Fam. Physician*, **31**:177–180 (1985).

DiPalma, J. R.: "Atrial Natruretic Factor," *Am. Fam. Physician*, **34**:174–176 (1986).

Hamer, J.: "The Modern Mangement of Congestive Heart Failure, in D. S. Rowlands (ed.), *Recent Advances in Cardiology-9*, Churchill-Livingstone, Edinburgh, 1984, pp. 275–288.

Hayward, R.: "Digitalis the Present Position," in J. Hamer (ed.), *Drugs for Heart Disease*, 2d ed., Chapman and Hall, London, 1987, p. 145.

Leien, J., et al.: "Improved Exercise Capacity and Differing Arterial and Venous Tolerance During Chronic Isosorbide Dinitrate Therapy for Congestive Heart Failure," *Circulation*, **67**:817–822 (1983).

LeJentel, T. H., E. Keung, E. H. Sonnenblick: "Amrinone: A New Non-glycosidic, Non-adrenergic Cardiotonic Agent Effective in the Treatment of Intractable Myocardial Failure in Man," *Circulation*, **59**:1098–1104 (1979).

Needleman, P.: "Atriopeptin Biochemical Pharmacology," *Fed. Proc.*, **45**:2096–2100 (1986).

Schocken, D. D. and J. D. Holloway: "Vasodilators in the Management of Congestive Heart Failure," *Rational Drug Therapy*, **22**:1–7 (1988).

Smith, T. W., et al.: "Treatment of Life-Threatening Digitalis Intoxication with Digoxin Specific Fab Antibody Fragments," *N. Engl. J. Med.* **307**:1357–1362 (1982).

Smith, T. W.: "Digitalis, Mechanisms of Action and Clinical Use," *N. Engl. J. Med*, **318**:358–365 (1988).

Weber, K. T., et al.: "Amrinone and Exercise Performance in Patients with Chronic Heart Failure," *Am. J. Cardiol.*, **48**:164–169 (1981).

C H A P T E R   **27**

Drugs for Tachyarrhythmias

Joseph R. DiPalma

The realization that sudden death due to cardiovascular disease has reached epidemic proportions in the western world has led to efforts to stem this seemingly avoidable tragedy. The cause is believed to be the sudden and sometimes unprovoked onset of ventricular fibrillation, which can occur even in young persons and quite often without obvious coronary artery disease. In cases which have occurred in fortuitous circumstances where cardioversion and resuscitative measures could be immediately applied, patients have gone on to live normal lives, and this lends credence to the idea that prophylactic measures could be successful. Of course, heart disease, depending on its severity, proportionally increases the risk of sudden death from ventricular fibrillation. Often it is preceded by lesser arrhythmias such as frequent ventricular premature beats and runs of ventricular tachycardia. Prevention of these premonitory arrhythmias is felt by most cardiologists to be useful prophylactically beyond the immediate relief of symptoms. Consequently there has been a much greater use of antiarrhythmic drugs in the last 10 years, and the demand for new and better ones has increased. This chapter covers those tachyarrhythmias (atrial flutter and fibrillation and ventricular tachycardia and fibrillation) which are most responsible for causing severe symptoms and sudden death. The few bradyarrhythmias which cause symptoms are handled in other chapters.

Meanwhile the comprehension of the mechanism of action of antiarrhythmic drugs has greatly advanced and has permitted an orderly classification. As shown in Table 27-1, the drugs are arranged according to

their actions on the excitable membrane of the cardiac myocyte. In order to understand the reasoning which led to this classification, it is necessary to review the excitation and recovery cycle of the various contractile and conducting cells of the heart. As in nervous tissue, excitation and conduction are phenomena which are related to the influx and efflux of sodium, calcium, and potassium with some contribution of chloride and magnesium. These are best studied by the technology of recording monophasic action currents in individual cardiac myocytes. In addition, it is necessary to have an appreciation of the gating mechanisms by which the channels in the membrane of the myocyte conduct these metallic ions into and out of the cell.

REVIEW OF CARDIAC ELECTROPHYSIOLOGY

When a cardiac cell is quiescent, its transmembrane potential varies from -80 to -90 mV (inside negative) and is called the *transmembrane resting potential*. On excitation the transmembrane potential reverses, and the inside of the membrane rapidly becomes positive with respect to the outside. On recovery from excitation, the resting potential is restored. The changes in potential following excitation are summarily referred to as the *transmembrane action potential*. These changes have been divided into five phases: depolarization and reversal of transmembrane potential, designated phase 0; three phases of repolarization, designated phases 1, 2, and 3; and the resting potential, designated phase 4.

TABLE 27-1   Classification of antiarrhythmic drugs based on their mechanism of action

Groups	Drugs	Main mechanism of action	Dominant electrophysiologic effects
IA	Quinidine Procainamide Disopyramide	Sodium-channel blockade	Depolarization depressed Repolarization prolonged Conduction slowed
IB	Lidocaine Tocainide Mexiletine Phenytoin	Sodium-channel blockade	Depolarization slightly depressed Repolarization shortened Conduction slowed
IC	Flecainide Encainide Propafenone	Sodium-channel blockade	Depolarization markedly depressed Repolarization slight effects Conduction slowed
II	Propranolol, others	Beta-adrenergic blockade	Action mainly on slow response fibers to suppress automaticity and delay conduction
III	Amiodarone Bretylium	Sodium-, calcium-, and probably potassium-channel blockade	Repolarization prolonged
IV	Verapamil Diltiazem	Calcium-channel blockade	Action mainly on slow-response fibers to suppress automaticity and delay conduction

However, not all cardiac action potentials show a clear separation between phases 1, 2, and 3. Also, there are quantitative differences between transmembrane potentials recorded from different types of cardiac fibers and between their responses to depolarization (Fig. 27-1*b*).

Fibers displaying two distinct types of responses have been identified; they have been named *slow-response fibers* and *fast-response fibers*. Fibers which normally display only slow-response characteristics include normal SA and AV nodal tissue and injured or partially depolarized fast-response fibers. Slow-response tissues have low resting membrane potentials (between −40 and −70 mV) and exhibit slower conduction of impulses than that seen in fast-response fibers. The slow response is dependent on the extracellular concentration of calcium ions and is initiated when membrane permeability to calcium is increased during membrane depolarization (phase 0). During this time calcium and possibly sodium ions enter the cell, elevating the transmembrane potential to approximately +10 mV. Because all cardiac cells possess slow-response characteristics and because nodal tissue is exclusively slow-response in nature, it has been suggested that the property of automaticity (see below), which is fundamental to all cardiac conduction tissue, may be linked to, among other factors, the slow response. An example of the monophasic action potential typical of slow-response tissue is illustrated in Fig. 27-1*a*.

Fibers which exhibit a fast response in addition to the slow response are found in normal atrial and ventricular muscle and specialized ventricular conduction tissue such as Purkinje fibers. The monophasic action potential of fast-response fibers is characterized by a very steep slope for phase 0 upstroke (also referred to as the *sodium spike*) resulting from a rapid inward movement of extracellular sodium ions. These tissues have high resting membrane potentials (-80 to -95 mV) which must be maintained for maximum upstroke velocity, i.e., maximum responsiveness. Consequently, impulse propagation through such tissues is sodium-dependent and rapid. The following is a description of events which occur during the monophasic action potential of fast-response fibers: As the wave of excitation spreads from neighboring cells, the permeability for sodium ions increases and sodium rapidly enters the cell, causing it to become depolarized, i.e., electrically positive relative to the exterior (phase 0).

This ionic shift creates an electrochemical and concentration gradient which reduces the rate of sodium influx but favors the influx of chloride and efflux of potassium (phase 1). Rapid sodium influx triggers the slow inward movement of calcium, which balances potassium leakage and holds the membrane potential fairly steady (phase 2 plateau). When calcium influx slows, the continued efflux of potassium restores the membrane potential to predepolarization levels. Finally, active pumping mechanisms restore the ions to their proper local concentrations (phase 4).

During injury or ischemia in fast-response fibers, the rapid influx of sodium is believed to be lost or inhibited. This results in an action potential which closely resembles that of a slow-response fiber exhibiting slowed impulse conduction, which may favor the development of certain arrhythmias (see below).

The monophasic action potential typical of fast-response tissue is illustrated in Fig. 27-1*b*.

The Gating Mechanisms

Recent work indicates that the movement of the ions across the cell membrane is not simply a question of the size of the ion versus the size of a hole in the mem-

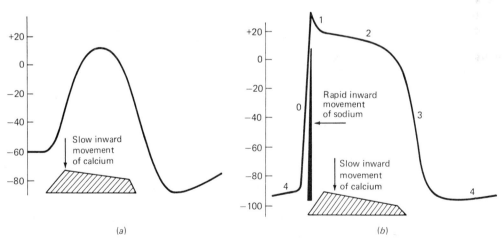

FIGURE 27-1   (*a*) Monophasic action potential recorded from a slow-response fiber (SA node) showing the relationship of calcium influx to depolarization in the absence of sodium influx. The ordinate is in millivolts. (*b*) Diagrammatic representation of a monophasic action potential recorded from a fast-response fiber showing the relationship between ionic movements and the phases of depolarization (0), repolarization (1, 2, 3), and the resting membrane potential (4). The ordinate is in millivolts.

brane. Rather there is a complex system of channels for each ion which are composed of highly structured proteins capable of acting as valves or gates to allow or to prevent the passage of ions.

The sodium channel, which has been most studied in the electric eel *Electrophorus electricus*, is voltage-gated and consists of a single polypeptide of 26,000 to 30,000 molecular weight. The polypeptide is composed of some 1800 amino acid residues and has four repeating homologous units so oriented that they form a channel and a gating mechanism. Of course, there is some variation in different species and organs, but it appears that the essential structure and design are the same. In mammalian counterparts the unit also contains 2 or 3 smaller polypeptides of molecular weight 37,000 to 45,000. DNA recombinant techniques have permitted cloning of DNA sequences complementary to the messenger RNA coding for the channel protein of the electroplax of *E. electricus*.

By use of binding assays using specific neurotoxins, such as tetrodotoxin, similar channels have been identified in rat brain and skeletal muscles as well as in chick cardiac muscle. In addition, specific neurotoxins have enabled an analysis of the mechanisms of the functioning sodium channel. Three states are described: (1) resting, but available for activation; (2) activated, channel open and conducting; (3) inactivated, channel closed and not available (see Fig. 27-2).

A postulated mechanism for the functioning of the sodium channel is as follows (review Fig. 27-2): the complex protein has at least three sensitive components which handle only sodium. Outside the membrane there is a free portion which identifies and allows only this ion to enter the channel (recognition site). The middle portion of the channel has a portion which is *voltage-sensitive* and serves as a gate to keep the channel closed at rest or diastole (M gate). Apparently the M gate is kept closed by the negativity of the electronic membrane potential. Any slight change toward positivity may trigger the M gate to open (a stimulus). This is known as a *threshold potential*. Inside the cell membrane a portion of the protein is apparently sensitive to the concentration of sodium (H gate). Normally in the resting state the H gate is open. Thus when the membrane is stimulated, sodium enters the channel and rapidly flows freely into the cytosol. Realize that there is a very large pressure behind the sodium because of the large differential concentration between the intercellular fluid and the cytosol. As the sodium rushes in, the membrane becomes com-

pletely depolarized and the potential rises toward positivity, causing the M gate to stay open (phase 0 of action potential). Meanwhile, as the concentration of sodium builds up in the cytosol, the H gate closes, preventing further inflow. This whole phase of the depolarization takes only 1 ms or less in the case of nerve and only several milliseconds in the case of heart so that the inward flow of sodium, although fast, is very small in amount. This allows many excitations or depolarizations to take place without exhausting the system and, of course, the Na^+, K^+-ATPase system gradually pumps out the accumulated sodium. Once the H gate closes, the channel is inactivated and must return to the resting state before it can again allow sodium to enter the cell. In normal tissue during diastole, recovery to the resting state is easily accomplished, and thus there are many channels available for the next excitation. In ischemic or damaged cells recovery is difficult, and fewer channels are readied for the next cycle.

It is important to point out that drugs which owe their antiarrhythmic properties to a blocking action in the sodium channel have differential effects because they have diverse physicochemical properties. For example, the M-gate region can be affected by drugs which enter the channel like sodium (more hydrophilic) or by drugs which dissolve in the membrane and enter the cytosol (more lipophilic). When the M gate is closed or in the resting state in normal tissues, hydrophilic drugs cannot affect the H gate. Nor can they be completely effective in the M gate, since the receptor area in the protein may be below the M gate and they must wait for the gate to open (activated state) to act. Therefore they will be most active in cases of fast rhythms where the ratio of open to closed channels is higher. Drugs which are more lipophilic will tend to be active on resting as well as inactivated channels. In ischemic myocytes such drugs are more effective, since the number of inactivated channels is greater than in normal tissues. For these reasons local anesthetics, i.e., group IB drugs in Table 27-1, have diverse actions on the sodium channel and are therefore useful in differing clinical situations.

It follows that the quality, number, physical state, and distribution of channels for sodium, potassium, and calcium mainly determine the contour and functional characteristics of the monophasic action potential of various myocytes in the heart. Thus the pacemaker regions of the heart (SA and AV nodes) have a monophasic action potential which has relatively slow

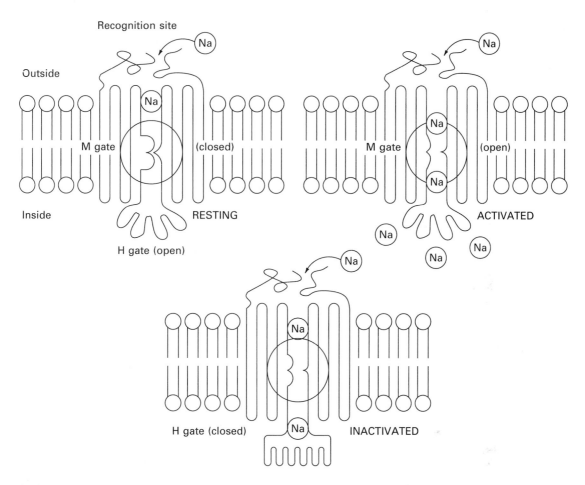

FIGURE 27-2 A highly schematic diagram of the sodium channel of a cardiac myocyte. The channel is composed of a large protein which is folded in the biomolecular lipid membrane in such a manner as to form four homologous units which in turn form a channel or pore. On the outside of the membrane the ends of the protein chain form a recognition site, or specificity gate, which identifies sodium. In the channel itself there is an area which is sensitive to stimuli and presumably by an allosteric mechanism can open or close the pore. This is the M gate. Inside the membrane, a portion of the protein forms an additional gate which can also block the passage of sodium (H gate). The channel is thought to exist in three states. In the fully polarized membrane the channel is at rest with the M gate closed and the H gate open. Upon stimulation, the M gate opens and sodium can enter the myocyte (activated state). A millisecond later the H gate closes, inactivating the channel and blocking the entrance of sodium into the myocyte. The area in the vicinity of the M gate is thought to be the receptor site for local anesthetics (circled). It is thought that the local anesthetic cannot easily reach this sensitive area when the M gate is closed. When the M gate is open, the local anesthetic can reach the receptor area both in the disassociated and undisassociated forms. Thus in most instances these agents are generally more effective on activated channels. On the other hand, highly lipid-soluble drugs such as lidocaine can read the M gate receptor area through the membrane or even the cytosol, and thus such drugs are effective on both activated and inactivated channels.

depolarization (phase 0), a small plateau (phase 2), while repolarization (phase 3) is comparable to that in other myocytes. However, the most remarkable difference is in the resting potential (phase 4). Instead of being isoelectric, it rises in a gentle slope, seemingly triggering the next depolarization (see Fig. 27-3). In fact, experimental conditions which favor and increase this slope cause tachycardia and conditions which flatten the slope bradycardia. Indeed, when an atrial or ventricular myocyte "takes over" pacemaker activity, the normal flat resting potential now becomes sloped, resembling that of pacemaker myocytes.

As shown in Fig. 27-3, atrial and ventricular myocytes have essentially the same contour of action potential except that the atrial potential is of smaller amplitude and shorter in duration. Atrial and Purkinje fibers have more overshoot (phase 1), which may be indicative of their conductive properties.

PATHOPHYSIOLOGY OF CARDIAC ARRHYTHMIAS

Many factors influence the normal rhythm of electrical activity in the heart, including automaticity, refractoriness, conduction velocity, excitability, and impulse conduction through the atrioventricular node. In general, however, all arrhythmias can be shown to result from defects in automaticity, which cause abnormal impulse formation, or defects in conduction, which allow abnormal impulse propagation, or both.

Automaticity

The term *automaticity* is used to describe the behavior by which cardiac fibers spontaneously generate action potentials. The property of automaticity is a feature common to all cardiac conduction tissue, and in some cells, e.g., nodal tissue, it is believed to be related to the slow inward movement of calcium ions.

Under normal circumstances, the task of impulse generation in the heart is under control of specialized cells that spontaneously depolarize during phase 4 (the resting phase). Once such depolarizations reach the threshold potential, an action potential is initiated which subsequently propagates throughout the myocardium. These specialized cells, by virtue of their rapid rate of spontaneous discharge, control impulse formation for the entire heart and are consequently known as *pacemaker cells*.

Other cells with a high degree of automaticity exist which discharge more slowly than the pacemaker cells. Normally, such cells are depolarized before they attain threshold potential by impulses originating in the pacemaker area (SA node). Pacemaker control of the heart, therefore, resides in those cells whose rate of spontaneous depolarization is most rapid. This rate of discharge can be increased by a number of mechanisms either singly or in combination: (1) increasing the slope of phase 4 of the myocardial action potential, (2) decreasing (making less negative) the resting membrane potential, and (3) increasing (making more negative) the threshold potential. Conversely, the rate of spontaneous depolarization can be decreased by changing these variables in the opposite direction. The relative decrease in the rate of spontaneous depolarization of the SA node or the relative increase in spontaneous depolarization rate of cells outside the SA node favors the loss of pacemaker control by the SA node to a new area of pacemaker activity called an *ectopic focus*. Ectopic foci typically arise in circumstances under activity of other automatic cells, for example, during vagal overtone or in the presence of drugs which depress the SA node. Ectopic foci can also assume pacemaker activity when the automaticity of nonnodal cells is stimulated, as occurs in ischemia, acidosis, digitalis toxicity, ionic imbalance, and catecholamine excess. Arrhythmias which appear to result from an increase in the automaticity of SA nodal tissue or ectopic pacemaker tissue include sinus tachycardia and atrial tachycardia. Arrhythmias produced by reductions in automaticity of these tissues include premature ventricular beats and AV junctional rhythm.

Conduction

The progressive movement of an action potential from one area of the myocardium to another is termed *conduction*. It is a property of excitable tissue which allows an impulse to pass from cell to cell, that is, to be propagated.

Disturbances in conduction also contribute to the development of arrhythmias. Slowing or loss of impulse propagation from the atria to the ventricles results in various degrees of AV block with subsequent dissociation of pacemaker control. Conduction is influenced by several factors: the *excitability* of cells which lie in the path of a propagated impulse, the *responsiveness* of these cells, and the *refractoriness* and

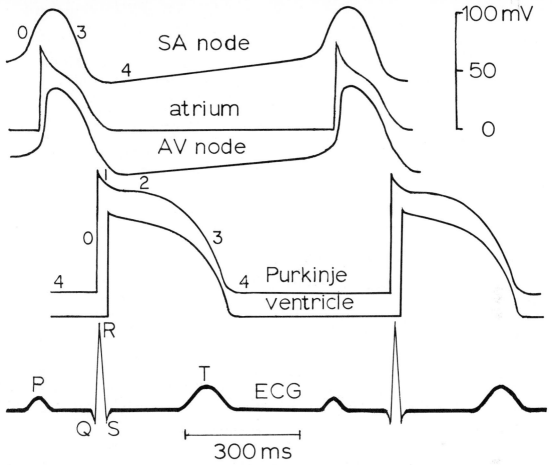

FIGURE 27-3 Schematic reconstruction of the monophasic action potentials of selected myocytes of the heart arranged in temporal sequence for two complete cycles. The clinical ECG is included to illustrate the relationship of this diphasic recording to the cyclic events which are occurring in pertinent parts of the heart. Note that the amplitude of the ECG has no relationship to that of the monophasic action potentials. The latter potentials have five phases: phase 0 = depolarization; phase 1 = early and brief repolarization; phase 2 = plateau; phase 3 = rapid repolarization; phase 4 = resting, or the diastolic, potential. The potentials of the SA node and the AV node myocytes differ from those of atrium, Purkinje, and ventricle myocytes by having slow depolarization and no phases 1 and 2. In addition, the resting potential slopes upward (becomes more positive) during diastole characteristic of pacemaker myocytes. The Purkinje and ventricular myocytes have potentials of greater amplitude and duration than the nodal and atrial myocytes. The SA node, because of its anatomic location, innervation, and inherent greater automaticity, sets the rhythm of the heart. The ECG reflects the temporal events of the cycle. Thus the P wave is related to atrial depolarization; the QRS complex to ventricular depolarization; the T wave to ventricular repolarization. It follows that the P-R interval measures atrial-ventricular conduction time; the QRS ventricular activation (depolarization plus conduction); the Q-T interval mainly duration of the ventricular action potentials. The ECG is, of course, a surface reflection of the electrical activity of the heart but as indicated can serve as an accurate diagnostic tool for changes brought about in rhythm and in the effects of antiarrhythmic agents.

response characteristics of the tissue which a propagated impulse encounters.

Excitability is defined as the reciprocal of the magnitude of an electric impulse required to change the resting membrane potential to the threshold potential at which an action potential is propagated. *Responsiveness* is the maximum rate of depolarization during phase 0 of the action potential, i.e., the slope of phase 0, and is influenced by the value of the transmembrane potential at the time of excitation. Higher resting membrane potentials increase responsiveness; conversely, lower (less negative) potentials reduce it. *Refractoriness* is defined as the inability to respond to a stimulus. For the most part, we restrict our consideration of refractoriness to the duration of the *effective refractory periods* (ERP). The ERP is the period during which a premature stimulus, regardless of strength, will fail to propagate an impulse (Fig 27-4).

These factors influence conduction in a number of ways. Generally, if an ectopic focus develops, the relatively more rapid rate of diastolic depolarization of the SA node will prevent impulses propagated by the ectopic focus from encountering any but refractory tissue. During the relative refractory period (RRP), a premature stimulus may, depending on strength, propagate an impulse but at a slower rate than when the stimulus occurs outside the refractory periods (Fig. 27-4).

Decreasing the ERP favors the propagation of premature impulses because the chances of encountering excitable tissue are increased. Conversely, lengthening the ERP decreases the chances that impulses from ectopic foci will be propagated. Since the ERP constitutes a portion of the action potential duration (APD), it is sometimes useful to determine its change relative to that of the APD. The ERP/APD ratio serves to express the relationship between these intervals and has been employed as an index of refractoriness.

Interference with conduction of propagated impulses may produce serious dysfunctions of the heart, including AV block, bundle branch block, and various tachyarrhythmias. Cardiac stretch and local tissue hypoxia may reduce the speed of impulse conduction through segments of the myocardium, resulting in the reexcitation of recently depolarized, but no longer refractory, tissue. This phenomenon, known as *reentry*, is often responsible for coupled beats, called *bigeminy*, and AV nodal and ventricular tachycardias.

Conduction of propagated impulses is also influenced by the response characteristics of the tissue which an impulse encounters. This is particularly true for slow-response tissues like SA and AV nodal tissue, which have long, time-dependent refractory periods. In these tissues, impulse conduction is very slow, and this can result in the unidirectional block of an impulse and subsequent reentrant arrhythmias.

TYPES OF CARDIAC ARRHYTHMIAS

Cardiac arrhythmias can arise at practically every level of the heart. Arrhythmias which develop at or above the level of the AV node are classified as *supraventricular arrhythmias*, whereas those which develop in the His-Purkinje system or the ventricles are called *ventricular arrhythmias*.

Supraventricular Arrhythmias

Paroxysmal Atrial Tachycardia   Paroxysmal atrial tachycardia (PAT) is characterized by atrial rates of 150 to 250 beats per minute and most often 180 to 200 beats per minute. This rhythm often occurs in the absence of demonstrable heart disease. In the absence of heart disease and drug therapy, it is common to see

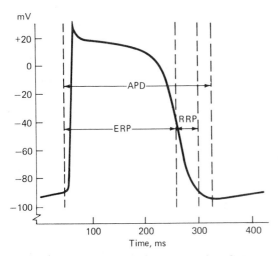

FIGURE 27-4   Diagrammatic representation of a monophasic action potential recorded from a Purkinje myocyte showing the durations of the effective refractory period (ERP), the relative refractory period (RRP), and the action potential (APD).

each atrial depolarization conduct to ventricles so that the atrial and ventricular rates are identical. Paroxysms often spontaneously terminate but also may be tenaciously persistent and cause severe anxiety and palpitations or induce heart failure even in otherwise normal hearts.

Atrial Flutter   Atrial flutter is characterized by regular beating of the atria at rates between 250 and 300 beats per minute; most commonly the atrial rate is precisely 300 beats per minute. In adults who have not been treated, every other atrial depolarization is usually conducted to the ventricles, producing a ventricular rate of 150 beats per minute. Unlike atrial fibrillation, atrial flutter produces effective contraction of the atria with less thrombosis in the atria. Subsequent embolization is consequently much less common.

Atrial Fibrillation   Atrial fibrillation is a rhythm characterized by irregular, disorganized depolarization of the atrium at rates of 350 to 600 beats per minute. These rapid depolarizations do not produce effective atrial contractions. The rapid atrial rate exceeds the ability of even the normal AV conducting system to trasmit impulses; therefore, the ventricular rate is much slower, 130 to 170 beats per minute in untreated cases, and is characteristically irregular. This rhythm diminishes the "cardiac reserve," produces palpitations, and is associated with an increased incidence of thromboembolization of the pulmonary or systemic arterial systems. The decrease in cardiac reserve commonly leads to the onset or aggravation of congestive heart failure, angina pectoris, or symptoms of cerebrovascular insufficiency.

Ventricular Arrhythmias

Premature Ventricular Contractions   Premature ventricular contractions (PVCs), or extrasystoles, originate in the ventricles and travel in unorthodox pathways, and the QRS complexes are thus wide and bizarre in configuration, prematurely interrupting the dominant rhythm. Premature ventricular contractions are very common both in individuals with normal hearts and in those with heart disease. Most of these cases require no treatment. If premature depolarizations are frequent or cause troublesome symptoms or signs, treatment should be considered. The decision to treat PVCs also may be based on the condition associated with the arrhythmia. For instance, digitalis in excessive doses may lead to frequent premature ventricular beats. If digitalis is continued, ventricular tachycardia or ventricular fibrillation may occur and can prove fatal. Another example is the occurrence of PVCs during acute myocardial infarction, where PVCs may presage ventricular tachycardia or fibrillation.

Ventricular Tachycardia   Ventricular tachycardia is a rapid rhythm (150 to 200 beats per minute) originating in the ventricles. This site of origin produces QRS complexes in the ECG which are slurred and widened. The configuration of the QRS complexes during ventricular tachycardia is the same as that of PVCs originating in either the right or left ventricle. The cycle length between beats is slightly irregular, and the QRS complexes are independent of the P waves. The etiologic factors and therapeutic goals are similar to those discussed under PVCs. However, ventricular tachycardia is much more likely to produce circulatory impairment than even frequent PVCs, and congestive cardiac failure or severe hypotension may ensue. When such catastrophic events are precipitated by ventricular tachycardia, it should be terminated immediately using appropriate drugs or electric countershock.

Ventricular Fibrillation   This tachyarrhythmia is exactly analogous to atrial fibrillation. However, while in the atrium the arrhythmia has relatively little consequence with respect to the pumping function of the heart, fibrillation in the ventricle results in an instantaneous drop in blood pressure to zero because of absence of cardiac output. Death is inevitable in a few minutes unless the arrhythmia is converted and the normal heart beat restored. No drug therapy is practical. The remedy is cardiac massage to restore some circulation, artificial respiration, and dc countershock (cardioversion). *The aim of drug therapy is to prevent this most common cause of sudden death by lessening the chance of its development.*

Unusual Tachyarrhythmias

Wolff-Parkinson-White   (WPW)   Syndrome   A reexcitation syndrome is one in which the impulse from the atrium reaches the ventricle by an abnormal route without the usual delay built into the normal conduction pathway. Hence the ventricle is "preexcited." Patients with this syndrome are subject to paroxysmal attacks of atrial tachycardia, flutter, and fibrillation. These are, of course, attended by rapid ventricular rates, even as rapid as 250 to 300 per minute which are life-threatening, especially if the individual does not have adequate cardiac reserve.

Torsade de Pointes   This literally means turning of the points (QRS complexes). It occurs in situations where the Q-T interval is prolonged (long action potential duration) and consists of ventricular tachycardia which undulates around the ECG isoelectric base. It usually begins with a single premature contraction superimposed on the T wave of the previous normal beat.

There are many causes including congenital long Q-T interval; drugs with quinidine-like properties such as type IA antiarrhythmics, tricyclics and others; electrolyte imbalance, especially hyperkalemia and hypomagnesemia; liquid protein diets; CNS lesions; myocarditis and myocardial ischemia; marked bradycardia; and mitral valve prolapse syndromes.

Fortunately torsade de pointes usually terminates spontaneously. However, it easily converts to ventricular fibrillation, and thus it must be recognized and treated properly to avoid sudden death.

ANTIARRHYTHMIC DRUGS

Few groups of drugs have been so well studied and understood from the viewpoint of the molecular, as well as the physiologic, mechanism of action. This has permitted a useful and logical classification based upon accurate data (review Table 27-1). Based upon the exquisite understanding of the mechanism of tachyarrhythmias and the knowledge of how the drugs affect these mechanisms, it is possible to prescribe with considerable accuracy a particular drug for a particular arrhythmia. In difficult cases it is necessary to actually invasively study the patient's electrophysiologic disturbance. In advanced cardiac clinics the patient who is subject to a tachyarrhythmia is sedated, electrodes are placed in the heart, and by electrical pacing the tachyarrhythmia is induced. Then by giving one drug after another intravenously the threshold for inducing the arrhythmia is measured. By this method the best available drug is determined which presumably will increase the chance that the arrhythmia will not occur

spontaneously and hence prevent sudden death. Selection of a specific drug by this method is believed to yield better results than empiric prescribing.

Such electrophysiologic testing in humans is possible only because cardioversion can rescue the patient in case a fatal type of arrhythmia such as ventricular fibrillation is induced. In fact, cardioversion is so effective that it has replaced antiarrhythmic drugs in many instances in the conversion of tachyarrhythmias to sinus rhythm. Thus the role of antiarrhythmic drugs has changed to become more prophylactic—that is, to prevent recurrence of an arrhythmia once sinus rhythm has been established by cardioversion. *Thus the ultimate proof of clinical efficacy of an antiarrhythmic drug must be not only in that it relieves signs and symptoms but also in that it prolongs life.*

There is no doubt that the central nervous system exerts some control over the rhythm of the heart. This is expressed by impulses over the autonomic nervous system. Therefore, the arrhythmogenic action of catecholamines and cholinomimetic substances on the heart is most important.

Catecholamines

It is certain that sympathetic stimulation of the heart either by nerve impulse or endogenous and exogenous catecholamines initiates and perpetuates both atrial and ventricular tachyarrhythmias. Particularly in prophylaxis therapy beta-adrenergic blockade seems effective, and actually this is the only group of drugs which has proven ability to reduce mortality and prolong life. It is to be noted that drugs in groups IA and III also enhance block of the sympathetics, but this is mainly an alpha-type block.

Cholinomimetic Action

Cholinergic stimulation of the atrium can lead to atrial tachycardia and even flutter and fibrillation. A classic experiment is the application of a pledget of cotton soaked with Mecholyl to the exposed atrium. Fibrillation usually follows. Innervation of the ventricle by parasympathetic fibers is absent, and so ventricular arrhythmias are not produced by this method. Drugs with anticholinergic action are used particularly in the prophylaxis of atrial arrhythmias. This seems to be especially true during anesthesia and surgery.

GROUP I DRUGS

All these drugs have local anesthetic properties and have a common major mechanism of action in blocking the sodium channel. Depending on which stage of sodium-channel activity is most severely blocked, the change in physiology of the myocyte is variously affected (see Table 27-1). All the drugs in this group have unequal actions on the physiologic properties described above. Table 27-2 provides a summary of these effects.

TABLE 27-2   Effects of antiarrhythmic drugs on the physiologic functions of heart muscle and the conduction system; comparison to the effects of digitalis

Function	Drugs in groups						
	IA	**IB**	**IC**	**II**	**III**	**IV**	**Digitalis**
Automaticity							
SA node	+/−	+/−	0	− − − −	− − − −	− − − −	− − − −
Ectopic foci	− − − −	− − − −	− − − −	− − − −	− − − −	− − − −	+ + + +
Conduction velocity							
Atrium	− − − −	0	− − − −	+/−	− − − −	0	+/−
AV node	− − − −	0	− − − −	− − − −	− − − −	− − − −	− − − −
His-Purkinje	− − −	0	− − − −	+/−	− − − −	0	+/−
Refractory period							
Atrium	+ + + +	0	0	+/−	+ + + +	0	− −
AV node	+ +	0	0	+ + + +	+ + + +	+ + + +	+ + + +
His-Purkinje	+ + + +	0	+ + + +	0	+ + + +	0	0
Ventricle	+ + + +	0	+ + + +	0	+ + + +	0	− − − −
Action-potential duration	+ + + +	− − − −	0	0	+ + + +	0	− − − −
Responsiveness (rate of depolarization)	− − − −	0	− − − −	0	− −	0	+ +
Catecholamine block	+ +	0	0	+ + + +	+ +	0	0
Anticholinergic	+ + + +	0	0	0	0	0	0
Local anesthetic activity	+ +	+ + + +	+ +	+	+	+	0
Sodium-channel block	+ + + +	+ + + +	+ + + +	+	+ + +	0	0
Calcium-channel block	0	0	0	0	+	+ + + +	0

Code: Increase = + to + + + +; Decrease = − to − − − −; effect varies with dose and circumstances = +/−; unknown or indefinite = 0.

Group IA

Quinidine

Quinidine is the dextro stereoisomer of quinine; it exerts all the pharmacologic actions of quinine, including antimalarial, antipyretic, and oxytocic effects. The actions of quinidine on cardiac muscle are relatively more intense than those of quinine. Conversely, quinidine, although less effective against malaria than quinine, can be used for this purpose.

Source and Chemistry Quinidine is one of the four most important alkaloids isolated from cinchona bark. Quinidine consists of a quinoline group attached by a secondary carbinol to a quinuclidine ring. There is a methoxy group on the quinoline ring and a vinyl group on the quinuclidine ring. Quinidine differs from quinine only in the configuration of the carbinol grouping (see Fig. 27-5).

Pharmacodynamics

Cardiovascular system The major effects of quinidine on the electrical activity of the heart have been described above. In addition, quinidine depresses contractility, especially in toxic doses. In therapeutic usage, however, it may actually increase cardiac output because of its vasodilatory properties. The depressant effect on contractility may be of real importance when myocardial disease is present. Large oral doses of quinidine reduce arterial pressure in humans. Considerably smaller intravenous doses have the same effect. Rapid intravenous injection may cause a precipitous decrease in blood pressure and cardiac output.

Many of the effects of quinidine on the electrical activity of the heart can be appreciated from the ECG. Patients in sinus rhythm may show an increase in sinus rate, which presumably is caused by anticholinergic action, a reflex increase in sympathetic activity, or both. High doses, particularly in patients with atrial disease, may produce sinus arrest or sinoatrial (SA) block. Because of its effects on conduction in the His-Purkinje system and ventricle, quinidine causes a progressive prolongation of the QRS complex. Prolongation of the QRS complex and serious conduction disturbances are more likely when abnormality of the conduction system is present before quinidine administration. Quinidine increases the QT interval corrected for rate. This effect, at low doses, is due primarily to the effects of quinidine on repolarization of ventricular muscle. At higher doses, changes in the QT interval and in the configuration of the T wave result also from the quinidine-induced disturbances of conduction. In usual therapeutic doses quinidine has little effect on the P-R interval. This may be due to the fact that an anticholinergic action is balanced by a direct depressant effect on AV conduction. In sufficiently high concentrations quinidine can produce heart block of any degree.

Central Nervous System Quinidine first stimulates and then depresses the higher nerve centers. In humans, intravenous administration of quinidine may produce a sensation of warmth, profuse diaphoresis, and nausea and vomiting. Rarely, it may produce psychosis-like symptoms.

Autonomic Nervous System Quinidine appears to interfere with the effects of the parasympathetic nervous system on the heart. A vagal blocking action would be expected to increase the heart rate. However, this is opposed by the direct action of quinidine on pacemaker and conduction tissue, which is to slow the heart rate. For this reason, variable effects are noted on heart rate dependent on the initial vagal tone (see Table 27-2). Note that it also causes some degree of catecholamine block.

Skeletal Muscle Quinidine, like the other cinchona alkaloids, increases the maximum tension developed by skeletal muscle in response to direct electrical stimulation. This action contrasts with its negative inotropic effect on cardiac muscle. Quinidine increases refractoriness of skeletal muscle. Quinidine also decreases the effectiveness of transmission across the neuromuscular junction and diminishes the response of skeletal muscle to intraarterial injections of acetylcholine. This had led to the use of quinidine (actually quinine) for "night cramps" or spasm of the leg skeletal muscle.

Pharmacokinetics Quinidine is approximately 80 percent absorbed from the gastrointestinal tract. A single oral dose produces peak plasma concentration within 1 to 2 h. Therapeutic plasma levels vary from 2.5 to 8.0 μg/mL.

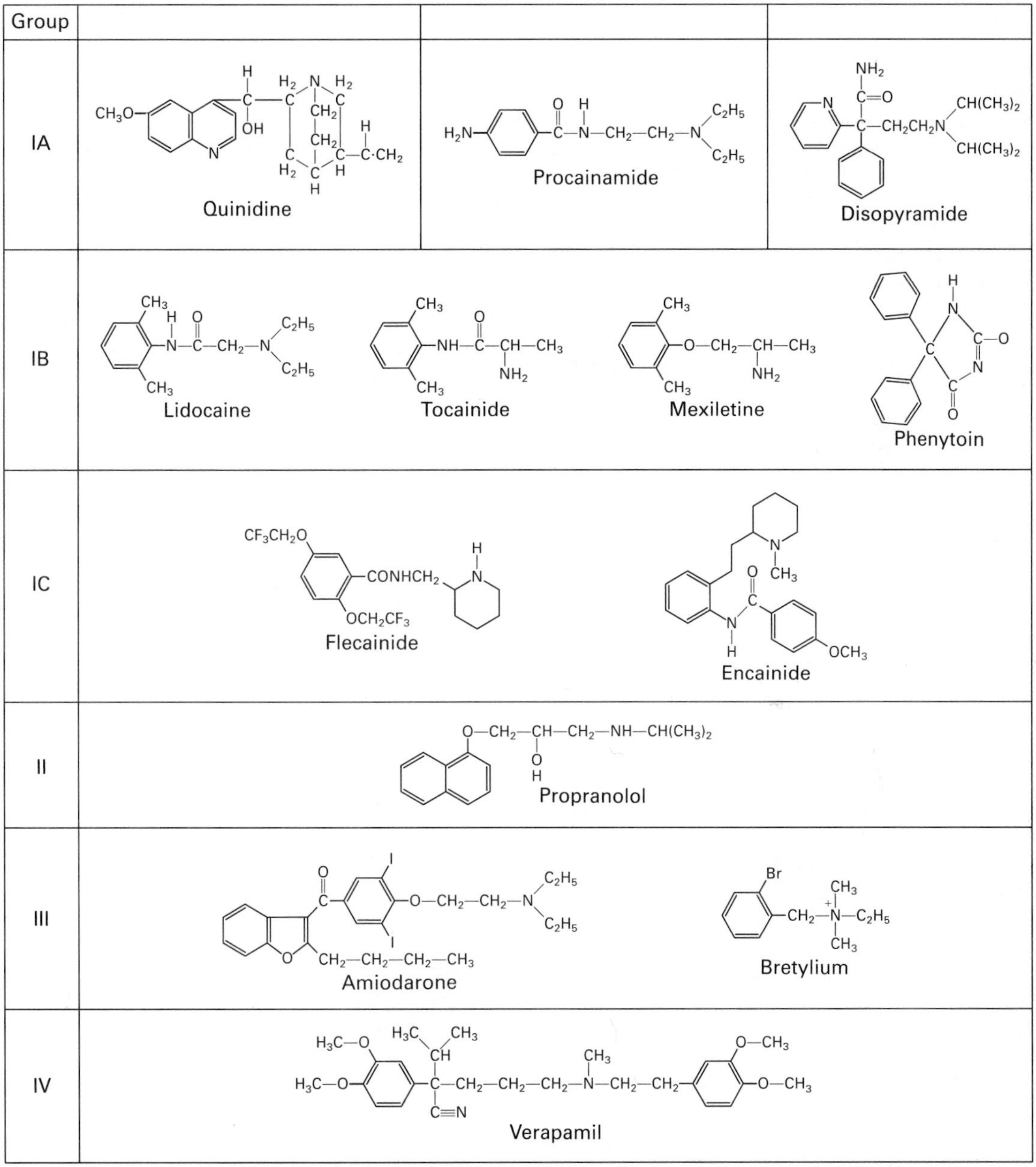

FIGURE 27-5 Chemical structures of the most commonly used antiarrhythmic drugs arranged by groups representing major mechanisms of action.

Quinidine disappears from plasma with a half-life between 6 and 7 h. The drug is biotransformed in the liver to an active derivative, dihydroquinidine, and inactive hydroxylated products. Approximately 85 percent of plasma quinidine is bound to blood proteins. The amount of unaltered quinidine excreted unchanged varies from 20 to 50 percent. About 95 percent of an administered dose can be recovered from the urine as the sum of quinidine and its biotransformation products.

Therapeutic Uses   Quinidine is commonly used to abolish atrial and premature ventricular contractions and to prevent paroxysmal supraventricular or ventricular tachycardia. Quinidine is also useful in converting atrial fibrillation to normal sinus rhythm. When used to eliminate atrial flutter, quinidine administration should not precede that of digitalis. In the absence of a digitalis-included AV block, quinidine can precipitate a 1:1 heart block and a dangerously rapid ventricular rate. Quinidine is not frequently administered parenterally because of adverse reactions such as hypotension.

Adverse Reactions   One of the major problems in the effective use of quinidine is its toxicity. Few patients find quinidine tolerable in long-term use, particularly in higher dosage ranges.

Cinchonism   Quinidine, like the other cinchona alkaloids, can induce cinchonism. Symptoms of mild cinchonism may include tinnitus, impaired hearing, headache, mild diarrhea, or slight blurring of vision. Symptoms of severe toxicity include severe tinnitus and hearing loss, blurred vision, diplopia, photophobia, and altered perception of color. Severe cerebral signs, such as confusion, delirium, or psychosis, may accompany the headache. Nausea, vomiting, and diarrhea may be severe and accompanied by abdominal pain. The skin is often hot and flushed.

Gastrointestinal Effects   Nausea, vomiting, and diarrhea each occur alone or in varying combinations and often in the absence of symptoms involving other systems. Quinidine administration is often continued even with mild gastrointestinal symptoms; more severe reaction may force discontinuing the drug.

Blood Pressure Effects   When given intravenously, and to a lesser extent intramuscularly, quinidine may cause significant and even profound arterial hypotension. In most instances this pressure drop is primarily due to a decrease in arteriolar resistance without marked reduction in cardiac output. Severe, protracted hypotension may be treated with catecholamines.

Cardiac Effects   Quinidine in concentrations above 2.0 μg/mL causes a progressive linear increase in duration of the QRS and Q-T intervals of the ECG; the change in QRS has a higher correlation with plasma drug concentration. This relationship is useful in monitoring the cardiac effects of quinidine; the dose administered is reduced if a normal QRS duration increases by 50 percent over the control value. The Q-T interval is also a useful measurement to follow, and changes in this interval are easy to detect at ordinary ECG recording speeds. At plasma concentrations that may be toxic (8 μg/mL), complete SA block, high-grade AV block, or total asystole may occur. Ventricular ectopic depolarizations may become frequent and occur repetitively; ventricular tachycardia or fibrillation may ensue. Although such severe myocardial toxicity may diminish as plasma concentration declines after withholding quinidine, the ECG and hemodynamic parameters of each patient should be closely monitored. Catecholamines, molar sodium lactate, and glucagon may be useful to counteract quinidine toxicity in cases which require more active intervention.

A frequently mentioned complication of quinidine therapy for atrial fibrillation is the so-called paradoxic increase in ventricular rate. In many cases of atrial fibrillation, when quinidine is used alone for conversion, the atrial rate slows markedly before the change to sinus rhythm occurs. However, in a few of these cases the ventricular rate may suddenly rise as atrial rate falls because of a decrease in concealed conduction of atrial impulses in the AV junction. Even though this event is uncommon in patients treated with quinidine alone, many physicians digitalize their patients prior to using quinidine to avoid this eventuality. Hypersensitivity reactions, including fever, thrombocytopenic purpura, and hepatitis, are not uncommon complications of quinidine therapy.

Drug Interactions   Quinidine can have additive effects when administered together with digitalis, phenytoin, procainamide, propranolol, phenothiazines, and other agents, and caution should be exercised when using such combination therapy. Quinidine potentiates the neuromuscular blockade produced by curariform drugs, depolarizing blocking agents, and certain antibiotics such as neomycin. Barbiturates and anticonvulsants which induce the drug-metabolizing microsomal system shorten the half-life of quinidine by about 50 percent, and therapy with agents in these classes should be started and stopped with great caution in patients receiving quinidine. Anticonvulsants and aluminum hydroxide antacids may reduce or delay quinidine absorption from the gastrointestinal tract. Other antacid agents which indirectly alkalinize the urine may potentiate quinidine via increased tubular reabsorption. Quinidine is known to increase serum digoxin concentrations. It has been suggested that quinidine displaces digoxin from tissue-binding sites; interference with renal digoxin excretion by quinidine has also been proposed. Quinidine may inhibit the formation of prothrombin and of other vitamin K–dependent clotting factors, heightening the effect of oral anticoagulants. Quinidine toxicity may be exaggerated by simultaneous use of pyrimethamine, quinine, and Rauwolfia alkaloids. Because of its anticholinergic nature, quinidine may antagonize the effects of cholinergic agents.

Procainamide

The actions of procainamide are qualitatively similar to those of procaine. Its effects on the electrical activity of the heart are almost identical to those of quinidine. Procainamide is superior to procaine as an antiarrhythmic agent because, in contrast to procaine, (1) it is well absorbed after oral administration, (2) it has a long duration of action because it resists hydrolysis by plasma esterases, and (3) its effects on the heart are relatively strong, while its effects on the central nervous system are relatively weak.

Chemistry Procainamide differs from procaine in that the ester linkage has been replaced by an amide bond. Its chemical structure is shown in Fig. 27-5.

Pharmacodynamics

Cardiovascular System The effects of procainamide on the electrical activity of the heart are qualitatively the same as those of quinidine. Like quinidine, procainamide has a negative inotropic effect, although at equivalent therapeutic doses this action may be less intense. Like quinidine, procainamide causes a decrease in systemic arterial pressure, which is particularly prominent with intravenous administration. Peripheral vasodilation and depression of cardiac contractility contribute to the hypotensive action.

The changes in the ECG produced by procainamide are similar to those caused by quinidine. Prolongation of the QRS complex is a most consistent change. Prolongation of the corrected Q-T interval, changes in the morphology of the T wave, and at high doses, prolongation of the P-R interval or production of heart block are less frequent. As in the case of quinidine, changes in the ECG may provide some guide to the doses of procainamide to be employed. The presence of abnormalities of conduction increases the likelihood that the drug will cause further conduction delay or block.

Pharmacokinetics Procainamide can be given orally, intramuscularly, or intravenously. Absorption is approximately 85 percent complete following oral administration, and peak plasma concentrations are reached in 45 to 90 min. Intramuscular injections produce peak levels within 15 to 45 min, but values are more variable than after oral or intravenous doses. Procainamide is only sparingly bound to plasma proteins (approximately 15 percent). However, it is bound in various body tissues in concentrations in excess of the plasma concentrations. Disappearance of procainamide from the plasma approximates a first-order process with a half-life of 2 to 3 h. Unlike its homolog procaine (an ester), procainamide (an amide) is highly resistant to esterases but is hydrolyzed by amidases. When it occurs, biotransformation takes place in the liver. Nearly 90 percent or procainamide and its biotransformation products are excreted in the urine. The major product is N-acetylprocainamide (NAPA), which appears as 10 to 12 percent of a single dose in slow acetylators and about 25 percent in rapid acetylators. This product is pharmacologically active and equal to procainamide in antiarrhythmic potency. Because NAPA is less likely to cause a lupus-like syndrome, it may be marketed as a substitute for procainamide. Urinary clearance of all products occurs by glomerular filtration and tubular secretion. Approximately 50 to 60 percent is excreted unchanged.

Therapeutic Uses Procainamide is indicated for the treatment of paroxysmal atrial tachycardia, atrial fibrillation, premature ventricular contractions, and ventricular tachycardia. Therapeutic plasma concentrations range from 4 to 8 μg/mL. Intravenous and oral dosage schedules may require adjustment upward in dialysis patients and downward in undialyzed individuals with renal failure. For rapid establishment of therapeutic concentrations, parenteral procainamide is superior to quinidine.

Adverse Reactions   Many of the undesirable effects of procainamide are related to the plasma concentrations, the rate of change of plasma concentration, and the route of administration. The intravenous route of administration is more often associated with cardiac toxicity than is widening of the QRS complex, ventricular ectopic beats, ventricular tachycardia and fibrillation, or asystole. High doses of procainamide may diminish myocardial contractility and cause hypotension or worsen cardiac failure.

Agranulocytosis and syndrome resembling systemic lupus erythematosus (SLE) may be produced by procainamide. Approximately 60 percent of patients receiving it develop a positive antinuclear antibody or anti-DNA antibody. Clinically, these patients may remain asymptomatic; however, those who exhibit symptoms resembling lupus more often than not are slow acetylators. Agranulocytosis may be severe and responsible for fatal infections. Arthralgia is the most prevalent symptom, and fever, pleuropneumonic involvement, and hepatomegaly are all common. This syndrome possesses features distinct from idiopathic SLE. There is no predilection for females. Renal and cerebral involvements are not seen.

Drug Interactions   Procainamide may potentiate the hypotensive effect of antihypertensive drugs and thiazide diuretics. Like quinidine and other antiarrhythmic drugs, procainamide may potentiate the neuromuscular blockade produced by skeletal-muscle relaxants, magnesium salts, and certain antibiotics. Also, like quinidine, procainamide has anticholinergic properties which antagonize cholinergic drugs and enhance the effects of other drugs with anticholinergic activity.

Individuals sensitive to procainamide will exhibit cross-sensitivity to lidocaine and other local anesthetic agents. Because of additive effects, procainamide should be combined with other antiarrhythmic agents cautiously. Although useful in treating digitalis-induced tachyarrhythmias, procainamide should be

administered with care to prevent the development of ventricular fibrillation or cardiac depression.

Disopyramide

Chemistry   Disopyramide is not structurally related to any other antiarrhythmic drug, as can be seen from the structure (see Fig. 27-5). This agent is extremely water-soluble (the lipid-to-water partition coefficient is approximately 3.0). The pK_a of the free base is 8.36.

Pharmacodynamics

Cardiovascular System   Therapeutic doses of disopyramide prolong the ERP of the atrium and the ERP of the ventricle. Unlike quinidine, disopyramide has little effect on impulse conduction through the AV node, bundle of His, and Purkinje fibers and consequently little effect on P-R or Q-T intervals or on QRS duration. In addition, recommended oral doses of disopyramide produce significant (10 percent) reductions in blood pressure with a minimum of cardiac depression.

Autonomic Nervous System   Disopyramide has relatively more anticholinergic activity than quinidine. Oral disopyramide has no effect on resting sinus rhythm, but it is likely that the anticholinergic actions have a role in the activity of this drug at the AV node. These anticholinergic actions are also responsible for the gastrointestinal and urogenital side effects cited below.

Pharmacokinetics   Orally administered disopyramide is absorbed well (80 percent) but slowly from the gastrointestinal tract. Peak plasma levels of disopyramide are attained within 2 h of, and last several hours after, a single oral dose.

Approximately 50 percent of the drug is bound to plasma proteins. The average half-life of disopyramide is about 7 h, with an apparent volume of distribution of about 0.8 L/kg. In patients with impaired renal function, the serum half-life is prolonged, ranging from 8 to 18 h. About one-half of a disopyramide dose is excreted unchanged in the urine, about 25 percent appears as the mono-N-dealkylated product, and the remainder appears as other products. The major biotransformation product of disopyramide is approximately 25 percent as active biologically as the parent compound and is present in the blood at about 10 percent of the concentration of the parent compound.

Therapeutic Uses Oral disopyramide is indicated to prevent and reduce the incidence of premature ventricular contractions and has been employed prophylactically to reduce the incidence of sudden death following myocardial infarction. However, there is no proof that this mission was accomplished. Indeed, elderly patients should not receive this drug because of its adverse effects. Because of the large contribution of renal excretion to the termination of disopyramide's action, patients with reduced renal function must be monitored carefully to avoid the adverse effects listed below, and dosing intervals must be increased accordingly. This drug is freely dialyzable and presents no elimination problems for the chronic hemodialysis patient. Normal therapeutic plasma concentrations range from 2 to 4 μg/mL.

Adverse Reactions Most often these effects are related to the anticholinergic activity of the drug and include xerostomia, blurred vision, and reduction in nasal and lacrimal secretions. Urinary retention, constipation, and nausea have also been reported. Other more serious adverse effects, including acute psychoses, cholestatic jaundice, hypoglycemia, and agranulocytosis, are reversible upon removal of the drug.

Because disopyramide elevates intraocular pressure, caution should be exercised in patients with narrow-angle glaucoma who are using this drug. Likewise, urinary retention may make the drug unsuitable for use in patients with prostatic hypertrophy. Disopyramide therapy should be undertaken and discontinued cautiously in patients stabilized on warfarin. A 200 percent increase in warfarin dosage was found to be necessary when disopyramide was precipitously withdrawn. The mechanism for this interaction is currently unknown.

Group IB

With the exception of phenytoin, the drugs in this group are chemically related to lidocaine. Actually, they represent oral forms of this primarily parenteral drug.

Lidocaine

Like procainamide, lidocaine is an amide with a local anesthetic effect. The chemistry of lidocaine and its effects on most organ systems are discussed in Chap. 24 ("Local Anesthetics") (see Fig. 27-5).

Cardiac Effects Lidocaine and its oral congeners differ substantially from the group IA drugs with respect to action on the sodium channel. Lidocaine is a true local anesthetic with a pK_a and lipophilic quality to penetrate membranes easily. Futhermore, its action is more easily reversible than quinidine and group IA drugs. Consequently, its ability to affect inactivated blocked sodium channels is greater than that of the group IA drugs (see explanation above, under "Gating Mechanisms"). Since in ischemic myocytes the proportion of blocked to unblocked sodium channels is greater than in nonischemic myocytes, lidocaine and its relatives have a greater effect in myocytes deprived of oxygen. This makes lidocaine and subgroup IB drugs most suitable in cases of acute myocardial infarction and in the recovery period following such injury. Furthermore, lidocaine does not lengthen repolarization and thus is inherently less apt to cause torsade de pointes. This fits in nicely with the fact that lidocaine is of most utility in ventricular tachyarrhythmias associated with myocardial infarction (ischemia) and those of digitalis toxicity.

Although it is the least arrhythmogenic of all drugs used for this purpose, lidocaine is still toxic to the circulation because it depresses contractility and may cause excessive vasodilation. Attention to proper dosage and blood levels is, therefore, important.

Pharmacokinetics Because of its extensive (70 percent) first-pass biotransformation, lidocaine is not given by the oral route. When used as an antiarrhythmic drug, lidocaine is administered almost exclusively via the intravenous route by intermittent bolus or continuous infusion. In emergencies it may be given intramuscularly. The half-life of lidocaine in plasma ranges from 1 to 2 h, but the actual duration of action is shorter (approximately 0.25 h) because the parent compound is redistributed rapidly out of the plasma to other tissues. Lidocaine is well distributed despite the fact that its binding to plasma proteins is in the range of 60 percent. It is concentrated in many tissues relative to the plasma, including heart muscle. Rapid biotransformation and redistribution of the drug cause the concentration in tissues to fall rapidly after a single dose. The liver is the primary site of biotransformation; the hepatic microsomal enzyme system initially oxidatively demethylates lidocaine; then the amide bond is hydrolyzed by amidases. Only about 5 percent of a dose is excreted in the urine without undergoing biotransformation. Plasma concentrations higher than expected can occur when usual doses are given to individuals with severe impairment of hepatic function.

Therapeutic Uses   Lidocaine disappears rapidly from the plasma compartment as it is redistributed to other tissues. A steady-state plasma concentration is quickly reached, however, using continuous constant-rate infusion, and this is the mode of administration most frequently employed. It is imperative that the infusion rate be meticulously controlled to avoid ineffective or toxic concentrations. Therapeutic plasma concentrations range from 1 to 5 μg/mL. Lidocaine is usually administered intravenously for the short-term therapy of life-threatening ventricular arrhythmias such as those which may accompany myocardial infarction and for ventricular arrhythmias which may arise during surgical manipulation of the heart.

Adverse Reactions   Most untoward effects of lidocaine are related to the central nervous system and are believed to be due to its biotransformation products. These undesirable effects can be seen at plasma lidocaine concentrations of 10 μg/mL or more. They include dizziness, excitement, drowsiness, psychosis, confusion, euphoria, and seizures. Respiratory acidosis and alkalosis, nausea, and vomiting may also occur. In normal therapeutic doses, hypotension, heart block, and sinoatrial arrest have been reported.

Drug Interactions   The half-life of propranolol is prolonged when used simultaneously with lidocaine probably as a result of altered hepatic blood flow reducing propranolol's biotransformation. Phenytoin, on the other hand, may decrease lidocaine's activity by speeding its enzymatic destruction in the liver or may exhibit additive effects on the myocardium. Like quinidine and procainamide, lidocaine interacts with muscle-relaxant drugs, enhancing their activity. Procainamide and lidocaine have an additive effect on the central nervous system, causing restlessness and visual hallucination.

Tocainide and Mexiletine

Both these drugs are close chemical congeners of lidocaine (see Fig. 27-5).

Pharmacokinetics   The oral bioavailability of both drugs is good, and both avoid the first-pass effect of lidocaine. Tocainide has a half-life of 11 to 15 h, whereas mexiletine's is 10 to 12 h. Protein binding of tocainide is 10 to 20 percent. That of mexiletine is 50 to 60 percent. Therapeutic serum levels, respectively, of tocainide and mexiletine are 4 to 10 and 0.5 to 2 μg/mL. Both have metabolic byproducts as 25 to 55 percent of tocainide and only 10 percent of mexiletine is excreted unchanged in the urine.

Clinical Use   Both drugs are indicated for symptomatic PVCs, couplets, or runs of ventricular tachycardia. They are ineffective in supraventricular arrhythmias. In practice where these drugs find the most usage is to replace IV lidocaine therapy with oral therapy in post-myocardial infarction accompanied by symptomatic ventricular arrhythmias.

Adverse Reactions   Both drugs have all the toxicities of lidocaine, including worsening of arrhythmias, conduction disturbances, and cardiogenic shock (cardiovascular) and nausea, vomiting, heartburn, diarrhea, dizziness, tremor, nervousness, and skin rash (GI). Tocainide may cause increased ANA (antinuclear antibodies), alopecia, and cinchonism. Both drugs in overdose cause CNS symptoms similar to all local anesthetics. Thus it is doubtful that these drugs are actually more tolerable than quinidine or procainamide in long-term usage.

Phenytoin

The chemistry of phenytoin and effects on most organ systems are discussed in Chap. 21. The major effects of phenytoin on the heart are similar to those of lidocaine. Actually its activity is limited, and it has been useful only because oral substitutes for lidocaine have not been available until recently. Its many adverse reactions do not favor its use in preference to the lidocaine substitutes which are orally bioavailable. In the past phenytoin has been useful in digitalis-induced arrhythmias. However, the more intelligent use of digitalis has supplanted even this use.

Group IC

This subset of sodium-channel blockers is the most powerful of the series presumably because they have a more marked effect on depolarization (see Table 27-1).

Flecainide

Chemically this is a fluorinated congener of procainamide. As can be seen in Fig. 27-5, it is created by insertion of trifluoroethoxy groups on positions 2 and 5 of the procaine benzene ring. The side chain ends in a piperidine ring. These changes alter the pharmacologic effects of procainamide considerably, but flecainide retains its local anesthetic and sodium channel blocking activity.

Electrophysiology Depolarization is markedly slowed, whereas repolarization is only slightly affected. Consequently, responsiveness is reduced and conduction is slowed. The refractory period of normal myocytes is not significantly depressed. High doses of intravenous flecainide easily produce conduction defects such as prolonged atrial-His and His-ventricular intervals, i.e., various degrees of heart block. Generally P-R and QRS intervals are increased by 25 percent, even with therapeutic doses. The J-T interval, measured from the end of the QRS complex to the end of T wave (equivalent to Q-T), is insignificantly prolonged as might be expected from the lack of effects on repolarization. As with other local anesthetics, these changes in membrane actions are more marked in ischemic myocytes, as compared to normal. Thus we have the picture of a powerful antiarrhythmic agent but one which also is potentially quite toxic.

Cardiovascular Effects Cardiac performance is depressed as shown by increases in pulmonary capillary wedge pressure and left ventricular end-systolic volume. Heart rate, blood pressure, and pulmonary vascular resistance ordinarily do not change. Where there is a reduced left ventricular ejection fraction, further depression must be expected. Consequent to the depressive actions, new or worsened heart failure occurs in 5 percent of patients receiving flecainide. In patients who already have considerable heart failure, flecainide therapy can be safely administered only in the hospital, with continuous cardiac monitoring.

Pharmacokinetics Oral bioavailability is 95 percent with peak plasma levels in 2 to 4 h. The plasma half-life is about 20 h. Protein binding is 30 to 40 percent. About 85 percent is excreted in urine as flecainide and metabolites. Obviously dosage must be reduced in patients with renal disease. Therapeutic plasma levels are from 0.2 to 1.0 μg/mL, which is associated with a 90 percent suppression of PVCs. Toxic levels are above 1.0 μg/mL and show a good correlation with adverse ECG changes.

Clinical Use Like other local anesthetics, flecainide is primarily for ventricular arrhythmias. Several studies have confirmed a superiority over quinidine in suppression of PVCs and of eliminating nonsustained ventricular tachycardia. Unfortunately, flecainide is not different from other antiarrhythmic agents because its efficacy is dependent on left ventricular function. Patients with poor function are less likely to have their arrhythmia controlled. In programmed electrical stimulation studies, however, flecainide prevented the induction of sustained ventricular tachycardia in 30 to 50 percent of patients, showing flecainide to be superior to other agents.

The only supraventricular arrhythmia which has been adequately studied is reentry tachycardia (Wolff-Parkinson-White syndrome) where flecainide is quite effective. No long-term studies are available, so the effectiveness of flecainide in preventing sudden death is unknown.

Adverse reactions As with most local anesthetics, CNS symptoms such as tremor, fatigue, and paresthesias can occur. Blurred vision, headache, and nausea have an incidence of about 12 percent.

The provocation of congestive heart failure is uncommon. Proarrhythmic effects are highest in patients with sustained ventricular tachycardia, particularly in patients with low cardiac output who are receiving high initial doses of flecainide.

Encainide

The chemical structure of encainide differs markedly from that of other antiarrhythmic agents. It is a benzanilide compound derived from analogues of lysergic acid (see Fig. 27-5). Oral absorption is good with peak plasma levels in 30 to 90 min and a half-life of 4 h after dosing. Pharmacokinetics are complicated because of two active metabolites, *O*-desmethyl encainide (ODE) and 3-methoxy-*O*-desmethyl encainide (MODE), which cause a nonlinear disposition. All these active elements bind to plasma proteins from 75 to 92 percent. A further complication is that due to genetic differences 7 percent of patients do not convert encainide to ODE and MODE; instead they convert it to *N*-desmethyl encainide. In this case elimination is prolonged to yield a plasma half-life of 6 to 12 h. Such patients require reduced dosage.

The electrophysiologic effects of encainide resemble closely those of flecainide. Some differences are due to the fact that ODE's effects resemble more closely those of group IA. Obviously ECG changes also resemble those described for flecainide.

Clinical use of encainide is primarily for serious ventricular tachyarrhythmias although, like flecainide, it is effective in some supraventricular arrhythmias. It has a tendency to cause proarrhythmia, and its adverse effects are similar to other class I agents. The important question of whether it is capable of preventing sudden death will be answered because it is one of the agents selected for an extensive long-term study in the Cardiac Arrhythmia Suppression Trial.

GROUP II DRUGS

Propranolol

In that all beta blockers decrease stimulatory sympathetic nervous impulses and endogenous catecholamine influences on the heart, they are inhibitory of both supraventricular and ventricular tachyarrhythmias. However, only propranolol and acebutolol have FDA approval for this purpose. Indeed acebutolol's approval is only for the management of PVCs.

Propranolol has been studied most extensively both experimentally and clinically. Unlike the majority of beta blockers available, propranolol has considerable sodium channel blocking activity, especially at higher doses. Some effect in potassium efflux is evident even at low doses. Thus propranolol may be the best choice, although practically all beta blockers can be used for antiarrhythmic action.

Automaticity suppression is the main action. Sinus rate is decreased when sympathetic stimulation is high as in emotional states or in exercise. Suppression of automaticity of Purkinje fibers can also be demon-

strated. There is little effect on the ERP, conduction, or excitability.

It must be emphasized also that propranolol and other β blockers can control arrhythmias by the relief of ischemia by lessening oxygen demand of the heart.

As might be expected, propranolol finds most utility for the control of supraventricular arrhythmias. Atrial premature beats are usually controlled by propranolol alone. In combination with digitalis, propranolol has been used for the control of atrial flutter and fibrillation. Here, however, the end object is not the conversion of the arrhythmia but the slowing of the ventricular rate. In cases refractory to digitalis alone, the addition of propranolol permits sufficient slowing of the ventricular rate apparently by further increasing the refractory period of AV conduction. The combination of quinidine and propranolol to convert atrial fibrillation to sinus rhythm may work when quinidine alone fails. Similarly, control of WPW syndrome may be achieved by this combination. In this case not only is supraventricular tachyarrhythmia suppressed but also the increase in refractory period of the AV nodal area prevents ventricular tachyarrhythmias by suppressing reentry pathways.

Ventricular tachyarrhythmias do not respond to propranolol alone. Premature ventricular beats which occur in the absence of demonstrated heart disease are well controlled and often even if not suppressed become asymptomatic. Tachyarrhythmias as a result of hyperthyroidism are usually well controlled by beta blockers. Here, of course, sympathetic stimulation is an obvious cause.

Beta blockers are often prescribed in ischemic heart disease for they have been proven to decrease mortality especially post-myocardial infarction. They are not a contraindication to the use of other antiarrhythmic agents. Thus, unwittingly, the clinician is currently using combination therapy to control arrhythmias. The complete pharmacology of beta blockers is discussed in Chap. 8.

GROUP III DRUGS

Amiodarone

Chemically amiodarone is quite different from other antiarrhythmics. It has a benzofuranyl cyclic ring with a hydrocarbon chain in addition to the usual benzene ring. The latter with iodine substitutes and chain structure is faintly reminiscent of a thyroxine-like molecule (see Fig. 27-5).

The electrophysiologic effects are also unique. A powerful blocker of sodium channels, it differs from quinidine in being most effective in the channels which are in the inactivated state. Thus it primarily affects tissues with long action potentials. Automaticity is depressed. The main result is a prolongation of action potential duration and ERP with little effect on conduction and responsiveness. There is also little effect on resting membrane potential. In addition, amiodarone is a weak calcium-channel blocker and may also block potassium channels. As a consequence of these complex actions the ECG may show decrease sinus rate, slowing of AV conduction, and slight increase of QRS duration, but the most marked action is prolongation of the Q-T interval.

Clinical use of amiodarone is limited because of its cardiac and extracardiac toxicity. There is agreement that it is the most effective of all antiarrhythmic agents. Both supraventricular and ventricular arrhythmias often respond when other drugs fail. It is particularly effective in WPW syndrome. Suppression of ventricular premature beats occurs in at least 80 percent of patients, while ventricular tachycardia responds in 70 percent of patients.

Cardiac toxicity consists of bradycardia, heart block, and induction of heart failure. As with other antiarrhythmics, proarrhythmia can be produced, although this is less likely than with other agents.

It is the extracardiac cardiac effects which actually limit amiodarone's use. These are due mainly to the deposition of amiodarone as microcrystals in various tissues. These are visible in the cornea as yellow-brown granules which rarely cause visual disturbance except as a halo effect at night in peripheral vision. On discontinuance of the drug, they resolve, but this may take many months. More serious is the deposition of crystals in the skin. This causes photosensitivity, and the sun must be avoided. In some patients a grayish-blue skin discoloration develops. In the lung amiodarone causes inflammation and fibrosis, and this is most limiting in long-term use and with higher doses. Fatalities have been reported. Hepatocellular necrosis may also occur. Less serious adverse reactions are constipation and peripheral neuropathy. Paradoxically amiodarone may cause either hyper- or hypothyroidism. The thyroid function must be monitored, particularly in patients with previous history of thyroid dysfunction.

In addition to these adverse reactions, amiodarone interacts with many other cardiac drugs. When administered together with either warfarin, digoxin, quinidine, procainamide, or phenytoin, the activity of these drugs is increased by 50 to 300 percent, presumably because their biotransformation is reduced.

The complex pharmacokinetics of amiodarone add to the difficulty of its use. The oral drug is slowly and variably absorbed, averaging about a 50 percent bioavailability. Peak plasma concentrations are observed 3 to 7 h after a single dose. There is a 2- to 3-day and sometimes longer lag between achievement of an adequate blood levels of 1 to 2 μg/mL and observable clinical effects. The volume of distribution is very large, averaging 60 L/kg. This fits in with its accumulation, including metabolites in fat, liver, lung, and spleen. Elimination is mainly by bile excretion with negligible renal removal. After discontinuance of the drug, antiarrhythmic effects may persist for weeks or months.

Because of these unusual pharmacokinetic parameters, amiodarone requires large loading doses (500 to 1600 mg for 1 to 3 weeks), which are then gradually adjusted to a maintenance daily dose of 400 mg.

Because of these toxicity restrictions, amiodarone is assigned only to the therapy of very serious tachyarrhythmias such as a recurrent ventricular fibrillation and hemodynamically unstable ventricular tachycardia. Therapy is usually started in a hospital where monitoring and resuscitation facilities are available.

Bretylium

This agent is unique in being a quaternary amine (see Fig. 27-5). As such it is poorly absorbed orally and is used only as an intravenous or intramuscular agent.

Like many quaternary amines, it initiates release of neuronal catecholamines followed by inhibition. This, however, is not its main antiarrhythmic action. In fact, the initial release of catecholamines can precipitate arrhythmias and requires caution. Bretylium has a direct action, especially on ischemic myocytes. The action potential of ischemic myocytes in particular is lengthened along with the ERP. Conduction and responsiveness are not affected. Automaticity is suppressed. The ECG shows decreased sinus rate and increased P-R and Q-T intervals.

Oral bioavailability is poor. Peak plasma concentrations are seen within 1 h of intramuscular administration. However, suppression of premature beats may not be seen until 6 to 9 h after administration. Intravenous administration results in immediate antiarrhythmia effects, but generally suppression of ventricular tachycardia may take 20 min to several hours to be clearly manifest. Elimination of the unchanged drug is mainly renal.

Adverse reactions to bretylium consist of transient hypertension followed by hypotension and postural effects. Syncope may occur. Nausea and vomiting are induced by rapid IV infusion. Initial worsening of arrhythmias may occur, and precipitation of angina is a possibility.

Bretylium is an emergency drug which is used in situations where other procedures and drugs have failed. It is clearly of utility only in ventricular tachyarrhythmias and there on an emergency basis.

GROUP IV DRUGS

Verapamil

The calcium-channel blockers are naturally of greater utility in supraventricular tachyarrhythmias where the slow calcium current has a greater influence on the action potential of nodal myocytes as compared with that on ventricular myocytes. The sinus rate is slowed, and the ERP of atrial myocytes and the AV node is prolonged. Thus calcium-channel blockers can effectively suppress atrial tachycardia. Also they can very effectively suppress the ventricular rate in atrial flutter and fibrillation. For these purposes the calcium-channel blockers have either supplemented or replaced digitalis, propranolol, and even cardioversion for these arrhythmias.

Verapamil has been the preferred agent, but diltiazem is also effective, whereas nifedipine has little antiarrhythmic activity. Other calcium-channel blockers under development may also be effective. The pharmacology of these agents is completely discussed in Chap. 28.

CLINICAL ASPECTS OF ANTIARRHYTHMIC THERAPY

Very few therapies match antiarrhythmic drug therapy with respect to the capacity to accurately pinpoint physiologic and anatomic defects and to select specific agents or devices for correction. Unfortunately, all antiarrhythmic drug therapy treats symptoms and not the cause of the membrane aberration which precipitates the arrhythmia. Therefore, the first guiding principle is to treat the cause rather than the symptoms. Since by far a great majority of arrhythmias are the result of ischemia, oxygen therapy, heart failure therapy, and attention to respiratory difficulties are the first line of attack. Ultimately surgical correction (coronary angioplasty, bypass surgery) may be needed. Drugs which aid coronary circulation such as beta blockers and nitrites have been shown to reduce mortality, and none of the antiarrhythmic drugs have this distinction.

Yet a patient with a tachyarrhythmia will surely die unless the arrhythmia stops spontaneously or is arrested by medical or surgical interventions. The tachyarrhythmias which require immediate intervention in ascending order of urgency are shown in Table 27-3. Those arrhythmias which are frequently treated because they cause symptoms or because it is felt that therapy will be prophylatic against sudden death are also shown in Table 27-3.

The currently available technology has refined antiarrhythmic therapy so that selection of the proper drug or procedure may depend on sophisticated diagnostic procedures such as clinical electrophysiologic testing. At the least, the minimal requirement to effectively prescribe antiarrhythmic therapy requires in and out of the hospital ECG rhythm monitoring. In addition, antiarrhythmic drugs have a narrow therapeutic range, and in many cases maintenance of plasma levels spells the difference between success, failure, and toxicity. This assumes that qualified laboratories are available. In addition, the fragile nature of rhythm maintenance in sick hearts requires that resuscitative measures be accessible at all times. Devices which are worn by the patient and continuously monitor the rhythm of the heart and diagnose the onset of a dangerous tachyarrhythmia, as well as immediately apply cardioversion, have been devised. The efficacy of these devices in preventing sudden death is being compared to that of drugs.

TABLE 27-3 Therapy of tachyarrhythmias

Arrhythmia	Drug or other therapy
Tachyarrhythmias requiring immediate therapy to prevent sudden death (in ascending order of urgency)	
Atrial tachycardia	Verapamil, digitalis, beta blockers.
Atrial flutter	Verapamil, digitalis, beta blockers, sodium-channel blockers.
WPW with ventricular tachycardia	Sodium-channel blockers, especially group IC; in desperate cases amiodarone.
Ventricular tachycardia	Sodium-channel blockers, bretylium, cardioversion, surgical removal of ectopic focus.
Ventricular fibrillation	Cardioversion with or without the prior use of drugs followed by prophylactic drug therapy usually sodium-channel blockers and in refractory cases amiodarone.
Tachyarrhythmias which are treated for the relief of symptoms and with the expectation that sudden death will be prevented	
WPW without ventricular tachycardia	Any group IA drugs such as quinidione or disopyramide.
Frequent atrial premature beats	Propranolol or other beta blockers and verapamil or diltiazem.

Ventricular premature beats
  Frequent with symptoms
 	
  With myocardial infarction
	Any of group I drugs
	  Quinidine, disopyramide, tocainide, and flecainide.
	  Group IB drugs are favored, lidocaine and congeners.

Ventricular tachycardia (unsustained)	Any of group I drugs which can be tolerated and which significantly reduce incidence. Group IC drugs are the most effective but also the most toxic.

BIBLIOGRAPHY

Anderson, G. J.: "Antiarrhythmic Actions of Amiodarone," *Am. Fam. Physician*, **25**:178–180 (1982).

DiPalma, J. R., and J. Schultz: "Antifibrillatory Drugs," *Medicine*, **29**:123–168 (1950).

DiPalma, J. R., and G. J. Anderson: in R. E. Rakel (ed.), *Premature Beats in Conn's Current Therapy*, Saunders, Philadelphia, 1984.

Hamer, J.: "Antiarrhythmic Drugs," in J. Hamer (ed.), *Drugs for Heart Diseases*, 3d ed., Chapman and Hall, London, 1987, pp. 1–28.

Hearse, D. J., A. S. Manning, and M. J. James: *Life-Threatening Arrhythmias during Ischemia and Infarction*, Raven, New York, 1987.

Muhiddin, K. A., and P. Turner: "Is There an Ideal Antiarrhythmic Drug? A Review—with Particular Reference to Class 1 Antiarrhythmic Agents," *Postgrad. Med. J.*, **61**:665–678 (1985).

Nestico, P. F., and J. Morganroth: Flecainide: "A New Antiarrhythmic Agent," *Am. Fam. Physician*, **34**:197–200 (1986).

Noda, M., et al.: "Primary Structure of *Electrophorus electricus* Sodium Channel Deduced from cDNA Sequence," *Nature*, **312**:121–127 (1984).

Noda, M., et al.: "Existence of Distinct Sodium Channel Messenger RNAs in Rat Brain," *Nature*, **320**:188–192 (1986).

Salkoff, L. B., and M. A. Tanouye: "Genetics of Ion Channels," *Physiol. Rev.*, **66**:301–320 (1986).

Scholtysik, G., and U. Quast: "Sodium Channel Pharmacology in Mammalian Cardiac Cells: Extension by DPI 201–106," *Triangle*, **25**:105–116 (1986).

Vaughan Williams E. M.: "A Classification of Antiarrhythmic Actions Reassessed after a Decade of New Drugs," *J. Clin. Pharmacol.*, **24**:129–147 (1984).

Vaughan Williams E. M.: *Antiarrhythmic Action and the Puzzle of Perhexiline*, Academic, New York, 1980.

Volosin K. J., and A. J. Greenspon: "Tocainide: A New Drug for Ventricular Arrhythmias," *Am. Fam. Physician*, **33**:233–235 (1986).

Woolsey, R. L., A. J. J. Wood, and D. M. Roden: "Encainide," *N. Engl. J. Med.*, **318**:1107–1115 (1988).

C H A P T E R 28

Antianginal Drugs

Joseph R. DiPalma

Angina pectoris, or pain in the chest, is a characteristic painful sensation which is reflective of ischemia of the myocardium. Usually it is precipitated by exercise, excitement, or a heavy meal. It is relieved by rest. This type of angina is classified as fixed, or stable angina, because it occurs under predictable circumstances. The cause is an obstruction in one or more of the major coronary arteries, and the lesion is usually arteriosclerotic. Generally narrowing of the vessel must be 50 percent or more before any appreciable ischemia occurs.

A second type of angina (so-called variant, or Prinzmetal, angina) is believed to be due to vasospasm. It occurs at rest or even during sleep and is unpredictable or unstable. An individual may have a mixture of both stable and unstable angina.

The heart has no pain fibers. Angina is, therefore, a referred type of pain mediated probably over autonomic nervous system fibers segmentally to the upper thoracic spinal segments. It is usually felt in the left shoulder and arm, the neck, and rarely in the right shoulder. Resection of the cervical sympathetic ganglia relieves the pain. So does any chest operation which disturbs the autonomic innervation of the heart. Sedatives, alcohol, opioids, and various CNS drugs also relieve the pain but obviously do nothing for the ischemia. The physician must recognize this and treat the ischemia primarily and not simply make the patient more comfortable. In fact, ischemia of the myocardium may occur without pain or any symptoms—so-called *silent ischemia*. It is even more important for

the physician to recognize the existence of this type of ischemia by appropriate diagnostic methods and to treat it in order to prevent myocardial infarction and possible sudden death.

The major drugs which have been found useful in the therapy of myocardial ischemia and the relief of the pain of angina pectoris are peripheral vascular and coronary vessel vasodilators. These include the nitrates and nitrites, beta-adrenergic blockers and calcium-channel antagonists.

THE NITRATES AND NITRITES

Pharmacologic Classification

This group includes both organic nitrites and organic nitrates. The names and formulas of four antianginal compounds are shown in Fig. 28-1. It is believed that all the compounds in this class have a similar mechanism of action. As antianginal agents, the nitrates may be classified into (1) rapidly acting agents used to terminate an attack of angina and (2) agents with prolonged action, which are employed to prevent attacks of angina. Nitroglycerin (glyceryl trinitrate) and amyl nitrite are rapidly acting agents with a short duration of action. Other organic nitrates used for prolonged action are erythrityl tetranitrate, isosorbide dinitrate, and pentaerythrityl tetranitrate. These agents are administered orally to prevent angina attacks. However, isosorbide dinitrate and erythrityl tetranitrate

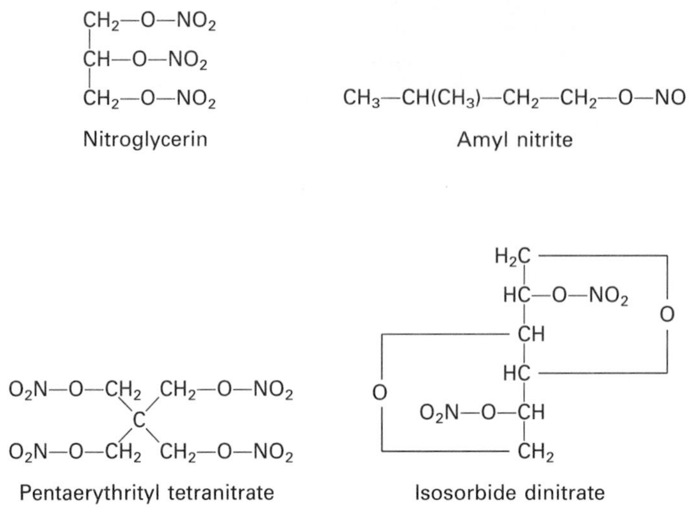

FIGURE 28-1 Structural formulas of nitrates and amyl nitrite.

have been administered sublingually to terminate acute attacks and obtain a more prolonged effect.

Mechanism of Action

At a molecular level, despite much investigation, there is still doubt about the intimate mechanism of action. Certain facts seem well established. Nitrates are converted to the nitrite form (NO) in the smooth-muscle cell. The receptor has sulfhydryl groups which apparently can convert NO_2 to NO. This free radical, in turn, reacts with guanylate cyclase to cause increased synthesis of guanosine 3′-5′-monophosphate (cyclic GMP). As a result cyclic GMP-dependent protein kinase is activated, and as a consequence there is less phosphorylation of muscle protein. Dephosphorylated muscle protein has less capacity to contract. In this manner nitrates relax all smooth muscle, including that of the biliary system, ureters, and bronchioles. However, the relaxing action is most active in blood vessels. It might be added that this mechanism of action is also that of sodium nitroprusside (Chap. 31).

Dilating the coronary vessels selectively cannot completely explain the beneficial actions of vasodilators. In the stable form of angina this does not work because the lesion in the vessel forms a rigid structure which is incapable of dilation. Moreover, the coronary circulation always operates under conditions of maxi-

mum dilation and responds to ischemia itself as a most powerful stimulation to dilate. Also the vessels not involved with the atherosclerotic lesion which are capable of dilating increase the blood flow to normal myocardium, thus relatively decreasing the flow to the ischemic area. This is commonly called *coronary steal* and is actually harmful rather than beneficial. There is one exception. In variant angina the atherosclerotic lesion is only partially developed, and the vessel is capable of spasm. This has been proven by the injection of small amounts of ergonovine into the involved coronary artery under direct visualization during catheterization. This produces spasm in sensitized vessels. Coronary vasodilators relieve this spasm and do benefit the ischemic area.

The consensus of most cardiologists is that it is mainly the effects of vasodilators on the peripheral circulation which produce the beneficial action in angina. This is best considered in terms of the oxygen supply/demand ratio. At each level of work the heart requires a definite amount of oxygen. Vasodilators reduce peripheral arterial resistance and thus afterload; they also dilate veins and reduce venous return, hence preload. The resulting decrease in left ventricular volume makes the heart more efficient. The demand for oxygen is thus reduced at a given level of cardiac output. It may also be said that the vasodilator agents used to relieve angina increase the tolerance of the individual to exercise. As will be seen when other agents are discussed, other factors such as heart rate enter into the equation, but it is important to appreciate that the main thrust in the drug therapy of angina is to reduce the work of the heart to the point where the diseased coronary vessels are still able to supply the required oxygen.

There is, however, considerable evidence that some vasodilator drugs such as the nitrates directly affect the coronary circulation beneficially. They are particularly effective in vasospastic angina, and there is no doubt about their ability to dilate coronaries as observed angiographically. In animal models nitrates also increase circulation in the ischemic zone. Nitrates appear to favor the development of collateral circulation and also improve the ratio of endocardial to epicardial flow. The latter is important, since most ischemic areas are more severe in the endocardial zone as compared with the epicardial zone. The direct cardiac effects of nitrates or indeed any vascular dilator undoubtedly depend also on individual differences. The number of coronary vessels involved, the degree of development of collateral circulation, and the nature of the arteriosclerotic lesion are all important factors.

Pharmacodynamics

Nitrates have been shown to have a general vasodilator effect. Their action is generally more prominent in the postcapillary vessels, which favors pooling of blood in the systemic peripheral circulation. Venous return is thus consistently decreased and becomes more dependent on positional changes. Nitrates produce relaxation of all vascular smooth muscle, but the magnitude of their effect varies in different vascular beds. In the skin, nitrates produce vasodilation often associated with "flushing" of the skin of the neck and face. This effect is more prominent with amyl nitrite than with the longer-acting compounds.

Nitrates tend to produce tachycardia and reflex increase in contractility, which increases the work of the heart and may reduce its efficiency. In those patients in whom tachycardia is a problem, it is wise to use other antianginal drugs such as beta blockers and calcium-channel blockers, which slow heart rate.

In the cerebral vessels, nitrates produce vasodilation and an increase in intracerebral pressure. This, coupled with the decrease in systemic pressure, results in a decrease in blood flow through the brain, which may account for the headaches that are usually associated with nitrate therapy.

Retinal vessels dilate following use of nitrates; this can be directly observed through the ophthalmoscope. As may be expected, intracular tension is also increased, but with the short-acting compounds, this effect is not considered to be significant in relation to the drainage of the anterior chamber. However, caution in the use of short-acting compounds is recommended in glaucoma.

The relationship of the smooth muscle of the ureter, bile duct, and gut requires high doses. Attempts to utilize nitrates as antispasmodics have met with little success.

Pharmacokinetics

Most of the nitrates used therapeutically are absorbed through the mucous membranes, and many are absorbed through the skin. Gastrointestinal absorption, however, is variable. Amyl nitrite, a highly volatile liquid, is rapidly absorbed from the lungs as well as through mucous membranes. Its onset of action is 0.5 min and duration is 3 to 5 min. It is partially eliminated from the lungs and partially hydrolyzed to nitrite ion. Amyl nitrite is little used in medical practice. It has become a drug of abuse imagined to increase sexual pleasure and prowess.

Nitroglycerin is absorbed from mucous membranes, from the lungs, and through the skin. It is less effective following oral administration than sublingual administration. It is biotransformed in the liver by action of a glutathione-organic nitrate reductase. The products are 1,3- or 1,2-glyceryl dinitrate, which are weakly active compared with nitroglycerin. Excretion is urinary after inactivation to mononitrates. The oral dose is 20 times the sublingual dose because of the inactivation by gastric juice and a liver first-pass effect.

Although most other organic nitrates are administered orally, absorption through the mucous membranes has been demonstrated in most cases. Some of these (for example, isosorbide dinitrate and erythrityl tetranitrate) are also available for sublingual administration. Oral preparations of organic nitrates are absorbed slowly from the gastrointestinal tract. The exact fate of these compounds is not entirely known, although most appear to be biotransformed and excreted in the form of various nitrites and nitrates. The half-life for isosorbide dinitrate is 30 min, and for pentaerythrityl tetranitrate it is 2 h.

There are now many forms of nitroglycerin available, from intravenous to transdermal (see Table 28-1). The translingual spray is the most recent addition with a spectrum of activity similar to that of sublingual tablets but somewhat more convenient to use. Transdermal patches are less reliable than the topical ointment.

Tolerance

Repeated administration of nitrates leads to the development of tolerance manifested by the need for higher doses to produce the same effect. There is cross-tolerance between various compounds of this class. The mechanism of nitrite tolerance may be associated with the inability to convert NO_2 to NO by sulfhydryl. Experimentally tolerance may be reversed by the administration of dithiothreitol, a sulfhydryl regenerating agent. In general, tolerance develops quickly, within 2 to 3 weeks, but also disappears quickly, so that lack of exposure to nitrates for several days reestablishes the original sensitivity. Tolerance to nitrate-induced headache appears to develop more quickly than other nitrate effects. Headache symptoms may disappear within a few days after onset of therapy. Some cardiologists use intermittent administration to avoid tolerance.

TABLE 28-1   Available dosage forms of nitroglycerin with estimates of onset and duration of action

Dosage form	Onset	Duration
Intravenous	Immediate	3–5 min
Sublingual	1–3 min	0.5–1 h
Translingual spray	2 min	0.5–1 h
Oral sustained release	30 min	4–8 h
Topical ointment	0.5–1 h	2–12 h
Transdermal	0.5–1 h	18–24 h

Therapeutic Use

The short-acting nitrates are the most potent agents known for terminating an acute attack of angina. Nitroglycerin is the most frequently used agent. Pain is relieved within 1 to 3 min after sublingual administration of nitroglycerin. A similar effect can be produced with inhalation of amyl nitrite, but side effects are usually more prominent. Sublingual preparations of long-acting nitrates (isosorbide dinitrate, erythrityl tetranitrate) are effective within 3 to 5 min, and their effect may last for 1 to 2 h. Orally administered nitrates require a longer period (up to 30 min) to produce an effect which may last from 4 to 8 h (see Table 28-1). In general, oral preparations of organic nitrates are used prophylactically to reduce the frequency of attacks of angina, especially prior to activities known to precipitate angina attacks in a patient (e.g., physical exertion or emotional stress). The value of such prophylactic use of nitrates apparently varies and has not been conclusively demonstrated.

Various other drugs have been combined for the treatment of angina. It is not unusual to combine nitrates, beta blockers, and calcium-channel blockers. Antianxiety agents may overcome the apprehension of heart disease and the resulting enforcement of pain sensation. In general, the use of various mild sedatives and tranquilizers is considered a valuable adjuvant therapy in the treatment of angina pectoris. Similarly, therapeutic management includes the exclusion of stimulants (e.g., tobacco), reassurance by the physician, and avoidance of excessive emotional or physical stress. Moderate exercise, however, is considered by some to be an important part of long-term treatment.

Adverse Reactions

Certain undesirable effects of nitrates are related to their effects on the cardiovascular system. Throbbing headaches, flushing of the face, and dizziness are common, especially at the beginning of treatment. Headache is particularly common with some of the longer-acting compounds. Usually its severity decreases with continued use, but occasionally it may be so severe as to preclude further treatment. Postural hypotension is another common reaction which is apparently due to pooling of blood in the veins of the dependent parts of the body. The hypotensive effect of nitrates is potentially dangerous in patients with renal insufficiency, since it can aggravate renal ischemia. The use of nitrates is also contraindicated in acute myocardial infarction. Similarly, administration of nitrates in patients who also receive potent antihypertensive agents requires particular caution. Marked hypotension has also been reported in patients under nitrate treatment following ingestion of alcoholic beverages.

Gastrointestinal disturbances, including nausea and vomiting, are not uncommon following orally administered nitrates. The inorganic nitrites may lead to the development of methemoglobinemia. This is due to oxidation of hemoglobin by the nitrite ion and is useful in cyanide poisoning because of the high affinity of CN^- for methemoglobin (see Chap. 49).

Acute nitrate poisoning in humans is manifest by flushing of the face, marked fall in blood pressure, vomiting, cyanosis, and collapse. Death may occur from circulatory collapse or from respiratory failure.

Preparations

Amyl nitrite is available in fragile ampuls containing 0.2 to 0.3 mL. Ampuls are crushed in a handkerchief, and the released vapor is inhaled.

Nitroglycerin is available as sublingual tablets of various strengths, as capsules, and as an ointment (Nitrol, NitroBid, Nitrong) containing 2% nitroglycerin in a lanolin-petrolatum base, 0.3 to 9 mg.

Other forms of nitroglycerin are *intravenous*, available in concentrations of 0.5 to 10 mg/mL in sterile ampuls; *transdermal*, available in special delivery systems with nitroglycerin release rates of 2.5 to 15 mg per 24 h.

Erythrityl tetranitrate (Cardilate) is available in tablets of 5, 10, and 15 mg.

Isosorbide dinitrate (Isordil, Sorbitrate) is available in tablets for oral (5, 10, 20 mg) or sublingual (2.5 and 5 mg) use and in sustained-release tablets (40 mg).

Pentaerythrityl tetranitrate (Peritrate, PETN) is available in tablets of 10, 20, and 40 mg and in sustained-release tablets of 30, 45, 60, and 80 mg.

BETA-ADRENERGIC BLOCKING DRUGS

A very considerable advance in the therapy of angina has been the use of beta-adrenergic blocking agents (Chap. 8). The hemodynamic effects of beta-blocking agents may be listed as decreased heart rate, reduced blood pressure and cardiac contractility without appreciable reduction in cardiac output. These effects are most evident at rest but also persist during exercise. There is in brief a modulating effect on the heart with a buffering action against sympathetic stimulation and the cardiac autoregulatory mechanism. The reduced heart rate improves efficiency, while the longer diastolic interval allows improved coronary blood perfusion. The decrease in contractility is the cause of the reduced blood pressure. The beta blocking agents do not directly cause a decrease in peripheral resistance.

Blockade of the adrenergic drive of the heart may account for the moderation of blood pressure and decrease in heart work. Patients complain of fatigue and lack of drive and not being able to perform heavy exercise. Also patients with poor cardiac reserve are susceptible to the induction of congestive heart failure. Attempts to correct this by producing beta blockers with some beta-agonist activity such as pindolol have not been entirely successful. Although only propranolol and nadolol have been approved by the FDA for the therapy of angina, the other available beta blockers appear to be equally effective.

Acute attacks of angina are best treated with nitroglycerin. Beta blockers are suitable for chronic therapy and are especially useful in the angina, which sometimes develops post-myocardial infarction. Indeed the beta blockers are complementary to nitrate therapy because they correct the tendency of these drugs to increase heart rate. They also allow the nitrates to be used intermittently, thus minimizing the development of tolerance to nitrates. On the other hand, nitrates can be said to counteract some undesirable effects of beta blockers.

While it does not seem to matter which beta blocker is selected to treat angina, the question of dose is an important one. It is wise to start with minimal effective doses and gradually build up the dose to a satisfactory level balancing beneficial actions against side effects. As a guide, the resting heart rate should be 50 to 60 beats per minute. Exercise should increase the heart rate to no more than 100 to 120 heartbeats per minute (for the complete pharmacology of beta blockers and preparations and doses see Chap. 8).

CALCIUM-CHANNEL BLOCKERS

The membranes of most cells, but especially those of smooth muscle, cardiac muscle, and nerve, contain channels for the conduct of calcium into the cell. These channels are of two types; one is voltage-sensitive like that of sodium. Other channels exist which are not voltage-sensitive. The calcium channels in contrast to sodium channels are slowly conducting, and hence the term "slow calcium channel." (See Chap. 27 for relationship to action potential.) As with sodium, calcium must be pumped out of the cell against a gradient, and as with sodium, this is accomplished by a calcium-sensitive ATPase. In addition, recall that there is a sodium-calcium exchange which further regulates the available amount of free calcium in the cytosol. This mechanism comes into play with the action of digitalis in heart muscle (see Chap. 26). Calcium is, of course, involved in many other important cellular metabolisms, not the least of which is the formation of bone. These concern hormonal mechanisms covered in Chap. 35. Here we are concerned with the role of calcium in the control of the tone of smooth muscle, especially that of the vasculature.

Originally this group of drugs was developed as coronary vasodilators, and they were used as such in Europe for some years before it was found that they inhibited the contractile action of calcium on smooth muscle and cardiac muscle. Originally known as *calcium antagonists*, their main action is on membrane calcium channels, as it has been only recently discovered. These include not only those that are voltage-sensitive but also those that are voltage-insensitive. The name *calcium-channel blockers* is, therefore, more aptly applied to this subset of calcium antagonists.

Chemistry

The calcium-channel blockers have a very diverse chemistry, and this may indicate that there are different receptor sites in calcium channels on the cell membrane and within the cell. *Verapamil* is a benzene acetonitrile and is the oldest of the currently available agents. *Diltiazem* is a thiodiazepine, and *nifedipine* is a dihydropyridine. Only diltiazem is freely water-soluble, the others being highly lipid soluble. Structural formulas are shown in Fig. 28-2. Nicardipine, a newer agent, is related to nifedipine.

Mechanism of Action

There is now ample evidence that contraction of vascular smooth muscle is controlled by the cytoplasmic concentration of calcium. Two main mechanisms regulate the cystolic calcium concentration. The first of

these involves voltage-dependent calcium channels which respond to depolarization of the membrane by opening. Extracellular calcium moves into the cells as a result. This mechanism is known as *electromechanical coupling*. A second mechanism exists which is independent of membrane polarization. This involves release of calcium from the sarcoplasmic reticulum, which secondarily causes an influx of extracellular calcium through non-voltage-linked calcium channels.

Transduction of the increased calcium concentration, by either mechanism, occurs by binding of calcium to calmodulin. In turn, the Ca^{2+}-calmodulin complex initiates phosphorylation of the light chain of myosin by activation of light-chain kinase. Contraction of smooth muscle results from the interaction of phosphorylated light-chain myosin and actin (see Fig. 28-3).

The calcium-channel blockers can block the influx of calcium by either mechanism. However, the voltage-dependent channels respond to a lower concentration than the non-voltage-dependent channels. It thus appears that the ratio of voltage-sensitive to non-voltage-sensitive channels determines the selectivity of response of veins and arteries. At the doses used clinically, calcium-channel blockers relax arterial smooth muscle with little action on veins.

It will be recalled that excitation-contraction coupling in cardiac myocytes depends more on sodium than calcium influx. Consequently calcium-channel blockers have relatively little effect on contractility at doses which relax smooth muscle. However, the cardiac myocytes at the sinoatrial and atrioventricular nodes are more importantly dependent on movement of calcium through slow channels. The calcium-channel blockers (especially verapamil and also diltiazem, but not nifedipine) impede recovery of the cardiac slow calcium channels. Consequently heart rate is slowed and conduction from atrium to ventricle is blocked (see Chap. 27).

Pharmacodynamics

The calcium-channel blockers tend to relax and reduce the tone of all smooth muscle. This has led to some attempts to use such agents as antispasmodics in gastrointestinal disorders and asthma. Clearly the relaxing action is most marked on vascular smooth muscle. Arterioles are much more affected than veins. Thus calcium-channel blockers lower blood pressure and reduce afterload without appreciable effect on pre-

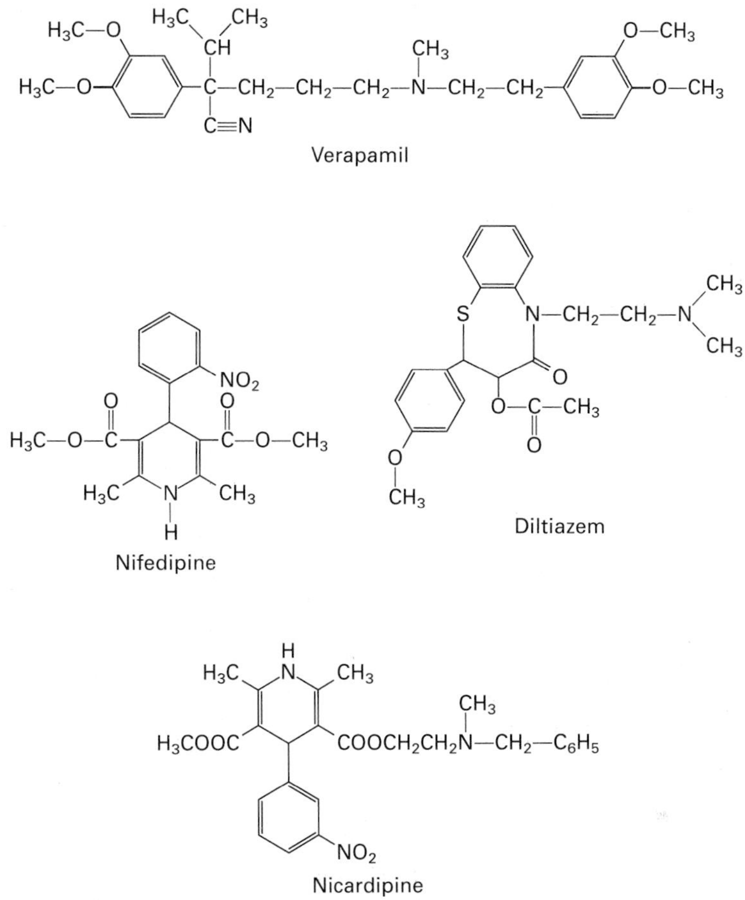

FIGURE 28-2 Structural formulas of calcium-channel blockers.

load. In this regard nifedipine is the most effective, followed by verapamil and then diltiazem (Table 28-2). Benefit in angina consists not only of the vasodilatory action on coronary vessels, especially vasospastic ones, but also in the reduction of afterload, hence oxygen requirements, of the heart.

Both the action potential and muscle contraction of the heart are calcium-related. A reduction in calcium entry into the myocytes, especially those of the SA and AV nodes, results in slowing of the rate of SA node and slowing of conduction in the AV node. Actual contractility of the ventricular muscle is usually not affected at therapeutic dose levels, and indeed cardiac output may actually increase as a result of the decrease in peripheral resistance. With toxic doses or in hearts already in failure, myocardial contractility may be severely com-

promised. The cardiac effects are useful. Verapamil and diltiazem are effective in blocking the numerous impulses to the ventricle in atrial flutter and fibrillation by effectively slowing the ventricular rate to an effective level. In this regard calcium-channel blockers can be used instead of, or in combination with, digitalis to control the ventricular rate in atrial flutter and fibrillation. They are also effective in arresting atrial tachycardia (see Chap. 27).

Skeletal muscle is not affected by calcium-channel blockers. Fortunately, there is a large intracellular pool of calcium in the skeletal muscle fiber so that dependence on transmembrane calcium influx is not required.

The excitation-coupling mechanism involving calcium also is operative in other organs such as glands

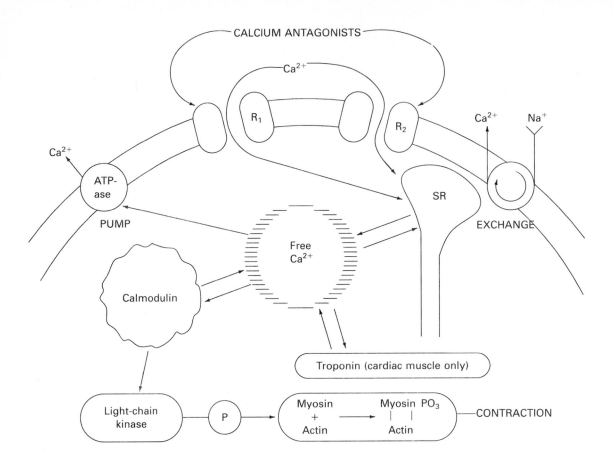

FIGURE 28-3 Schematic diagram of the mechanism of action of calcium-channel blockers. A section of cell membrane is shown with calcium channels R_1 (voltage-dependent) and R_2 (non-voltage-dependent). Calcium influx occurs through both channels and is stored in the sarcoplasmic reticulum (SR). There is a small pool of free calcium, which is a second messenger. It is in equilibrium with the calcium in SR and also with calcium bound to calmodulin. The level of free calcium is crucial to muscle tone and contraction. In heart muscle which has troponin the action of calcium is direct to remove the barrier between the interaction of myosin and actin to cause contraction. In smooth muscle free calcium attaches to a small protein, calmodulin, which in turn activates light-chain kinase which promotes the phosphorylation (P) of myosin, which again permits the myosin actin interaction and muscle contraction. (It might be recalled that nitrates through cyclic GMP, and also beta-adrenergic antagonists through cyclic AMP, inhibit light-chain kinase.) Calmodulin-calcium stimulates, and it is in this manner that the level of cytosolic free calcium controls the tonus of smooth muscle. It must also be mentioned that calcium is pumped out of the cell by an ATPase system in the membrane similar to that of sodium. There is also a sodium/calcium exchange during depolarization: with sodium influx some calcium leaves the cell. Thus the receptors for calcium antagonists are the calcium influx channels. These have gates and have activated and resting states similar to the sodium channels, but their workings are less well understood. (Modified from Opie and Thadani, 1987.)

TABLE 28-2 Comparative cardiovascular actions of calcium-channel blockers

Drug	FDA indications	Reduction of vascular resistance (peripheral)	Reduction of heart block	Cardiac contractility
Nifedipine	Vasospastic and stable angina	+ + + +	0	+
Verapamil	Vasospastic and stable angina, atrial flutter and fibrillation, paroxysomal atrial tachycardia, essential hypertension	+ + +	+ +	+ +
Diltiazem	Vasospastic and stable angina	+ +	+ +	+

and the functioning of nerve endings. Experimental demonstration has been made of inhibition of secretion by the pituitary and pancreas of peptide hormones by calcium-channel blockers. Depression of release of transmitters from synaptosomes has also been revealed. Although verapamil has been shown to inhibit insulin release in humans, generally the dose is higher for these glandular and nervous effects than is required in the management of angina.

Pharmacokinetics

Calcium-channel blockers are oral drugs with reasonable oral bioavailability (Table 28-3). The onset of action is evident within 30 min, and peak effect varies

from 30 to 180 min. Elimination half-lives are from 3 to 6 h. Urinary excretion is the primary mode for nifedipine and verapamil, while diltiazem is excreted in the feces. All are protein-bound in the blood (80 to 90 percent). Metabolism of all the available compounds is extensive. Indeed verapamil and diltiazem undergo extensive first-pass hepatic metabolism. For emergency situations an intravenous preparation of verapamil is available.

Clinical Use

The most intensive use of calcium-channel blockers has been for angina and particularly the vasospastic variety. The FDA-approved uses are listed in Table

TABLE 28-3 Some pharmacokinetic parameters of calcium-channel blockers

Drug	Oral bioavailability absolute, %	Onset of action (oral), min	Time to peak effect, min	Half-life, h
Nifedipine	45–70	20	30	2–5
Verapamil	10–35	30	60–80	3–7
Diltiazem	40–65	30	120–180	3–5+

28-2. Actually all three drugs can be and are used for hypertension (see Chap. 31). As antiarrhythmic drugs, verapamil and diltiazem are superior (see Chap. 27). Nifedipine has a selectivity for vascular smooth muscle and has little affinity for myocardial receptors.

Adverse Reactions

The most serious toxic effects of calcium-channel blockers stem from their pharmacologic actions. With higher doses, or in especially sensitive cardiac muscle, reduction in calcium influx can cause severe reduction in contractility with consequent abrupt fall in cardiac output. In addition, excessive slowing and heart block can also precipitate heart failure. Actually severe and fatal episodes have been rarely reported; nevertheless, as shown in Table 28-4, the most frequent adverse reactions are cardiovascular. These include episodes of hypotension due to excessive vasodilation.

The central nervous system adverse effects may be due to the hypotensive effects but are more likely the result of a direct action. They are more frequent with nifedipine, which has the most effect on vascular resistance. Adverse reactions are summarized in Table 28-4.

Drug Interactions

As might be expected from a drug group that affects so vital a mechanism as calcium control of cellular functions, there are many drug interactions which have clinical significance. Some of the most important may be listed as follows:

1. Physiologic-Pharmacologic basis
   a. Beta-adrenergic blockers have negative inotropic and chronotropic cardiac effects. These are additive to similar actions of calcium-channel

TABLE 28-4   Adverse reactions generally encountered with the use of calcium-channel blockers

Adverse reaction	Nifedipine, %	Verapamil, %	Diltiazem, %
Cardiovascular			
Peripheral edema	10–12	1–2	2–3
Hypotension	5	3	1
Bradycardia		1	1
Congestive heart failure	2–7	1–2	1
Pulmonary edema	2	1–2	1
Central nervous system			
Dizziness	10–12	3–4	1–2
Lightheadness	10–12		
Headache	10–12	1–2	2
Weakness, shakiness	2–10		1
Gastrointestinal			
Nausea	10	2–3	2
Dermatologic			
Rash	2		1+
Pruritis	2		1
Hair loss		1	
Photosensitivity	[a]		1

[a]Can occur but has not been reported.
Source: Adapted from *Facts and Comparisons*, J. B. Lippincott Company, St. Louis, 1988.

blockers. While both groups of drugs can be used together, caution is required to prevent excessive depression of myocardial function.

    b. Simultaneous administration of calcium salts and vitamin D may lower the effectiveness of calcium-channel blockers. Calcium can be used to treat verapamil overdose.

    c. Antihypertensive drugs such as prazosin, methyldopa, clonidine, and other hypotensive agents can add to the hypotensive effects of calcium-channel blockers to cause dangerous hypotensive effects.

    d. Nondepolarizing muscle relaxants may have increased action due to calcium-channel blockers ability to block pre- and postjunctional channels. Caution is to be exercised in using these agents together.

2. Metabolic effects

    a. Verapamil and possibly diltiazem inhibit hepatic biotransformation of carbamazepine. Increased effects of carbamazepine are noted.

    b. Cimetidine decreases the first-pass effect of calcium-channel blockers. This may require a lower dose of these agents.

    c. Lithium plasma levels are decreased by verapamil. Monitoring of lithium levels is necessary to maintain therapeutic effects of lithium.

3. Protein binding

    a. Verapamil is highly protein-bound. It may displace other drugs such as warfarin and oral hypoglycemics.

Preparations and Doses

Diltiazem HCl (Cardizem) tablets 30, 60, 90, 120 mg; 180 to 360 mg daily in divided doses.

Nifedipine (Adalat, Procardia) capsules 10, 20 mg. Initial dose 10 mg twice a day. Titrate dose upward over 7 to 14 days. Do not exceed 180 mg/day.

Verapamil (Calan, Isoptin) tablets 80, 120 mg, sustained release 240 mg. Injection 5 mg per 2 mL.

MISCELLANEOUS DRUGS

Angina pectoris is so common a disease syndrome that over the years many different remedies have been used. Unfortunately, verification that seems to work most comes from anecdotal evidence. Modern techniques of measuring vascular dynamics have weeded out the less effective drugs. There are a few that merit mention.

Papaverine

This is an alkaloid which is present in crude opium but not related chemically to morphine and lacking euphoric and analgesic properties. It is a peripheral vasodilator with a direct action on blood vessels. However, its overall effect is weak at therapeutic doses relative to a fall in blood pressure or decrease in venous tone. Larger doses can cause arrhythmias.

In spite of definite evidence of efficiency, papaverine is widely prescribed for peripheral vascular disease, cerebral vascular accidents, and in general any condition which might benefit from vasodilation. A closely related drug is *ethavarine*.

Dipyridamole

This is a dipiperdino-pyrimidol compound which has had more than 20 years of use, especially in Europe, as a coronary vasodilator. As a vasodilator, dipyridamole pharmacologically resembles papaverine. At usual doses there is little change in blood pressure or peripheral blood flow. It does increase coronary flow but mainly in normal myocardium, and the benefit in this regard is considered minimal.

Dipyridamole has been recommended as prophylaxis for angina pectoris, but there is no substantial evidence that this goal is accomplished.

Because of its antiplatelet effects, dipyridamole has been widely used in conjunction with warfarin to prevent embolization from prosthetic heart valves. In combination with aspirin dipyridamole prolongs the survival of platelets in thrombotic disease. By itself dipyridamole has little effect. The mechanism of its antiplatelet effect may be inhibition of cyclic nucleotide phosphodiesterase activity. Concerning prevention of coronary thrombosis, several large studies have shown that aspirin alone is as effective as the combination of dipyridamole and aspirin.

Dipyridamole (Persantine) is available in 25-, 50-, and 75-mg tablets. Usual dose 50 mg two times a day.

BIBLIOGRAPHY

Braunwald, E.: "Mechanism of Action of Calcium Channel Blocking Agents," *N. Engl. J. Med.*, **307**:1618 (1982).

Cavin, C., R. Loutzenbieser, and C. Van Breeman: "Mechanisms of Calcium Antagonist Induced Vasodilation," *Annu. Rev. Pharmacol. Toxicol.*, **23**:373–396 (1983).

Fishman, W. H., et al.: "Antianginal Drug Therapy for Silent Myocardial Ischemia," *Am. Heart J.* **114**:140–147 (1987).

Gerthoffer, W. T., M. A. Trevethick, and R. A. Murphy: "Myosin Phosphorylation and Cyclic Adenosine 3′,5′-Monophosphate in Relaxation of Arterial Smooth Muscle by Vasodilators," *Circ. Res.*, **54**:839 (1984).

Janis, R. I., and A. Scriabine: "Commentary: Sites of Action of Ca^{2+} Channel Inhibitors," *Biochem. Pharmacol.*, **32**:3499–3507 (1983).

Nordlander, R.: "Use of Nitrates in the Treatment of Unstable and Variant Angina," *Drugs*, **33 Suppl. 4**:131–139 (1987).

O'Hara, M. J., et al.: "Diltiazem and Propranolol Combination for the Treatment of Chronic Stable Angina Pectoris," *Clin. Cardiol.*, **10**:115–123 (1987).

Opie, L. H.: *The Heart, Physiology, Metabolism, Pharmacology and Therapy*, Grune and Stratton, London, 1986.

Opie, L. H., and U. Thadani: in J. Hamer (ed.): *Antianginal Vasodilators in Drugs for Heart Disease*, 2d ed., Chapman and Hall, London, 1987, pp. 103–143.

Parker, J. O.: "Nitrate Therapy in Stable Angina Pectoris," *N. Engl. J. Med*, **316**:1635–1642 (1987).

Pepine, C. J., et al.: "Usefulness of Nicardipine for Angina Pectoris," *Am. J. Cardiol.*, **59**:13J–19J (1987).

Rodrigues, E. A., et al.: "Improvement in Left Ventricular Diastolic Function in Patients with Stable Angina after Chronic Treatment with Verapamil and Nicardipine," *Eur. Heart J.* **8**:624–629 (1987).

Samuelsson, O., et al.: "Angina Pectoris, Intermittent Claudication and Congestive Heart Failure in Middle-Aged Male Hypertensives. Development and Prediction Factors during Long-Term Antihypertensive Care." The Primary Preventive Trial, Goteborg, Sweden, *Acta Med. Scand.*, **221**:23–32 (1987).

Thompson, R. H.: "The Clinical Use of Transdermal Delivery Devices with Nitroglycerin," *Angiology*, **34**:23–31 (1983).

C H A P T E R 29

Agents Used
in Hyperlipoproteinemia

Joseph R. DiPalma

There used to be doubt that the level of blood cholesterol per se was clearly linked to arteriosclerotic disease, but recent large-scale studies have established a definite relationship. Indeed, a National Institutes of Health Consensus Development Conference has recommended that blood cholesterol determinations be obtained in all adult Americans. Those with elevations of 200 mg/dL should be treated with dietary measures and drugs as necessary to lower their cholesterol levels. Most authorities do not go this far, but meanwhile the discovery of new and active drugs and widespread publicity have greatly increased awareness in this area.

The disease arteriosclerosis is much more complicated than the association with high blood cholesterol and serious narrowing of crucial blood vessels such as the coronaries or carotids. A brief sequence of events in the formation of arteriosclerotic plaque is as follows: Over time, many years in most cases, at a point in a blood vessel where there is turbulence some injury to the endothelium occurs. Platelets are attracted to the injured site, possibly because of an endothelial factor. Combined action of endothelial growth and platelet-derived growth factors attracts macrophages, causing an inflammatory response leading to hypertrophy of the medial muscle of the artery, which does not appreciably narrow the vessel. The constriction of the artery is brought about by the deposition of cholesterol in a plaque formation. The endothelium never fully recovers and may be the site of thrombus formation in the narrowed vessel. The macrophages play a crucial role in this process for they have receptors for low-density lipoprotein LDL (see Table 29-1). This particle has a high content of cholesterol and apoprotein B. Hence the most appropriate name for the disorder is lipoproteinemia, indicating not only the fat content but also the protein content of the various particles which transport fat from dietary and synthesis sources to the other tissues.

CHOLESTEROL TRANSPORT

Cholesterol is transported as various size particles composed of triglycerides, proteins, cholesterol esters, and phospholipids. In Table 29-1 listed are the major blood particles whose function is to carry fats from one tissue to another. It appears that the various size particles are each designed for a particular purpose. For example, the chylomicrons are the largest particles composed mostly of triglycerides, and their function is to transport fat from the intestine to the liver. Chylomicrons contain little cholesterol and are not involved in the arteriosclerotic process. In contrast, LDL particles contain the most cholesterol, and they are the source of this sterol for synthesis of bile salts and adrenal and sex hormones, and also for the arteriosclerotic lesion. High-density lipoprotein (HDL) particles contain less cholesterol and little triglycerides and a large amount of protein. They are believed to remove excess cholesterol from the tissues.

The amount of cholesterol as represented by the above particles in the liver (where it is mainly synthesized), in the blood, and in the tissues is determined by many factors. The crucial element appears to be the

TABLE 29-1   Composition of the human plasma lipoproteins[a]

Lipoprotein macromolecules	Size, Å	% Triglyceride	% Cholesterol	% Phospholipids	% Protein	Major apoproteins	Predominant function
Chylomicrons	2000–5000	85	7	6	3	A1, A4, B, C, E	Transport of fat from intestine to liver
Very low density (VLDL)	500–800	60	16	14	9	B, C1, E	Transport of lipoprotein lipids to adipose tissue and muscle from the liver
Low density (LDL)	200	11	46	22	21	B	Transport of cholesterol LDL to the liver for bile acid synthesis and to adrenals and ovaries
High density (HDL)	80	8	20	22	50	A1, A2	Transport of cholesterol from tissues to liver for excretion

[a] Table partially adapted from S. Weis and A. G. Lacko: "Role of Lipoproteins in hypercholesterolemia," *Practical Cardiology* (special issue), May 1988, p. 12.

kind and quantity of receptors present in the various organs and tissues. This is genetically determined because the lipid particles which are produced by the body are composed of specific proteins (see Table 29-1). These serve as agonists for the receptors which are also proteins and also genetically determined. The function of LDL is to carry cholesterol to the tissues. Its role in the arteriosclerotic lesion has already been described. The amount of LDL available is a primary determinant factor in atherogenesis, and this serves as a basis for diagnosis and therapy, as discussed later.

Very-low-density lipoprotein (VLDL) is a large particle produced by the liver, which has a high concen-tration of triglycerides and considerable cholesterol. Its main function is to transport fat and be a source of the other particles in the bloodstream (Table 29-1).

As shown in Fig. 29-1, the amount of very-low-density lipoprotein in the blood is determined by (1) the production of VLDL by the liver; (2) the for-mation of an intermediate density lipoprotein (IDL) or remnants of VLDL which condense into LDL; (3) the amount of HDL which comes from the tissues and contributes to the formation of LDL; (4) the rate of utilization of LDL by the tissues; (5) the number of active receptors for LDL in the liver. Since HDL is considered to remove cholesterol from the tissues, a

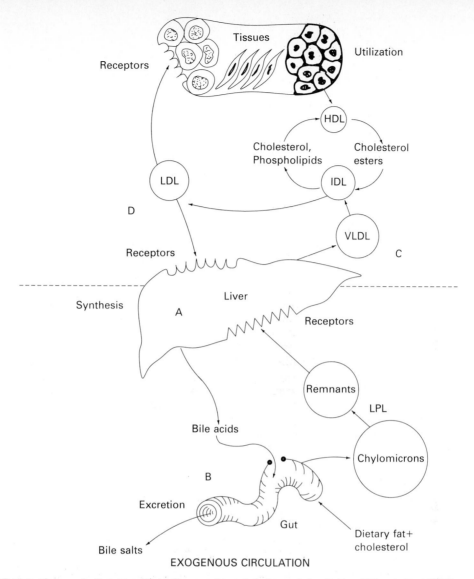

FIGURE 29-1 Schematic diagram of lipid, lipoprotein, and cholesterol circulation. Abbreviations: HDL = high-density lipoprotein; IDL = intermediate-density lipoprotein; LDL = low-density lipoprotein; VLDL = very-low-density lipoprotein; LPL = lipoprotein lipase. Dietary fat and cholesterol are ingested. From the gut, fatty acids and cholesterol are absorbed to enter the portal circulation as chylomicrons composed mostly of triglycerides but also containing protein and cholesterol. These break up into smaller remnants, due to the action of lipoprotein lipase, which are handled by the liver at various receptor sites. The liver synthesizes bile acids as well as cholesterol *de novo*. The bile acids are secreted into the intestine; most are reabsorbed, and only a small amount is excreted. From the liver, triglycerides and cholesterol enter the systemic circulation and form VLDL. This particle breaks up into intermediate particles, which further form LDL and are contributed to by HDL from the tissues. Special receptors are present in the tissues and the liver for LDL, which contains the largest amount of cholesterol.

Sites of action of cholesterol-lowering agents are as follows: (A) inhibition of synthesis by lovastatin in the liver by blocking HMG-CoA reductase; (B) increased excretion of bile salts by blocking reabsorption by bile acid sequestrants; (C) decreased production of VLDL by the liver caused by nicotinic acid; (D) probucol increased degradation of LDL cholesterol.

high blood level is perceived to be favorable and vice versa.

The formation and disposition of the various lipoproteins are imperfectly understood. Empiric observations have established some other parameters which must be taken into consideration in the diagnosis and therapy of hyperlipoproteinemias:

1. Dietary intake of fatty acids and cholesterol.
2. Rate of liver synthesis of cholesterol.
3. Ratio of saturated to unsaturated fatty acids in the diet. A well-established observation is that a diet high in saturated fats (meats) is associated with high levels of plasma cholesterol; similarly, a diet high in unsaturated fats (vegetable oils) is associated with low levels of plasma cholesterol.
4. Rate of utilization of cholesterol. Exercise, for example, increases the burning of fats for energy and also decreases plasma cholesterol. Growth increases and senescence decreases utilization of fats and cholesterol.
5. Endocrine diseases. Diabetes or insulin insufficiency leads to poor utilization of fat and early arteriosclerosis. Hyperthyroidism decreases and hypothyroidism increases the level of plasma cholesterol and atherogenic tendency. Changes in growth and adrenal and sex hormones are more tenuous factors but still important.

These are gross observations. There are many other causes of secondary hyperlipoproteinemia. These are listed in Table 29-2. On the whole, the diagnosis and treatment of hyperlipoproteinemias are based upon an accurate estimation of the level of plasma cholesterol,

TABLE 29-2   Causes of secondary hyperlipoproteinemia

Hypercholesterolemia	Hypertriglyceridemia
Nephrosis	Obesity
Biliary cirrhosis	Diabetes mellitus
Hypothyroidism	Alcoholism
Hypopituitarism	Estrogens
Extreme starvation	Uremia
Immunoglobulin-lipoprotein disorders	Corticosteroids
Beta blockers	Thiazide diuretics
	Isotretinoin

the ratio of LDL and HDL in the plasma, and the plasma triglyceride level.

CLASSIFICATION OF THE HYPERLIPOPROTEINEMIAS

Based upon electrophoretic patterns of the plasma of persons with clinical disease, it has been possible to separate the hyperlipoproteinemias into categories which represent genetic phenotypes (see Table 29-3). These familial hyperlipoproteinemias are usually severe and are represented by obvious clinical diseases such as xanthomas of various types and early atherogenesis (before age 40). In the general population of middle-aged persons about 15 percent have elevated blood cholesterol levels. Of these only 2 percent are of a familial type. The metabolic basis of the rest (polygenic, type II) remains unexplained except for those which are secondary to severe alcoholism, endocrine disease, or uremia.

CHOLESTEROL METABOLISM

Very briefly the pathway of synthesis of cholesterol is as follows:

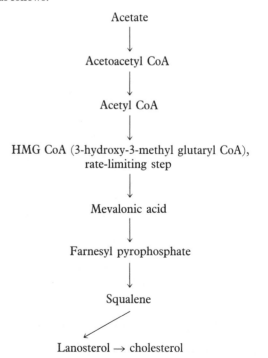

Acetate
↓
Acetoacetyl CoA
↓
Acetyl CoA
↓
HMG CoA (3-hydroxy-3-methyl glutaryl CoA), rate-limiting step
↓
Mevalonic acid
↓
Farnesyl pyrophosphate
↓
Squalene
↓
Lanosterol → cholesterol

TABLE 29-3   Characterization of the hyperlipoproteinemias

Phenotype	Descriptive name	Prevalence	Cholesterol	Triglycerides	Lipoprotein abnormalities	Risk of atherogenesis
I	Familial lipoprotein lipase deficiency	Rare	Normal	Markedly elevated	Increased chylomicrons	None
IIa, IIb	Familial hypercholesterol-emia	Relatively common	Marked elevation	Normal or slightly increased	LDL increased VLDL normal or slightly increased Low HDL	High
II	Polygenic hypercholesterol-emia	Most common	Marked elevation	Normal	LDL increased	Moderate
III	Familial dysbetalipopro-teinemia	Relatively uncommon	Elevated	Elevated	Abnormal beta-bound LDL increased	High
IV with IIa, IIb	Familial combined hyperlipocholes-terolemia	Common	Elevated	Elevated	VLDL increased	Moderately high
V	Familial hypertriglycer-idemia	Uncommon	Normal or elevated	Elevated	Increased chylomicrons, increased VLDL	Low

Cholesterol can be synthesized by many cells in the body, but, of course, the largest source is the liver. Dietary cholesterol contributes significantly to the body pool. The average American diet contains 1500 mg of daily cholesterol. It is important to point out that the rate-limiting step in synthesis is concerned with HMG-CoA reductase. Cholesterol itself inhibits by feedback HMG-CoA reductase and apparently promotes its inactivation by mechanisms as yet unknown. It is a logical control step where influence of cholesterol synthesis may be achieved. The only available excretion pathway is via the intestine as bile salts. Of course some cholesterol is utilized for conversion to adrenal and sex hormones and vitamin D. The endog-

enous and exogenous pathways of circulation of cholesterol are shown in Fig. 29-1. There are obviously many points where disturbance of synthesis, circulation, or excretion may result in a decrease of blood cholesterol levels. Measures which have proven most feasible and effective are enhancement of excretion as with the bile sequestrant resins and at the rate-limiting step in synthesis involving HMG-CoA reductase. Now that more is known about tissue and liver receptors for cholesterol and the specific protein content of the various cholesterol particles, new opportunities exist for the creation of drug antagonists which might be particularly effective to prevent athero-genesis.

HYPERTRIGLYCERIDEMIA

As shown in Table 29-3, which characterizes the hyperlipoproteinemias, elevated levels of triglycerides occur in phenotypes I, III, IV, and V and sometimes in IIa and IIb. In phenotype I, or familial lipoprotein lipase deficiency, the cholesterol is normal and only the triglycerides are elevated. It is of interest that there is no increased risk of atherogenesis and thus no need to treat the cholesterol level. In the other cases of hypertriglyceridemia, the cholesterol is also elevated. Therapy here aims to lower both cholesterol and triglycerides.

DIAGNOSIS

Establishment of clinically significant hyperlipoproteinemia is based on the plasma levels of total cholesterol, the LDL/HDL ratio, and triglycerides. The LDL/HDL ratio is important because the risk of atherogenesis is the higher the greater the amount of LDL as compared to HDL. Recall that HDL carries cholesterol from tissues, while LDL is the main particle bringing cholesterol to organs. In addition, there are instances where the elevated total cholesterol is composed mainly of increased HDL. Such individuals are not at risk of atherogenesis and need not be treated.

Other risk factors are considered. These are hypertension, smoking, alcohol, age, obesity, and most important, family history of early onset of arteriosclerotic lesions.

DIETARY MANAGEMENT

Therapy is always initiated first with dietary measures. Some mild cases may need no further therapy, but dietary measures at the least will diminish the dose of required drug medication.

The aim of dietary therapy is to reduce the daily intake of cholesterol to 200 mg and even to 100 mg in more severe cases. Another aim is to reduce the total fat intake, at the same time decreasing the amount of saturated fat and increasing the amount of unsaturated fat. If the individual is obese, the total caloric content of the diet is reduced to attain ideal weight. Dietary therapy is to be continued and insisted upon even if cholesterol levels appear not to respond, although in many cases a 10 to 15 percent reduction in total cholesterol levels is to be expected.

DRUG MANAGEMENT

The decision to use drugs to control cholesterol levels should not be taken lightly. Therapy must be continued for the rest of the individual's life. None of the drugs is without toxicity, and all incur considerable expense. Selection of a specific drug depends on the nature of the lipidemia. It is not logical to use a drug designed to lower cholesterol when the patient's disease is hypertriglyceridemia. Selection of patients for drug therapy depends on the total blood cholesterol level, the LDL/HDL ratio, family history of arterosclerotic disease, presence of arteriosclerosis (coronary heart disease for example), and other risk factors such as hypertension and unwillingness to give up smoking and alcohol.

SPECIFIC DRUGS

Bile Acid Sequestrants

At the present time two drugs are available which bind bile acids in the intestinal tract. These are colestipol and cholestyramine, and although they differ chemically, they have essentially the same actions. Both are large polymers classed as resins which are capable of cationic exchange. Being insoluble in water, they are not absorbed. They bind bile acids in the intestinal lumen at their quaternary ammonium biding sites releasing chloride in exchange for the bile acids. Since the complexed bile acids cannot be reabsorbed, they are excreted along with the resin in the feces.

Mechanism of Action Bile acids are byproducts of cholesterol and are ordinarily almost completely reabsorbed in the small intestine. Thus the essential structure of cholesterol is preserved for reuse by conversion of bile acids back to cholesterol in the liver. The bile acid sequestrants increase greatly the excretion of cholesterol (as bile acids), and thus the body must rely on increased synthesis to maintain cholesterol levels (see Fig. 29-1). The overall effect is a decrease in the body pool of cholesterol resulting in about a 10 to 20 percent decrease in total cholesterol mostly reflected in decreased LDL. VLDL may actually increase as does HDL. The number of LDL receptors in the liver increases, thus enhancing the uptake of LDL from the blood. Consequently the resins are not effective in patients who have homozygous familial hypercholesterolemia, because they do not have functioning receptors for LDL. Triglyceride levels are not significantly affected by resin therapy.

Since the resins are not absorbed or significantly metabolized, they have little systemic toxicity. However, by binding bile acids they affect the normal digestive process, and the most common complaints are constipation and bloating sensation. Bran and a high fiber diet offer relief. Some patients with sensitive bowels or cholestasis may have steatorrhea. At best many patients find the resins hard to take because of the many gastrointestinal side actions, and compliance is often inadequate.

In addition, since the resins may bind to many other essential nutrients and drugs, deficiencies and interactions are frequent and must be taken into account in each patient. Malabsorption of vitamin K may occur, and great care is required in patients taking both resins and dicoumarol-type anticoagulants. Among other drugs whose absorption may be impaired by the resins are digitalis glycosides, thiazides, antibiotics, thyroxine, iron salts, and folic acid. To forestall such interactions, other medications should be given at least an hour before the resin.

Therapeutic Use   The bile acid sequestrants are indicated in patients with primary hypercholesterolemia who have not responded adequately to diet. Patients who also have hypertriglyceridemia in addition to cholesterol elevation may also respond, but the resins are not indicated when the triglycerides alone are elevated. The long-term effectiveness of bile acid sequestrants and their safety have been established. In cases where the lowering of LDL is short of a desirable goal, the resins may be combined with other drugs such as probucol or lovastatin to obtain decreases of up to 50 percent in blood cholesterol levels.

The resins may also be used to reduce pruritis in partial biliary obstruction. Other uses are to bind the bacterial toxin in pseudomembranous colitis. Cholestyramine has also been used to bind the pesticide chlordecone (Kepone) in cases of poisoning. In this manner recirculation through the liver and bile is prevented and fecal excretion is increased.

Cholestyramine is available in 4-g packets and in bulk, colestipol in 5-g packets and in bulk. Generally starting doses are 20 g daily in three doses taken with meals. The powder is never taken dry. It should be mixed with water, fruit juice, or soup and allowed to hydrate before ingestion. Doses are individualized and can be moved upward to 30 to 32 g daily.

Nicotinic Acid

Niacin, or vitamin B_3, in the form of nicotinic acid in large doses lowers both cholesterol and triglycerides. Despite its troublesome side actions, it has had a long and successful history as an antihyperlipoproteinemic drug. These uses and functions of nicotinic acid have no relationship to the use and purposes of niacin as a vitamin. Yet either form of the vitamin satisfies vitamin requirements as the body nicotinic acid is converted to niacinamide and used in the nicotinamide adenine nucleotide (NAD) cycle. Nicotinic acid is well absorbed in the gut and is excreted as such along with smaller quantities of other metabolites.

Niacinamide   Nicotinic acid

Mechanism of Action   The locus of action is a reduction of production of VLDL by the liver, which in turn results in lower amounts of IDL and LDL. The reduction in VLDL production is thought to be related to inhibition of lipolysis in adipose tissue, decreased esterification of triglycerides in the liver, and increased activity of lipoprotein lipase. It is important to point out that nicotinic acid does not affect the total body synthesis of cholesterol.

The usual dose of niacin as a vitamin is about 20 mg a day. The required dose of nicotinic acid to lower blood cholesterol is 2 to 8 g daily, a dose of 100 to 400 times greater. At these high doses nicotinic acid reduces the level of cholesterol and triglycerides in types II, III, IV, and V hyperlipoproteinemia.

Adverse Actions   At the high doses nicotinic acid produces an intense cutaneous flush and pruritis. This has been related to the production of local prostaglandins and may be relieved by taking an aspirin 30 min before each dose of nicotinic acid. Considerable tolerance develops in time to the cutaneous flush. Various GI dysfunctions such as vomiting, diarrhea, and dyspepsia are common, and even peptic ulceration has been reported. Rarely there have been instances of hyperpigmentation of the skin and the formation of acanthosis nigricans. The most serious toxicity is confined to the liver. Elevations of plasma transaminase may be severe, and jaundice has occurred. In addition, hyperglycemia and decreased glucose tolerance can happen in nondiabetic individuals. Plasma uric acid can increase, and gouty arthritis has been reported. Consequently, nicotinic acid should not be used in persons with liver disease, diabetes, or gout.

Therapeutic Use　Nicotinic acid alone or in combination with bile acid sequestrants can lower both cholesterol and triglycerides from 10 to 30 percent. As one of the drugs compared in the Coronary Drug Project, it was successful in reducing the overall incidence of recurrent myocardial infarction. However, there was no effect on overall cardiovascular mortality. Compliance is a major difficulty, and the drug is reserved for patients who do not respond to other measures.

Clofibrate

This derivative of aryloxylisobutyric acid was the most active of a series of compounds which were found in the early 1960s capable of reducing plasma concentrations of total lipid and cholesterol. The chemical structure is shown.

Clofibrate

Although widely used in hypercholesterolemia and as a test drug in the Coronary Drug Project, at the present time the use of clofibrate is mainly restricted to familial dysbetalipoproteinemia (type III).

Mechanism of Action　The site of action of clofibrate is uncertain. It does increase the activity of lipoprotein lipase, which intravascularly enhances the rate of conversion of VLDL to IDL and LDL. Hepatic synthesis and delivery of VLDL are apparently not affected by clofibrate.

Clofibrate decreases plasma triglyceride concentrations by reducing levels of VLDL. Most patients also have a fall in levels of LDL and plasma cholesterol.

Unfortunately, a large fall in VLDL can also result in an increase in LDL, and the net effect on cholesterol is reduced. It is a common experience that only modest reductions in levels of cholesterol (5 to 10 percent) are experienced. In contrast, triglyceride levels are reduced by about 20 to 25 percent. HDL levels are not affected. An exception is familial dysbetalipoproteinemia where cholesterol may be lowered by as much as 50 percent.

Adverse Actions　Clofibrate is deceptively well tolerated by most patients in the initiation of therapy. With long-term use there may occur weight gain (increased appetite), skin rash, alopecia, weakness and impotence, breast tenderness, and loss of libido. A disturbing action is a flu-like syndrome of muscle aches, cramps, stiffness, and weakness, which is associated with elevations of creatinine phosphokinase activity in the plasma. Patients who have elevation of this enzyme and other enzymes (transaminases) of liver and muscle origin should not receive clofibrate. With long-term use the incidence of gallstones and cholecystitis increases.

Clofibrate is available as capsules containing 500 mg. The usual daily dose is 2 g in two to four doses taken with food.

Gemfibrozil

Related to clofibrate chemically, gemfibrozil has similar pharmacologic and clinical usefulness. As can be seen in the chemical structure, gemfibrozil differs from clofibrate in having methyl substitutions in the phenyl ring, and the aliphatic chain is longer and ends as a carboxylic acid.

Gemfibrozil

Absorption from the intestinal tract is good. Peak plasma levels occur at 1 to 2 h following a single dose. Despite enterohepatic circulation and reabsorption in the intestine, there is no tendency for the drug to accumulate. Excretion is urinary with about 70 percent eliminated unchanged.

Clinical Use Gemfibrozil has an indication for hypertriglyceridemia in adults with serum triglyceride levels greater than 750 mg/dL (types IV and V hyperlipoproteinemia) who are at risk of pancreatitis and who do not respond to dietary therapy.

The main action of gemfibrozil like clofibrate is to decrease VLDL in the plasma. Only modest decreases in LDL levels occur while HDL is elevated moderately. Clofibrate does not elevate HDL levels and this may be an important difference between the older and the new agent.

Adverse Actions Gemfibrozil appears safe in long-term use. However, because it has not been in use as long or as extensively as clofibrate, there has been less chance of encountering toxicity. Nevertheless, those adverse reactions which have been experienced are similar to those seen with clofibrate. It is reasonable to expect that the long-term toxic effects of gemfibrozil might be the same as those of clofibrate.

Gemfibrozil is available as 300-mg capsules. The usual dose ranges from 500 to 1500 mg/day in two divided doses 30 min before meals.

Probucol

Introduced relatively recently as an antihypercholesteremic agent, probucol differs chemically from the other agents. Chemically probucol is a bis-phenol containing sulfur and many methyl groups. It is as a result highly lipophilic, distributes into adipose tissue, where it persists with as much as 20 percent of peak blood levels remaining after 6 months.

Probucol

Probucol lowers serum cholesterol with little or no effect on triglycerides. The LDL fraction is decreased, but there is a proportionally greater decremental effect on the HDL fraction. From an epidemiologic viewpoint, this is harmful because a decrease in HDL signifies less removal of cholesterol from the tissues, and patients who respond favorably to anticholesteremic

therapy generally have a decrease in LDL and a rise in HDL fractions. In any event the fall in plasma total cholesterol is a modest 10 to 15 percent when probucol is used alone.

The mechanism of action of probucol is obscure (see Fig. 29-1). It appears that the LDL fraction is more rapidly degraded, but there is no increase in LDL receptors in the liver. An increase in excretion of bile acids is observed, which may be related to the LDL action. Probucol decreases the synthesis of apoproteins A1 and A2, which may account for the decrease in HDL.

The indication for probucol therapy is type IIa familial hypercholesterolemia. There have been limited large-scale studies which have compared probucol with other agents. The best results are reported when probucol is used in conjunction with the bile acid sequestrants. An advantage of the combined use is that probucol antagonizes the constipating action of the resins. The decrease in HDL fraction is considered a risk factor for atherogenesis, and thus probucol is usually reserved for patients who do not respond or cannot tolerate the other agents.

Adverse reactions to probucol include Q-T prolongation. In animals probucol is cardiac arrhythmogenic, and this limits probucol use to patients who have no evidence of heart disease. Diarrhea and loose stools are a common complaint. Other GI complaints such as nausea, abdominal pain, vomiting, and flatulence disappear with continued use. Less frequent are skin rashes, thrombocytopenia, peripheral neuritis, and angioneurotic edema. Probucol does not appear to be liver toxic but there have been mild elevations of serum transaminases.

Probucol is available as 250-mg coated tablets. The usual dose is 500 mg taken twice daily with morning and evening meals.

Lovastatin

The latest introduction is lovastatin, which is one of a series of unique compounds isolated from a fungus *Aspergillus terreus*. These agents are potent competitive inhibitors of HMG CoA reductase, which is the rate-limiting step in cholesterol synthesis. They are, when properly used, the most effective agents for lowering plasma cholesterol. Chemically, lovastatin is an inactive lactone which is converted in the body by hydrolysis to the corresponding β-hydroxy-acid form.

The chemical structure is shown, and the features which allow it to inhibit HMG CoA reductase can be noted:

Lovastatin

HMG–CoA

Mechanism of Action   The decrease in synthesis of cholesterol initiates in the liver a compensatory increase in the assembly of LDL receptors. Thus LDL levels are diminished in the blood, and there is an increased utilization of body cholesterol by the liver for conversion to bile acids. It follows that if dietary intake of cholesterol is not restricted, the liver will use exogenous cholesterol to make up for the deficit in synthesis (see Fig. 29-1). There is a corresponding increase in HDL levels in the blood. This is favorable and interpreted to signify an increased movement of cholesterol from the tissues to the liver. The blood level of apolipoprotein B also falls, and this suggests that lovastatin actually reduces the concentration of LDL particles rather than just lowering the cholesterol content. The triglyceride blood level is also lowered, and this reflects diminished level of VLDL, which has been confirmed in clinical studies. The degree of effect of lovastatin is comparable to and exceeds all other agents including the resins.

Pharmacokinetics   In ^{14}C-labeled studies in humans after a single oral dose, 10 percent of the dose was excreted in the urine and 83 percent in the feces. In the dog it has been observed that there is extensive first-pass extraction in the liver limiting availability to general circulation. Since the site of action of the drug is in the liver and there is little need to inhibit synthesis of cholesterol in peripheral tissues, this is not a disadvantage. Lovastatin is highly bound to plasma proteins. It crosses the blood-brain barrier and the placenta.

Major active metabolites are the 6′-hydroxy derivative and the beta hydroxy acid plus two other unidentified moieties. While the blood level of lovastatin peaks at 2 to 4 h after a single dose and declines thereafter, it has been found that a single daily dose given with the evening meal achieves satisfactory responses. Interestingly, the drug is more effective at night than during the day.

Therapeutic Use   Lovastatin is indicated in types IIa and IIb hyperlipoproteinemias. It should only be used after diet and other nondrug measures have failed to achieve a satisfactory lowering of total cholesterol blood level. In addition, other correctable causes of hypercholesterolemia such as hyperthyroidism, diabetes mellitus, and the nephrotic syndrome should be managed. It is important to determine the actual LDL and HDL levels, as there are a subset of patients with high total cholesterol who do not have elevated LDL. Instead they apparently have non-LDL fractions, and these do not put them at increased risk for atherogenesis.

With diet and lovastatin therapy, as much as 30 percent lowering of total blood cholesterol may be achieved. Combined with cholestyramine or colestipol, the lowering may be as much as 50 to 60 percent.

Adverse Reactions   In about 2 percent of patients receiving lovastatin for a year or more, elevations of serum transaminases as much as 3 times normal occurred. When lovastatin was terminated, the levels gradually fell to normal. Patients receiving lovastatin should have liver function tests before and every 4 to 6 weeks for the first 15 months of therapy. Liver disease of any kind and alcoholism are contraindications to the use of lovastatin.

Lovastatin can cause myalgia. About 0.5 percent of patients develop myositis, which is associated with elevated levels of creatinine phosphokinase (CPK). Elevated levels of enzyme or active clinical myositis require termination of lovastatin therapy. In fact therapy should be withheld in any patient at risk from renal failure as a result of rhabdomyolysis (severe infection, shock, trauma, electrolyte disturbances, and uncontrolled seizures).

Because of a high prevalence of baseline lenticular opacities and the appearance of new opacities, there is an indication that lovastatin may cause this defect. Slit lamp studies should be done before therapy is started and at yearly intervals thereafter.

The risk of carcinogenesis is not known. Lovastatin should not be used in pregnancy or in children. No significant drug interactions have been reported.

Lovastatin is available as 20-mg tablets. The usual dose is 20 mg daily with the evening meal. Maximum dose is 80 mg.

Dextrothyroxine

It has been known for many years that hyperthyroidism is associated with hypocholesteremia. Although thyroid hormone enhances cholesterol biosynthesis, it reduces LDL concentrations and has a greater effect on catabolism; the end result is a reduction of serum cholesterol levels. Dextrothyroxine has substantially less calorigenic activity than the natural hormone L-thyroxine.

Dextrothyroxine has been recommended in hyperlipoproteinemia, types II and III. Its mechanism of action is to increase degradation of cholesterol and lipoproteins, resulting in a lowering of plasma cholesterol.

The side effects observed with dextrothyroxine therapy are generally related to increased metabolism and cardiotoxicity. These include palpitations, loss of weight, nervousness, insomnia, excessive sweating, glucose intolerance, and diarrhea. As can be expected, this drug is contraindicated in patients with organic heart disease or cardiac arrhythmias and with advanced liver or kidney disease. In addition, dextrothyroxine may potentiate the effect of oral anticoagulants.

Dextrothyroxine (Choloxin) is available in 1-, 2-, 4-, and 6-mg tablets. Initial dose is 1 to 2 mg/day, increased at monthly intervals to 4 to 8 mg/day.

Neomycin

Many other drugs have had a trial in an attempt to lower blood cholesterol. Among them is neomycin, which, when combined with bile acid sequestrants or

with nicotinic acid, has had some degree of success. Apparently neomycin is able to block the absorption of cholesterol as well as bile acids. It may be considered as an alternative for patients who tolerate the resins poorly (see Chap. 43 for a fuller description of neomycin).

Neomycin sulfate is available as 500-mg tablets. The usual dose is 4 to 12 g daily in divided doses.

BIBLIOGRAPHY

Brown, M. S., P. T. Kovaneu, and J. L. Goldstein: "Regulation of Plasma Cholesterol by Lipoprotein Receptors," *Science*, **212**:628 (1981).

Brown, M. S., and A. Goldstein: "Receptor-Mediated Pathway for Cholesterol Homeostasis," *Science*, **232**:34–47 (1986).

Canner, P. L., et al.: "Fifteen Year Mortality in Coronary Drug Project Patients. Long Term Benefits with Niacin," *J. Am. Coll. Cardiol.*, **8**:1245–1255 (1986).

Consensus Conference: "Lowering Blood Cholesterol to Prevent Heart Disease," *JAMA*, **253**:2080–2086 (1985).

DiPalma, J. R.: "Lovastatin: Cholesterol-Lowering Agent," *Am. Fam. Physician*, **36**:189 (1988).

Goldstein, J. L., T. Kita, and M. S. Brown: "Defective Lipoprotein Receptors and Aterosclerosis: Lessons from an Animal Counterpart of Familial Hypercholesterolemia," *N. Engl. J. Med.*, **309**:288 (1983).

Havel, R. J.: "Lowering Cholesterol, 1988," *J. Clin. Invest.*, **81**:1653–1660 (1988).

Lovastatin Study Group II: "Therapeutic Response to Lovastatin (Mevinolin) in Nonfamilial Hypercholesterolemia," *JAMA*, **256**:29–34 (1986).

Repka, F. J., and R. F. Leighton: "Step Management of Hypercholesterolemia," *Am. Fam. Physician*, **36**:236–248 (1987).

"Report of the National Cholesterol Educational Program Expert Panel on Detection, Evaluation and Treatment of High Blood Cholesterol in Adults," *Arch. Intern. Med.*, **148**:36 (1988).

"The Lipid Research Clinic Coronary Primary Prevention Trial, Results 1. Reduction in Incidence of Coronary Disease," *JAMA*, **251**:351–364 (1984).

Tyroler, H. A.: "Review of Lipid Lowering Clinical Trials in Relation to Observational Chemical Studies," *Circulation*, **76**:515–522 (1987).

Vega, G. L., and S. M. Grundy: "Mechanisms of Primary Hypercholesterolemia in Humans," *Am. Heart J.*, **113**:493 (1987).

Diuretics

Andrew P. Ferko

The development of effective oral diuretic agents began in the 1950s with the introduction of chlorothiazide. Diuretics are a widely prescribed group of drugs used primarily in the management of edema and hypertension. They are drugs which increase urine flow by promoting a net loss of sodium ions and water from the body by interfering with ionic transport. The principal site of action for the diuretics in the removal of edematous fluid from the body is the nephron unit of the kidney. These agents are classified according to their proposed mechanism of action in the nephron (Table 30-1).

RENAL PHYSIOLOGY

In the kidney the nephron unit can regulate reabsorption of electrolytes and water at several sites: the proximal tubule, loop of Henle, distal tubule, and collecting duct (Fig. 30-1). The glomerulus permits filtration of most of the essential constituents of the extracellular fluid and waste products. However, it prevents passage of plasma proteins, lipids, and substances bound to proteins.

The nephron unit normally reabsorbs 99 percent of the glomerulus filtrate. In the first segment of the nephron, the proximal tubule, 50 to 60 percent of ions and water are reabsorbed. Sodium is actively reabsorbed from the lumen through the tubule cell into the blood; chloride and water diffuse passively. Also, the majority of bicarbonate transport into the blood occurs in this portion of the nephron and is mediated by the

enzyme carbonic anhydrase. The fluid in the proximal tubule is similar in osmolality to that of the interstitial fluid and plasma.

The proximal tubule contains the secretory processes for organic acids and bases by which these compounds enter the renal tubular fluid from the blood. Not only does this secretory system provide a means for the renal elimination of certain diuretics but it also allows these diuretics (e.g., furosemide, triamterene)

TABLE 30-1 Classification of diuretic drugs

I. Agents which increase renal solute excretion

   A. Inhibit reabsorption of sodium and chloride ions
      Thiazides, chlorthalidone, indapamide, metolazone
      Bumetanide, ethacrynic acid, furosemide

   B. Potassium-sparing diuretics
      Amiloride
      Spironolactone
      Triamterene

   C. Depress carbonic anhydrase activity
      Acetazolamide

II. Agents used as osmotic nonelectrolytes

    Mannitol

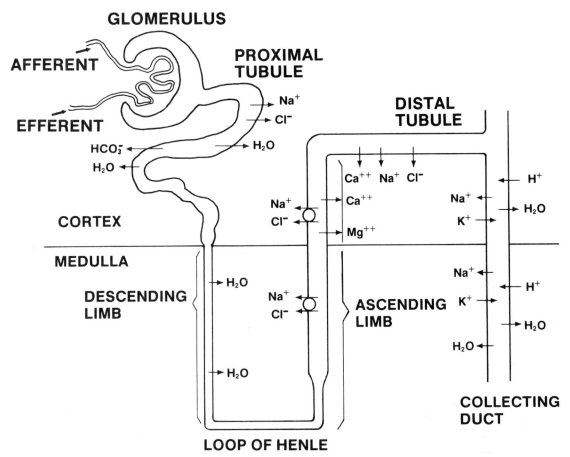

FIGURE 30-1 Diagrammatic representation of nephron unit showing sites of electrolyte and water reabsorption.

to gain access to their site of action in the lumen of the nephron.

As the remaining portion of the glomerular filtrate, approximately 40 percent, enters the descending limb of the loop of Henle, a concentrating mechanism operates. Water is removed passively, and the tubular fluid becomes hypertonic as it approaches the curvature.

In the ascending limb of the loop of Henle, the tubular fluid becomes hypotonic. This area is divided into medullary and cortical portions. In the medullary segment of the thick ascending limb it appears that a sodium-chloride cotransport system is responsible for the reabsorption of sodium and chloride. In this region magnesium and calcium ions are also removed from the tubular luminal fluid. However, water does not

follow sodium and chloride, since the entire ascending limb is impermeable to water. The sodium entering the medullary interstitium maintains the hypertonicity of this tissue and is responsible for the free-water reabsorption from the collecting duct. Since sodium is removed and water remains in the lumen, the tubular fluid becomes hypotonic. For didactic purposes, the hypotonic fluid formed may be said to consist of two hypothetical compartments: one isosmotic with plasma and the other free of solute, or so-called free water.

In the cortical segment of the ascending limb, more sodium and chloride are reabsorbed from the lumen by a sodium-chloride cotransport mechanism, and further formation of free water occurs. The sodium chloride reabsorbed from the cortical area, however, does not contribute to the hypertonicity of the interstitium. In total, about 20 to 30 percent of filtered sodium chloride is reabsorbed in the ascending limb of the loop of Henle.

The tubular fluid entering the distal convoluted segment is hypotonic. Sodium chloride is reabsorbed out of this region. Calcium is actively transported from the tubular fluid under the influence of parathyroid hormone. In addition, the distal tubule appears to be impermeable to water even when antidiuretic hormone is present.

When fluid enters the last segment of the nephron unit, the collecting duct, sodium is actively reabsorbed. This active transport mechanism is mediated by the mineralocorticoid aldosterone. In response to the removal of sodium, potassium and hydrogen ions are secreted passively. Water movement out of the collecting duct is controlled by antidiuretic hormone (ADH), which increases the permeability of the duct to water. The concentrations of ADH are highest in dehydration or water deprivation. Free water which is formed in the ascending limb of the loop of Henle can be reabsorbed in this area. The amount of reabsorption depends on the concentration of ADH and the degree of hypertonicity of the medullary interstitium.

The hypertonicity of the medullary interstitium plays an important part in the hypothesis of the countercurrent multiplier mechanism. According to this theory, sodium is transported from the ascending limb of Henle's loop into the descending limb. This establishes a small concentration gradient between the fluid contents of the ascending and descending limbs at successive levels along the course of the loop. Sodium concentration increases progressively down the descending limb because of countercurrent flow, and each unit of filtrate becomes more concentrated until it reaches the loop itself. This process establishes the medullary hypertonicity, which provides the osmotic gradient necessary to abstract water from the lumen of the collecting duct in the final concentration of urine.

The high concentration of solute in the medulla is maintained by the vasa recta acting as a countercurrent exchanger. This process, which depends on the slow rate of medullary blood flow, maintains the 300/1200-mOsm/kg concentration differential between the cortex and the tip of the medulla. Only the water and sodium necessary to maintain the normal electrolyte concentrations of the body pass into the systemic circulation. The countercurrent exchange system thus prevents excessive loss of sodium from the medulla and papillae.

THIAZIDE DIURETICS

The thiazides are sulfonamide derivatives which (1) promote the renal excretion of sodium and chloride, (2) remain effective in the presence of acidosis or alkalosis, (3) inhibit carbonic anhydrase in vitro, and (4) lower arterial blood pressure in hypertensive patients. Qualitatively, the thiazide diuretics are the same. The structures of chlorothiazide and other thiazide diuretics are presented in Table 30-2.

Hydrochlorothiazide causes less inhibition of carbonic anhydrase but produces 5 to 10 times more sodium diuresis than does chlorothiazide at equal milligram doses. The hydrogenated ring of hydrochlorothiazide permits many possible substitutions, and the structure-activity relationships have been extensively studied in this series of compounds.

Mechanism of Action

Thiazides promote urinary excretion of sodium, chloride, potassium, water, and, in the case of chlorothiazide, bicarbonate. Urinary loss of bicarbonate, when it occurs, is due to a weak inhibition of carbonic anhydrase by the thiazides in the proximal convoluted tubule. This effect of chlorothiazide is insignificant at usual dose levels. The thiazide diuretics cause sodium excretion even in the presence of systemic alkalosis or acidosis and, therefore, do not exhibit the phenomenon of refractoriness.

The principal site of action for the diuretic effect of the thiazides is the distal tubule of the nephron. They inhibit the reabsorption of sodium and chloride. The exact mechanism of action responsible for the inhibition of sodium chloride transport is not fully known. In addition, the thiazides enhance the reabsorption of calcium ion in the distal tubule. When the increased load of sodium in the renal tubular fluid reaches the collecting duct, some sodium is actively reabsorbed and potassium is secreted, resulting in an increased urinary potassium concentration. If thiazides evoke sufficient potassium excretion, hypokalemia is produced. The thiazides may also promote the loss of magnesium from the body.

In addition to the action of removing edematous

TABLE 30-2   Structure and therapeutic dose of various thiazide diuretics

Generic name	X	Y	R	Δ 3,4	Oral dose, mg/day
Chlorothiazide	Cl	H	H	Yes	500–1000
Hydrochlorothiazide	Cl	H	H	No	50–150
Bendroflumethiazide	CF_3	H	$-CH_2-\bigcirc$	No	5–15
Polythiazide	Cl	CH_3	$CH_2SCH_2CF_3$	No	2–4

fluid from the body, the thiazides are used clinically to reduce elevated blood pressure. This antihypertensive effect of the thiazides is not entirely explained by their diuretic effect and the consequent decrease in circulating blood volume. It appears that relaxation of the peripheral vascular smooth muscle may also be involved in the antihypertensive effect of the thiazides, particularly when they are used for longer than 2 weeks.

Pharmacokinetics

These drugs are well absorbed from the gastrointestinal tract, except for chlorothiazide. The thiazides appear in the bloodstream and remain there in active concentrations for several hours, the exact length of time depending on the derivative. After intravenous injection, diuresis begins promptly but lasts only about 2 h. These drugs are therefore more suitable for oral rather than intravenous administration. After oral administration of chlorothiazide and hydrochlorothiazide, diuresis begins in 2 h and lasts about 6 to 12 h.

The half-life for chlorothiazide is 1 to 2 h, whereas the half-life for hydrochlorothiazide is 6 to 15 h. Bendroflumethiazide and polythiazide have durations of action for 6 to 12 and 24 to 48 h, respectively. The thiazides are highly bound to plasma proteins (>90 percent) and are excreted primarily by the kidney and to lesser extent by the liver. In the kidney these diuretics are excreted both in the glomerular filtrate and by proximal tubular secretion.

Adverse Reactions

Most adverse effects which develop during thiazide therapy are due to hypotension or electrolyte abnormalities such as hyponatremia, hypokalemia, and hypomagnesemia. Lassitude, weakness, and vertigo occur with large doses of thiazides. Anorexia, heartburn, nausea, vomiting, cramps, diarrhea, and constipation have all been reported, but they usually disappear when the dose is lowered and plasma electrolyte abnormalities are corrected.

A common toxic reaction to thiazide diuretics is a maculopapular skin rash. This occurs in about 1 percent of patients treated with chlorothiazide. Blood dyscrasias from chlorothiazide are rare. The drugs may also cause photosensitivity.

Thiazide diuretics tend to precipitate digitalis intoxication in patients receiving any of the cardiac glycosides. The development of digitalis toxicity under these conditions is attributable to the enhanced excretion of potassium, which creates hypokalemia. The development of hypokalemia seems to enhance the binding of digitalis glycosides to Na^+, K^+-ATPase. Restoration of normal serum potassium levels usually eliminates the toxicity. Also, individuals with ische-

mic heart disease may be predisposed to serious arrhythmias if hypokalemia occurs while on thiazides.

A gradual increase in blood uric acid level is commonly recorded during thiazide therapy. Acute attacks of thiazide-induced gout, however, are less common. This effect, which is caused by the thiazides as a
class, is apparently due to an inhibition of renal tubular secretion of uric acid and an increased urate
reabsorption in the distal tubule as a result of the diuretic-induced volume depletion. These drugs do not
increase the rate of production of uric acid. Thiazide
administration causes an increase in urinary excretion
of phosphate and a reduction in calcium excretion.

Hyperglycemia may develop occasionally from the
thiazide diuretics and may be due to interference with
the release of insulin from the pancreas. However, this
effect should not prevent the use of these compounds
in patients with diabetes mellitus if therapy is carefully
monitored. Also, thiazides may produce pancreatitis.

It has been shown that this group of diuretic agents
reduces the hypertensive action of pressor amines and
increases the skeletal muscle paralysis caused by tubocurarine and other antidepolarizing agents. The latter
interaction may be related to the hypokalemic effect of
the thiazides. Additionally, increased lithium intoxication has been noted with diuretic therapy, since the
diuretic agents reduce renal lithium clearance from the
body.

The thiazides should be used with caution in pregnancy, since they may produce adverse reactions such
as jaundice, thrombocytopenia, and possibly other
adverse effects, mentioned above, on the fetus and
newborn infant.

Clinical Uses

The thiazide drugs are used extensively in treating
hypertension, either alone or as baseline drugs to
which are added the more potent antihypertensive
agents. For further information, see Chap. 31.

The thiazide diuretics can be used in the day-to-day
management of chronic congestive heart failure when
renal function is normal. However, their use does not
reduce the importance of other factors in the management of congestive heart failure, such as bed rest and
controlled salt and fluid intake. Digitalis therapy may
be continued in patients with cardiac failure who are
receiving thiazide drugs. However, the serum potas-

sium level should be monitored, since low serum potassium concentration potentiates digitalis toxicity.
Use of potassium supplements may be necessary.

Thiazide may cause a diuretic response in patients
with nephrosis and other types of renal disease. In general, the efficiency of a thiazide is directly related to
the remaining functional properties of the kidney. In
such circumstances, the therapeutic efficacy of thiazide diuretics is less than that of a loop diuretic. Surprisingly, thiazides are also effective for palliative
treatment of the polyuria of nephrogenic and neurohy-
pophyseal diabetes insipidus. The mechanism by
which diuretic agents exert this antidiuretic action is
not completely known, but it is postulated that they
indirectly decrease urinary volume by depleting body
sodium and thus may enhance the action of antidiuretic hormone.

Other conditions which may respond to thiazide
therapy include liver disease with ascites, premenstrual fluid retention, and the positive salt balance associated with glucocorticoids and some estrogens.

It has been suggested that the use of thiazide diuretics in pregnancy should be limited. In pregnancy
edema is common and usually needs no treatment.
However, thiazides are recommended in pregnancy
when edema is due to pathologic causes. The use of
thiazides in pregnant women necessitates that the expected benefit be weighed against possible risks to the
fetus.

THIAZIDE-RELATED COMPOUNDS

Metolazone and chlorthalidone are classified as diuretic
and antihypertensive drugs. Chemically they resemble
the thiazides in that both are sulfonamide derivatives.
The mechanism of action of these compounds is similar to that of the thiazides; however, they do not inhibit carbonic anhydrase.

Metolazone

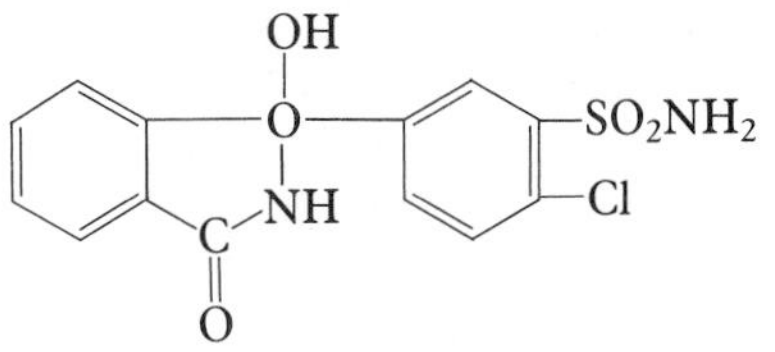

Chlorthalidone

Following oral administration of metolazone, the onset of diuresis occurs in about 1 h and lasts from 12 to 24 h. Chlorthalidone is orally effective with an onset of action at 2 h and a duration of action from 24 to 72 h. Its long duration of action is attributed to a high degree of protein binding and enterohepatic recirculation of the drug. Both diuretics are excreted by the kidney through glomerular filtration and proximal renal tubular secretion.

Indapamide is chemically a benzene-sulfonamide derivative, and its mechanism of action for the diuretic response appears to be similar to the thiazides.

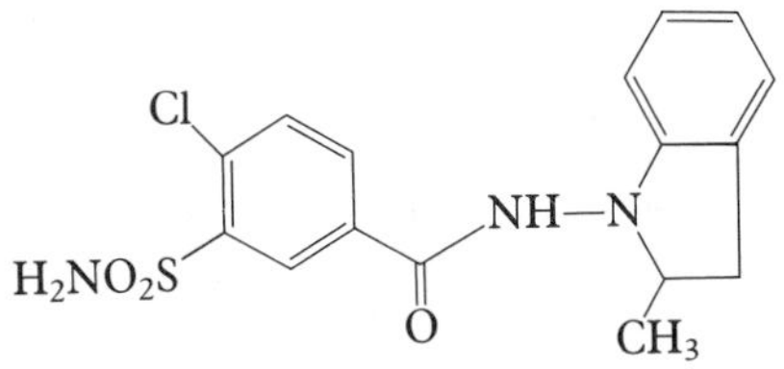

Indapamide

The drug is well absorbed (>90 percent) following oral administration and attains peak plasma concentration at 1 to 2 h. A duration of action of up to 36 h has been reported. Plasma protein binding is approximately 75 percent. Indapamide is extensively biotransformed in the liver, and about 7 percent appears in the urine as unchanged drug. The half-life of indapamide is 14 h.

The ability of indapamide, metolazone, and chlorthalidone to remove edematous fluids is equivalent to that of the thiazide diuretics but less than that of furosemide. These agents are useful in the management of edema associated with liver, kidney, or heart disease and in the treatment of essential hypertension either alone or in combination with other antihypertensive drugs.

Adverse reactions encountered with indapamide, metolazone, and chlorthalidone are similar to those of the thiazides as described previously.

LOOP DIURETICS

Bumetanide (a monosulfamoyl metanilamide derivative), ethacrynic acid (an aryloxyacetic acid derivative), and furosemide (a monosulfamoylanthranilic acid derivative) have greater diuretic efficacy than chlorothiazide when used at maximal therapeutic doses. Administered orally or intravenously, these diuretics produce a prompt increase in renal sodium and chloride excretion and urine volume.

The structural formulas of the loop diuretics are shown in Fig. 30-2.

Mechanism of Action

Loop diuretics cause their potent diuretic response primarily by inhibiting the cotransport of sodium and chloride from the renal tubular fluid into the cortical and medullary portions of the ascending limb of the loop of Henle. Along with the increased urinary sodium and chloride excretion, there is an increase in the excretion of potassium, hydrogen, magnesium, and calcium. Renal chloride and potassium excretion is greater than that of sodium. Urinary titratable acidity

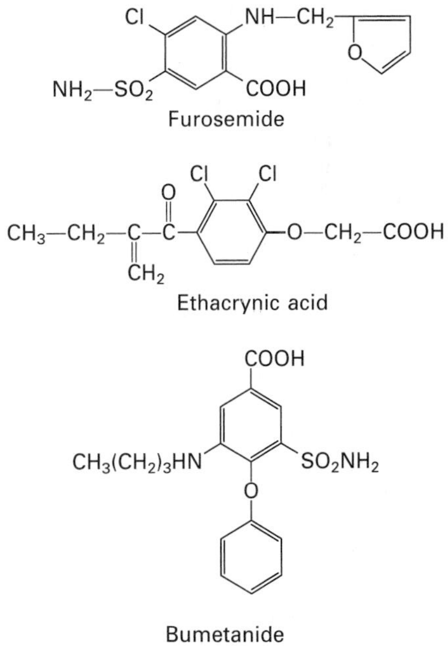

Furosemide

Ethacrynic acid

Bumetanide

FIGURE 30-2 Structural formulas of loop diuretics.

increases after a loop diuretic and ammonium concentration and pH fall. Hypochloremic alkalosis can be produced.

Since the loop diuretics decrease the reabsorption of sodium and chloride in the medullary portion of the loop of Henle, there occurs a reduction in the hypertonicity of the medullary interstitium. Also, free-water reabsorption is reduced in the collecting duct.

Pharmacokinetics

When given orally, the loop diuretics have an onset of action in about 30 min to 1 h, and the diuretic response may last for 6 h; with intravenous or intramuscular injection, the effect is almost immediate with a duration of 2 h. Some other pharmacokinetic data are presented in Table 30-3. About 90 percent of the administered dose of furosemide is excreted by the kidney. Furosemide is both filtered through the glomerulus and secreted by the cells of the proximal convoluted tubule. The remainder of the dose is present in the feces.

Approximately 60 percent of an intravenous dose of ethacrynic acid is excreted in the urine by filtration and active proximal tubular secretion. The remaining portion of the drug is eliminated in the bile. In both the urine and bile, ethacrynic acid is excreted unchanged and in a conjugated form (e.g., cysteine).

Bumetanide is mainly eliminated from the body in the urine as unchanged drug (45 percent) and oxidative metabolites.

Adverse Reactions

Bumetanide, ethacrynic acid, and furosemide produce adverse reactions that are largely the same and are usually related to excessive fluid and electrolyte loss. Side effects include thirst, urinary frequency, nocturia, muscle weakness and cramps, headache, and mental confusion. Hypokalemia, prehepatic coma, hypotension, hyperuricemia, hyperglycemia, blood dyscrasias, and shock have been reported.

In the presence of hypokalemia the toxicities of digitalis glycosides, e.g., digoxin, may be increased. The development of hyperuricemia is due to the interference of the active secretion of uric acid in the proximal tubule by the loop diuretic. The elevation of blood glucose, glucosuria, or alteration in glucose tolerance tests may be related to a decreased release of insulin from the pancreas by the loop diuretics.

Other adverse reactions are transient hearing loss, tinnitus, irreversible hearing impairment, jaundice, and gastrointestinal disturbances such as anorexia, nausea, vomiting, abdominal pains, and diarrhea. In addition, lowering of serum calcium and magnesium concentrations have been observed. Individuals sensitive to sulfonamides may show similar allergic reactions to furosemide and bumetanide.

Drug Interactions

The loop diuretics can exhibit drug-drug interactions when they are administered concomitantly with other therapeutic agents. Bumetanide, ethacrynic acid, and furosemide may increase the toxicities of lithium because they reduce the renal clearance of lithium. These diuretics may enhance the ototoxic potential of aminoglycoside antibiotics and may increase the nephrotoxicity of cephaloridine and other drugs that possess potential nephrotoxicity. The loop diuretics augment the therapeutic effect of antihypertensive agents. It has been shown that nonsteroidal anti-inflammatory agents, e.g., indomethacin, can decrease the natriuretic and antihypertensive effect of these diuretics. This action of the nonsteroidal anti-inflammatory

TABLE 30-3 Pharmacokinetic data of the loop diuretics

Drug	Duration of action, h	Half-life, h	% Absorption (oral)	Protein binding
Bumetanide	3–6	1–1.5	70–95	95
Ethacrynic acid	6–8	1.0	100	95
Furosemide	6–8	1.0	65	97

agents is related to inhibition of prostaglandins, which appear to have a role in sodium excretion.

In addition, furosemide may increase the toxicities of high doses of prescribed salicylates because of competition at renal excretory sites. Furosemide may decrease the hypertensive response of pressor amines, e.g., norepinephrine. This diuretic also attenuates the neuromuscular blockade of tubucurarine and may potentiate the effect of succinylcholine.

Clinical Uses

The loop diuretics are recommended in the treatment of fluid retention because of their high therapeutic efficacy (Fig. 30-3). Maximum therapeutic doses produce a greater diuretic response than the thiazide diuretics. Bumetanide, ethacrynic acid, and furosemide are useful in treating edema associated with congestive heart failure, cirrhosis of the liver, nephrotic syndrome, chronic heart failure, and renal failure. These diuretics are frequently employed in patients who do not respond to thiazides, e.g., in patients who show evidence of hypervolemia and decreased glomerular filtration rates, manifested in elevated serum creatinine or blood urea nitrogen (BUN) concentrations. Furosemide and ethacrynic acid are used in the therapy of acute pulmonary edema. Furosemide is also indicated for the treatment of chronic hypertension alone or with other antihypertensive drugs. The safety and efficacy of ethacrynic acid and bumetanide for the treatment of chronic hypertension have not been established. It is reported that the loop diuretics are effective in the acute treatment of hypercalcemia.

POTASSIUM-SPARING DIURETICS

Spironolactone

Spironolactone is an aldosterone antagonist which interferes with the action of the hormone at the target organ and is most effective when circulating aldosterone levels are high.

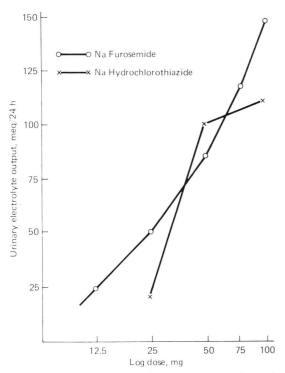

Spironolactone

Mechanism of Action Spironolactone exerts its diuretic effect by interfering with the aldosterone-mediated sodium reabsorption in the collecting duct, thereby increasing sodium loss in the urine and allowing for retention of potassium in the body. Spironolactone acts presumably by binding to the cytoplasmic aldosterone receptor complex in a competitive manner. The binding of spironolactone prevents the conversion of the receptor complex to its active form, and this eventually leads to a reduction in the synthesis of a transport protein that is required for the reabsorption of sodium in the collecting duct.

Canrenone, an active biotransformation product of spironolactone, has the same mechanism of action as spironolactone and, therefore, adds to the pharmaco-

FIGURE 30-3 Comparative efficacy of furosemide and hydrochlorothiazide.

logic effect of spironolactone. Both compounds are competitive antagonists of aldosterone.

Pharmacokinetics Spironolactone is well absorbed from the gastrointestinal tract (Table 30-4). Its onset of action is delayed, and the maximum effect may not be observed for several days after initiating therapy. The drug is biotransformed by the liver to an active metabolite, canrenone. Canrenone and other metabolites are excreted by the kidney and bile.

Adverse Reactions Spironolactone is contraindicated in the presence of hyperkalemia, since it may cause further elevation of plasma potassium concentrations. Potassium supplements should not be continued during spironolactone therapy.

Lethargy, drowsiness, ataxia, headache, and mental confusion have been observed during spironolactone therapy, and a few patients have developed a transient maculopapular or erythematous rash while receiving the drug. These eruptions usually disappear within 48 h after discontinuing the drug. Diarrhea and other gastrointestinal disturbances may occur during spironolactone therapy. Spironolactone may produce metabolic acidosis. Androgenic side effects of the drug include hirsutism, irregular menses, and deepening of the voice. It is reported that spironolactone may induce gynecomastia, which appears to be related to dose and duration of therapy. Generally, this effect is reversible on discontinuation of therapy. Spironolactone may increase the effects of digoxin, since it decreases the renal excretion of the cardiac glycosides. In addition, this diuretic may increase the blood levels of lithium and decrease the effects of pressor amines, e.g., norepinephrine.

Clinical Uses Spironolactone increases renal sodium excretion when prescribed alone or in combination with hydrochlorothiazide. Spironolactone diminishes the kaliuresis induced by thiazide diuretics. It is therefore a useful adjunct in the management of patients with intractable edema in whom hypokalemia is a frequent complication. It is also indicated for the treatment of primary hyperaldosteronism, hypertension, and edematous conditions associated with cirrhosis of the liver, nephrotic syndrome, and congestive heart failure. Most patients with chronic congestive heart failure, however, are satisfactorily maintained with the proper use of thiazides or a loop diuretic.

Triamterene

Triamterene is a pyrazine derivative which inhibits sodium reabsorption and, consequently, prevents potassium secretion in the collecting duct. Such a potassium-sparing diuretic causes a moderate increase in sodium and bicarbonate excretions in the urine and decreases urinary potassium and ammonia. It has little effect on urine volume, but when combined with thiazides or loop diuretic, it enhances the diuretic response without increasing the output of potassium in the urine.

Triamterene

Its principal effects appear to be on the collecting duct, where, as mentioned above, it inhibits sodium reabsorption and potassium secretion. Although triamterene behaves like an aldosterone antagonist, its action is due to a direct effect on the collecting duct and is not due to competitive aldosterone inhibition.

Pharmacokinetics Triamterene is absorbed from the gastrointestinal tract and has an onset of action in 2 to 4 h. The drug is eliminated from the body by the liver and kidney. In the liver triamterene is biotransformed by hydroxylation and then conjugated to a sulfate. In the kidney the drug is excreted by proximal tubular secretion. Other pharmacokinetic data are presented in Table 30-4.

Clinical Uses and Adverse Reactions Triamterene causes a moderate increase in sodium and bicarbonate excretion and a decrease in urinary potassium and ammonia. It is a weak diuretic when used alone, but when combined with the thiazides, the combination is more effective than either drug alone. Triamterene is usually recommended in combination with other diuretics for the treatment of edema due to congestive heart failure, cirrhosis of the liver, and nephrotic syndrome. When used with hydrochlorothiazide in treating hypertension, triamterene produces a positive potassium balance and a rise in plasma potassium concentrations.

TABLE 30-4 Pharmacokinetic data of K$^+$-sparing diuretics

Drug	% Absorption	Half-life, h	Protein binding	Duration of action, h
Amiloride	15–20	6–9	23	24
Spironolactone	90	20	98	48–72
Triamterene	30–70	3	50–70	12–16

Triamterene either alone or with thiazide diuretics may cause hyperkalemia, electrocardiographic changes, and death. Renal function must be known before the drug is administered, and it should not be used in the presence of renal failure. Triamterene has also been reported to decrease glomerular filtration rate and to increase blood urea concentrations. This diuretic is contraindicated in hyperkalemia.

Amiloride

Amiloride is a potassium-sparing diuretic that exhibits mild diuretic activity.

$$\text{Cl}-\underset{\text{H}_2\text{N}-\overset{\displaystyle N}{\underset{\displaystyle N}{\quad}}-\text{NH}_2}{\overset{\displaystyle N}{\quad}}-\text{CO}-\text{NH}-\underset{\parallel\text{NH}}{\text{C}}-\text{NH}_2$$

Amiloride

The drug is absorbed from the gastrointestinal tract but shows low bioavailability (Table 30-4). The onset of action is approximately 2 h. Unlike spironolactone and triamterene, this diuretic is not biotransformed by the liver. It is excreted by the kidney and undergoes active secretion in the proximal tubule of the nephron.

Mechanism of Action Amiloride has its site of action in the collecting duct of the nephron unit. The drug appears to directly inhibit the reabsorption of sodium and promote the conservation of potassium. This potassium-sparing diuretic is not a direct aldosterone antagonist.

Adverse Reactions and Clinical Uses Adverse reactions for amiloride include headache, weakness, fatigability, muscle cramps, and dizziness. Gastrointestinal effects such as nausea, vomiting, anorexia, and diarrhea have been reported. Less frequently there are occurrences of orthostatic hypotension, dry mouth, paresthesia, mental confusion, and insomnia. Amiloride is contraindicated in hyperkalemia.

Amiloride is rarely used alone, and its main indication is in combination with the thiazide or loop diuretics in congestive heart failure or hypertension. Amiloride is incorporated into the treatment of these patients to prevent or correct the condition of hypokalemia.

ACETAZOLAMIDE

Acetazolamide, an aromatic sulfonamide with a free sulfamyl group ($-SO_2NH_2$), is a carbonic anhydrase inhibitor. The drug produces an alkaline urine with increased concentrations of sodium, potassium, and bicarbonate ions. Patients may exhibit refractoriness to the diuretic response of acetazolamide.

Mechanism of Action

The diuretic action of acetazolamide is due to inhibition of carbonic anhydrase in the renal tubule, mainly in the proximal tubule. Following administration of acetazolamide, reabsorption of sodium ions in exchange for hydrogen ions is depressed, sodium bicarbonate excretion is increased, and chloride output is decreased. Bicarbonate excretion is increased because of the lack of hydrogen ions to neutralize urinary bicarbonate.

Chloride ions are retained by the kidney to offset the loss of bicarbonate and maintain ionic balance. Because of decreased availability of hydrogen ions, potassium is excreted in exchange for sodium and urinary potassium output increases.

The renal electrolyte excretion pattern of patients receiving a carbonic anhydrase inhibitor is characterized by increased amounts of sodium, potassium, and bicarbonate output, with only moderate increases in water output. The urine becomes alkaline, and the plasma bicarbonate concentration decreases. If therapy is continued, the patient develops a metabolic acidosis. Plasma chloride levels increase. Urinary ammonia concentrations drop when hydrogen ions present in the tubule are insufficient to convert ammonia to NH_4^+.

Pharmacokinetics

Acetazolamide is absorbed rapidly from the gastrointestinal tract; peak plasma levels are reached within 2 h after oral administration. Acetazolamide is excreted unchanged in the urine by proximal tubular secretion, about 80 percent of a single oral dose appearing in the urine within 8 to 12 h.

Adverse Reactions

Acetazolamide produces reversible side effects, which include flushing, headache, drowsiness, dizziness, fatigue, irritability, and excitability. Instances of polydipsia and polyuria, paresthesias, ataxia, hyperpnea, anorexia, vomiting, and gastrointestinal distress have been reported during therapy with carbonic anhydrase inhibitors. Such manifestations disappear when dosage is reduced.

Like antibacterial sulfonamides, acetazolamide may cause fever and blood dyscrasias such as leukopenia, agranulocytosis, thrombocytopenia, and aplastic anemia. Allergic skin reactions, including exfoliative dermatitis, may develop during acetazolamide administration. Genitourinary complications of acetazolamide therapy include crystalluria, calculus formation (chiefly calcium phosphate and citrate) with renal colic, and secondary renal lesions.

Clinical Uses

Acetazolamide is a weak diuretic with limited use since the introduction of the thiazides. However, there are five indications for a carbonic anhydrase inhibitor: (1) in edema, to promote a diuretic response, (2) in glau-

coma, (3) in absence seizures, (4) in premenstrual tension, and (5) in acute mountain sickness.

SUMMARY

The comparative effects of the various diuretic agents which have been discussed individually thus far are listed in Table 30-5. A relative comparison of urinary excretion patterns, urinary pH, alteration in the blood acid-base balance, and refractoriness is indicated.

OSMOTIC NONELECTROLYTES

Today the most clinically used member of this category is mannitol. In the presence of normal cardiorenal function, mannitol causes a decrease in water reabsorption in the nephron unit and promotes an osmotic diuresis, generally without significant sodium excretion. This agent is not metabolized or reabsorbed by the tubular cells; it is excreted by the glomeruli and, being osmotically active, retains water in the tubular fluid to increase urine volume.

Adverse Reactions

Mannitol does not penetrate the cells, and its only method of excretion is via the glomerular filtrate. Intravenous infusions of mannitol, therefore, increase blood volume. Expansion of blood volume in patients with congestive heart failure may cause further decompensation. When given to patients with renal failure, mannitol produces vascular overfilling with hyperosmolality and hyponatremia. Clinically, there is a picture of tissue dehydration accompanied by signs of congestive heart failure. Hyperosmolality has been reported after mannitol infusions in patients with cirrhosis and ascites. Peritoneal dialysis may correct the overhydration produced by mannitol infusions, but deaths due to vascular overfilling, hyperosmolality, and hyponatremia have also been reported.

Clinical Uses

Mannitol is used as an adjunct in the prevention or treatment of oliguria and anuria. It may also be employed to reduce intraocular pressure pre- and postop-

TABLE 30-5   A comparison of various diuretic drugs: Urinary excretion patterns, pH, acid-base alterations, and refractoriness

Drugs	Urinary excretion[a]					Blood acid-base balance[c]	Refractoriness
	Na^+	Cl^-	K^+	HCO_3^-	pH[b]		
Thiazides	↑	↑	↑	→ ↑ [d]	↓	Hypochloremic alkalosis	No
Thiazide-related	↑	↑	↑	→	↓	Hypochloremic alkalosis	No
Loop diuretics	↑	↑	↑	→	↓	Hypochloremic alkalosis	No
K^+-sparing diuretics	↑	↑	↓	↑	↑	Metabolic acidosis	No
Acetazolamide	↑	↓	↑	↑	↑	Metabolic acidosis	Yes

[a] Key: increase (↑); decrease (↓); no change (→).
[b] Urinary pH.
[c] Possible alterations.
[d] Chlorothiazide may produce slight increase.

eratively in ophthalmic procedures and in the treatment of brain edema.

PREPARATIONS AND DOSE

Thiazides

Chlorothiazide (Diuril) is available in 250- and 500-mg tablets and in a suspension containing 250 mg per 5 mL. Chlorothiazide is administered orally, the usual dose range varying between 0.5 and 2.0 g once or twice daily. A lyphilized powder of chlorothiazide sodium is prepared in vials of 500 mg for intravenous injection or slow intravenous infusion.

Hydrochlorothiazide (Esidrix, HydroDiuril, Oretic) is supplied in 25-, 50-, and 100-mg tablets. The usual dosage range is between 25 and 200 mg/day.

Bendroflumethiazide (Naturetin) is supplied in 2.5-, 5-, and 10-mg tablets. The usual dose range is between 5 and 15 mg/day.

Polythiazide (Renese) is supplied in 1-, 2-, and 4-mg tablets. The usual dose range is between 1 and 4 mg/day.

Thiazide-Related Agents

Chlorthalidone (Hygroton) is supplied in tablets of 50 and 100 mg. The usual dose is 50 to 100 mg/day.

Metolazone (Zaroxolyn) is supplied in tablets of 2.5, 5, and 10 mg. The usual dose is 5 to 20 mg/day.

Indapamide (Lozol) is supplied in tablets of 2.5 mg. The usual dose is 2.5 to 5 mg daily.

Loop Diuretics

Bumetanide (Bumex) is supplied in 0.5-, 1-, and 2-mg tablets. A solution of 0.25 mg/mL in 2-mL containers is available. The usual oral dose is 0.5 to 2 mg/day. The usual intramuscular or intravenous dose is 0.5 to 1 mg.

Ethacrynic acid (Edecrin) is supplied in 25- and 50-mg tablets and in an oral solution of 10 mg/mL. The usual oral dosage of up to 200 mg may be required. Sodium ethacrynate is available in vials containing 50 mg/mL to be injected intravenously. The usual dose is 50 to 100 mg.

Furosemide (Lasix) is supplied in 20-, 40-, and

80-mg tablets. The usual dose of furosemide is 40 to 80 mg orally as a single daily dose. The total daily dose may be increased to 200 mg, administered as a single dose or in two divided doses. Furosemide is available in 2-, 4-, and 10-mL ampuls, each milliliter containing 10 mg/mL. The usual intramuscular or intravenous dose is 20 to 40 mg.

Potassium-Sparing Diuretics

Amiloride (Midamor) is supplied in 5-mg tablets. The recommended initial dose is 5 mg daily.

Spironolactone (Aldactone) is supplied in 25-mg tablets. An initial schedule of 25 mg two to four times daily is recommended.

Triamterene (Dyrenium) is available in 50- and 100-mg capsules. The recommended initial dose is 100 mg twice daily.

Other Agents

Acetazolamide (Diamox) is available in 125- and 250-mg tablets and in 500-mg sustained-release capsules. The usual oral dose is 250 mg two to four times daily. Sodium acetazolamide is supplied in 500-mg vials. The usual intravenous or intramuscular dose range is 0.5 to 1.0 g daily.

Mannitol is a polyhydric alcohol which must be infused intravenously to produce a diuretic response. The usual dose is 25 to 100 mg/day, prepared in a 10% aqueous solution.

BIBLIOGRAPHY

Beermann, B., and M. Groschinsky-Grind: "Clinical Pharmacokinetics of Diuretics," *Clin. Pharmacokinet.*, 5:221–245 (1980).

Cannon, P. J.: "Diuretics: Their Mechanism of Action and Use in Hypertension," *Cardiovas. Rev. Rep.*, 4:649–666 (1983).

Hackett, P. H., and D. Rennie: "Incidence, Importance, and Prophylaxis of Acute Mountain Sickness," *Lancet*, 2:1149–1154 (1976).

Hendry, B. M., and J. C. Ellory: "Molecular Sites for Diuretic Action," *Trends in Pharmacol Sci*, 9:416–420 (1988).

Herbert, S. C., and T. E. Andreoli: "Control of NaCl Transport in Thick Ascending Limb," *Am. J. Physiol.*, 246:F745–F756 (1984).

Koechel, D. A.: "Ethacrynic Acid and Related Diuretics: Relationship of Structure to Beneficial and Detrimental Actions," *Annu. Rev. Pharmacol. Toxicol.*, 21:265–293 (1981).

Kokko, J. P.: "Site and Mechanism of Action of Diuretics," *Am. J. Med.*, 77:11–17 (1984).

Lant, A.: "Diuretics: Clinical Pharmacology and Therapeutic Use," *Drugs*, 29:57–87, 162–188 (1985).

Rybak, L. P.: "Drug Ototoxicity," *Annu. Rev. Pharmacol. Toxicol.*, 26:79–100 (1986).

Velazquez, H., and F. S. Wright: "Control by Drugs of Renal Potassium Handling," *Annu. Rev. Pharmacol. Toxicol.* 26:293–310 (1986).

Warren, S. E., and R. C. Blantz: "Mannitol," *Arch. Intern. Med.*, 141:493 (1981).

Warnock, D. G., and J. Eveloff: "NaCl Entry Mechanism in Luminal Membrane of the Renal Tubule," *Am. J. Physiol.*, 242:F561–F574 (1982).

CHAPTER 31

Antihypertensive Drugs

Joseph R. DiPalma

Hypertension is a syndrome characterized by elevated blood pressure. The pathophysiologic basis for 90 to 95 percent of the cases of the disease remains unexplained, and therefore the condition is called *primary*, or *essential*, *hypertension*. The remaining 5 to 10 percent may be due to a number of known causes, including renal artery stenosis, aortic coarctation, Cushing's syndrome, and pheochromocytoma. This is called *secondary hypertension*. Although the cause of primary hypertension is unknown, empirical treatment is generally effective and should be instituted until the etiology of the disease is defined and more specific therapy is employed. This chapter deals with the treatment of primary hypertension.

Sustained elevated blood pressure causes vascular alterations throughout the body. Many studies have concluded that the higher the arterial pressure, whether systolic or diastolic, the higher the morbidity and mortality. Classification of hypertension on the basis of severity is presented in Table 31-1.

Diastolic pressure is the basis for confirming primary hypertension. Virtually all patients with a diastolic pressure of at least 105 mmHg should be treated with antihypertensive drugs. For patients with lower diastolic pressures, treatment should be individualized, with consideration of other risk factors, e.g., the family history or sex of the patient.

PRINCIPLES OF DRUG THERAPY

One traditional principle of antihypertensive therapy is that patients may require multiple drugs, affecting the major sites which control changes in peripheral vascular resistance: the central vasomotor sympathetic center, the peripheral sympathetic nervous system, the heart, and the arteriolar smooth muscle. Three classes of drugs are used—depending on the severity of hypertension (Table 31-1)—which are introduced in a specific sequence, based on the pharmacologic profiles on the drugs and clinical experience. This sequence should be flexible and should provide several alternatives. It is important to remember that the therapeutic regimen for the hypertensive patient must be individualized. However, some general principles should be followed. Traditionally all patients are started on an oral antihypertensive diuretic as the first line of therapy. Although the mechanism by which diuretics lower blood pressure is not fully delineated, they certainly have proven to be the most useful antihypertensive drugs. Generally well tolerated, these drugs enhance the effectiveness of all other antihypertensive therapy. The second group of drugs constitutes the sympatholytic agents (sympathetic nervous system depressants), given either after a diuretic has been started or concurrently with it. Finally, after sympathetic blockade has been established, peripheral vasodilators may be added. Therapy with peripheral vasodilators should be initiated only after sympathetic blocking agents have been employed. The former drugs cause two troublesome side effects, increased cardiac output and tachycardia, which occur when blood pressure falls in response to peripheral vasodilation in the presence of an intact sympathetic nervous system.

TABLE 31-1 Classification of diastolic hypertension by degree of severity

Degree	Diastolic pressure, mmHg	Outlook
Severe	130 or above; grade III or IV retinopathy	Medical emergency
Moderately severe	115–129	40% of the patients can be expected to have morbid events within 20 months
Moderate	105–114	One-half of the patients may have morbid events within 5 years
Mild	90–104	Excessive cardiovascular disease over long term

Because long-term diuretic therapy may lead to hypokalemia, uricemia, hypercholesteremia, and other side effects, a more recent approach is *monotherapy* with either a sympathomimetic blocker, an angiotensin converting enzyme (ACE) inhibitor, or a calcium-channel blocker. Most experience with monotherapy has accrued with beta blockers, but ACE inhibitors are gaining popularity. Calcium-channel blockers are still in the experimental stage but may prove to be superior agents for monotherapy. Generally monotherapy is reserved for mild to moderate hypertension and is less successful in moderate to severe hypertension. Monotherapy is becoming increasingly popular because of its simplicity, fewer side effects, and improved patient compliance. Peripheral vasodilators are not used for monotherapy.

ORAL ANTIHYPERTENSIVE DIURETICS

The mechanism of the antihypertensive effect of diuretics has not been completely elucidated. It appears, however, to be related to a reduction in both total body sodium and extracellular fluid volume. Diuretics reduce elevated blood pressure by enhancing sodium and water excretion via the kidney, with a consequent reduction in extracellular fluid and plasma volume. Although certain diuretics, i.e., the thiazides, relax vascular smooth muscle by a direct action, many anti-hypertensive diuretics do not. Therefore, it appears that this action is not primarily responsible for the hypotensive response to these drugs.

The various diuretics and the usual doses employed in patients with hypertension are listed in Table 31-2. As a rule, patients are started on a diuretic from the thiazide or thiazide-related group. The effects of these drugs are quite similar; milligram dose and duration of action vary. The three main side effects associated with this group are (1) hyperuricemia, (2) hyperglycemia, and (3) electrolyte abnormalities characterized by hypokalemia, metabolic alkalosis, and hypochloremia.

Furosemide, although a more efficacious diuretic, has not demonstrated a more potent antihypertensive action than the standard thiazide-like group. Furosemide is used for those patients who show evidence of hypervolemia and decreased glomerular filtration rates, manifested in elevated serum creatinine or blood urea nitrogen (BUN) concentration. Occasionally a patient with renal insufficiency, on a thiazide diuretic, will exhibit deterioration of renal function and a rising BUN; this has not been noted with furosemide.

Spironolactone is a competitive inhibitor of aldosterone but does not have side effects such as potassium wasting, hyperuricemia, or deterioration of glucose tolerance. Spironolactone is used as a first-line diuretic for patients with gout or diabetes mellitus or for those who have shown hypokalemic responses to the thiazide group of diuretics.

SYMPATHOLYTIC AGENTS

Centrally Acting Sympathetic Inhibitors

It has been established that central catecholaminergic neurons are an important factor in the regulation of systemic arterial blood pressure. Stimulation of α-adrenergic receptors in specific areas of the CNS leads to hypotension and bradycardia. These effects appear to be mediated through the activation of an inhibitory neuronal system in the medullary vasomotor center which decreases sympathetic outflow from this area to the periphery.

A few clinically useful antihypertensive drugs, e.g., clonidine and methyldopa, appear to act principally by alteration of central sympathetic function. Reserpine, propranolol, and hydralazine also have actions on the CNS which may be important to their antihypertensive effects. However, these compounds have significant peripheral actions; therefore, these drugs are discussed in other sections of this chapter.

Clonidine Clonidine is structurally related to the imidazoline derivative tolazoline, a peripheral vasodilator and α-adrenergic-receptor blocker.

Clonidine

These actions have not been attributed to clonidine; in fact, the drug may produce mild, transient peripheral α-adrenergic-receptor stimulation, evidenced by a transient rise in arterial blood pressure, especially after intravenous administration. However, the central antihypertensive action quickly predominates as clonidine accumulates in the CNS.

TABLE 31-2 Oral antihypertensive diuretics

Classification and generic name	Trade name	Total daily doses, mg, oral	Duration of action, h
Thiazides			
Chlorothiazide	Diuril	500–1000	6–12
Hydrochlorothiazide	HydroDiuril, Esidrix	50–100	6–12
Benzthiazide	Exna	50–200	12–18
Hydroflumethiazide	Saluron, Diucardin	50–100	12–24
Bendroflumethiazide	Naturetin	2.5–20	18–24
Methylothiazide	Enduron	5–20	24
Trichlormethiazide	Naqua, Metahydrin	2–4	24
Polythiazide	Renese	2–4	24–36
Cyclothiazide	Anhydron	1–2	18–24
Thiazide-related			
Chlorthalidone	Hygroton	25–100	48–72
Metolazone	Diulo, Zaroxolyn	2.5–20	12–24
Indapamide	Lozol	2.5	24–36
Furosemide	Lasix	80–320	4–8
Ethacrynic acid	Edecrin	50–200	6–8
Bumetanide	Bumex	0.5–10	3–6
Spironolactone	Aldactone	50–100	2–8
Triamterene	Dyrenium	50–100	12–16
Amiloride	Midamor	5–10	18–24

Mechanism of Action The mechanism of action of clonidine is not completely understood. However, from the accumulated experimental data, it appears that the antihypertensive effects of the drug result mainly from potent stimulation of either postsynaptic alpha-adrenergic receptors in the vasomotor center of the medulla, or presynaptic alpha receptors in the nucleus tractus solitarii, or both. Central alpha-receptor activation causes decreased sympathetic tone from the medullary vasomotor center to the heart and the vasculature.

Effects on Organ Systems The cardiovascular effects of oral clonidine include decreased arterial blood pressure, heart rate, cardiac output, and peripheral vascular resistance. Orthostatic hypotension is mild and infrequent. There is little effect on renal blood flow and glomerular filtration rate. Renin secretion is suppressed.

In addition to the antihypertensive actions in the CNS, clonidine may produce drowsiness and sedation. Tolerance to the sedative effect of the drug has been noted during chronic administration. Clonidine reduces salivary flow and causes xerostomia, which appears to be due to a central effect of the drug.

Pharmacokinetics The drug is adequately absorbed after oral administration. Blood pressure falls within 30 to 60 min, with the maximum effect occurring within 2 h. The duration of the antihypertensive effect is at least 6 h, and estimates of the mean biologic half-life range between 8 and 13 h. The plasma clearance of clonidine is between 200 and 500 mL/min. The exact biotransformation fate of the compound is not known; it is eliminated primarily in the urine.

Therapeutic Use In combination with an oral diuretic such as hydrochlorothiazide, chlorthalidone, or furosemide, clonidine is a drug of choice for the management of various degrees of hypertension. If blood pressure is not adequately controlled with a diuretic-clonidine combination, a peripherally acting sympathetic inhibitor or a vasodilator may be added to the therapeutic regimen without significant adverse drug-drug interactions. Clonidine can be employed in uncomplicated mild to severe hypertensive states or when hypertension is complicated by cerebrovascular insufficiency, ischemic heart disease, or congestive heart failure.

Adverse Reactions The most common adverse reactions to clonidine include dry mouth, drowsiness, sedation, and constipation. Generally, these side effects diminish as therapy is continued. Serious organ toxicity is rare.

When discontinuing the drug, the dose should be reduced gradually over 2 to 4 days to avoid the potential of a withdrawal syndrome, observed when clonidine therapy is stopped abruptly. Symptoms include headache, nervousness, abdominal pain, sweating, tachycardia, and a rapid rise in blood pressure. The pathophysiology of this syndrome is unknown but can be reversed by resumption of clonidine therapy or by a combination of phentolamine and propranolol.

The antihypertensive effects of clonidine will be diminished if given concurrently with tricyclic antidepressants. The mechanism responsible for this drug-drug interaction has not been established.

Preparation *Clonidine hydrochloride* (Catapres) is available in tablets of 0.1 and 0.2 mg. A transdermal preparation is available containing 2.5, 5, or 7.5 mg.

Methyldopa Methyldopa is the α-methylated derivative of levodopa.

$$HO-\underset{HO}{\bigcirc}-CH_2-\underset{NH_3}{\overset{CH_3}{\underset{|}{\overset{|}{C}}}}-CO_2H$$

Methyldopa

Mechanism of Action Several mechanisms have been proposed in attempts to explain the antihypertensive effects of methyldopa. These include (1) inhibition of the decarboxylation of dopa in sympathetic neurons, which would decrease norepinephrine stores and vasomotor tone, and (2) biotransformation of methyldopa to methylnorepinephrine, which displaces norepinephrine from storage granules and acts as a weak "false neurotransmitter."

At present, it is generally accepted that the major antihypertensive action of methyldopa is on the CNS. Using a modification of the false-neurotransmitter hypothesis, it is believed that the drug enters the CNS, is biotransformed to and is stored as methylnorepinephrine in adrenergic neurons, and upon release activates the α-adrenergic-receptor mediated inhibitory system in the vasomotor center. Methylnorepinephrine is a potent stimulatory of α-adrenergic receptors in the CNS; however, its action on peripheral α receptors is rather weak.

Effects on the Cardiovascular System The cardiovascular effects of this drug are similar to those observed with clonidine. Methyldopa produces less bradycardia and greater orthostatic hypotension than comparable antihypertensive doses of clonidine. Methyldopa has no direct cardiac action and generally does not alter glomerular filtration rate or renal blood flow. Normal or elevated plasma renin activity may be decreased by the drug.

Pharmacokinetics The drug is incompletely absorbed following oral administration. The peak antihypertensive effect occurs at about 6 h, and the duration of action is 12 to 24 h. Methyldopa is widely distributed throughout the body; however, this is not reflected in its calculated apparent volume of distribution (0.5 L/kg). Since the drug accumulates in adrenergic nerve endings of the brain and periphery and is not in equilibrium with the circulation, classic pharmacokinetic parameters are of little value.

Plasma protein binding of methyldopa is between 0 and 20 percent. Circulating drug is biotransformed in the liver to the sulfate conjugate, which appears to be inactive. As mentioned previously, methyldopa taken up into adrenergic neurons is biotransformed to the active product, methylnorepinephrine. The parent compound and all biotransformation products are excreted in the urine.

Therapeutic Use The only indication for methyldopa is hypertension.

Adverse Reactions and Precautions Common adverse reactions include transient drowsiness, headache, and fatigue, which usually diminish as therapy is continued. Paresthesias, parkinsonism-like symptoms, depression, and psychic disturbances including nightmares and mild psychosis may occur.

Cardiovascular reactions may include bradycardia, aggravation of angina pectoris, fluid retention, and orthostatic hypotension.

Drug-related fever, a lupus-like syndrome, and myocarditis have been reported. In addition, gastrointestinal symptoms including nausea, vomiting, abdominal distention, constipation, and diarrhea may occur.

A positive Coombs' test will occur in approximately 20 percent of patients; however, hemolytic anemia is rare (0.2 percent). At the initiation of methyldopa therapy, blood counts should be performed, and periodic blood counts should be done to detect hemolytic anemia.

Methyldopa is contraindicated in active hepatic disease (e.g., hepatitis and cirrhosis) since the drug may cause jaundice and result in abnormal liver function.

Preparations *Methyldopa* (Aldomet) is available in tablets of 125, 250, and 500 mg. Methyldopate hydrochloride (Aldomet ester HCl), 250 mg per 5 mL, is a soluble salt available for parenteral use.

Guanabenz and Guanfacine These are two centrally acting alpha-adrenergic agonists. As with clonidine and methyldopa, stimulation of these receptors causes inhibition of central nervous system sympathetic outflow. Both drugs reduce both supine and standing blood pressure and heart rate.

The chemistry of these drugs is similar.

Guanabenz

Guanfacine

Pharmacokinetics Guanabenz is about 75 percent orally bioavailable. There is extensive biotransformation with less than 1 percent of the unbound drug being present in the urine. Half-life is 7 to 10 h.

Guanfacine is 90 percent orally bioavailable. With a large volume of distribution, it has a long half-life of 16 to 20 h. It is eliminated both by renal and liver biotransformation.

Both drugs have adverse reactions similar to those of clonidine. Sedation and dryness of the mouth are most common. Weakness and orthostatic hypotension are a natural consequence of this type of drug. Headache, palpitations, bradycardia, nasal congestion, blurred vision and gastrointestinal disturbances occasionally occur. Also, as with clonidine, withdrawal reactions (rebound hypertension) may happen when the drug is withdrawn abruptly.

Preparations *Guanabenz* (Wytensin) is available in 4- and 8-mg tablets. Adult dose 4 mg twice a day.

Guanfacine (Tenex) is available in 1-mg tablets. Adult dose 1 mg at bedtime to minimize somnolence.

Both drugs are started at the lowest dose and titrated upward carefully to achieve the desired blood pressure lowering. The concomitant use of a diuretic lowers the effective dose.

Peripherally Acting Sympathetic Inhibitors

Beta-Adrenergic Sympathetic Blockers The most commonly utilized antiadrenergic substances for the therapy of hypertension are the beta-adrenergic blockers. They are discussed in detail in Chap. 8. Despite years of use, the mechanism of action by which adrenergic beta blockers lower blood pressure is not completely understood. Agreement is certain that they depress myocardial function and decrease cardiac output. Heart rate is slowed, and the catechol autoregulator drive is moderated and reduced. Peripheral resistance is not directly affected, but as the cardiac output falls, there is reflexly an increase. The ability of beta blockers to inhibit plasma renin activity may be significant in a subset of patients. Theories concerning presynaptic beta-blockade blocking norepinephrine release and thus reducing vasoconstriction as well as effects on the prostaglandin and kinase systems are less certain. At the present time there are eight beta blockers commercially available which are used as antihypertensives. They are listed in Table 31-3 along with the features which might make them more likely candidates for antihypertensive therapy. Actually all of them are equally efficacious as antihypertensives, but in a subgroup of hypertensive patients

TABLE 31-3   Features of beta-adrenergic blockers which apply to antihypertensive therapy

Drug	Cardio-selectivity	ISA	MSA	Alpha blockade	Lipid solubility	Effect on serum lipids	Compliance doses per day
Acebutolol	+	+	+	−	Moderate	Minimal	1–2
Atenolol	+	−	−	−	Lowest	+	1
Metoprolol	+	−	+	−	Moderate	+	1–2
Nadolol	−	−	−	−	Low	+	2
Pindolol	−	++	+	−	Moderate	Minimal	2
Propranolol	−	−	++	−	High	+	1–2[a]
Timolol	−	−	−	−	Moderate	+	2
Labetalol	−	−	+	+	Moderate	Small	2

Notes: Cardioselectivity = relatively greater effect on β_1 than β_2 receptors; ISA = intrinsic sympathomimetic activity; MSA = membrane-stabilizing action; alpha blockade = ability to block α_1 as well as β_1 and β_2 receptors; effect on serum lipids = decrease in HDL cholesterol, increase triglycerides.
[a] Propranolol is available in a sustained-release tablet, which allows once a day dosage.

there may be a preference based on the following features of each beta blocker.

Cardioselectivity Acebutolol, metoprolol, and atenolol which are primarily beta$_1$-blocking agents would presumably at ordinary antihypertensive doses have less effect on beta$_2$ receptors. This would make these drugs more suitable for patients with some degree of sensitivity to bronchospasm. Actually all beta blockers are contraindicated in persons with asthma and significant chronic obstructive pulmonary disease, because the cardioselectivity is relative rather than absolute.

Intrinsic Sympathetic Activity (ISA) Acebutolol and pindolol have the ability to stimulate as well as block beta-adrenergic receptors. A number of claims are made for this feature. Theoretically there should be less bradycardia, less risk of congestive heart failure, less increase in peripheral resistance, and more ease of withdrawal of the therapy. Whether these advantages are substantial in clinical practice is still uncertain. Another claimed advantage of beta blockers with ISA is a less or absent tendency to decrease HDL cholesterol and increase triglycerides. Thus the possession of ISA would make this type of beta blocker attractive for use in patients especially at risk for coronary heart disease.

Lipid Solubility Only atenolol has a lipid solubility low enough to allow a claim that it does not significantly cross the blood-brain barrier. All beta blockers cause varying degrees of dizziness, vertigo, fatigue, mental depression and headache. This has been attributed at least in part to the ability to cross the blood-brain barrier and have a CNS depressant effect. More likely the CNS symptoms are due to the lowering of blood pressure and blood supply to the brain. In any event, it sometimes happens that some of the CNS symptoms disappear on the substitution of a less lipophilic agent.

Membrane Stabilizing Activity (MSA) Propranolol especially and metoprolol have MSA. This has main utility in the control of arrhythmias, mainly ventricular premature contractions. Actually all beta blockers have the ability to suppress minor arrhythmias by virtue of their sympatholytic activity. Whether MSA is a real advantage at therapeutic doses has not been finally determined. Nevertheless, beta blockers with MSA might be advantageous in hypertensive patients who also have premature ventricular contractions.

Compliance It is claimed with some justification that once-a-day dosage leads to greater compliance. Only atenolol has a pharmacokinetic profile that allows this feature. Other beta blockers such as acebutolol and metoprolol can sometimes be used once daily but in any event none need be administered more than twice a day. A special sustained release preparation of propranolol allows once a day dosage, as compared to the twice-a-day ordinary tablet.

Alpha-Receptor Blockade

Drugs which block alpha-adrenergic receptors such as phentolamine and phenoxybenzamine (see Chap. 8) have not been successful in treating hypertension. In part, this is because of their side actions but also because of development of tolerance. Labetalol has alpha-blocking capacity in addition to its beta-blocking main action. In contrast to the other beta blockers, labetalol lowers blood pressure by lowering peripheral resistance rather than depressing myocardial function alone. Heart rate is slowed as with other beta blockers. Labetalol is useful for the parenteral therapy of hypertensive crises and as a step 2 drug in the oral therapy of hypertension.

Reserpine, and related *Rauwolfia* alkaloids, may be employed in the therapy of hypertension (see Chap. 8). Although the antihypertensive effect of reserpine is mild, its use may be advantageous in that it is effective in both the supine and erect postures and adverse reactions are generally mild. The most common side effect of reserpine is psychic depression, occasionally progressing to severe disturbances, including nightmares and severe depressive reactions. Nasal stuffiness, retention of sodium and water with edema, and increased gastric acid secretion also commonly occur.

Guanethidine (see Chap. 8) is a potent long-acting antihypertensive agent; its action is almost exclusively orthostatic, with very little effect on blood pressure when the patient is in a supine position. The most common side effects are related to the orthostatic hypotension, i.e., dizziness, weakness, and syncope. Bradycardia, edema, nasal stuffiness, mild diarrhea, and inhibition of ejaculation may occur. The drug has a notable lack of severe organ toxicity or effects on the central nervous system.

Although guanethidine is occasionally used in monotherapy, most often it is a step 2 or 3 drug in severe hypertension.

Guanadrel, a chemical relative of guanethidine, has similar pharmacologic actions and indications. Both guanethidine and guanadrel should not be used in patients with pheochromocytoma, as they render the patient extremely sensitive to circulating norepinephrine. Both drugs should not be combined with tricyclic antidepressants or phenothiazines either, which can reverse their effects.

Prazosin   Originally believed to be a direct acting vasodilator, it is now known that prazosin is a selective blocker of peripheral postsynaptic (alpha$_1$) receptors (see Chap. 8). In contrast to phentolamine and phenoxybenzamine, which block both presynaptic (alpha$_2$) and postsynaptic (alpha$_1$) receptor sites, prazosin leaves the inhibitory pathway intact and is thus far more effective as an antihypertensive agent than nonselective adrenergic alpha blockers. Prazosin slows the heart rate—an important distinction compared to direct vasodilators which cause tachycardia. Prazosin does not affect serum lipids, which is considered to be an advantage over the beta blockers.

Prazosin is a guinazoline derivative with the following structure:

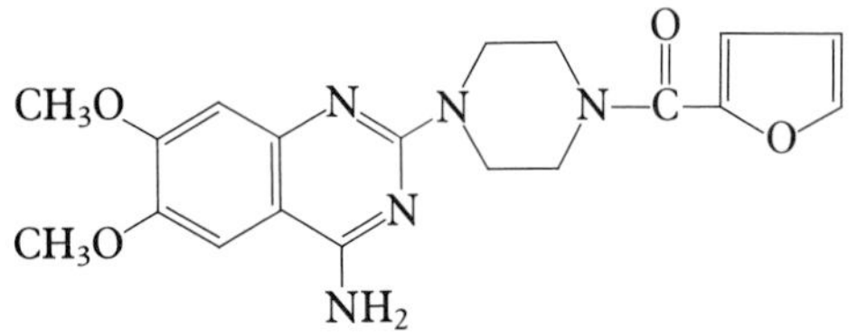

Prazosin

Terazosin is a closely related compound. It has the advantage of once-a-day dosage.

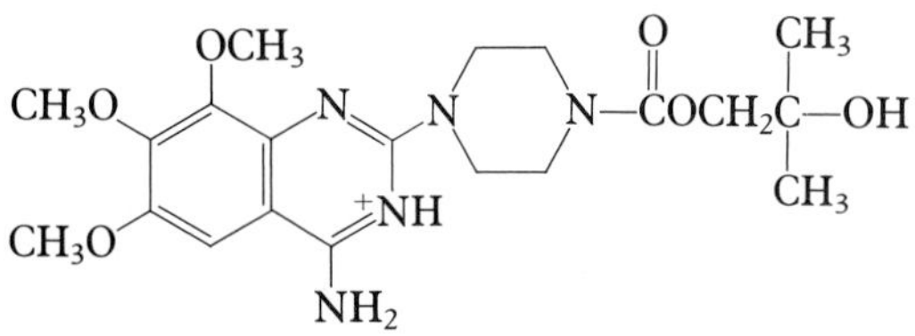

Terazosin

Pharmacokinetics   The drug is well absorbed after oral administration; significant plasma levels have been obtained within half an hour, with peak plasma concentration occurring at 2 h. The half-life of prazosin has been estimated at 2.5 h. The drug is highly bound to plasma proteins ($>$95 percent) at therapeutic concentrations, extensively biotransformed in the liver, and primarily excreted via the bile and feces.

Therapeutic Use   Prazosin is indicated for mild to moderate hypertension. Blood pressure (mainly diastolic) is reduced in both the supine and standing positions and is unaccompanied by significant changes in cardiac output, heart rate, or renal blood flow.

Adverse Reactions   The most common adverse reactions are dizziness, headache, drowsiness, weakness, palpitations, and nausea. Postural hypotension, resulting in loss of consciousness, has occurred in some patients within 2 h of the first few doses of the drug. Tolerance occurs to this effect, which can be minimized by starting with the lowest dose and gradually increasing to the maintenance dosage regimen.

Preparations   *Prazosin hydrochloride* (Minipress) is available in capsules of 1, 2, and 5 mg.

Terazosin HCL (Hytrin) is available in 1-mg tablets.

Pargyline   Although the monoamine oxidase inhibitor (MAOI) pargyline has substantial potency and the advantage of no soporific side effects, it has proved difficult to use in clinical practice because of two major problems: (1) a considerable orthostatic effect and (2) an extremely long duration of action. This leads to cumulative drug effect and, occasionally, severe orthostatic hypotension, even though the dose is not increased. Because it is a potent MAOI, patients must be warned against ingestion of cheese, wines, and beers, which may contain tyramine and cause severe paradoxic hypertensive responses.

Available sympatholytic drugs, their doses, and their mechanisms of action are listed in Table 31-4.

ARTERIAL VASODILATORS

Hydralazine

The structure of hydralazine is as follows:

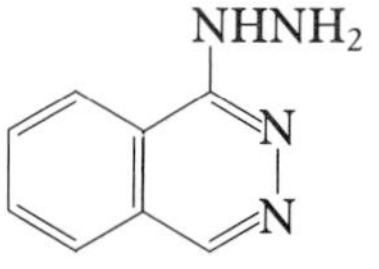

Hydralazine

TABLE 31-4 Sympatholytic antihypertensive drugs

Mechanism	Drugs	Trade name	Initial dose/maximum dose, mg/day
Decreased cardiac output; inhibition of renin release	Acebutolol	Sectral	200/800
	Atenolol	Tenormin	25/100
	Metoprolol	Lopressor	50/300
	Nadolol	Corgard	20/480
	Pindolol	Visken	10/60
	Propranolol	Inderal	40/480
	Timolol	Blocadren	10/60
In addition to above, some peripheral vasodilation	Labetalol	Normodyne Trandate	200/1200
Central inhibition of sympathetic outflow	Clonidine	Catapres	0.1/2.4
	Guanabenz	Wytensin	4/32
	Methyldopa	Aldomet	250/2000
Depletion of peripheral catecholamines	Guanadrel	Hylorel	10/150
	Guanethidine	Ismelin	10/300
Selective blocker of alpha, postsynaptic receptors	Prazosin	Minipress	2/20
	Terazosin	Hytrin	1/5
Suppression of CNS sympathetic activity; depletion of peripheral catecholamines	Reserpine	Serpasil Sandril	0.1/0.5

Cardiovascular Effects Hydralazine exerts an antihypertensive effect by direct relaxation of vascular smooth muscle. Vasodilation is not uniform; the drug primarily affects arteriolar (resistance) vessels with minimal effects on the venous (capacitance) vessels. These actions result in decreased blood pressure (diastolic more than systolic) and decreased peripheral vascular resistance.

The drug has no significant effects on nonvascular smooth muscle or cardiac tissue. Homeostatic circulatory reflexes remain intact; hydralazine-induced hypotension activates cardiovascular reflexes, resulting in increased sympathetic discharge, heart rate, stroke volume, and cardiac output. Therefore, the drug is most effectively employed in combination with a beta blocking agent to counteract these cardiac effects.

Pharmacokinetics Hydralazine is well absorbed (80 percent) after oral administration; peak serum levels are reached 1 to 2 h after a dose. Approximately 85 percent of the circulating drug is bound to serum proteins. The apparent volume of distribution is low (0.3 to 0.7 L/kg). The biologic half-life is between 2 and 8 h. A major biotransformation pathway involves acetylation in the liver. In addition, the compound is hydroxylated and biotransformed by unidentified processes; therefore, only 1 to 3 percent is excreted unchanged in the urine.

Therapeutic Use Hydralazine may be employed in a regimen with other drugs in the treatment of primary hypertension. Hydralazine alone is not a drug of choice for chronic therapy even in mild hypertensive states.

Adverse Reactions Common adverse reactions include headache, palpitations, flushing, anginal pain, anorexia, nausea, vomiting, and diarrhea. Chronic administration of hydralazine can lead to an acute rheumatoid state which can develop into a clinical picture simulating acute systemic lupus erythematosus, e.g., arthralgia, myalgia, fever, dermatoses, and anemia. This syndrome occurs more frequently with high doses (greater than 200 mg daily) and long exposure to the drug and in "slow acetylators." The hydralazine lupus-like syndrome is reversible when the drug is stopped.

Preparations *Hydralazine hydrochloride* (Apresoline) is available as tablets of 10, 25, 50, and 100 mg and for injection as ampuls containing 20 mg/mL.

Minoxidil

Minoxidil is a direct-acting peripheral vasodilator that acts on all vascular smooth muscle and decreases systolic and diastolic blood pressure. Reflex responses to the hypotension include tachycardia, increased renin secretion, and sodium and water retention. Orthostatic hypotension does not commonly occur.

Minoxidil

Pharmacokinetics Minoxidil is almost completely absorbed (90 percent) from the gastrointestinal tract. Blood pressure begins to decline within 30 min; the peak effect occurs in 2 to 3 h. The average plasma half-life is 4.2 h; however, the duration of the antihypertensive effect is approximately 75 h. Therefore, the time course of the effect does not correspond to the drug concentration in the plasma.

Minoxidil does not bind to plasma proteins. The drug is biotransformed predominantly by glucuronide conjugation at the *N*-oxide position in the pyrimidine

ring. Minoxidil and its biotransformation products are excreted in the urine.

Therapeutic Use Because of potential serious adverse reactions, this compound is indicated only for severe hypertension that is not controllable by a diuretic plus two other antihypertensive drugs.

Adverse Reactions and Warnings Adverse reactions associated with minoxidil therapy include salt and water retention, pericardial effusion and tamponade, hypertrichosis, ECG abnormalities, and reduced hematocrit, hemoglobin, and erythrocyte count. In experimental animals cardiac lesions were observed after short-term use of minoxidil. One cannot rule out the possibility of cardiac lesions in humans.

One of the less common adverse effects of minoxidil is hirsutism, especially with long-term use. This has led to the local application of a 2% solution of minoxidil to the scalp in male pattern baldness. After 3 to 4 months of daily application in about 50 percent of patients, a very modest increase of hair growth is noted. After 8 months, dense growth may occur in 8 percent of patients. Minoxidil as a 2% solution (Rogaine) is now marketed for this purpose. Systemic toxicity may occur from absorption of the drug and patients must be carefully monitored.

The drug is contraindicated in pheochromocytoma because it may stimulate catecholamine release from the tumor.

Minoxidil must usually be used in conjunction with a diuretic and a beta-adrenergic blocking agent to reduce sodium and water retention and tachycardia, respectively.

Preparations *Minoxidil* (Loniten) is available as tablets containing 2.5 and 10 mg.

ANGIOTENSIN CONVERTING ENZYME (ACE) INHIBITORS

Renin

Renin, a proteolytic enzyme produced by the juxtaglomerula apparatus of the kidney, acts like a hormone in the sense that it initiates control of physiologic functions of other organs. Increased secretion is stimulated by a fall in renal perfusion pressure as occurs in renal artery stenosis, hemorrhage, dehydration, and sodium depletion. It is also under control of the nervous system (beta stimulation and block) and, probably by an atrial natriuretic factor, a newly discovered cardiac peptide hormone.

Angiotensin I is a prohormone which is produced by the action of renin on a peptide substrate produced by the liver. Angiotensin I is relatively inactive and is activated by conversion to angiotensin II by a converting enzyme present in the lungs and other tissues. Receptors present on the membrane of smooth-muscle cells of arterioles and the adrenal cortex cells (aldosterone secretion) are specifically stimulated by angiotensin II. Increases in peripheral resistance, heart rates, cardiac output, and sodium and water retention result. By a feedback loop induced by the rise in blood pressure and renal perfusion, the secretion of renin is reduced.

The renin-angiotensin system's role in normotensive individuals is probably minor. In hypertensives it is an important mechanism that maintains the elevated arterial pressure by increasing fluid volume and causing arteriolar constriction. Although it might be attractive to surmise that the etiology of essential hypertension is a disturbance of the renin-angiotensin system in every case, the proof of this has never been established. Certainly in renal artery stenosis, reestablishment of flow or removal of the affected kidney cures the hypertension, but a vast majority of hypertensive patients have no demonstrable pathology which might lead to increased production of renin. Nevertheless, ACE inhibitors have proven to be a group of very effective antihypertensive agents and are beginning to replace the beta blockers especially as monotherapy.

Early attempts to block the renin-angiotensin system produced angiotensin II competitive antagonists. These are variations of the angiotensin peptide by substitution of the phenylalanine in position 8 with another amino acid. The most studied has been *saralasin*, in which sarcosine is substituted. Saralasin is a partial antagonist, and when given intravenously to normal subjects, it causes a transient rise in blood pressure which is followed by a fall. Saralasin is useful diagnostically because in renin-dependent hypertensive patients there is a sustained fall in blood pressure, whereas in individuals with low-renin hypertension there is a sustained pressor response. Saralasin remains an interesting and important investigative tool. It is not available as a commercial drug.

Angiotensin II itself is a potent pressor agent which has the advantage of not constricting capacitance ves-

sels and not stimulating the sympathetic system. However, it has limited therapeutic use in view of the many pressor agents available which are cheaper and for practical purposes just as effective.

Captopril, Enalapril, and Lisinopril

The inhibitors of the renin-angiotensin system which have proven to be clinically successful are those which compete for the converting enzyme of angiotensin I and angiotensin II.

Chemistry   The original inhibitor of converting enzyme was a nonpeptide known as *teprotide*. By analysis of the amino acid sequence and some ingenious deductions, an orally effective relatively simple chemical which is essentially a modified and substituted proline was produced. The structure of *captopril* is as follows:

Captopril

Note that captopril has a sulfur atom, which contributes to some of its adverse effects. Another successful compound is *enalapril*, which also has a proline moiety differing from captopril in being a tripeptide instead of a dipeptide analog.

Enalapril

Actually enalapril is a prodrug and must be biotransformed in the body to the active metabolite enalaprilat. Also it does not contain sulfur.

The most recent introduction is *lisinopril*. Chemically it resembles enalapril. However, it does not rely on biotransformation for the production of an active metabolite. Lisinopril is itself active and has a long duration of action. Like enalapril it lacks a sulfur atom.

Mechanism of Action   It turns out that the ACE inhibitors are very specific in their action. They do not interact with other components of the angiotensin-renin system. In addition to inhibiting the conversion of angiotensin I to angiotensin II, they reduce responsiveness to angiotensin II and also inhibit the inactivation of *bradykinin*. Both these actions would tend to augment the vasodilator properties of ACE inhibitors. In addition the cessation of angiotensin II synthesis leads to a compensatory adjustment of extra production of renin and angiotensin I. This apparently does not contribute to any adverse effect.

Cardiovascular System A single oral dose of captopril in a normal subject results in only a slight fall in blood pressure. Repeated doses over several days result in a more sustained fall and a slight blunting of postural reflexes. However, if the individual is sodium-depleted, even a single dose causes a distinct fall in blood pressure. After taking captopril, the pressure response to angiotensin II is absent, while that to angiotensin I is unchanged. The ability of angiotensin II to stimulate secretion of aldosterone is also depressed.

In hypertensive patients, whether caused by increased renin or not, ACE inhibitors satisfactorily lower arterial, both systolic and diastolic, blood pressure. The action of ACE inhibitors is enhanced by diuretics.

Pharmacokinetics On the whole the ACE inhibitors are excellent oral drugs with good bioavailability (see Table 31-5). Captopril's absorption is interfered with by food, and therefore oral dosing is done 1 h before meals. Enalapril itself has a short half-life. However since it is converted in the body to enalaprilat, which has a half-life of 11 h, it is long-acting and can be given in once-a-day dosage. Lisinopril is also long-acting, and once-a-day dosage is possible. Extending the dose beyond the recommended range does not result in increased antihypertensive effect. Adding a diuretic does and is recommended when it proves impossible to control pressure with ACE inhibition alone.

Adverse Effects All the ACE inhibitors have the usual side effects of gastrointestinal, CNS, and cardiovascular minor complaints in an incidence of about 0.5 to 2 percent. Most experience has been with captopril,

TABLE 31-5 Pharmacokinetic properties of ACE inhibitors

Drug	Dose[a]	Time to peak serum levels, h	Percent absorbed	Half-life, h	Elimination
Captopril (Capoten)	25 mg bid or tid	0.5–1.5	75 Food inhibits	2	95% in urine
Enalapril (Vasotec)	5 mg to 20–40 mg daily	0.5–1.5	60	1.3[b]	94% in urine and feces
Lisinopril (Prinivil) (Zestril)	10 mg to start, 20–40 mg daily	Approximately 7	25	12	Mainly in urine

[a]Initial dosage is without diuretics. If a satisfactory blood pressure response is not obtained, diuretic may be added. Patients with renal failure, as evidenced by elevated creatinine clearance, require reduction in dosage.
[b]Long half-life of enalapril results from the conversion of enalapril to enalaprilat, an active ACE inhibitor which has a half-life of 35 h.

but its toxicities generally apply to the other ACE inhibitors. Transient elevations of BUN and creatinine may occur, especially in patients with volume depletion or renovascular hypertension. In patients with renal impairment, elevations in serum potassium occur. There is a small incidence of proteinuria and other signs of renal failure. Early in the use of captopril, nephrotic syndrome occurred in about 20 percent of cases. However, the dose was too high and reduction in dosage greatly reduced this complication. Neutropenia and agranulocytoses occur in a small incidence and, of course, obviate therapy with ACE inhibitors. The incidence is highest in patients who already have collagen diseases. Cholestatic jaundice is a rare occurrence.

Angioedema occurs in an incidence of 0.1 to 0.1 percent. When life-threatening because of laryngeal edema, epinephrine is to be given. Excessive hypotension may occur, which requires careful attention to reduction of the initial doses.

Clinical Use The ACE inhibitors are beginning to replace the beta blockers as first-line monotherapy of mild to moderate essential hypertension. They also have gained prominence as vasodilator therapy of congestive heart failure (see Chap. 26).

CALCIUM-CHANNEL BLOCKERS

Although nifedipine has been used most frequently for antihypertensive therapy, verapamil and diltiazem appear to be equally efficacious antihypertensive drugs. These drugs are discussed in detail in Chap. 28. They are also used as vasodilators in congestive heart failure (Chap. 26) and as antiarrhythmic drugs (Chap. 27).

THERAPEUTIC APPROACHES TO ANTIHYPERTENSIVE THERAPY

Over the past 30 years the therapy of hypertension has evolved gradually in a pattern of stepped diet and drug therapy which has been eminently satisfactory. Most cases of hypertension are mild to moderate (see Table 31-1) and can be treated on an ambulatory basis. Often the patient may have fever or minor symptoms so that compliance with drug therapy is difficult especially if the drugs used have many side actions.

The traditional stepped therapy of hypertension is as follows:

1. Restrict dietary sodium to 2 g daily. Eliminate risk factors such as obesity, smoking, alcohol. Encourage exercise.
2. Diuretics.
3. Sympatholytic drugs, either centrally or peripherally acting. Beta blockers have been most popular, although clonidine, prazosin, and methyldopa are widely used.
4. Add a third drug, usually a peripherally direct acting vasodilator such as hydralazine or minoxidil. ACE inhibitors and calcium-channel blockers have also been used as a fourth step.

In the past 5 years there has been a strong movement toward monotherapy with one of three groups of drugs, namely, beta blocker, ACE inhibitors, and calcium-channel blockers. Diet therapy and reduction of risk factors is, of course, first advised. However, the drug chosen for monotherapy is titrated to the maximum dose before other therapy is considered. A diuretic is added only after failure to adequately control the blood pressure. Monotherapy will be satisfactory therapy for many mild to moderate hypertensives and appears to be simpler, to be less apt to have adverse drug effects and interactions, and to increase compliance.

At the present time there is an intensive effort to determine which is the superior group of drugs for antihypertensive monotherapy. The beta blockers have been used for the longest time, and consequently there is more experience with their use. They are the only group of drugs with a proven record of reduction of mortality. However, the other two groups may be equally effective in this regard.

No therapy thus far developed has succeeded in reducing the incidence of coronary heart disease. This is a paradox in view of the observed reduction in treated hypertensive patients of the incidence of stroke and renal disease. For this reason, attention to the lipid profile of each hypertensive patient must be examined and treated if abnormal.

Finally this chapter does not deal with secondary hypertension such as that caused by pheochromocytomia, aldosteronism, coarctation of the aorta, and renal disease. Therapy used in these diseases is covered under the drugs themselves such as phentolamine, phenoxybenzamine, and metyrosine.

HYPERTENSIVE EMERGENCIES

The patient with hypertensive emergencies requires constant monitoring of blood pressure in an intensive-care setting or its equivalent. The availability of diazoxide and nitroprusside has considerably enhanced the ability to deal with hypertensive emergencies. Other drugs which are valuable for certain hypertensive emergencies are listed in Table 31-6.

Diazoxide

Diazoxide is a nondiuretic thiazide derivative that produces a prompt reduction in blood pressure by directly relaxing smooth muscle of the arterioles. Like hydralazine, this agent has little direct effect on the venous system or the heart.

Diazoxide

In addition to the hypotensive action, diazoxide produces a prompt elevation of blood glucose levels,

primarily because of inhibition of insulin release from the pancreas.

Pharmacokinetics   The oral bioavailability of diazoxide is 100 percent. Greater than 90 percent is bound to plasma proteins, resulting in a low apparent volume of distribution (0.2 L/kg). The drug is biotransformed to inactive alcoholic and carboxylic acid products, which are subsequently conjugated by sulfate prior to excretion via the kidney. The half-life of the parent compound is 20 to 40 h, largely because of a high degree of renal tubular reabsorption.

Routes of Administration   Taking advantage of its rapid onset of action, this drug is employed as a bolus intravenous injection for the emergency reduction of blood pressure. Administered orally, the drug is employed for its hyperglycemic effects.

Therapeutic Uses   Diazoxide has been employed orally in the management of hypoglycemia due to hyperinsulinism associated with islet-cell adenoma of carcinoma. However, its major use is in hypertensive emergencies, always administered by the intravenous route for a prompt, effective, and prolonged response. By this route the onset of action is within 32 s, the peak effect occurs between 2 and 5 min, and the dura-

TABLE 31-6   Some drugs for hypertensive emergencies

Drug	Dose and method of administration	Onset
Trimethaphan	1 mg/mL in intravenous infusion; titrate	Instantaneous
Sodium nitroprusside	5–100 mg/L intravenous infusion; titrate	Instantaneous
Diazoxide	300–600 mg as rapid intravenous push	Instantaneous
Nifedipine	10–20 mg sublingual or chewed	5–30 min
Labetalol	20–80 mg IV at 10-min intervals (maximum dose 300 mg)	Immediate

tion of action is 3 to 8 h. Diazoxide is not generally employed for primary hypertension because of its side effects.

Adverse Reactions The major effects of diazoxide on water and electrolyte balance are opposite to those of the diuretic thiazides. Diazoxide causes marked sodium and water retention, expands plasma volume, and can produce edema in patients with inadequate myocardial function. In common with the structurally related diuretics, diazoxide produces hyperglycemia and hyperuricemia.

Preparations *Diazoxide* is available as a sterile solution (Hyperstat) in an ampul containing 300 mg per 20 mL for intravenous use in hospitalized patients and as capsules (Proglycem) containing 50 and 100 mg and a suspension containing 50 mg/mL.

Sodium Nitroprusside

Sodium nitroprusside, $Na_2Fe(CN)_5NO \cdot 2H_2O$, is a potent, immediately acting intravenous hypotensive agent which is used for reduction of blood pressure in hypertensive crises. Hypotensive effects are caused by peripheral vasodilatation as a result of a direct action on both arteriolar and venular blood vessels.

The effects of the drug occur rapidly but are of short duration (ending when IV infusion is stopped). Adverse reactions that have been noted by too rapid administration include nausea, apprehension, headache, restlessness, muscle twitching, palpitations, and abdominal pain. These effects are self-limiting because of the short metabolic half-life of the drug. Nitroprusside is biotransformed to cyanide and to thiocyanate. If excessive amounts are used, thiocyanate toxicity (e.g., tinnitus, blurred vision, delirium) may result. With gross overdosage, cyanide intoxication is possible.

Preparations *Sodium nitroprusside* (Nipride) is available in a 5-mL vial containing 50 mg of drug to be used as an intravenous infusion with sterile 5% dextrose in water.

BIBLIOGRAPHY

Epstein, M. and J. R. Oster: *Hypertension, A Practical Approach*, Saunders, Philadelphia, 1984.

European Working Party on High Blood Pressure in the Elderly: "Efficacy of Antihypertensive Drug Treatment According to Age, Sex, Blood Pressure and Previous Disease in Patients at the Age of 60," Lancet, **2**:589–592 (1986).

Freis, E. D.: "Veterans Administration Cooperative Study on Nadolol as Monotherapy and in Combination with a Diuretic," *Am. Heart J.*, **108**:1087–1091 (1984).

Gifford, R. W., Jr.: "Role of Diurectics in Treatment of Hypertension," *Am. J. Med.*, **77**:102–106 (1984).

Haber, E., and E. E. Slater: "High Blood Pressure," *Sci. Am. Med.*, **1**:1, **VII**:1–30, 1988.

Helgeland, A., R., et al.: "Enalapril, Atenolol and Hydrochlorothiazide in Mild to Moderate Hypertension: A Comparative Multicenter Study in General Practice in Norway," *Lancet*, **1**:872–875 (1986).

Kaplan, N. M.: "Non-drug Treatment of Hypertension," *Ann. Intern. Med.*, **102**:359–373 (1985).

Kaplan, N. M., A. Carnegie, P. Raskin, et al.: "Potassium Supplementation in Hypertensive Patients with Diuretic-Induced Hypokalemia," *N. Engl. J. Med.*, **312**:746–749 (1985).

"Labetalol for Hypertension," *Med. Lett. Drugs Ther.*, **26**:83 (1984).

McChesney, J. A., and W. J. C. Amend, Jr.: "Minoxidil in the Treatment of Refractory Hypertension Due to a Spectrum of Causes," *J. Cardiovasc. Pharmacol.*, **2**:S131–134 (1980).

Multiple Risk Factor Intervention Trial Research Group: "Multiple Risk Factor Intervention Trial: Risk Factor Changes and Mortality Results," *JAMA*, **248**:1465–1477 (1982).

Sassano, P., G. Chatellier, A. M. Amiot, et al.: "A Double-Blind Randomized Evaluation of Converting Enzyme Inhibition as the First Step Treatment of Mild to Moderate Hypertension," *J. Hypertens.*, **2** (**suppl**):575–581 (1984).

Spivack, C., S. Ocken, and W. H. Frishman: "Calcium Antagonists: Clinical Use in Treatment of Systemic Hypertension," *Drugs*, **25**:154–165 (1983).

Drugs for Chronic Obstructive Pulmonary Diseases

David M. Ritchie and Michael P. Wachter

Asthma is a clinical syndrome characterized by increased responsiveness, narrowing of the airways, and subsequent episodes of breathlessness, wheezing, and cough. Associated with narrowed airways may be changes in ciliary activity and mucus secretion. Cough may be a major factor during an asthmatic attack. An acute attack can be brought on by external stimuli such as airborne antigen, exercise, cold air, or other unknown triggers. Most studied of these stimuli are exercise and antigen. Clinically, asthma is usually graded as either mild, moderate, or severe. Mild asthma does not usually interfere with normal activities and is controlled by bronchodilators. Moderate asthma may occasionally interfere with normal routine, and it may require steroids for control. Severe asthma limits normal activity considerably and can at times result in life-threatening episodes.

Patients with asthma may quite often demonstrate signs of chronic bronchitis and/or emphysema as well. Chronic bronchitis is characterized by excessive mucus production and is associated with chronic productive cough. Emphysema is defined as a condition of the lung characterized by an abnormal and permanent enlargement of respiratory airspaces accompanied by destruction of their walls without fibrosis. All these disease syndromes lead to episodes of wheezing and coughing. Since the molecular mechanisms of these pathologic changes are largely unknown, therapy for asthma and other chronic obstructive pulmonary diseases (COPDs) is directed toward symptomatic relief of the acute bronchospasm or, in the case of prophylactic drugs like cromolyn, prevention of an attack.

To understand the rationale behind the therapeutic agents of this class, a physician must have a basic understanding of the pathophysiology involved in an acute or chronic allergy-induced bronchospasm. Our understanding of the mechanism of allergic bronchospasm involves mediation by reaginic antibodies, that is, IgE. IgE is synthesized by plasma cells in response to an initial exposure of allergen in a susceptible individual (Fig. 32-1). These newly synthesized IgE molecules fix themselves to mast cells in the airway mucosa and basophils and mast cells throughout the body. These fixed IgE molecules are antigen-specific. On reexposure to the same antigen, an antigen-antibody interaction takes place which involves one antigen molecule cross-bridging two IgE molecules, resulting in a perturbation of the cell membrane. Membrane perturbation, or cell activation, is followed by a series of biochemical events including the rapid influx of calcium into the cell and subsequent activation of phospholipase enzymes within the cell (see Fig. 32-1). Phospholipase metabolizes membrane phospholipids to arachidonic acid, which is subsequently metabolized via cyclooxygenase to prostaglandins (PGs) and lipoxygenase to leukotrienes (LTs) and hydroxyeicosatetrenoic acids (HETEs) (Fig. 32-2). Some of the cyclooxygenase products, i.e., $PGF_{2\alpha}$ and thromboxanes, and the sulfidoleukotrienes (LTC_4, LTD_4, and LTE_4), are potent bronchospastic agents. Along with the PGs, LTs, and HETEs, phospholipid metabolism

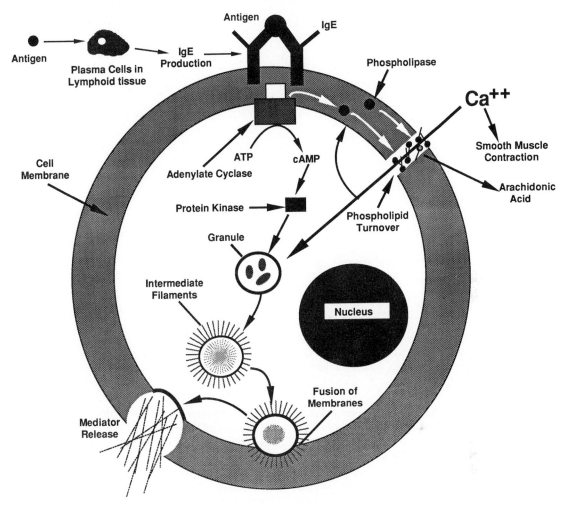

FIGURE 32-1 Schematic representation of sensitization and reexposure to antigen and the resultant mast cell activation.

by phospholipase also leads to the production of platelet activating factor (PAF), another potent bronchospastic agent which may contribute to the airway narrowing seen in asthma. These newly synthesized mediators are released from the cell along with stored mediators such as histamine and cause smooth-muscle contraction, edema, cellular infiltration, and mucus secretion.

Although the immunologic response described above may be responsible for cases of allergic asthma, it is not the only mechanism resulting in broncho-

spasm. Acute attacks of bronchospasm may be caused by a sensitivity to aspirin, by exercise, or by heat loss from the airways and from other undefined mechanisms. These cases are sometimes referred to as *bronchial hyperreactivity cases* rather than allergic bronchospasm. Airway hyperreactivity appears to be universal in individuals with respiratory disease.

The mechanism behind bronchial hyperreactivity is unknown. However, whatever the mechanism, it appears to be related to released mediators and the interaction of these mediators with neural and humoral

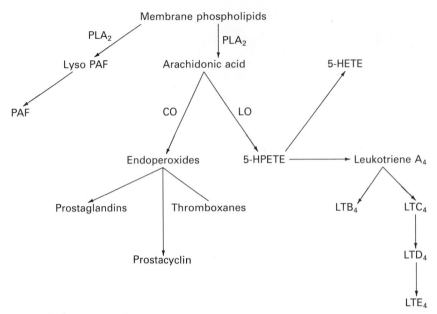

FIGURE 32-2   Metabolism of membrane phospholipids to products of arachidonic acid metabolism and platelet activating factor (PAF). PLA_2 = phospholipase A_2; CO = cyclooxygenase; LO = lipoxygenase; 5-HPETE = 5-hydroperoxyeicosatetrenoic acid; 5-HETE = 5-hydroxyeicosatetrenoic acid; LT = leukotriene.

pathways involved with homeostatic control of respiratory smooth muscle. With this interaction in mind, it becomes understandable why a variety of types of pharmacologic interventions may have an effect on asthma, albeit not afford a cure. This appears to be the case clinically, since mediator release inhibitors (cromolyn) calcium entry blockers, lipoxygenase-cyclooxygenase inhibitors, specific receptor antagonists (LTs, histamine, PAF, PGs), as well as physiologic antagonists like theophylline or beta-receptor agonists may all have some effect in asthma, yet none offers a cure.

BRONCHODILATORS

Methylxanthines

The three best known naturally occurring methylxanthines are theophylline, theobromine, and caffeine. Major sources of these compounds are tea, cocoa, and coffee, respectively. For example, an average cup of coffee contains approximately 60 to 100 mg of caffeine. For use as a bronchodilator, theophylline is the compound of most interest.

The xanthines belong to a family of compounds which contain the purine ring system, one of the most important heterocyclics found in nature. Purines can be derived from the fusion of a pyrimidine and imidazole rings. Theophylline is 1,3-dimethylxanthine, and its structure, along with other analogs, is shown in Table 32-1. The three major xanthines all exert similar biologic effects but differ in their potencies.

The mechanism of action of theophylline as a bronchodilator is unknown. However, several theories have been suggested based on the close structural similarity of theophylline with adenosine and 3'5'-cyclic adenosine monophosphate (cAMP). Theophylline inhibits a cyclic AMP phosphodiesterase, which leads to an increase in cytosolic cyclic AMP and a subsequent relaxation of airways (and other) smooth muscle. However, theophylline is not a potent phosphodiesterase inhibitor, and the necessary concentrations may be unattainable in vivo. Theophylline inhibits the reuptake of catecholamines, which can elevate cyclic AMP and result in subsequent bronchodilation.

More recently, theophylline has been shown to be an adenosine receptor antagonist, and this action may

TABLE 32-1   Commonly used xanthines: structures and pharmacologic comparisons

$$
\begin{array}{c}
\text{R--N} \quad \overset{O}{\underset{O}{\bigcirc}} \quad \text{N--R}_2 \\
\text{R}_1
\end{array}
$$

Compound	R	R_1	R_2	CNS stimulation	Bronchodilation	Diuresis	Cardiac stimulation	Skeletal-muscle stimulation
Caffeine	Methyl	Methyl	Methyl	+++	+	+	+	+++
Theobromine	H	Methyl	H	+	+	++	++	+
Theophylline	H	Methyl	Methyl	++	+++	+++	+++	++
Enprofylline	H	Propyl	H	+	++++	+	++++	−−

be responsible for its bronchodilating properties. Adenosine is an endogenous mediator which, when interacting with membrane receptors, may cause bronchoconstriction. Theophylline is known to antagonize the binding of adenosine to these cell surface receptors and thus prevent the bronchospasm produced. Although this mechanism may be important to the action of theophylline, newer methylxanthines (enprofylline) have demonstrated as good or better bronchodilating properties than theophylline while being essentially devoid of adenosine receptor-binding properties.

Pharmacologic Effects Theophylline and the other methylxanthines exert pharmacologic effects on a variety of organ systems (Table 32-1). One of their most pronounced effects is the relaxation of respiratory smooth muscle. Additionally, theophylline is a CNS stimulant, decreases mean arterial blood pressure, increases diuresis, possesses cardiotonic activity, and causes effects on the gastrointestinal system, which may be related to its CNS effects. The action of theophylline on the CNS, cardiovascular, and gastrointestinal systems are the most commonly observed side effects of the use of theophylline as a bronchodilator.

The effect of theophylline on the CNS is directly related to the dose of compound administered and can be exhibited as restlessness, anxiety, tremors, and even convulsions at sufficiently high doses. Theophylline also stimulates the medullary respiratory centers, an effect sometimes used therapeutically in cases of respiratory apnea. The nausea and vomiting associated with theophylline usage are also thought to be centrally mediated and dose-dependent. Nausea is a particularly common side effect seen with initial theophylline use.

On the cardiovascular system, the methylxanthines exert direct positive inotropic and chronotropic effects on the heart. In the periphery, methylxanthines cause a decrease in peripheral vascular resistance, except in the cerebral vasculature where theophylline causes vasoconstriction. The inotropic effects of the methylxanthines are thought to be mediated via increased calcium influx modulated by cyclic AMP and the effect of the xanthines on cardiac specific phosphodiesterases.

In the gastrointestinal tract, methylxanthines stimulate secretion of both gastric acid and digestive enzymes. On the kidney, the methylxanthines possess diuretic activity, albeit weak. Diuresis may be due to an increased glomerular filtration rate as well as a decreased tubular absorption of sodium. The bronchodilating properties of theophylline are due to direct effects on respiratory smooth muscle. Theophylline also affects skeletal muscle to improve contractile responses. This effect may provide therapeutic effects in cases of diaphragm fatigue.

Pharmacokinetics   Theophylline is generally administered orally in sustained release preparations. Aminophylline (the theophylline-ethylenediamine complex) is available for oral, intravenous, or suppository use. A wide variety of preparations of theophylline are available, and the pharmacokinetics are dependent on which preparation is used. Generally, theophylline is rapidly and completely absorbed from the gastrointestinal tract. Methylxanthines are distributed throughout the body and are able to cross the placenta. Metabolism occurs primarily in the liver by oxidation and demethylation with up to 15 percent excreted unchanged in the urine. The half-life of theophylline averages about 3.5 h in children and 8 or 9 h in adults. In smokers, the half-life of theophylline is decreased to approximately half that of nonsmokers. The effectiveness of theophylline as a bronchodilator is usually achieved with attained blood levels of 10 to 20 μg/mL. Nausea, vomiting, and restlessness may be associated with these levels. Blood levels higher than 20 μg/mL may be associated with greater toxicity. Toxic effects associated with elevated serum levels are ventricular arrhythmias, convulsions, and possible death, which may occur without previous warning. It is for this reason (low therapeutic index) that blood levels should be monitored individually to establish a safe and effective dose of theophylline.

Drug Interactions   Theophylline interacts with a variety of other therapeutic agents. Most notable are the agents which increase the effects of theophylline, since these agents may lead to severe theophylline toxicity when administered concurrently. Cimetidine, an H_2-receptor antagonist; erythromycin and troleandomycin, antibiotics; and some oral contraceptives may increase theophylline blood levels into the toxic range. It is important to monitor theophylline levels frequently whenever one of these other medications is required. Other interactions with theophylline may occur with lithium, phenytoin, barbiturates, and beta blockers, leading to decreased effectiveness of one or both drugs. Additionally, concurrent administration of halothane to persons receiving theophylline may result in cardiac dysrhythmias. With such a potential for drug interactions, it is important for the physician to be aware of any other medications being taken by the patient receiving theophylline.

Clinical Use   The methylxanthines are indicated for use as bronchodilators in cases of acute or chronic obstructive pulmonary disease. Since theophylline is only marginally soluble in water, many different salts have been prepared. Initial loading doses of theophylline correspond to a total dose of approximately 5 mg/kg. Intravenous dosage should be administered by infusion to prevent achieving toxic levels. It is important to emphasize the importance of monitoring blood levels of theophylline during changes in dose levels. For acute intravenous use, aminophylline is generally employed at a loading dose of approximately 5 mg/kg infused over 30 min with monitoring of blood levels to prevent acute toxicity. For maintenance therapy, 0.6 to 0.7 mg/kg/h should be sufficient, with the dose decreased to 0.3 mg/kg/h in patients with heart or liver disease.

Preparations   *Theophylline* is available for oral use in a variety of preparations from rapid acting to 12-h capsules. The dose and frequency of administration may be different for each preparation, and the package literature should be consulted.

Beta-Receptor Agonists (Sympathomimetics)

The beta-receptor agonists are discussed in Chap. 7. However, one of their most important uses is in the treatment of obstructive airways disease. These agents relax smooth muscle and inhibit allergic mediator release, presumably by elevation of cAMP as a result of activation of adenylate cyclase. The activation of beta-adrenergic receptors results in the relaxation of airways smooth muscle, skeletal muscle tremor, and positive inotropic and chronotropic effects on the heart. Nonselective stimulation of beta receptors by agents such as epinephrine and isoproterenol makes these drugs effective bronchodilators with limited use owing to cardiac side effects. Newer beta$_2$-selective adrenergic receptor agonists have been developed which provide effective bronchodilation with lessened cardiac side effects.

One of the earliest beta-receptor agonists used for bronchodilation was epinephrine. Epinephrine is an effective bronchodilator when given subcutaneously or as an aerosol. It is not a selective beta$_2$ agonist and thus possesses various cardiac side effects, including tachycardia, arrhythmias, and worsening of angina.

Ephedrine is another nonselective beta-receptor agonist which has been used for many years in the treatment of asthma. It has a longer duration, greater oral activity, and more central nervous system effects than epinephrine. With the advent of newer selective agents, current use of ephedrine is generally limited to combination use in fixed-dose preparations of various over-the-counter remedies.

Isoproterenol is a potent bronchodilator and is generally used by aerosol to determine reversibility in the diagnosis of obstructive respiratory disease. Isoproterenol has a short duration of action (60 to 90 min), and cardiac effects are common.

The development of the newer beta$_2$-receptor agonists has considerably lessened the incidence of cardiac side effects with aerosol administration for bronchodilation. The relative selectivity for beta-adrenergic receptors as compared with that of epinephrine and isoproterenol is shown in Table 32-2. Generally, these compounds are longer-acting than epinephrine or isoproterenol, and most are available as aerosol and oral preparations. Aerosol administration results in the greatest local effect on airways smooth muscle while minimizing or eliminating side effects (skeletal muscle tremor, CNS activity, cardiac effects).

There has been discussion in the literature concerning the development of tolerance to the beta-receptor agonists. It is not clear whether actual tolerance develops, that is, a decrease in beta-receptor responsiveness, or whether the apparent observation of tolerance is due to a worsening of the clinical condition. In either case, the increased use of beta-agonist bronchodilators should suggest to the patient and physician that a reevaluation of therapy should be initiated. If increased dosages of the beta-agonist bronchodilators are being used, then the clinical objective of controlling symptoms with a minimum of medication has no longer been achieved.

Adverse Reactions As discussed previously, the major side effects associated with the nonselective beta-adrenergic receptor agonists are cardiac and central nervous effects. Cardiac effects consist of positive inotropic and chronotropic effects, which are easily noticeable to the patient, and the chance of arrhythmias. Central nervous system effects can generally be classified as stimulatory. With the newer beta$_2$-selective agents, skeletal muscle tremor is a relatively common, dose-related side effect. The patient generally becomes tolerant of this effect with continued use.

Clinical Use The beta-receptor agonists are approved as bronchodilators for use in a wide variety of obstructive airways diseases. Since the compounds are physiologic antagonists, they relax airways smooth muscle regardless of the responsible mechanism. Albuterol and the other beta$_2$-selective compounds are currently mainstays of asthma therapy as both prophylactics and for use in acute bronchospastic episodes. Their prophylactice use also extends to use in exercise-induced asthma.

Anticholinergics

Anticholinergics (covered in detail in Chap. 10) have been used for centuries in the treatment of obstructive lung disease. Cholinergic blocking drugs affect a variety of tissues and systems and thus have the potential for a wide array of side effects. By inhibiting the action of acetylcholine on respiratory smooth muscle, anticholinergics prevent bronchospasm resulting from vagus nerve discharge. The vagus nerve is thought to play a role in some types of obstructive airways disease, and the effectiveness of anticholinergic agents in some patients adds credence to this theory.

Clinically, these agents have been shown to produce bronchodilation in some cases and also to normalize a hyperreactive airway. In many cases of obstructive lung disease the airways become hyperreactive, that is, they constrict to an irritant that has no effect on a nonasthmatic. This response is apparently due to the airways hyperreactivity or lower threshold to response of asthmatics, compared to nonasthmatics. Anticholinergics appear to reestablish the airways to a nonasthmatic state, alleviating the hyperreactivity.

Clinically, these agents are generally used by inhalation for the treatment of airways disease. Atropine has been shown to be an effective bronchodilator by aerosol, and its effect can persist for over 4 h. Local side effects by aerosol atropine can include drying of the mouth and the resultant discomfort. Systemic adverse reactions may include urinary retention, tachycardia, and agitation. Systemic side effects can be minimized by the use of a quaternary ammonium derivative, ipratropium bromide (Atrovent). This compound is

TABLE 32-2　Comparative adrenoceptor selectivity and pharmacologic effect of selected sympathomimetic bronchodilators

Name	β_1	β_2	α	Duration	Advantages, disadvantages
Albuterol (Ventolin)	+	++++	−	Long-acting 6 h	Highly potent; orally active, safer than isoproterenol IV.
Epinephrine	++++	+++	+++	Short-acting <1 h	Rapid onset; side effects due to nonselective β_2-agonist activity.
Isoproterenol (Isuprel)	++++	++++	(+)	Short-acting <1 h	Both β_1 and β_2 effects cause tachycardia and arrhythmias.
Metaproterenol (Alupent)	++	++	−	Long-acting 4–5 h	Less effective and less β_2-selective than albuterol.
Terbutaline (Bricanyl)	+	+++	−	Long-acting >6 h	More side effects than albuterol; lesser tendency for drop in Pa_{O_2}.
Fenoterol (Berotec)	+	++++	−	Long-acting >6 h	By aerosol, ≈2 × potency of albuterol.
Pirbuterol (Exirel)	+	++++	−	Long-acting 6 h	More selective for lung tissue than cardiac, compared to albuterol and isoproterenol; improved cardiac performance.
Procaterol (Mucodine)	+	++++	−	Long-acting	More potent and more effective than albuterol in controlling bronchial asthma.

poorly absorbed and does not cross the blood-brain barrier easily, thus allowing the administration of higher doses to the lung. Ipratropium is an effective bronchodilator in some patients and can be a valuable agent for use in those individuals who cannot tolerate the beta-receptor agonists. Approved uses for these agents include emphysema and chronic bronchitis, although work continues for an asthma indication.

MEDIATOR RELEASE INHIBITORS

Cromolyn Sodium

The prototype mediator release inhibitor is cromolyn sodium (Intal), and the history of cromolyn reflects the history of this class of drugs. Many compounds have been synthesized which have similar activity profiles in animal studies, but none has proven as efficacious as cromolyn in the clinic. Cromolyn was first discovered during investigations of khellin, a derivative isolated from the Middle Eastern plant *Ammi visnaga*. Many of these derivatives have smooth-muscle-relaxing properties causing vasodilation and relaxation of airways smooth muscle. Based on the activity of khellin, many analogs, directed toward a more soluble chromone with greater potency, were synthesized in the late 1950s and early 1960s.

Early on, the chromone-2-carboxylic acids were recognized as not having smooth-muscle-relaxant properties; however, in human volunteers, they inhibited antigen-induced bronchospasm if given prior to antigen as an aqueous aerosol. Animal models showed these compounds to be essentially inactive, so further screening was conducted in humans.

Studies continued with this series, looking for greater potency and longer duration. Significant progress was made when two carboxychromone molecules were attached by an alkylenedioxy chain forming a bischromone. One of the early compounds in this series, cromolyn was found to be active by aerosol as a prophylactic and to have a duration of several hours.

The essential chemical features of cromolyn are the planar chromone rings linked by a 2-hydroxy-trimethylenedioxy group at the 5 position(s) with carboxyl groups in the 2 position(s). Cromolyn is soluble in water up to approximately 5%. It is stable in dilute acids but labile in alkali.

Cromolyn

The mechanism of action of cromolyn has received much interest since its introduction. Cromolyn is referred to as a *mediator release inhibitor (MRI)*, that is, it stabilizes mast cell membranes and prevents release of mediators in response to various stimuli. Blockade of mediator release (stabilization of membranes) is evident in allergic subjects where cromolyn inhibits both the early and late phase reactions to antigen exposure. Additionally, the release of histamine and leukotrienes from human lung fragments is inhibited by cromolyn in vitro.

Cromolyn differs from most medicaments used in obstructive airways disease in that it is useful only as a prophylactic. It inhibits antigen- or exercise-induced bronchospasm if administered prior to exposure but has no bronchodilating properties. Cromolyn lacks oral activity and thus must be administered by inhalation. It is available as a dry powder (Spinhaler), in a metered dose inhaler or as a solution for use in a nonmetered nebulizer. Cromolyn is also available as a nasal or opthalmic preparation for use in seasonal rhinitis.

Clinical use of cromolyn in airways disease is restricted to prophylactic use. In asthma, cromolyn is not universally efficacious; however, it is effective in a percentage of patients as measured by a decrease in attack severity or decrease in the use of concomitant medications. Patient variability makes it necessary to try cromolyn therapy for at least 4 weeks to determine a therapeutic effect. The usual dose of cromolyn is 20 mg inhaled four times daily. With the exception of local irritant effects in the mouth and airways, and occasionally a powder-induced bronchospasm, adverse reactions to cromolyn are rare. Some of the local irritant effects can be prevented by prior treatment with a beta$_2$-adrenergic receptor agonist.

Corticosteroids

Corticosteroids (see Chap. 39) have been used extensively in the treatment of obstructive airways disease. The myriad of side effects associated with their use systemically has limited their use to those patients whose symptoms were uncontrolled by other therapies. Corticosteroids are not bronchodilators, and it is generally believed that their beneficial effects in chronic airways disease are due to their anti-inflammatory effect. One action may be to inhibit phospholipase activity, thus inhibiting the production of a variety of inflammatory mediators (see introductory text to this chapter).

Except in extreme cases, corticosteroids can be used for the treatment of airways disease by the inhaled route of administration. Those agents available for topical use include beclomethasone, triamcinolone, and flunisolide. The use of aerosols decreases the systemic toxicity associated with oral use of these agents, but it does not eliminate it. Some of the more severe adverse effects associated with steroid use, aerosol or oral, include reduced hypothalamic-pituitary-adrenal functions, osteoporosis, cataract formation, and stunting of growth. Of course, the occurrence of these effects varies widely among patients on this type of ther-

TABLE 32-3   Corticosteroids available as aerosol products for respiratory disease

Generic name	Structure (hydrocortisone)	Commercial name	Dosage regimen
Flunisolide	6α-Fluoro, 16, 17-dihydroxy acetonide	AeroBid	250 μg/dose 2 doses bid
Beclomethasone diproprionate	9α-Chloro, 16β-methyl	Beclovent	42 μg/dose 2 doses qid
		Vanceril	42 μg/dose 2 doses qid
Triamcinolone acetonide	9α-Fluoro, 16, 17-dihydroxy acetonide	Azmacort	100 μg/dose 2 doses qid

apy. The individual agents available for aerosol use in pulmonary disease are listed in Table 32-3 along with their structures and recommended dosages.

POTENTIAL THERAPEUTIC CATEGORIES

Antagonists of Mediator Receptor Sites Leukotrienes are a family of compounds which are potent chemotactic factors (primarily LTB_4) and potent bronchospastic agents (LTC_4, LTD_4, LTE_4). These agents act via membrane receptors on cells or smooth muscle. Therefore, the potential to inhibit their action by specific receptor blockade offers a possible therapeutic approach to inhibiting the bronchospasm and the cellular infiltration associated with their action. Several pharmaceutical companies are currently evaluating specific LTD_4 receptor antagonists for their effects in asthma or acute bronchospasm. To date, they have proven to be antagonists of LT-induced bronchospasm and have demonstrated mild effects in the bronchospasm associated with asthma. It is important to remember that there are a variety of mediators associated with asthma, and several specific receptor blockers may be needed to cause the desired therapeutic effect.

Similar to the studies with leukotrienes, various pharmaceutical companies around the world are currently evaluating PAF antagonists in the same way.

Clinical trials have been somewhat disappointing with these compounds as well, but as our experience with specific antagonists grows, studies may demonstrate greater efficacy in combination than with single entities alone.

Inhibitors of Allergic Mediator Synthesis Another approach to prevent the effect of inflammatory mediators is to inhibit their synthesis. An excellent example of this approach is the inhibition of cyclooxygenase by nonsteroidal anti-inflammatory agents to prevent production of pro-inflammatory prostaglandins. Like the work being done on receptor antagonists, this is another area of research being pursued both in the pharmaceutical industry and academia. To date, obtaining potent, orally active lipoxygenase and phospholipase inhibitors has been difficult; however, a number of potential chemical leads have been described. Several lipoxygenase inhibitors have been discovered that are not orally active but are active with topical administration. These compounds are being evaluated in diseases like psoriasis and atopic dermatitis, where oral activity is not a prerequisite. Further studies may uncover agents active orally or by aerosol which would be of use in respiratory disease.

Calcium Entry Blockers A third approach to block the effect of inflammatory-bronchoconstrictory mediators is to inhibit the reaction one step above phospholipase, that is, prevent the influx of calcium into the cell with calcium blocking agents (refer to Fig. 32-1). One of the problems with these agents is their vascular liability, since systemic absorption of these compounds leads to decreases in heart rate and blood pressure. Aerosol administration of calcium blockers may offer a significant advantage toward utilizing these agents for asthma. Also, the development of bronchial-tissue-selective calcium blockers may provide a means of using this mechanism for pharmacologic intervention. Research is just beginning in this area, and whether it will produce therapeutically useful agents remains to be seen.

Clinical Pharmacology

The major goal of pharmacologic intervention in asthma is to maintain the patient as symptom-free as possible on the least amount of medication. The first line of therapy for an acute bronchospasm in a previously asymptomatic patient consists of either one to two inhalations of a sympathomimetic bronchodilator or administration of a rapid-onset theophylline preparation. In less severe bronchospasm an oral sympathomimetic bronchodilator may be adequate if tolerated by the patient. The onset of action for the oral bronchodilators may be 30 to 60 min.

If symptoms persist or recur, around-the-clock oral bronchodilator therapy should be initiated. This may include theophylline, a sympathomimetic, or both, usually beginning with a long-acting theophylline preparation every 12 h. Should the patient have problems tolerating theophylline, the dose may be decreased and supplemented with the sympathomimetic. There have been some suggestions of adverse myocardial effects with the use of theophylline—sympathomimetic bronchodilator combinations. Clinical evidence supporting these suggestions is rare; however, the physician should be aware of the possibility, especially when treating patients with cardiovascular disease.

If the patient tolerates the theophylline but symptoms are not controlled, the dose of theophylline may be increased every 2 to 3 days while monitoring blood levels to achieve and maintain adequate serum theophylline levels (10 to 20 μg/mL). As an alternative to increasing the theophylline dose or if symptoms are still not controlled with increased theophylline, again the patient may be supplemented with oral or inhaled sympathomimetics. If necessary, both routes, oral and aerosol, may be used to achieve the necessary bronchodilator effect. If the sympathomimetics are not well tolerated, ipratropium can be used as an alternative or as a supplement. Once the symptoms are controlled, medication is continued at that dosage level for two to three asymptomatic days. The doses of bronchodilators can then be gradually decreased until the minimum dose of these agents necessary to control symptoms is reached.

If the patient fails to respond to the therapy described above, corticosteroid therapy should be initiated. Therapy should be started aggressively with high doses over 3 to 4 days. Response to steroid therapy may occur within 6 to 24 h but could also take up to 3 days. If the effect is favorable in less than 5 days, discontinue the corticosteroids abruptly while continuing the oral bronchodilators for an additional week before adjusting the dose. When the steroids are used longer than 5 days, taper off the dose over the same number of days as the maximum dose was given. If the patient fails to respond to these therapies, hospitalization may be required for more intensive care.

In the patient with an acute, severe asthmatic attack, emergency measures may be indicated. An assessment of the severity of the disease must be accomplished, including blood-gas determinations. Administration of oxygen may be necessary to maintain the Pa_{O_2} at 60 to 65 mmHg. Subcutaneous epinephrine may be required or may be supplemented or replaced with a nebulized bronchodilator. As a next step, intravenous administration of fluids and aminophylline may be initiated if a suitable response is not achieved. If patients have a prior history with corticosteroids or if they are on maintenance corticosteroid therapy, corticosteroids should be administered as an oral "burst" of high dose or an intravenous infusion followed by an oral burst.

For the maintenance therapy of the chronic asthmatic patient, the physician should try to control the symptoms with nonpharmacologic measures such as avoidance, if possible. If not, several alternatives could be used for chronic therapy. Long-acting oral theophylline should be tried initially. Dosage should be adjusted to maintain serum levels of between 10 and 20 μg/mL. If the patient does not tolerate theophylline or if symptoms are not controlled, a sympathomimetic may be added or substituted, either as an aerosol or oral preparation. If symptoms are still not controlled, corticosteroid therapy is usually indicated.

Corticosteroids should be initiated by inhalation in an attempt to control symptoms while minimizing adverse reactions. Once symptoms are controlled, the dose of corticosteroids should be reduced to the minimum dose required to maintain the patient symptom-free. If the corticosteroid preparation causes airway irritation or bronchospasm, pretreatment with a sympathomimetic bronchodilator may help prevent or lessen these effects.

If theophylline and/or sympathomimetic bronchodilators and/or inhaled corticosteroids are ineffective, the patient must be treated with systemic corticosteroids. If acute symptoms are present, give a high dose of corticosteroid and then taper the dose to the least dose necessary to control symptoms. Alternate-day therapy with the corticosteroids will help to control the side effects associated with their use.

During the treatment of the chronic asthmatic patient, cromolyn sodium represents an alternative that may be tried at any time. In patients who do not respond well to bronchodilator therapy, cromolyn may offer a viable therapeutic approach, without resorting to corticosteroids. A 4- to 8-week trial with cromolyn by Spinhaler, metered dose inhaler, or nebulized solution is usually necessary to define a clinical effect, which could be reduction in symptoms and/or reduction in concomitant medications. Cromolyn represents a unique compound which can be very effective in some patients, particularly those with exercise-induced asthma.

BIBLIOGRAPHY

Altounyan, R. E. C.: "Review of Clinical Activity and Mode of Action of Sodium Cromoglycate," *Clin. Allergy*, **10** (**Suppl**):481–489 (1980).

Chu, S. S.: "Bronchodilators. Part 1: Adrenergic Drugs," *Drugs of Today*, **20**:439–464 (1984).

Chu, S. S.: "Bronchodilators. Part II: Methylxanthines," *Drugs of Today*, **20**:509–527 (1984).

Church, M. K.: "Cromoglycate-like Antiallergic Drugs: A Review," *Drugs of Today*, **14**:281–341 (1978).

Church, M. K.: "Biochemical Basis of Pulmonary and Antiallergic Drugs," in J. P. Devlin (ed.), *Pulmonary and Antiallergic Drugs*, Wiley, New York, 1985, pp. 43–122.

Daniels, T. C., and E. C. Jorgensen: "Central Nervous System Stimulants," in R. F. Doerge (ed.), *Wilson and Grisvold's Textbook of Organic Medicinal and Pharmaceutical Chemistry*, Lippincott, Philadelphia, 1982, pp. 383–400.

Graft, D. F., and M. D. Valentine: "Immunotherapy," in A. P. Kaplan (ed.), *Allergy*, Churchill-Livingstone, New York, 1985.

Hendeles, L., and M. Weinberger: "Improved Efficacy and Safety of Theophylline in the Control of Airway Hyperactivity," *Pharmacol. Ther.*, **18**:91–105 (1982).

Katz, D. H.: "Regulation of the IgE System: Experimental and Clinical Aspects," *Allergy*, **39**:81–106 (1984).

Lawlor, G. J., Jr., and D. P. Tachkin: Asthma, in G. J. Lawlor Jr. and T. J. Fischer (eds.), *Manual of Allergy and Immunology*, Little Brown, Boston, 1988, pp. 115–165.

Long, J. W.: *The Essential Guide to Prescription Drugs*, Harper & Row, New York, 1987.

Nijkamp, F. P.: "The Pharmacology of Anti-Asthmatic Drugs," in P. K. Saxena and G. R. Elliott (eds.), *Pathophysiology and Treatment of Asthma and Arthritis, Agents & Actions*, **14**(**Suppl**.): 84–103 (1984).

Rall, T. W.: "Evolution of the Mechanism of Action of the Methylxanthines: From Calcium Mobilizers to Antagonists of Adenosine Receptors," *Pharmacologist*, **24**:277–287 (1982).

Rocklin, R. E., A. L. Sheffer, D. F. Greineder, and K. L. Melmom: "Generation of Antigen-Specific Suppressor Cells during Allergy Desensitization," *N. Engl. J. Med.*, **302**:1213–1219 (1980).

Snider, G.: "The Interrelationships of Asthma, Chronic Bronchitis and Emphysema" in D. B. Weiss and M. S. Segal (eds.), *Bronchial Asthma: Mechanisms and Therapeutics*, Little Brown, Boston, 1976, pp. 31–42.

"Standards for the Diagnosis and Care of Patients with Chronic Obstructive Pulmonary Disease (COPD) and Asthma. Official Statement of the American Thoracic Society," *Am. Rev. Resp. Dis.*, **136**:225–243 (1987).

Toogood, J. H., and D. W. Moote: "Steroid Therapy and Allergic Reactions," in A. P. Kaplan (ed.), *Allergy*, Churchill-Livingstone, New York, 1985.

PART VI

Hematopoietic System

SECTION EDITOR
Andrew P. Ferko

CHAPTER 33

Antianemia Agents

David L. Topolsky and Sigmund B. Kahn

Anemia is a clinical sign indicating a reduction in the red blood cell mass. *Anemia* is defined by a lowered hemoglobin concentration, a reduced red blood cell count or a reduction in the hematocrit (packed cell volume, PCV). Functionally, anemia may result in tissue hypoxia because of hemoglobin's key role in oxygen transport. Patients with anemia may complain of a variety of nonspecific symptoms, including fatigue, dyspnea, lightheadedness, pallor, or palpitations. The clinical complaints of the patient often do not define the etiology of the anemia. In other words, the cause of anemia is rarely ascertained merely by eliciting signs and symptoms from the patient.

The causes of anemia are quite varied, but several different classification systems are clinically useful. Anemia may be classified pathophysiologically in the following manner: (1) deficiency of building blocks or growth factors needed for normal red blood cell development, (2) deficiency of, or defect in, stem cell proliferation, (3) excessive loss of red blood cells. Another schema views anemia as a morphologic entity. This classification is described in Table 33-1 and is based on the morphologic characteristics of the red blood cells. In this case pathophysiology is implied by the red blood cell morphology. These two different classification schemas are by no means mutually exclusive, and often in practice both are used in trying to define the precise cause of the anemia.

A third system of classification is based entirely on etiology. Since many different etiologies can produce anemia via similar pathophysiologic mechanisms [i.e.,

impaired globin synthesis (thalassemia) and iron deficiency, both cause anemia by interfering with the building blocks of hemoglobin], this method may be quite cumbersome. In practice it is best to classify the anemia morphologically, then define its pathophysiology, and finally, it is essential to understand and to determine etiology before any treatment is suggested.

MICROCYTIC ANEMIA: IRON DEFICIENCY

Iron in the Body

Of the elements found in the body, iron is one of the most multifunctional and essential. Iron is found in hemoglobin, myoglobin, storage compounds (ferritin and hemosiderin), transferrin, and enzymes such as the cytochromes (Fig. 33-1).

Hemoglobin Hemoglobin contains the major portion of body iron. It is a protein that has a molecular weight of 64,658 and has approximately 0.35 percent iron by weight. Divalent iron is bound in stable covalent linkage within the porphyrin ring of heme, with additional coordination positions attached to the globin peptide chains. Molecular oxygen is bound reversibly by the iron (ferrous) of hemoglobin. Oxidation of the iron to the ferric state (as in methemoglobin) causes hemoglobin to lose its capacity to carry oxygen. A single molecule of hemoglobin consists of four atoms of iron each inserted into a molecule of proto-

TABLE 33-1   Morphologically classified anemias

Class	Number of red blood cells	Size of red blood cells	Amount of Hb/RBC	Usual pathophysiologic mechanism	Some causes
Macrocytic	Decrease	Increase	Slight increase	Megaloblastosis vs. reticulocytosis	Vitamin B$_{12}$ or folate deficiency; hemolytic anemia
Normocytic	Decrease	No change	No change	Marrow failure (usually)	Aplastic anemia; anemia of chronic disease
Simple microcytic	Decrease	Slight decrease	Slight decrease	Marrow failure	Chronic inflammation
Hypochromic microcytic	Slight decrease	Decrease	Marked decrease	Decreased hemoglobin production	Iron deficiency; thalassemias

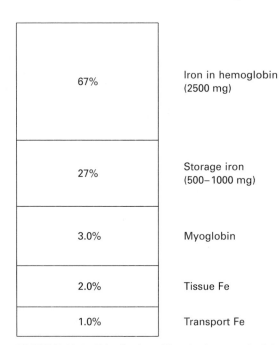

67%	Iron in hemoglobin (2500 mg)
27%	Storage iron (500–1000 mg)
3.0%	Myoglobin
2.0%	Tissue Fe
1.0%	Transport Fe

FIGURE 33-1   Distribution of iron in the normal adult subject.

porphyrin to yield heme. Each of these heme molecules is attached to one of four globin chains, two alpha and two beta. Deficiency of any component (iron, porphyrin, globin) leads to a hypochromic microcytic anemia.

Myoglobin   Myoglobin, with a molecular weight of 16,500, is the protein-bound heme of skeletal and cardiac muscle. The concentration of this protein varies greatly in different muscles and is only about 1 percent of the concentration of hemoglobin in blood. The affinity of myoglobin for oxygen is much greater than that of hemoglobin, especially at low oxygen tensions, thus facilitating the acceptance of oxygen carried by hemoglobin.

Transferrin   Transferrin, which is a beta globulin of molecular weight 90,000, has the specific property of binding iron; each transferrin molecule combines with two atoms of ferric iron. The combination is reversible. Transferrin serves to *transport* iron from the gastrointestinal tract to the bone marrow, to other tissue storage sites, and to the cells of the body that require iron. Under physiologic circumstances, about 20 to 35 percent of all available binding sites on the transferrin molecule are occupied by iron atoms. When there is a pathologic increase in body content, the saturation of transferrin increases. Conversely, in iron deficiency the saturation of transferrin falls below 15 percent. Both the serum iron and, indirectly, the serum transferrin level can be measured clinically. In practice, these tests serve as rough estimates of the state iron stores.

Ferritin and hemosiderin Ferritin and hemosiderin are the storage forms of iron in the body. Ferritin, a soluble iron-containing complex, is composed of a protein, apoferritin, within whose matrix iron, in amounts up to about 23 percent by weight, is bound in the form of hydroxide and phosphate complexes. Its major function is as a storage compound, although with its iron in the reduced form it has vasodepressive and antidiuretic properties. Ferritin can now be easily measured in the serum, and this has been shown to correlate with total body iron stores. This makes the serum ferritin test very important in the diagnosis of disease related to abnormalities of iron metabolism. Hemosiderin, an iron protein complex, the chief storage form of iron within the reticuloendothelial system, is distinguishable from ferritin by its lack of solubility in water and its increased iron concentration—up to 35 percent iron by weight. Evaluation of bone marrow hemosiderin is a clinically available test which is helpful in the diagnosis of iron deficiency.

Enzymes and Cofactors In cells, iron is an integral part of the heme enzymes (catalases, peroxidases, the cytochromes, and cytochrome oxidase) and of the ferroflavoproteins (succinic dehydrogenase, xanthine oxidase, and NADH cytochrome reductase). Iron also serves as a necessary cofactor for other enzymes. Iron is present in small amounts in a variety of other cell components, including red hair pigment, the muscle proteins (myosin and actin), a protein of human milk, and some compounds found in the brain.

Iron Absorption, Transport, and Storage

Iron is presented to the gastrointestinal tract in a variety of forms. Iron may be ingested in the form of simple inorganic salts derived primarily from cooking and food processing or in the form of heme compounds such as hemoglobin or myoglobin found within meat.

The average American diet contains about 6 mg of elemental iron per 1000 kcal. Thus the average daily intake of iron is 6 to 24 mg daily, provided a balanced diet is being ingested. Only about 5 to 10 percent of the ingested iron, rarely more, is actually absorbed, which closely matches the need, since in the average adult only 0.5 to 1.8 mg of iron is actually lost daily. Factors which tend to increase iron absorption include an acid pH of the gastric contents, ionization of food iron, solubility of the ingested iron salts, and iron ingested as heme or as other water-soluble chelates. Iron absorption increases in iron deficiency or when the rate of hematopoietic activity in the marrow increases for any cause. It is important to remember that the body has very limited ability to increase the absorption of ingested iron, even in the face of severe iron deficiency.

Absorption of iron can be accomplished at almost any level of the gastrointestinal tract, but it is most efficient in the duodenum and proximal jejunum. Virtually all iron that is absorbed by the intestine enters the body via the bloodstream rather than by lymphatics. Uptake into the mucosal cell is unidirectional with no excretion of iron into the intestinal lumen except by cell desquamation. Absorption of iron normally balances excretion, with maintenance of fairly constant body composition. Iron absorption depends on a metabolically active two-stage process which is normally at a maximum in the proximal duodenum. Ferrous iron is better absorbed than is the ferric form. The initial rapid stage involves the binding of low-molecular-weight iron compounds to the cell surface and is virtually complete within an hour. The second, slower stage involves the binding of iron to intracellular proteins, one of which is ferritin. The ferritin actually acts as an intracellular storage depot. By means of signals generated by the body in response to need (the nature of these signals has not been completely defined), the intracellularly absorbed iron is then transferred to the plasma protein transferrin. The iron, now bound to transferrin, is transferred to tissues for utilization or to reticuloendothelial stores for later use. Cells that require iron have transferrin receptors on their surfaces. By a process of endocytosis, the iron-transferrin complex is ingested, the iron removed intracellularly, and the transferrin returned to the circulation.

Iron not transferred to transferrin with the 2- to 3-day life span of the gastrointestinal mucosal cell is maintained within the cell bound to ferritin and is lost to the body by desquamation of the cell from the villous tip. This tightly regulated process, in the past called the mucosal block, prevents excessive accumulation of iron within the body. Iron stores are located in the reticuloendothelial systems and in hepatocytes. About two-thirds of storage iron is in the form of ferritin, and one-third is in the form of hemosiderin. In cases of excessive storage of iron, hemosiderin becomes the chief storage form.

Table 33-2 outlines the changes that occur in iron metabolism in various conditions.

Iron Excretion

The capacity of the body to excrete iron is limited. Most excretion is by desquamation of iron-containing cells from the bowel, skin, and genitourinary tract, although some iron is contained in fluids such as bile, urine, and sweat. The total daily iron loss for an adult male or nonmenstruating female is about 0.5 to 1.0 mg; an additional daily increment of 0.5 to 0.6 mg is added for normal menstrual loss.

Iron loss as hemosiderin granules in the urinary sediment is found in many patients with massive iron overload and in some patients with brisk intravascular hemolysis. During pregnancy iron is lost from the mother to the fetus and the placental tissues; there is further loss of iron at delivery, and normal iron excretion (minus menstrual losses) continues. The point to stress here is that in cases of iron overload, the ability of the body to excrete the excess iron is very limited.

Iron Requirements

Requirements for iron vary during different periods of life and reflect the demands of growth, menstruation, or pregnancy. The effects of these variations superimposed on the baseline excretion are listed in Table 33-3. Men and postmenopausal women ingesting a balanced diet normally maintain an adequate iron balance. Women during their reproductive years and adolescent girls, who must cope with both growth and menstruation, are constantly in precarious iron balance and readily become iron-deficient, since the ability to increase iron absorption is very limited. Similarly, infants from 6 to 24 months of age, during the period of rapid increase in body size, often outstrip their dietary iron supply.

The kinetics of the daily turnover of iron bound to plasma transferrin for a normal subject is schematically summarized in Fig. 33-2. As indicated in Fig. 33-2, all iron exchange among the various sites within the body must occur via the plasma, mediated by the binding of the elemental iron to transferrin. In the normal state the amount of iron entering the plasma is equal to the amount leaving the plasma. The major exchange of iron occurs from the red blood cell (RBC) to the marrow. The erythropoietic labile pool refers to the iron available to RBC marrow precursors for hemoglobin synthesis. Of the 35 mg of iron turned over each day, 21 mg is used to produce hemoglobin for

TABLE 33-2   Changes in clinically measured parameters of various iron anemias

Condition	Serum iron	Serum transferrin	Serum ferritin
Iron deficiency (i.e., blood loss)	↓	↑	↓
Normal pregnancy	↓	↑	↓
Hemosiderosis/ Hemochromatosis	↑	→	↑
Anemias not directly by changes in iron metabolism			
Aplastic anemia	↑	↓	↑
Hemolytic anemia	→	→	→
Megaloblastic anemia	↑	→	→

Note: ↑ = increased; ↓ = decreased; → = unchanged or normal.

TABLE 33-3 Estimated dietary iron requirements

	Absorbed iron requirement, mg/day	Daily food iron requirement,[a] mg/day
Normal men and nonmenstruating women	0.5–1	5–10
Menstruating women	0.7–2	7–20
Pregnant women	2–4.8	20–48[b]
Adolescents	1–2	10–20
Children	0.4–1	4–10
Infants	0.5–1.5	1.5 mg/kg[c]

[a] Assuming 10% absorption.
[b] This amount of iron cannot be derived from diet and should be met by iron supplementation in the latter half of pregnancy.
[c] To a maximum of 15 mg.

circulating RBC, 11 mg is used to maintain the labile pool, and the remainder is distributed within stores and intracellular fluid. The reader should note that only 1 mg of iron is lost daily and 1 mg is absorbed daily. Should there occur a loss of RBC from the body through bleeding, the amount of iron lost would be made up by storage iron. Conversely, if absorption of iron is in excess of utilization, the storage pool would increase.

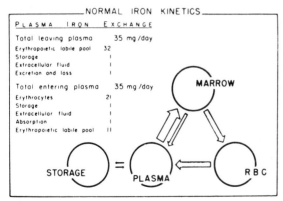

FIGURE 33-2 Summary of iron kinetics of a normal adult subject.

Iron-Deficiency States

In iron-deficiency states, regardless of the etiology, there is an orderly progression of iron depletion, most of which occurs long before clinical signs or symptoms become apparent. The earliest identifiable change is manifest by a loss of storage iron, but with maintenance of normal hemoglobin concentration, iron-dependent enzyme function, and transport iron. This phase is termed *iron store depletion*. Assessment of the patient at this time would be expected to yield low levels of serum ferritin and no stainable iron in the marrow, but normal serum iron concentration, transferrin levels (clinically measured as the total plasma iron-binding capacity, TIBC), hemoglobin concentration, and RBC morphology. As further depletion occurs, there occurs a slow decline in the serum iron concentration, a rise in the TIBC, and a fall in hemoglobin concentration, followed by the development of characteristic microcytic hypochromic red blood cells. It will be at some point along this spiral that the clinical symptoms of anemia would occur.

The diagnosis of iron-deficiency anemia is based on the finding of small erythrocytes (microcytes) filled poorly with hemoglobin (hypochromia). Only late in the course are cells of bizarre shape (poikilocytosis) and variable size (anisocytosis) sometimes seen. The diagnosis is confirmed by finding a low serum iron concentration coupled with a normal or high TIBC, with the total saturation of the iron-binding protein of less than 15 percent. Other confirmatory tests would be a low serum ferritin and absence of stainable marrow iron. Iron-deficiency anemia constitutes the major cause of hypochromic anemia, the others being the thalassemia syndromes (globin deficiency) and the anemia caused by impaired porphyrin synthesis.

Clinically, iron-deficiency anemia is a sign rather than a disease. In adult males and postmenopausal females iron deficiency usually signifies the presence of significant blood loss, the cause of which must be diligently sought, most often by careful examination of the gastrointestinal tract. For women of childbearing age, excessive menstrual flow and multiple pregnancies are the most common causes. Infants and children with rapid growth demands on limited dietary iron intake may suffer from iron deficiency. Bleeding related to laboratory testing will add to their iron depletion. Malabsorption of iron as a result of gastrointestinal diseases or surgical alteration of the gastrointestinal tract may be an additional cause of iron-deficiency anemia. Rarely in the United States is pure dietary insufficiency of iron the sole cause of iron-deficiency anemia in adults.

In the treatment of iron-deficiency anemia there are two basic points to consider: (1) recognition and correction of the underlying cause and (2) repletion of body iron. The second of these is usually quite easily achieved, but it is probably the first which is most important in the long run. It is common to find that iron-deficiency anemia is the first sign of a potentially more serious clinical condition (i.e., colon cancer, chronic gastrointestinal bleeding, or genital-urinary bleeding). The task of the clinician is to become aware of the etiology of the iron deficiency and correct this problem before prescribing any of the iron compounds listed below.

Iron Compounds for Oral Administration

Ferrous Sulfate   Over the years ferrous sulfate has been the standard to which new iron preparations have been compared. Two forms of ferrous sulfate are generally used therapeutically: (1) the hydrated salt ($FeSO_4 \cdot 7H_2O$) contains 20 percent elemental iron by weight and (2) the exsiccated form (80% anhydrous $FeSO_4$) contains 30 percent elemental iron.

Most ferrous sulfate tablets contain 60 mg of elemental iron, and the usual adult with iron deficiency will require between 150 to 200 mg of elemental iron per day. Given an absorption rate of 5 to 20 percent, in order to replete body iron completely, 3 to 6 months of continuous oral therapy are usually required.

Liquid forms of ferrous sulfate are available. Ferrous sulfate syrup contains 40 mg of ferrous sulfate per milliliter (8 mg of iron per milliliter). The usual pediatric dose for treatment of iron-deficiency anemia is 5 mL two or three times a day.

Ferrous Gluconate   Ferrous gluconate was introduced in an effort to reduce the side effects of ferrous sulfate. It is supplied as tablets of 320 mg containing 11.5 percent iron, as capsules of 435 mg containing 50 mg of iron, and as an elixir containing 300 mg per teaspoon, equivalent to 36 mg or iron. In order to administer an adequate dose of elemental iron, four to six tablets per day of this preparation would have to be taken.

Ferrous Fumarate   Ferrous fumarate is a redbrown iron salt of fumaric acid containing 33 percent elemental iron. It is relatively resistant to oxidation, even in uncoated tables, and is relatively insoluble in aqueous solution except as low pH.

The most common reason for failure of oral iron to correct iron deficiency is patient noncompliance, provided the etiology of the blood loss has been corrected. Noncompliance is usually a result of the side effects of the iron preparations. Most troublesome to the patient are the gastrointestinal symptoms of constipation, pyrosis, or loose stool.

Placebo-controlled studies indicate that gastrointestinal intolerance ascribed to medicinal iron ingestion occurs only in 5 to 10 percent of patients given the usual therapeutic doses listed above.

Iron Compounds for Parenteral Use

The great majority of patients with iron-deficiency anemia can best be treated with orally administered iron. However, the use of parenteral preparation of iron may be desirable for certain patients: (1) those who are unable to tolerate or unwilling to take iron orally, e.g., those with ulcerative colitis, regional enteritis, colostomies, or extensive bowel resections, as well as those who for various reasons cannot be relied upon to take medications prescribed for them; (2) those who are unable to absorb iron given orally, e.g., patients with idiopathic or postresection malabsorption syndromes; and (3) those with severe iron deficiency for whom it is impossible to provide iron quickly enough by the oral route.

Iron Dextran   This is a complex of ferric hydroxide and low-molecular-weight dextran (5000 to 20,000 average molecular weight). The compound contains 50 mg of elemental iron per milliliter. The preparations can be given either by deep intramuscular or intravenous injection. It is recommended that no more than 2 mL be given by either route per day. Total intravenous dose infusion has been used but is not at this time approved in the United States. Intravenous iron therapy has been associated with the infrequent occurrence of anaphylaxis, so it is recommended that a 0.5-mL test dose be given 1 to 2 days prior to the institution of parenteral therapy. Other toxicities include skin staining at the injection site, local thrombophlebitis, arthralgias, fever, hypotension, bradycardia, myalgias, headaches, abdominal pain, nausea, vomiting, and dizziness.

Acute Iron Toxicity

The ingestion of large doses of soluble iron compounds, especially by small children, often results in acute iron intoxication, leading to severe symptoms and death in a high proportion of cases. Lethal doses of ferrous sulfate have varied from 3 to 18 g, although survival has been reported after doses as high as 15 g.

The clinical effects of ingesting toxic doses of iron have been divided into four phases chronologically. The first phase begins with abdominal pain, nausea, and vomiting about 30 to 60 min after the iron tablets are taken. Partially dissolved iron tablets may be vomited together with brown or bloody stomach contents. Irritability, pallor, and drowsiness appear along with frequent black or bloody diarrhea. Signs of acidosis and cardiovascular collapse may become prominent; coma and death ensue within 4 to 6 h in about 20 percent of children taking large doses of iron. The second phase is a period of improvement with subsidence of the initial signs and symptoms spontaneously or in response to treatment. This period, lasting 8 to 16 h, may herald the onset of progressive improvement. Often, however, this lull in symptoms is shattered by a third phase of progressive cardiovascular collapse, convulsions, coma, and high mortality about 24 h after iron ingestion. Finally, a fourth phase of gastrointestinal obstruction from scarring of the stomach or small intestine may occur weeks or months after the recovery from the initial episode of iron intoxication. The most important aspect of management of acute iron toxicity is prevention. Especially in children, in whom accidental ingestion is most common, prevention cannot be overemphasized. In the event of either intentional or accidental ingestion of large amounts of iron, the following is a rational approach to the treatment of the patient: (1) Rid the stomach of its contents by inducing emesis and by lavage with a large-bore tube to remove undissolved iron tablets. With the tube still in place, instill a 1% solution of sodium bicarbonate. Deferoxamine (see below), an iron-chelating compound, may also be instilled in a dosage of 5 to 10 g to bind residual iron in a poorly absorbable form. Deferoxamine mesysalate (Desferal Mesylate) should also be administered by an intravenous infusion. Follow the gastric lavage with an enema to remove iron from the lower bowel. (2) Institute measures to combat peripheral vascular collapse, including early replacement of body fluids and electrolytes, using isotonic saline solution, Ringer's lactate solution, plasma, dextran, or whole blood. (3) Additional measures of value include treating metabolic acidosis with appropriate solutions of sodium bicarbonate and using oxygen and vasopressor substances to help combat shock. The use of barbiturates or benzodiazepines may be required to control convulsions.

Iron Chelation Therapy: Deferoxamine

Deferoxamine is a powerful iron-chelating agent derived from *Streptomyces pilosus*. The compound's affinity for iron is high ($K_a = 10^{31}$), whereas its affinity for calcium is much less ($K_a = 10^2$). Deferoxamine will bind iron from transferrin, ferritin, and hemosiderin, but not from hemoglobin or the cytochromes.

Pharmacokinetics Deferoxamine is poorly absorbed from the gastrointestinal tract, making parenteral administration mandatory for removal of excess body iron. The drug is metabolized by as yet undefined pathways. It is degraded by plasma enzymes. Metabolites and unchanged drug are excreted in the urine.

Deferoxamine binds ferric iron to form the water-soluble chelate, ferroxamine. Whereas ionized heavy metal ions such as iron salts are highly toxic to tissues, chelates of heavy metals are usually harmless. The newly formed ferroxamine is excreted into the urine.

Toxicities and Contraindication Allergic reactions occur commonly and include pruritus, urticaria, skin rashes, and much less commonly, anaphylaxis. Other toxicities include dysuria, abdominal pain, diarrhea, and cataract formation. This drug is contraindicated in pregnancy and renal dysfunction.

Preparations Deferoxamine is available in liquid form as Desferal Mesylate.

Chronic Iron Overload

Excessive amounts of iron may accumulate in the body under a variety of conditions. The following lists the major types of iron-storage diseases:

1. Idiopathic hemochromatosis
2. Transfusion iron overload
3. Medicinal iron overload
    a. Oral
    b. Parenteral
4. Hemolytic iron overload
    a. Refractory anemias
    b. Thalassemia
5. Dietary iron overload
    a. Bantu siderosis
    b. Kaschin-Beck disease

Much confusion results from the nomenclature of clinical disorders of iron overload which reflects an incomplete understanding of the pathogenesis of excessive body-iron storage and associated tissue damage. For the sake of discussion, *hemosiderosis* is defined as an increase in reticuloendothelial cell iron without any associated tissue damage. The term *hemochromatosis* is used to denote increased storage iron with associated tissue damage.

Idiopathic Hemochromatosis and Transfusional Hemosiderosis

Idiopathic hemochromatosis is an uncommon disease that is a result of a regulatory abnormality that involves both the intestinal absorption of iron and the reticuloendothelial cells' ability to handle the iron that is absorbed. Excessive absorption over many years leads to accumulation of reticuloendothelial iron with eventual "spillover" into the plasma and the tissues. Particular organs damaged by excessive iron storage are the liver, pancreas, thyroid, adrenals, heart, and the stomach. This disorder has been found to be inherited and linked to a specific human leukocyte antigen CHLA-A3. It appears that the homogenous condition must be present to have the full-blown disease. It is theoretically possible, however, that people homogenous for the A3 linked gene may be more susceptible to the secondary causes of hemochromatosis mentioned above. The disease occurs primarily in men 50 to 70 years of age and is only one-tenth as prevalent in women (presumably because menstrual loss rids these women of excess iron).

The diagnosis is usually established by the demonstration of cirrhosis and excessive iron deposits on biopsy of the liver. Increased iron in skin, gastric mucosa, or urine sediment are confirmatory findings. Elevated plasma iron level with almost completely saturated iron-binding capacity is generally observed. The serum ferritin level is usually found to be greater than 500 ng/mL and is often even greater than 1000 ng/mL. Bone marrow iron may not show any significant increase, however.

Removal of excess iron by repeated phlebotomy prevents further tissue damage. Patients must be monitored by the serum ferritin level for the remainder of their life.

Transfusion hemosiderosis is a complication of the multiply transfused patient. Each 1 mL of packed red blood cells delivers 1 mg of elemental iron which the body cannot excrete. After 100 or more units of blood the tissue iron stores become fully saturated and parenchymal organ damage may occur. The picture resembles hemochromatosis. Phlebotomy, as used in idiopathic hemochromatosis, is not feasible, for obvious reasons, in these anemic patients receiving blood transfusions. Alternate means of iron removal involves the use of deferoxamine. A single dose of 500 to 1000 mg of deferoxamine can mobilize up to 50 mg of iron, which is then excreted in the urine. Deferoxamine is usually given daily intravenously or via continuous intravenous or subcutaneous infusion over a 6- to 9-h period. Treatment is repeated periodically after the initial removal of as much excess iron as possible.

THE MEGALOBLASTIC ANEMIAS: FOLIC ACID (FOLATE) AND VITAMIN B$_{12}$ DEFICIENCY

Deficiency of either vitamin B$_{12}$ or folate will cause macrocytic anemia characterized by a peculiar morphologic appearance of red blood cell precursors in the marrow called the *megaloblastic change*. Megaloblastic change was a term coined by Paul Ehrlich in the 1880s. He described bone marrow red blood cell precursors which were larger than normal and which demonstrated nuclear-cytoplasmic maturation dyssynchrony. In such cases, the appearance of the cytoplasm seemed more mature than the nucleus. Actually, it has been shown that nuclear maturation lags behind the maturation of the cytoplasm. After repletion of the missing vitamin, the bone marrow morphology is restored to normal and the anemia is corrected.

Occasionally other deficits in cellular building blocks may give rise to a morphologic picture very similar to vitamin B_{12} or folate deficiency. Examples include blockage of active building block synthesis with antimetabolite therapy (i.e., 6-mercaptopurine, 5-fluorouracil or methotrexate), hereditary orotic aciduria, and certain refractory anemias. In these instances, vitamin B_{12} and folate replacement will not improve the anemia, nor will administration of these vitamins correct the abnormal morphology. The bone marrow abnormalities noted in the above instances are termed *bone marrow megaloblastoid changes* to distinguish them from true megaloblastosis.

Current evidence suggests that the megaloblast is a cell in a state of "unbalanced growth" due to impaired synthesis of one or more deoxyribonucleotides, the precursors of DNA. Hence the RNA/DNA ratio rises, since the replication of DNA and cell division are blocked, while the synthesis of cytoplasmic components proceeds normally. The roles of vitamin B_{12} and folate in deoxyribonucleotide synthesis are discussed later.

Folic Acid

Chemistry and Nomenclature Folic acid, the common name of pteroylglutamic acid, is a parent compound of a large group of growth factors and coenzymes collectively referred to as *folates*. The folic acid molecule contains three structural units: (1) a pteridine derivative, (2) *p*-aminobenzoic acid, and (3) glutamic acid (see Fig. 33-3). Pteroylglutamic, or folic, acid (F) is metabolically active only after conversion to its coenzyme form, 5,6,7,8-tetrahydrofolic acid (FH_4). Reduction of F to FH_4 is believed to occur in two steps: F is reduced to 7,8-dihydrofolic acid (FH_2), and FH_2 is reduced further to FH_4, both reactions being catalyzed by a single NADPH-linked enzyme, dihydrofolate reductase (DHRF).

Because reduced derivatives of folic acid are extremely sensitive to oxidation in air, they are unstable and difficult to preserve. A notable exception is the stable compound N^5-formyl FH_4, which was isolated from liver and yeast soon after the discovery of folic acid. It was first recognized as a growth factor for *Leuconostoc citrovorum* (since renamed *Pediococcus cerevisiae*) and, thus, it was named *citrovorum factor*. Leucovorin and folinic acid are the currently used names for this compound.

Sources The many different forms of folates are widely distributed in nature. Green leaves, presumed to be sites of active folate synthesis, are especially rich in the vitamin. Though the vitamin is also synthesized by many bacteria, the principal sources in the average diet are leafy vegetables, liver, and fruits. Excessive cooking, particularly with large amounts of water, may remove or destroy a large fraction of the folate in foods. Most food folate exists as polyglutamates with up to six glutamate moieties added to the parent molecule. In nature, folates always exist in a reduced form, but as soon as food folates are exposed to air, oxidation to folic acid occurs.

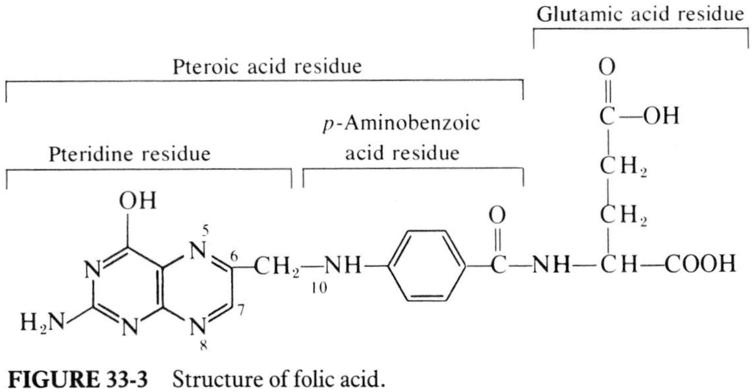

FIGURE 33-3 Structure of folic acid.

Absorption and Fate Even though the minimum daily requirement of folate is 50 μg, when 0.2 to 2.0 mg of folic acid is administered orally to a normal person, more than 65 percent is usually absorbed. About 5 percent of the 0.2 mg dose and 15 percent of the 2.0 mg is excreted in the urine. After a 1 mg oral dose, serum levels can be detected within minutes and reach a peak in about 1 h.

Gastrointestinal absorption occurs primarily in the upper small bowel and requires dihydrofolate reductase (DHFR), which is found in high concentrations in the mucosal cells of the duodenum and proximal jejunum. Therefore, any disease process that affects this area of the gut will have an adverse impact on folate absorption. Although various folates are synthesized by intestinal bacteria, little of the vitamin derived from this source is absorbed, since most of the synthesis of bacterial folate occurs in the colon, which is distal to the major area of folate absorption.

Reduced monoglutamates are absorbed rapidly by simple diffusion, while most food polyglutamated folate is absorbed by an active process. First, the absorbed polyglutamates must be broken down to monoglutamate forms. After passage into the intestinal cell as polyglutamate, a lysosomal enzyme known as conjugase removes the extra glutamatic acid moieties yielding monoglutamate folate. DHFR then reduces the compound to FH_4, and other enzymes add a single carbon fragment reduced to its methyl form to produce N^5-methyl FH_4. The latter compound then passes to the circulation.

Once the folate is absorbed, it is transported via a nonspecific binding protein to the tissues, where it is either stored or used. Folate is used by all dividing tissues and is stored in the liver. Folate is stored intracellularly in a polyglutamate form. While most folate coenzymes are monoglutamates, some of their coenzymatic activity involves polyglutamate forms, also. Body stores are maintained by food intake and an active enterohepatic circulation of the vitamin. The liver secretes folate into the bile, which is then reabsorbed by the intestinal cells. Most of the folate lost from the body is through the urine, and some is lost through the feces.

Metabolic Functions In metabolism, FH_4 is a catalytic self-regenerating acceptor-donor of 1-carbon units in reactions involving 1-carbon transfers from a carbon-containing donor compound, X—C, to an acceptor, Y:

$$
\begin{array}{l}
X{-}C \ \ + FH_4 \longrightarrow X \ \ \ + C{-}FH_4 \\
C{-}FH_4 + Y \ \ \longrightarrow Y{-}C + FH_4 \\
\hline
\text{Sum: } X{-}C \ \ + Y \ \ \longrightarrow Y{-}C + X
\end{array}
$$

The varieties of C—FH_4 differ only in the identity to the 1-carbon unit and the site of its attachment to FH_4: 1-carbon units can attach to either N^5, N^{10} or to both nitrogens (Fig. 33-3).

Figure 33-4 demonstrates the metabolic action of FH_4. Methylene, methenyl, and methyl groups are found among the 1-carbon units carried by FH_4. Specific enzymes are known which interconvert many of these compounds. In human folate deficiency, the reaction, whose impairment produces the major clinical manifestations, is that which catalyzes thymidylate synthesis. The methylation of deoxyuridylate (dUMP) to thymidylate (dTMP), catalyzed by the thymidylate synthetase, is an essential preliminary step in the synthesis of DNA. The coenzyme of reaction, N^5, N^{10}-methylene FH_4, transfers a 1-carbon group and also acts as a hydrogen donor in reducing the transferred group to a methyl group. This reaction generates FH_2, which dihydrofolate reductase must reduce to FH_4 before it can again be utilized as a folate coenzyme. Limitation of thymidylate synthesis in folate deficiency results in the defective DNA synthesis manifested by megaloblast formation.

Impairment of folate metabolism occurs in vitamin B_{12} deficiency. In Fig. 33-4 the only reaction in which N^5-methyl FH_4 may be utilized is by the donation of its methyl group to homocysteine to form methionine. Since this reaction depends on vitamin B_{12} coenzyme, when there is vitamin B_{12} deficiency (see section on vitamin B_{12}), the N^5-methyl FH_4 remains unutilizable (i.e., it "piles up" and is "trapped"). Since only N^5, N^{10}-methylene FH_4 can be used for DNA synthesis, the FH_4 trapped as N^5-methyl FH_4 is unavailable for synthesis of N^5, N^{10}-methylene FH_4 (and for other FH_4 reactions). This creates relative "folate deficiency." This mechanism may account for the megaloblastosis seen in vitamin B_{12} deficiency. Evidence supporting this mechanism includes the fact that intracellular folates are low in vitamin B_{12} deficiency, while serum folate, whose major form is N^5-methyl FH_4, is raised in vitamin B_{12} deficiency.

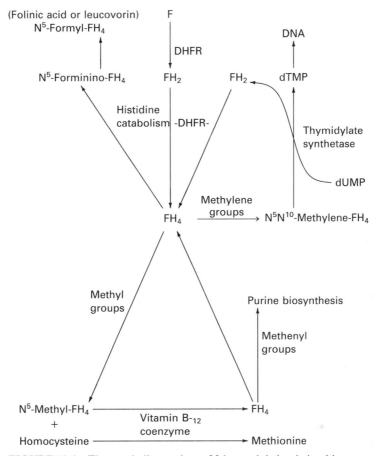

FIGURE 33-4 The metabolic reactions of folate and their relationship to vitamin B_{12}.

Requirements and Distribution The minimum daily requirement for folic acid in the normal adult is approximately 50 μg. Although the average diet contains several times this amount in the form of various food folate compounds, body reserves of folic acid are relatively smaller than are those of vitamin B_{12}. Reducing folate acid intake from a normal to a low daily intake of 5 μg/day results in the development of megaloblastic anemia in about 4 months. The majority of folate is stored within the liver.

Folate Deficiency The principal causes of folate deficiency are inadequate dietary intake, defective intestinal absorption, abnormally increased requirements, and impaired utilization in the tissues. In contrast to the vitamin B_{12}–deficiency syndromes, malnutrition is an important cause of folate deficiency. This is often associated with chronic alcoholism.

Various forms of malabsorption, tropical sprue, and nontropical sprue (adult and infantile celiac disease) are also causes of folate deficiency. In tropical sprue, treatment with folate alone may reverse all abnormalities, including the defective absorption of the vitamin itself. In nontropical sprue, as in most other forms of malabsorption, folate treatment corrects only the folate deficiency, without affecting the absorptive defect. Low serum folate levels in patients receiving phenytoin and other anticonvulsants have been attributed to a reversible drug-induced malabsorption of folate.

Increased requirements for folate occur in chronic hemolytic anemias, leukemia, other malignant diseases, and pregnancy, which increases requirements threefold to sixfold.

Finally, a major mechanism of folate "deficiency" is the inhibition of folate reduction caused by administration of various pharmacologic agents. The 4-aminofolic acid analogs, such as methotrexate, are powerful inhibitors of DHFR. Other, weaker inhibitors of DHRF in widespread use are trimethoprim and dyrenium.

Diagnosis of Folate Deficiency   If there is a clinical suspicion of folate deficiency (i.e., chronic alcholism, malabsorption, etc.), or a macrocytic anemia, or findings on peripheral smear suggestive of deficiency (e.g., hypersegmented polymorphonuclear leukocytes), the diagnosis should be confirmed with a serum folate. This should always be done before any replacement therapy is given, as even a small amount of oral folate may increase serum values appreciably.

It is essential to distinguish between folic acid and vitamin B_{12} deficiencies so that the pathogenetic mechanism may be understood and appropriate therapy given. (Gastrointestinal features of folate deficiency may also be similar to those of pernicious anemia.) Neurologic abnormalities are said to occur only in vitamin B_{12} deficiency, although scattered recent reports have suggested that neurologic changes may occur in pure folate deficiency. It should be remembered that neuropathies may result from deficiencies of other vitamins that may accompany a deficiency of folate (i.e., alcoholic polyneuropathy often accompanies folate deficiency).

Therapy of Folate Deficiency   The sole indication for folic acid therapy is folate deficiency or, as in pregnancy, anticipated folic acid deficiency. All therapeutic effects are attributable to reversal of the deficiency state.

The vitamin is available as 1.0-mg tablets. The sodium salt of folic acid (folate sodium) is available as a parenteral solution of 5 mg/mL and may be given by intramuscular, intravenous, or deep subcutaneous injection. Although the parenteral administration of folic acid has no advantage over oral administration, this route may be preferred when the folate deficiency is caused by malabsorption rather than by ingestion of inadequate amounts. Doses of 0.5 to 1.0 mg daily are considered adequate for parenteral therapy. The oral replacement dose of folic acid is 0.25 to 1.0 mg daily. Daily doses greater than 1 mg do not appear to enhance the hematologic effect.

Calcium leucovorin, tablets or injection, the clinically available preparation of N^5-formyl FH_4, is used in the presence of severe intoxication by folic acid antagonists (such as methotrexate), which act by blocking the reduction of FH_2 to FH_4. No purpose is accomplished in ordinary folate deficiency by giving this compound in place of folic acid. Suggestions that impaired reduction of folate in liver disease may respond to leucovorin have not been clinically proved. Leucovorin is available as a sterile solution containing 5 mg/mL of the calcium salt. The usual dose is 3 to 6 mg/day administered intramuscularly. Tablets containing 5 to 25 mg are also available. The absorption of this compound is similar to that of folic acid.

Adverse reactions caused by folic acid have not been observed even with doses 100 times higher than the usual minimum daily requirement (MDR). In patients on phenytoin or primidone, folate administration may cause seizures, probably because of concomitant changes in serum levels of the anticonvulsant.

Vitamin B_{12}

Chemistry and Nomenclature   Chemically, the structure of vitamin B_{12} relates it to the corrinoid compounds; the term *cobalamin* (introduced before the structure was known) is frequently used to refer to the vitamin B_{12} molecule minus the cyano group (Fig. 33-5). Vitamin B_{12} itself then becomes cyanocobalamin. The cyanomoiety of cyanocobalamin may be replaced by a hydroxyl group to yield hydroxycobalamine. Cobalamin, in either the cyano or hydroxy form, is readily converted to deoxyadenosylcobalamin in tissues by a coenzyme synthetase system. This compound is known as vitamin B_{12} coenzyme. In this reaction, the deoxyadenosyl moiety of ATP is transferred intact to the vitamin to form the coenzyme. Most natural sources of vitamin B_{12} contain the coenzyme or hydroxycobalamine.

Sources   Only bacteria can synthesize vitamin B_{12}. Vitamin B_{12} is required by all living cells. Plants obtain their supply from soil bacteria, while animals attain their supply by diet. Foods especially rich in vitamin B_{12} include liver, seafood, meat, eggs, and milk.

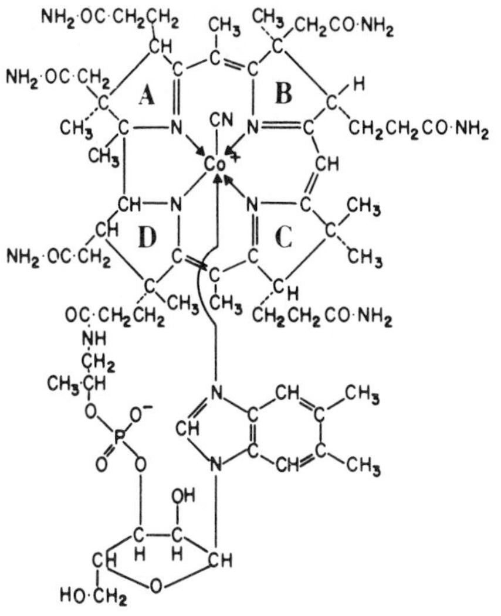

FIGURE 33-5 Chemical structure of vitamin B_{12}.

The average daily dietary intake of vitamin B_{12} is between 5 and 30 μg. The MDR is 1 to 3 μg. The vitamin is widely distributed throughout body tissues. In the human being, the total body content is 4 to 5 mg, about 1 mg being in the liver.

Absorption and Fate Human gastric intrinsic factor (IF) binds dietary vitamin B_{12} and small oral doses of pure cyanocobalamin. Intrinsic factor is a glycoprotein with a monomeric molecular weight of 50,000 to 60,000. When it binds vitamin B_{12}, it forms a dimer of molecular weight 114,000 to 119,000. The dimeric molecule binds two molecules of vitamin B_{12}. Vitamin B_{12} must be released from various food proteins to which it is bound by pancreatic proteases.

The intrinsic factor B_{12} complex is carried through the intestine to the terminal ileum, where the complex attaches to specific receptors on the microvilli of the terminal ileum. The vitamin B_{12} is then internalized by an active metabolic process, while the IF is released to be lost with the fecal contents. This accounts for the delay of several hours in the appearance of the vitamin in the bloodstream. Small physiologic doses of vitamin B_{12} are absorbed very efficiently in this fashion, while larger oral doses are absorbed by simple diffusion, both in normal and pernicious anemia subjects (*vide infra*). In these instances, the vitamin appears almost immediately in the blood. The range of blood levels of vitamin B_{12} is 200 to 1000 pg/mL.

Normal plasma contains at least two vitamin B_{12}–binding proteins, termed *transcobalamin I* and *transcobalamin II* (TC I and TC II). The former, an alpha$_1$ globulin, binds most of the circulating endogenous vitamin B_{12}. TC I is derived from the white blood cells and their precursors. TC II, a beta globulin, normally one-third to two-thirds saturated, is derived from the reticuloendothelial system and mediates the transfer of vitamin B_{12} to other cells in the body. Thus, TC II binds most of the ingested or injected vitamin B_{12}. Small injected doses of vitamin B_{12} are almost completely retained, while doses of more than 50 μg are lost in the urine, since this dose exceeds the binding capacity of the TC II. Free vitamin B_{12} is filtered by the glomerulus and is lost in the urine, since there is no tubular reabsorption.

Vitamin B_{12} is excreted in the bile. There is an active enterohepatic circulation of vitamin B_{12}. The total amount of vitamin B_{12} in feces exceeds the sum of that excreted in the urine plus the unabsorbed vitamin because there is new synthesis by colon bacteria. Vitamin from the latter source is not available to the human host. As yet, there is little information concerning the degradation of vitamin B_{12} in human tissues.

Metabolic Functions As currently understood, the biochemical systems impaired in human vitamin B_{12} deficiency are (1) the metabolism of methylmalonyl CoA and, thus, propionate catabolism, and (2) methionine synthesis and, thus, N^5-methyltetrahydrofolate demethylation (see section on folate). While the exact role for vitamin B_{12} in the maintenance of neurologic function is unknown, it has been suggested that impairment of methylmalonyl CoA conversion accounts for the neurologic damage of human vitamin B_{12} deficiency. The cobamide-dependent isomerization of methylmalonyl CoA is a step in the catabolism of propionic acid. Propionic acid metabolism resulting from fatty-acid oxidation in animal tissue involves the biotin-dependent carboxylation of propionyl CoA to methylmalonyl CoA. After a racemization step, methylmalonyl CoA mutase catalyzes the reversible conversion of methylmalonyl CoA to succinyl CoA (Fig. 33-6), which can then enter the tricarboxylic acid cycle after conversion to succinate. Nondividing nerve cells are not engaged in DNA synthesis, but they do synthesize myelin and other lipids. Vitamin B_{12}–deficient humans excrete abnormal quantities of methylmalonate and acetate. Data suggest that the presence

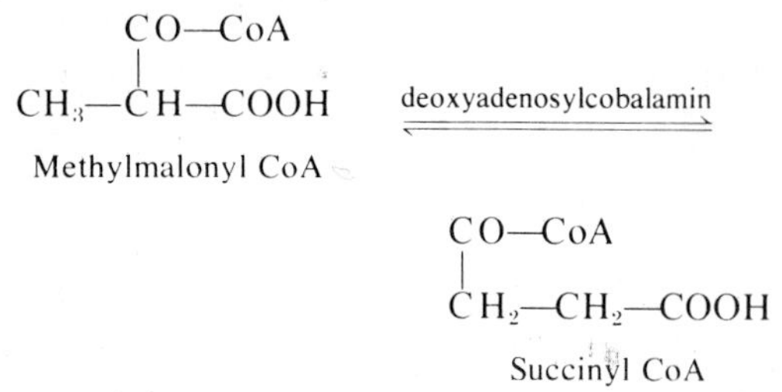

$$CO—CoA$$
$$CH_3—CH—COOH$$ deoxyadenosylcobalamin

Methylmalonyl CoA

$$CO—CoA$$
$$CH_2—CH_2—COOH$$

Succinyl CoA

FIGURE 33-6   The conversion of methylmalonyl CoA (MMA) to succinyl CoA. The source of the MMA is propionate.

and severity of neurologic symptoms correlate with the degree of acetic aciduria, but not of methylmalonic aciduria. These results, as well as evidence from isotopic studies of propionate metabolism in human vitamin B_{12} deficiency, are compatible with the view that distorted lipid metabolism may be responsible for neurologic damage.

The interrelationship between folate and vitamin B_{12} metabolism has been discussed previously. The trapping of folate caused by vitamin B_{12} deficiency has been presented as an explanation for the megaloblastic anemia seen in vitamin B_{12}–deficient patients (Fig. 33-4).

Vitamin B_{12} Deficiency States   Deficiency of vitamin B_{12} may be caused by the following mechanisms: (1) decreased ingestion, (2) decreased absorption, (3) increased requirement, (4) impaired utilization and increased loss. Vitamin B_{12} deficiency secondary to decreased ingestion occurs in persons who are strict ovo-lacto-vegetarians and is quite rare because all organisms require vitamin B_{12} and, therefore, most food supplies contain vitamin B_{12}. The most common cause of vitamin B_{12} deficiency is decreased absorption secondary to the loss of the intrinsic factor. The deficiency may be manifest by degenerative changes of the dorsal and lateral columns of the spinal cord and peripheral nerves yielding disturbances of vibratory sense, proprioception, and pyramidal-tract function. Mental aberrations, ranging from mood changes to frank psychosis, may occur. Optic atrophy and toxic amblyopia (usually associated with tobacco use) may be associated with vitamin B_{12} deficiency. Neurologic symptoms may dominate the clinical picture, occurring sometimes in the absence of anemia.

Diagnosis of Vitamin B_{12} Deficiency   In the proper clinical setting and with the characteristic peripheral blood findings, in all regards similar to that seen in folate deficiency, a serum vitamin B_{12} level should be obtained. A low value supports the diagnosis of vitamin B_{12} deficiency. Then, an assessment of the cause of the vitamin B_{12} deficiency must be undertaken. If the history suggests no obvious etiology (e.g., malabsorption syndrome), the usual first step is the Schilling test, which involves measuring the amount of absorption of an orally administered tracer dose of radioactive vitamin B_{12} (^{60}Co-labeled). There is reduced absorption of the radioactive vitamin B_{12} in instances where vitamin B_{12} absorption is impaired. If the results of the first Schilling test show low absorption of the vitamin, the test is repeated with orally administered IF given with the tracer vitamin B_{12}. If the second test is normal, then the cause of the deficiency is an absence of IF.

It is important to note that anyone suspected of having vitamin B_{12} deficiency should also be evaluated for concomitant folate deficiency, since the two may coexist. It should again be stressed that the hematologic picture of vitamin B_{12} is the same as that of folate deficiency.

Therapy of Vitamin B_{12} Deficiency   Vitamin B_{12} is usually administered intramuscularly or subcutaneously as cyanocobalamin (vitamin B_{12}) injection, preparations of which are marketed in multidose or single-dose ampuls containing 100 or 1000 $\mu g/mL$. These routes of administration are used, since in most cases vitamin B_{12} deficiency is due to intestinal malabsorption. The absence of intrinsic factor (IF) is commonly the result of the disease pernicious anemia (PA), in which gastric atrophy and parietal cell loss occur. IF deficiency may also be caused by surgical gastrectomy, destruction of the gastric lining secondary to ingestion of corrosives, and rarely anti-IF antibodies in the gastric secretions. In addition, many different intestinal diseases as well as the ingestion of *para*-aminosalicylic acid, colchicine, neomycin, ethanol, and KCl impair the absorption of the vitamin. Other causes of decreased absorption of vitamin B_{12}, not involving IF, include infestation with the vitamin B_{12}–devouring fish tapeworm *Diphyllobothrium latum*, intestinal bacterial overgrowth syndromes, blind loop syndromes, and chronic pancreatitis. Increased requirements for the vitamin include multiple pregnancies, malignancies, and chronic hyperthyroidism. Impaired utilization is the least frequent cause and may be seen in certain rare enzyme deficiencies or chronic nitrous oxide administration. Increased loss is quite rare and occurs in congenital absence of transcobalamin II.

About 90 percent of the total body stores of vitamin B_{12} must be depleted before hematologic evidence of a deficiency state develops. Since the daily requirement of vitamin B_{12} is 1 to 3 μg, an interval of many years must elapse before deficiency symptoms develop after abrupt loss of vitamin B_{12} absorption from any cause.

The major clinical manifestations of vitamin B_{12} deficiency are (1) megaloblastic anemia and its many sequelae, (2) gastrointestinal symptoms, including glossitis and the dyspepsia caused by gastric mucosal atrophy, and (3) diverse neurologic abnormalities with degenerative changes of the dorsal and lateral columns of the spinal cord and peripheral nerves.

To replete a deficient patient, a dose of 500 to 1000 μg daily for 10 to 30 days followed by a similar weekly dose for 2 months is usually sufficient to saturate stores. Many different dosing schemes exist and are equally effective, as long as stores are repleted and all reversible signs and symptoms are corrected. Actually, more than half of the pharmacologic dosages listed above are lost in the urine.

The monthly maintenance dose of vitamin B_{12} in patients with pernicious anemia is 500 to 1000 μg. In order to guarantee the retention of the average monthly requisite of 30 to 60 μg, dosage of 1000 μg monthly is usually given. There are many different oral vitamin B_{12} preparations available. Except for the rarely seen dietary deficiency of vitamin B_{12}, oral preparations have no use in the management of vitamin B_{12} deficiency (e.g., pernicious anemia, malabsorption), since absorption of these materials is not predictable. It also is axiomatic that use of vitamin B_{12} in the management of anemia not caused by vitamin B_{12} deficiency is contraindicated.

Adverse reactions to vitamin B_{12} are rare. Doses in excess of 1000 μg are well tolerated.

Patients with intrinsic heart disease who become anemic due to deficiency of vitamin B_{12} may develop heart failure following vitamin B_{12} therapy if their blood volume expands rapidly. Rarely, a patient with vitamin B_{12} deficiency may develop polycythemia vera, which had been masked by the vitamin B_{12} lack.

BIBLIOGRAPHY

Chanarin, I.: "Management of Megaloblastic Anemia in the Very Young," *Br. J. Haematol.*, **53:**1–3 (1983).

Dallman, P. R.: "Manifestation of Iron Deficiency," *Semin. Hematol.*, **19:**19–20 (1982).

Dallman, P. R.: "Iron Deficiency and the Immune Response," *Am. J. Clin. Nutr.*, **46:**329–334 (1987).

Das, K. C., and V. Herbert: "Vitamin B-12 and Folate Interrelations," *Clin. Haematol.*, **5:**697–725 (1976).

English, E. C.: "Anemia," *J. Fam. Pract.*, **24:**521–527 (1987).

Finch, C. A., and H. Huebers: "Perspectives in Iron Metabolism," *N. Engl. J. Med.* **306:**1520–1528 (1982).

Hallberg, L.: "Bioavailability of Dietary Iron in Man," *Annu. Rev. Nutr.*, **1:**123–147 (1981).

Howe, R. B.: "Current Concepts of Anemia in Elderly Patients," *Compr. Ther.*, **13:**30–36 (1987).

Kellermeyer, R. W.: "General Principles of Evaluation and Therapy of Anemias," *Med. Clin. North Am.*, **68:**533–543 (1984).

Ritchey, A. K.: "Iron Deficiency in Children. Update on an Old Problem," *Postgrad. Med.*, **82:**59–63 (1987).

Scott, J. M., J. J. Dinn, P. Wilson, and D. G. Weir: "Pathogenesis of Subacute Combined Degeneration: A Result of Methyl Group Deficiency," *Lancet*, **2:**334–337 (1981).

Anticoagulant and Procoagulant Drugs

Carl Barsigian and José Martinez

Blood coagulation is an important physiologic process which, when properly regulated, provides the body with a patent hemostatic defense mechanism. Under normal conditions, the formation of microscopic clots is responsible for repair of damaged vessels throughout the body. Such repair prevents bleeding that may occur as a result of the wear and tear of normal life. Once the damaged vessel is restored by renewal of its endothelial surface, the insoluble clot is efficiently removed by the fibrinolytic mechanism, which proteolytically degrades it into a series of soluble fragments that are cleared from the circulation by as yet undefined pathways. A precisely regulated balance between the coagulative and fibrinolytic pathways, along with the nonthrombogenic nature of intact normal epithelium, maintains the homeostatic state of the vascular system.

Perturbation of the endogenous controls of the coagulative and fibrinolytic pathways may have dire consequences. On the one hand, inappropriate initiation of coagulation or defective disassembly of the clot may lead to thrombosis with subsequent ischemia, infarction, or death. On the other hand, failure of coagulation to occur normally or the presence of an overactive clot resolution mechanism may result in hemorrhage. Depending on the location of the thrombotic or hemorrhagic lesion within the vascular tree, a wide range of clinical problems of diverse severity may result.

Treatment of thrombotic or hemorrhagic disorders often involves drug therapy. The rational use of drugs that influence clot formation and resolution is based on an understanding of the fundamental concepts of the coagulative and fibrinolytic pathways. As a result of the power of modern technology, our understanding of the basic biochemistry of these processes is rapidly expanding. The discussion that follows below outlines current concepts of these mechanisms as a foundation for understanding the pharmacology of the anticoagulant and procoagulant drugs.

THE COAGULATIVE PATHWAY

Hemostasis (i.e., the arrest of bleeding) involves a complex interplay between formed elements—platelets and endothelial cells—and soluble plasma proteins—clotting factors—that proceeds in an orchestrated manner and culminates with the formation of a stable blood clot. Within seconds after injury to the vascular endothelium, platelets (thrombocytes) adhere to the damaged area via interactions between specific platelet-membrane receptors and proteins of the exposed subendothelium. One well-characterized mechanism is mediated by the von Willebrand factor (vWF), a glycoprotein that functions as a molecular bridge between subendothelial matrix components (e.g., collagen fibrils) and a specific vWF receptor—glycoprotein Ib—present on platelet plasma membranes. Adhesion is rapidly followed by platelet aggregation (the clumping of platelets to each other), resulting in formation of the primary hemostatic plug. Aggregation is mediated by the binding of fibrinogen to a receptor—glycoprotein IIb/IIIa—which is exposed on the platelet plasma membrane following platelet activation by agonists such as collagen, thrombin, and adenosine diphosphate (ADP). The latter agonist, which is released from platelets that have been activated by contact with subendothelial collagen, subsequently binds to its platelet receptor, resulting in the synthesis of thromboxane A_2 (Chap. 23), a potent platelet-activating agent that initiates a secondary wave of aggregation with subsequent enlargement of the primary hemostatic plug.

The primary hemostatic plug is fragile and can be disrupted by the shear stress imposed by the flowing of blood. With time, however, the platelet plug undergoes stabilization due to biochemical platelet-platelet interactions and to the localized initiation of the coagulative pathway involving the blood-clotting factors. The consequence of these events is the formation of the secondary hemostatic plug consisting of a network of covalently cross-linked fibrin overlying and intermingled with aggregated platelets and other entrapped vascular cells.

The formation of cross-linked fibrin is the end result of the intricate and tightly regulated series of enzymatic and nonenzymatic reactions and interactions depicted in Fig. 34-1. The clotting factors (Table 34-1) involved in coagulation can be classified either as enzymes (most of which are serine proteases) or cofactors (nonenzymes). A vast majority of the enzymes circulate as inactive proenzymes or zymogens, which are converted to the active proteases when coagulation is initiated via either the intrinsic or extrinsic pathways. In the intrinsic pathway, all elements necessary for coagulation to occur are present within the blood. In contrast, the extrinsic pathway requires the exposure or expression of a glycoprotein (tissue factor) on the surface of perturbed endothelial cells. Tissue factor (III), which is not expressed on normal endothelium, is also present on fibroblasts and smooth muscle cells, which may initiate coagulation in areas where the subendothelium has been denuded due to physical or chemical injury. Furthermore, the presence of tissue factor in tumor cells and leukocytes suggests that it may also be involved in the initiation of extravascular coagulation at sites of malignancy, inflammation, or tissue injury.

For didactic purposes, the coagulative pathway may be represented as occurring in three stages (Fig. 34-1): (1) the activation of factor X to factor Xa (via the intrinsic and/or extrinsic pathways), which then acti-

vates the final "common pathway," (2) the conversion of prothrombin (factor II) to thrombin (factor IIa), and (3) the thrombin-mediated transformation of fibrinogen to fibrin. The biochemistry of each of these stages will now be discussed in greater detail.

The first stage of coagulation can be mediated either via the intrinsic or extrinsic pathways and involves signal amplification, which occurs in the classic "cascade" fashion, with one molecule of activated factor activating many molecules of the next zymogen in the pathway. Normally, the intrinsic and extrinsic pathways interact to culminate in the activation of factor X to factor Xa. Blood coagulation initiated via the intrinsic pathway involves surface or contact activation and four major plasma proteins: high-molecular-weight kininogen, prekallikrein, factor XII, and factor XI. A major feature of contact activation is the initiating effect of negatively charged surfaces such as certain extracellular matrix components (possibly operative in vivo) or kaolin or dextran or glass (as nonphysiologic in vitro activators). These early events involve the binding of the contact-activation factors to the negatively charged surfaces, resulting in activation and amplification of the procoagulant biochemical reactions. None of these reactions are Ca^{2+}-dependent, in contrast to the majority of those that follow.

In the first Ca^{2+}-dependent step of the intrinsic pathway, factor XIa activates factor IX to factor IXa. Factor IXa then activates factor X to factor Xa by a

TABLE 34-1 Clotting factors

International nomenclature	Common name
I	Fibrinogen
II	Prothrombin
III	Tissue factor (thromboplastin)
IV	Calcium
V	Proaccelerin
VII	Proconvertin
VIII	Antihemophilic factor
IX	Christmas factor
X	Stuart-Prower factor
XI	Plasma thromboplastin antecedent
XII	Hageman factor
XIII	Fibrin-stabilizing factor

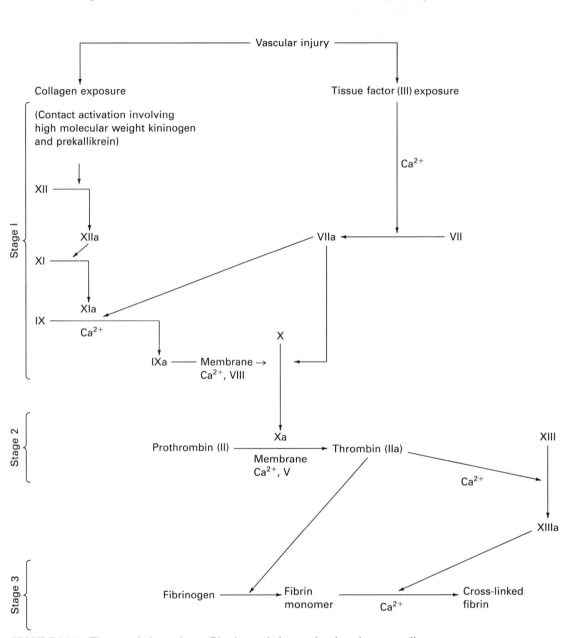

FIGURE 34-1   The coagulative pathway. Blood coagulation can be viewed as proceeding through three stages: (1) the activation of factor X to factor Xa (which can be initiated via either the intrinsic or extrinsic systems), (2) the conversion of prothrombin to thrombin, and (3) the transformation of fibrinogen into fibrin. Fibrin monomers then spontaneously polymerize and undergo factor XIIIa-mediated cross-linking to form a stabilized fibrin clot.

unique mechanism in which a cofactor (factor VIIIa) binds to the platelet surface and serves as a receptor for the Ca^{2+}-dependent binding of factors IXa and factor X on the platelet surface and dramatically increases the rate at which factor IXa converts factor X to the serine protease factor Xa. In the extrinsic pathway, perturbation of vascular endothelial cells or denudation of the subendothelium results in the expression of tissue factor (factor III) that binds and activates factor VII. The tissue factor–factor VIIa complex can directly activate factor X without the involvement of the factor IXa-VIIIa-platelet complex, or it can activate factor IX, thereby mediating factor Xa generation through the intrinsic pathway, as discussed above. Though the relative contribution of the intrinsic and extrinsic pathways in vivo remains unresolved, both pathways converge to generate factor Xa in the first stage of the coagulative mechanism.

When factor Xa is generated, the second stage of coagulation is initiated, and prothrombin (factor II) is converted to the active serine protease thrombin (factor IIa). At this step, factor Va (a nonenzyme) serves as a cofactor much in the same manner as does factor VIIIa in the formation of factor Xa. By binding to the surface of activated platelets, factor Va acts as a receptor for factor Xa and prothrombin, thereby greatly accelerating factor Xa-mediated conversion of prothrombin to thrombin. The thrombin formed is released from the platelet surface and activates additional factor V and factor VIII, resulting in a marked increase in further thrombin generation.

When thrombin becomes available in the blood, the third stage in clot formation can proceed. This reaction is the transformation of fibrinogen to fibrin, a unique proteolytic modification that is not Ca^{2+}-dependent. The action of thrombin as a catalyst promotes the conversion of fibrinogen to fibrin monomers that spontaneously polymerize, resulting in the formation of insoluble fibrils and fibers of fibrin. Simultaneously, thrombin activates factor XIII to factor XIIIa (a transglutaminase, as opposed to a serine protease), which in the presence of Ca^{2+} covalently cross-links the polymerized fibrin, resulting in the formation of a stable fibrin clot.

Thrombin plays a central role in the coagulative pathway in that it manifests both procoagulant and anticoagulant properties. As a procoagulant, thrombin functions by promoting platelet aggregation, by activating factors VIII and V, by transforming fibrinogen to fibrin, and by converting factor XIII to factor XIIIa, which promotes covalent cross-linking of fibrin polymers. In addition to these coagulative properties, thrombin also displays significant anticoagulant activity, which is initiated when it binds to a receptor (thrombomodulin) present on endothelial surfaces (Fig. 34-2). Once bound to thrombomodulin, thrombin is rendered inactive as a procoagulant, but is transformed into a potent anticoagulant by virtue of its ability to activate protein C to protein Ca, which, together with its cofactor protein S, inactivates the two major clotting cofactors (factors VIIIa and Va) thus depressing the coagulative mechanism.

THE FIBRINOLYTIC PATHWAY

Fibrinolysis (i.e., clot resolution) is mediated principally by plasmin, a plasma serine protease derived from the inactive zymogen known as *plasminogen*. Conversion of plasminogen to plasmin involves cleavage of a single peptide bond (Arg 560–Val 561), resulting in generation of a two-chain sulfide-linked molecule (Fig. 34-3). The heavy chain (*N* terminus) contains five disulfide-bonded loops, or "kringles," which act as lysine-binding sites and are responsible for the binding of plasminogen and plasmin to specific lysine residues in polymerized fibrin. The light chain (*C* terminus) contains the active catalytic site of the molecule. Plasminogen activation to plasmin can be mediated via endogenous or exogenous activators. Similar to endogenous activation of the coagulative mechanism, endogenous activation of the fibrinolytic mechanism involves factors present in the blood or released into the blood from extravascular tissue. One mechanism involves contact activation of factor XII to factor XIIa with subsequent factor XIIa-mediated conversion of prekallikrein to kallikrein, which may result in kallikrein-mediated activation of plasminogen. Alternatively, kallikrein may convert plasma prourokinase (also called single-chain urokinase-type plasminogen activator; scu-PA), an endogenous plasminogen activator derived from extravascular cells such as fibroblasts, to urokinase (also called two-chain urokinase-type plasminogen activator; tcu-PA), which is approximately 20,000 times more active than kallikrein in activating plasminogen. The conversion of prourokinase to urokinase can also be mediated by a tissue-type plasminogen activator (t-PA), which is syn-

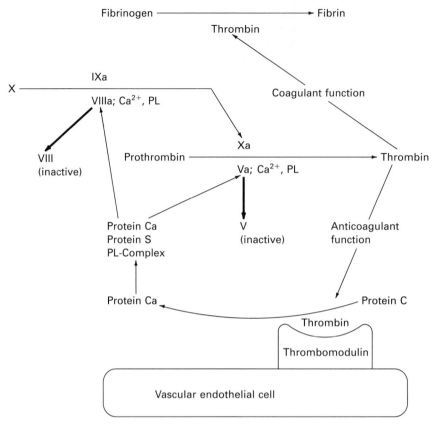

FIGURE 34-2   The protein C–thrombomodulin anticoagulant pathway. Upon binding to thrombomodulin, a vascular endothelial cell receptor, thrombin is rendered inactive as a procoagulant and transformed into a potent anticoagulant by virtue of its ability to activate protein C to protein Ca, which, in complex with protein S and membrane phospholipids (PL), inactivates factors VIIIa and Va, thereby retarding procoagulant mechanisms.

thesized by vascular endothelial cells and thought to be the principal plasminogen activator in vivo. The primary exogenous plasminogen activator, streptokinase, does not occur endogenously in humans, hence the term *exogenous*. Each of these plasminogen activators, with the exception of streptokinase, is a serine protease that activates plasminogen by selective cleavage of the Arg 560–Val 561 peptide bond. Plasmin itself can also cleave this bond and act, in positive feedback fashion, as a plasminogen activator. Once formed, plasmin degrades the insoluble fibrin clot into a series of soluble proteolytic fragments, resulting in the dissolution of the clot (Fig. 34-4). The ability of

plasminogen and plasmin to bind to fibrin is important in limiting the proteolytic degradation of circulating fibrinogen and other plasma proteins.

Localized fibrinolysis is a finely tuned homeostatic mechanism much in the same sense as the coagulative mechanism. As mentioned earlier; plasminogen binding to fibrin serves to confine the proteolytic action of plasmin in areas of thrombosis. However, should plasmin become free in plasma, it is normally rapidly inactivated by a specific inhibitor, α_2-antiplasmin, so that circulating fibrinogen (and factors VIII and V) is protected. However, should plasmin generation exceed the capacity of the α_2-antiplasmin neutralizing system, a systemic "lytic state" may result, leading to consumption of fibrinogen, factor VIII, factor V, and other plasma proteins. Localization of fibrinolysis is also mediated by endothelial cells, which synthesize and secrete t-PA, which binds to fibrin and selectively activates the fibrin-bound plasminogen. However, significant amounts of t-PA do not appear to be released at the early stages of clot formation. During this phase, a plasminogen activator inhibitor is released from platelets and endothelial cells, thereby allowing

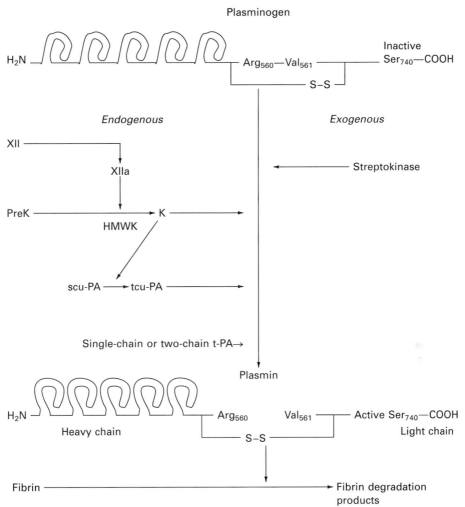

FIGURE 34-3   The fibrinolytic pathway. Fibrinolysis is mediated by the serine protese plasmin, which is derived from the inactive precursor plasminogen. Endogenous plasminogen activators include the enzyme kallikrein (K), single-chain and two-chain urokinase-type plasminogen activators (scu-PA and tcu-PA, respectively), and single-chain or two-chain tissue-type plasminogen activators (t-PA). Streptokinase is a nonhuman protein, and is therefore classified as an exogenous plasminogen activator. Each of these plasminogen activators (with the exception of streptokinase) functions by cleaving the Arg 560–Val 561 bond of plasminogen, thus generating the two-chain disulfide-linked plasmin molecule.

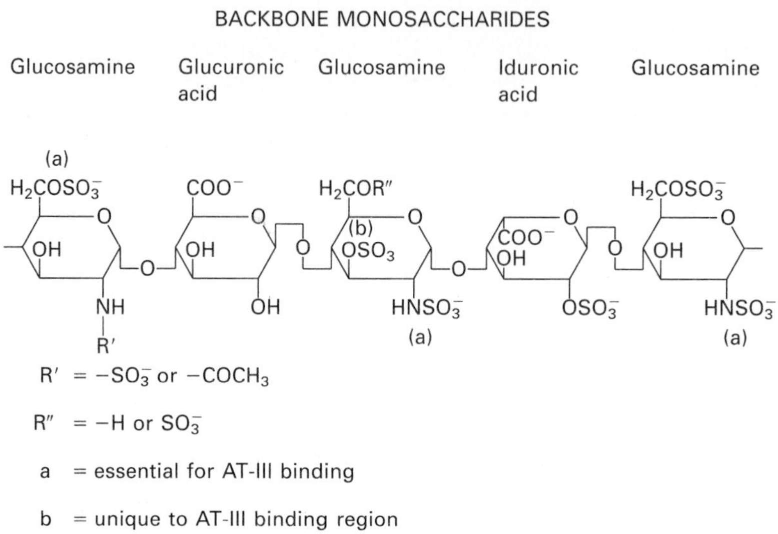

BACKBONE MONOSACCHARIDES

| Glucosamine | Glucuronic acid | Glucosamine | Iduronic acid | Glucosamine |

R' = $-SO_3^-$ or $-COCH_3$

R" = $-H$ or SO_3^-

a = essential for AT-III binding

b = unique to AT-III binding region

FIGURE 34-4   The antithrombin III binding sequence of heparin. A pentasaccharide sequence consisting of substituted moieties of glucosamine, glucuronic acid, glucosamine, iduronic acid, and glucosamine functions as the antithrombin III binding structure within the heparin molecule. The critical substitutions to these monosaccharides that are involved in the binding of antithrombin III (AT-III) are depicted in the figure.

the assembly of a functional hemostatic clot. Subsequently, inhibitor production decreases and t-PA production increases, with the end result being the breakdown of the fibrin clot and recanalization of the damaged vessel. Several of the plasmin-derived degradation products of cross-linked fibrin—the fibrin-split products—can be assayed in plasma as evidence of active coagulative and fibrinolytic mechanisms.

ANTICOAGULANT DRUGS

Heparin   Heparin is a naturally occurring sulfated polysaccharide found principally in the mast cell granule. During synthesis within the mast cell, polysaccharide chains of molecular weights up to 100,000 are covalently linked to polypeptide core proteins forming proteoglycan structures. The polysaccharide chains undergo extensive postsynthetic modifications, and the resulting highly sulfated proteoglycans are stored within basophilic granules. The lysosomes of the mast cell contain proteases and glycosidases which, presumably upon release of granular contents, degrade the

heparin-proteoglycan, resulting in the generation of a diverse heterogeneous population of sulfated oligosaccharides (molecular weights from 5000 to 30,000), which constitute the heparin present in extracellular tissue spaces and in the purified preparations that are used clinically. Commercial sources of heparin include porcine intestinal mucosa and bovine lung. The final extracts must be standardized by biologic assay, and the potency of each preparation must be expressed in terms of USP units of heparin activity. Currently, all heparin preparations contain at least 120 USP units per milligram.

Chemistry   The heparin molecule is composed of three monosaccharides that occur as repeating disaccharide units of D-glucosamine linked with either D-glucuronic acid or L-iduronic acid (Fig. 34-4). Individual heparin molecules vary considerably in length, and therefore commercial heparin is a molecularly heterogeneous preparation. A majority of the monosaccharides are modified by being either N-acetylated, N-sulfated, or O-sulfated, thereby accounting for the strong negative charge of heparin molecules. Sulfation at critical positions is essential for functional activity (Fig. 34-4), as discussed later.

Mechanism of Action The anticoagulant action of heparin requires the presence of the plasma serine protease inhibitor, antithrombin III (AT-III). The ability of this natural inhibitor to inactivate thrombin is increased markedly in the presence of heparin. A specific pentasaccharide sequence (Fig. 34-4) within the heparin molecule mediates the high-affinity binding of AT-III by heparin. Only about one-third of the molecules present in unfractionated heparin preparations contain this pentasaccharide structure. These molecules are primarily responsible for the antithrombin activity of commercially available heparin.

Binding of AT-III to the pentasaccharide sequence is essential but not sufficient for thrombin neutralization by heparin, as evidenced by the finding that the synthetic pentasaccharide, though still exhibiting high-affinity AT-III binding, fails to inhibit thrombin activity. Because larger oligosaccharides, greater than 14 monosaccharides, containing the pentasaccharide structure exhibit both thrombin binding and neutralizing activity, it has been proposed that heparin acts as an anticoagulant by serving as a template for the assembly of AT-III and thrombin. Once bound to heparin, a stable bond is rapidly formed between the active center serine of thrombin and a specific arginine residue of AT-III. The thrombin–AT-III complex dissociates from the heparin molecule, freeing the latter to interact with other AT-III molecules and to inactivate additional thrombin.

Experimentally, the heparin–AT-III complex can also neutralize the activity of factors IXa, Xa, XIa, and XIIa. In fact, certain low-molecular-weight heparins may act as anticoagulants primarily through neutralization of factor Xa rather than thrombin. Theoretically, therefore, heparin can be considered to retard all three stages of blood coagulation: (1) the formation of factor Xa, (2) the factor Xa-mediated conversion of prothrombin to thrombin, and (3) the thrombin-mediated transformation of fibrinogen to fibrin.

Pharmacokinetics Because heparin is a largely negatively charged molecule, it is not absorbed via the oral, sublingual, or rectal routes and is therefore administered parenterally. Intravenous or subcutaneous administration is preferred, since intramuscular injection commonly results in hematomas at the injection site. Heparin is highly bound to plasma proteins (approximately 95 percent), and its apparent volume of distribution is 0.05 to 0.2 L/kg. Depending on the dose, the half-life of heparin varies considerably among patients. The half-life after commonly employed doses of the drug can vary between 1 and 5 h. Because of its extensive binding to plasma proteins, heparin is only minimally available for passive excretion by the kidney. Heparin is biotransformed, by liver heparinase, to inactive products which are excreted in the urine. Heparin itself appears in the urine only after the intravenous administration of large doses. Low urinary excretion, however, fails to account for the rapid loss of heparin from the peripheral blood. The latter observation may be due to extensive binding of heparin to the surface of endothelial cells throughout the vascular tree. Also, it is hypothesized that mast cells may act as a storage depot for exogenously administered heparin. Heparin does not cross the placenta or pass into maternal milk, and thus it has theoretical advantages over warfarin as an anticoagulant in pregnancy. Unfortunately, experience has shown that approximately one-third of all pregnancies will terminate in premature delivery or stillbirth. Heparin therapy also carries significant risk of hemorrhage for the mother, and the rational use of anticoagulants during pregnancy remains a controversial area.

Adverse Reactions The major toxicity of heparin is bleeding, which may frequently occur from mucous membranes or open wounds. Intracranial hemorrhage can also occur and represents one of the most serious toxicities of heparin therapy. Because of the short duration as action of aqueous heparin, treatment of such hemorrhagic phenomena usually involves decreasing the dose or frequency of injections. Alternatively, the anticoagulant action of heparin can be directly antagonized by the intravenous administration of protamine sulfate, a strongly basic, low-molecular-weight protein that reacts directly with acidic heparin thus forming an inactive complex. When protamine is used, it is essential to determine the amount of heparin remaining in the patient and to administer equimolar amounts of protamine, because excess protamine can itself induce bleeding by virtue of its ability to bind to platelets, fibrinogen, and other plasma proteins. To minimize hypotension, bradycardia, or dyspnea, which may result from histamine release from mast cells, protamine should be administered intravenously at a very slow rate of not more than 50 mg in a 10-min period.

Long-term use of heparin (3 months or more of therapy) may cause osteoporosis with spontaneous fractures. Mild to severe thrombocytopenia can occur, which appears to be due to heparin-induced platelet aggregation (mild thrombocytopenia) or to the production of heparin-dependent antiplatelet antibodies (severe thrombocytopenia). The severe form of thrombocytopenia occurs only after several days of therapy and is not dose-related. Platelet aggregation resulting from this mechanism may result in venous or arterial thrombosis, such as stroke or gangrene. Heparin therapy in these patients should therefore be discontinued. Hemorrhage may also result due to the development of thrombocytopenia. Transient and reversible alopecia represents an undesirable but less serious adverse reaction to heparin therapy.

Clinical Use Heparin is indicated as an anticoagulant in the prevention and treatment of deep venous thrombosis (DVT), pulmonary embolism, and arterial thrombosis. For the prophylactic prevention of DVT, the ability of the heparin–AT-III complex to neutralize factor Xa appears to be more important than its inhibitor effect on thrombin. Low-dose heparin (5000 units given subcutaneously two to three times a day) is used prophylactically to prevent thromboembolic complications following surgery, in certain cases of trauma such as fractures, and in patients with acute coronary thrombosis. Whether prophylactic treatment is instituted depends on many factors, such as the age of the patient, the degree of bed rest, the presence of a history of previous thromboembolic disease, and the absence of specific contraindications. Heparin therapy is monitored by using the activated partial thromboplastin time (aPTT), which normally varies between 20 and 35 s. Low-dose prophylactic therapy does not require that the aPTT be prolonged. For the therapeutic treatment of established acute thrombotic episodes, larger doses of heparin are used, and the marked inhibitory action of the heparin–AT-III complex on preformed thrombin is central. In the aggressive treatment of DVT or pulmonary embolism, the daily administration of 16,000 to 30,000 units of heparin by continuous intravenous infusion is required so that the aPTT is prolonged 1.5 to 2 times that of baseline. After the initial thrombotic episode is resolved, long-term therapy with adjusted-dose heparin (i.e., subcu-

taneous injections of increasing doses of heparin every 12 h until the midinterval aPTT is prolonged 1.5 times over baseline) is very effective in preventing the recurrence of venous thrombosis and is associated with a low incidence of bleeding.

Heparin may also be useful as an adjunct in the treatment of coronary occlusion with acute myocardial infarction, especially after fibrinolytic therapy or angioplasty. Anticoagulant therapy reduces the frequency of arterial embolism in patients with arterial fibrillation, mitral stenosis, or prosthetic heart valves.

Since heparin exerts its anticoagulant effect by combining with preformed factors present in plasma, it is effective not only in vivo but also in vitro. In this context, it is utilized to prevent coagulation during extracorporeal oxygenation of blood, during hemodialysis, and in blood samples drawn for laboratory analysis. Moreover, it is used routinely in maintaining the patency of indwelling vascular catheters. Heparin, as the sodium salt, is available as sterile solutions for injection in a variety of concentrations ranging from 250 to 40,000 units/mL.

Oral Anticoagulants

Warfarin In contrast to heparin , warfarin (and all other currently employed oral anticoagulants) is effective only in vivo, since it acts by altering the hepatic synthesis of several essential blood-clotting factors.

Chemistry Warfarin, the most commonly employed oral anticoagulant, and dicumarol, the first oral anticoagulant used clinically, are both structural analogs of 4-hydroxycoumarin (Fig. 34-5.) Dicumarol (bishydroxycoumarin) is a dimeric derivative of 4-hydroxycoumarin, which was isolated from spoiled sweet clover and shown to be the causative agent of "sweet clover disease," a fatal hemorrhagic diathesis of cattle prevalent in the 1920s. Dicumarol has been largely replaced by warfarin, which is prepared as the sodium salt of the racemic mixture. Interestingly, the levorotatory isomer of warfarin is several times more potent than the dextrorotatory form. Other coumarin derivatives include phenprocoumon and acenocoumarol.

Mechanism of Action The therapeutic action of warfarin depends on its ability to suppress the formation of biologically functional factors II, VII, IX, and

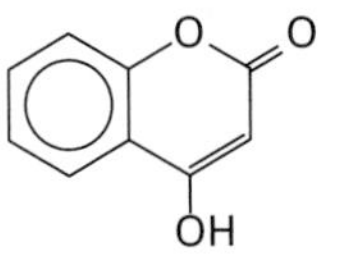

4-Hydroxycoumarin
(nucleus required for activity)

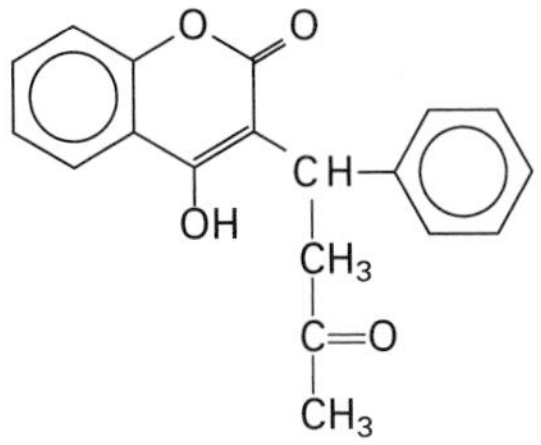

Warfarin

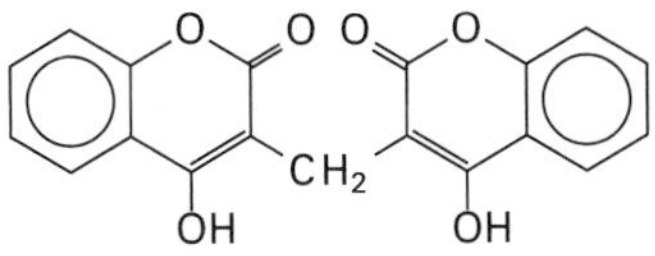

Dicumarol
(Bishydroxycoumarin)

FIGURE 34-5 Structure of oral anticoagulants. The intact 4-hydroxycoumarin nucleus is essential to the anticoagulant activity of warfarin and dicumarol. Commercial warfarin is supplied as the racemic mixture; however, the levorotatory isomer is severalfold more potent than the dextrorotatory form.

X by the liver. These factors (along with protein C and protein S) are referred to as the *vitamin K–dependent clotting factors*, since their biosynthesis by the hepatocyte is partially linked to hepatic vitamin K metabolism. Vitamin K can be supplied to the liver either from dietary plant sources (vitamin K_1; phylloquinone) or as a metabolite of gut flora (vitamin K_2; menaquinone). Though the relative contribution of either form in vivo is unknown, it is clear that the quinone form of the vitamin must be reduced to the hydroquinone, which functions as a cofactor in the synthesis of active vitamin K–dependent proteins. Conversion of the hydroquinone to the epoxide form of vitamin K is catalyzed by vitamin K epoxidase and is coupled to vitamin K–dependent carboxylase-

mediated γ-carboxylation of glutamic acid residues present in the *N*-terminal regions of the polypeptide backbones of each of the vitamin K–dependent factors (Fig. 34-6). The exact nature of the coupling between epoxidation and γ-carboxylation remains elusive, but it is well established that γ-carboxylation contributes Ca^{2+}-binding properties of these proteins, conferring on them the capacity to bind to phospholipid surfaces such as platelet membranes and endothelial cell membranes. It appears that a single Ca^{2+} serves as an ionic bridge between 2 (or possibly 3) intramolecular γ-carboxyglutamic acid residues present in the proteins, thereby exposing membrane-binding domains. Whether Ca^{2+} actually serves to link the vitamin K–dependent proteins to the cell membranes remains unknown. However, in the absence of adequate γ-carboxylation, the vitamin K–dependent factors cannot bind to membranes and therefore are nonfunctional in coagulation, even though present at near normal concentrations in plasma.

Warfarin acts as a vitamin K antagonist primarily by blocking the reduction of the epoxide to the quinone form of vitamin K. This reaction is mediated by a poorly characterized vitamin K epoxide reductase that utilizes an unknown endogenous dithiol, in vivo, or dithiothreitol ($DTTH_2$), in vitro, as cofactor. Conversion of the quinone form to the active hydroquinone appears to be mediated by two enzymes: (a) a warfarin-sensitive enzyme that may be identical or very similar to the dithiol-dependent vitamin K epoxide reductase and (b) a warfarin-insensitive vitamin K reductase that utilizes NAD(P)H, rather than a dithiol, as cofactor (Fig. 34-6). Though the pathway mediated by the latter enzyme is only minimally active in vivo, the inhibitory effects of warfarin on synthesis of the vitamin K–dependent factors can be overcome by the administration of large doses of the vitamin, which increase vitamin K shunting through this pathway.

Pharmacokinetics Warfarin is absorbed rapidly and completely from the gastrointestinal tract, whereas dicumarol is absorbed more slowly and erratically. Under certain circumstances, sodium warfarin may be administered parenterally. The coumarin anticoagulants are largely confined to the circulation. Binding of warfarin to serum albumin, for example, is approximately 99 percent, resulting in a low apparent volume of distribution (0.1 L/kg). Warfarin is completely biotransformed by the liver drug-metabolizing

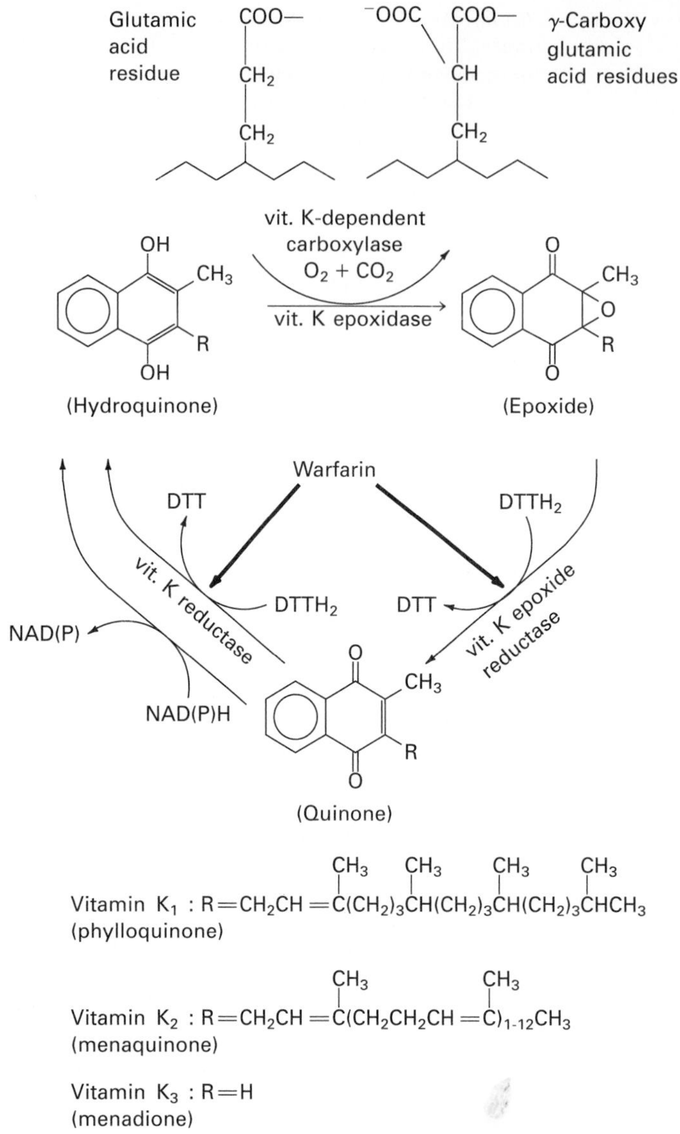

FIGURE 34-6   The vitamin K cycle and the mechanism of action of warfarin. Conversion of the hydroquinone form of vitamin K to the epoxide is catalyzed by vitamin K epoxidase and is coupled to γ-carboxylation of glutamic acid residues present in vitamin K–dependent proteins. The γ-carboxylation reaction is catalyzed by vitamin K–dependent carboxlase. Neither epoxidation nor carboxylation is affected by warfarin. Rather, warfarin inhibits the dithiol ($DTTH_2$)-dependent conversion of the quinone to the hydroquinone. See text for further details.

microsomal system to hydroxylated derivatives that have weak anticoagulant activity. The metabolic half-life of warfarin is approximately 2 days, but the hydroxylated biotransformation products may be excreted in the urine for up to 4 weeks after a single dose.

Adverse Reactions   The principal toxicity of warfarin is the direct effect of overdosage, resulting in marked hypoprothrombinemia manifest as ecchymo-

ses and, if not recognized and corrected, fatal hemorrhage. The hypoprothrombinemia can be treated with fresh plasma, which supplies functional vitamin K–dependent blood coagulation factors. In extreme emergency, vitamin K–dependent factor concentrates may be used. Large doses of vitamin K_1 may also help by increasing shunting through the warfarin-insensitive NAD(P) H-dependent reductive pathway (Fig. 34-6). Vitamin K_3 (menadione) is less effective in this regard. The action of vitamin K begins within half an hour following intravenous administration; however, there is a latent period of several hours before its effect on the prothrombin time is obtained. Therefore, when hemorrhage occurs (and depending on its severity), the dose of the anticoagulant should be reduced or discontinued, and vitamin K_1 or fresh plasma may be administered.

Adverse reactions of warfarin, other than hemorrhage, are uncommon and may include alopecia, urticaria, dermatitis, nausea, diarrhea, abdominal cramps, and, on rare occasions, skin necrosis. It is also contraindicated in the first 10 weeks of pregnancy due to potential embryopathy, which most commonly involves the development of nasal hypoplasia and stippled epiphyses. This type of classic warfarin embryopathy may be due to the biosynthesis of a nonfunctional acarboxy form of the vitamin K–dependent protein osteocalcin, which plays a role in bone ossification. Independent of embryopathy, central nervous system abnormalities have been described when warfarin is used between 10 and 40 weeks of gestation.

Perhaps no other group of drugs is more subject to drug interactions than are the oral anticoagulants. The reason is that the hypoprothrombinemic effect is directly related to the free-plasma level, which is determined not only by the dose but also by the extent of plasma protein binding and by the rate of biotransformation. Table 34-2 lists drugs that may alter the activity of the anticoagulants. In general, the mechanisms responsible for enhanced anticoagulant effects include (1) decreased absorption of vitamin K from the gastrointestinal tract, (2) displacement of the anticoagulant from binding sites on plasma proteins, (3) inhibition of hepatic biotransformation of the anticoagulant, (4) inhibition of platelet aggregation, and (5) reduction in the production of clotting factors. On the other hand, decreased anticoagulant effects may result from (1) induction of the drug-metabolizing microsomal system or (2) enhancement of the production of clotting factors. These interactions become especially problematic after a patient has become stabilized on an anticoagulant dosage regimen. For example, all the drugs that induce increased activity of the liver microsomal enzyme system cause an increased inactivation of the oral anticoagulants. This decreases their effect for a given dose, so the clinician observing this effect may tend to increase the dose. If at this point the inducing drug is discontinued, the anticoagulant will have a

TABLE 34-2 Drug interactions with oral anticoagulants

Enhanced oral anticoagulant activity	
Mechanism	**Drugs**
Decreased vitamin K absorption	Antibiotics Mineral oil
Displacement from plasma proteins	Salicylates Phenylbutazone Chloral hydrate Clofibrate
Inhibition of biotransformation	Allopurinol Disulfiram Metronidazole Chloramphenicol
Inhibition of platelet aggregation	Aspirin Indomethacin Sulfinpyrazone Dipyridamole
Decreased clotting factor production	Quinidine
Depressed oral anticoagulant activity	
Enzyme induction	Barbiturates Glutethimide Griseofulvin
Increased clotting factor production	Vitamin K, oral Contraceptives

much greater effect and hemorrhage may result. Conversely, the coumarin derivatives are known to increase the blood level of phenytoin and to increase the effect of oral hypoglycemic drugs.

Clinical Use Warfarin and other oral anticoagulants are routinely used for the prophylaxis and treatment of DVT (deep venous thrombosis) and pulmonary embolism. As a result of the mechanism of action of the oral anticoagulants, the therapeutic action of these agents only occurs in vivo and requires several days to become manifest. The anticoagulant action of warfarin is monitored by measuring the prothrombin time (PT), which has a normal range of 11 to 13 s. Although synthesis of the vitamin K–dependent factors by the liver is decreased almost immediately following absorption of the drug, some time is required before blood levels of the preformed factors fell as a result of normal utilization. Factor VII activity falls rapidly (within 1 day) due to its short biologic half-life (5 to 6 h). This affects the PT but may not prevent thrombosis. Factor IX activity is depressed within about 2 days and also affects the PT. Most importantly though, patients are not adequately anticoagulated until 4 or 5 days, at which time the activities of all factors are sufficiently depressed to provide clinically apparent therapeutic anticoagulation (PT of 1.4 to 2 times control, depending on the nature of the clinical disorder). For this reason, when rapid anticoagulation is required—such as in cases involving active thrombosis—heparin is preferred, since it inhibits coagulation almost instantaneously. The time required for the PT to return to normal when oral anticoagulant therapy is discontinued varies more than the time required to produce an effect, and, depending on the drug, may be from 1 to 8 days.

Current therapeutic regimens to treat thrombosis usually start with the immediate administration of heparin to establish immediate anticoagulation during the 4 to 5 days required for the anticoagulant effects of warfarin to reach therapeutic levels. Warfarin therapy is usually continued, under close medical supervision, for 4 to 6 months following an episode of DVT or pulmonary embolism. In patients with DVT, the PT should be maintained at about 1.4 times baseline. In the treatment of arterial embolization in patients with mitral valve disease, warfarin therapy is usually continued for the life of the patient. Warfarin is also indicated for most patients with mechanical prosthetic heart valves.

Phenindione   Like the coumarin derivatives, phenindione acts by altering the biosynthesis of the vitamin K–dependent coagulation proteins by the liver. Phenindione, as well as anisindione, is well absorbed following oral administration. Adverse reactions to the indandiones are similar to those produced by the coumarin agents. In addition, large doses or excessively rapid rate of administration may produce polyuria, polydipsia, and tachycardia. Granulocytopenia and a

jaundice-producing liver dyscrasia have been reported as additional adverse effects. These drugs are rarely used in the United States.

FIBRINOLYTIC DRUGS

Heparin and oral anticoagulants are ineffective in reducing the size of preformed fibrin clots. For this purpose, activation of the endogenous fibrinolytic mechanism via the administration of plasminogen activators such as streptokinase and urokinase is most frequently employed. However, since these first-generation fibrinolytic agents activate plasminogen that is free in plasma, their use is associated with a significant risk of bleeding due to plasmic degradation of fibrinogen and other coagulation factors. The discovery of endothelial cell tissue type plasminogen activator (t-PA), a potent activator of fibrin-bound plasminogen (but not of soluble plasmonogen), has generated tremendous interest in the potential development of this agent as a clot-specific fibrinolytic drug.

Streptokinase   Streptokinase (SK), a protein secreted by group C hemolytic streptococci, was the first clinically useful fibrinolytic agent. Unlike other plasminogen activators, SK is not an enzyme and does not itself cleave any bonds within the plasminogen molecule. Rather, it forms an equimolar complex with plasminogen, resulting in SK-plasminogen. The SK then can induce a conformational change within the plasminogen that results in exposure of the active site within the molecule and forms SK-plasminogen activator complex. This SK-plasminogen activator complex can convert SK-plasminogen to SK-plasmin. Both the SK-plasminogen activator complex and the SK-plasmin can degrade fibrin or can activate soluble plasma plasminogen to plasmin, the net result of all reactions being the degradation of fibrin. The drug, which has a plasma half-life of 15 to 30 min, is used intravenously to treat patients with acute massive pulmonary embolism and extensive thrombi of deep veins. It is also employed via the intracoronary or intravenous routes in the treatment of acute myocardial infarction. In this regard, it is crucial to begin fibrinolytic therapy very early (if possible, within 1 h following the onset of symptoms) in order to achieve maximum therapeutic benefit (i.e., increased survival). It is quite clear that fibrinolytic therapy begun later than 6 h following the onset of symptoms is associated with a much lower success rate.

The major complication associated with streptokinase therapy is bleeding due to the dissolution of hemostatic plugs and to the consumption of fibrinogen and other coagulation factors. When used via the intracoronary route in the treatment of acute myocardial infarction, however, the incidence and severity of bleeding are lower, due to the smaller doses used compared with the therapeutically equivalent intravenous dose. On the other hand, intravenous streptokinase therapy is easier to initiate within the crucial first few hours following the onset of symptoms of acute myocardial infarction. Because streptokinase is a foreign protein, it is pyrogenic and antigenic and therefore allergic reactions, including anaphylaxis, may occur.

Recently, various streptokinase derivatives have been introduced and are being evaluated for their potential use as fibrinolytic agents. The best characterized of these are the acylated plasminogen-streptokinase activator complexes (APSAC). In these products, the conformationally altered plasminogen molecule of the SK-plasminogen activator complex is acylated at its active center serine and is therefore inactive as such. Theoretically, this would prevent the in vivo inactivation by α_2-antiplasmin and the activation of plasma plasminogen, but not the binding of the APSAC to fibrin. The fibrin-bound APSAC would then undergo spontaneous deacylation with concurrent local generation of active SK-plasminogen activator complex and a more fibrin-selective lytic activity. The half-life of APSAC is also much longer than that of streptokinase, thereby allowing administration by intravenous bolus injection (as opposed to continuous infusion), which provides sustained fibrinolytic activity and greater protection against rethrombosis. However, these theoretical advantages of APSAC over SK have yet to be firmly established in large-scale clinical trials.

Urokinase Urokinase (UK) is a two-chain disulfide-linked enzyme extracted from human urine or human kidney cells, which directly cleaves the Arg 560–Val 561 peptide bond in the plasminogen molecule, thus activating plasminogen to plasmin. As with streptokinase, urokinase can produce systemic plasminogen activation with development of the lytic state. Prourokinase (i.e., scu-PA), an endogenous plasminogen activator, is relatively more clot-specific than urokinase and therefore produces less systemic plasminogen activation with a lower incidence of bleeding.

The indications for these intravenous products are similar to those for streptokinase. Since they are endogenous proteins, they are not antigenic. Nevertheless, mild allergic reactions such as skin rash, bronchospasm, and febrile reactions have been reported.

Tissue-Type Plasminogen Activator Tissue-type plasminogen activator is a glycoprotein of molecular weight 68,000 which is synthesized by vascular endothelial cells. In contrast to most other serine proteases, t-PA does not appear to occur in zymogen form. The enzymatic activity of t-PA can be increased by treatment with plasmin, which cleaves a single peptide bond converting the single-chain t-PA to a disulfide-linked two-chain form. In the presence of fibrin, however, both forms exhibit similar activity.

Serving as the major endogenous promotor of fibrinolysis, t-PA binds avidly to fibrin, where it proteolytically cleaves the Arg 560–Val 561 bond of fibrin-bound plasminogen, converting the latter to the active disulfide-linked two-chain plasmin molecule, which mediates the degradation of the cross-linked fibrin clot (Fig. 34-3). The t-PA molecule is extremely inefficient at activating plasminogen which is not bound to fibrin. Consequently its action is preferentially localized to areas of thrombosis, and the tendency of t-PA to produce systemic fibrinogenolysis is much lower than that of either streptokinase or urokinase.

Experimentation has revealed a significant dose-related fibrinolytic action of t-PA. Furthermore, clinical trials using t-PA have demonstrated recanalization of occluded coronary arteries within 30 to 60 min. However, clinically significant bleeding occurs in some patients (presumably due to lysis of good clots in areas of vascular injury), and the ultimate usefulness of t-PA in coronary artery disease, though very promising, remains to be established.

The t-PA molecule was originally purified from the media of a cultured human melanoma cell line, but is now available as the genetically recombinant form (rt-PA). Both natural t-PA and rt-PA have very short biologic half-lives (approximately 3 min) and are removed from the circulation mainly by the liver. For this reason, they are administered by continuous intravenous infusion. In the treatment of acute infarction, the intravenous route of administration is as efficacious as the intracoronary route. This is due to the clot-specific nature of t-PA.

PROCOAGULANT DRUGS

Systemic Procoagulants

The systemic procoagulant drugs currently employed act either by replacement of deficient clotting factors (antihemophilic factor; factor IX complex), by increasing the plasma concentrations of endogenous clotting factors (Desmopressin), or by inhibition of the natural fibrinolytic mechanism (aminocaproic acid; tranexamic acid).

Antihemophilic Factor Hemophilia A is an X-linked genetic disorder characterized by a deficiency of factor VIII (antihemophilic factor). As a consequence of this major disturbance of the intrinsic coagulative pathway, these patients experience episodic bleeding disorders such as hemarthroses, intramuscular hematomas, hematuria, and intracranial hemorrhage.

Factor VIII, which is present in plasma at about 100 ng/mL and manifests a half-life of 8 to 12 h, can be supplied as fresh (or fresh frozen) plasma, cryoprecipitate, or lyophilized concentrates. Fresh or fresh-frozen plasma contains, by definition, 1.0 international unit (IU) of factor VIII coagulant activity per milliliter, and is therefore frequently unsuitable for replacement therapy due to potential volume overload, which may result if administration of high levels of factor VIII activity is required. Cryoprecipitate, a product prepared from fresh-frozen plasma thawed at 4°C, offers an advantage in this regard, since it contains approximately 7 to 10 IU of factor VIII activity per milliliter. The various concentrates prepared from large batches of pooled human plasma are convenient for self-administration by the patient and can be stored at ambient temperatures. Cryoprecipitate, which must be stored frozen, is the agent of choice in the treatment of von Willebrand's disease because it contains large amounts of high-molecular-weight vWF multimers that are not present in the concentrates but are essential to restoring normal hemostasis in patients with von Willebrand's disease. The foregoing preparations are effective in reducing spontaneous hemarthroses, deep hematomas, and bleeding after trauma or surgery.

A major problem with the administration of factor VIII-containing products is the risk of iatrogenic non-A, non-B hepatitis and acquired immune deficiency syndrome (AIDS). The risk for transmission of these diseases to hemophiliacs is greatest when the lyophilized concentrates are used, since these products are prepared from pooled plasma obtained from very large donor populations. Various modalities of heat treatment have been employed to irradicate the AIDS virus from factor VIII concentrates; however, the risk of non-A, non-B hepatitis still poses a significant clinical problem. Very recently, factor VIII has been highly purified by using monoclonal antibody immunoaffinity chromatography to von Willebrand factor. Since factor VIII circulates in plasma complexed with the von Willebrand Factor, purified factor VIII can be eluted from the antibody-bound factor VIII/vWF complex, concentrated, subjected to dry heat treatment, and prepared as a sterile lyophilized powder. Factor VIII prepared in this manner is 99.9 percent pure and is virtually free of infectious hepatitis or AIDS viruses. Currently, this product is undergoing clinical trials and may represent a remarkable advance in the safety of the therapy of hemophilia A. The future development of genetically recombinant factor VIII will also add a new dimension to the treatment of this disease.

Factor IX Complex Factor IX complex is a dried human plasma fraction containing factors II, VII, IX, and X, which may be used when the activity of one or more of these factors is low due to genetic or acquired deficiencies. The most frequent use of factor IX complex is in patients with hemophilia B, who suffer from an X-linked genetic deficiency of factor IX.

Desmopression Desmopression functions by increasing the titers of endogenous clotting factors. This agent, which is a structural analog of the pituitary hormone vasopressin, functions by stimulating the release of endogenous pools of factor VIII and vWF into the circulation. As a result of this action, it is used to promote hemostasis in mild classic hemophiliac patients or patients with von Willebrand's disease who undergo minor surgery such as tooth extraction or tonsillectomy. It is ineffective in patients with severe classic hemophilia, since these patients do not have sufficient endogenous pools of factor VIII. Only patients with baseline titers of 5 to 10 percent of normal usually respond. The antidiuretic action of desmopressin may lead to electrolyte imbalance and fluid overload, though this is rare. Desmopressin is administered intravenously.

Aminocaproic Acid   Aminocaproic acid, though not a procoagulant per se, is effective in decreasing hemorrhage with surgical procedures. Aminocaproic acid is a structural analog of lysine, differing only by the absence of the α-amino group. Because binding of plasminogen or plasmin to fibrinogen or fibrin is mediated by lysine groups present within the fibrin or fibrinogen structure, aminocaproic acid functions as a competitive inhibitor of plasmin(ogen) binding to fibrin, thus reducing the activity of the fibrinolytic mechanism and shifting the homeostatic balance in favor of coagulation. Aminocaproic acid can be administered orally or intravenously. It is rapidly absorbed from the gastrointestinal tract, has a serum half-life of 1 to 2 h, and is excreted unchanged in the urine (greater than 90 percent within 24 h). Its concentration in urine can be up to 100-fold greater than in plasma, and it is therefore very useful for treating bleeding from the urinary tract.

Tranexamic Acid   Like aminocaproic acid, tranexamic acid is a lysine analog that functions as a competitive inhibitor of plasmin(ogen) binding to fibrin(ogen). Tranexamic acid lacks the α-amino group of lysine, but contains two additional carbon atoms that form a six-membered ring structure. As a result of these molecular differences, it is 6 to 10 times more potent than aminocaproic acid is, but overall the two drugs manifest very similar pharmacokinetic profiles.

Topical Procoagulants

Thrombin   Thrombin is prepared from bovine plasma and is used topically to arrest bleeding from abraded or otherwise open vessels when it is impractical to use ligation or pressure techniques or when these techniques are unsuccessful.

Absorbable Gelatin   Absorbable gelatin is a specially prepared form of gelatin (denatured collagen) that has been processed so that it is porous, nonantigenic, and completely absorbed after application. The material is available as a sterile film and sterile sponge for topical use in many fields of surgery and as a sterile

powder for decubitus ulcers and chronic leg ulcers. A nonsterile powder of absorbable gelatin, used with thrombin, is occasionally useful by the oral route for gastroduodenal hemorrhage, although its clinical use in this situation is limited.

Microfibrillar Collagen Hemostat   Microfibrillar collagen hemostat is an absorbable, sterile, topical preparation of bovine collagen that allows platelets to adhere and aggregate, thereby promoting coagulation. It is used in surgical procedures as an adjunct to hemostasis when control of bleeding by other procedures is ineffective or impractical.

Oxidized Cellulose   Oxidized cellulose is surgical gauze that has been treated with nitrogen dioxide. When it comes in contact with tissue fluid, it forms a sticky and gummy artificial clot that provides mechanical hemostasis.

PREPARATIONS

Alteplase (Activase), a tissue-type plasminogen activator made by recombinant DNA technology, is available as a powder (lyophilized) in 20- and 50-mg vials.

Anisindione (Miradon) is available as 50-mg tablets.

Dicumarol is available as 25- and 50-mg tablets.

Heparin, as the sodium salt, is available as sterile solutions for injection in a variety of concentrations, ranging from 1000 to 40,000 units per milliliter. It is also available as a calcium salt (Calciparine) for injection (5000 to 20,000 USP heparin units).

Phenprocoumon (Liquamar) is available as 3-mg tablets.

Streptokinase (Streptase) and *urokinase* (Abbokinase) are available as powders for reconstitution.

Warfarin sodium (Coumadin Sodium, Panwarfin) is available as 2-, 2.5-, 5-, 7.5-, and 10-mg tablets and in 50-mg vials.

Warfarin potassium (Athrombin-K) is available as 5-mg tablets.

BIBLIOGRAPHY

Collen, D.: "Human Tissue-type Plasminogen Activators: From the Laboratory to the Bedside," *Circulation*, 72:18–20 (1985).

Collen, D., and H. R. Lijnen: "Fibrinolysis and the Control of Hemostasis," in *The Molecular Basis of Blood Diseases*, G. Stamatoyannopoulos, A. W. Nienhuis, P. Leder, and P. W. Majerus (eds.), Saunders, Philadelphia, 1987, pp. 662–668.

Collen, D., D. C. Strump, and H. K. Gold: "Thrombolytic Therapy," *Ann. Rev. Med.*, **39**:405–423 (1988).

Furie, B., and B. C. Furie: "The Molecular Basis of Blood Coagulation," *Cell*, **53**:505–518 (1988).

Hull, R., and J. Hirsh: "Long-term Anticoagulant Therapy in Patients with Venous Thrombosis," *Arch. Int. Med.*, **143**:2061–2063 (1983).

Jorgensen, M. J., B. C. Furie, and B. Furie: "Vitamin K-Dependent Blood Coagulation Proteins," I. M. Arias, W. W. Jakoby, H. Popper, D. Schachter, and D. A. Shafritz, (eds.), in *The Liver: Biology and Pathobiology*, 2d ed., Raven Press, New York, 1988, pp. 495–503.

Lindahl, U., and L. Kjellen: "Biosynthesis of Heparin and Heparin Sulfate," in *Biology of Proteoglycans*, T. N. Wight and R. P. Mecham (eds.), Academic Press, Orlando, 1987, pp. 59–104.

Marder, V. J., and S. Sherry: "Thrombolytic Therapy: Current Status: 1," *N. Eng. J. Med.*, **318**:1512–1520 (1988). "Thrombolytic Therapy: Current Status: 2," *N. Eng. J. Med.*, **318**:1585–1595 (1988).

Miescher, P. A., and E. R. Jaffe (eds.): "Human Factor VIII:C Purified Using Monoclonal Antibody to von Willebrand Factor," *Seminars in Hematology*, **25** (Suppl. 1): 1–45 (1988).

Nemerson, Y.: "Tissue Factor and Hemostatis," *Blood*, **71**:1–8 (1988).

Rosenberg, R. D.: "The Heparin-Antithrombin System: A Natural Anticoagulant System," R. W. Colman, J. Hirsh, V. J. Marder, and E. W. Salzman (eds.), in *Hemostasis and Thrombosis: Basic Principles and Clinical Practice*, 2d ed. J. B. Lippincott, Philadelphia, (1987), p. 1373–1392.

Schafer, A. I.: "Focusing on the Clot: Normal and Pathologic Mechanisms," *Ann. Rev. Med.*, **38**:211–220 (1987).

Verstraete, M., and D., Collen: "Thrombolytic Therapy in the Eighties," *Blood*, **67**:1529–1541 (1986).

Walsh, P. N.: "Oral Anticoagulant Therapy," *Hosp. Prac.*, **Jan**:101–120 (1983).

PART VII

Endocrines

SECTION EDITOR

Gerald H. Sterling

Thyroid and Parathyroid Drugs

Elizabeth L. Helfer and Leslie I. Rose

THYROID HORMONES AND ANTITHYROID DRUGS

The thyroid gland exerts a profound metabolic control over the body through two iodine-containing amino acid hormones, triiodothyronine (T_3) and thyroxine (tetraiodothyronine, T_4). These hormones regulate general body metabolism by controlling the rate of the cellular oxidative processes. The activity of the thyroid gland is directly regulated by the pituitary thyroid-stimulating hormone (TSH) thyrotropin.

Anatomically, the thyroid is a bilateral organ in the neck. It consists of vesicles lined by cuboidal epithelium surrounding a follicular cavity containing the colloidal iodinated protein thyroglobulin. In addition to follicular cells which secrete thyroid hormones, the thyroid gland has other cells which secrete a third hormone, calcitonin, which is involved in calcium homeostasis and is discussed later.

Normal Thyroid Function

The absorption of iodide, as well as biosynthesis, secretion, and degradation of active thyroid hormones, occurs by means of complex metabolic pathways. The major steps are described here and summarized in Table 35-1.

Dietary Intake Molecular inorganic iodine is reduced in the gastrointestinal tract to iodide which is absorbed. Dietary inorganic iodide (I^-) is absorbed as such. Organic iodine compounds are absorbed and then biotransformed by reductive dehalogenation in the liver, yielding inorganic iodide to the iodide pool.

Human dietary intake varies considerably, according to the local iodine content of the soil and water and the variations among culturally determined eating habits. The euthyroid individual may ingest 150 to 250 μg of iodine daily (up to 700 μg daily in the United States) and eliminate the same amount in the urine and feces. About 80 to 90 percent of the iodine is excreted in the urine, while 10 to 20 percent is eliminated in the feces. The metabolic products of the thyroid hormones are excreted in the feces.

Iodide Uptake by Thyroid Usually about half of the daily intake of iodine is "trapped" by the thyroid gland, while most of the remainder is excreted by the kidney. In the normal thyroid, this active transport system is capable of sustaining an intracellular iodide concentration 25 to 40 times higher than that of the extracellular fluid; TSH stimulates this uptake. The iodide "trapping mechanism" of the thyroid requires energy, which is supplied by actively respiring thyroid cells and has been linked to potassium transport. Since there is little free iodine in the thyroid gland (less than 0.2 percent of the total thyroidal iodine), this trapping process can be regarded as the rate-limiting step in thyroid hormone formation.

Iodide Oxidation and Organification The sequential reactions involved in iodide oxidation and organification are (1) oxidation of iodide ion to a form that serves as an iodinating reagent, (2) iodination of

TABLE 35-1   Steps in iodide oxidation, organification, and secretion

Step	Stimulated by	Inhibited by
1 Uptake of circulating iodide ion by thyroid	TSH	Thiocyanate, nitrite, and perchlorate ions
2 Enzymatic oxidation of iodide ion to active iodine		Propylthiouracil, methimazole
3 Reaction of active iodine with tyrosine groups on thyroglobulin to form MIT and DIT		
4 Combination of MIT and DIT groups on thyroglobulin to form T_4 and T_3		
5 Storage of the iodinated thyroglobulin in the colloid of the thyroid gland		
6 Proteolysis of iodinated thyroglobulin and secretion of T_4 and T_3	TSH	Iodide ion (high concentrations)
7 Conversion of T_4 to T_3 by liver and kidney		Glucocorticoids, amiodarone, Inderal, propylthiouracil
8 Circulating T_4 and T_3 on alpha-globulin and prealbumin inhibits TSH secretion by anterior pituitary		

tyrosyl groups in preformed thyroprotein to form iodotyrosines, and (3) coupling of two iodotyrosines to form iodothyronines.

The oxidation of iodide is catalyzed by a thyroid peroxidase in the microsomal fraction. The reaction requires molecular oxygen and a source of hydrogen peroxide. The product of this peroxidation has not been identified because of its extreme reactivity, which results in instantaneous iodination of the tyrosyl groups. Hypoiodite (IO^-) or iodinium ion (I^+) has been postulated as the intermediate. Tyrosine groups of thyroglobulin readily react with the highly active iodine, forming monoiodotyrosine (MIT) and diiodo-tyrosine (DIT) (see Fig. 35-1). Two DIT molecules or one DIT molecule and one MIT molecule aerobically condense to form T_4 and T_3 (Fig. 35-1), respectively, in the approximate ratio of 4:1. Two MIT molecules do not condense because the nature of the biosynthetic reaction is such that DIT must remain in peptide linkage during the coupling reaction; consequently, DIT

must be at least one of the two reaction partners. T_3 and T_4 are stored in the colloid of the follicular cavity as a moiety of the thyroglobulin molecule.

Thyroglobulin is a large protein (MW 670,000) containing 5900 amino acid residues, of which 110 to 120 are tyrosyl residues. As the thyroglobulin molecule is folded, only about 10 percent of the tyrosines are iodi-nated, and of these only a few are coupled to form thy-ronine. Thus there are only about three thyronines per molecule of thyroglobulin. The iodine in thyroglobu-lin is distributed approximately as follows: 30 percent in T_4, 3 percent in T_3, 20 percent in MIT, and 40 per-cent in DIT.

Circulating Thyroglobulin   It has been customary to believe that thyroglobulin, which is a prohormone and a very large molecule, remains in the thyroid gland. The development of radioimmunoassay, and particularly a double-antibody technique, enabled the detection of the minute amounts present in the bloodstream of euthyroid subjects (5.1 ng/mL average, range 1.6 to 20.7 ng/mL). Patients with Graves' disease show elevated thyroglobulin blood levels. This is consistent with the finding that a thyroid-stimulating immunoglobulin is the etiological cause of hyperthyroidism in these patients. What role, if any, thyroglobulin plays as a thyroid hormone in the peripheral tissues is not clearly defined.

Secretion of T_3 and T_4   Thyroglobulin is stored as colloid droplets within the thyroid gland. Upon stimulation for hormone synthesis, the thyroglobulin is first hydrolyzed, separating out iodotyrosines (MIT and DIT) and T_3 and T_4. The iodotyrosines are deiodinated within the thyroid gland, and their iodide rejoins the general iodide pool where it can be reused to synthesize new hormone. The iodothyronines, T_3 and T_4, are released into the circulation. Normally, 80 μg of T_4 is secreted daily. Approximately 33 μg of T_3 is produced daily, of which 20 percent is the result of direct secretion by the thyroid gland; the remaining 80 percent is produced by peripheral conversion of T_4 to T_3 (mainly by the liver and kidney).

Plasma Binding and Transport of Thyroid Hormones T_4 and T_3 are transported into the blood-stream bound firmly but reversibly to plasma proteins. Most of the thyroid hormones are bound to an alpha$_2$-globulin, thyroxine-binding globulin (TBG) or to a prealbumin, thyroxine-binding prealbumin (TBPA). Only 0.02 percent of T_4 and 0.3 percent of T_3 circulate unbound. The binding protects the thyroid hormones from loss in the urine and also serves as a reservoir which regulates the peripheral supply of hormone in the active free form. Tissue utilization of thyroid hormones results in a reduction in the peripheral level of T_3 and T_4, shifting the balance to favor dissociation of the protein-bound complex. By this mechanism, it is possible for the free hormone to be delivered to the peripheral tissues at rates proportional to the metabolic requirement of each tissue.

Degradation of Thyroid Hormone   The liver is the major site of biotransformation of T_3 and T_4; however, kidney and muscle are other sites where conjugation to glucuronides and sulfates occurs. In the liver, T_4 is conjugated mainly as the glucuronide, while T_3 is conjugated mainly as the sulfate. After excretion via the bile duct, the conjugates are hydrolyzed in the intestine, and most of the T_4 and T_3 reenter the bloodstream via the hepatic portal circulation. Approximately 10 to 20 percent of thyroid hormone conjugates are excreted in the feces.

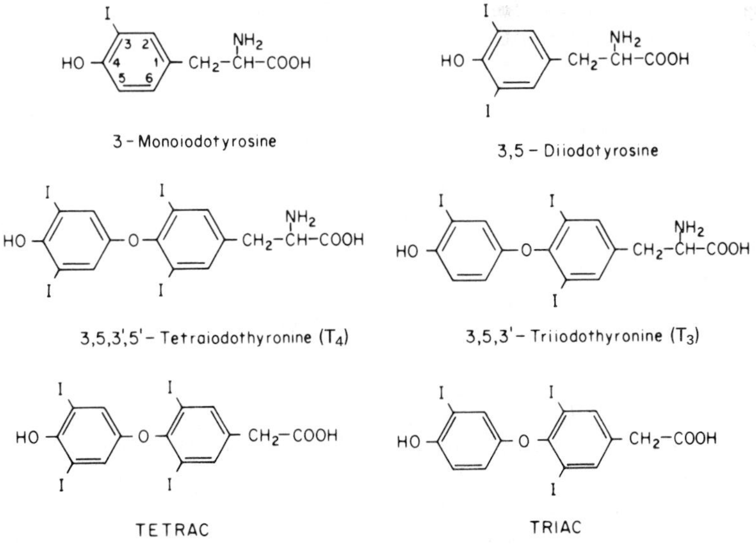

FIGURE 35-1   Thyroid iodoamino acids and metabolites.

Tetraiodothyroacetic acid (TETRAC) and triiodo-thyroacetic acid (TRIAC) are two other metabolites produced by the liver and kidney by oxidative deamination and transamination of the alanine side chains of T_4 and T_3 (see Fig. 35-1). They are subject to conjugation and deiodination as are the parent compounds.

Regulation of Synthesis and Release of Thyroid Hormones The hypothalamus secretes thyrotropin-releasing hormone (TRH), which stimulates the pituitary to produce and secrete thyrotropin-stimulating hormone (TSH). Studies in humans indicate that TSH induces the synthesis and release of thyroglobulin. Thyroid hormones inhibit the release of both thyroglobulin from the thyroid gland and TSH from the pituitary.

Hormonal Actions of T_3 and T_4 Consistent with present theories of hormone action, receptors in the cell nucleus are postulated for thyroid hormones. Measurements of hormone-receptor binding both in vivo and in vitro suggested that T_3 rather than T_4 is the physiologically active ligand. Other metabolites do bind, but their contribution appears to be minor. Solubilized T_3-receptor complex also binds to DNA, and this may explain the nuclear localization. Histones also participate in the localization of T_3 receptors in chromatin material. In contrast to steroid hormones, where the hormone-receptor complex has to translocate to the nucleus, thyroid hormone receptors are already allied to chromatin material and translocation is unnecessary (Fig. 35-2).

Extranuclear modes of action for thyroid hormone are still a valid concept, and some of the actions of this hormone may be apart from the regulation of macromolecular synthesis. Thus the transport of amino acids is enhanced in the presence of thyroid hormone when protein synthesis is blocked.

The actions of thyroid hormone may now be described. At very low concentrations, the thyroid hormones initiate normal growth and development. The mechanism of this growth-promoting quality is thought to be initiation of the incorporation of amino acids into specific proteins. At higher concentrations, the thyroid hormones have been shown to induce many oxidative enzymes and to uncouple oxidative phosphorylation. This results in increased heat production and oxygen consumption. Although liver, muscle, kidney, and heart, among others, are in-

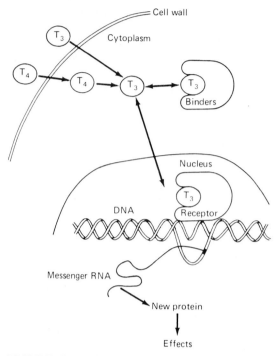

FIGURE 35-2 Highly schematic diagram of a tissue cell response to thyroid hormone. Circulating T_4, the predominant form of thyroid hormone, enters the cell where, in the cytoplasm, halogenases convert it to T_3 and other metabolites. Binders for T_3 are present in the cytoplasm. Receptors bind the T_3 which enters the nucleus. This hormone-receptor complex is in close conjunction with DNA. By a little-understood mechanism this brings about changes in specific mRNAs which in turn are involved in the synthesis of new protein which reflects the thyroid hormone response. [Modified from J. D. Baxter and J. W. Funder, "Hormone Receptors," *N. Engl. J. Med.*, **301**:1149–1161 (1979).]

volved, some, such as the brain, lymph nodes, spleen, and testes, are apparently not stimulated in this manner by the thyroid hormones.

Many aspects of carbohydrate and lipid metabolism are affected by thyroid hormones, either alone or in combination with other hormones. These affect many biologic events and include

1. Increased intestinal absorption of glucose and galactose

2. Potentiation of the glycogenolytic-hyperglycemic and lipolytic actions of epinephrine
3. Potentiation of insulin-induced glycogen synthesis and glucose utilization
4. Reduced serum cholesterol level
5. Increased uptake of glucose by adipose tissue
6. Increased mobilization of free fatty acids from adipose tissue (in part through potentiation of epinephrine)
7. Maturation of the CNS

Thyroid hormones decrease the level of serum cholesterol by stimulating cholesterol degradation in excess of biosynthesis. These hormones also increase coenzyme and vitamin requirements probably indirectly through increased metabolic demand.

Disorders of Thyroid Function

Thyroid hormone disease states may be the result of overproduction of thyroid hormone, *hyperthyroidism*, or underproduction of thyroid hormone, *hypothyroidism*. In either case, goiter may be present.

Hypothyroidism Hypothyroidism may be due to failure of the thyroid gland to develop or to synthesize thyroid hormones appropriately, damage to the thyroid gland (e.g., surgery, scarring from irradiation or autoimmune disease), or failure of the pituitary and/or hypothalamus to secrete the stimulatory hormones necessary for thyroid hormone secretion, TSH, and TRH. At birth, cretins (babies with congenital hypothyroidism) may be recognized by a puffy expressionless face, decreased muscle tone, coarse features, and a large tongue. Irreversible mental retardation will occur unless thyroid hormone replacement therapy is instituted promptly. Hypothyroidism (myxedema) in adults can be recognized by coarse, dry skin, bradycardia, anemia, and delayed relaxation of the deep tendon reflexes, especially prominent in the Achilles tendon. While findings may be subtle in early hypothyroidism, in later stages of disease, if untreated, coma may ensue. Juvenile hypothyroidism (postinfancy) presents similarly to adult hypothyroidism, with concurrent growth retardation.

Drugs Used in Hypothyroidism *Therapy* consists of thyroid hormone replacement. Levothyroxine (L-T_4) is the preferred form of therapy. It is converted in vivo to T_3, which is the active form of the hormone.

Thyroxine therapy provides constant serum levels of both T_4 and T_3 and is therefore the treatment of choice for hypothyroidism. T_3 and T_4/T_3 combination preparations have no advantage over thyroxine. Administration produces rapid peaks and nadirs of serum T_3 concentrations, as contrasted to the stable hormone concentrations achieved with thyroxine therapy. These preparations are less accurately titrated and stabilized in individual patients than is levothyroxine. These preparations contain high levels of T_3 and probably should not be used.

Levothyroxine Sodium (L-T_4) is pure synthetic T_4. The oral absorption of L-T_4 is approximately 81 percent. A single dose will be eliminated in 6 to 7 days. The usual replacement dose is 25 to 200 μg given orally once daily. L-T_4 is also available in a parenteral form for treatment of myxedema coma. The usual dose is 200 to 500 μg given intramuscularly or intravenously once. Daily therapy may then be instituted with 50 μg L-T_4 daily parenterally until enteral intake is possible. Some improvement in condition may be seen 6 h after the initial dose; the full therapeutic benefit may not be evident for over 24 h. Serum T_4 concentrations usually return to normal within 24 h.

Liothyronine Sodium (L-T_3) is a pure synthetic hormone. The oral absorption is approximately 90 percent. It has a more rapid onset of action and elimination than does L-T_4, peaking within several hours of administration. Its major indication is in patients who must be withdrawn from L-T_4 therapy for weeks (e.g., for thyroid scans) to provide temporary hormonal therapy that may be rapidly withdrawn while avoiding the side effects of hypothyroidism. The usual replacement dose is 25 to 50 μg daily. L-T_3 is also available in a parenteral form for emergency treatment of myxedema coma. The usual dose is 100 μg intravenously or intramuscularly followed by 25 μg daily.

Desiccated Thyroid (made mainly of bovine, ovine, and porcine thyroid glands) is standardized by its organic iodine content. Both T_3 and T_4 are present. The usual replacement dose is 15 to 300 mg/day.

Thyroglobulin (Proloid) is a purified extract of porcine thyroid glands. It, like desiccated thyroid, is standardized by its organic iodine content. The usual replacement dose is 15 to 300 mg/day.

Liotrix is a 4:1 mixture of synthetic L-T_4 and L-T_3. It has no advantage over pure L-T_4. The usual replacement dose is 150 to 200 mg/day. Each Liotrix tablet contains 60 μg L-T_4 and 15 μg L-T_3.

In addition to these thyroid hormone preparations that are commonly used, dextrothyroxine (D-T_4), the dextrorotatory (optical) isomer of L-T_4, deserves comment. It was introduced as a cholesterol-lowering agent. However, it is usually contaminated with up to 1 percent L-T_4. It should not be used for therapy of hypothyroidism. In addition, the Coronary Drug Project discontinued the use of D-T_4 as a cholesterol-lowering drug.

Iodine deficiency is a cause of goiter and hypothyroidism in some countries but is virtually nonexistent in the United States due to the addition of iodide to table salt and bread. Therefore, iodine has no role in treating hypothyroidism in this country, and it may cause hyperthyroidism if given to patients with goiters (Jod-Basedow syndrome).

Adverse Reactions Untoward effects of thyroid hormone therapy may result from overdosage. These effects take the form of symptoms of hyperthyroidism variably accompanied by psychotic behavior, angina pectoris, cardiac decompensation, myalgia, and severe diarrhea. In addition, acute Addison's crisis may occur in patients with undiagnosed and/or untreated concomitant adrenal insufficiency. Once the patient is euthyroid on replacement therapy, there are no drug interactions of note.

Hyperthyroidism Excessive production of thyroid hormones may be due to the presence of autoantibody which binds to the TSH receptor and stimulates it. Rarely, it may be due to a TSH-secreting pituitary neoplasm. Symptoms include weight loss, increased appetite, perspiration, fever, tachycardia, diarrhea, muscle weakness, anxiety, tremors, and eyelid retraction, causing a typical stare. Signs and symptoms may be subtle, especially in elderly patients.

Treatment of hyperthyroidism consists of drugs to inhibit excessive thyroid hormone synthesis, radioactive iodine to destroy the overactive gland, or surgery, to remove the overactive thyroid gland. Because surgery is very dangerous and may result in a potentially lethal episode of acute hyperthyroidism (thyroid storm), it is usually reserved for pregnant women in whom other therapeutic modalities are contraindicated.

Drugs Used in Hyperthyroidism: Thioamide (Thiocarbamide) Drugs Thioamides are the pri-

mary agents useful in the long-term therapy of mild to moderate hyperthyroidism. They are similar structurally in that they all contain a thiourea functional group (Fig. 35-3). Propylthiouracil and methimazole are preferred over the original drugs in the class, due to their much lower incidence of toxicity.

Mechanism of action Thioamides are reducing agents. They inhibit the synthesis of thyroid hormones by inhibiting organification of iodine and the coupling of iodotyrosines. In addition, propylthiouracil, but not methimazole, inhibits peripheral conversion of T_4 and T_3. Once stores of preformed thyroid hormones are depleted, concentrations of circulating thyroid hormones fall.

Pharmacokinetics These drugs are about 75 percent absorbed after oral administration. Propylthiouracil has its onset of action 20 to 30 min after administration. Serum levels peak approximately 1 h after administration. Its half-life is 2 h. Methimazole has a longer duration of action than does propylthiouracil, with a half-life of 6 to 13 h and serum concentrations peaking 2 h after administration.

Therapeutic use Thioamides may be employed as the sole therapeutic agent in the treatment of hyperthyroidism. There is a delay in the patient's therapeutic response to the drugs until circulating levels of thyroid hormones are reduced. The drugs may be taken for years, as recent studies indicate that less than 25 percent of people with hyperthyroidism will have spontaneous remission within 2 years, and many of these will

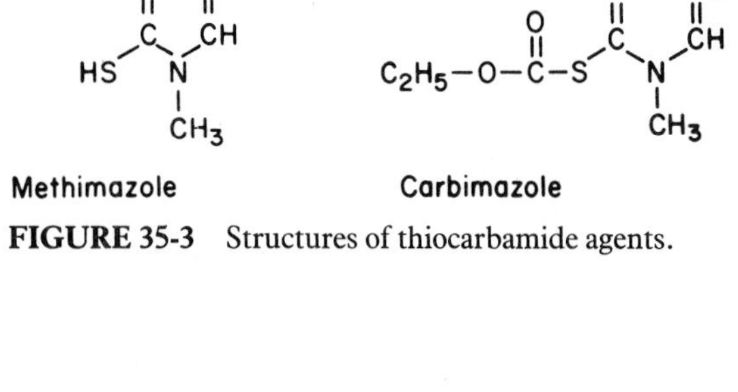

FIGURE 35-3 Structures of thiocarbamide agents.

relapse. These drugs may also be used in conjunction with iodide to prepare patients for surgery, and they may be used following radioactive iodine administration until the latter takes effect. Overtreatment may result in hypothyroidism.

Adverse reactions Adverse reactions consist of fever, skin rash, urticaria, myalgia, jaundice, edema, gastrointestinal upset, hepatitis, nephritis, lymphadenopathy and arthralgia. In addition, potentially fatal agranulocytosis may occur in less than 1 percent of patients. This occurs without warning, and may occur immediately, within months of starting therapy or even after more than a year of treatment. Patients should be warned of this complication and should have emergent white blood cell counts checked if fever or sore throat develops. These drugs cross the placenta, and maternal overdose may result in the birth of a goitrous cretin. They are secreted into breast milk and therefore should not be given to nursing mothers.

Preparations and dosages Propylthiouracil (PTU) is available in 50-mg tablets. The usual dose for initiation of therapy is 300 to 600 mg/day (given in divided doses four times daily) for suppression of hyperthyroidism. The usual maintenance dose is 50 to 200 mg/day in divided doses given four times daily.

Methimazole (Tapazole) is available in 5- and 10-mg tablets. Due to its longer duration of action (half-life 6 to 13 h) than PTU, methimazole may be given on a once or twice daily dosage schedule. The usual dose for initiation of therapy is 30 to 60 mg/day, and 5 to 20 mg/day for maintenance therapy. Administration to pregnant women has been associated with congenital scalp defects (aplasia cutis) in their offspring.

Iodide in large doses inhibits the release of thyroid hormones as well as their synthesis by blocking the organification of iodine. These effects are short-lived, however, and hyperthyroidism may be exacerbated by outpouring of preformed thyroid hormones as well as new synthesis of thyroid hormones. Thyroid storm may result. Iodide is usually used in conjunction with thioamide drugs to prepare patients for surgery. The usual doses used are Lugol's solution (5 g iodine + 10 g potassium iodide per 100 mL solution, yielding 6 mg iodine per drop) 5 drops daily, or SSKI (saturated solution of potassium iodide, 100 g potassium iodide per 100-mL solution yielding 50 mg iodide per drop) 1 drop three times daily. Sodium iodide (0.5 to 1.0 g daily) may be administered intravenously. Side effects include acute hypersensitivity reactions with angioedema, hemorrhagic skin lesions, and serum sickness and chronic toxicity (*iodism*). Iodism is characterized by unpleasant taste, burning in mouth, swelling of parotid and submaxillary glands, rhinitis, increased salivation, headache, productive cough, gastric irritation, bloody diarrhea, depression, and skin lesions; these symptoms usually resolve several days after discontinuation of iodine.

Radioactive iodine (^{131}I) has been used to partially or totally destroy the thyroid gland for treatment of hyperthyroidism. It has a half-life of 8 days, and it emits both beta particles and gamma rays. The beta particles have ionizing properties and thus destroy cells, but they have poor penetration (1 to 2 mm) and are undetectable outside the body. Gamma rays penetrate further and can be used for diagnostic purposes. Radioactive iodine is also used as an adjuvant to surgery for treatment of many types of thyroid cancer. The major side effect is permanent hypothyroidism (which is treated with replacement thyroid hormone therapy). Radiation-induced thyroiditis may occur in some patients but is of limited duration. Resultant hypoparathyroidism is exceedingly rare.

Beta blockers, such as propranolol, are frequently useful in temporarily blocking the peripheral manifestations of hyperthyroidism while the patient undergoes definitive therapy. They do not inhibit thyroid gland function, but they mask the adrenergic manifestations of tremor, stare, and tachycardia. The usual starting dose of propranolol is 40 mg every 6 h; it may be titrated to the desired heart rate. These drugs are discussed in Chap. 8.

Protirelin is a synthetic TRH (Fig. 35-4). The sole indication for protirelin is the assessment of thyroid gland function as an adjuvant to other diagnostic procedures. Patients with hyperthyroidism will not re-

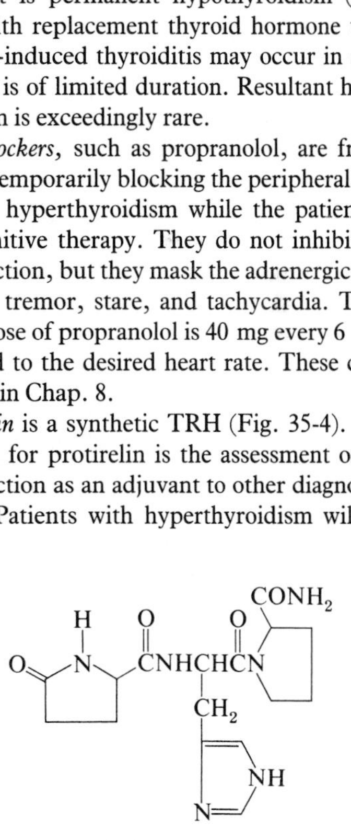

FIGURE 35-4 Protirelin.

spond to administration with elevated TSH levels. Patients with hypothyroidsm due to hypothalamic disease or to intrinsic thyroid disease (primary hypothyroidism) show a greater response than do those with pituitary dysfunction. The supersensitive TSH assay, which is able to distinguish low from normal TSH levels, often makes this test unnecessary.

Protirelin is given intravenously; its half-life is 5 min. TSH levels peak in 20 to 30 min following administration in normal individuals and fall to baseline over the next several hours. Side effects include marked changes in blood pressure (both hypo- and hypertension), headache, flushing, nausea, the urge to urinate, a bad taste in the mouth, and chest pressure. Rarely, pituitary apoplexy has occurred when protirelin was given to a patient with a pituitary adenoma.

CALCIUM, PARATHYROID HORMONE, CALCITONIN, AND VITAMIN D

Calcium

An adult human contains approximately 1200 g of calcium; about 10 g is found in the extracellular fluid and soft tissues, while the remainder (approximately 99 percent) is deposited in bone. The normal concentration of total plasma calcium, which is divided about equally between free ionic calcium and calcium loosely bound to plasma proteins (Table 35-2), is 8.8 to 10.3 mg per 100 mL of plasma. This range of concentrations of calcium in plasma also is apparently ideal for normal growth and development of the skeleton and for the maintenance of healthy bone.

One of the principal functions of calcium is at the cellular membrane: a decrease causes less stability, an increase causes greater stability. For instance, nerve fiber membranes in the presence of low calcium become partially depolarized and therefore transmit repetitive and uncontrolled impulses. Spasm or tetany of skeletal muscles may result. Very high concentrations of calcium ions depress neurons in the CNS presumably because membranes will not depolarize.

Calcium Homeostasis Despite the many functions of calcium described above, its main role is the preservation of the integrity of bone. Certainly the main signs and symptoms of disorders of calcium metabolism relate to bony defects and calcification of soft tissues. For these reasons, the homeostasis of calcium is of critical importance to the bodily economy. Unfortunately calcium homeostasis involves many interrelating factors which are difficult to compose into a conceptual model. At the least, calcium metabolism is controlled by three main hormones: parathyroid hormone (PTH), vitamin D, and calcitonin (CT). If the intake is adequate (15 mg/kg body weight in the young adult), the concentration of blood calcium will depend on the rate of intestinal absorption, deposition or resorption in bone, and renal excretion. Thus it is the control of these latter factors by vitamin D, PTH, and CT which determines calcium metabolism at any given moment.

A model, called the "butterfly" model, has been devised which aids the comprehension of the interaction of the main factors and elements in calcium metabolism (Fig. 35-5). The critical factor in the butterfly model is the serum calcium level (SCa^{2+}). If for any reason it falls (lower central point of loops), there will be induced an increased secretion of PTH and a decrease in the secretion of CT. This brings about increased bone resorption (1A); 1,25-$(OH)_2D_3$, the active form of vitamin D, causes increased intestinal absorption of calcium and also, by a minor feedback loop, increases the resorption of bone (2A). Meanwhile the renal excretion of calcium is decreased (3A) while the serum phosphate (SP) declines as a result of increased renal excretion of urinary phosphate (UP). This results in an increase in serum calcium. Should the serum calcium attain a level above the normal, the opposite events will occur (loops 1B, 2B, and 3B).

Obviously, such a model oversimplifies a very complicated series of events. Unfortunately, neither the time constants of the various events nor the magnitude of the response are known. Both PTH and CT respond relatively rapidly compared with vitamin D. However, the potential contribution of vitamin D (reserve capac-

TABLE 35-2   Distribution of calcium in human plasma

Form	Percent of total
Ionized	48
Protein-bound	46
Complexed	3
Unidentified	3

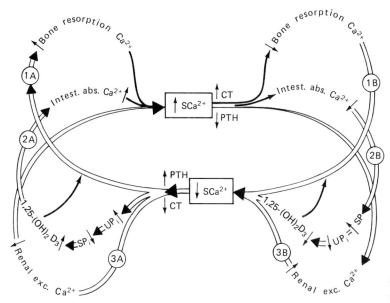

FIGURE 35-5 The "butterfly" model of calcium homeostasis depicted by three overlapping loops operating by negative feedback. The loops relate to one another through the blood concentration of ionic calcium (Ca^{2+}), parathyroid hormone (PTH), and calcitonin (CT). Loop 1 represents bone resorption; on the left, limb 1A indicates increased bone resorption and limb 1B decreased bone resorption. Loops 2 and 3 deal in a similar manner with intestinal absorption and renal excretion of calcium, respectively. Also shown are the relationships of $1,25\text{-}(OH)_2D_3$ (the active form of vitamin D) and the role of the concentration of serum phosphate (SP) and urinary phosphate (UP). The influence of $1,25\text{-}(OH)_2D_3$ in stimulating bone resorption is shown by a minor feedback loop (2A to 1A and 2B to 1B). (See text for further details.) [Modified by C. D. Arnaud, "Calcium Homeostasis: Regulatory Elements and Their Integration," *Fed. Proc.*, **37**:2557–2560 (1978).]

ity) is much greater than that of PTH or CT. That is, over a period of time vitamin D can have a dominant effect simply because, although slower, its capacity to achieve a determinate action is greater. The components of the model can now be examined in detail.

Parathyroid Hormone

Source and Chemistry Parathyroid hormone is a polypeptide hormone secreted by the parathyroid glands. There are usually four parathyroid glands, but supernumerary glands are common. Each gland normally weighs 25 to 75 mg. They are generally situated near the thyroid gland. Histologically, normal parathyroid glands consist of sheets of chief cells, measuring 4 to 8 μm in diameter. These cells contain secre-

tory granules and secrete PTH. Oxyphil cells, larger (6 to 10 μm in diameter) with eosinophilic cytoplasm, are also present. These cells are believed to be a degenerative form of chief cells and generally do not secrete PTH.

PTH is an 84-amino-acid chain polypeptide. It is biosynthesized in the form of a larger precursor, prepro-PTH (115 amino acids), which is then converted to pro-PTH (90 amino acids). Pro-PTH is then cleaved to PTH in the parathyroid glands. Pre-pro-PTH and pro-PTH have little biologic activity. The first (*N*-terminal) 34 amino acids of PTH confer its biologic activity.

Effects The major physiologic function of PTH is to raise the plasma calcium ion concentration to the optimum level for efficient neuromuscular activity. After total parathyroidectomy, plasma calcium concentrations may fall below 6 mg/dL; without therapy seizures, tetany, and death may ensure. In hyperparathyroidism, excess circulating PTH causes hypercalcemia. The sites of action of PTH are bone, kidney, and intestine.

Bone   PTH increases the resorption of bone, the chief reservoir of calcium within the body. It increases osteoclast activity while inhibiting osteoblastic function. In normal adults, osteoclastic and osteoblastic functions are balanced. In states of excess PTH secretion, the rate of bone resorption increases without an increase in bone formation, and serum calcium levels rise. In states of PTH deficiency, bone resorption decreases without a decrease in bone formation, and serum calcium levels fall.

Kidney   PTH enhances the fractional reabsorption of calcium from the glomerular filtrate. It inhibits phosphate reabsorption by the renal tubules.

Intestine   PTH stimulates intestinal absorption of calcium indirectly by stimulating renal 1-hydroxylation of 25-hydroxycholecalciferol (25-OH-D) to 1,25-dihydroxycholecalciferol (1,25-$(OH)_2$-D). Vitamin D is the principal factor responsible for promoting the absorption of calcium from the intestine.

Preparation and Administration   There is a very limited clinical use for PTH because of the length of time required to reach the peak effect, the short duration of action, and the possible antigenicity of the animal preparations. In addition, calcium infusions can substitute more effectively where a rapid increase in serum calcium is necessary; for long-term treatment the vitamin D derivatives are more effective, since they can be given orally and antigenicity is not a factor. PTH may be used as a diagnostic aid in patients with hypocalcemia. Patients with hypoparathyroidism generally respond to PTH administration by increasing urinary cyclic adenosine monophosphate (AMP) and phosphate excretion; patients with pseudohypoparathyroidism (target-organ resistance to PTH) shows a blunted response.

Pharmacokinetics and Pharmacological Effects PTH must be given parenterally. When given subcutaneously or intramuscularly, an elevation of serum calcium is usually evident within 4 h if at all, reaching a maximum in 8 to 16 h and returning to the control level in 20 to 24 h. If continued effect is desired, the dose may be repeated at intervals of 12 h. Parathyroid Injection may also be administered intravenously for more rapid onset of action, but the duration of the effect is much shorter than after subcutaneous or intramuscular injection.

Adverse Reactions   Adverse reactions to PTH administration include nausea, abdominal cramps, the urge to defecate, diarrhea, tingling of the extremities, and a metallic taste. Patients may experience pain at the injection site. Allergic reactions to the animal preparations have been observed.

Preparations and Dosages   *Parathyroid Injection, USP,* is made from bovine parathyroid glands. The usual dose for the diagnosis of pseudohypoparathyroidism is 200 units intravenously.

   Synthetic human parathyroid hormone 1-34 (teriparatide acetate) has recently been introduced for clinical use. The dose for the diagnosis of pseudohypoparathyroidism is 200 units intravenously.

Calcitonin

When hypercalcemic blood is perfused through the thyroid gland, a hypocalcemic hormone, calcitonin (thyrocalcitonin), is secreted by the parafollicular, or C, cells of the thyroid gland. Calcitonin has been isolated from humans and other mammals, as well as birds and fish. In all species, it is a 32 amino acid polypeptide with an *N*-terminal seven-membered disulfide ring and a *C*-terminal proline-amide. The individual amino acids differ from species to species. Salmon calcitonin is the most potent.

Mechanism of Action   Calcitonin's action is hypocalcemic and hypophosphatemic. However, the normal output of calcitonin by the thyroid gland is not sufficient to produce hypocalcemia. Removal of the thyroid gland does not result in hypercalcemia in usual circumstances.

   The major site of action of calcitonin is bone, where it inhibits osteoclastic function. It also inhibits PTH-stimulated bone resorption. In pharmacologic doses, it has a direct calciuric effect. These effects are mediated by cyclic AMP, which is formed through activation of adenylate cyclase by calcitonin.

Regulation of Secretion The rate of secretion of calcitonin is regulated by the ionic calcium concentration of blood flowing through the thyroid gland, increasing as the calcium concentration increases, and falling as it decreases.

Preparation, Dosage, and Administration Calcitonin is ineffective if given orally. It is active when administered parenterally.

Synthetic human and salmon (Calcimar) preparations are available as lyophilized powder, 400 MRC (Medical Research Council) units per vial. Calcitonin may be used to treat hypercalcemia of various causes. While the hypocalcemic effect is rapid (within 24 to 48 h), it is short-lived, because tachyphylaxis may develop within several days. Glucocorticoids may prevent this. The usual starting dose for treatment of hypercalcemia is 4 MRC units per kilogram of body weight subcutaneously every 12 h; for treatment of Paget's disease, the dose is 100 MRC units subcutaneously daily.

Adverse Reactions Nausea and vomiting are the most frequent side effects and may occur in 50 percent of patients. These symptoms are usually mild and do not necessitate discontinuation of therapy. Facial flushing is also common. Local inflammatory reactions at the site of injection may develop. Less commonly, abdominal cramps, diarrhea, itching, urinary frequency, and urticaria may develop.

Vitamin D

Precursors of vitamin D are present in many foods of vegetable and animal origin. The liver of fish is especially rich in vitamin D, and cod liver oil has been a traditional source. Much confusion has existed as to the most desirable preparation, since the active form of vitamin D was not known. Nor was it realized that vitamin D acts as a hormone in the body rather than as a vitamin. It does so because it is capable of being synthesized, in contrast to classic vitamins, and also because it actually functions as a messenger substance with control action rather than entering into a critical metabolic step of synthesis or as a cofactor for an enzyme.

Present understanding of the pathway of biotransformation of vitamin D includes the following. Provitamin D_3 (7-dehydrocholesterol) is converted to previtamin D_3 by the action of ultraviolet light on the skin. In turn, the photoisomer previtamin D_3 is thermally converted to vitamin D_3 (cholecalciferol). With the aid of a plasma-binding protein (vitamin D–binding globulin), vitamin D_3 is transported to the liver. Here vitamin D, 25-hydroxylase stimulates hydroxylation of carbon-25 to produce the major circulating form of vitamin D, 25-OHD_3, which is inactive at physiologic concentrations. Again with the aid of a plasma-binding protein, 25-OHD_3 is transported to the kidney. In this organ, it is converted to 1,25-$(OH)_2D_3$ when hypocalcemia and hypophosphatemia are present. This is the most active form of vitamin D, and it is highly effective in causing increased intestinal absorption of calcium and also resorption of calcium from bone. PTH is also a tropin for the renal synthesis of 1,25-$(OH)_2D_3$. On the other hand, in the absence of stimulation by PTH and with normal serum calcium and phosphate, the kidney converts D_3 to 24,25-$(OH)_2D_3$, which is only weakly active. Table 35-3 summarizes these events.

Historically, the substances designated as vitamin D_1 were later shown to be a mixture of antirachitic substances. A commonly prescribed form of vitamin D in commercial preparations is ergosterol, which is also present in irradiated bread and milk. Ergosterol is the provitamin for vitamin D_2 (ergocalciferol). Ergocalciferol and cholecalciferol are metabolized by the same pathway and have similar biologic activities.

The major storage form of vitamin D in the body is D_3. Ordinarily, with average daily intake of milk, meat, and fish and with some exposure to sunlight, supplemental amounts of vitamin D are not needed. Poor diet, malnutrition, infancy, pregnancy and lactation, and lack of exposure to sunlight are generally considered indications for supplementation. Even under these circumstances, the recommended daily allowance (RDA) of 400 IU of vitamin D should not be exceeded.

Hypervitaminosis D This is perhaps the most common of the vitamin toxicity syndromes. It is easily caused by overenthusiastic medication, either professionally or self-prescribed. The syndrome in mild form consists of hypercalcemia with nausea, weakness, weight loss, vague aches and stiffness, constipa-

TABLE 35-3   Functional metabolism of vitamin D

Organ	Metabolic effect		
Skin, UV light	7-Dehydrocholesterol $\longrightarrow$		Vitamin D_3 (cholecalciferol) $\downarrow$
Liver			25-OHD_3 $\downarrow$
Kidney	Influence of PTH, low serum P_i, low serum Ca^{2+}		$1,25\text{-(OH)}_2D_3$
	Influence of normal serum P_i, normal serum Ca^{2+}	$24,25\text{-(OH)}_2D_3$ (inactive)* $\downarrow$ $1,24,25\text{-(OH)}_3D_3$ (inactive)*	$\downarrow$
Intestine	Increases absorption of Ca^{2+}		$1,25\text{-(OH)}_2D_3$ (active) $\downarrow$
Bone	Causes resorption of Ca^{2+}		$1,25\text{-(OH)}_2D_3$ (active)

tion or diarrhea, anemia, and mild acidosis. Eventually impaired renal function results with polyuria, nocturia, polydipsia, hypercalcinuria, and azotemia. If allowed to progress, eventual nephrocalcinosis takes place along with calcification of other soft tissues. Marked CNS symptoms such as mental retardation and convulsive states occur. Osteoporosis may cause fractures in adults; in children there is a decreased rate of linear growth.

Treatment of hypervitaminosis D consists of withdrawal of vitamin therapy, a low calcium diet, increased fluid intake, and acidification of the urine. A loop diuretic may aid in the elimination of calcium. In desperate cases, dialysis may have to be used. Recovery is the rule if irreversible damage has not occurred.

Pharmacologic Doses of Vitamin D   In severe hypocalcemic states, large doses of vitamin D preparations are indicated. For example, in fully developed rickets 1000 IU daily for 10 days will usually reverse the disorder. Certainly 3000 to 4000 IU of vitamin D should be reserved for the most severe cases.

Vitamin D–dependent rickets (pseudo-vitamin D–deficiency rickets), an inherited autosomal recessive defect, responds only to $1,25\text{-(OH)}_2D_3$. Hypoparathyroidism requires doses of vitamin D of 50,000 to 200,000 IU daily. This turns out to be far more effective therapy than the use of PTH, because intestinal absorption of calcium is the most crucial factor in reversing a calcium deficiency (see Table 35-4). For patients with hypocalcemia due to chronic renal dialysis, $1,25\text{-(OH)}_2D$ (calcitriol) is available. In all instances, additional calcium should be given in the diet (at least 1 g daily). There is danger of precipitation of hypercalcemia with all intensive vitamin D therapy. This is especially true of calcitriol, and monitoring of serum calcium levels is advisable.

Paget's Disease   Paget's disease is a bone disorder characterized by rapid uncontrolled increase in bone resorption, the new bone formed being structurally abnormal. Symptoms may include bone pain, thickening of the skull, compression of spinal and cranial nerves, and hearing loss. Serum alkaline phosphatase and urinary hydroxyproline are usually elevated. This disease is common and is often treated with calcitonin alone or in combination with etidronate. Calcitonin administered subcutaneously or intramuscularly may relieve symptoms. The drug is given for prolonged periods. Sodium etidronate, a diphosphonate, is useful in patients not responding to calcitonin.

Etidronate *Pharmacologic effects* Etidronate inhibits hydroxyapatite crystal formation, growth, and dissolution. It inhibits bone resorption. A significant drop in serum calcium is usually seen by the third day after intravenous administration. Oral etidronate has been shown to maintain normal serum calcium concentrations.

Pharmacokinetics The plasma half-life is approximately 6 h after intravenous administration. Etidronate is excreted unchanged in the urine. Approximately half the administered dose is taken up by bone; the half-life of the dose in bone is over 90 days. Orally administered etidronate is approximately 1 to 6 percent absorbed.

Adverse reactions Patients may experience a metallic taste during and after infusion. Hyperphosphatemia may be observed; this generally resolves after therapy is discontinued and has not been of clinical significance. Hypersensitivity reactions have been reported. Diarrhea and nausea may occur.

Preparations and Dosage *Calcitriol* [Rocaltrol, 1,25-$(OH)_2D_3$] is available in capsules of 0.25 μg. The usual dose is 0.25 μg daily; up to 1 μg daily may be required. This preparation is indicated in patients with impaired ability to convert 25-OHD$_3$ to 1,25-$(OH)_2D_3$. Because it is the active hormone, it has the most rapid onset of action of all vitamin D preparations and is useful in treating acute hypocalcemia and hypoparathyroidism. Serum calcium levels should be closely monitored while on this preparation.

Dihydrotachysterol (Hytakerol) is available in 0.125-mg tablets and 0.25-mg/mL solution. The usual adult dosage is 0.75 to 2.5 mg/day. Unlike vitamin D and ergocalciferol compounds, dihydrotachysterol is active in nephrectomized patients and does not require 1-hydroxylation in the kidney.

Vitamin D (various) is available in multivitamin preparations, 400 IU. Usual dose is one capsule daily for supplementation or for prophylaxis of rickets.

Ergocalciferol (vitamin D$_2$, Deltalin, Drisdol, Geltabs) is available in 0.625-mg (25,000 units) and 1.25-mg (50,000 units) capsules and 0.250-mg/mL (10,000 units/mL) solution. The usual adult dosage range is 1.25 to 25 mg daily.

Calcifediol (25-hydroxycholecalciferol) is available in 20- and 50-μg capsules. The usual adult dosage range is 50 to 100 μg daily.

Hypercalcemia Hypercalcemia may be caused by malignancy, granulomatous diseases, endocrinologic diseases, genetic disorders, prolonged immobilization, and drugs. Hyperparathyroidism is usually treated

TABLE 35-4 Effect of vitamin D preparations compared with PTH on calcium and phosphate homeostasis

Preparation	Calcium absorption	Phosphate excretion	Bone resorption	Onset of action
Vitamin D (D$_2$ or D$_3$) (physiologic dose 500–1000 units/day)	3+*		+	2+
Vitamin D$_2$ or D$_3$ (pharmacologic dose 50,000–250,000 units/day)	4+	2+	3+	2+
Dihydrotachysterol (1 mg/day)	3+	3+	3+	+
PTH	+	4+	4+	4+

*Key: 4+ = high; 3+ = moderate; 2+ = low; + = slight.

surgically; in other cases, removal of the cause should be attempted. Frequently, other therapeutic interventions are necessary to control the hypercalcemia in the acute setting.

Saline hydration is important, and all patients with hypercalcemia should be kept well hydrated. Saline hydration promotes renal excretion of calcium. Furosemide may be added to saline hydration to increase renal calcium excretion. This agent is discussed elsewhere.

Phosphates may be administered as neutral phosphate or potassium phosphate. Phosphate forms complexes with calcium, resulting in a fall of serum calcium. These are generally given orally, because rapid intravenous administration may result in extraskeletal precipitation of calcium salts; if these precipitate in the kidneys, renal failure may result. The usual initial dose is 1 to 2 g of elemental phosphorus daily in divided doses. Gastrointestinal side effects include diarrhea and nausea.

Calcitonin may be useful in acutely controlling hypercalcemia. This is discussed above.

Plicamycin (Mithramycin) is a cytotoxic antibiotic often used as a cancer chemotherapeutic agent. It blocks calcium resorption from bone. Side effects include hepatic and renal toxicity, nausea, vomiting, and thrombocytopenia. The usual dose for the treatment of hypercalcemia is 25 μg per kilogram of body weight, intravenously. Serum calcium concentrations usually fall within a few days; however, they may fall within hours of Plicamycin administration. The duration of the response is variable. Plicamycin may be administered again should hypercalcemia recur.

Etidronate is available as an intravenous preparation for the treatment of hypercalcemia. The usual dose is 7.5 mg per kilogram of body weight daily for three days. It must be diluted in at least 250 mL of saline and should be infused over at least 2 h. Oral etidronate is available in 200- and 400-mg tablets. The dosage range is 5 to 20 mg per kilogram of body weight per day given as a single oral dose.

BIBLIOGRAPHY

Arnaud, C. D.: "Calcium Homeostasis: Regulatory Elements and Their Integration," *Fed. Proc.*, **37**:2557–2560 (1978).

Baxter, J. D., and J. W. Flunder: "Hormone Receptors," *N. Engl. J. Med.*, **301**:1149–1161 (1979).

Cooper, D. S., and E. C. Ridgway: "Clinical Management of Patients with Hyperthyroidism," *Med. Clin. North Am.*, **69**:953–971 (1985).

Fish, L. H., et al.: "Replacement Dose, Metabolism and Bioavailability of Levothyroxine in the Treatment of Hypothyroidism," *N. Engl. J. Med.*, **316**:764–770 (1987).

Habener, J. F., and H. M. Kronenberg: "Parathyroid Hormone Biosynthesis: Structure and Function of Biosynthetic Precursors," *Fed. Proc.*, **37**:2561–2566 (1978).

Habener, J. F., and J. T. Potts, Jr.: "Biosynthesis of Parathyroid Hormone," *N. Engl. J. Med.*, **299**:580–585, 635–644 (1978).

Haussler, M. R., and T. A. McCain: "Basic and Clinical Concepts Related to Vitamin D Metabolism and Action," *N. Engl. J. Med.*, **297**:974–983, 1041–1050 (1977).

Hennessey, J. V., et al.: "L-Thyroxine Dosage: A Reevaluation of Therapy with Contemporary Preparations," *Ann. Int. Med.*, **105**:11–15 (1986).

Kanis, J. A., et al.: "Effects of Intravenous Etidronate Disodium on Skeletal and Calcium Metabolism," *Am. J. Med.*, **82**(suppl. 2A):55–70 (1987).

Kumar, R., and B. L. Riggs: "Vitamin D in the Therapy of Disorders of Calcium and Phosphorus Metabolism," *Mayo. Clin. Proc.*, **56**:327–333 (1981).

Martin, J. K., et al.: "The Peripheral Metabolism of Parathyroid Hormones," *N. Engl. J. Med.*, **301**:1092–1098 (1979).

Sterling, K.: "Thyroid Hormone Action at the Cell Level," *N. Engl. J. Med.*, **300**:117–122, 173–177 (1979).

Van Herle, A. J., G. Vassart, and J. E. Dumont: "Control of Thyroglobulin Synthesis and Secretion," *N. Engl. J. Med.*, **301**:239–248, 307–314 (1979).

Insulins and Oral Hypoglycemic Agents

Jeffrey L. Miller and Gerald H. Sterling

Insulin and oral hypoglycemics are agents useful in the treatment of diabetes mellitus. Diabetes mellitus is a metabolic disease associated with high blood glucose levels and alterations in carbohydrate, lipid, and protein metabolism. Ketoacidosis is its most severe acute biochemical disturbance. The vascular complications of diabetes mellitus consist of progressively advancing microangiopathies involving the extremities, eyes, kidneys, and heart. The clinical manifestations of this vascular degeneration include gangrene of the foot, blindness, uremia, and coronary artery disease.

CLASSIFICATION OF HUMAN DIABETES

Diabetes mellitus is classified by the American Diabetes Association according to whether the patient is insulin-dependent (IDDM, type I) or noninsulin dependent (NIDDM, type II). Type I diabetes is caused by an absolute deficiency of insulin; the patient, therefore, requires insulin for maintenance of life. In its classic form, type I diabetes usually commences in the early teen years, though symptoms may first occur in adults and may present with weight loss. It is the most severe type of diabetes; ketoacidosis is common. Type II diabetes classically affects obese adults and often in the early stages is associated with a state of insulin resistance (i.e., high circulating concentrations of insulin which are ineffective due to an insulin receptor or postreceptor defect secondary to the obesity). Nonobese type II diabetes is due to a relatively low level of insulin secretion. Hyperglycemia may not be

as severe, and ketoacidosis less common, than in type I diabetes. Controlled diet and exercise may control the hyperglycemia in a type II diabetic patient. Oral hypoglycemic agents and insulin are available if the patient does not respond to diet therapy alone. Sometimes the type II diabetic patient requires insulin for adequate glucose control but not for maintenance of life. A majority of diabetics are type II.

Secondary causes of diabetes include syndromes of endocrine overactivity (acromegaly and Cushing's disease, etc.) and drug-induced diabetes (e.g., thiazide diuretics and thyroid hormones). Finally, gestational diabetes (onset during pregnancy, usually late second trimester) is well recognized. There is a high incidence of diabetes developing again postgestationally in these individuals.

The clinical symptoms of diabetes are usually those due to hyperglycemia (nocturia, polyuria, polydipsia, and polyphagia). In the type II diabetic there is also usually a history or evidence of recent weight gain. Although diabetes was originally defined as a hyperglycemia with subsequent glycosuria, it was subsequently recognized that not only were the metabolic alterations of fats and proteins interrelated with those of carbohydrates, but they were of profound importance. These metabolic alterations (Fig. 36-1) include overproduction of glucose from glycogen and other sources in the liver, underutilization of glucose peripherally, depression of oxidation of glucose in muscle and adipose tissue, and the almost complete disappearance of lipogenesis.

Glucose metabolism is decreased in regard to both Embden-Meyerhof and pentose phosphate pathways.

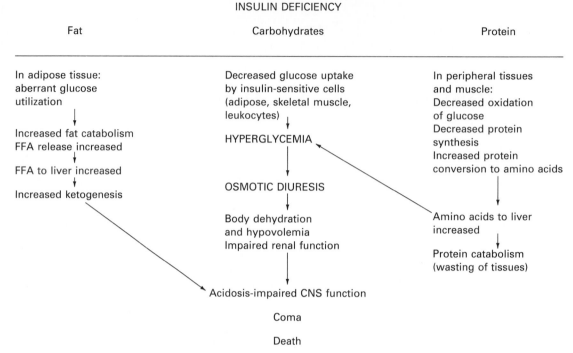

FIGURE 36-1   Metabolic alterations due to insulin deficiency.

Protein in peripheral tissues is broken down excessively, and the amino acids are taken into the liver and converted into glucose (gluconeogenesis). Similarly, there is a decrease of protein synthesis from amino acids in muscle, with eventual inhibition of growth. Fat synthesis is blocked at one or more sites early in the normal sequence of reactions. Conversion of glucose to α-glycerolphosphate is inhibited in adipose tissue, with defective esterification of fat and a rise in serum-free fatty acids. The inability of liver and muscle to cope with this defect in lipid metabolism results in excess fat metabolism and excess production of ketone bodies, leading to ketonemia and ketonuria.

The hyperglycemia and ketonemia eventually result in profound water and electrolyte disturbances and cause alterations of acid-base balance of blood as well as losses of total fixed bases, which clinically constitute diabetic ketoacidosis. With acidosis, the proper functioning of the brain tissue is impossible, and coma and death may result.

INSULIN

Insulin was discovered in 1921 by Banting and Best, who extracted the active product from the pancreas and demonstrated its therapeutic effectiveness in diabetic dogs and humans. Insulin is a protein (MW 6000) composed of 51 amino acids arranged in two chains (A and B) (Fig. 36-2). The tertiary structure is held together by disulfide bonds between cysteine residues. Insulin is synthesized as preproinsulin, containing the A and B chains connected by a large peptide (35 amino acids) and an additional sequence of 16 amino acids. The 16 amino acids are cleaved to form proinsulin. When proinsulin is hydrolyzed to insulin, the connecting peptide in humans, called *C-peptide* (31 amino acids), which links the threonine of the B chain to the glycine of the A chain is produced. Proinsulin and C-peptide have no known physiologic function. However, since C-peptide is secreted along with insulin, measurement of C-peptide in addition to insu-

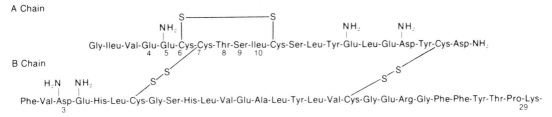

FIGURE 36-2 Structural formula of human insulin. Porcine insulin differs in position 30, and bovine in positions 8, 10, and 30.

lin can be useful in the diagnosis of diabetes. A nondiabetic may excrete approximately 30 μg/day of C-peptide in the urine. A type I diabetic would excrete much less (10 μg/day), whereas a type II diabetic's output would vary from less than 30 μg/day in those patients with low insulin production to greater than 60 μg/day in patients who are insulin-resistant. The amino acid composition of the A and B chains may differ in different species and may explain the various antigenicities and serum binding of insulin derived from human, porcine, or bovine pancreas (see Fig. 36-2).

Secretion and Metabolism

Insulin is synthesized and secreted from the beta cells of the pancreas by exocytosis. Preproinsulin is synthesized in the endoplasmic reticulum, where it is converted to proinsulin. Proinsulin is stored in the granules of the Golgi apparatus, where it is gradually cleaved to form insulin. As the granules secrete insulin, some proinsulin and C-peptide are also released. The rate of insulin secretion is affected by (1) food products, (2) gastrointestinal hormones, and (3) neuronal control. In humans, glucose is the most potent stimulus for insulin biosynthesis and release. Insulin concentration in the blood varies from approximately 20 μU/mL during fasting to 100 μU/mL after consumption of a meal or glucose infusion. Since insulin promotes the storage of all fuels, amino acids, fatty acids, and ketone bodies may also stimulate insulin release. Several gastrointestinal hormones (e.g., secretin, cholecystokinin, and gastrin) have also been shown to stimulate insulin release.

Autonomic and central neurons innervate the pancreas and can regulate insulin secretion. Norepinephrine and epinephrine inhibit insulin secretion through alpha-adrenergic receptors. Selective stimulation of beta$_2$-adrenergic receptors enhances insulin secretion. Stimulation of the vagus nerve also enhances insulin secretion through muscarinic receptors.

Circulating insulin has a very short biologic half-life of approximately 5 min. The compound is rapidly destroyed by enzymatic degradation and removed from the blood primarily by the liver and kidney. The enzymes responsible include insulinase, which cleaves the disulfide bonds, and proteases, which further degrade the insulin.

Mechanism of Action

Insulin acts by binding to specific receptors on the surface of insulin-sensitive tissue. The receptor is composed of four functional subunits, two alpha and two beta. The alpha subunit binds insulin, whereas the beta subunit is a tyrosine-specific kinase. The insulin-receptor complex can be internalized by endocytosis, which may be the means of inactivation. Stimulation of the receptor by insulin causes phosphorylation of the beta subunit and endogenous substrates, initiating a number of biochemical events (e.g., facilitation of glucose transport into cells, enhancement of amino acid incorporation into proteins, increased lipid synthesis).

Physiologic and Biochemical Effects

Binding of insulin to its receptor produces a change in membrane structure to facilitate the penetration of monosaccharides, primarily glucose, amino acids, and fatty acids, through the cell membrane of insulin-sensitive tissues. These tissues include skeletal and heart muscle, fat, and leukocytes. Other tissues, such as liver, are less sensitive to this action of insulin. In liver and peripheral tissue, insulin also acts to regulate the enzymes of glucose metabolism. The brain is not considered to be insulin-dependent.

Insulin acts on skeletal muscle to facilitate the uptake of glucose and amino acids. The glucose uptake enhances glycogen synthesis and storage. Uptake of amino acids promotes protein synthesis and tissue growth.

Adipose tissue is the largest store of energy in the body. Insulin acts to facilitate the production and storage of triglycerides. This is accomplished by enhanced uptake of glucose which is metabolized to 2-glycerophosphate, the backbone of triglycerides, and enhanced uptake of free fatty acids.

As already mentioned, uptake of glucose, amino acids, and fatty acids by the liver is not insulin-dependent. However, insulin does have profound effects on several enzyme systems. Insulin acts to enhance glycogen synthesis and to increase the synthesis of enzymes unique to glycolysis. In addition, insulin suppresses the enzymes of gluconeogenesis. Thus, an insulin-induced signal will stimulate glycolysis and glycogenolysis while reducing glucose production; lack of insulin will produce the opposite, as characterized in diabetes.

Pharmacokinetics and Preparations Used in Diabetes

Because of its protein nature, insulin is destroyed if administered orally; therefore it must be administered parenterally, usually by the subcutaneous route. In order to delay absorption and prolong its action, insulin is combined with certain proteins and/or precipitated or crystallized in specific buffers (Table 36-1).

All preparations of insulin are now supplied in 10-mL vials and marketed in concentrations of 40 and 100 units/mL. These preparations are from bovine or porcine sources. Additionally, human insulin is now available and marketed. It is produced either by recombinant DNA technology or chemical conversion of porcine insulin. Some of these preparations are available as purified insulins that have been subjected to ion exchange chromatography, which reduces the amount of proinsulin and noninsulin protein present in the finished product to miniscule amounts (equal to or less than 10 parts per million). Insulin injection is also supplied at 500 units/mL for emergency use or in

treatment of diabetic patients with insulin resistance (i.e., those with daily requirements of greater than 200 units/day).

Insulin Injection (Crystalline Zinc Insulin, Regular Insulin)   The first insulin developed for clinical use was the amorphous form of insulin. The preparation is a clear solution. Rapidly acting insulin (regular, crystalline zinc insulin) is purified, crystallized, and stabilized at neutral pH. The addition of zinc also contributes to the stability. Regular insulin is usually administered subcutaneously 15 to 30 min before each meal so that availability will coincide with need (see Fig. 36-3). It is also used in the management of diabetic coma, where it is administered by intravenous injection. The duration of action is 6 to 8 h; this short duration of action constituted the rationale for the 6-h management program, whereby the diabetic administered insulin and consumed a meal every 6 h. Regular insulin is the only type useful in insulin infusion pumps.

Protamine Insulins

Protamine Zinc Insulin (PZI) Suspension   Mixing insulin, protamine, and zinc in a phosphate buffer (pH 7.4) yields protamine zinc insulin suspension.

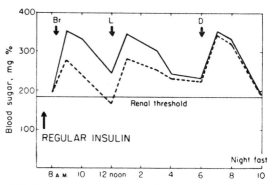

FIGURE 36-3   The duration of action of regular insulin. One moderate-size dose of regular insulin was given in the morning to a patient with moderately severe untreated diabetes who was eating three meals a day: breakfast (Br), lunch (L), and dinner (D). The solid line indicates the blood sugar curve before insulin, and the broken line the curve after the single dose of regular insulin. Note the limited effectiveness of one dose of this type of insulin.

TABLE 36-1 Insulin preparations

Types of insulin	Action*			Added protein	
	Onset, h	Maximum effect, h	Duration, h	Type	Amount, mg per 100 units of insulin
Insulin injection (regular, crystalline zinc)	0.5–1	2–4	6–8	None	
Isophane insulin suspension (NPH)	1–2	8–10	18–26	Protamine	0.3–0.5
Protamine zinc insulin suspension (PZI)	4–6	14–20	26–36	Protamine	1–1.5
Prompt insulin zinc suspension (semilente)	1–2	3–7	12–16	None	
Insulin zinc suspension (lente)	2	8–10	18–26	None	
Extended insulin zinc suspension (ultralente)	4–8	16–18	30–36	None	

*The time action is an estimate and varies from one patient to another. Human insulin may be quicker acting than pork and beef sources. Increasing doses produces a longer time-action curve.

When the basic protamine molecule is combined with the acidic insulin, the complex flocculates out as a fine suspension containing 1 to 1.5 mg of protamine and 0.2 mg of zinc per 100 units of insulin. This represents a 150 percent excess of protein. The addition of the zinc stabilizes the preparation and prevents clumping. Its onset of action is slow (4 to 6 h), and its duration of action is long (26 to 36 h). The clinical response to PZI is shown in Fig. 36-4.

Isophane Insulin Suspension (NPH Insulin)
This preparation is an example of a type of insulin with intermediate action. It is a suspension of a crystalline form of protamine zinc insulin which contains only 0.3 to 0.5 mg of protamine per 100 units of insulin.

This is just enough protamine to bind the regular insulin. Its action is similar to a mixture having one part protamine zinc insulin and two parts regular insulin. The action of NPH (neutral protamine Hagedorn) insulin starts in about 1 to 2 h, reaches a peak of activity in 8 to 10 h, and wanes by 18 to 26 h.

Insulin Zinc Suspension (Lente Insulins) In order to prolong the therapeutic effectiveness of insulin without combining it with protamine, which may produce an antigenic response, an alternative purification method was developed. By this method, insulin crystals are formed in various sizes, each giving a different time-action response. At present there are three available forms:

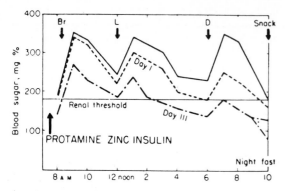

FIGURE 36-4 The duration of action of protamine zinc insulin. A moderate-size dose of protamine zinc insulin was given to a patient with moderately severe untreated diabetes who was eating three meals a day as in Fig. 36-3. The solid line indicates the blood sugar curve before treatment, and the broken lines the curve on the first and third days of treatment. The progressive effect of this type of insulin upon the blood sugar curve during a given day may be noted, with a maximum effect at night. A small amount of food (snack) is interposed at bedtime to avoid hypoglycemia. The progressive improvement in the blood sugar curve from the first day to a maximum effect on the third day is a characteristic response of this type of insulin.

1. Prompt insulin zinc suspension (semilente insulin) is a crystalline form with small crystals which dissolves rapidly, producing a prompt, short action of 12 to 16 h (Table 36-1).
2. Extended insulin zinc suspension (ultralente insulin) is composed of large crystals and hence is long-acting (duration of 30 to 36 h).
3. Insulin zinc suspension (lente insulin) is an intermediate-acting preparation (duration of 18 to 26 h), which is a mixture of 30 percent prompt insulin zinc suspension and 70 percent extended insulin zinc suspension. Variations can be custom-mixed from the prompt and extended insulin zinc suspensions to suit the individual needs of patients.

Dosage

The dose of insulin to be used is ultimately determined by clinical trial in a given patient on a given diet as the amount which accomplishes the therapeutic objective set by the physician. Such objectives vary from a minimum of eliminating diabetic symptoms to a maximum of attaining normoglycemia. The normal pancreas produces from 30 to 50 units of insulin per day, so most diabetics with insulin deficiency require somewhat less than this dosage of insulin. Usual nonpregnant adults theoretically require 0.6 units/kg of insulin every 24 h.

Factors that may increase insulin requirements include (1) metabolic needs of the body, for example, thyrotoxicosis and fever; (2) stress conditions, for example, surgery, injury, myocardial infarction, anesthesia, and infection; (3) development of insulin resistance; (4) reduced muscular exercise; (5) psychic stress; and (6) drugs administered which increase plasma glucose levels. A list of factors is given in Table 36-2.

Coadministration of other drugs may greatly alter the effectiveness of insulin. Those agents which reduce the effect of insulin, thus increasing the insulin requirement, include corticosteroids, dextrothyroxine, epinephrine, oral contraceptives, thiazides, and thyroid hormones. Most of these act by increasing plasma glucose levels. The thiazide diuretics also reduce insulin secretion. The mechanism of dextrothyroxine is not completely known. Agents enhancing the

TABLE 36-2   Factors which increase the need for insulin

Gain in weight
Increased caloric intake
Hyperthyroidism
Stress
Fever
Ketosis
Infections
Pregnancy
Extensive burns
Deep roentgen-ray therapy
Cessation of exercise
Epinephrine
Corticosteroids
Thiazides
Estrogens
Progestogens

effect of insulin include ethanol (acute), guanethidine, and oral hypoglycemics, all of which decrease plasma glucose by altering carbohydrate metabolism.

Adverse Reactions

Hypoglycemia is the major adverse reaction of insulin therapy. Regularity in eating and avoidance of wide variations in diet are important in maintaining normoglycemia. Warning symptoms of milder degrees of hypoglycemia such as fatigue, headache, and drowsiness must be watched for, and the insulin dose reduced or food interposed at such times. Hypoglycemia can be anticipated to occur at the time of peak action of the insulin. A severe prolonged hypoglycemic reaction can, if untreated, lead to permanent cerebral damage, coma, or death.

The prime clinical manifestations of insulin overdosage are due to the effects of hypoglycemia on the nervous system. Once the blood sugar drops below 50 to 60 mg per 100 mL, symptoms of hunger, faintness, sweating, tremors, muscular weakness, nausea, psychic disturbances, and finally loss of consciousness (insulin shock) may occur.

Fortunately, the mammalian body has corrective factors available to counteract hypoglycemia by providing glucose from the liver through gluconeogenesis from noncarbohydrate sources and by glycogenolysis. These factors include adrenal corticosteroids, epinephrine, and pituitary growth hormone. All these hormones also decrease peripheral utilization of glucose. Glucagon secreted by pancreatic alpha cells also has glycogenolytic action. These hormonal factors are elicited promptly in response to hypoglycemia.

Allergic reactions to insulin can be either local or systemic. Local allergic reactions include the formation of an erythematous area at the site of injection. This reaction appears within an hour and may persist for several days; it usually occurs within the first few days after initiation or reinstitution of insulin therapy, suggesting prior sensitization to beef or pork protein. Systemic allergy consists of angioedema, nausea, vomiting, diarrhea, bronchial asthma, and dyspnea. Hypotension, shock, and death are also produced occasionally. Systemic manifestations from therapeutic doses of insulin usually occur in patients having a history of allergic reactions to other drugs or those being treated with insulin intermittently. Occasionally, the patient must be desensitized with repeated injections of small amounts of insulin. Atrophy or hypertrophy of fat tissue at the site of frequent injections also may occur. To reduce the incidence of allergic reactions, it may be necessary to change to an insulin from a different source or to human insulin.

Adverse reactions attributable directly to insulin administration are due to two factors: (1) impurities in insulin preparations and (2) species of origin. These two factors are particularly important with respect to insulin allergenicity. Highly purified insulins are far less antigenic than impure insulins, and human insulin is less antigenic than porcine, which in turn is less antigenic than bovine. Price is still a factor; less pure bovine preparations are currently cheaper than highly purified human insulin, which is cheaper than highly purified porcine. With the commercial availability of human insulin, one would anticipate little clear evidence for the use of porcine insulin. Because of the high purity and the antigenicity, human insulin should categorically be prescribed to the following groups of patients: patients with true insulin allergy, patients with lipoatrophy, patients with insulin resistance states due to insulin antibodies, newly diagnosed patients, and pregnant diabetic patients.

Local infections due to improper sterilization of the injection site can also occur. However, local infections at injection site are uncommon today due to numerous bacteriostatic agents in commercially available insulin preparations.

Several hormones such as growth hormone, corticotropin, glucocorticoids, thyroid hormones, estrogens, progestogens, and glucagon act in various ways to inhibit the action of insulin. Also, epinephrine inhibits insulin secretion and stimulates glycogenolysis. Therefore, raising the plasma levels of these substances either endogenously or exogenously will increase the need for insulin.

Differential Diagnosis and Treatment of Hypoglycemia The symptoms of diabetic acidosis due to ketone-body production resulting from lack of effectiveness of insulin may be confused with those of severe insulin hypoglycemia, especially that due to the long-acting varieties of insulin. Intravenous glucose therapy should not be delayed while waiting for the results of laboratory findings. After withdrawal of blood for analysis, the first mode of therapy for an unconscious diabetic is glucose solution (50 percent) intravenously. If the patient does not improve and exhibits hyperglycemia and acidosis, this can be followed by insulin injection intravenously.

When a patient suffering from insulin-induced hypoglycemia is conscious, the patient should be given sugar-containing foods such as orange juice, sweet drinks, or lump sugar. It may take 30 to 45 min for an effect. For more severe degrees of hypoglycemia with unconsciousness, glucose intravenously is the treatment of choice. Glucagon, by injection, may also be used therapeutically for hypoglycemia. It is most often kept at home, so a family member may give the glucagon intramuscularly in an emergency.

GLUCAGON

Another pancreatic hormone, glucagon, is a protein composed of a single chain of amino acids. It is secreted by the alpha cells of the pancreas in response to hypoglycemia, is detectable in blood by radioimmunoassay at a level of about 500 pg/mL in the fasting state, and is destroyed by the liver. The main function of glucagon is to help maintain blood sugar levels by hepatic glycogenolysis. The marked hepatic overproduction of glucose and ketones that characterize uncontrolled diabetes appears to require both a deficiency of insulin and a relative excess of glucagon. When injected for hypoglycemia, glucagon acts by stimulating hepatic phosphorylases, and is effective within 15 min after intravenous infusion at a dosage level of 2 μg/min or 1 to 2 mg administered by the deep subcutaneous route.

Glucagon is also indicated as a diagnostic aid in the radiologic examination of the gastrointestinal tract when a hypotonic state is advantageous.

ORAL HYPOGLYCEMIC AGENTS

The sulfonylureas are orally effective hypoglycemic agents which may be useful in individuals with NIDDM (type II) who have some endogenous insulin secretion. When the sulfonylureas are employed, concomitant dietary regulation is of utmost importance in order to decrease obesity, which of its own accord will diminish insulin resistance.

Sulfonylurea Agents

The six sulfonylurea hypoglycemic agents in current use are subdivided into two groups. The first-generation agents, those exclusively available until the early 1980s, include tolbutamide, acetohexamide, tolazamide, and chlorpropamide. The second-generation agents, glyburide and glipizide, became commercially available in the United States in 1984. The sulfonylureas all have a common structure (Table 36-3). They therefore have the same mechanism of action. Various side chains alter their potency and pharmacokinetic profile.

Mechanism of Action   The action of the sulfonylurea drugs is to promote increased insulin secretion from pancreatic beta cells. In *acute* experiments, it has been shown repeatedly that the sulfonylureas markedly increase the plasma insulin level. This insulin rise results from direct stimulation of pancreatic beta cells to release insulin. This stimulating effect is dependent on the functional state of beta cell reserve. Since the action of the drugs requires a minimum amount of functioning beta cell tissue (at least 30 percent of normal), this effect does not occur in pancreatectomized individuals or in patients with an absolute deficiency of insulin (that is, type I diabetes). This mechanism appears to be the major factor early on for their therapeutic effectiveness in type II diabetes. In chronic therapy, the drugs also appear to reset the postreceptor defect. Another mechanism which may contribute to the hypoglycemic effect of these agents is suppression of glucagon release.

Pharmacokinetics   When administered orally, the sulfonylurea drugs are completely absorbed from the small intestine and appear in the systemic circulation within 1 to 2 h. However, these drugs have differences in their rates of absorption, biotransformation, and duration of action (Table 36-4). Close to 100 percent of tolbutamide is absorbed after oral administration, with 88 percent bound to plasma protein. Tolbutamide is rapidly biotransformed to inactive products. Most of the drug is excreted in the urine as carboxy- or hydroxymethyltolbutamide.

Acetohexamide is hydroxylated to a metabolite having 2.5 times the hypoglycemic activity. Therefore, its duration of action is considerably prolonged.

TABLE 36-3 Sulfonylureas

Generic name	Structural formula
Tolbutamide	
Chlorpropamide	
Acetohexamide	
Tolazamide	
Glyburide	
Glipizide	

Tolazamide is metabolized to products having weak hypoglycemic effect.

In contrast to tolbutamide, chlorpropamide is only slowly biotransformed to hydroxylated and hydrolyzed products and is mostly (80 to 90 percent) excreted in the urine unchanged. The amount excreted unchanged depends on the pH of the urine; alkalinization increases urinary excretion.

The second-generation oral hypoglycemic glipizide is biotransformed to inactive products, whereas glyburide yields weakly active metabolites. Glipizide's products are excreted primarily in the urine. Unlike other sulfonylureas, glyburide's products are excreted equally in the urine and bile. This is advantageous in patients with renal impairment to prevent buildup of the drug, which would produce excessive hypoglycemic effects.

Adverse Reactions The effectiveness and safety of the oral sulfonylureas has been questioned based on a study published in 1970. A group of 800 diabetics on tolbutamide and/or diet therapy compared with insulin and diet therapy were studied at 12 university medical centers for up to 8 years. The results of the controversial University Group Diabetes Program (UGDP) study were as follows: (1) combinations of diet plus tolbutamide are no more effective than diet alone in prolonging life; and (2) a higher mortality by cardio-

TABLE 36-4 Dose and pharmacokinetic properties of the sulfonylureas

	Tolbutamide	Acetohexamide	Tolazamide	Chlorpropamide	Glyburide	Glipizide
Usual dose, mg/day	1500	500	250	250	10	10
Dose range, mg/day	500–3000	250–1250	100–500	100–500	1.25–20	2.5–20
Biotransformation/ excretion	Liver inactive products	Liver active products	Liver mildly active	Liver inactive products	Liver weakly active	Liver inactive products
	Renal	Renal	Renal	Renal	Renal and bile	Renal
Biologic half-life, h	4–5	6–8	7	36	10	2–4
Onset of action, h	1–4	1–2	4–6	1–3	2–4	1–1.5
Peak hypoglycemic activity, h	4–6	3	4–8	4–6		
Duration of action, h	6–12	12–24	12–24	24–60	16–24	12–24

vascular disease from diet plus tolbutamide occurs than from diet alone or diet plus insulin. Though the study has been criticized by diabetologists for defective design, a warning of increased possibility of cardiovascular disease is included in the package insert of these agents.

Hypoglycemia is the most common untoward reaction to the sulfonylureas and occurs more frequently with chlorpropamide, the longest-acting agent. It is more prominently observed in patients given large doses, with impaired hepatic or renal function, and in patients failing to maintain a proper diet. The milder the diabetes and the more elderly is the patient, the greater is the possibility of hypoglycemia. A central nervous system syndrome of muscular weakness, vertigo, ataxia, and mental confusion has been described following administration of very high doses of these drugs. However, these effects on the CNS are reversible on withdrawal of the drug and are definitely related to dose. Gastrointestinal symptoms in susceptible individuals consist of heartburn, upper abdominal discomfort, nausea, lower abdominal cramps, and diarrhea. Exacerbation of peptic ulcer may occur. Accordingly, a history of gastrointestinal disease re-

quires low dosage or avoidance of sulfonylurea drug therapy.

Hypersensitivity reactions have been described with all the sulfonylurea drugs. The incidence is about 1 to 5 percent and may involve a variety of systems. Skin reactions consist of photosensitivity, erythema, and morbilliform or maculopapular rashes. The hematopoietic effects consisting of leukopenia, thrombocytopenia, pancytopenia, agranulocytosis, hemolytic anemia, and aplastic anemia have been rarely reported. The hepatic reaction may be a simple elevation of alkaline phosphatase (which may occur without drug therapy in diabetes) or cholestatic jaundice. These reactions usually occur within the first 6 to 8 weeks of therapy.

Drug Interactions Several drugs may antagonize or potentiate the hypoglycemic action of the sulfonylureas. Drugs that impair glucose tolerance by a variety of mechanisms antagonize the effectiveness of the sulfonylureas. These include corticosteroids, thyroid hormones, thiazide diuretics, furosemide, and oral contraceptives. Other drugs, such as phenylbutazone, clofibrate, dicumarol, and salicylates, potentiate the action of sulfonylureas, such as tolbutamide, by displacing them from plasma proteins or interfering with their biotransformation or excretion. Monoamine oxidase inhibitors (e.g., phenelzine, tranylcypromine) increase the hypoglycemic effect by reducing plasma glucose and by reducing hepatic metabolism of the drugs.

Minor disulfiram-like symptoms may develop when alcohol is ingested in the presence of sulfonylureas, because of the inhibition of intermediary biotransformation of alcohol. There can be an increased hypoglycemic effect with ingestion of alcohol, particularly in fasting individuals, as a result of the suppression of gluconeogenesis. Also, a decreased hypoglycemic effect may occur with chronic alcohol abuse because of the increased biotransformation of the sulfonylurea.

The sulfonylureas also interact with insulin, producing an exacerbated hypoglycemic effect.

Therapy of Diabetes Mellitus In type I, insulin-dependent diabetics, insulin must be administered to maintain life. In addition, maintenance of proper body weight through low-calorie diet and physical exercise is important and must be regimented to maintain a normoglycemic state, reducing complications of the disease. In type II, noninsulin-dependent diabetics, an effort must be made to regulate the disease through diet and weight reduction alone. If a drug must be added, the physician has a choice of insulin or one of the sulfonylureas.

Warnings The sulfonylurea drugs should not be used alone for the management of patients with an absolute or severe deficiency in endogenous insulin action. Such patients are prone to ketoacidosis and constitute the type I diabetics. The use of sulfonylureas is contraindicated in the presence of ketosis or complications likely to increase severity of the diabetes. Following surgical intervention, except for minor procedures, sulfonylureas must be supplemented by or replaced with insulin. The long half-life of chlorpropamide makes it necessary to stop the drug at least 2 days prior to a major surgical procedure. If an emergency surgical procedure precludes this, provision must be made for continuous postoperative intravenous therapy with glucose-containing solutions for a similar period. The sulfonylureas should not be used in nondiabetic patients with renal glycosuria because of hyperresponsiveness causing prolonged or fatal hypoglycemia. They are also contraindicated in the treatment of prediabetes and subclinical diabetes. The sulfonylurea drugs should be used with great caution or not at all in the presence of peptic ulcer, extensive hepatic disease, or renal disease. Though these drugs have not yet been found to be teratogenic, they may not be used in pregnancy, since their safety has not yet been established. Similarly, consideration should be given to the possible hazards of their use in women of childbearing age who might become pregnant.

Preparations and Doses *Chlorpropamide* (Diabinese) is supplied in tablets of 100 and 250 mg for oral use. The recommended dose is 100 to 500 mg/day given as a single dose.

Tolazamide (Tolinase) is supplied in tablets of 100, 250, and 500 mg for oral use. The recommended dose is 100 to 500 mg/day.

Acetohexamide (Dymelor) is supplied in tablets of 250 and 500 mg for oral use. The recommended dose is 250 to 1250 mg/day.

Tolbutamide (Orinase) is supplied in tablets of 250 and 500 mg for oral use. The recommended dose is 500 to 300 mg/day in divided doses.

Glyburide (Diabeta, Micronase) is supplied in 1.25-, 2.5-, and 5.0-mg tablets for oral use. The recommended dose is 1.25 to 20 mg/day.

Glipizide (Glucotrol) is supplied in 5- and 10-mg tablets for oral use. The recommended dose is 2.5 to 20 mg/day.

BIBLIOGRAPHY

Binder, C., et al.: "Insulin Pharmacokinetics," *Diabetes Care,* **7:**188 (1984).

Boyden, T., and R. Bressler: "Oral Hypoglycemic Agents," *Adv. Intern. Med.,* **24:**53–70 (1979).

Cader Asmal, A., and A. Marble: "Oral Hypoglycaemic Agents: Update," *Drugs,* **28:**62–78 (1984).

Fajans, S. S., and J. W. Con: In B. S. Leibel and S. G. Wrenshall (eds.), *On the Nature and Treatment of Diabetes,* Excerpta Medica Foundation, New York, 1965, pp. 641–656.

Feldman, J. M.: "Glyburide: Second-Generation Sulfonylurea Hypoglycemic Agent; History, Chemistry, Metabolism, Pharmacokinetics, Clinical Use and Adverse Effects," *Pharmacotherapy,* **5:**43–62 (1985).

Freinkel, N., et al.: "Care of Pregnant Woman with Insulin-Dependent Diabetes Mellitus," *N. Engl. J. Med.,* **313:**96–101 (1985).

Jacobs, S., and P. Cuatrecasas: "Insulin Receptors," *Ann. Rev. Pharmacol. Toxicol.*, **23**:461 (1983).

Karam, J. H.: "Pancreatic Hormones and Antidiabetic Drugs," in B. C. Katzung (ed.), *Basic and Clinical Pharmacology*, pp. 484–496. American Diabetes Association: "Policy Statement: Glycemic Effects of Carbohydrates," *Diabetes Care*, **7**:607–608 (1984).

Kreisberg, R. A.: "The Second-Generation Sulfonylureas: Change or Progress?," *Ann. Intern. Med.*, **102**:126 (1985).

Lebovitz, H. E.: "Glipizide: Second-Generation Sulfonylurea Hypoglycemic Agent: Pharmacology, Pharmacokinetics and Clinical Use," *Pharmacotherapy*, **5**:53–77 (1985).

Lockwood, D. H., J. E. Gerich, and I. Goldfine (eds.): "Symposium on Effects of Oral Hypoglycemic Agents on Receptor and Postreceptor Actions of Insulin," *Diabetes Care*, **7** (**Suppl. 1**):1 (1984).

Melander, A., and E. Wahlen-Bohl: "Clinical Pharmacology of Glipizide," *Am. J. Med.*, **75** (**Suppl. 5B**):41 (1983).

Paice, B. J., et al.: "Undesired effects of Sulphonylurea Drugs," *Adv. Drug React. Acc. Pois. Rev.*, **1**:23–36 (1985).

Pedersen, O., and H. Beck-Neilsen: "Insulin Resistance and Insulin-Dependent Diabetes Mellitus," *Diabetes Care*, **10**:516–523 (1987).

Seltzer, H. S.: "Efficacy and Safety of Oral Hypoglycemic Agents," *Ann. Rev. Med.*, **31**:261–272 (1980).

Shen, S. W., and R. Bressler: "Clinical Pharmacology of Oral Antidiabetic Agents," part 2, *N. Engl. J. Med.*, **296**:787–793 (1977).

Teutsch, S. M., et al.: "Mortality among Diabetic Patients Using Continuous Subcutaneous Insulin-Infusion Pumps," *N. Engl. J. Med.*, **310**:361–368 (1984).

University Group Diabetes Program Study: *Diabetes*, **19** (**Suppl. 2**):747–830 (1970).

Williams, H. E., and C. E. Becker (eds.): *Endocrine Disorders: Clinical Pharmacology*, MacMillian, New York, 1978, pp. 515–546.

C H A P T E R **37**

Female Sex Hormones, Oral Contraceptives, and Fertility Agents

Delphine B. Bartosik

Few areas in biology offer such an intuitively obvious picture of drug effects as is apparent with the effects of steroid sex hormones. In this chapter, basic features of estrogens, progestins, and their combined effects, as seen in oral contraceptives, will be reviewed. In addition, several fertility agents of disparate mechanisms will be discussed: hypothalamic peptides (LHRH and congeners), gonadotropins (human menopausal gonadotropins, HMG, and human chorionic gonadotropin, HCG), antiestrogens (clomiphene and tamoxifen), and inhibitors of prolactin secretion (bromocriptine). In order to understand more fully the pharmacology of the female sex hormones and related compounds, we review the physiology of the monthly menstrual cycle.

MENSTRUAL CYCLE

The menstrual cycle is a repetitive ovulatory sequence with a mean duration of 28 days. It is commonly divided into two phases, a *follicular* (proliferative) phase commencing on the first day of menstruation and a *luteal* (secretory) phase beginning just prior to ovulation. The pituitary hormones involved with ovarian stimulation and function are follicle-stimulating hormone (FSH) and luteinizing hormone (LH). Figure 37-1 illustrates the variation in hormonal levels during a typical cycle.

Pituitary gonadotropin secretion is regulated by the episodic pulsatile release of hypothalamic LH-releasing hormone (LHRH) into the hypophyseal portal veins. There are LHRH receptors on pituitary cells

specialized to secrete the glycoprotein hormones FSH and LH. These gonadotropic hormones, in turn, promote both steroid hormone production and the requisite growth and delivery of gametes to achieve reproduction, including follicular growth, ovulation, corpus luteum maintenance, and maintenance of early pregnancy. Overall control mechanisms are homologous in males and females. This discussion will be confined to the female.

The first events in the ovarian cycle are initiated by FSH. Early in the cycle FSH brings about stimulation of follicle growth and enlargement of the ovum itself, along with increased proliferation of granulosa and theca cells. The theca interna cells produce estrogen under the influence of LH. In addition, FSH increases the amount of fluid in the graafian follicle to form the mature follicle.

As the follicle matures, it secretes increasing amounts of estrogen; when the appropriate level of estrogen is achieved, a brief excessive release of LH occurs. Ovulation takes place on day 14, approximately 36 h after the onset of the LH surge. The combined action of FSH and LH is needed for rupture and liberation of the ovum from the follicle. The liberated follicle then undergoes certain changes to form the corpus luteum; this is followed by the elaboration of progesterone by the granulosa cells. Again, estrogen continues to be released from the theca cells.

LH maintains the functioning of the corpus luteum for approximately 10 days postovulation. If fertilization does not take place, the corpus luteum will begin

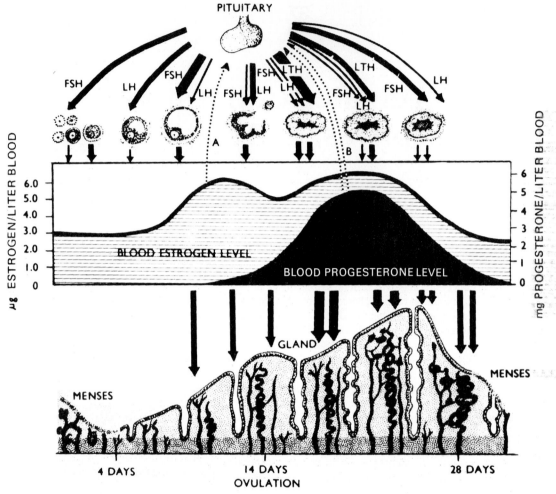

FIGURE 37-1 Variations in pituitary and ovarian hormone secretion, and endometrial morphology during the menstrual cycle. The top graph demonstrates the alterations in FSH and LH concentrations during the cycle in relation to effects on the follicle. The bottom graph shows the level of blood estrogen and progesterone as related to glandular secretions.

to reduce hormone production and eventually cease functioning altogether. The onset of menses will then follow at about the twenty-eighth day of the cycle.

Simultaneously with ovulation in the ovary, the endometrium of the uterus manifests cyclic alterations. These changes result from the influence of estrogen and progesterone on the tissues. In the first part of the cycle, as estrogen is being secreted, the endometrium enters its proliferative phase (approximately

11 days). During this phase the tissue increases in thickness, with progressive growth of glandular and vascular elements. Under the combined influence of estrogen and progesterone on the endometrium following ovulation, the secretory phase (approximately 13 days) is established. During this period there is further development of blood vessels and glandular structures, and an elaboration of the contents of the glandular epithelial cells. If implantation of a fertilized ovum

does not occur, the levels of progesterone and estrogen gradually decrease. The endometrium then begins to undergo desquamation, and menses ensue.

If the egg is fertilized, the syncytiotrophoblast is the source of production of a new series of protein substances, among which is HCG. One of the many effects of HCG is to prolong the secretory life span of the corpus luteum for the duration of pregnancy. Beyond the first trimester of pregnancy, the progesterone production by the placenta is many times that produced by the corpus luteum, the latter being unnecessary for the maintenance of normal pregnancy in the human being.

The entire ovary is capable of synthesizing three classes of steroid hormones: progesterone (C-21), androstenedione (C-19), and estradiol (C-18). Plasma low-density lipoprotein (LDL) cholesterol is the major source of steroidogenic cholesterol from which the steroids are derived. The overall steroidogenic pathways are presented in Fig. 37-2.

Cholesterol liberated from LDL apoproteins is transported to mitochondria, where side-chain cleavage takes place, releasing pregnenolone (C-21). This occurs in all steroidogenic tissue and is, in general, regulated by LH in the gonads and adrenocorticotrophic hormone (ACTH) in the adrenal cortex.

Progesterone is derived from pregnenolone by the action of Δ5-3β-ol-dehydrogenase-Δ4-5-isomerase (3β-HSD). The enzymes which subsequently metabolize progesterone are found in interstitial cells and theca cells. There is a dual enzyme complex which produces 17α-hydroxyprogesterone and Δ4-androstenedione. The Δ4-androstenedione can be metabolized either to testosterone or to estrone. Aromatase catalyzes the conversion of androstenedione to estrone and testosterone to estradiol.

ESTROGENS

Chemistry and Synthesis

Estrogen is a general term used to describe chemical compounds which have estrogenic activity. Estrogens can be divided into two chemical categories: those with a steroid nucleus and those without one. Endogenous estrogens, some synthetic estrogens, the nonsteroidal estrogens, and antiestrogens of major interest are illustrated in Fig. 37-3.

17β-Estradiol is an 18-carbon, cyclopentanophenanthrene molecule with an aromatic ring and a hydroxyl group in the C-17 position. It is the major estrogen synthesized and secreted by the normal human ovary. The oxidized derivative, estrone, is also secreted by the premenopausal ovary, but in much smaller quantities.

Biosynthesis of 17β-estradiol from cholesterol takes place in both granulosa and theca cells of the follicular ovary and in the human corpus luteum. The complete enzymatic pathway for estrogen biosynthesis (cholesterol to estrogen) is not present in the placenta. Nevertheless, it can transform C-19 steroids of fetal and maternal origin to estrogen.

Gonadotropic regulation of ovarian estrogen production involves the "steroidogenic" hormone LH, which enhances the rate of cholesterol conversion to pregnenolone. Within the follicular apparatus, the theca interna cells produce the C-19 precursors which are aromatized to estradiol. The granulosa cell aromatase enzyme system is induced by FSH. The capacity to aromatize (C-19) androgens efficiently determines which follicle will become the dominant follicle and, therefore, ovulate.

A variety of tissues such as fat, muscle, liver, skin, endometrium, and even hypothalamus also have the aromatase enzyme system necessary to transform C-19 steroids to estrogen. Fat is an important locus of total estrogen production in obese postmenopausal patients. Androgens secreted by the adrenals are aromatized in fat to estrone.

Estriol is a major metabolite of estradiol in which an additional hydroxyl group is added in the 16 position of the steroid nucleus. This takes place in the liver. In the fetoplacental unit, estriol is produced through a series of steps in which dehydroepiandrosterone, produced by the fetal adrenal gland is hydroxylated in the fetal liver and aromatized to estriol in the placenta.

Conjugating estradiol with straight-chain fatty acids results in a marked prolongation of the half-life of these estrogens and, therefore, in the marked enhancement of their biologic activity. Parenteral administration of short-chain fatty acid conjugates of estradiol (cypionate and valerate) have been used for many years for long-term estrogen replacement therapy.

Mechanism of Action

The hormonal actions of estrogens on target tissues are based on a multistep mechanism involving specific estrogen receptors. Estrogen is transported to target tis-

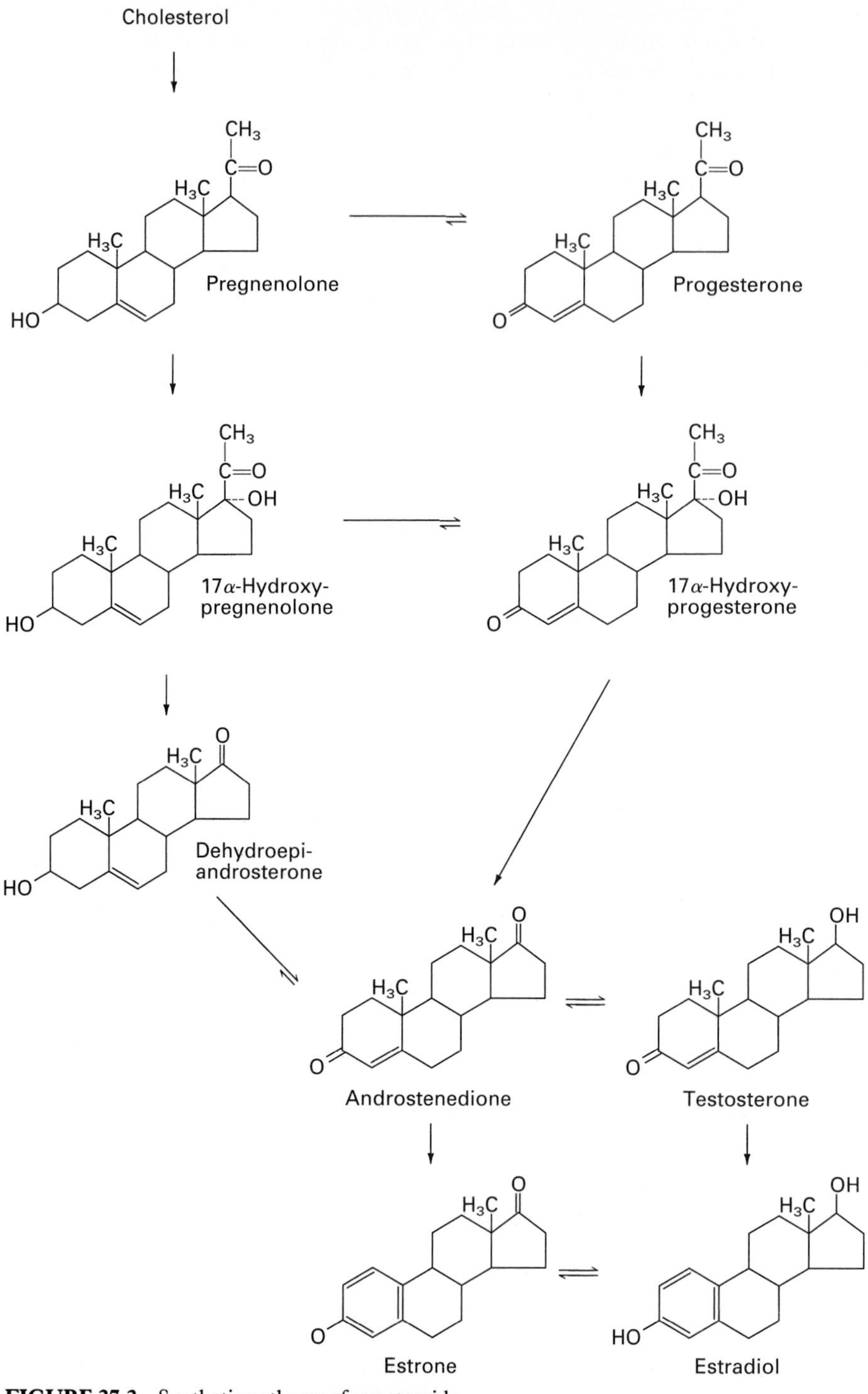

FIGURE 37-2 Synthetic pathway of sex steroids.

ENDOGENOUS ESTROGENS

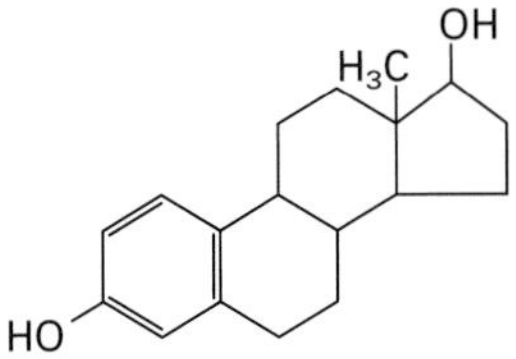

Estradiol

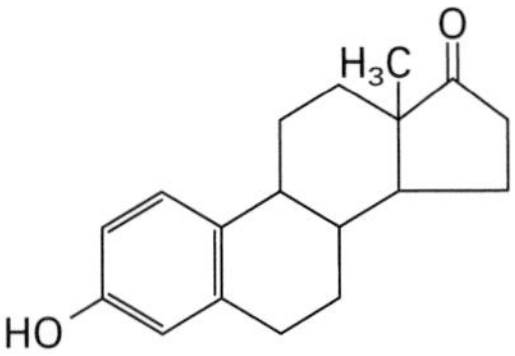

Estrone

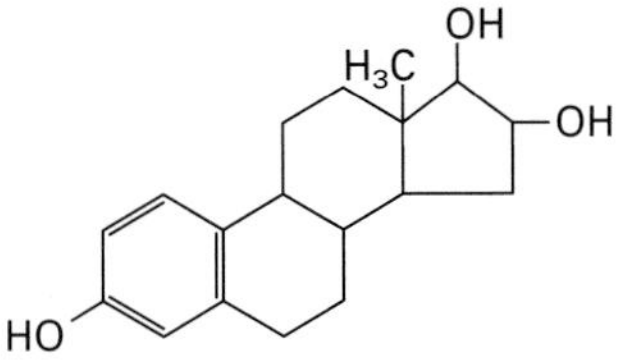

Estriol

SYNTHETIC, STEROIDAL

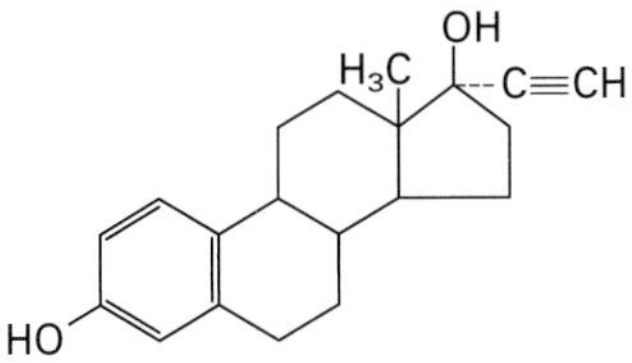

Ethinyl estradiol

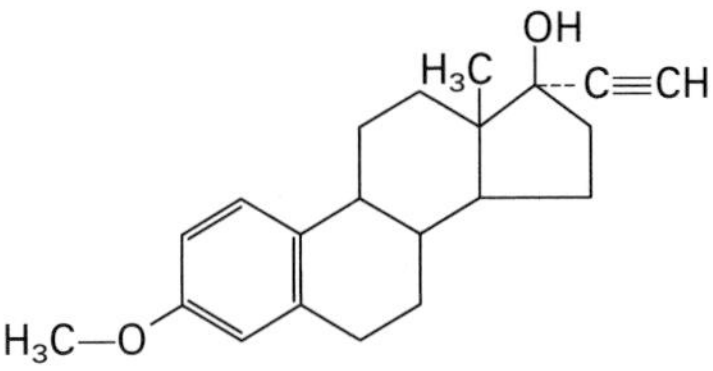

Mestranol

SYNTHETIC, NONSTEROIDAL

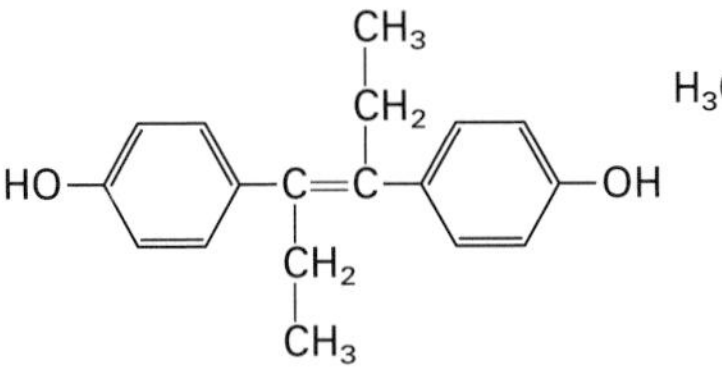

Diethylstilbestrol

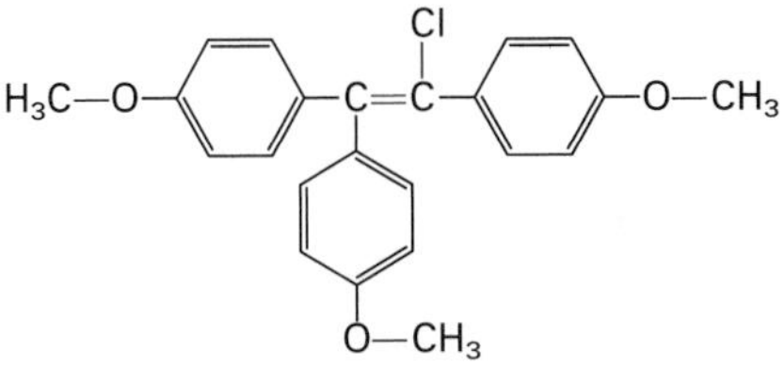

Chlorotrianisene

ANTIESTROGENS

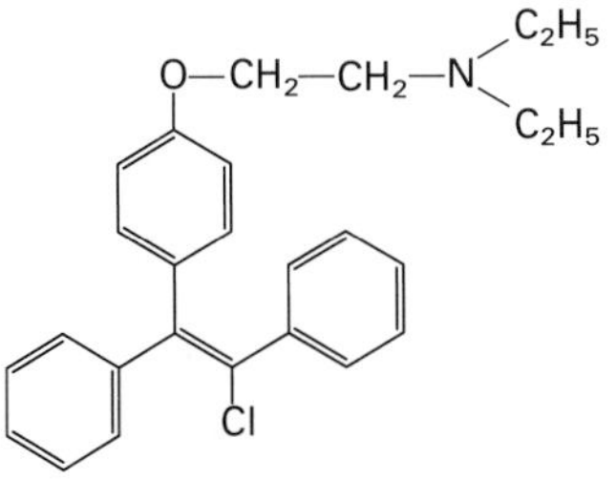

Clomiphene

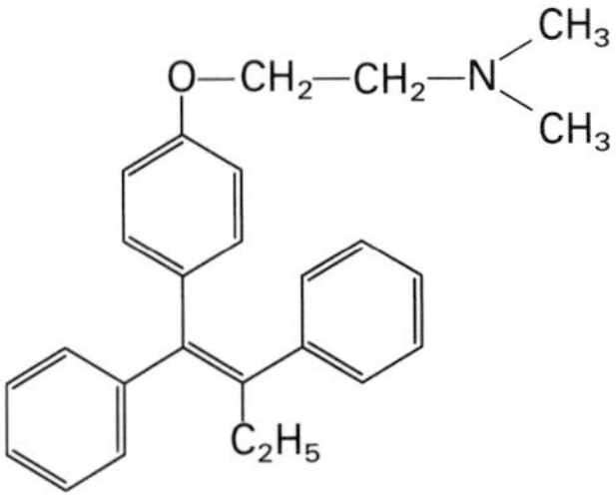

Tamoxifen

FIGURE 37-3   Structural formulas of endogenous and clinically important estrogens and antiestrogens.

sues in a protein-bound form and subsequently diffuses into the cell as free estrogen. The estrogen then binds to cytoplasmic estrogen receptors, each containing two receptor subunits (A and B). When estrogen binds to both subunits, a conformational change occurs, resulting in translocation of the estrogen-receptor complex to the nucleus.

Upon entering the nucleus, the complex binds through the B subunit to a nonhistone protein on specific nuclear DNA acceptor sites which are important for gene regulatory effects. This newly formed complex allows for dissociation of the two subunits, transport of the A subunit to DNA, which activates the RNA polymerase to transcribe new messenger RNA and hence new protein synthesis. The steroid receptor complex eventually dissociates from the acceptor sites, with some of the receptors being reused.

Effects of Estrogen on Organ Systems

Estrogen has divergent actions on different tissues in the body. The endometrium is the most dramatically responsive of the tissues affected by cyclical changes of ovarian hormones. The secretion of estradiol during the ovarian follicular phase induces proliferation of the glands and stroma of the endometrium. At puberty, the fallopian tubes, uterus, cervix, and vagina each respond to estrogen by growth and maturation of the muscle and epithelial elements.

Also at puberty, estrogen induces an increase in size of the breasts by stimulating growth and development of the epithelial ducts. Estrogen acts by binding to breast tissue in a manner analogous to its binding in the uterus. Prolactin is necessary for the development of estrogen receptors in the breast. In addition to important effects at puberty, estrogens help maintain secondary sex characteristics and influence plasma lipids in adults.

The role of steroid sex hormones in the pubertal growth of bone is poorly understood. Estrogen is believed to stimulate pubertal growth by increasing production of an insulin-like growth factor. Estrogen deprivation, either because of ovarectomy or menopause, results in accelerated osteoporosis.

The synthesis of many proteins is markedly increased by estrogens. Among these are hormone-binding globulins, including thyroid-, corticosteroid-, vitamin D–, and sex hormone–binding globulins.

Each of these globulins increase in a dose-dependent manner. Several clotting factors, renin substrate (angiotensinogen), and renin are also increased by estrogen administration.

Lipid metabolism and fat deposition are affected by estrogens; high-density lipoprotein (HDL) concentrations in plasma are elevated. The fact that HDL cholesterol levels are higher in premenopausal females as compared to similarly aged males is believed to contribute to the protected state of younger women from coronary heart disease.

Finally, estrogens can promote sodium retention, with associated fluid retention and edema. This is more likely to occur when only high doses of estrogen are used. However, the effects of estrogen upon fluid retention are less severe than are those following testosterone or glucocorticoid therapy.

Pharmacokinetics

Estrogens are absorbed via the skin and mucous membranes as well as from subcutaneous and intramuscular sites. Esterification of estrogen can be used to delay the rate of absorption from parenteral sites. Systemic effects may occur from direct absorption through the skin.

Oral administration of estrogens results in rapid absorption from the gastrointestinal tract. However, the hormone is carried directly to the liver, where it is readily inactivated. Minor structural changes, such as the presence of an ethinyl group at position 17 results in decreased rate of liver inactivation. When estradiol is administered (as the micronized preparation), it is almost completely converted to estrone prior to absorption. The transdermal route is being used in estrogen replacement therapy and appears to be a safe and effective method.

The physiologically active and major estrogen in the body is 17β-estradiol. Estrogens circulate in the blood in both conjugated and unconjugated forms. Estrogenic steroids are generally conjugated through the hydroxyl group at C-3 with inorganic sulfate or glucuronic acid. Conjugation takes place in the liver.

The estrogens are highly bound to plasma proteins (50 to 80 percent). Only the unbound or "free" estrogens are biologically active. Conjugated steroids are more water-soluble, and thus their excretion into the urine is facilitated.

Large amounts of estrogen in the free form are also excreted by the liver in the bile. An enterohepatic circulation of estrogens exists in which estrogens conjugated in the liver are excreted in the bile, hydrolyzed within the gastrointestinal tract, and reabsorbed.

There are many other transformations of estradiol which take place in the liver, such as hydroxylation in the 2 position of estrogen, resulting in dramatic decreases in the bioactivity of estrogen. Hydroxylation in the 16 position of estriol maintains a bioactive compound. These factors have been shown to be of considerable biologic and clinical significance.

Conjugating estrogens with straight-chain fatty acids results in a marked prolongation of the biologic activity of these estrogens. These "conjugated estrogens," because of their extremely long half-lives and increased bioactivity, may be involved in the development of endometrial and/or breast cancer.

Diethylstilbestrol, a nonsteroidal compound, is orally active and has a relatively long duration of action. Following oral administration, it is slowly biotransformed in the liver, with its metabolites excreted by the kidney.

Adverse Reactions

The adverse effects of estrogens are either dose-related or dependent on prolonged estrogen administration without concomitant use of cyclic progestogens. Adverse reactions include nausea, chloasma, vaginal infections, mucoid leukorrhea, and edema. Therapy can result in endometrial hyperplasias and carcinomas, but much more frequently will result in abnormal vaginal bleeding. The major lethal effects of estrogens are related to their effects on the coagulation-fibrinolytic system with resultant thromboembolic phenomena. Estrogens enhance coagulation by promoting synthesis of factors II, VII, IX, and X. Other adverse reactions will be discussed in conjunction with the use of oral contraceptives.

It has been reported that diethylstilbestrol (DES), given in large doses to women early in pregnancy, leads to vaginal adenocarcinoma in female offspring after puberty. It is not known whether other estrogens may cause similar effects. However, this has limited the use of DES to treatment of cancer and is contraindicated in pregnant women.

There are several strong contraindications to estrogen replacement therapy; these include estrogen-dependent malignancy, undiagnosed abnormal vaginal bleeding, thrombophlebitis, thromboembolic phenomena, cerebral vascular disease or coronary occlusive disease, estrogen-induced hypertension, markedly impaired liver function, history of obstructive jaundice of pregnancy, and congenital hyperlipidemias. These conditions are discussed in more detail in the section on oral contraceptives.

Therapeutic Uses

Estrogen replacement therapy is used in agonadal, menopausal, and hypothalamic amenorrheic states (i.e., in primary hypogonadism and hormonal therapy in postmenopausal women). Estrogens commonly used for hormone replacement therapy are presented in Table 37-1.

As in other clinical endocrine disorders, once the diagnosis of hypoestrogenism is established, replacement therapy is recommended. There are several special considerations for estrogen replacement therapy. First, in the normal younger woman estrogen is secreted on a daily basis. Therefore, administration of estrogens for only 21 to 25 days can frequently result in estrogen deprivation symptoms, such as hot flashes, irritability, and insomnia. Optimal physiologic estrogen replacement therapy should utilize daily estrogen administration, in conjunction with monthly 14-day courses of progestins. Any abnormal vaginal bleeding is investigated by physical examination, pap smear, and endometrial sampling.

A special indication exists for the administration of very large doses of intravenous estrogens; an occasional patient with dysfunctional uterine bleeding may have life-threatening hemorrhage. The problem may be controlled by intravenous administration of "conjugated estrogen."

In patients being treated for acute painful osteoporosis, large doses of estrogen are started. There will be a clinical response in terms of decreased back pain within days and/or weeks. Once this effect is accomplished, the dose can be decreased.

Ethinyl estradiol, in extremely large doses, is used as a "morning after" contraceptive. There is a significant reduction in the expected pregnancy rate when estrogen is administered within 24 to 72 h after an isolated unprotected coital exposure has been reported.

TABLE 37-1 Estrogens of clinical importance for hormone replacement therapy

Orally active preparations	
"Conjugated estrogens"*	0.3–2.5 mg/day
Estrone sulfate*,†	0.3–2.5 mg/day
Ethinyl estradiol	0.02–0.05 mg/day
Mestranol‡	0.02–0.05 mg/day
Micronized estradiol	1–2 mg/day

Parenteral preparations	
"Conjugated estrogens"	25 mg once only (IV)
Estradiol cypionate	2–5 mg every 2–4 wks (IM)
Estradiol valerate	2–20 mg every 2–4 wks (IM)

Vaginal estrogen preparations	
Estradiol vaginal cream	2–4 g/day
Dienestrol vaginal cream	1–2 applicators full/day

Nonsteroidal estrogens	
Diethylstilbestrol	0.1–0.5 mg/day
Quinestrol	0.1–0.2 mg/day

Transdermal ("the patch")	
Estradiol	0.5 or 0.1 mg/patch (change twice/week)

*Average replacement dose is 0.9 to 1.25 mg/day.
†This preparation is available as the piperazine salt. It is also called estropipate.
‡Available in the United States only in oral contraceptives.

ANTIESTROGENS

Clomiphene citrate and tamoxifen are orally active, nonsteroidal compounds related to diethylstilbestrol (Fig. 37-3). In some bioassays these are weak estrogens but, more importantly, they act as antiestrogens.

Tamoxifen (Nolvadex) Tamoxifen is a competitive inhibitor of estradiol. It is used in the palliative treatment of estrogen-receptor positive breast cancer. It should be used in conjunction with chemotherapeutic agents more effective in killing rather than suppressing the cancer cells.

Tamoxifen is absorbed from the gastrointestinal tract following oral administration. Peak plasma levels are reached in 4 to 7 h. The initial plasma half life is 7 to 14 h. Most of the drug is conjugated in the liver, then excreted by the kidney. Less than 30 percent is excreted unchanged or hydroxylated. The drug undergoes enterohepatic recirculation. Tamoxifen is given in doses of 10 to 20 mg twice a day. The most common adverse reactions include nausea or vomiting and hot flashes. Other estrogen-type side effects occur, but are much less common.

Clomiphene (Clomid) Clomiphene acts by enhancing new follicular growth with resultant ovulation. The drug attaches to cytosolic estrogen receptors, but the clomiphene-receptor complex does not bind to nuclear acceptors for estrogen. This is interpreted by the hypothalamus as a hypoestrogenic state. The hypothalamic response is the increased secretion of LHRH, which enhances gonadotropin secretion. The increased FSH and LH secretion initiates sequential follicular growth and ovulation.

Clomiphene is administered orally. It has a long half-life; only about one-half of an ingested dose is excreted in 5 days. The drug is eliminated primarily in the feces, with small amounts in the urine. Some of its antiestrogenic effects may persist for weeks.

The major indication for clomiphene use is ovulation induction on anovulatory women who have some basal estrogen production. It works much less effectively in hypoestrogenic anovulatory disorders such as hypothalamic amenorrhea. Clomiphene is used to enhance the fertility of women who are oligo-ovulators; that is, if a woman has three or four ovulatory cycles per year, her fertility will be enhanced by ovulating on a monthly basis. Clomiphene is also used to gain predictability of ovulations in women undergoing artificial insemination. Ovulation induction is most commonly accomplished by administering 50-mg tablets per day from the fifth through the ninth day of the menstrual cycle.

Since an expected effect of clomiphene is follicular growth, higher doses may induce the growth of multicystic ovaries. There is a reported 8 to 10 percent incidence of twins with this drug, but multiple births of more than two babies are considered rare. Ovarian cysts may occur in 5 to 15 percent of patients. Massive cystic enlargement of the ovaries is a rare but serious side effect. When clomiphene induces ovulation, it has been shown to reduce the length of the luteal phase in some patients. This luteal-phase deficiency can be treated by administration of human chorionic gonadotropin or progesterone.

Other adverse reactions include menopausal-type hot flashes, headaches, occasional reversible hair loss, and less commonly gastrointestinal distress and breast engorgement. Symptoms are reversible when therapy is discontinued.

PROGESTINS

The term *progestin* (or progestogen) includes progesterone and other compounds which share its physiologic action.

Progesterone is the active hormone secreted by the steroidogenic tissues, corpus luteum and placenta. It is ineffective when given orally because of extensive metabolism before reaching the peripheral circulation. It must therefore be administered parenterally or transvaginally, usually in the form of suppositories.

The major orally active progestins were developed for use in oral contraceptives. Subsequently, these effects were shown to be mediated through suppression at the hypothalamic-pituitary level.

Progestins induce secretory changes in the uterine glandular epithelium and decidual changes in the stroma. Normal menstruation ensues when the corpus luteum stops producing progesterone approximately 14 days after ovulation. Progestational agents given about 6 to 7 days after ovulation and continued for 3 or more weeks will result in a delay of menstruation until 2 to 3 days after the hormone is stopped.

Chemistry

The structures of several progestins are presented in Fig. 37-4. Progesterone loses much of its biologic activity by adding a hydroxyl group to the C-17 position.

Esterifying this hydroxyl group with a long-chain fatty acid such as caproic acid results in a long-acting progestin by parenteral administration (27-hydroxyprogesterone caproate).

Progestins derived from nortestosterone may have higher androgenic properties than those derived from the C-21 steroid nucleus. Norethindrone, the C-17 ethinyl derivative, is a very powerful progestin.

Mechanism of Action

Progesterone acts on steroid receptors similarly to the way estrogens do. The progesterone-receptor complex translocates to the nucleus, where it stimulates production of specific mRNA and, hence, specific protein synthesis. Estrogen appears to induce an increase in the number of progesterone receptors. Conversely, progesterone decreases the content and/or the biologic efficacy of estrogen receptors in the target tissues.

Pharmacokinetics

Progesterone is absorbed following oral administration but is extensively metabolized and conjugated in the liver. Its metabolic clearance rate is approximately 2100 L/day, while the hepatic blood flow is about 1500 L/day, suggesting an extrahepatic clearance. Progesterone binds to corticosteroid-binding globulin; the physiologic significance of this is unclear. It is also bound to plasma albumin.

The major metabolites of progesterone are 2-α-dihydroprogesterone and pregnanediol. The latter is excreted in the urine as the monoglucosiduronate, and its measurement has been used to assess corpus luteum function because it reflects about 10 percent of the progesterone production rates.

The clinical situations in which progesterone itself must be given, instead of other progestins, are those in which an embryo or fetus could be affected or harmed by the other drugs. In these situations, progesterone must be given either as an intramuscular injection or as a vaginal suppository.

Pharmacodynamics

The physiologically important effects of progesterone occur on estrogen primed tissues. These effects include the induction of secretory endometrium and

A. Progestins derived from (C-21) progesterone

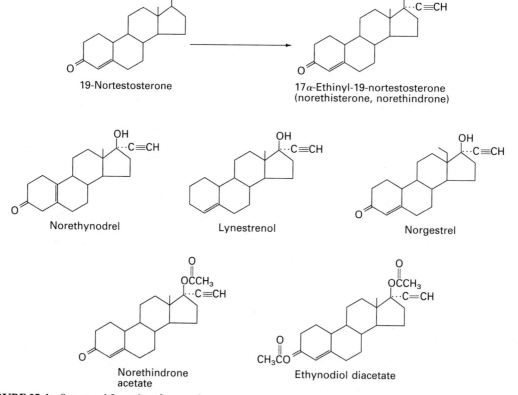

B. Progestins derived from (C-18) 19-nortestosterone

FIGURE 37-4 Structural formulas of progestins.

decreased myometrial contractility of the uterus. They are essential for early implantation of the embryo and maintenance of pregnancy to term. Progesterone withdrawal is an important part of the mechanism necessary for the initiation of labor.

Progesterone induces an elevation of basal body temperature, a thermogenic action which is clinically useful in detecting ovulation. In the breast, progesterone stimulates growth of alveolar epithelium and is necessary for the prolactin-mediated postpartum induction of lactation. Progesterone stimulates respiration and reduces the arterial P_{CO_2}.

The role of progesterone in fluid and water balance is contradictory, since many patients describe "fluid retention" with progestins, yet progesterone appears to stimulate urinary sodium excretion by antagonizing the effects of aldosterone on the distal tubule of the kidney.

The effects of individual progestins are best considered in conjunction with coadministration of estrogens in oral contraceptive medications.

Clinical Uses

Many progestins are of clinical importance (Table 37-2). Their uses are discussed below.

The "progestin challenge test" is extremely useful in the differential diagnosis of "amenorrhea" in a wide variety of clinical conditions. Once pregnancy is excluded, progestin is administered daily for 10 to 14 days. As in physiologic menstruation, vaginal bleeding begins 1 to 3 days after blood progestin levels fall. However, if estrogen production is absent or if the endometrium has been destroyed by disease, progestin is ineffective in inducing vaginal bleeding.

Progestins are also useful in therapy of dysfunctional uterine bleeding. Anovulatory women will not have a luteal phase in their menstrual cycles: this presents as "dysfunctional uterine bleeding" during adolescence and perimenopausal times of life. Dysfunctional uterine bleeding during adolescence is a chronic condition in which the patient fails to have an LH surge and does not ovulate. This may self-correct as

TABLE 37-2   Progestins of clinical importance

Progesterone and derivatives	Preparations available
Progesterone	Aqueous suspension, 25 & 50 mg/mL; in oil, 25 & 50 mg/mL; suppositories, 25–200 mg
17 α-Hydroxy-progesterone caproate	125 & 250 mg/mL
Medroxyprogesterone acetate	2.5- & 10-mg tablets in oil, 50 & 100 mg/mL
Megestrol acetate	20- & 40-mg tablets

19-Nortestosterone derivatives	
Norethindrone	0.35- & 5-mg tablets
Norethindrone acetate	5-mg tablets
Norethynodrel	Only available in oral contraceptives
Ethynodiol diacetate	Only available in oral contraceptives
dl-Norgestrel	0.075-mg tablets and oral contraceptives
l-Norgestrel	Only available in oral contraceptives

the patient's hypothalamic-pituitary-ovarian axis matures. The patient may exhibit irregular and often heavy vaginal bleeding. This bleeding can be completely controlled by administering orally active progestins. In patients with occasional dysfunctional uterine bleeding and life-threatening vaginal hemorrhage, one of two therapies of progesterone may stop bleeding and could avoid a surgical D & C (dilatation and curretage).

The mechanism for perimenopausal dysfunctional uterine bleeding is probably inadequate follicular growth, perhaps insufficient FSH receptors present on the follicles, and decreasing numbers of primary follicles within the aging ovary. Once cancer of the cervix or endometrium is excluded, this condition can be controlled by cyclic progestin therapy.

When postmenopausal estrogen replacement therapy is begun in a woman with an intact uterus, cyclic progestin therapy must also be started. This results in regular shedding of a progestin-matured endometrium and reduces the development of endometrial hyperplasia and carcinoma which occurs in an unacceptably high proportion of women given "unopposed" cyclic estrogen therapy.

Certain patients with premenstrual syndrome experience substantial symptomatic improvement with the administration of cyclic progestin. Cyclic therapy with vaginal progesterone suppositories is the most commonly used. However, medroxyprogesterone acetate or norethindrone acetate may also be tried. Symptoms of premenstrual syndrome in occasional patients may be markedly worsened by any of these individual progestins.

In contrast to the cyclic progestin therapy described above, continuous progestin therapy has been used in the treatment of two conditions: endometriosis and endometrial carcinoma. Endometriosis is a condition in which endometrial tissue is growing in ectopic or abnormal places, most commonly in the cul-de-sac or on the uterosacral ligaments. This condition is associated with menstrual pain, other pelvic pain, and infertility. The ectopic endometrial tissue is dependent for its proliferation on ovarian estrogen production or, after ovarectomy, on exogenous estrogen. Long-term administration (at least 6 months) of continuous progestin induces prolonged amenorrhea, resulting in resorption of the ectopic endometrium, presumably by peritoneal macrophages. Although there is some controversy as to whether this "pseudopregnancy" is the most efficient way of restoring fertility, there is no controversy over the fact that both pelvic pain and menstrual pain are dramatically reduced.

With respect to endometrial carcinoma, only the highly differentiated and hormonally dependent forms of endometrial carcinoma can be somewhat controlled by high-dose, continuous progestin therapy. Megestrol acetate is recommended. Hormonally dependent breast cancers have been treated with megestrol acetate as an adjunct and not as primary chemotherapy.

Vaginal or parenteral progesterone is used for treatment of luteal-phase defects and the associated phenomena of habitual abortion. The current practice is to begin vaginal progesterone therapy on the third or fourth day after the LH surge. This may delay the onset of spontaneous menses. Blood HCG is measured about the 14th day after the LH surge; if this is negative, the progesterone is discontinued. If it is positive, the progesterone is continued, usually through the ninth to twelfth week of pregnancy, by which time placental production of progesterone should be more than ample to continue the pregnancy.

Medroxyprogesterone acetate (Depo-Provera) and norethindrone enanthate (Noristerat) provide highly effective contraception for women in many countries. Depo-Provera is approved for other indications in the United States, but not for contraception. Its major disadvantage is that it may remain in the body for several months after the medication is discontinued. Norplant implants, nonbiodegradable silastic capsules which release Levonorgestrel for up to 3 years, are currently available in Europe.

DANAZOL (DANOCRINE)

Danazol

Danazol is an isoxazole derivative of 17α-ethinyltestosterone. It works directly on the hypothalamic-pituitary axis to inhibit gonadotropin secretion.

Danazol inhibits the midcycle secretion of gonadotropins, LH and FSH, in a dose-dependent manner; the higher doses induce a marked hypoestrogenic state. During this hypoestrogenic state, the ectopic endometrium of endometriosis undergoes resolution. There is a dramatic reduction in the menstrual and pelvic pain associated with endometriosis following a prolonged course of danazol.

The benefits of danazol in the treatment of symptomatic endometriosis are greater than can be accounted for by the single mechanism described above. Other mechanisms include prevention of the postcastration increase in circulating gonadotropins. Danazol binds to androgen, progesterone, and glucocorticoid receptors, but only the danazol-androgen–receptor complex binds to the nuclear-acceptor DNA complex with resultant initiation of androgen-receptor–specific RNA synthesis. It does not bind to intracellular estrogen receptors. Danazol binds to both sex hormone– and corticosteroid-binding globulins, with resultant increased metabolic clearance of progesterone. Finally, danazol acts directly on ovarian enzyme complexes to inhibit ovarian steroidogenesis.

The side effects of danazol are multiple and are related both to the hypoestrogenic and androgenic effects of the compound. The most common side effects are weight gain, acne, oily skin, atrophic vaginitis, hot flashes, and muscle cramps. It also has profound androgenic effects.

The most serious side effects of danazol are related to an occasional allergic reaction, manifested by a pruritic and erythematous rash of the upper body; hypertension, which may take several months to develop; and depression, which can develop during the first week of treatment. The depression can be associated with a great deal of anxiety, and all patients should be warned of its possible occurrence.

For treatment of endometriosis, danazol is administered orally in high doses; the dose can usually be lowered within the first 1 to 3 months. Patients much be warned that once the dose of danazol is lowered to 200 to 400 mg/day, they might begin to ovulate again, with the possibility of an unwanted pregnancy. For long-term maintenance of a patient with an established tendency to get endometriosis, cyclic administration of oral contraceptives is extremely beneficial.

Although there is some controversy as to whether a course of danazol improves the fertility of patients with endometriosis, there is virtually universal agreement that danazol dramatically relieves the pain associated with endometriosis.

Danazol in much lower doses, 25 to 200 mg/day, is FDA approved for the treatment of painful fibrocystic breast disease. Other conditions improved by danazol include angioneurotic edema, systemic lupus erythematosus (in some patients), and hemophilia or premenstrual syndrome (in some patients).

ORAL CONTRACEPTIVES

One of the most important uses of synthetic estrogens and progestins has been as oral contraceptives. The agents can be classified according to their steroid content and are listed in Table 37-3: (1) Fixed combinations contain constant amounts of estrogen (ethinyl estradiol) and progestin (e.g., norethindrone); (2) multiphasic combinations contain constant amounts of estrogen combined with variable doses of progestin. The dose of progestin changes from one week to the next; (3) "minipills" consist only of progestin at a constant dose.

The major mechanism of action of combined oral contraceptives is to inhibit the mid-cycle LH surge and thereby inhibit ovulation. Additionally, the oral contraceptives thicken the cervical mucus, thereby inhibiting sperm penetration; alter secretory changes in the endometrium, which interferes with implantation; and alter fallopian tubal transport, which discourages implantation.

Adverse Effects

Breakthrough bleeding is frequently reported during the first several cycles after beginning oral contraceptive use. Most commonly, this resolves within several cycles; however, it may be necessary to use a different formulation. When breakthrough bleeding begins after many oral contraceptive cycles in which it does not occur, the patient should be completely evaluated for organic causes, which may include pelvic inflammatory disease, endometriosis, adenomyosis, and uterine leiomyomata.

Amenorrhea occurs less frequently but can be quite alarming to the patient who is concerned about an unwanted pregnancy. Careful history will usually reveal a gradual decrease of menstrual flow over many cycles. The anxiety caused in patients with this condition usually warrants changing the formulation.

TABLE 37-3   Representative formulations of oral contraceptives

	Estrogen (ethinyl estradiol), mg	Progestin, mg	Progestational potency, relative units
Fixed doses of estrogen and progestin			
Ortho-Novum 1/35 Norinyl 1/35	0.035	Norethindrone (1.0)	2.0
Ovcon 35	0.035	Norethindrone (0.4)	0.8
Brevicon Modicon	0.035	Norethindrone (0.5)	1.0
Loestrin 1.5/30 Zorane 1.5/30	0.30	Norethindrone acetate (1.5)	6.0
Loestrin 1/20 Zorane 1/20	0.02	Norethindrone acetate (1.0)	4.0
Lo/Ovral	0.03	*dl*-Norgestrel (0.3)	18
Nordette Levlen	0.03	*l*-Norgestrel (0.15)	18
Demulen 1/35	0.035	Ethynodiol diacetate (1.0)	30
Multiphasics: variable amounts of estrogen and progestin			
Ortho-Novum 7/7/7	0.035	Norethindrone (0.5/0.75/1.00)	1.5
Ortho-Novum 10/11	0.035	Norethindrone (0.5/1.0)	1.5
Tri-Norinyl	0.035	Norethindrone (0.5/1.0/0.5)	1.33
Tri-Levlen	6D × 0.03 5D × 0.04 10D × 0.03	*l*-Norgestrel × 0.05 × 0.075 × 0.125	11.0
Triphasil	6D × 0.03 5D × 0.04 10D × 0.03	*l*-Norgestrel × 0.05 × 0.075 × 0.125	11.0

TABLE 37-3 (*continued*) **Representative formulations of oral contraceptives**

	Estrogen (ethinyl estradiol), mg	Progestin, mg	Progestational potency, relative units
Progestin only			
Micronor	0.000	Norethindrone (0.35)	0.7
Nor-QD	0.000	Norethindrone (0.35)	0.7
Ovrette	0.000	*l*-Norgestrel (0.075)	9.0

Headache, depression, and loss of libido may occur and may warrant changing the oral contraceptive formulation and/or changing to a different type of contraception. Serum hormone assays may be elevated because of the increased hormone-binding globulins induced by the bolus effect of estrogen on liver protein synthesis.

Several vitamins such as pyridoxine, folic acid, and ascorbic acid show decreased serum concentrations. Serum levels of vitamin A are increased. The significance of these observations remains obscure.

Potential complications of oral contraceptives based on their components are as follows:

Estrogen
  Nausea
  Chloasma
  Monolia vaginal infections
  Mucoid leukorrhea
  Increase in pigment of areolae
  Increase in size of leiomyoma
  Edema

Progestogen (with androgenic potential)
  Increased appetite with weight gain
  Acne
  Hirsutism
  Seborrhea
  Cholestatic jaundice (also with estrogens)

Progestogen (without androgenic potential)
  Decreased libido
  Delayed onset of menses
  Fatigue
  Decreased menstrual flow
  Depression
  Uterine cramps

Estrogen and progestogen deficiency
  Vasomotor symptoms
  Irritability
  Decreased menstruation
  Breakthrough bleeding and spotting

Several absolute contraindications to oral contraceptive administration have been deeply entrained in the public mind. Few practitioners would permit women with such risks as thrombophlebitis or thromboembolic phenomena to take oral contraceptives. In addition, careful screening has resulted in the exclusion of patients with high-risk factors before oral contraceptives would even be considered. Accordingly, there is a lower incidence of serious problems in women taking the low-dose oral contraceptives as compared to earlier formulations.

Many of the conditions for which oral contraceptives are contraindicated are actually contraindications to the estrogen component. The most important risk factors to which estrogens contribute are those associated with thrombosis or thromboembolic phenomena. Progestin-only formulations may be prescribed in some of these situations.

Absolute Contraindications to Oral Contraceptives

Thrombophlebitis, Thromboembolic Disorder A common consensus is that risk of development of thrombophlebitis or thromboembolic disorders is related to the amount of estrogen in the oral contraceptive formulation. Even though the presently used formulations have very low hormone contents of both estrogen and progestin, this remains an absolute contraindication to oral contraceptive usage.

Cerebrovascular Accident or History Smoking, hypertension, and age are independent risk factors for development of cerebrovascular accidents. Aside from these factors, the risks are increased in relation to the dose of estrogen in the formulation.

Coronary Artery Disease and Ischemic Heart Disease There is an increased risk of myocardial infarction associated with smoking, hypertension, hypercholesterolemia, and diabetes mellitus. All of these risk factors are worsened by the concomitant use of oral contraceptives.

Known or Suspected Breast Cancer Many epidemiologic studies have failed to implicate the use of either oral contraceptives or estrogen replacement therapy with the development of breast cancer. In fact, most studies on oral contraceptive use have shown a dramatic decrease in the incidence of benign breast disease. Nevertheless, our understanding of the possible stimulatory effects of hormones on estrogen-receptor positive breast cancers precludes the use of oral contraceptives in patients with breast cancer.

Known or Suspected Estrogen-Dependent Neoplasia Aside from breast cancer, the major estrogen-dependent neoplasia is adenocarcinoma of the endometrium. The estrogen component of oral contraceptives would be a strong contraindication to their use in patients with known or suspected endometrial carcinoma.

Known or Suspected Pregnancy There is absolutely no indication for beginning oral contraceptive therapy in a woman who is known or suspected of being pregnant.

Hypertension Many women experience small elevations of blood pressure while taking oral contraceptives (5 mm systolic and 1 to 2 mm diastolic), and these are neither absolute nor relative contraindications to continued use. However, occasionally women develop significant hypertension ($>140/90$), which mandates discontinuance. The hypertensive mechanism involves the renin-angiotensin-aldosterone system with increased angiotensinogen and angiotensin. The elevated blood pressure normalizes within 1 to 2 months following discontinuation.

Active Gallbladder Disease There is a discrepancy on the associated risks of gallbladder disease and oral contraceptive use. Nevertheless, if a patient has had a demonstrable attack of acute cholecystitis, it would be imprudent to allow oral contraceptive use.

Sickle Cell Disease Sickle cell disease is associated with an increased risk of thrombophlebitis and thromboembolic phenomena. Accordingly, this diagnosis would present a strong contraindication to oral contraceptive use.

Elective Surgery within Four Weeks Elective surgery puts patients at increased risk for thrombophlebitis and thromboembolic phenomena. Accordingly, this would present a strong relative contraindication to oral contraceptive use.

Long-Term Cast or Leg Paralysis These factors result in immobilization which predisposes to thrombophlebitis.

Forty Years Old and a Second Risk Factor for Cardiovascular Disease As discussed above, combined oral contraceptives synergize with other risk factors for cardiovascular disease. Consequently, if a second risk factor were present, this would mandate using local contraceptives.

Thirty Years Old and Smoking More than 15 Cigarettes per Day Heavy cigarette use presents a major risk factor in women over the age of 30.

Other contraindications include benign or malignant liver tumors, undiagnosed abnormal genital bleeding, and mononucleosis.

Relative Contraindications

Diabetes, Prediabetes, or a Strong Family History There is an impaired glucose tolerance in 15 to 40 percent of women using oral contraceptives. Women with insulin-dependent diabetes are also at increased risk for thrombosis. Previous cholestasis during pregnancy, congenital hyperbilirubinemia, or oral contraceptive–induced cholestasis, and/or current impairment of liver function tests (or within the past year) are relative contraindications.

Most steroids are extensively excreted in the bile. In addition, conjugation, especially with glucuronic acid is common to most sex steroid hormones. An entero-hepatic circulation of estrogens and probably progestins exists in which these steroids are conjugated in the liver and excreted in the bile.

The parenchymal cells of the liver take up and excrete various other organic anions, including bile salts. The capacity of the liver to excrete all organic anions is significantly altered by steroid hormones and pregnancy. Partial or complete interruption of the enterohepatic circulation of estrogens and progestins occurs in the syndrome of recurrent intrahepatic cholestatic jaundice of pregnancy. Susceptible individuals will also develop intrahepatic cholestatic jaundice in response to oral contraceptive administration.

Family History of Myocardial Infarction in People under 50 Years of Age   This should be considered a relatively strong contraindication because of the unknown effects of oral contraceptives in this group of patients.

Severe Headaches (Especially Vascular or Migraine)   There is considerable variation in the occurrence of migraine headaches. They may be made worse, made better, or be unaffected by oral contraceptive use (whether combined or progestin-only formulations). Currently, migraine headache, per se, is not a contraindication to prescribing oral contraceptives.

May Warrant Use of Progestin-Only Oral Contraceptives   There are several situations in which many clinicians would use neither fixed nor multiphasic oral contraceptives. However, use of the progestin-only formulations may be acceptable. These situations include age greater than 45 years; recent delivery; any cardiac or renal disease; lactation, depression, chloasma, or hair loss during pregnancy; asthma; epilepsy; varicose veins.

Noncontraceptive Indications for Oral Contraceptive Use

There are a great variety of clinical situations in which oral contraceptives have been given with significant improvement in the patient's well-being. These conditions include menstrual pain (dysmenorrhea), menstrual irregularities of any kind, osteoporosis associated with hypothalamic amenorrhea syndromes, recurrent functional ovarian cysts, iron deficiency anemia (when caused by heavy menstrual flow), premenstrual syndromes, breast swelling, pain and nodularity of fibrocystic breast disease, acne, and cyclic edema. In addition, there is evidence that oral contraceptive use may induce long-term protection from endometrial and ovarian carcinoma, ectopic pregnancy, and pelvic inflammatory disease. Oral contraceptives improve the symptoms of endometriosis, but cyclic administration of oral contraceptives does not cure this condition.

Drug Interactions

Antibiotics alter the gastrointestinal flora and can result in a decreased potency of oral contraceptives. The mechanism is believed to be via an altered enterohepatic circulation of the hormones, resulting in decreased hormone efficacy.

Drugs which induce liver microsomal enzymes will cause a more rapid metabolism of the hormones and therefore decrease their efficacy. Such drugs include barbiturates, primidone, carbamazine, phenytoin, piperidinediones, rifampin, and benzodiazepines such as chlordiazepoxide and diazepam.

Anticoagulant therapy for any indication requires discontinuation of oral contraceptives because they can cause a hypercoagulable state.

FERTILITY AGENTS

Gonadotropins

Human chorionic gonadotropin (HCG) is purified extract of human placental tissue. It has predominantly LH-like activity in that it binds to all LH receptors. It is more widely and cheaply available than human pituitary luteinizing hormone. HCG differs from LH in that it has a different B chain, has higher sugar content, and has a longer half-life. Its use is limited to ovulation induction, for which it is administered intramuscularly as a bolus to replace the LH surge. In smaller daily doses, it is used to support corpus luteum function in patients with luteal-phase defects.

Human menopausal gonadotropin (HMG) is a purified extract of human menopausal urine. The final product has very similar amounts of FSH and LH. The bioactivity is determined by bioassay. More recently, a preparation with predominantly FSH activity has been FDA approved. In females, the only use for these preparations is to stimulate folliculogenesis in infertile patients. This requires daily intramuscular injections of the hormone. The number of follicles stimulated is correlated with the amount of HMG used. However, each cycle must be monitored with daily estrogen determinations and serial ultrasound measurements of the diameter of each follicle. When the largest follicle reaches a diameter between 1.8 and 2.2 cm, ovulation is induced with a single IM injection of HCG.

The purified FSH preparation is used for ovulation induction in select patients with high endogenous LH secretion.

The indications for ovulation induction with HMG include hypopituitarism and hypothalamic amenorrhea unresponsive to clomiphene. Unexplained infertility and patients with polycystic ovarian disease who are resistant to ovulation induction with clomiphene are also candidates for HMG. Obviously, normal patient fallopian tubes and adequate numbers of sperm should be demonstrated before using HMG.

Most practitioners use HMG to induce multiple follicles or superovulation for the newer reproductive technologies of in vitro fertilization and gamete intrafallopian transfer (GIFT). The standard for these technological procedures is that a minimum of three fertilized eggs should be implanted in the uterus for each attempt. Extra fertilized eggs may be frozen for implantation in future cycles.

Inhibitors of Prolactin Secretion

The major known function of pituitary prolactin in human beings is its fundamental role in normal postpartum lactation. A variety of pathological conditions associated with hyperprolactinemia will result in anovulatory, hypoestrogenic amenorrhea. The excess prolactin secretion is believed to cause direct inhibition of the hypothalamic LHRH secretory neurons by a short-loop negative feedback mechanism. It is generally agreed that hypoestrogenic amenorrhea must be treated to prevent premature osteoporosis. However, the usual estrogen replacement therapy in these situations causes some concern when given to hyperprolactinemic patients because estrogen directly stimulates hypertrophy of pituitary lactotropes.

Bromocriptine

Bromocriptine (2-bromo-α-ergocryptine mesylate) is a dopamine agonist drug which binds to the dopamine receptors on pituitary lactotropes. The net effect is to decrease pituitary prolactin secretion in a dose-dependent manner.

Side effects include nausea, anorexia, hypotension, headaches, nasal stuffiness, and depression. Peripheral prolactin levels are followed with the dose increased until normal prolactin levels are obtained. The drug is as effective in pituitary prolactin-secreting tumors as it is in pituitary hyperplasia. The drug can be stopped as soon as pregnancy is established. In very large pituitary tumors, therapy is continued throughout pregnancy.

Bromocriptine is also used to suppress postpartum lactation. The older treatment of this condition with huge doses of estrogen should no longer be recommended.

Bromocriptine is also useful for treating most pituitary tumors, whether they are actively secreting hormones or simply causing symptoms because of mass effect. This antitumor effect frequently results in reduction of tumor size and/or symptoms within weeks of beginning therapy.

LHRH Agonists and Antagonists

Luteinizing hormone-release hormone (LHRH) is a linear decapeptide found in highest concentrations in nerve endings of the median eminence of the hypothalamus. The secretion of LHRH is influenced by catecholaminergic, serotonergic, cholinergic, and peptidergic (e.g., opioid peptides) mechanisms as well as by various hormones. The final common pathway of these stimuli can be conceptually visualized as a "pulse generator" with which LHRH induces the pulsatile secretion of the gonadotropins FSH and LH.

The most important physiologic concept of the role of LHRH on pituitary FSH and LH secretion is that pulsatile LHRH is necessary for normal ovulatory function. Conversely, constant infusion of LHRH induces "down-regulation" of the LHRH receptors, resulting in a cessation of gonadotropin secretion and a profound hypogonadal state.

LHRH has a very short half-life. It is used clinically in two situations. It is used in a "stimulation or provocative test" to help distinguish pituitary from hypothalamic hypogonadism. Following basal LH and FSH determination, an IV bolus of LHRH (100 to 150 μg) is given with blood FSH and LH assayed. It is also commonly used to induce ovulation. LHRH is administered in a pulsatile manner, preferably intravenously. Several pumps are commercially available, which are worn by the patient during the several weeks required to induce ovulation.

Leuprolide acetate is an LHRH agonist, FDA approved for inducing a profound hypogonadal state in males with metastatic prostate carcinoma. Leuprolide and other LHRH agonists are being extensively investigated in a variety of clinical conditions such as treatment of endometriosis, treatment of sex hormone–dependent malignancies, suppression of precocious puberty, shrinkage of leiomyomata uteri, and suppression of endogenous gonadotropin secretion prior to HMG/HCG induction of ovulation in anovulatory patients with high endogenous LH secretion (such as patients with polycystic ovarian disease). These hormones must be given as daily subcutaneous injections.

The side effects of treatment include profound nausea, which resolves after several months, hypogonadal osteoporosis, which will worsen as a function of the duration of treatment, and profound "menopausal" hot flashes in both men and women.

BIBLIOGRAPHY

Benson, M. D., and R. W. Rebar: "Relationship of Migraine Headache and Stroke to Oral Contraceptive Use," *J. Reprod. Med.* **31**:1082–1088 (1986).

Breckenridge, A.: "Drug Interactions with Oral Contraceptives: An Overview," in S. Garattini and H. W. Berendes (eds.), *Pharmacology of Steroid Contraceptive Drugs*, Raven Press, New York, 1977, pp. 307–311.

Breuer, H.: "Metabolic Pathways of Steroid Contraceptive Drugs," in S. Garattini and H. W. Berendes (eds.), *Pharmacology of Steroid Contraceptive Drugs*, Raven Press, New York, 1977, pp. 73–88.

Chetkowski, R. J., M. D. Meldrum, K. A. Steingold, D. Randle, J. K. Lu, P. Eggena, J. M. Hershman, N. K. Alkjaersig, A. P. Fletcher, and H. L. Judd: "Biologic Effects of Transdermal Estradiol," *N. Engl. J. Med.*, **314**:1615–1620 (1986).

Hatcher, R. A., F. Guest, F. Stewart, G. K. Stewart, J. Trussell, S. C. Bowen, and W. Cates: *Contraceptive Technology 1988–89*, 14th ed., Irvington, New York, 1988.

Henzl, M. R.: "Contraceptive Hormones and Their Clinical Use," in S. S. C. Yen and R. B. Jaffe (eds.), *Reproductive Endocrinology, Physiology, Pathophysiology and Clinical Management*, 2d ed, Saunders, Philadelphia, 1986, pp. 643–682.

Heuson, J.-C., and A. Coune: "Hormone-Responsive Tumors," in P. Felig, J. D. Baxter, A. E. Broadus, and L. A. Frohman (eds.), *Endocrinology and Metabolism*, 2d ed, McGraw-Hill, New York, 1987, pp. 1736–1767.

Miller, D. R., L. Rosenberg, D. W. Kaufman, D. Schottenfeld, P. D. Stolley, and S. Shapiro: "Breast Cancer Risk in Relation to Early Oral Contraceptive Use," *Obstet. Gynecol.*, **68**:863–868 (1986).

Speroff, L., R. H. Glass, and N. G. Kase: *Clinical Gynecologic Endocrinology and Infertility*, 4th ed., Williams and Wilkins, Baltimore, 1988, pp. 461–498.

Vickery, B. H., and J. J. Nestor, Jr.: In L. Speroff (ed.), *Seminars in Reproductive Endocrinology*, Thieme Medical Pub., New York, 1986, 5:353–370.

Vorys, N.: "The Effects of Sex Steroids on the Liver," in J. R. Givens (ed.), *Clinical Use of Sex Steroids*, Chicago: Year Book Medical Pub., 1980, pp. 257–291.

Yen, S., C. C. Hsieh, and B. MacMahon: "Extrahepatic Bile Duct Cancer and Smoking, Beverage Consumption, Past Medical History and Oral Contraceptive Use," *Cancer*, **59**:2112–2116 (1987).

Zimmerman, A. W.: "Hormones and epilepsy," *Neurol. Clin.*, **4**:853–861 (1986).

Male Sex Hormones and Anabolic Steroids

Judith L. Albert and Steven J. Sondheimer

Androgens are steroid hormones which are principally secreted by the male gonad. The female ovary and the adrenals also secrete appreciable amounts of these hormones, but to a much lesser degree than do the testes. Androgens have both masculinizing and anabolic or growth-stimulating effects; hence their designation as male sex hormones and/or anabolic steroids.

CHEMISTRY

All androgens possess the cyclopentanophenanthrene nucleus (three benzene rings and a five-carbon ring). Testosterone is the major naturally occurring androgen. The structures of testosterone and selected clinically available compounds are shown in Fig. 38-1. Structural analogs of testosterone were synthesized for clinical use for maximal absorption from various routes of administration and prolongation of androgenic effects.

PHYSIOLOGIC REGULATION

Testosterone is synthesized by the Leydig cells in the testes. Men produce between 2.5 and 10 mg of testosterone daily, in a circadian pattern with highest amounts in the early morning. Synthesis of testosterone is under control of the hypothalamopituitary system. Steroidogenesis in the Leydig cell is stimulated by the anterior pituitary hormone, *luteinizing hormone* (LH), previously called *interstitial cell-stimulating hormone* (ICSH).

Follicle-stimulating hormone (FSH) is also necessary for spermatogenesis. Testosterone, in a classic negative feedback system, suppresses secretion of LH and FSH. Estrogen, also secreted by the testes or by peripheral conversion of testosterone, also inhibits secretion of FSH and LH.

MECHANISM OF ACTION

The androgenic effect of testosterone in many tissues depends on conversion to its more active metabolite dihydrotestosterone (DHT) by the enzyme 5-α-reductase in target tissues. All steroids including testosterone exert their effects by binding to receptors in target tissues; dihydrotestosterone binds 10 times more tightly to the androgen receptor than does testosterone. The androgen receptor has been demonstrated to belong to a group of steroid-receptor proteins which reside in the cell nucleus. The androgen-receptor gene has recently been localized to the X chromosome, and cloning of androgen-receptor complementary DNA has been accomplished. The receptor protein is thought to contain several regions which have different functions, namely, an area involved with DNA binding, one responsible for binding to the androgen, and another that activates transcription of messenger RNA (mRNA). Thus the hormone-receptor complex resides in the nucleus and causes its target tissue effect by activating the transcription of specific mRNAs, which in turn direct the synthesis of specific proteins involved in regulation of growth and cell division. The

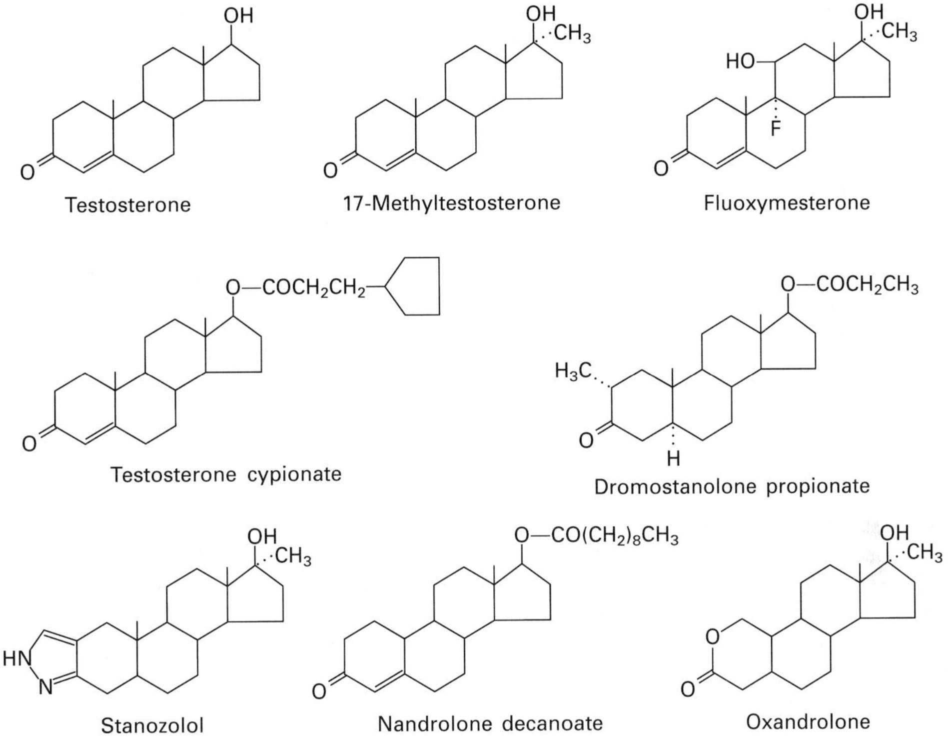

FIGURE 38-1   Structures of selected clinically used androgenic and anabolic steroids.

androgen receptor has been widely thought to be cytosolic in location. However, recent evidence indicates that the predominance of androgen-receptor binding takes place in the nucleus.

PHARMACOKINETICS

As indicated, endogenous androgens are primarily produced in the testes. Androgens may also be produced by the theca cells in the ovarian cortex. Most of these androgens are aromatized to estrogens by the granulosa cells of the ovary; some are secreted into the peripheral circulation as androgens. Androgens and androgenic precursors secreted by the ovary can be converted to testosterone in peripheral tissues. The adrenal cortex also is responsible for the production of androgens and androgenic precursors. When an enzyme defect exists in the adrenal cortex, such as in congenital adrenal hyperplasia, large quantities of androgens and androgen precursors may be secreted

with masculinizing effects. Although little testosterone is actually secreted by the adrenal, peripheral conversion of androgens to testosterone is again important. Once testosterone is released to the peripheral circulation, 98 to 99 percent of testosterone is bound to sex hormone—binding globulin, while 1 to 2 percent is in the free form. Testosterone reduces hepatic synthesis of sex hormone–binding globulin, while estrogen increases production. It is the free form of testosterone which exerts an effect on target tissues. The half-life of endogenous testosterone is 10 to 20 min. Metabolism of endogenous testosterone results in production of an active metabolite, DHT, as well as estrogenic compounds (e.g., estradiol). See Fig. 37-2 for details of the interrelationship of testosterone to other steroid hormones.

When testosterone is administered orally or parenterally, it is rapidly absorbed and inactivated by the liver. Biochemical modifications of testosterone are necessary for its clinical pharmacologic use to reduce its biotransformation and prolong its duration of action. Modifications to protect the compound from biotransformation include esterification of the 17-β-hydroxy group (e.g., testosterone cypionate), methylation of the 17-α position (e.g., methyltestosterone), halogenation of the ring (fluoxymesterone), and alterations of ring structure. In addition to side-chain modifications, solutions for parenteral injection can be placed in aqueous solution to delay absorption. Esterification of androgens followed by suspension in oil for intramuscular injection can also delay absorption and allow for continued availability of the steroid over a period of several days. Thus, drugs such as testosterone cypionate can be given for intervals of 2 to 4 weeks. The prolonged bioavailability of the modified injectable androgens makes them particularly attractive for replacement therapy in the hypogonadal male. The various testosterone esters available for intramuscular injection have different absorption properties but prolonged action. The oral preparations are primarily methylated compounds. See Table 38-1 for a list of available drugs.

Biotransformation of androgens occurs primarily in the liver. Testosterone is converted to androstenedione, which can then be reduced to the 17-ketosteroids, androsterone or etiocholanolone. These products have significantly less androgenic potency. The 17-ketosteroids are then secreted in the urine. Since adrenal and gonadal androgens share a common metabolite in the 17-ketosteroids, urinary ketosteroid determinations may not accurately reflect plasma levels of gonadal or exogenous androgens. In fact, a majority of urinary 17-ketosteroids are adrenal metabolites.

EFFECTS OF ANDROGENS ON ORGAN SYSTEMS

Male

Physiologic effects of testosterone and other androgens are seen throughout development, beginning in early fetal life and varying as growth and development of the organism proceed in the male. Androgens produced by the testes cause masculinization of the genital tract of the male fetus early in gestation. In puberty, androgens are responsible for the increase in the size of the penis and testes, growth of the beard, and growth of the pubic and axillary hair. Androgens are also necessary for spermatogenesis and sperm matura-

tion. Androgens cause proliferation of sebaceous glands and increase the secretion from these glands. Other effects at puberty in the male include growth of the larynx, which results in deepening of the voice, and increase in skeletal muscle mass, especially of the shoulder girdle. This increase in skeletal muscle mass is a manifestation of the anabolic effects of androgens. Testosterone also has a growth-promoting effect on bone, which is mediated by growth hormone. In studies of boys with constitutional delay of growth, testosterone has been shown to increase endogenous growth hormone levels as well as increase rates of linear growth. Androgens also stimulate epiphyseal maturation and closure, which ultimately limit the phase of accelerated linear growth that occurs in puberty. The stimulatory effect on epiphyseal growth by androgens is much less than that seen with estrogens.

Female

Androgens produced by the ovary and adrenal glands are important in the pubertal development of the female also. Growth of pubic and axillary hair is attributed to androgenic stimulation. In the normal female the total rate of production of the weaker androgens, androstenedione and dihydroepinandrosterone, far exceeds the rate of production of testosterone, the more potent androgen.

In both males and females, androgens have a negative feedback effect on the secretion of gonadotropins for the pituitary. This is an important aspect of the function of the hypothalamic-pituitary-gonadal axis in pubertal development as well as in adult life. Pharmacologic doses of androgens certainly suppress pituitary gonadotropin secretion, which may have adverse effects on normal gonadal function.

Hematopoietic Effects

Androgens have a stimulatory effect on normal hematopoietic cells, which is mediated by erythropoietin. Steroids may enhance the effects of erythropoietin as well as increase its production. Steroids may also have a direct growth-promoting effect on erythroid stem cells. The higher levels of circulating androgens in males are responsible for the normal difference in hemoglobin, hematocrit, and red blood cell mass between males and females.

TABLE 38-1   Androgen preparations in clinical use

		Relative activity		Dosage	
	Trade name	Androgenic	Anabolic	Androgenic	Anabolic
For intramuscular injection					
Testosterone (aqueous suspension)	Testoject-50	1	1	10–50 mg 3 times/week	
Testosterone esters (in oil suspension)					
Testosterone propionate	Testex	1	1	10–25 mg 2–3 times/week	
Testosterone cypionate	Depo-Testosterone	1	1	50–400 mg every 2–4 weeks	
Testosterone enanthate	Delatestryl	1	1	50–400 mg every 2–4 weeks	
Dromostanolone propionate (oil suspension)	Drolban	1	3		100 mg* 3 times/wk
Nandrolone phenpropionate (oil suspension)	Durobolin	1	3–5		25–50 mg* weekly
Nandrolone decanoate (oil suspension)	Deca-Durabolin	1	3–4		50–100 mg every 3–4 wks
For oral or buccal administration (as tablets)					
Methyltestosterone	Metandren	1	1	10–40 mg/day PO† 5–20 mg/day buccal	
Fluoxymesterone	Halotestin	1	1–2	2–10 mg/day PO	
Methandrostenolone	Dianabol	1	3		2.5–5 mg/day
Oxymetholone	Anadrol	1	3		1–5 mg/kg/day‡
Stanozolol	Winstrol	1	3–5		6 mg/day‡
Oxandrolone	Anavar	1	3–13		5–10 mg/day

*For treatment of breast cancer.
†PO = oral.
‡For treatment of anemia.

THERAPEUTIC USES

Male Hypogonadism

The use of androgenic steroids is clearly indicated as replacement therapy for the male with gonadal failure. Testicular deficiency can be a congenital or an acquired condition. In either case, the treatment is the same. In congenital hypogonadism in the male, puberty will not occur unless androgens are administered. Masculinizing features as well as the pubertal growth spurt are lacking without replacement therapy.

Testosterone esters (e.g., testosterone enanthate, testosterone propionate, testosterone cypionate) are usually administered parenterally in these cases, with careful monitoring of the response of penile and testicular growth. Although patients with hypogonadotropic hypogonadism (hypothalamic-pituitary dysfunction) can be treated with exogenous gonadotropins to stimulate the gonads, frequently the administration of synthetic androgens is a simpler and less expensive means of achieving the same results.

Anemia

Androgens have been reported to enhance red blood cell production by increasing the production of erythropoietic-stimulating factor. Androgens have thus been used for treatment of various forms of anemia. For example, some patients with anemia based on lack of bone marrow proliferation of red blood cell precursors and some patients with anemia of chronic renal failure respond to therapy with androgens. Unfortunately, the response of these patients is unpredictable and may not be sustained. Patients often do not tolerate the side effects of the steroids; therefore, studies have been undertaken in anemic patients to identify factors which may predict response to androgen therapy. Some studies indicate that testosterone esters administered by injection have better results in the treatment of anemia than orally administered agents.

Breast Cancer

Androgens have been used secondarily in the treatment of breast carcinomas, particularly in women who are 1 to 5 years postmenopausal. Their effect seems to be primarily palliative and may be a result of the an-

tiestrogen properties of androgens. This type of therapy only benefits women with a hormone-sensitive tumor. Use of specific antiestrogens such as tamoxifen may be equally effective and better tolerated by the patient with an estrogen-responsive breast tumor.

Endometriosis

Danazol is a derivative of the synthetic steroid 17-ethinyltestosterone (ethisterone). It has weak androgenic potential and multiple endocrine effects, which combine to make it an effective medical therapy for endometriosis in women. It is capable of binding to androgen, progesterone, and glucocorticoid receptors. Danazol also has significant antigonadotropin activity.

In addition, danazol is also used for the treatment of angioneurotic edema, an autosomal dominant immune disorder that results in random activation of the complement cascade and release of local factors responsible for angioedema. Danazol is the preferred steroid for treatment of angioedema because of its weak androgenic potential. Its effect is mediated through synthesis of inhibitory proteins by the liver that prevent activation of the complement system. A complete discussion of danazol is found in Chap. 37.

ADVERSE REACTIONS AND PRECAUTIONS

The most frequent side effect of androgenic steroids is virilism. Signs of virilism in the prepuberal male include growth of pubic hair, increase in penile size, and increase in frequency of erections. Prolonged use in males can lead to feminization by reducing release of endogenous gonadotropin. In females, untoward effects of androgen therapy include hirsutism, clitoral enlargement, acne, deepening of the voice, and menstrual irregularities. Other undesirable effects associated with these agents are premature epiphyseal closure, liver dysfunction, hypercalcemia, and retention of sodium and water, which may cause edema. Androgenic compounds are contraindicated in pregnant women and in patients with prostatic or breast carcinoma. It should be noted that the 17-α-methylated androgens available for oral administration have a higher incidence of hepatic side effects such as jaundice. These compounds should be avoided in patients with liver disease.

USE OF ANABOLIC STEROIDS BY ATHLETES

Anabolic steroids are closely related structurally to testosterone and thus possess both androgenic and anabolic activities. They were originally designed to induce weight gain and improve nitrogen balance in individuals with recent illness. However, the widespread use of androgens and anabolic steroids by athletes is a major concern of both the athletic and medical communities. Because of their known growth-promoting properties, many athletes, both male and female, use androgens in alarmingly high doses to improve performance and enhance muscle strength. A comparison of androgenic and anabolic activity of these compounds is shown in Table 38-1. Although some studies document improvements in muscle strength associated with steroid use, these findings are not consistently reproduced. Well-controlled studies of this area are difficult to design and carry out. Most investigators agree that significant weight gain results from self-administration of oral and injectable androgens by athletes. However, the weight gain may be the result of fluid retention and not increased tissue growth. Steroids also improve appetite, and weight may simply result from the combined effects of athletic training and increased intake of nutrients.

Changes in athletic performance may be related to the psychologic effects of steroids. Androgens have long been linked to the behavioral changes that take place in puberty. Athletes report increased aggression and mood changes during steroid usage, which may be looked upon as beneficial in competitive performance.

Many athletes obtain anabolic steroids from black-market sources, but a surprising number may get the drugs from legitimate sources such as pharmacists, physicians, and trainers. Drug-use regimens may combine oral and parenteral agents over a period of weeks to months, and usually have a 4- to 6-week drug holiday prior to competitions when drug testing is carried out.

Regardless of the benefits perceived by athletes who self-administer androgens, the adverse effects can be quite significant. Females can become obviously virilized, as evidenced by hirsutism, voice changes, and clitoral hypertrophy. Conversely, males may exhibit feminization because high levels of circulating androgens can inhibit release of gonadotropins from the hypothalamopituitary system, resulting in higher than normal peripheral production of estrogen enzymatically in some tissues. The most common effect of increased estrogen in males is gynecomastia. When androgens are administered to young male athletes who have not completed the pubertal transition to adulthood, premature epiphyseal closure can occur, causing reduction in adult height. Although total circulating androgen levels rise with steroid administration, endogenous testosterone production by the testes is probably decreased with large drug doses. Exogenous androgens also decrease baseline gonadotropin levels. These two effects may result in decreased spermatogenesis. Although this is a reversible side effect, resumption of baseline testicular function may not be seen until up to 4 to 6 months after the drugs are stopped.

Liver damage may also result from androgen usage, especially when orally active preparations with methyl substitutions are used. The damage may be mild, resulting in jaundice, or severe enough to result in hepatocellular carcinoma.

Reports of mental disorders, ranging from depression to psychoses, are becoming more frequent in association with androgen usage by athletes. Psychiatrists clearly recognize that these steroids can commonly cause mental disturbances.

Finally, steroids have known effects on lipid and cholesterol metabolism. Androgens decrease HDL levels while they increase total cholesterol. This theoretically has an adverse effect on the risk of cardiovascular disease. It is unclear whether temporary alterations in lipid metabolism secondary to steroid usage by athletes actually have long-term effects.

All of these side effects can potentially occur when androgens are used for the other indications previously mentioned. The risks of serious complications of drug therapy are generally more acceptable in a disease state. Performance athletes represent specimens of human health, not disease. Although efforts have been made to develop steroids with low androgenic potential and high anabolic potential, they have been largely unsuccessful. All anabolic steroids currently in use have androgen properties.

BIBLIOGRAPHY

Fotherby, K. and F. James: "Metabolism of Synthetic Steroids," *Adv. Steroid Biochem. Pharmacol.*, **3**:67–165 (1972).

Link, K., R. M. Blizzard, W. S. Evans, D. L. Kaiser, et al.: "The Effect of Androgens on the Pulsatile Release and the Twenty-Four Hour Mean Concentration of Growth Hormone in Peripubertal Males," *J. Clin. Endocrin. Metabol.*, **62**:159–164 (1986).

Lubahn, D. B., D. R. Joseph, P. M. Sullivan, H. F. Wittard, et al.: "Cloning of Human Androgen Receptor Complementary DNA and Localization to the X Chromosome," *Science*, **240**:327–339 (1988).

Neff, M. S., J. Goldberg, R. F. Slifkin, A. R. Eiser, et al.: "A Comparison of Androgens for Anemia in Patients on Hemodialysis," *N. Engl. J. Med.*, **304**:871–875 (1980).

Kalmanti, M., N. Dainiak, J. Martino, M. Dewey, et al.: "Correlation of Clinical and in Vitro Erythropoietic Responses to Androgens in Renal Failure," *Kidney Int.*, **22**:383–391 (1982).

Barbieri, R. L., and K. J. Ryan: "Danazol: Endocrine Pharmacology and Therapeutic Applications," *Am. J. Obstet. Gynecol.*, **141**:454–463 (1981).

Perlmutter, G., and D. T. Lowenthal: "Use of Anabolic Steroids by Athletes," *AFP*, **32**:208–210 (1985).

Hurley, B. F., D. R. Seals, J. M. Hagberg, A. C. Goldberg, et al.: "High-Density-Lipoprotein Cholesterol in Bodybuilders vs. Powerlifters," *J. Am. Med. Assoc.*, **252**:507–513 (1984).

Ruokonen, A., M. Alen, N. Bolton, and R. Vihko: "Response of Serum Testosterone and Its Precursor Steroids, SHBG and CBG to Anabolic Steroid and Testosterone Self-Administration in Man," *J. Steroid Biochem.*, **23**:33–38 (1985).

C H A P T E R   **39**

Corticotropin and Corticosteroids

Karl Salman and Leslie I. Rose

The term *corticosteroids* designates those steroid hormones normally secreted by the adrenal cortex: glucocorticoids, mineralocorticoids, and sex steroids. Production of these hormones is under direct control of adrenocorticotropic hormone (ACTH, corticotropin) originating from the anterior pituitary. The first section deals with the pharmacology and clinical applications of ACTH. Glucocorticoids and mineralocorticoids are addressed in the second section. Sex steroids were discussed in the preceding chapters.

CORTICOTROPIN

Source and Chemistry

ACTH is a polypeptide hormone secreted by the corticotropic cells of the anterior pituitary gland. It is derived by proteolytic cleavage from a precursor glycoprotein, pro-opiomelanocortin.

Human ACTH is composed of 30 amino acids with a molecular weight of 4500. Its structure is shown in Fig. 39-1. It differs from the ACTH of various animal species in the sequence between amino acids 29 and 33. However, ACTH (1–24) is 100 percent conserved in mammalian species and retains its biologic activity. Its synthetic form, cosyntropin (Cortrosyn) is used clinically to assess adrenocortical function. Other sources of ACTH include extraction from animal pituitary glands of chromatographic or electrophoretic techniques and synthesis of the entire human ACTH polypeptide, but there are few clinical indications for their use.

Regulation of Secretion and Effects of ACTH

Regulation of Secretion Secretion of ACTH is regulated by corticotropin-releasing factor (CRF), a 41 amino acid peptide formed in the median eminence of the hypothalamus. CRF reaches the pituitary corticotropic cells through the hypothalamic portal venous system.

Plasma cortisol (hydrocortisone) modulates ACTH secretion by a negative-feedback mechanism both at the hypothalamic and pituitary level. This simple negative feedback can be overridden in periods of stress such as exercise, surgery, hypovolemia, hyperthermia, and hypothermia as well as psychologic stress. ACTH secretion also occurs in bursts 7 to 13 times a day, independent of plasma cortisol levels and in a pattern reproducible for any given person. This diurnal rhythm is under hypothalamic control and does not submit to negative feedback.

Action on the Adrenal Cortex Some of the actions of ACTH on the adrenal cortex occur within minutes, whereas others become apparent only after several hours or days of exposure. Within 1 min of administration of a bolus of ACTH, the concentration of adenosine-3′,5′-monophosphate (cyclic AMP) rises within the adrenal. This in turn stimulates the formation of the labile protein which activates the conversion of cholesterol to pregnenolone. Pregnenolone will then be converted by various enzyme systems to other steroid hormones. This entire process requires about 3 min. More prolonged exposure to ACTH promotes

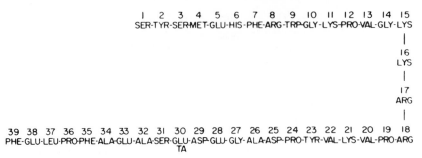

FIGURE 39-1 Amino acid sequence of human ACTH.

adrenal growth, stimulates protein and cholesterol synthesis, increases the functional capacity of the enzyme systems, and leads to depletion of adrenal ascorbic acid.

Extra Adrenal Effects Corticotropin can affect lipid and carbohydrate metabolism. These effects have been demonstrated mostly in vitro and with pharmacologic doses of ACTH. It stimulates lipolysis by activation of a "hormone-sensitive lipase" in adipose tissue, mediated by cyclic AMP. This leads to a rise in plasma-free fatty acids, an increase in hepatic fat, and accelerated ketogenesis. ACTH improves glucose tolerance and increases muscle glycogen by stimulating insulin secretion. Prolonged exposure to ACTH, on the other hand, can induce insulin resistance as well as cutaneous hyperpigmentation.

Pharmacokinetics

ACTH is destroyed by proteolytic enzymes and thus cannot be given orally. Similarly, when administered subcutaneously or intramuscularly, much of it is inactivated before reaching the circulation. When given intravenously, its half-life is about 15 min. The amount of ACTH in the urine is negligible, indicating inactivation in the tissues. Maximal stimulation of the adrenal cortex can be obtained with more prolonged exposure, and corticosteroid secretion shows a linear increase with the duration of ACTH infusion.

Bioassay

Commercial corticotropin is obtained from the pituitary glands of various mammalian species. Its potency, expressed in USP units, is determined by injecting it subcutaneously in hypophysectomized rats and measuring the depletion of adrenal ascorbic acid.

Therapeutic and Diagnostic Applications

At present corticotropin has no therapeutic usefulness, with the possible exception of multiple sclerosis. Adrenal insufficiency, its main potential indication, is better treated with oral synthetic corticosteroids. Its important use is in the diagnosis of adrenal insufficiency. The rapid ACTH stimulation test measures the rise of plasma cortisol 30 to 50 min after intramuscular or intravenous injection of ACTH or cosyntropin. In the event of a subnormal response, a more prolonged stimulation can be done by infusing cosyntropin over 6 to 24 h. Primary adrenal insufficiency (Addison's disease) is characterized by the absence of a cortisol response to ACTH or cosyntropin. A mild increase in cortisol is seen in secondary adrenal insufficiency (hypopituitarism).

Adverse Reactions

Adverse reactions are mostly a result of the increased rate of secretion of corticosteroids and include fluid retention, hypokalemic alkalosis, and glucose intolerance. Hypersensitivity reactions are rare. They range from fever to life-threatening anaphylactic reactions. Synthetic ACTH, though less antigenic than the natural peptide, also rarely induces hypersensitivity.

Preparations and Doses

Corticotropin injection, USP (Acthar) is a lyophilized powder for injection, derived from mammalian pituitaries. Ordinarily 25 USP units are infused over 8 h.

Repository corticotropin injection, USP (H.P. Acthar Gel) is a highly purified ACTH in gelatin solution for prolonged release after intramuscular or subcutaneous injection. Average dose is 40 USP units once daily.

Corticotropin zinc hydroxide suspension, USP (Cortrophin Zinc) is purified corticotropin absorbed in zinc hydroxides, for intramuscular injection. Typical dose is 40 USP units once daily.

Cosyntropin (Cortrosyn) is a synthetic peptide consisting of the first 24 amino acid residues of human ACTH. It is a lyophilized powder for intramuscular or intravenous injection and is approved for diagnostic purposes: A dose of 0.25 mg (about 25 units) is injected in the rapid ACTH stimulation test.

CORTICOSTEROIDS

This section deals with two groups of corticosteroids: (1) glucocorticoids, which influence carbohydrate, lipid, and protein metabolism and possess anti-inflammatory properties; and (2) mineralocorticoids, which affect fluid and electrolyte balance. However, the biologic properties of the various corticosteroids are within a spectrum that ranges from strict glucocorticoid to strict mineralocorticoid activity.

Source and Chemistry

The naturally occurring steroid hormones originate from cholesterol. The rate-limiting step is the side-chain cleavage of cholesterol to form pregnenolone and isocaproic aldehyde. This reaction occurs in the mitochondria and requires molecular oxygen and NADPH. All corticosteroids are pregnane derivatives (Fig. 39-2) with ketone groups on C-3 and C-20, an unsaturated bond between C-4 and C-5 (denoted as Δ^4); and a 17β-CO—CH$_2$OH side chain. They vary in the presence or absence of an 11-keto, 11β-hydroxyl, 17α-hydroxyl group, and/or 18-oxygen function. These differences determine the main physiologic and pharmacologic actions of the end products and of some of their precursors. The main endogenous glucocorticoid is cortisol (hydrocortisone), and the main endogenous mineralocorticoid is aldosterone. Figure 39-3

Pregnane

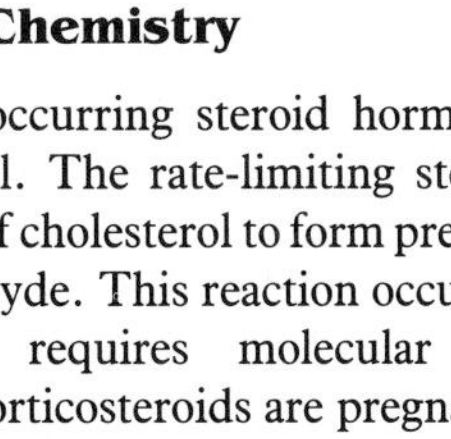

FIGURE 39-2 Backbone structure of corticosteroids.

shows the structural formulas of the main endogenous steroids. Figure 39-4 shows the structural formulas of commonly used synthetic corticosteroids.

Relation of Structure to Function

The relationship of chemical structure to function for corticosteroids is extremely complex, but a number of basic generalizations can be made. Generally, structural modifications alter receptor affinity, the rate of biotransformation of the compounds, and the degree of glucocorticoid or mineralocorticoid action. For glucocorticoid activity, the 11β-hydroxyl and 17α-hydroxyl groups are important. For adequate mineralocorticoid activity, the presence of oxygen at C-11 and C-18, or absence of oxygen at both C-11 and C-17, is required. In general, glucocorticoid binding occurs on the surface of the molecule, especially involving the 11β-hydroxyl and 17β-CO—CH$_2$OH groups, which project above the plane of the ring. Since the 11β-hydroxyl group is generally essential for glucocorticoid activity, it seems likely that this group is involved in the primary steroid-receptor combination with a secondary combination with the 17β-CO—CH$_2$OH side chain. Thus bulky beta substitutes would interfere with binding and decrease activity, while equatorial or alpha substitutes would not.

Since 11-desoxycorticosterone has no glucocorticoid activity but is a potent mineralocorticoid and has only two potentially reactive substitutes, receptor combination must involve the 3-keto and/or the 17β-CO—CH$_2$OH groups. Some association with the alpha surface of the molecule of rings A,C, and D may also be involved. The fact that the modifications affecting the D ring markedly affect mineralocorticoid activity suggests that the 17β-CO—CH$_2$OH side chain may be more important. 9α-Fluorination increases the mineralocorticoid potency of both 11-hydroxy (cortisol) and 11-desoxy (desoxycorticosterone) compounds. Furthermore, the influence of the 18-aldehyde group as in aldosterone is unknown. Conceivably it influences the reactivity of the 11-oxygen function, but it could also change the D ring or influence the 17β side chain.

Mechanism of Action

Steroids are reversibly bound in plasma to two proteins: corticosteroid-binding globulin (CBG, transcortin), a specific, high-affinity α_2-globulin; and albu-

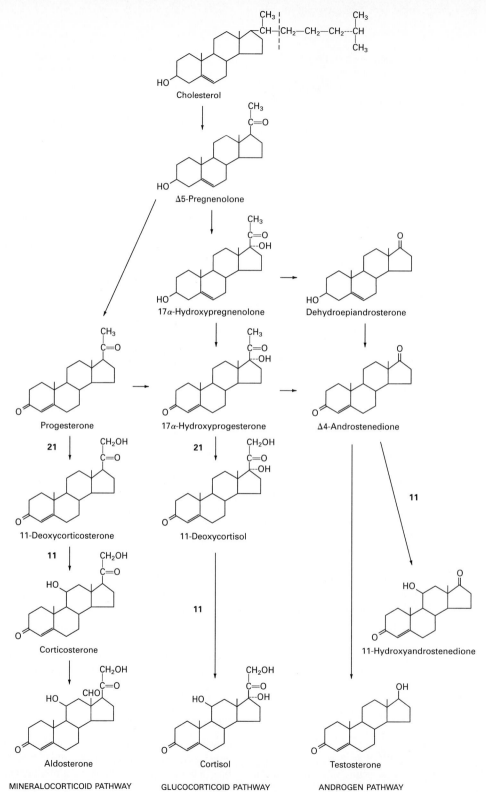

FIGURE 39-3 Biosynthetic pathways of adrenal corticosteroids. 21 = C−21 hydroxylase; 11 = C−11 hydroxylase.

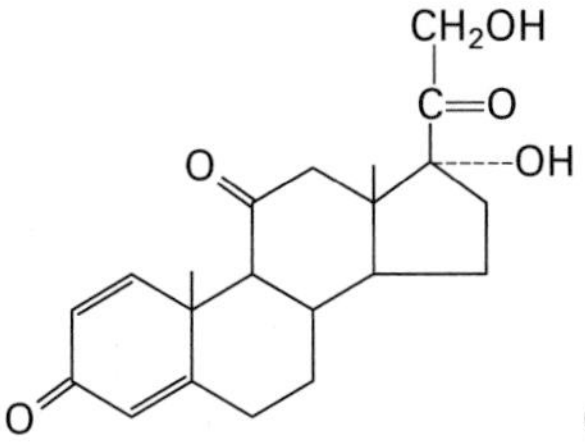

Prednisone
(Δ^1, cortisone)

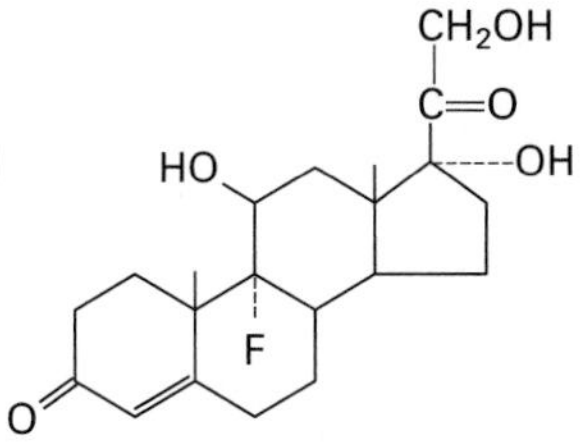

9α-Fluorohydrocortisone

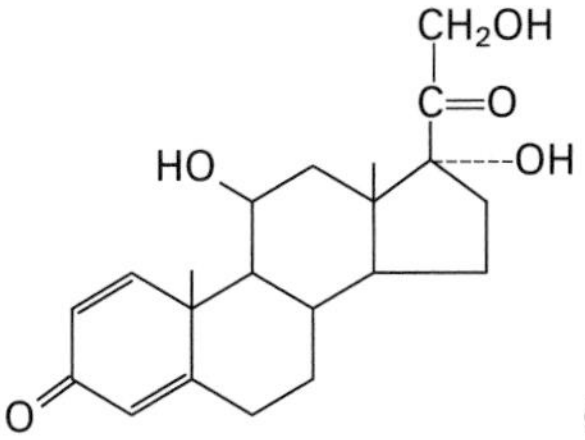

Prednisolone
(Δ^1, cortisol)

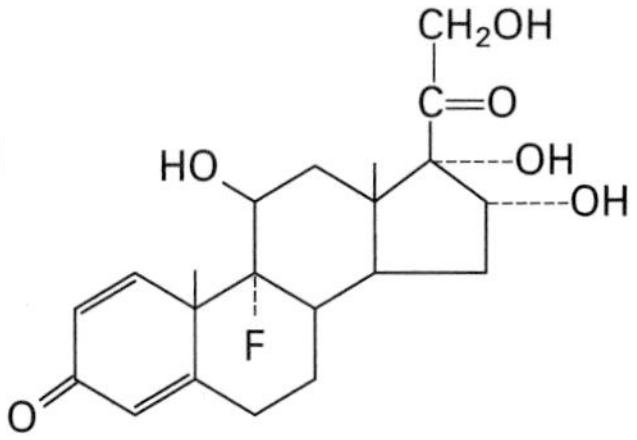

Triamcinolone
(9α-fluoro, 16α-hydroxy, prednisolone)

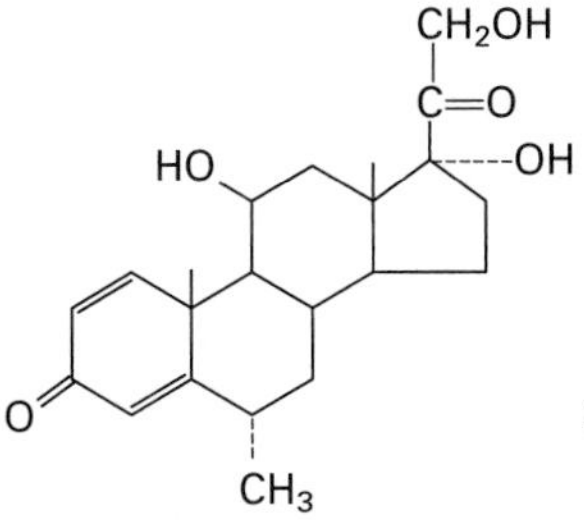

6α-Methyl prednisolone

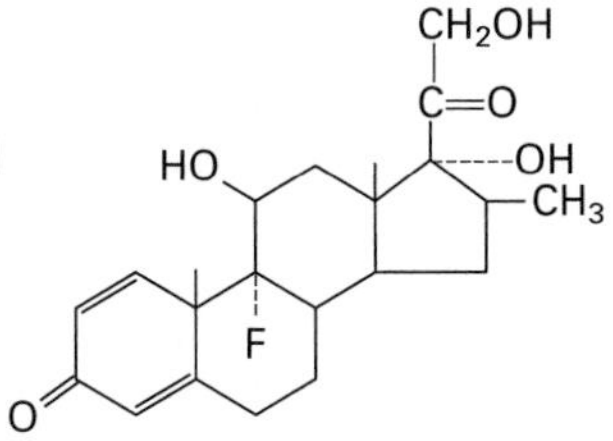

Betamethasone
(9α-fluoro, 16β-methyl, prednisolone)

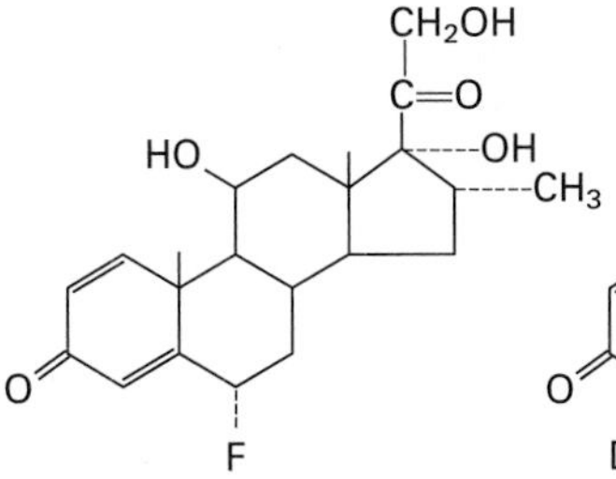

Paramethasone
(6α-fluoro, 16α-methyl, prednisolone)

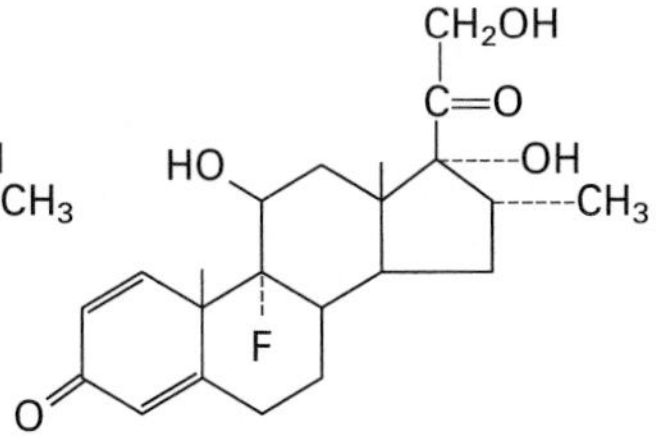

Dexamethasone
(9α-fluoro, 16α-methyl, prednisolone)

FIGURE 39-4 Structural formulas of commonly used synthetic corticosteroids.

min, which has nonspecific, low-affinity binding properties. Plasma-free steroids enter target cells by passive diffusion and bind to a cytoplasmic soluble-binding protein (acceptor site), forming a steroid-acceptor protein complex. This complex undergoes a conformational change and migrates to the nucleus, where it interacts with steroid receptors on chromatin. This induces transcription of new mRNA and new protein synthesis.

Effects on Organ Systems

Glucocorticoids influence virtually every tissue and organ in the body. The end result of their action is the induction (anabolism) or suppression (catabolism) of protein synthesis. For example, there is a marked increase in the concentration and activity of liver enzymes such as glucose-6-phosphatase, fructose-6-diphosphatase, and phosphoenolpyruvate carboxykinase following glucocorticoid administration. But glucocorticoids can also suppress DNA synthesis, induce protein breakdown in muscle, suppress inflammatory responses, and inhibit cell proliferation in epithelial, lymphoid, connective, and bone tissue. In lymphatic cells, glucocorticoids stimulate the synthesis of an "inhibiting protein" responsible for the catabolic action.

Mineralocorticoids (e.g., aldosterone) facilitate the transport of sodium across the distal renal tubule epithelium. They increase the activity of enzymes involved in the generation of adenosine triphospate (ATP), which will act as an energy source for the sodium pump. They also increase phospholipase activity, fatty-acid synthesis, and acyltransferase activity. These actions play a role in the regulation of the sodium transport.

Carbohydrate and Protein Metabolism When glucocorticoids are administered acutely to normal fasting humans, their catabolic action mobilizes amino acids from protein in muscle and plasma, increasing their flow to the liver, where they serve as substates for gluconeogenesis. Glucose utilization by peripheral tissues is inhibited. Fatty acids are mobilized from adipose tissue and replace glucose as an energy source for muscle. This results in a rise in plasma glucose, stimulating insulin release to prevent ketogenesis. More prolonged exposure to glucocorticoids stimulates release of glucagon, which promotes gluconeogenesis and decreases sensitivity to insulin. The overall effect of glucocorticoids on energy metabolism is the conservation of carbohydrate in the form of glycogen and the use of proteins and lipids as alternative sources of fuel.

Lipid Metabolism Lipogenesis is normally initiated when glucose, under the action of insulin, enters the adipocytes. It is then metabolized to acetyl CoA, which will be used for fatty-acid synthesis. Fatty acids, in turn, are esterified with glycerol phosphate to form triglycerides. This anabolic cascade is inhibited by glucocorticoids; this blockade can be overcome by large doses of insulin. Lipolysis occurs with stimulation of an adipocyte "hormone-sensitive lipase" by catecholamines and various hormones such as ACTH, glucagon, and TSH. However, the presence of glucocorticoids is usually necessary for this activation. Insulin blocks this effect. Thus the antagonistic actions of glucocorticoids and insulin participate in the regulation of lipid metabolism. Clinically, patients with glucocorticoid excess exhibit a characteristic redistribution of fat, which accumulates in the face ("moon face"), interscapular area ("buffalo hump"), supraclavicular fossae, and omentum (truncal obesity).

Electolyte and Water Metabolism Aldosterone is the most potent endogenous mineralocorticoid. It acts on the distal renal tubules, where it promotes sodium reabsorption and increases urinary excretion of potassium and hydrogen ions. Adrenal insufficiency is characterized by hyponatremia, hyperkalemia, acidosis, contraction of extracellular volume, cell hydration, and increased urinary excretion of sodium. In the absence of exogenous mineralocorticoid, most patients can be maintained alive with sodium chloride solution.

Hypercorticism results in a positive sodium balance, normal or increased plasma sodium concentration, hypokalemic hypochloremic alkalosis, and increased extracellular volume. If this state persists, sodium excretion eventually increases until it equals sodium intake, thus averting gross edema. However, despite this poorly understood "escape phenomenon," the excessive urinary excretion of potassium and hydrogen ions continues.

Glucocorticoids also possess mineralocorticoid activity and can cause salt and water retention, but they are 1000 times less potent than aldosterone, thus limiting the amount of free cortisol available to compete for mineralocorticoid-binding sites.

Central Nervous System In states of hypercorticism (Cushing's syndrome), there are profound effects on the CNS. Up to 20 percent of patients are psychotic. Other psychologic manifestations include irritability, insomnia, difficulty in concentrating, and hallucinations. When Cushing's syndrome is drug-induced, the most common manifestation is euphoria.

Patients with Addison's disease commonly exhibit apathy, depression, and fatigue. There is a lowered threshold for the senses of taste, smell, and hearing. An EEG shows diffuse high-amplitude slowing of activity.

The exact mechanism of glucocorticoid action on the central nervous system is not well understood. Glucocorticoids regulate cerebral blood flow and the movement of sodium and potassium across cell membranes. They also modulate neural conduction by their stimulatory effect on neurotransmitter release; in high doses they increase neuronal excitability and lower the seizure threshold.

Cardiovascular System The effect of mineralocorticoids on sodium and water retention, hence on plasma volume, has already been discussed. However, the cardiovascular actions of corticosteroids are complex and still poorly understood. Adrenal insufficiency is characterized by hypotension and decreased cardiac output. Heart size is reduced and myocardial contractility is depressed. Arteriolar tone is diminished, partly through decreased inhibition of prostacyclin (PGI_2) synthesis. Capillary permeability is increased. These phenomena do not respond to volume expansion or administration of catecholamines, but they respond dramatically to intravenous cortisol.

Cushing's syndrome is also accompanied by depressed cardiac output. This effect, however, is a result of prolonged arterial hypertension and is not totally reversible after treatment of the hyperadrenocortical state.

Gastrointestinal System High-dose glucocorticoids are associated with an increased incidence of gastric and duodenal ulcers. However, the incidence of such ulcers in patients with natural Cushing's syndrome is the same as in the normal population. High-dose steroids increase gastric secretion of acid and pepsin, but this effect is probably not a major contributing factor, since patients with achlorhydria can also develop steroid-induced ulcers. More importantly, glucocorticoids decrease the rate of gastric mucous secretion and reduce the rate of renewal of gastric surface epithelial cells, thus weakening the physical barrier and delaying the healing of mucosal lesions.

Musculoskeletal System Excess glucocorticoids cause muscle weakness and can, with chronic use, lead to muscle atrophy. This steroid-induced myopathy is a result of increased protein breakdown. Adrenal insufficiency is associated with weakness and fatigability, but this may be due to the compromised cardiovascular state rather than to a primary effect on muscle. In primary aldosteronism, the observed weakness is secondary to hypokalemia.

Children treated with supraphysiologic doses of glucocorticoids exhibit a delay in linear growth and skeletal maturation. Osteopenia is a frequent complication of chronic steroid therapy and is the end result of two distinct mechanisms: (1) direct inhibition of osteoblasts and (2) inhibition of intestinal calcium absorption, leading to secondary hyperparathyroidism and consequently to stimulation of osteoclastic activity. Cartilage breakdown may occur, leading to joint degeneration. The analgesic properties of glucocorticoids might facilitate the prolonged, painless traumatization of the joint and development of a severe arthropathy. Avascular necrosis of bone is another complication of glucocorticoid excess. Its mechanism remains poorly understood.

Skin and Connective Tissue The main cutaneous finding in adrenal insufficiency is the slow development of a diffuse hyperpigmentation, more pronounced over exposed areas of skin, areas subject to pressure and friction such as the knees and axillae, and, more characteristically, in the creases of palms and soles. Normally pigmented areas such as the nipples and genital skin appear darker. This phenomenon is a result of increased plasma levels of melanocyte stimulating hormone (MSH, melanocortin) which, along with ACTH, is derived by proteolytic cleavage from a common precursor glycoprotein, preopiomelanocortin. Vitiligo may appear, interspersed with hypermelanosis, indicating the presence of "idiopathic" adrenal insufficiency, an acquired autoimmune disorder. Body hair is diminished and at times absent.

Excessive glucocorticoids inhibit fibroblast activity, resulting in decreased collagen formation. Patients with Cushing's syndrome exhibit thinning of skin and the development of purplish striae, predominantly on the lower abdomen and hips. The loss of collagen support around subcutaneous blood vessels lead to easy bruising and purpura. Skin ulcers may develop as a result of minor trauma and wound healing is delayed. The changes in fat distribution have been described earlier. Women may display mild hirsutism and acne secondary to increased production of androgens by the adrenals. Hyperpigmentation, such as in Addison's disease, can be seen in Cushing's disease, in which a pituitary adenoma secretes large amounts of ACTH.

Hematologic Effects Glucocorticoids display both anti-inflammatory and immunosuppressive characteristics through complex and, at times, shared mechanisms, some of which remain poorly understood. They act on the different components of the inflammatory process, which includes various cell types, enzymes, and vascular responses. They increase the polymorphonuclear count by accelerating the transfer of mature neutrophils from the bone marrow and inhibiting their passage from blood to the site of inflammation. Glucocorticoids also cause lymphocytopenia, monocytopenia, and eosinopenia by several mechanisms, which probably include redistribution of these cells into other compartments, including the bone marrow and spleen. In addition, there is a delayed release of monocyte precursors from the bone marrow. The end result is decreased influx of leukocytes to the inflammatory site. Cells within this site release the enzymes stored in their lysosomes. The stabilizing effect of steroids on lysosomal membranes remains controversial and is thought to be of little significance with the usual pharmacologic doses. Macrophages have been demonstrated in vitro to exhibit decreased bactericidal and fungicidal activity. Clearance of opsonized and nonopsonized materials by the reticuloendothelial system is decreased. Finally, glucocorticoids suppress the vasodilatation which is responsible for increased capillary permeability and edema.

Most immunologic processes display an inflammatory component upon which glucocorticoids can act following the above mechanisms. Although all subpopulations of lymphocytes are decreased, the depression of cell-mediated immunity is probably not the sole result of direct action of corticosteroids on T lymphocytes; rather, steroids seem to act preferentially, by direct or indirect means, on the macrophages. Thus, decreased recruitment of the latter leads to blunted cutaneous delayed hypersensitivity. The effect of macrophage migration inhibitory factor (MIF) and macrophage aggregating factor (MAF) is suppressed, resulting in decreased access of these cells to the sites of inflammatory and immunologic processes. The effect of glucocorticoids on humoral immunity is less well understood. Corticosteroids inhibit the passage of immune complexes across basement membranes and decrease the levels of complement. However, there is so far no convincing evidence of a more direct effect on autoimmune processes such as the suppression of antibody production.

Endocrine Effects The hypothalamic-hypophyseal-adrenal axis, like many other endocrine systems, is regulated by a negative-feedback mechanism. Glucocorticoids inhibit release of ACTH. Administration of exogenous corticosteroids for more than 3 weeks causes decreased stimulation of the adrenals by ACTH, resulting in atrophy of the adrenal cortex. The degree of atrophy is dose-dependent. Even a low-dose regimen, such as prednisone, 5 mg/day, or its equivalent, can induce detectable adrenal suppression. The fascicular and reticular zones are most affected. The zona glomerulosa, which secretes aldosterone, is minimally dependent on ACTH and thus is least sensitive to pituitary suppression. The clinical implication of adrenal atrophy is the development of primary adrenal insufficiency. The exogenous corticosteroids are sufficient to replace output by the deficient gland under basal conditions. However, in stressful situations such as surgery, major illness, or trauma, when a normal adrenal would increase in production by up to tenfold, larger doses of steroids should be administered to avoid development of a state identical to adrenal crisis. When chronic steroid therapy is discontinued, increased production of ACTH stimulates the adrenal once again. However, during the first 9 to 12 months following interruption of therapy, the gland, which has not fully recovered from its prolonged suppression, remains in a state of relative insufficiency and is unable to meet the increased demands in conditions of stress. Such patients are at risk of developing acute adrenal insufficiency and should be covered with large doses of exogenous steroids throughout the duration of their illness.

Functional Tests

Dexamethasone Suppression Test Hypercortisolism (Cushing's syndrome) can be the result of abnormal adrenal hyperactivity secondary to adrenal adenoma or carcinoma, an ACTH-secreting pituitary adenoma, or ectopic production of ACTH or CRF. However, hypercortisolism can also be a normal physiologic response to stress.

Dexamethasone is a potent synthetic glucocorticoid which can suppress the pituitary-adrenal axis at a dose which will not affect plasma or urinary concentrations of endogenous steroids. Its structural formula is shown in Fig. 39-4.

Overnight Dexamethasone Suppression Test
Dexamethasone 1.0 mg is given orally at 11:00 P.M. The plasma cortisol level at 8:00 A.M. the next day should be less than 5 μg/dL, indicating normal negative feedback. Higher cortisol levels are suggestive but not diagnostic of hyperadrenocorticism. In Cushing's syndrome, levels are usually greater than 20 μg/dL. This is a rapid test, frequently used for screening purposes, with the knowledge that false positive results are not infrequent.

Low-Dose and High-Dose Dexamethasone Suppression Tests These tests are done consecutively over a 6-day period. During the first 2 days, 24-h urine samples are collected for free cortisol and creatinine. On days 3 and 4, dexamethasone (0.5 mg) is given orally every 6 h, starting at 8:00 A.M., as urine collection continues. On days 5 and 6, dexamethasone (2.0 mg) is given orally every 6 h, while urine collection proceeds. Plasma cortisol is measured at 4:00 P.M. on days 4 and 6. A normal suppression on low-dose dexamethasone is indicated by a greater than 50 percent drop in urine cortisol or a plasma cortisol level less than 5 μg/dL. On high-dose dexamethasone, a greater than 50 percent fall in urine cortisol or a plasma cortisol less than 10 μg/dL indicates partial suppression and is suggestive of an ACTH-producing pituitary adenoma (Cushing's disease). Failure to suppress suggests adrenal tumor or ectopic production of ACTH or CRF.

False positive results can be seen in some patients with endogenous depression. Patients on phenytoin or phenobarbital also fail to suppress, secondary to the accelerated rate of metabolism of dexamethasone. Other drugs such as sympathomimetics, nasal decongestants, and oral contraceptive agents can also inhibit dexamethasone suppression. Finally, as mentioned earlier, stress is a frequent cause of false positive results, especially among hospitalized patients.

ACTH Stimulation Test The secretory reserve of the adrenal cortex can be determined by its response to exogenous ACTH. A 24-h infusion of synthetic 1–24 ACTH (cosyntropin, Cortrosyn) is initiated with a concomitant 24-h urine collection for 17-hydroxycorticosteroids. A partial rise in 17-hydroxycorticosteroids is suggestive of secondary adrenal insufficiency (hypopituitarism); failure to respond is characteristic of primary adrenal failure (Addison's disease). Sometimes, a more prolonged, 48-h, infusion is necessary to separate those two entities. A quicker alternative is the rapid Cortrosyn test; 0.25 mg (about 25 units) Cortrosyn is injected intravenously or intramuscularly. Plasma cortisol and aldosterone are measured before and 30 or 60 min after injection. Normally, cortisol should rise by more than 7 μ/dL from baseline with a peak level greater than 20 μ/dL. Primary adrenal insufficiency is characterized by a subnormal response of cortisol and aldosterone. A normal rise in aldosterone with a subnormal cortisol response is indicative of secondary adrenal insufficiency.

Metyrapone Test Metyrapone is one of several drugs designed to block steroidogenesis.

Metyrapone

Metyrapone inhibits 11-hydroxylase, the enzyme which catalyzes the addition of a hydroxy group on position 11 of 11-deoxycortisol (compound S) and 11-deoxycorticosterone (DOC) to form cortisol and corticosterone, respectively. Administration of metyrapone causes a transient deficiency in cortisol, thereby decreasing negative feedback on the pituitary. ACTH release is increased, causing a rise in 11-deoxycortisol and of its metabolites in the form of urinary 17-hydroxycorticosteroids (17-OHCS). This test studies the secretory potential of the pituitary, after an ACTH stimulation test has determined adequate adrenocortical function. It is conducted over a 3-day period. On day 1, a 24-h urine collection is obtained for baseline concentrations of 17-OHCS and creatinine. On day 2, metyrapone (Metopirone) is administered at a dose of 750 mg orally every 4 h (total dose 4.5 g) while urine collection continues. A final 24-h urine collection is performed on day 3. Normally, the urinary 17-OHCS should demonstrate a threefold or greater increase from their baseline value or attain a concentration of 18 mg per 24 h or more on day 3. Plasma 11-deoxycortisol should rise above 290 nmol/L. Hyperthyroidism, phenytoin, or barbiturate therapy can blunt the response to metyrapone by increasing the rate of metabolism of the drug.

Spironolactone

Mineralocorticoids such as aldosterone increase renal tubular reabsorption of sodium and chloride and augment potassium excretion. Spironolactone is a synthetic compound which belongs to the group of 17-spirolactone steroids.

Spironolactone

It has no positive intrinsic activity. It is a competitive aldosterone antagonist, binding to the same receptor sites as the natural hormone. Spironolactone (Aldactone) thus is only effective in the presence of aldosterone and is indicated in the treatment of primary and secondary hyperaldosteronism. Its pharmacology is discussed in the chapter on diuretics since spironolactone is used as a potassium-sparing diuretic.

Clinical Uses of Corticosteroids

Corticosteroids do not cure any disease, but they are nevertheless used in a variety of conditions where their anti-inflammatory, immunosuppressive, and mineralocorticoid properties are applied. They also serve as replacement therapy in patients with adrenal insuffi-

ciency. Corticosteroids can be life-saving in status asthmaticus, severe allergic reactions, and transplantation rejection. They are available as nasal sprays for allergic rhinitis. They are effective in noninfectious granulomatous diseases, such as sarcoid, and in many collagen vascular diseases, particularly rheumatoid arthritis and systemic lupus erythematosus. Intra-articular injection is indicated in some rheumatologic disorders. They have been used in treatment of leukemia. They can also be applied topically as ointments, creams, lotions, and sprays for treatment of dermatologic and ophthalmologic diseases.

Adverse Reactions

Corticosteroids are very potent drugs, and it is virtually impossible to achieve clinical improvement on pharmacologic doses of steroids without inducing side effects. Consequently, they should be used at the smallest effective dose and over the briefest period (in short-lived illnesses). There are no absolute contraindications for their use, especially in life-threatening situations. However, continued use of large doses can result in iatrogenic Cushing's syndrome. Corticosteroid therapy can also lead to peptic ulceration with or without hemorrhage and increased susceptibility to infection. Osteoporosis may be induced by chronic use in the elderly. Myopathy is an uncommon but serious complication. Psychosis can also occur. Therefore, caution should be exercised when administering corticosteroids to patients with peptic ulcer disease, osteoporosis, tuberculosis, and other chronic infections and psychological disorders.

In intensive corticosteroid therapy, sudden cessation results in withdrawal symptoms consisting mainly of signs of adrenal insufficiency, but they may also include fever, myalgia, arthralgia, and malaise. It is advisable to reduce corticosteroid doses gradually rather than terminate therapy abruptly.

Dosage

By far the most serious complication of chronic steroid therapy (more than 3 weeks duration) is suppression of the hypothalamic-pituitary-adrenal axis (HPA axis). Dosage should thus be frequently adjusted according to disease activity to avoid overtreatment. Moreover, the choice of steroids is important, since preparations with long half-lives, such as dexamethasone, cause more suppression than those preparations with shorter half-lives such as hydrocortisone or prednisone. Similarly, the more potent drugs have more potential for suppression (Table 39-1). During full-blown disease activity, patients are placed on a several-times daily, relatively large dose corticosteroid regimen. If clinical improvement occurs but the primary stimulus for the disease process is still present, steroid administration is reduced to one daily morning dose. As remission is maintained, an alternate-day regimen is substituted, whereby double the daily dose is given as a single dose every other day. This method is thought to minimize inhibition of the HPA axis while keeping disease activity in a stable subclinical state. If relapse occurs, a temporary return to divided-dose daily corticosteroids will be necessary. Daily physiologic replacement doses of glucocorticoids are standard: cortisone acetate, 37.5 mg; hydrocortisone, 30 mg; prednisone, 7.5 mg; or dexamethasone, 0.5 to 0.75 mg.

Preparations

Glucocorticoids can be administered orally, parenterally (intramuscular, intravenous, intra-articular, and intralesional), by inhalation, and topically (ophthalmic solutions, dermal preparations, and retention enemas). All routes of administration may lead to a certain degree of systemic absorption and induce suppression of the hypothalamopituitary axis. Structures of some chemically useful agents are shown in Fig. 39-4. The compounds are classified based on their duration of action, relative potency, and ratio of anti-inflammatory to mineralocorticoid activity (see Table 39-1).

Beclomethasone dipropionate is available in metered-dose aerosol units which deliver 42 μg per actuation nasally (Vancenase, Beconase) or orally (Vanceril, Beclovent).

Bethamethasone (Celestone, etc.) is available as various salts for oral administration, as creams, oint-

TABLE 39-1 Relative potencies of some natural and synthetic corticosteroids

Drug	Relative anti-inflammatory effect	Relative sodium-retaining effect	Equivalent dose for anti-inflammatory activity, mg
Glucocorticoids			
Short-acting (biologic half-life, 8–12 h)			
Hydrocortisone (cortisol)	1.0	1.0	20
Cortisone	0.8	0.8	25
Prednisone	4.0	0.8	5
Prednisolone	4.0	0.8	5
Methylprednisolone	5.0	0.5	4
Intermediate-acting (biologic half-life, 12–36 h)			
Triamcinolone	5.0	0	4
Paramethasone	10.0	0	2
Long-acting (biologic half-life, 36 h)			
Dexamethasone	30.0	0	0.75
Betamethasone	30.0	0	0.6
Mineralocorticoids			
Aldosterone	0	300–900	
Fludrocortisone	10.0	250	

ments, and lotions for topical use, and as a topical aerosol.

Cortisone acetate is available as tablets of 25 mg and as a suspension for injection containing 25 and 50 mg/mL.

Hydrocortisone is available as tablets of 10 and 20 mg; as single-dose retention enema bottles containing 100 mg per 60 mL; as a topical cream, 1 and 2.5%; as an ointment, 1 and 2.5%; as a lotion, 0.5, 1, and 2.5%; and as a 0.5% topical aerosol.

Hydrocortisone sodium succinate (Solu-Cortef) is a sterile powder for intramuscular or intravenous injections. Available in vials of 100, 250, 500, and 1000 mg.

Fludrocortisone acetate (Florinef Acetate) is available in 0.1-mg tablets.

Dexamethasone (Decadron) is available as tablets of 0.25, 0.5, 0.75, 1.5, 4, and 6 mg; as an elixir containing 0.5 mg/mL; as a topical cream of 0.1%; and as a 0.01% topical aerosol.

Dexamethasone sodium phosphate (Decadron) is available as a suspension for IM or IV injection containing 4 mg/mL, and in a concentration of 24 mg/mL for IV administration only; as a 0.05% ophthalmic ointment; and as an inhaler which delivers approximately 0.1 mg per actuation.

Prednisone is available as tablets of 2.5, 5, 10, 20, and 50 mg and as a syrup containing 1 mg/mL.

Methylprednisolone (Medrol) is available as tablets of 2, 4, 8, 16, 24, and 32 mg and as a topical solution in a concentration of 2.5 mg (0.25%) and 10 mg (1.0%) per gram.

Methylprednisolone sodium succinate (Solu-Medrol) is available as a powder for IM or IV injection in vials of 40, 125, 500, 1000, and 2000 mg.

Triamcinolone (Aristocort) is available as 1-, 2-, 4-, and 8-mg tablets.

Triamcinolone diacetate (Aristocort) is available as a syrup containing 0.4 mg/mL; as a suspension for IM injection at a concentration of 40 mg/mL; and as a suspension for intralesional injections at a concentration of 25 mg/mL.

Triamcinolone acetonide (Aristocort, Kenalog) is available as a 0.025, 0.1, and 0.5% cream and ointment; as a 0.025 and 0.1% lotion; as a spray which delivers up to 0.2 mg per 2-s application; and as a suspension for intramuscular and intralesional injection at a concentration of 10 and 40 μg/mL.

BIBLIOGRAPHY

Dluhy, R. G., T. Himathongkam, and M. Greenfield: "Rapid ACTH Test with Plasma Aldosterone Levels: Improved Diagnostic Discrimination," *Ann. Intern. Med.,* **80:**693–696 (1974).

Fainer, A. S., D. C. Dale, and J. E. Balow: "Glucocorticoid Therapy: Mechanisms of Action and Clinical Considerations," *Ann. Intern. Med.,* **84:**304–315 (1976).

Fraser, R., J. J. Brown, A. F. Lever, P. A. Mason, and J. I. S. Robertson: "Control of Aldosterone Secretion," *Clinical Sci.,* **56:**389–399 (1979).

Graber, A. L., R. L. Ney, W. E. Nicholson, D. P. Island, and G. W. Liddle: "Natural History of Pituitary-Adrenal Recovery following Long-Term Suppression with Corticosteroids," *J. Clin. Endocrin. Metabol.,* **25:**11–16 (1965).

Makman, M. H., B. Dvorkin, and A. White: "Evidence for Induction by Cortisol in Vitro of a Protein Inhibitor of Transport and Phosphorylation Processes in Rat Thymocytes," *Proc. Natl. Acad. Sci. USA,* **68:**1269–1273 (1971).

Melby, J. E.: "Systemic Corticosteroid Therapy: Pharmacology and Endocrinologic Considerations," *Ann. Intern. Med.,* **81:**505–512 (1974).

O'Malley, B. W.: "Mechanisms of Action of Steroid Hormones," *N. Engl. J. Med.,* **284:**370–377 (1971).

Rose, L. I., and C. Saccar: "Choosing Corticosteroid Preparations," *Am. Family Physician,* **17:**198–204 (1978)

Rose, L. I., G. H. Williams, P. I. Jagger, and D. P. Lawler: "The 48-Hour Adrenocotrophin Infusion Test for Adrenocortical Insufficiency," *Ann. Intern. Med.,* **73:**49–54 (1970).

Streek, W. F., and D. H. Lockwood: "Pituitary Adrenal Recovery following Short-Term Suppression with Corticosteroids," *Am. J. Med.,* **66:**910–914 (1979).

Taylor, A. L., and L. M. Fishman: "Corticotropin-Releasing Hormone," *N. Engl. J. Med.,* **3419:**213–222 (1988).

Thorn, G. W., and D. P. Lawler: "Clinical Therapeutics of Adrenal Disorders," *Am. J. Med.,* **53:**673–684 (1972).

PART VIII

Antineoplastic Agents

SECTION EDITOR
Joseph R. DiPalma

C H A P T E R **40**

Cancer Chemotherapy

Isadore Brodsky, Pamela Crilley, and Allen E. Lord Terzian

The cure of a patient with cancer depends on the success of removal or destruction of every cancer cell within the body. Currently, even with the best and most efficiently applied detection procedures, only 50 percent of all newly diagnosed cancer patients will be cured of their disease. The reason for failure to cure is not delay in diagnosis. It is because cancer has spread beyond the confines of its primary location, making local form of therapy inadequate. In essence, these patients need some form of systemic treatment.

Surgery, chemotherapy, and radiation constitute the three forms of treatment for cancer, but only chemotherapy can effectively treat systemic disease.

Cancer chemotherapy is totally nonspecific. By that we mean that the drugs kill not only cancer cells but also normal cells that happen to be dividing. Because of the nonspecificity of killing, strategies have been developed to increase relatively the cancer-killing potential of these agents by lessening the toxic impact on normal tissues. These strategies require a knowledge of the pharmacology of the drugs as well as a knowledge of tumor cell kinetics.

It has been recognized for decades that cancers grow at different rates than the tissues from which they are derived. Paradoxically, and contrary to that which is expected, normal tissues often grow faster than the cancerous ones. Thus normal tissues may recover from the cytoinhibitory effects of cancer chemotherapy faster than the cancer being treated. By "cycling" the drug therapy being given, differential cytotoxicity favoring cancer cytoreduction may occur. Then it is incumbent upon the clinician to recognize these patients for optimum therapy to be given.

Much has been written about the side effects and toxicities of cancer therapy. One ought to distinguish the difference between a noncytotoxic toxicity (i.e., nausea and vomiting) and a cytotoxic effect on normal tissue (bone marrow suppression). Similarly, the clinician ought to recognize why chemotherapy may fail. Cytokinetic failure and lethal side effects created in normal tissues are obvious reasons. Repair of cellular damage, impaired cellular drug penetrance, increased cellular drug excretion, and drug detoxification are other mechanisms for failure of therapy. A molecular biology approach in which specific drug receptors are identified and where cellular metabolisms are defined has made possible a more efficient selective toxicity for the cancerous cell, as compared to the normal cell.

THE CELL CYCLE

Cell division by both normal and neoplastic cells progresses through an orderly sequence of events collectively called the *cell cycle*. The biochemical changes that occur within growing cells during the cell cycle have been divided into four major phases (Fig. 40-1). The M phase is the period of mitosis (cell division); the S phase is the time during which DNA is synthesized. The G_1 phase is usually the longest phase and is the interval during which RNA synthesis, protein synthesis, and cellular growth occur. The G_2 phase is the interval during which formation of specialized proteins, in preparation for mitosis, occurs. Cells that are dormant or in a resting state, but retain the potential to divide, are said to be in phase G_0.

549

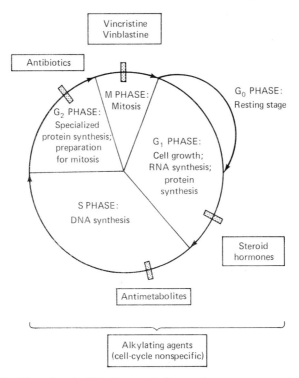

FIGURE 40-1   The cell cycle. This diagram indicates where some cancer chemotherapeutic agents act during the cell growth cycle. Antibiotics, for example, are cell-cycle-specific for the G_2 phase; alkylating agents are cell-cycle-nonspecific and affect cell growth during all phases.

Most cancer chemotherapy drugs cause cell death by affecting the ability of cells to divide. This means the drugs inhibit one or more of the phases of the cell cycle or prevent a cell in G_0 from entering into the cycle. Drugs that inhibit cell replication during a phase of the cycle are termed *cell-cycle–specific cytotoxic agents*. Methotrexate (an antimetabolite), for example is a cell-cycle–specific antimetabolite that inhibits DNA synthesis during the S phase. Because its cytotoxic action is restricted to one phase of the cell cycle, methotrexate is termed a *phase-specific cytotoxic agent*. Agents that are active while the cancer cells are dividing but whose action spans more than one phase of the cycle are termed *cycle-specific agents*. Cell-cycle–nonspecific drugs (e.g., mechlorethamine, an alkylating agent) affect cellular division at all phases of the cell cycle as well as cells within G_0. Figure 40-1 shows an outline of the site of action of various cancer chemo-

therapeutic agents in the cell cycle. Cells that are in the G_0 phase are relatively resistant to most chemotherapy drugs requiring increased dosages to attain any response. The toxicity of cycle-specific drugs is proportional to the length of exposure, whereas the toxicity of the cycle-nonspecific drugs is purely dose-related. Therefore cycle-specific drugs given by continuous infusion become much more toxic than the same total dose given as an intravenous bolus. This is because during increased exposure time, an increased proportion of cells will pass through the specific phase affected by the drug.

Malignant neoplasms are composed of *dividing cells, nondividing cells* (G_0), and *end-stage cells*, which have permanently lost the capacity to divide and will eventually die. The *growth fraction* relates the fraction of cells in cell cycle to the portion of nonproliferating cells (G_0 and end-stage cells). Chemotherapy is most effective against dividing cells. As cancers enlarge, the growth fraction usually decreases, and consequently the number of cells sensitive to chemotherapy decreases. Chemotherapy also tends to be more cytotoxic against cells with a short cycle length (e.g., lymphoma and leukemia) than those with a long cycle length (e.g., colon cancer and lung cancer).

Mathematical models have been developed to describe the complex growth of neoplasms. At low tumor burden (<10,000 cells), growth of cancers is exponential. This rapid growth phase reflects a short cycle length, minimal cell loss, and a high growth fraction. These facts mean that the time it takes for the total number of cells within a given neoplasm to double (doubling time) is short. With time, however, the doubling time increases, the growth fraction decreases, and a graph of tumor size versus time demonstrates a plateau. The equation for this type of growth pattern was originally described by the eighteenth-century mathematician Gompertz and is known as *Gompertzian growth*. For these reasons advanced cancers are generally less responsive to chemotherapy than those treated earlier.

In order for chemotherapy to be effective for neoplasms with a low growth fraction, the noncycling (G_0) cells need to be forced back into cycle where they will be more vulnerable. A combination of drugs, usually including cycle-nonspecific agents, are given initially. The cycle-nonspecific drugs usually reduce tumor bulk and recruit resting cells into cycle. After a rest period of several weeks to allow recovery of normal tissues, a different combination of drugs (i.e., phase- or cycle-specific) is administered. This strategy enhances tumoroidal effectiveness, reduces clinical side effects, and decreases the emergence of multiple drug-resistant clones.

Chemotherapy is often administered in cycles every 3 or 4 weeks to allow recovery of normal tissues. Each cycle kills malignant cells by first-order kinetics; that is, a constant *fraction* of cells is killed each month, not a constant *number* of cells. Therefore the ability to reduce the tumor cell number to zero (and cure the patient) is related to the *fraction* of cells killed per cycle, the number of cells initially present (which may also predict the number of inherently resistant cells), the length of time between cycles (which allows for regrowth of tumor cells), and the number of cycles given.

GENERAL TOXICITIES TO NORMAL TISSUES

Chemotherapeutic agents are not selectively toxic to neoplastic cells. Therefore, inhibition of cell division of normal cells also occurs. Toxicity to normal tissues often is proportional to dose and/or duration of therapy. In general, the most common dose-limiting toxicities of chemotherapy drugs relate to their inhibition of rapidly proliferating tissues such as bone marrow and gastrointestinal (GI) tract epithelium.

Most chemotherapy drugs cause dose-related reversible bone marrow suppression, resulting in leukopenia and thrombocytopenia, which is most pronounced 10 to 14 days after administration. Bone marrow recovery is complete by 3 to 4 weeks. This places some patients at a temporary risk of severe infection and bleeding.

Nausea and vomiting are also common and are caused by both a central nervous system (CNS) effect at the chemoreceptor trigger zone and through GI irritation. Many chemotherapy drugs cause temporary arrest of the cellular proliferation of the GI mucosa necessary to maintain the integrity of the lining of the GI tract. This can cause severe oral and esophageal pain (i.e., mucositis). If mucosal damage is severe, abdominal pain, diarrhea, GI bleeding, gram-negative sepsis, and bowel perforation can result.

DRUG CLASSIFICATION

Drugs discussed in this chapter are divided into six major groups, as shown in Table 40-1. This arbitrary division provides a convenient basis both for describing the action of the drugs and for helping choose drugs for particular clinical circumstances.

Antimetabolites

Antimetabolites are structural analogs of naturally occurring substances. They interfere with various metabolic processes and disrupt cell function and proliferation. These drugs may act in two ways: (1) by incorporation into a metabolic pathway and formation of a "false" metabolite which is nonfunctional or (2) by inhibition of the catalytic function of an enzyme or enzyme system. Included in the antimetabolite group are the folic acid analogs (methotrexate and tri-

TABLE 40-1   Some examples of cancer chemotherapeutic agents

1. Antimetabolites
    Folate antagonists: methotrexate, trimetrexate
    Purine derivatives: mercatopurine, thioguanine
    Pyrimidine derivatives: fluorouracil, floxuridine, cytarabine

2. Alkylating Agents
    Nitrogen mustards: mechlorethamine, chlorambucil, cyclophosphamide, mephalan, ifosfamide
    Nitrosourease: lomustine, carmustine, streptozocin
    Triazine: dacarbazine
    Alkyl Sulfonate: busulfan
    Platinum Derivatives: cisplatin, carboplatin
    Methylhydrazine: procarbazine

3. Antibiotics
    Dactinomycin (actinomycin D)
    Plicamycin (mithramycin)
    Bleomycin
    Anthrocyclines: doxorubicin, daunorubicin
    Mitomycin (mitomycin C)
    Mitoxantrone

4. Plant Derivatives
    Alkaloids: vincristine, vinblastine
    Epipodophyllotoxins: etoposide (VP-16), teniposide (VM-26)

5. Miscellaneous
    Amsacrine (m-AMSA)
    Asparaginase
    Hydroxyurea

6. Hormones
    Estrogens: estradiol, diethylstilbesterol, estramustine (see Chap. 37)
    Progestines: hydroxyprogesterone, megestrol, hydroxyprogesterone (see Chap. 37)
    Adrenocorticoids: prednisone, prednisolone (see Chap. 39)
    Androgens: testosterone, fluoxymesterone (see Chap. 38)
    Antiestrogen: tamoxifen (see Chap. 37)
    Gonadotropin analogue: leuprolide

metrexate), purine derivatives (mercaptopurine and thioguanine), pyrimidine derivatives (fluorouracil, floxuridine, and cytarabine), and the substituted urea (hydroxyurea). Figure 40-2 shows some useful antimetabolites, which are discussed below, compared structurally with their corresponding metabolite.

Folate Antagonists

Methotrexate   Mechanism of action   The principal action of methotrexate is to compete with folic acid for the active binding sites on the enzyme dihydrofolate reductase (DHFR). This enzyme's function is to keep folic acid in its reduced state, 5,6,7,8-tetrahydrofolic acid (FH_4) (Fig. 40-3). This reduction occurs in two steps: the first is an NADPH-dependent reduction of folic acid to 7,8-dihydrofolic acid (FH_2), and the second is an NADH- or NADPH-dependent reduction of FH_2, to FH_4. The reduced folates are the active forms, and they function as carriers of one-carbon groups which are required during the synthesis of purines and the pyrimidine thymidylate. Specifically, FH_4 is required for methylation of deoxyuridine monophosphate to deoxythymidine monophosphate and for the addition of formate to the purine precursor inosinic acid. The FH_4 is oxidized to inactive FH_2 during this reaction. Therefore during the S phase a constant supply of DHFR is needed to maintain a pool of reduced folates within the cell. After methotrexate exposure, oxidized folates build up and DNA synthesis is inhibited. The affinity of dihydrofolate reductase for the antimetabolite is far greater than its affinity for the normal substrates, folic acid, and FH_2. Because of the marked affinity of the enzyme for methotrexate, even very large doses of folic acid given simultaneously fail to reverse the effects of methotrexate. If folic acid is given 1 h prior to methotrexate, the drug effects can be prevented, since this allows time for the reduction of folic acid to the active derivatives. Leucovorin (folinic acid, citrovorum factor), if given with or shortly after methotrexate, also prevents its effects, since leucovorin (N^5-formyl FH_4) is a derivative of the product (FH_4) of the blocked reaction. (Fig. 40-3) and can directly supply a source of reduced folates. There is, however, no selective block of toxic effects, and except in special circumstances (see "Therapeutic Uses," below), the use of leucovorin can prevent both the therapeutic and toxic effects of methotrexate.

METABOLITE | ANTIMETABOLITE

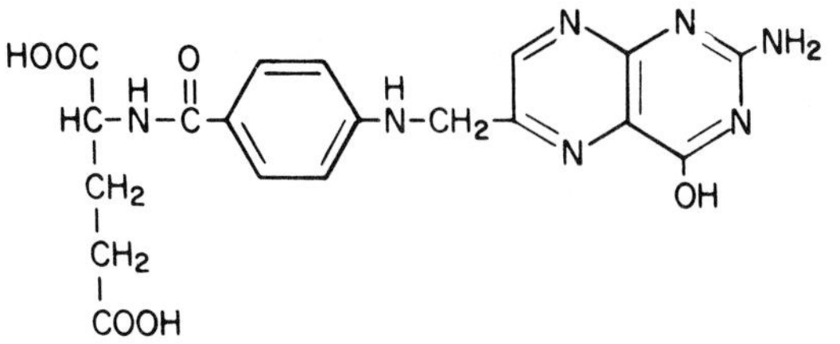

Folic acid (Pteroylglutamic acid)

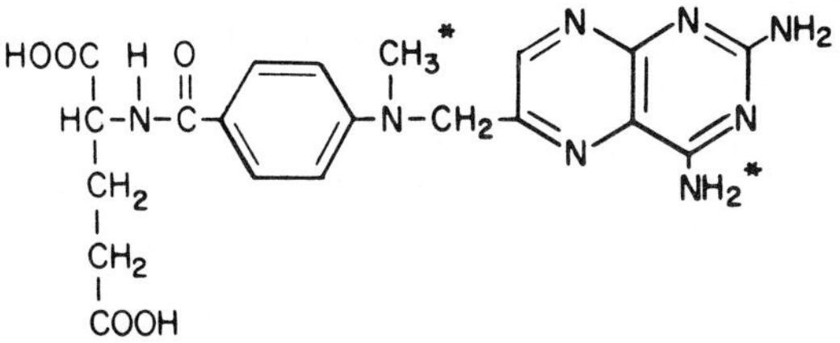

Methotrexate
(4-Amino-N^{10}-methylpteroylglutamic acid)

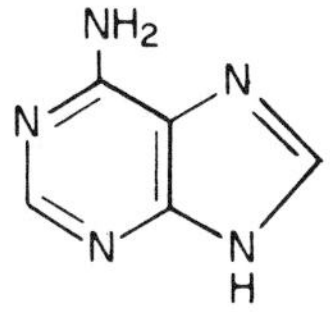

Adenine

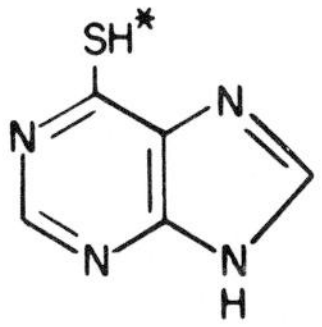

Mercaptopurine

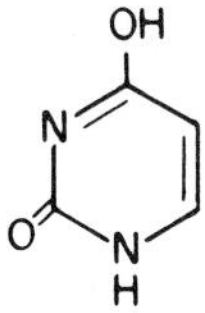

Uracil

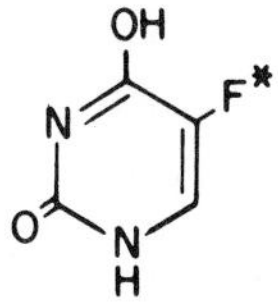

Fluorouracil

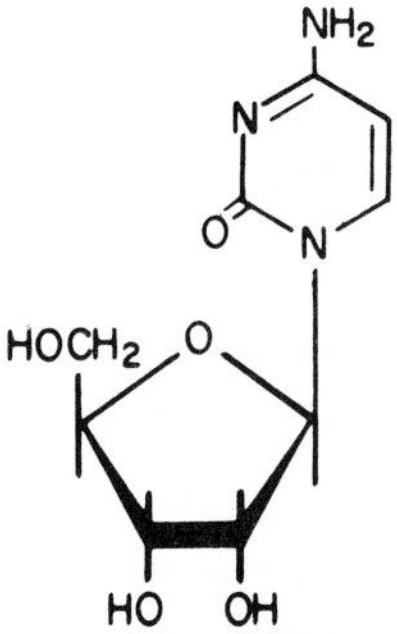

Ribosylcytosine

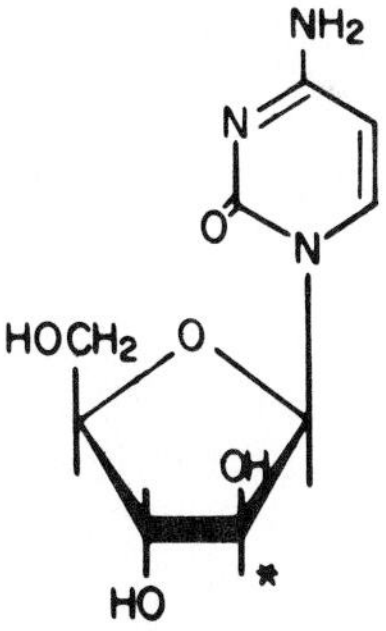

Cytarabine

FIGURE 40-2 Examples of antimetabolites compared with the corresponding metabolites. (The asterisk indicates structural change.)

Pharmacokinetics Methotrexate is well absorbed from the GI tract in doses less than 25 mg. Erratic absorption is seen with larger doses. Peak blood concentration occurs after 1 h. After intravenous or intramuscular injection, the drug rapidly distributes in the extracellular fluid. Methotrexate enters cells by carrier-mediated active transport, although passive diffusion may occur with very large doses. Its half-life is biphasic after a short distribution phase. The primary half-life is 2 to 3 h and is followed by a terminal half-life of 8 to 10 h. Increased toxicity due to prolongation of either half-life occurs with renal disease. Accumula-

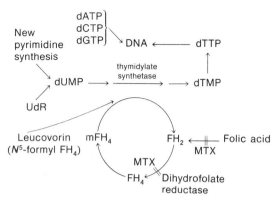

FIGURE 40-3 A schematic representation of the formation of DNA from precursors. The relationship of the generation of thymidylate synthetase cofactor is shown FH$_2$ = dihydrofolate; FH$_4$ = tetrahydrofolate; mFH$_4$ = N^5, N^{10}-methylenetetrahydrofolate; MTX = methotrexate; UdR = uridine; dUMP = deoxyuridylate; dTMP = thymidylate; dATP, dCTP, dGTP, dTTP = deoxyribonucleotidetriphosphates of adenine, cytosine, guanine, and thymine.

tion of drug in pleural or peritoneal fluid can increase toxicity by prolongation of the terminal half-life. The highest tissue levels are found in the kidney and liver. The drug is approximately 50 percent bound to plasma proteins.

Methotrexate penetrates the blood-brain barrier poorly, and when used in conventional doses its concentration in the cerebrospinal fluid (CSF) is less than 10 percent of that in the blood. When given intrathecally, the drug's concentration can be maintained in the CSF for long periods of time. Transport of the drug from the CSF to the systemic circulation does occur. Although methotrexate can be biotransformed in the liver to much less active metabolites, its major route of elimination is the kidney. Methotrexate should be used cautiously in the presence of renal insufficiency.

Therapeutic uses Methotrexate is indicated for the treatment of acute lymphatic leukemia (ALL), choriocarcinoma, non-Hodgkin's lymphoma (NHL), mycosis fungoides, sarcoma of the bone, and cancer of the head and neck and breast and lung. It is also used intrathecally for the treatment of meningeal involvement by cancer, lymphoma, or leukemia.

In an attempt to overcome resistant cells, very high dose regimens have been used with "rescue" by leucovorin 18 to 36 h after the start of the methotrexate infusion. These regimens have achieved cytotoxic CNS levels. They require vigorous hydration to avoid acute renal failure and careful monitoring of methotrexate blood levels to avoid life-threatening toxicity.

Adverse reactions The most common adverse reactions are myelosuppression, nausea, vomiting, abdominal pain, ulceration, and severe mucositis. Hepatic fibrosis can occur with chronic maintenance therapy for ALL or psoriasis. Acute liver atrophy and allergic pneumonitis may be seen rarely. With high-dose regimens, acute renal failure can occur due to precipitation of methotrexate and its metabolites in the renal tubules.

Trimetrexate   (5-methyl-6-[[(3,4,5-trimethoxy-phenyl) amino]methyl]-2,4-quinazolinediamine) Trimetrexate was originally synthesized as an antimalarial agent. It is available as an investigational drug.

Mechanism of action It is a potent inhibitor of DHFR and thus causes inhibition of DNA synthesis in a manner similar to methotrexate.

Pharmacokinetics It is well absorbed orally and can be used intravenously. Elimination is through liver metabolism. The cellular uptake is different from that for methotrexate with less reliance on active transport. It has a biphasic half-life. The initial half-life is 3 h followed by a terminal half-life of 15 to 20 h. Intracellular levels may be 10- to 100-fold higher than those of methotrexate.

Therapeutic uses Trimetrexate has activity against breast, non-small-cell lung cancer and head and neck tumors. It may be useful against some tumors resistant to methotrexate. It also has been used as an antiprotozoa in *Pneumocystis carinii* pneumonia.

Adverse reactions Myelosuppression, mild mucositis, nausea, and skin rash have been described.

Purine Derivatives Among the many purine analogs which have been synthesized, mercaptopurine and thioguanine have proven to be the most clinically effective in cancer chemotherapy. Two other purine analogs are allopurinol, an inhibitor of xanthine oxidase, and azathioprine, and immunosuppressive agent. The structures of these purine analogs are shown in Fig 40-4.

Mercaptopurine (6-MP) and Thioguanine (6-TG)

Mechanism of action   These compounds inhibit the *de novo* synthesis of the purine nucleotides which are composed of a purine base and a phosphorylated ribose sugar. Both compounds need to be converted to the nucleotide level by attaching them to a phosphoribosyl moiety.

This moiety converts 6-MP to the nucleotide 6-thioinosine-5-phosphate (T-IMP), the active form of the drug. *De novo* purine synthesis involves the building of a purine ring step by step on the framework of an activated form of D-ribose-5-phosphate through an inosinic monophosphate (IMP) intermediate. T-IMP through a negative-feedback-like mechanism inhibits the first step in the synthesis of IMP and inhibits the conversion of IMP to adenine and guanine nucleotides, which are necessary for DNA synthesis. Also the triphosphate form of 6-MP is incorporated into DNA and may produce delayed cytotoxicity.

6-TG is converted to its active form 6-thioguanine-5-phosphate (6-thio-GMP). Its major mechanism of action involves the incorporation of the triphosphate form into DNA, replacing the guanine nucleotide and inhibiting DNA synthesis.

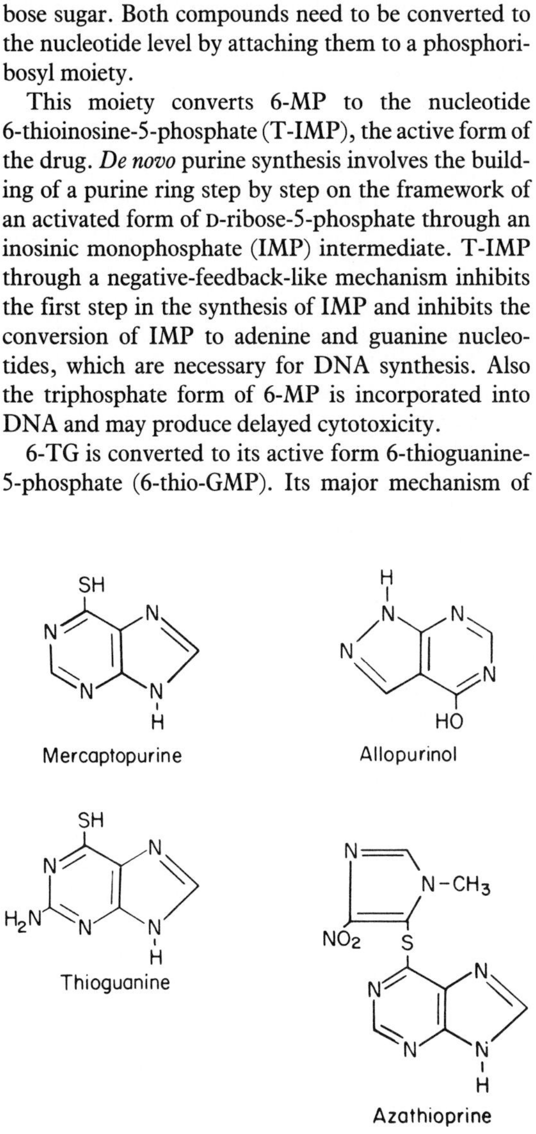

Pharmacokinetics   The absorption of both 6-MP and 6-TG is variable and incomplete and averages 30 to 50 percent of an orally administered dose. Both have half-lives of approximately 1.5 h. Protein binding for 6-MP is approximately 19 percent when given in large doses. 6-MP is liver-metabolized by two pathways. The first involves oxidation by xanthine oxidase, and the second involves methylation of its sulfhydryl group followed by oxidation. 6-T6 is excreted by kidneys primarily as methylated metabolites.

Therapeutic uses   Mercaptopurine has been of value in the treatment of ALL in children and adults. It is of particular use for maintenance therapy. Thioguanine may have some clinical utility when combined with other agents for acute myelogenous leukemia.

Adverse reactions   Some patients, after continued treatment with mercaptopurine or thioguanine, complain of nausea and epigastric distress, probably due to an early toxic effect on the intestinal tract. However, thioguanine causes fewer gastrointestinal side effects than does mercaptopurine. Bone marrow depression is the chief toxic action of both drugs, and excessive dosage produces leukopenia and thrombocytopenia. Although jaundice occurs frequently in patients taking mercaptopurine, permanent liver damage is rare. Nevertheless, liver function tests should be monitored and the drug should be discontinued if liver function tests become abnormal.

Drug interaction: Allopurinol   Allopurinol is a potent inhibitor of xanthine oxidase, which is responsible for the conversion of hypoxanthine and xanthine to uric acid. Consequently, allopurinol is used to treat the excessive production of uric acid seen in gout, leukemia, and lymphoma, particularly where treatment results in the rapid dissolution of neoplastic cells with liberation of their nucleic acid purines and subsequent oxidation of these purines to uric acid. Since mercaptopurine is also a substrate for xanthine oxidase, the concurrent administration of allopurinol delays the oxidative degradation of mercaptopurine and markedly increases its toxicity. The dose of mercaptopurine should therefore be reduced to one-third to one-fourth

FIGURE 40-4   Purine antimetabolites.

of the usual dose if allopurinol is to be given concurrently. Since thioguanine is degraded by other pathways not dependent on xanthine oxidase, its toxicity is not enhanced by allopurinol and, therefore, it may be used more safely than mercaptopurine in clinical situations where allopurinol is needed. Allopurinol produces few adverse reactions, although about 5 percent of patients develop an allergic rash, which is promptly responsive to withdrawal of the medication.

Pyrimidine Derivatives Numerous fluorinated pyrimidine analogs were synthesized as potential anticancer drugs. The most intensively studied of these have been fluorouracil and floxuridine. The structure of flourouracil is shown in Fig. 40-2, and the structure of floxuridine is as follows:

Floxuridine

Fluorouracil (FU, 5-FU) and Floxuridine (FUDR, 5-FUDR) *Mechanism of action* Probably the most important mechanism of action of the fluorinated pyrimidines is the inhibition of thymidylate synthetase and thus interference with DNA production. See Fig. 40-3. This action is accomplished by formation of an active metabolite, 5-fluorodeoxyuridinemonophosphate (FdUMP), from both fluorouracil and floxuridine. FdUMP forms a complex with the reduced folate N^5, N^{10} methylene tetrahydrofolate. This complex inhibits thymidylate synthetase and decreases the methylation of 2-deoxyuridylic acid to form thymidylic acid. The thymidine deficiency which results interferes with cell division and causes cellular injury and death. Also, the triphosphated form of fluorouracil can be incorporated into RNA and interfere with protein synthesis.

Pharmacokinetics Fluoruracil is absorbed irregularly from the GI tract and is degraded by the liver when ingested. Its bioavailability is less than 15 percent when taken orally. For these reasons it is only used intravenously. After an intravenous bolus, it rapidly distributes throughout the body and enters cells by passive diffusion; it has a half-life of only 10 min. Eighty percent is metabolized by the liver, and the metabolic products appear in the urine. Although fluorouracil has a short half-life, the active metabolite FdUMP may persist intracellularly for an extended period.

Therapeutic uses Fluorouracil administered intravenously is indicated in the management of carcinomas of the head and neck, colon, rectum, breast, stomach, bladder, and pancreas. Topical application of the drug is effective for multiple actinic or solar keratoses. This method of administration is also useful in the treatment of superficial basal cell carcinomas.

The combination of high-dose leucovorin followed by fluorouracil has been effective in the treatment of metastatic colon and stomach cancer. Leucovorin supplies a source of reduced folates which may occur in insufficient quantities within neoplastic cells. Leucovorin enhances the formation of the FdUMP IN5-10 methylene tetrahydrofolate

Floxuridine (FUDR) is used for hepatic artery infusion of patients with colon cancer metastatic to liver. Its rapid first-pass metabolism allows greater dosage with lessened systemic toxicity.

Adverse reactions The effects of fluorouracil and floxuridine are most prominent on the rapidly proliferating tissues of the bone marrow and GI tract. Toxicity includes bone marrow suppression, glossitis, diarrhea, and gastrointestinal ulceration and bleeding. The use of leucovorin in combination with 5-FU results in increased toxicity to the normal GI tract. However, the toxicity is more than compensated for by the enhanced tumoricidal effect of the combination.

Cytarabine (Cytosine Arabinoside, Ara-C) *Mechanism of action* Cytarabine is an antimetabolite (Fig 40-2) effective in the treatment of the leukemias. Similar to the other pyrimidine antimetabolites, cytarabine must be "activated" by biotransformation to the corresponding nucleotide. Ara-cytosine triphosphate (ara-CTP) is the active form of the drug. Cytarabine inhibits DNA polymerase and ara-CTP is incorporated into DNA, which inhibits DNA synthesis.

Pharmacokinetics Less than 20 percent of cytarabine is absorbed after oral administration; therefore it is administered intravenously or intramuscularly. Plasma levels with intramuscular use are much lower than those with intravenous use. It has a biphasic half-life. The initial half-life is approximately 10 to 20 min, the terminal half-life about 1 h. About 75 to 90 percent of the drug is excreted in the urine as an inactive metabolite ara-uracil.

Therapeutic use Ara-C is useful for ALL and acute nonlymphatic leukemia (ANLL). When administered by continuous infusion in combination with an anthracycline, remissions of 70 to 80 percent are achieved in ANLL. Resistant leukemia has been treated successfully with very high dose intermittent schedules (usually every 12 h). These doses yield cytotoxic CSF levels.

Adverse reactions Ara-C produces bone marrow depression and gastrointestinal toxicity. When high-dose regimens are used, cerebellar toxicity, conjunctivitis, and elevated liver enzymes can result.

Alkylating Agents

Bis(β-chloroethyl)sulfide (mustard gas) was the most effective war gas used during World War I. In 1935, a nitrogen-containing analog of sulfur mustard, tris(β-chloroethyl)amine, was prepared. This and the related series subsequently prepared have been called *nitrogen mustards*. Many analogs of nitrogen mustard and related agents (e.g., the nitrosoureas) have been synthesized and tested in various biologic systems.

Mechanism of Action The alkylating agents are highly reactive compounds with the ability to form covalent bonds with nucleophilic (electron-rich) sites on molecules such as nucleic acids, phosphates, amino acids, and proteins. Alkylation refers to the formation of a new covalent bond between the above molecules and one of the carbon atoms of an alkylator. This is usually accomplished through the formation of a positively charged carbonium ion ($-Ch^{2+}$). This unstable intermediate may attack any electron-rich site, but it has a predilection for the N-7 position of guanine. The cytotoxic effects of these agents most likely reflect their ability to bind to the nucleotides of DNA. This results in DNA misreading, single- and double-strand breaks, and DNA interstrand cross-linking. Cell death occurs through interference with DNA replication and mitosis. The bifunctional alkylators have the capacity to form DNA interstrand cross-linkages, which makes them more cytotoxic than the monofunctional alkylators. The alkylators have an effect during any part of the cell cycle (cell-cycle nonspecific), but cells in the late G_1 or S phases (especially if rapidly dividing) are most susceptible. Representative chemical reactions are shown in Fig. 40-5.

General Properties

Chemistry The structures of the alkylating agents used most commonly in cancer chemotherapy are shown in Fig. 40-6. Note that all but CCNU contain two or three alkylating groups and are thus known as *bifunctional* or *polyfunctional* alkylating agents. Although the alkylators share a common mechanism of action, their clinical utility varies because of differences in pharmacokinetics, metabolism, lipid solubility, ability to cross cell membranes, and toxicities. They can be classified into (1) nitrogen mustard derivatives (2) nitrosoureas, (3) triazene derivatives, (4) alkyl sulfonates, (5) platinum derivatives, and (6) methyl hydrazines.

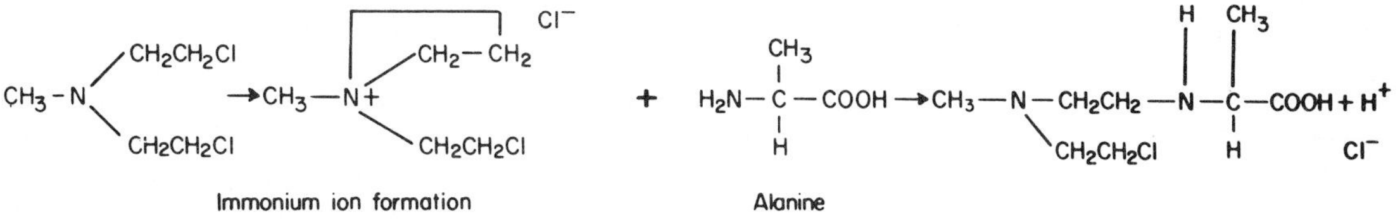

Immonium ion formation   Alanine

FIGURE 40-5 Reactions of an alkylating agent (meehlorethamine) with an amino acid.

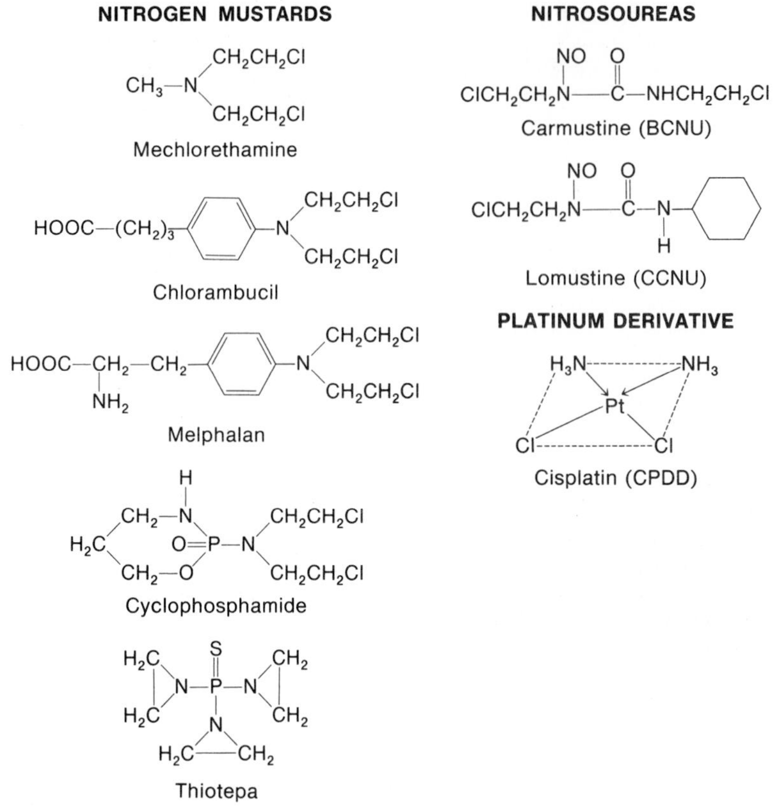

NITROGEN MUSTARDS

$$CH_3—N \begin{smallmatrix} CH_2CH_2Cl \\ \\ CH_2CH_2Cl \end{smallmatrix}$$

Mechlorethamine

$$HOOC—(CH_2)_3— \underset{}{\bigcirc} —N \begin{smallmatrix} CH_2CH_2Cl \\ \\ CH_2CH_2Cl \end{smallmatrix}$$

Chlorambucil

$$HOOC—CH_2—\underset{\underset{NH_2}{|}}{CH_2}— \bigcirc —N \begin{smallmatrix} CH_2CH_2Cl \\ \\ CH_2CH_2Cl \end{smallmatrix}$$

Melphalan

Cyclophosphamide

Thiotepa

NITROSOUREAS

$$ClCH_2CH_2N \overset{NO}{\underset{}{}} \overset{O}{—C—NHCH_2CH_2Cl}$$

Carmustine (BCNU)

$$ClCH_2CH_2N \overset{NO}{\underset{}{}} \overset{O}{—C—}\underset{H}{N}— \bigcirc$$

Lomustine (CCNU)

PLATINUM DERIVATIVE

$$H_3N\text{------}NH_3$$
$$Pt$$
$$Cl\text{------}Cl$$

Cisplatin (CPDD)

FIGURE 40-6   Alkylating agents.

Pharmacokinetics   Generally, the alkylators are eliminated by metabolic pathways with partial excretion of those metabolites through the kidney. The nitrosoureas and cisplatin, however, are excreted in the urine predominantly unchanged.

Adverse Reactions   The adverse reactions of the alkylators as a group include

1. Myelosuppression manifested by a dose-related leukopenia and thrombocytopenia.
2. Gastrointestinal toxicity including nausea, vomiting, mucositis, diarrhea, and possible intestinal mucosal ulceration.
3. Alopecia.
4. Reproductive toxicity with impairment of spermatogenesis, menstrual irregularities, and possible irreversible sterility.

5. Pulmonary fibrosis has been a rare complication of almost all alkylators.
6. Teratogenic effects. An increased incidence of fetal birth defects has been associated with the use of alkylators during the first trimester of pregnancy.
7. Carcinogenic effects. The use of alkylating agents has been shown to increase the incidence of AML, NHL, and other secondary tumors. Although this was first recognized with the use of cyclophosphamide, melphalan, and chlorambucil, most alkylating agents have been implicated. A marked increase in AML has been demonstrated, for example, in patients with polycythemia vera treated with chlorambucil and with the use of nitrogen mustard (the M in MOPP) for Hodgkin's disease. In Hodgkin's disease, the incidence of AML at 10 years varies between 2 and 10 percent in dif-

ferent reports. The use of combined mode (chemotherapy and radiation) appears to be most leukemogenic. A vast majority of cases occur 2 to 9 years after treatment.

8. Drug-specific toxicities are mentioned below.

Individual Agents

Nitrogen Mustards Mechlorethamine (Nitrogen Mustard) Mechlorethamine is commonly used intravenously in combination with other drugs for Hodgkin's disease and for mycosis fungoides. It is very irritating and cannot be administered orally. Its cytotoxic and vesicant properties make it useful for intrapleural administration for malignant pleural effusions. It is a potent vesicant and can cause severe tissue damage and necrosis, requiring skin grafting if given through an extravasated intravenous line. Local venous thrombosis and thrombophlebitis may occur after intravenous use.

Chlorambucil Chlorambucil is well absorbed after oral use. The plasma half-life is approximately 90 min. It is used for chronic lymphatic leukemia (CLL), multiple myeloma, and NHL. It is used orally and is well tolerated. Chlorambucil is usually given over a period of several weeks or more. The therapeutic response may be gradual, and the effect may be sustained by maintenance therapy.

Cyclophosphamide Cyclophosphamide is available for intravenous or oral use. It requires metabolism by the liver to phosphoramide mustard, the active form of the drug. It is well absorbed after oral administration and is approximately 55 percent protein-bound. It has an average half-life of 6 h. Ten to 20 percent of a dose is excreted unchanged in the urine. Cyclophosphamide is useful for chronic lymphatic leukemia (CLL), Hodgkin's disease and NHL, Burkitt's lymphoma, ALL, multiple myeloma, breast, ovarian, and lung cancers, and as part of a preparative regimen for bone marrow transplantation. It is thus one of the most frequently used chemotherapeutic agents. It is not a vesicant but can cause severe hemorrhagic cystitis, especially with high intravenous doses or with prolonged oral administration. With very high doses syndrome of inappropriate antidiuretic hormone (SIADH) can occur, and myocardial necrosis has rarely been reported.

Melphalan Melphalan, also known as L-phenylalanine mustard (L-PAM), can be administered orally or intravenously. With oral use, plasma levels vary from 25 to 90 percent of those by the intravenous route, due to incomplete absorption and/or first-pass hepatic metabolism. Plasma half-life is approximately 90 min. Ten to 15 percent of unchanged drug is excreted in the urine. It is used for multiple myeloma, breast, and ovarian cancers. Its side effects are similar to those of other alkylating agents.

Triethylenethiophosphoramide Triethylenethiophosphoramide is used intravesicularly for the early stages of carcinoma of the bladder. It is also occasionally used for carcinomas of the ovary and breast. When used intravenously, 85 percent is excreted unchanged in the urine.

Ifosfamide Ifosfamide is an investigational drug. It is a derivative of cyclophosphamide with different metabolic and pharmacologic properties. It has activity against soft tissue sarcomas, lung cancer, NHL, and testicular carcinoma. Adverse reactions are similar to those of cyclophosphamide, except for less bone marrow depression and more bladder toxicity. It has also been reported to cause cardiac necrosis and central nervous system effects.

Nitrosoureas Lomustine (CCNU) Lomustine is available for oral use only. It is very lipid-soluble and is rapidly and completely absorbed after oral administration. Peak levels occur in 3 h. CSF levels may approach 50 percent of plasma levels. Plasma half-life is variable, with a range of 16 to 72 h. Sixty percent is excreted through the kidneys as metabolites. Lomustine is active against NHL, brain tumors, small-cell lung cancer, and gastrointestinal cancers. It can cause delayed cumulative bone marrow toxicity white blood count (WBC) nadir 4 to 6 weeks, so 6-week intervals or more are recommended between doses to allow for adequate bone marrow recovery. Kidney damage can occur with prolonged administration, particularly with a large cumulative dose.

Carmustine (BCNU) Carmustine is available for intravenous use only. It is highly lipid-soluble and crosses well into the CSF where levels are at least 50 percent of plasma level. Plasma half-life is 15 to 30 min. Sixty to 70 percent of a dose is excreted in the urine. Carmustine is useful for NHL, multiple myeloma, and brain tumors. Delayed bone marrow toxicity is also seen. Pulmonary fibrosis has been associated with its use and is usually dose-related. Renal toxicity can occur as with lomustine.

Streptozocin Streptozocin is available for intravenous use. Plasma half-life is 35 min. Sixty to 70 percent is excreted by the kidney, of which 20 percent is the unchanged drug. Streptozocin has a predilection for the beta cells of the pancreatic islets. It is active against pancreatic islet cell tumors and carcinoid. It may cause mild glucose intolerance. It commonly causes severe dose-related kidney damage. Myelosuppression is mild.

The Triazine Derivative *Dacarbazine* (DTIC) Dacarbazine is available for intravenous use and is only 5 percent protein-bound. It has a biphasic half-life of 5 H. Forty percent of an administered dose is excreted unchanged in the urine. Metabolic products are also excreted in the urine. It is active against Hodgkin's disease, soft tissue sarcomas, and melanoma. Toxicity includes severe nausea and vomiting, a flulike syndrome, and rare hepatic necrosis.

Alkyl Sulfonates

$$CH_3-\overset{\overset{O}{\|}}{\underset{\underset{O}{\|}}{S}}-O-(CH_2-CH_2)_2-O-\overset{\overset{O}{\|}}{\underset{\underset{O}{\|}}{S}}-CH_3$$

Busulfan

Busulfan Although busulfan is classified as a bifunctional alkylating agent, it binds poorly to DNA and has not been shown to cause interstrand cross-linking. Unlike other alkylators, it has little effect on lymphocytes and is much less immunosuppressive. It has potent cytotoxic properties and the ability to kill stem cells and cells in the G_0 phase of the cell cycle. Busulfan is available for oral use. It is well absorbed after oral administration and is completely metabolized. It is used for myeloproliferative disorders [primarily chronic myelogenous leukemia (CML) and polycythemia vera (p. vera)], and as part of a preparative regimen for bone marrow transplantation. Because it has a significant effect on stem cells, it can produce smooth, long-term control of CML and p. vera. It has

not been shown to increase the incidence of secondary leukemia, in contrast to other alkylating agents. It produces little mucositis or gastrointestinal disturbance in conventional doses. If blood counts are not carefully followed during prolonged use, irreversible marrow depression can occur. A clinical syndrome resembling adrenal insufficiency has been rarely reported.

The Platinum Derivatives *cis-Diamminedichloroplatinum (cis-DDP)* cis-DDP is an inorganic platinum-containing compound which functions like an alkylator. It produces interstrand and intrastrand cross-linking of DNA. cis-DDP is available for intravenous use only. It is 90 percent protein-bound. It has a biphasic half-life. The initial half-life is 8 to 10 min, and the terminal half-life is approximately 45 min. It is renally excreted, highly active against testicular and ovarian carcinomas, and useful for carcinoma of the head and neck, esophagus, bladder, cervix, and lung. Nephrotoxicity is common and dose-related; its incidence can be decreased with vigorous hydration. Severe nausea, vomiting, peripheral neurophathy, ototoxicity, and anaphylaxis can be seen. Myelosuppression is mild.

cis-Diammine (1,1-cyclobutanedicarboxylato)platinum (carboplatin) Carboplatin is an investigational drug developed in order to decrease the toxicity of the parent compound cis-DDP. It has much less nephrotoxicity and less neurotoxicity and ototoxicity than cis-DDP. Its dose-limiting side effect is myelosuppression. Carboplatin has a clinical spectrum similar to cisplatin.

Methylhydrazine *Procarbazine* Procarbazine was initially synthesized as a monoamine oxidase (MAO) inhibitor. It is thought to act as an alkylating agent. Procarbazine is completely absorbed after oral administration and crosses well into the CSF. It has a half-life of only 7 min after intravenous use. It is liver-metabolized and renally excreted as *N*-isopropylterephthalamic acid. Procarbazine can be used intravenously or orally and is indicated for the treatment of brain tumors, lung cancer, and Hodgkin's disease. Adverse reactions include myelosuppression, peripheral neuropathy, and CNS toxicity. Since it is a weak MAO inhibitor, foods with a high tyramine content should be avoided.

Antibiotics

Dactinomycin (Actinomycin D)

Mechanism of Action The actinomycins were the first antibiotics to be isolated from a species of *Streptomyces*. Dactinomycin is a chromopeptide with a phenoxazone-ring and two cyclic polypeptides. Dactinomycin forms a complex with DNA involving selective binding to and intercalation between the guanine-cytosine segments, with a specific block in DNA-dependent RNA synthesis. The greatest effect of the drug occurs in early S phase. Another cytotoxic effect of dactinomycin is to cause single-stranded breaks in DNA.

Pharmacokinetics Dactinomycin is available for intravenous use. It is rapidly concentrated in nucleated cells and minimally metabolized. The plasma half-life is approximately 36 h. Most of the drug is excreted in the urine and bile unchanged. It does not penetrate into the CSF.

Therapeutic Uses Dactinomycin is effective against Wilms's tumor, Ewing's sarcoma, rhabdomyosarcoma, testicular carcinoma, gestational choriocarcinomas, lymphoma, and Kaposi's sarcoma.

Adverse Reactions The most frequent toxicity is myelosuppression. Gastrointestinal toxicities can include stomatitis, nausea, vomiting, and diarrhea. Abnormalities of liver and kidney functions have been reported. Dactinomycin can enhance radiation injury. Extravasation can produce significant tissue necrosis.

Plicamycin (Mithramycin)

Mechanism of Action Plicamycin is a cytotoxic antibiotic from *Streptomyces plicatus*. Its mechanism of action is similar to dactinomycin in that it inhibits the synthesis of DNA-dependent RNA synthesis.

Pharmacokinetics Plicamycin is available for intravenous use only. Its metabolism and excretion is poorly understood. Caution should be used in the presence of liver or kidney disorders.

Therapeutic Uses Plicamycin is useful in the treatment of malignant hypercalcemia and testicular germ cell neoplasms.

Adverse Reactions The major side effects of plicamycin include nausea and vomiting, hepatic and renal toxicities, and a hemorrhagic diathesis associated with severe thrombocytopenia and decreased synthesis of certain clotting factors.

Bleomycin Sulfate

Mechanism of Action Bleomycin is an antibiotic complex derived from a strain of *Streptomyces verticillus*. Bleomycin has antitumor, antiviral, and antibacterial activity. Bleomycin binds with DNA to produce single- and double-strand breaks. DNA is cleaved at the guanine-cytosine and guanine-thymine sequences.

Pharmacokinetics Bleomycin is administered via the parenteral route. After intravenous use, its initial plasma half-life is 10 to 20 min. After intramuscular use, peak levels occur in 30 to 60 min and are approximately one-third of those achieved with intravenous administration. Bleomycin is metabolized and renally excreted. Approximately 30 to 40 percent is excreted in the urine as unchanged drug. It is advisable to decrease the dose of bleomycin by at least 50 percent in the presence of renal insufficiency.

Therapeutic Uses Bleomycin is active in testicular cancer, Hodgkin's lymphoma and non-Hodgkin's lymphoma and squamous cell carcinomas of the head and neck, cervix, esophagus, and lung.

Adverse Reactions An important toxicity of bleomycin is interstitial pneumonitis, which may progress to pulmonary fibrosis. This pulmonary toxicity is dose-related. Abnormalities in the diffusion capacity of the lungs are most commonly seen with total doses above 250 mg. Mucocutaneous reactions are common and include skin ulceration, hyperpigmentation, erythema, and stomatitis. Myelosuppression is rare. Pyrexia, which is particularly common in lymphoma patients, may occur either alone or in combination with wheezing, hypotension, and vomiting.

The Anthracyclines

Mechanism of Action Doxorubicin and daunorubicin are antibiotics derived from a *Streptomyces*. The structure of the anthracyclines includes the amino sugar daunosamine with a planar naphthacenequinone nucleus. Doxorubicin differs from daunorubicin by a single hydroxyl group on carbon-14. These drugs cause DNA intercalation, participate in oxidation-reduction reactions, impair DNA repair, chelate divalent cations, and interfere with cell membranes to alter their function.

Pharmacokinetics   Doxorubicin and daunorubicin are given intravenously and are both extensively protein-bound. They are cleared from the plasma with triphasic half-lives of 10 to 30 min, 3 h, and 25 h. Doxorubicin and daunorubicin are metabolized by carbonyl reduction to the active alcohols doxorubicinol and daunorubicinol, respectively. Although a minor amount is excreted by the kidneys, most of the inactive metabolites are recovered in the bile. Doses need to be decreased in the presence of liver disease.

Therapeutic Uses   Doxorubicin is extremely active in acute leukemia, lymphoma, breast and ovarian cancers, sarcoma, and several other solid tumors. Daunorubicin is highly effective in acute myelogenous leukemia.

Adverse Reactions   Bone marrow suppression and mucositis are the major side effects of the anthracyclines. Nausea, vomiting, and alopecia will occur in the majority of patients. Drug extravasation of doxorubicin and daunorubicin can cause severe tissue injury. A dose-limiting side effect of the anthracyclines is cardiac toxicity. One form of cardiotoxicity is acute arrhythmia, which is not dose-dependent, and the other is a cumulative dose-dependent cardiomyopathy, which can occur at doses greater than 550 mg per square meter of body surface area. Endocardial biopsy can identify pathologic features of the latter. Studies are under way to develop new, less cardiotoxic anthracyclines.

Mitomycin (Mitomycin C)

Mechanism of Action   Mitomycin is an antibiotic isolated form *Streptomyces calspitosus*, and contains a quinone, a urethrane, and an aziridine. This compound becomes activated to behave as an alkylating agent and inhibits DNA synthesis. Mitomycin is most active in the cell cycle in late G and early S phases.

Pharmacokinetics   Mitomycin is administered via the intravenous route, is minimally protein-bound, and has a half-life between 10 and 30 min. The liver is the major site of metabolism.

Therapeutic Uses   Mitomycin has primarily been used in combination with other chemotherapeutic drugs in the treatment of carcinomas of the colon, pancreas, breast, lung, prostate, and head and neck.

Adverse Reactions   The major side effect of mitomycin is a cumulative delayed myelosuppression. Infrequently renal failure with microangiopathic hemolytic anemia may be seen. Interstitial pneumonitis is rare but may be fatal. Mitomycin may potentiate doxorubicin cardiotoxicity. Drug extravasation may cause significant local tissue injury.

Mitoxantrone   1,4-Dihydroxy-5,8-bis[[2-[(2-hydroxyethyl)amino]ethyl]amino]-9,10-anthracenedione dihydrochloride is structurally related to doxorubicin.

Mechanism of Action   Mitoxantrone's cytotoxicity may involve DNA binding through intercalation, causing DNA strand breakage.

Pharmacokinetics   Mitoxantrone is used intravenously with a biphasic half-life. The initial half-life is 13 min; the terminal half-life is 37 h. It is probably metabolized largely by the liver.

Therapeutic Uses   Mitoxantrone has activity in breast cancer, ANLL, and NHL.

Adverse Reactions   Adverse reactions include myelosuppression, nausea, vomiting, and mucositis. Cardiotoxicity has been reported, but appears to be less frequent than with the anthracyclines.

Plant Derivatives

Vinblastine and Vincristine

Mechanism of Action   Vinblastine and vincristine are *Vinca* alkaloids derived from the periwinkle plant (*Vinca rosea*). These agents cause the arrest of cell division in metaphase and inhibit the assembly of microtubules and thus the failure of the mitotic spindle. Cells in S phase appear to be most sensitive to the effects of these alkaloids.

Pharmacokinetics   Both vinblastine and vincristine are administered intravenously and are approximately 75 percent protein-bound. Both are metabolized by the liver. After an initial distribution phase, the plasma half-life of both drugs is biphasic with 2.3 and 84 h for vincristine and 1.5 and 24 h for vinblastine. Vincristine is partially metabolized by the liver and is excreted in the bile. Vinblastine is partially metabolized to deacetyl vinblastine, a more active form of the drug. Most of the drug is excreted unchanged in the bile. Dose modification is advisable for both drugs in the presence of liver disease.

Therapeutic Uses Vincristine is effective in combination with other chemotherapeutic agents in the treatment of ALL, Hodgkin's disease, and NHL. Vinblastine has found its major use in advanced testicular cancer as well as in lymphoma.

Adverse Reactions A significant and often dose-limiting effect of vincristine is neurotoxicity or peripheral neuropathy, which can manifest itself as muscular weakness or sensory impairment. Constipation and paralytic ileus can also occur. An advantage of vincristine for combination chemotherapy is its lack of myelosuppression.

Vinblastine has as its major toxicity profound myelosuppression. Neurotoxicity is rarely seen.

Epipodophyllotoxins

Mechanism of Action Etoposide (VP-16) and teniposide (VM-26) are two synthetic derivatives of the extract of the American mandrake plant. The mechanisms of actions of these two compounds have not been fully elucidated, but they appear to arrest cells in G_2 phase and to cause dose-dependent breaks in DNA strands.

Pharmacokinetics Both drugs are primarily given by the intravenous route, although etoposide is now available for oral use. Etoposide is 95 percent protein-bound. Its terminal half-life is 7 h. It is partially metabolized and excreted in the urine mainly as unchanged drug. Doses of both drugs should be reduced in the presence of severe hepatic dysfunction or significant renal insufficiency.

Therapeutic Uses Etoposide has shown significant activity against such tumors as testicular and small-cell lung cancer, lymphoma, leukemia, and Kaposi's sarcoma. Data on teniposide are more limited.

Adverse Reactions The most common toxicity for both etoposide and teniposide is leukopenia. Mild gastrointestinal complaints such as nausea, vomiting, diarrhea, and mucositis may occur.

Miscellaneous

Amsacrine (m-AMSA)

Mechanism of Action Amsacrine is an investigational acridine derivative which has undergone extensive trials in acute leukemia and lymphoma, and appears to have significant activity in both pediatric and adult acute leukemias. Amsacrine is a cytotoxic agent which binds to DNA through intercalation and has base specificity for A-T pairs. Amsacrine is more effective in cycling cells.

Pharmacokinetics It appears to be bioactivated in the liver and excreted in the bile. The half-life is approximately 7 h after intravenous administration over a 60 to 120 min period except in hepatic dysfunction where it is prolonged.

Therapeutic Uses The major benefit of amsacrine appears to be in pediatric and adult acute leukemias.

Adverse Reaction The major dose-limiting side effect is severe myelosuppression. An important side effect is cardiac toxicity which can be manifested as congestive heart failure, ventricular arrhythmia, abnormal echocardiogram, or sudden death. The exact mechanism for cardiac toxicity is not yet clear, but both prolonged Q-T intervals and hypokalemia have been observed in some cases of ventricular fibrillation. Correction of hypokalemia and cardiac monitoring during administration of amsacrine is recommended. Other adverse reactions of amsacrine include transient liver function abnormalities (particularly hyperbilirubinemia), nausea and vomiting, grand mal seizures, skin rash, gastrointestinal upset, and local phlebitis and tissue irritation.

Asparaginase (L-Asparaginase)

Mechanism of Action Asparagine is a nonessential amino acid and can be synthesized by a reaction catalyzed by the enzyme L-asparagine synthetase. Asparaginase is an enzyme which can hydrolyze L-asparagine to L-aspartic acid and cause depletion of L-asparagine. Asparaginase derived from *Escherichia coli* and *Erwinia carotovora* can be highly effective against acute lymphocytic leukemia by intracellular depletion of L-asparagine and subsequent inhibition of protein and nucleic acid synthesis.

Pharmacokinetics   Asparaginase can be given by the intravenous route, but the intramuscular route is preferred because of a decreased frequency of hypersensitivity reactions. Intramuscular peak plasma levels are approximately 50 percent of intravenous levels. Systemic absorption is slow. The half-life ranges from 11 to 22 h. Minimal urinary or biliary excretion occurs.

Therapeutic Uses   Asparaginase is particularly effective in the treatment of acute lymphocytic leukemia and may be effective in T-cell and other lymphomas.

Adverse Reactions   Asparaginase is an unusual chemotherapeutic agent in that it does not cause significant bone marrow or gastrointestinal toxicity. Nausea and vomiting may occur but are usually transitory and easily managed. Asparaginase inhibits protein synthesis and can cause liver toxicity in the form of hypoalbuminemia, decreased production of clotting factors and subsequent bleeding, and elevated bilirubin and transaminases. Dysfibrinogenemia can occur on the basis of a shortened fibrinogen survival due to the production of an intrinsically abnormal fibrinogen. Hypersensitivity reactions such as urticaria, bronchospasm, and hypotension may occur. Less frequent side effects include acute pancreatitis and encephalopathy.

Hydroxyurea   *Mechanism of action*   Hydroxyurea is a substituted derivative of urea. It inhibits the enzyme ribonucleotide reductase. This enzyme reduces ribonucleotides to deoxyribonucleotides, a necessary step prior to their insertion into DNA.

Pharmacokinetics   Hydroxyurea is well absorbed orally, with peak levels within 2 h and a half-life of 1 to 2 h. Fifty percent of an oral dose is metabolized by the liver to urea and excreted in the urine. The remainder is excreted in the urine unchanged.

Therapeutic Uses   Hydroxyurea is useful for the treatment of myeloproliferative disorders and can rapidly decrease the white blood cell count in acute leukemias. In combination with other drugs, it has been used for colon cancer.

Adverse reactions   Mild gastrointestinal side effects and bone marrow depression are its only common side effects.

Hormones

The hormones commonly used as adjuncts in cancer chemotherapy are listed in Table 40-1. Their pharmacology is not discussed in this chapter, as it is covered in their respective chapters. Adrenocorticosteroids can be quite effective in the treatment of neoplastic disorders as well as the palliation of such diverse complications of cancer as hypercalcemia, intracranial metastases, anorexia, and fever. The exact mechanisms involved in antitumor activity are not completely understood, but glucocorticoid receptors have been shown to be present on the malignant cells in some breast cancers.

Side effects include fluid retention, muscle weakness, glucose intolerance, and immunosuppression. The major uses of glucocorticoids in the treatment of cancer include ALL, NHL, Hodgkin's disease, and breast cancer. Steroids are also helpful in hypercalcemia, cerebral or spinal cord edema, and as a potent antiemetic.

Tamoxifen is an antiestrogen with the ability to bind to estrogen receptors on certain tumor cells and to compete for these receptor sites and inhibit DNA. Tamoxifen is administered through the oral route and has a biphasic plasma clearance with a primary half-life of several hours and a terminal half-life of about 1 week. Tamoxifen is excreted in the stool.

The side effects, though infrequent, are nearly always manageable and include mild nausea, fluid retention, thrombocytopenia, skin rash, and vaginal bleeding.

The major use of tamoxifen is for the palliation of the postmenopausal female with metastatic breast cancer. A role may also be present for this drug in the premenopausal female.

Androgens are occasionally effective for hormone-responsive advanced breast cancer. The exact mechanism of action is unclear.

Side effects include cholestatic jaundice, alteration in libido, virilization, and hypercalcemia.

Estrogens, including diethylstilbestrol, estradiol, and estramustine, are available for use in advanced breast cancer in receptor-positive postmenopausal females and in men with advanced prostatic carcinoma. The presence of estrogen and progesterone receptor positivity in breast cancer tissue will predict those women most likely to benefit from estrogen therapy. The antiestrogens have largely replaced estrogens for the treatment of advanced breast cancer. In prostatic carcinoma the estrogens will antagonize the androgen effect.

Side effects of estrogens include gastrointestinal upset, phlebitis, hypercalcemia flare, and gynecomastia in men.

Progestational agents may be helpful in certain advanced breast and endometrial malignancies. In patients with endometrial carcinoma, progestins may inhibit leutinizing hormone as well as DNA and RNA synthesis. Side effects include fluid retention and weight gain.

Gonadotropin-Releasing Hormone Analogs
Leuprolide is a peptide analog which has recently demonstrated clinical benefit in some patients with prostatic carcinomas. Leuprolide is a synthetic analog of a gonadotropin-releasing hormone which causes an initial increase followed by a marked decrease in circulating levels of gonadotropins and testosterone. Inhibition of follicle-stimulating hormone and leutinizing hormone occurs. Side effects include edema thromboembolism, nausea, and gynecomastia.

BIBLIOGRAPHY

Ackland, S. P., and R. L. Schilsky: "High-Dose Methotrexate: A Critical Reappraisal," *J. Clin. Oncol.*, **5**(12):2017–2031 (1987).

Berk, P. D., J. D. Goldberg, M. N. Silverstein, et al.: "Increased Incidence of Acute Leukemia in Polycythemia Vera Associated with Chlorambucil Therapy," *N. Engl. J. Med.*, **301**:441 (1987)

Brodsky, I.: "Busulfan: Effects on Platelet RNA Dependent DNA Polymerase Implications in the Treatment of Polycythemia Vera, Thrombosis and Atherosclerosis," *Biomedicine*, **36**:125–127 (1982).

Calabrese, P., P. S. Schein, and S. A. Rosenberg: *Medical Oncology: Basic Principles and Clinical Management of Cancer*, MacMillan, New York, 1985.

Chabner, B. A.: *Pharmacologic Principles of Cancer Treatment*, Saunders, Philadelphia, 1982.

Devita, V. T., S. Hellman, and S. A. Rosenberg: *Cancer Principles and Practice of Oncology*, J. B. Lippincott, Philadelphia, 1985.

Evans, B. D., I. E. Smith, M. E. Gore, M. D. Vincent, L. Repetto, J. R. Yarnold, and H. T. Ford: "Carboplatin (Paraplatin; JM8) and Etoposide (VP-16) as First-Line Combination Therapy for Small-Cell Lung Cancer," *J. Clin. Oncol.*, **5**(2):185 (1987).

Forastiere, A. A., R. B., Natale, B. J. Takasugi, M. P. Goren, W. C. Vogel, V. Kudla-Hatch: "A Phase I-II Trial of Carboplatin and 5-Fluorouracil Combination Therapy for Small-Cell Lung Cancer," *J. Clin. Oncol.*, **5**(2):190 (1987).

O'Dwyer, P. J., et. al.: "Etoposide (VP-16-213) Current Status of an Active Anticancer Drug," *N. Engl. J. Med.*, **312**(11):692–700 (1985).

Shenkenberg, T. D., D. D. Von Hoff: "Mitoxantrone: A New Anticancer Drug with Significant Clinical Activity," *Ann. Intern. Med.*, **105**:67–81 (1986).

Smith, T. T.: "Luteinizing Hormone-Releasing Hormone (LH-RH) Analogs in Treatment of Prostatic Cancer," *Urology* (Suppl.) **27**:9 (1986).

Tucker, M. A., C. N. Coleman, R. S. Cox, A. Varghese, and S. A. Rosenberg: "Risk of Second Cancers After Treatment for Hodgkin's Disease," *N. Engl. J. Med.*, **318**(2):76–81 (1988).

Von Hoff, D. D.: "Editorial: Whither Carboplatin?—A Replacement for or an Alternative to Cisplatin?," *J. Clin. Oncol.*, **5**(2):172 (1987).

Weinstein, G. B.: "Methotrexate," *Ann. Intern. Med.*, **86**:199–204 (1977).

Young, C. W., and J. H. Burchenal: "Cancer Chemotherapy," *Ann. Rev. Pharmacol.*, **11**:369–386 (1971).

Immunopharmacologic Drugs

Joseph R. DiPalma

The immune system is vital to the protection of the organism against invaders, both organic and inorganic. It also is the disposal system for sick, dead, or unwanted cells, and it is also the major protection against cancer. What is regarded as inflammation is in reality a major part of the immune reaction. In this sense all the drugs and mechanisms involved in inflammation which have been described in other chapters, such as histamine and antihistamines, prostaglandins and NSAIDs, kinins, serotonin, and many others belong to immunopharmacology. It would be impractical to include an interrelation of these agents to the immune process in this chapter. Rather it is wiser to concentrate on those drugs which have a direct effect on the cells that have immune functions such as lymphocytes, plasma cells, and subtypes of these cells. The products of these cells such as lymphokines, interferons, and interleukins are also important as drugs in their own right. Based on these considerations, a reasonable classification of immunopharmacologic drugs is shown in Table 41-1. It is apparent that immunopharmacologic drugs are of greatest utility for transplantation of organs, autoimmune diseases, and viral infections, especially AIDS. The drugs belong to groups which kill or prevent development of immune cells, specifically modify their functions, have a general suppressant effect (such as corticosteroids), are specific antibodies, or actually stimulate or modulate immune cells.

CYTOTOXIC AGENTS

Azathioprine

One of a series of analogs of mercaptopurine, azathioprine proved eventually to be more effective as an immunosuppressive than as a cytotoxic drug for cancer (see Chap. 40). Chemically it is an imidazolyl derivative of 6-mercaptopurine.

Azathioprine   6-Mercaptopurine

Actually azathioprine is a prodrug in that it is converted in the body to mercaptopurine, which reaction can occur in the tissues themselves in a nonenzymatic fashion with the aid of glutathione or other sulfhydryl compounds. Perhaps it is this attribute that makes it superior to mercaptopurine as an immunosuppressant. As a cytotoxic drug, azathioprine does not have a mechanism of action different from any of the other antimetabolites. Therefore, its action in suppression of the growth of lymphoid cells is not selective. With

TABLE 41-1 Classification of immunopharmacological drugs

Class	Agents	FDA approved indications	Unlabeled and experimental uses
Cytotoxic	Azathioprine	Renal homotransplantation Rheumatoid arthritis	Cardiac and other transplants, chronic ulcerative colitis, and other autoimmune diseases
	Cyclophosphamide	Cancer chemotherapy of lymphomas, multiple myeloma, leukemias	Wegener's granulomatosis, systemic lupus erythematosus, polyarthritis nodosa, multiple sclerosis, bone marrow transplants
	Vincristine Methotrexate Cytarabine	Cancer chemotherapy	Variety of autoimmune diseases
Specific T-cell inhibitor	Cyclosporine	Prophylaxis of organ rejection in renal, liver, and heart transplants	Other transplants such as bone marrow, pancreas, and heart/lung. Various autoimmune diseases such as uveitis, aplastic anemia, psoriasis, sarcoidosis, myasthenia gravis, Behçet's disease
Hormonal	Corticosteroids, prednisone	Many (see Chap. 39), including rheumatic disorders, collagen diseases, respiratory diseases	Transplants of all types, often in conjunction with other agents. All autoimmune disorders.
Antibodies	Antilymphocyte antibodies (ALG)		Renal transplants. Purge marrow in vitro prior to infusion
	Muromonab-CD3	Treatment of acute allograph rejection in renal transplant patients	
	$Rh_0(D)$ immune globulin	Prevention of sensitization to $Rh_0(D)$ factor to avoid hemolytic anemia	

TABLE 41-1 (*continued*) **Classification of immunopharmacological drugs**

Class	Agents	FDA approved indications	Unlabeled and experimental uses
Immunomodulating	Interferons alpha	Hairy cell leukemia	Many carcinomas, including bladder, Kaposi's sarcoma, leukemias, and lymphomas. Many viral infections, including AIDS
	beta and gamma		AIDS and Kaposi's sarcoma
	Interleukin 2 (IL-2)		Phase I AIDS Therapy of melanoma and other chemotherapy-resistant cancers
	Ampligen		Phase III AIDS

respect to renal homograph survival, azathioprine must be given in advance or at least simultaneously with the graft insertion. It has little effect on established graft rejections. Azathioprine also suppresses the severity of reaction to adjuvant arthritis, delayed hypersensitivity, and lymph node hyperplasia seen in animal models of immune activity. The mechanism of these effects is not known, but they are dose-related.

Pharmacokinetics Azathioprine is well absorbed in the gastrointestinal (GI) tract, with a peak level at 1 to 2 h after administration. The half-life of 5 h, measured by radioactive technology, does not reflect the duration of action of azathioprine, which is much longer. This is because after being cleaved into 6-mercaptopurine, further conversion into inactive 6-thiouric acid occurs catalyzed by xanthine oxidase. Proportions of metabolites are different in individual patients. As a consequence, blood levels of azathioprine have little significance, for it is the tissue levels that determine its effectiveness. Clearance is renal, and patients with poor renal function may need to have a reduction in dose.

Clinical Use Azathioprine has been the mainstay drug in all types of transplantation but especially in renal grafts. Under the best circumstances it can achieve a 50 to 70 percent graft take of 1 year or more. It has also been used in classical rheumatoid arthritis which is severe and erosive and nonresponding to conventional therapy. Unlabeled uses include ulcerative colitis and other autoimmune diseases. Cyclosporine has replaced azathioprine in most circumstances. Azothioprine, however, is useful in combination with cyclosporine or even replaces it in selected cases.

Toxicity Azathioprine has all the potential toxicity of cytotoxic drugs. These include the induction of severe leukopenia and thrombocytopenia because of severe bone marrow depression. Weekly blood counts are mandatory during the first month of therapy. Later, bimonthly and monthly blood counts may suffice.

The immunosuppression makes the patient susceptible to multiple infections. Patients must be carefully monitored for viral, fungal, and bacterial infections. Reduction of dose and rigorous antibiotic therapy is often necessary.

The risk of malignancy is greatly increased by immunosuppressive therapy. Renal transplant patients maintained on azathioprine have shown an increased incidence of the development of skin cancers and reticulum cell and lymphomatous tumors. Azathioprine must be avoided in pregnant patients because it is distinctly teratogenic.

Drug Interactions Xanthine oxidase inhibitors such as allopurinol arrest the degradation of azathioprine and hence increase its action. Patients on both drugs need to have the dose of azathioprine reduced to one-third to one-half the usual dose.

Azathioprine may decrease or even reverse the action of nondepolarizing muscle relaxants. The combination of azathioprine and prednisone is often salutary. However, the combination of azathioprine with gold, antimalarials, or penicillamine is unsatisfactory because of combined toxicity.

Azathioprine (Imuran) is available as tablets 50 mg or as an injection 100 mg per vial.

Cyclophosphamide

The alkylating agent cyclophosphamide is widely used in cancer chemotherapy. Its complete pharmacology is discussed in Chap. 40 and will not be repeated here.

As an immunosuppressant, cyclophosphamide is unique. First of all, it is probably the most potent of all such agents. Second, it destroys proliferating cells but also appears to alkylate a portion of resting cells. Third, its effect on T cells is such that, although overall suppressive, it may in some circumstances actually increase the response of these cells to antigen.

It has been successfully used in bone marrow transplants. A disadvantage in this type of graft is that cyclophosphamide does not prevent the graft-versus-host syndrome.

In relatively small doses cyclophosphamide has been effective in autoimmune disorders, including systemic lupus erythematosus, polyarthritis nodosa, Wegener's granulomatosis, and certain cases of aplastic anemia.

Large doses of cyclophosphamide cause pancytopenia. Gastrointestinal symptoms are usually severe. Cystitis occurs in about 25 percent of the cases, including the hemorrhagic variety in a lesser percentage. Alopecia, pulmonary fibrosis, and cardiac toxicity (hemorrhagic myocarditis) add to the adverse reactions. It is thus clear that cyclophosphamide benefits must be seriously balanced against the risks of therapy. In addition, there is also the risk of the induction of cancer and teratogenicity.

Miscellaneous Cytotoxic Agents

Presumably any cytotoxic drug that destroys bone marrow and lymphoid tissue can be used as an immunosuppressant. Among the drugs described in Chap. 40, vincristine, methotrexate, and cytarabine have been the most used as immunosuppressants, mainly in autoimmune diseases that have been refractory to other forms of therapy. Among the diseases treated with some success have been refractory renal transplants and thrombocytopenic purpura. However, the use of such immunosuppressants must be considered at the present time to be largely experimental. Methotrexate therapy of rheumatoid arthritis as a primary agent has recently gained favor.

SPECIFIC T-CELL INHIBITORS

Cyclosporine (Cyclosporin A)

With the discovery and development of cyclosporine, a new era in immunopharmacology was born. Cyclosporine is the first agent that affects a specific cell line of the body's immune defenses. It is suppressive mainly to T cells, in contrast to the generally cytotoxic agents that affect all cell lines at the same time. Of course, the fact that it has markedly improved the "take" of transplants and increased the potential of treating autoimmune diseases has amplified the interest of scientists and clinicians. The hope is to now find other agents, related or unrelated, that can specifically dissect out and treat other specific components of the immune system.

Chemistry Cyclosporine was originally isolated from the cultural broths of the fungus *Tolypocladium inflatum Gams*. The structure of cyclosporine is unique, being composed of 11 amino acids arranged in a cyclic fashion.

All are known aliphatic amino acids except number 1, which has never been isolated before. N-Methylleucine occupies positions 4, 6, 9, and 10, valine is in position 5, alanine in position 7, d-alanine in position 8, α-aminobutyric acid in position 2, sarcosine in position 3, and N-methylvaline in position 11. All are levo with the exception of positions 8 and 3. The structure lends itself to hydrogen bonding and is, therefore, quite rigid.

The complete synthesis of amino acids and cyclosporine itself has been accomplished. There are many analogs of cyclosporine, and some structural activity relationships have been found. It is known that cyclosporine's unique activity resides in a large portion

Cyclosporine

of the structure and not in a characteristic small segment. It is believed that the amino acid in the number 1 position is an important factor in its activity.

Cyclosporine is hydrophobic. It is soluble in methanol, ethanol, acetone, ether, and chloroform, and only slightly soluble in water and saturated hydrocarbons.

Mechanism of Action   Although a relatively large molecule, cyclosporine passes through cell membranes easily. Apparently there are no surface recognition receptors. There is a cytosolic cyclosporine-binding protein known as *cyclophilin*, with a molecular weight of about 15,000. Cyclophilins are present especially in T cells, but they are also in other tissues such as brain and kidney. Their exact function is unknown. It is conjectured that they have controlling action on the expression of an RNA in the synthesis of lymphokines. However, there is ample evidence that cyclosporine blocks the production of interleukin 2 by activated T cells; the acquisition of receptors for interleukin 2 by cytotoxic cells (killer cells) is inhibited, and the responsiveness of helper/inducer T cells to other lymphokines is reduced. Other actions which might be important are reduced production of interferon by lymphocytes and inhibited production of other lymphokines specific for macrophages.

While the mechanism of action of cyclosporine is still under intense investigation, it is important to point out what it does and does not do. It is not cytotoxic in the ordinary sense and hence does not depress bone marrow. Because it does not encourage (in fact, it suppresses) graft-versus-host immune reactions, it is especially useful in bone marrow transplants. Cyclosporine also has antiparasitic actions against schistosoma and malarial parasites. It also appears to be effective in reducing multidrug resistance in patients receiving cancer chemotherapy. The mechanism of action of these effects is unknown.

Pharmacokinetics   Oral absorption is variable. Based on patient studies, oral bioavailability as compared to IV administration is about 30 percent. Peak blood levels are achieved in about 3.5 h. Cyclosporine is extensively metabolized. No major pathway appears to exist. Only 0.1 percent appears in the urine unchanged. Hydroxylation of some of the amino acids constitutes some of the major metabolites.

Although highly bound to lipoproteins in the blood (90 percent), cyclosporine is largely distributed outside the blood volume. The half-life is approximately 19 h. Elimination is primarily biliary, with only about 6 percent excreted in urine.

Clinical Use Although in clinical use for only a decade, cyclosporine has established itself as the prime drug for organ transplantation. First used mainly in renal cadaveric transplants, it has improved the take in most clinics to 95 percent in the best series. In bone marrow transplants cyclosporine's better record in graft-versus-host reaction has made it the drug of choice. Results are generally better in heart transplantations than in the previous combination of prednisone, azathioprine, and other immune modulators. The most brilliant area of cyclosporine activity is the improved success of liver transplantation. It has even been possible to transplant heart and lung in the same patient.

For the purposes of transplantation, cyclosporine has been used alone successfully in some series. Experience has, however, indicated that the dose and hence the toxicity of cyclosporine can be reduced by the simultaneous use of prednisone. Cyclosporine must be continued indefinitely to prevent rejection, and attempts to reduce its long-term toxicity have included replacement by other immunosuppressants.

In autoimmune diseases, as might be anticipated, cyclosporine is most effective in those which are T-cell mediated. These include severe forms of psoriasis, rheumatoid arthritis refractory to all other therapy, uveitis, nephrotic syndrome, and type I diabetes mellitus. The last deserves mention, since for the first time it has been possible to prevent the development of insulin-dependent diabetes by inhibiting the self-destruction of the beta cells of the pancreas. Treatment must be started early, preferably even before insulin dependence begins, and must be continued indefinitely.

In antibody-mediated autoimmune diseases such as myasthenia gravis, systemic lupus erythematosis, autoimmune thrombocytopenic purpura, and Crohn's disease, the role of cyclosporine is less clear, although promising results have been reported. Trials in multiple sclerosis show a lack of efficacy.

The antiparasitic properties of cyclosporine have not been exploited clinically. However, experimental work with congeners in a murine model of schistosomiasis demonstrates prophylactic effectiveness. The use of cyclosporine in malaria may be in the direction of overcoming the resistance which malarial protozoa, particularly falciparum, develop against standard drugs.

Toxicity Cyclosporine is, unfortunately, a very toxic drug, although perhaps not more so than other antiimmune agents. Nephrotoxicity is the most consistent and significant risk. Other adverse reactions include hypertension, hirsutism, tremors, rarely convulsions, gum hyperplasia, and rarely hepatitis.

The mechanism of the cyclosporine-induced nephritis is unknown. Pathologists have difficulty distinguishing between a kidney which is undergoing graft rejection or one with cyclosporine toxicity. In all cases, including normal kidneys, there is some degree of reduction of creatinine clearance. Constant monitoring is required to avoid serious renal damage. Reduction of the dose often reduces the renal toxicity, but sometimes the cyclosporine therapy has to be terminated.

Like all immunosuppressants, cyclosporine increases the risk of development of neoplastic disease. It also renders the individual susceptible to all kinds of infections.

Drug Interactions Cyclosporine is biotransformed by the mixed oxidase microsomal enzyme system. Consequently, any drug that induces this system increases the elimination of cyclosporine and may require an increase in dose. These drugs include phenobarbital, carbamazepine, phenytoin, isoniazid, and rifampin. In contrast, diltiazem, erythromycin, ketoconazole, danazol, methyltestosterone, and oral contraceptives, which tend to repress the microsomal liver enzyme system, will increase the blood level of cyclosporine.

The nephrotoxicity of cyclosporine is increased by the simultaneous use of aminoglycosides and nonsteroidal anti-inflammatory drugs. Since cyclosporine already causes some potassium retention, potassium-sparing diuretics should not be given in order to avoid dangerous hyperkalemia.

Cyclosporine is available as an oral liquid containing 100 mg/mL alcohol 12.5% by volume, olive oil, and polyoxyethylated oleic glycerides as a vehicle. An intravenous solution contains 50 mg/mL cyclosporine, alcohol 32.9% by volume, and polyoxyethylated castor oil.

HORMONES

Corticosteroids

Since they first came into general use, the glucocorticoids were recognized to have actions on the immune mechanisms of the body. The lymphoid content of the lymph nodes and spleen is reduced. Proliferation of stem cells in the bone marrow is not inhibited. The glucocorticoids inhibit the synthesis of prostaglandins and leukotrienes, and this is probably one of the main actions in suppressing inflammation. This in part explains the immunosuppressant action of corticosteroids, for the response of the body to foreign invaders is an inflammatory response.

Whether corticosteroids are directly suppressive of specific immune cells is important. There is some evidence that corticosteroids can lyse T cells. Certainly precursor cells of all types are suppressed, and this leads to the diminished ability to produce antibodies and immune agents. Continual administration of corticosteroids causes increased catabolism of gamma G immunoglobulin (IgG).

It is customary to separate the metabolic actions of corticosteroids from the immunologic effects. On the whole, this is a reasonable assumption. On the other hand, the changes in carbohydrate, fat, and protein metabolism are certain to have an effect, albeit indirect, on the immune process. The overall clinically observable effect of corticosteroid therapy is that the individual has diminished ability to withstand infections and to heal wounds and that any disease process tends to be slowed but the eventual course is unchanged.

The complete pharmacology of corticosteroids is discussed in Chap. 39. Of the many preparations available, prednisone and prednisolone have been found to be the most useful in immune therapy from the viewpoint of efficacy and cost. Prednisone therapy attenuates, but does not cure, practically all autoimmune diseases. Especially satisfactory responses are obtained in rheumatoid arthritis, idiopathic thrombocytopenic purpura, lupus erythematosus, and many other less common autoimmune and collagen diseases. Were it not for the unacceptable toxicity of prednisone in long-term high-dose therapy, it would, in effect, be curative in these diseases. Withdrawal syndrome due to adrenal cortical suppression is not the least of these difficulties.

In transplantation, prednisone has an important effect, but by itself does not ensure a successful take. Prednisone is therefore used as an adjunct which has a valuable sparing effect on the dose of more toxic but more effective drugs such as azathioprine and cyclosporine.

ANTIBODIES

Antilymphocyte Antibodies

The production of antisera against a cell type is one of the oldest effective methods of achieving a specific immune action. Ideally this methodology is particularly suited to homologous organ transplantation. The technology ranges from the old method of injecting large animals with human lymphoid cells and collecting the serum to the more modern hybridoma techniques for the generation of monoclonal antibodies.

The most useful and most frequently used is antilymphocyte antibody (ALG). This antibody acts primarily on lymphocytes that are mature and which circulate in the blood and lymph. These lymphocytes are "thymus dependent" and are a main component of delayed hypersensitivity and cellular immunity reactions. This selectivity of ALG makes it useful in preventing transplant organ rejection.

The hybridoma technique is particularly useful for the production of anti–T-cell antibodies. Such antibodies are now being produced and in clinical evaluation. Of special value to prevent graft-versus-host syndrome is the procedure of "purging" the donor marrow in vitro with one or more monoclonal anti–T-cell antibodies prior to marrow infusion in the recipient.

Currently available is Anti-Thymocyte Globulin (Equine), Atgam. Precise methods of determining potency have not been developed. Anaphylactic and serum sickness do occur, especially when prednisone and azathioprine are stopped, and may require cessation of therapy. Patients are to be skin-tested for horse-serum sensitivity. The exact effectiveness of antithymocyte globulin cannot be predicted because it is used in conjunction with azathioprine and prednisone. With the advent of cyclosporine the need for ALG has declined.

Muromonab-CD3

A murine monoclonal antibody to the T-3 (CD3) antigen of human T cells known as muromonab-CD3 (Orthoclone OKT3) has recently become commercially available. It functions as an immunosuppressant, blocking graft rejection especially in renal transplants. T-cell function is blocked by interfering with CD3, a molecule in the membrane of these cells. CD3 is associated with antigen recognition and signal transduction. The number of circulating CD3 positive, CD4 positive, and CD8 positive T cells is decreased within minutes of administration of muromonab-CD3. It is indicated in the treatment of acute allograft rejection in renal transplant patients.

Administered intravenously as a bolus (not infused), muromonab-CD3 is usually given in conjunction with azathioprine and prednisone. Pyrexia, chills, dyspnea, chest pain, and vomiting are complications. Infections may be precipitated. Lymphoma has on rare occasion followed this treatment.

Whether muromonab-CD3 alone or in conjugation with other immunosuppressant drugs makes a substantial contribution to the treatment of acute allograph rejection in renal transplant patients remains to be decided. Clinical comparative trials because of ethical considerations are difficult to perform.

$Rh_0(D)$ Immune Globulin

One of the triumphs of immunopharmacology is the ability to anticipate and effectively treat the immune response which occurs when a nonsensitized $Rh_0(D)$- or $Rh_0(D^u)$-negative individual receives $Rh_0(D)$- or $Rh_0(D^u)$-positive blood. This ordinarily occurs as a result of fetomaternal hemorrhage or a transfusion mismatch.

$Rh_0(D)$ immune globulin is prepared by extraction from selected plasma from $Rh_0(D)$, D^u-negative mothers previously sensitized by Rh-incompatible pregnancies or from Rh-negative volunteers who have been deliberately immunized for this purpose.

The consequence of not administering $Rh_0(D)$ immune globulin to an Rh-negative mother is the development of erythroblastosis fetalis in the newborn. Requirements for administration of $Rh_0(D)$ immune globulin to the mother are as follows: (1) the mother must be $Rh_0(D)$- or $Rh_0(D^u)$-negative; (2) the mother must not have been previously sensitized to the $Rh_0(D)$ factor; (3) the infant must be $Rh_0(D)$- or $Rh_0(D^u)$-positive and direct antiglobulin negative.

$Rh_0(D)$ immune globulin is also required in incomplete pregnancy in all nonsensitized Rh-negative women after spontaneous abortions, ruptured tubal pregnancies, amniocentesis and other abdominal trauma, and transplacental hemorrhage. Exception is made only if the blood of the father is known to be $Rh_0(D)$- or $Rh_0(D^u)$-negative.

$Rh_0(D)$ immune globulin (Gamulin Rh, HypRh$_0$-D, Rh$_0$GAM) is available in prefilled sterile syringes or vials. It is given intramuscularly, not intravenously.

IMMUNOMODULATING AGENTS

Interferons and Interleukins

It is now known that there are many growth stimulants and growth inhibitors which are manufactured by various tissues upon appropriate conditions. Among these are interferons, which were first characterized as antiviral proteins produced by host cells. Later it was found that interferons had antiproliferative activity and also served as modulating agents for macrophages and natural killer cells. Interleukin 1 (IL-1) is considered to be an endogenous pyrogen, while interleukin 2 (IL-2) acts as a hormone which appears to stimulate the proliferation of T lymphocytes. The interleukins have important immunomodulary and regulatory functions.

The interferons are classed according to the cells of origin and the agents that cause induction (see Table 41-2). More recent technology allows interferons to be produced by recombinant DNA, usually by using a genetically engineered *Escherichia coli* bacterium containing DNA coded for human interferon. Thus it is possible to further classify alpha interferon as being associated with 11 functional and 5 pseudogenes; beta interferon is associated with only 2 genes, and gamma interferon with 1 gene.

Alpha interferon is now available commercially as a highly purified glycoprotein containing 165 amino acids. The mechanism of action of interferons is not completely understood. Their anticancer activity has been mainly studied in vitro by use of clonogenic cell assays and the regression of cancers implanted in nude

TABLE 41-2 Classification of human interferons

Type	Cells of origin	Inducing agents
Alpha (leukocytes)	Leukocytes or lymphoblasts	Viruses
Beta (fibroblast)	Fibroblasts	Double-stranded RNAs or viruses
Gamma (immune)	Leukocytes or lymphoblasts	Mitogens Concanavalin A phytohemagglutinin staphylococcal enterotoxins

mice. Unfortunately, the laboratory predictions do not always agree with clinical experience. Nevertheless, there is sufficient evidence to state that alpha interferon may induce remissions in 90 percent of cases of hairy cell leukemia. Certain cases of chronic myelogenous leukemia seem to respond well, but the response rate in Kaposi's sarcoma and hypernephroma is much smaller. Furthermore, the remission is seldom complete. A few cases of multiple myeloma, malignant lymphoma, and breast cancer have shown complete or partial responses. Interferons are seldom used as the sole agent, so it is difficult to assign exact values to effectiveness. Indeed, the effectiveness of interferons seems to be enhanced when it is used in conjunction with other cancer chemotherapeutic agents. It is believed that interferons enhance the host's defenses against tumor cells. Natural killer cells (large granular lymphocytes) which can recognize and kill tumor cells are enhanced by interferons. The activity of these cells can also be increased by double-stranded RNAs, which can induce the production of endogenous interferons.

Adverse reactions to interferons are common. Flulike syndromes, fever, fatigue, myalgia, headache, and chills occur in the majority of patients. Gastrointestinal symptoms (mainly anorexia, nausea, and diarrhea) are fairly common, while CNS symptoms such as dizziness and confusion are relatively uncommon. These symptoms tend to disappear with continued use.

More serious are skin rashes and alopecia. There is usually leukopenia and decreased hemoglobin, and some rise in liver function tests and proteinuria. Hypocalcemia is also induced.

These toxicities discourage the use of interferon except where the benefit is clearly greater than the risk. The use of interferon in viral diseases has been disappointing, although in cases which are desperate it may be worth a try. Some virus diseases which appear to respond are chronic non-A hepatitis, non-B hepatitis, herpes keratoconjunctivitis, rhinoviruses, varicella zoster, and viral hepatitis B.

Interferon Alfa-2a

Interferon alfa-2a (rl FN-A; lFLrA) (Roferon-A) is available as an injection solution containing 3 million IU per vial and as a powder for injection.

Interferon Alfa-2b

Interferon alfa-2b (lFN-alpha 2:rl FN-α2; α-2-interferon) (Intron-A) is available as an injection with 3.5 million, 10 million, and 25 million IU units per vial plus diluent.

Beta and gamma interferons are investigational drugs being tried in various cancers and virus diseases. Of particular interest is the effectiveness of gamma interferon in AIDS phase 1. Interleukin 2 is also an investigational drug. It is receiving trials in resistant types of cancers such as melanoma and in AIDS patients.

Ampligen

The induction of lymphokines which mediate cellular immunity is apparently brought about by RNAs. Double-stranded RNAs are most effective in inducing the production of all types of interferons and other intracellular mediators. Unfortunately, double-stranded (ds) RNAs are too toxic for clinical use.

Ampligen is a form of ds RNA which is not as toxic but which retains its ability to induce the production of lymphokines. Chemically it is a mismatched ds RNA, designated poly(I):poly(C_{12}U) or rI_n-r(C_{12}U)$_n$. Auridylic acid (U) creates a distortion which changes the conformation of RNA in one portion of the molecule. However, the trigger region for inducing interferons and lymphokines is preserved.

Ampligen in experimental studies when compared with ordinary RNA produces a 100-fold reduction in pyrogenicity, 25- to 10-fold reduction in mitogenicity, and a reduction in ds RNA antibody formation. Despite this much-reduced toxicity, ampligen retains its ability to induce interferons, stimulate killer cell activity, and activate a specific protein kinase.

Early studies with human clonogenic cell assays have shown promise in treating solid tumors such as glioblastoma, renal cell carcinoma, carcinoid tumors, and even melanoma. Clinical evaluation in its early stages has borne out the promise of the in vitro studies. Clinical studies in AIDS patients also show early clinical promise consisting of a reduction of symptoms, clearing of yeast infections, reduction of lymph node enlargements, and an increase of helper T_4 lymphocytes.

While later studies do not seem to confirm the beneficial effects, ampligen remains a potential therapeutic agent of great promise.

BIBLIOGRAPHY

Assan, R., G. Fleutren, and J. Sirmai: "Cyclosporine Trails in Diabetes: Update Results of the French Experience," *Transplant Proc.*, **20(3, Suppl. 4)**:178–183 (1988).

Borel, J. F.: "Immunosuppression: Building on Sandimmune (Cyclosporine)," *Transplant Proc.*, **20(1, Suppl. 1)**:149–153 (1988).

Borel, J. F.: "Basic Science Summary," *Transplant Proc.*, **20(2, Suppl. 2)**:722–730 (1988).

Brodsky, I., and H. R. Hubbell: "Interferons as Anticancer Agents," *Am. Fam. Physician*, **29**:146–248 (1984).

Brodsky, I. and D. R. Strayer: "Therapeutic Potential of Ampligen," *Am. Fam. Physician*, **36**:253–256 (1987).

Carter, W. A., D. R. Strayer, I. Brodsky, et al.: "Clinical, Immunological, and Virological Effects of Ampligen, a Mismatched Double-Stranded RNA in Patients with AIDS or AIDS-Related Complex," *Lancet*, **1(B545)**:1286–1292 (1987).

Dale, M. M., and J. C. Foreman (eds.): *Textbook of Immunopharmacology*, Blackwell Scientific, Boston, 1984.

DiPalma, J. R.: "Cyclosporine: An Immunologic Breakthrough," *Am. Fam. Physician*, **36**:245–247 (1987).

Ferguson, R. M., and B. G. Sommer (ed.): *The Clinical Management of the Renal Transplant Recipient with Cyclosporine*, Grune and Stratton, New York, 1986.

Fries, D., C. Hiesse, J. P. Santelli, et al.: "Triple Therapy with Low-Dose Cyclosporine, Azathioprine, and Steroids: Long-Term Results of a Randomized Study in Cadaver Donor Renal Transplantation," *Transplant Proc.*, **20(3, Suppl. 3)**:130–135 (1988).

Hess, A. D., A. H. Esa, and P. M. Colombani: "Mechanisms of the Action of Cyclosporine. Effects on Cells of the Immune System and on Subcellular Events in T Cell Activation," *Transplant. Proc.*, **20(2, Suppl. 2)**:29–40 (1988).

Kahan, B. D. (ed.): *Cyclosporine*. Vol. I. *Biological Activity and Clinical Applications*, Grune and Stratton, New York, 1983.

Kahan, B. D. (ed.): *Cyclosporine*. Vol. III. *Diagnosis and Management of Associated Renal Injury*, Grune and Stratton, New York, 1985.

Penn, I., and M. E. Brunson: "Cancers after Cyclosporine Therapy," *Transplant Proc.*, **20(3, Suppl. 3)**:885–892 (1988).

Tilney, N. L., T. B. Strom, and J. W. Kupliec-Weglinski: "Pharmacologic and Immunologic Agonists and Antagonists of Cyclosporine," *Transplant Proc.*, **20(3, Suppl. 3)**:13–22 (1988).

PART IX

Anti-Infective Agents

SECTION EDITOR

G. John DiGregorio

Antimicrobials I: Beta-Lactam Antibiotics

Abdolghader Molavi

GENERAL CONCEPTS

Antibiotics are compounds that are produced by microorganisms and have the capacity to kill or to inhibit the growth of bacteria and other microorganisms. This definition distinguishes between antimicrobial agents produced by microorganisms and those that are totally synthetic. The distinction is rather academic, and the word antibiotic is now often used to include both groups of antimicrobials.

The central concept of antimicrobial action is that of *selective toxicity*—that is, growth of the infecting organism is inhibited or the organism is killed without damage to the cells of the host. All clinically useful antimicrobials are selectively toxic to microorganisms. The nature and degree of this selectivity determines whether an antimicrobial is essentially nontoxic for mammalian cells or exhibits definite toxic potentials for certain specific mammalian tissues.

The antimicrobial agents exert their antibacterial effects through one of the following mechanisms: (1) inhibition of cell-wall synthesis (beta-lactam antibiotics, vancomycin, and cycloserine), (2) inhibition of protein synthesis (aminoglycosides, erythromycin, clindamycin, chloramphenicol, and the tetracyclines), (3) inhibition of nucleic acid synthesis or function (sulfonamides, trimethoprim, metronidazole, quinolones, and rifampin), and (4) inhibition of outer and/or cytoplasmic membrane function (polymyxins).

Determination of Antimicrobial Susceptibility

The rational approach to antimicrobial therapy of infections is based on the isolation and identification of the infecting organism and determination of its susceptibility to antimicrobial agents. The most widely used methods for in vitro sensitivity testing are the disk-diffusion and broth-dilution methods.

In the disk-diffusion method, paper disks containing specific amounts of antimicrobials are placed on the surface of an agar plate that has been completely streaked with a standard inoculum of the bacterium. After an overnight incubation, the diameters of clear zones around the disks indicating no bacterial growth are measured. These diameters are interpreted as *susceptible*, *intermediate*, or *resistant* for the individual drugs by referring to standardized values. The limitation of the disk-diffusion method is that it provides only qualitative data on the inhibitory activity of antimicrobial agents.

Quantitative susceptibility testing is performed most commonly by broth-dilution method. Serial twofold dilutions of the drug in broth are inoculated with a standardized suspension of the organism. The results are expressed as the *minimum inhibitory concentration* (MIC), which is the lowest concentration of the drug that inhibits visible growth after an overnight incubation. The *minimum bactericidal concentration* (MBC) can be determined by subculturing tubes that show no bacterial growth onto agar plates and reincubating overnight. It is the lowest concentration of the drug that kills at least 99.9 percent of the original bacterial inoculum. The results of quantitative susceptibility tests, MIC and MBC, should be correlated with the concentrations of the drug achieved in plasma and various body tissues and fluids.

Bactericidal versus Bacteriostatic

A bacteriostatic agent inhibits bacterial growth but does not kill the organism at concentrations that are achieved clinically. As might be expected, the MBCs of such an agent are substantially higher than the corresponding MICs. A bactericidal agent causes microbial cell death and lysis at concentrations that are achieved clinically. For these agents the MBCs are identical or very close to the corresponding MICs.

Treatment with a bacteriostatic drug stops bacterial growth, thereby allowing neutrophils and other host defenses to eliminate the pathogen. In cases where almost total reliance must be placed on a chemotherapeutic effect that is unaided by host defenses, such as endocarditis and infection in neutropenic hosts, bactericidal agents are more effective than bacteriostatic compounds. This difference, however, is nonexistent when the host defense mechanisms (local and systemic) are intact.

Resistance to Antimicrobial Drugs

Bacterial resistance to antimicrobial agents can be classified into two types: *intrinsic* and *acquired*. Intrinsic resistance of an organism is a stable genetic property encoded in the chromosome and shared by all strains of the species. Acquired resistance means that certain strains of a bacterial species have developed the ability to resist an antimicrobial drug to which the species as a whole is naturally susceptible. Acquired resistance implies a change in the DNA of the bacteria so that a new phenotypic trait is expressed. There are two ways by which resistance can be acquired: (1) by mutation in the chromosome of the bacterium or (2) by acquisition of new DNA sequences (plasmids) that encode a resistance function.

The biochemical mechanisms of intrinsic and acquired resistance are quite similar and can be divided into four basic categories: (1) drug inactivation or modification by bacterial enzymes, (2) formation of a permeability barrier so that the drug cannot reach the target site of its action, (3) alteration of the target so that it no longer binds or is affected by the drug, and (4) development of an altered metabolic pathway that bypasses the reaction inhibited by the drug.

Antimicrobial Combinations

When an organism is exposed simultaneously to two antimicrobial agents, the effect of the combination may fall into one of three patterns: additive effect, synergism, or antagonism. Two drugs are said to be additive when the activity of the drugs in combination is equal to the sum of their independent activities. The combined effect of two antimicrobials may be less than (antagonism) or greater than (synergism) the additive effect. Synergism can occur by different mechanisms such as sequential blockade of an essential metabolic pathway or increasing the bacterial cell permeability.

CHEMISTRY

Beta-lactam antibiotics include penicillins, cephalosporins, monobactams, and carbapenems. All have a four-membered beta-lactam ring (Fig. 42-1), which is essential for their antibacterial activity. The beta-lactam ring is fused to a five-membered thiazolidine ring in the penicillins and to a six-membered dihydrothiazine ring in the cephalosporins. In carbapenems, the beta-lactam ring is attached to a five-membered ring, as in penicillins. Substitution of carbon for sulfur and the presence of unsaturation in the five-membered ring account for the name *carba*penem. The monobactams lack the bicyclic structure characteristic of the other beta-lactam antibiotics; a sulfonic acid grouping is attached to the nitrogen of the beta-lactam ring.

MECHANISM OF ACTION

The basic mechanism of action of beta-lactam antibiotics is inhibition of cell-wall synthesis. This primary action triggers bacterial autolytic enzymes, which then disrupt the cell wall and cause bacterial lysis.

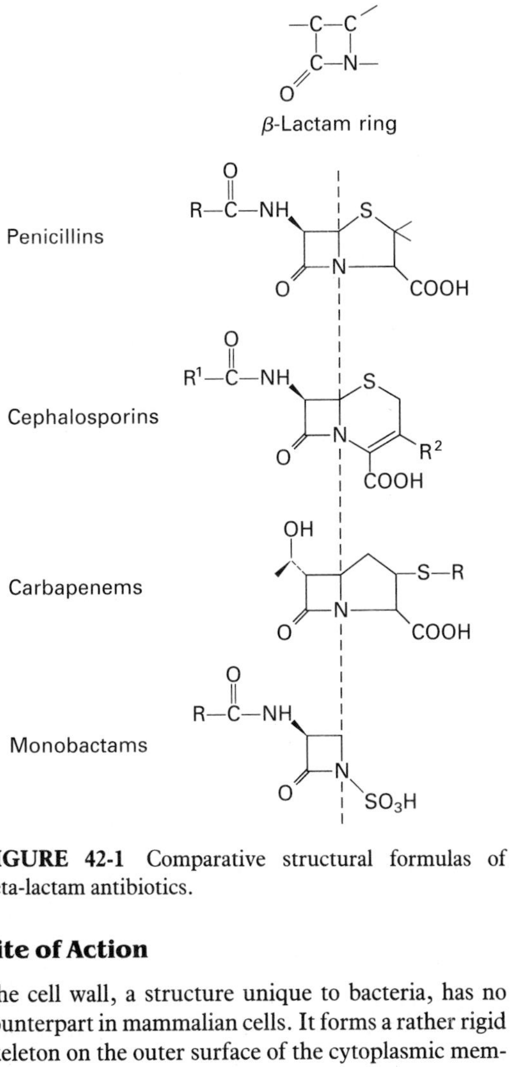

FIGURE 42-1 Comparative structural formulas of beta-lactam antibiotics.

volume hypertonic to the environment of the organism. Although this membrane is critical to the maintenance of the osmotic gradient between the bacterium and its environment, it is not strong enough in itself to keep the hypertonic sac from rupturing by osmotic shock. The cell wall encases the cytoplasmic membrane and protects the bacterial cell against lysis due to osmotic pressure differences between the cytoplasm and the external environment.

The basic component of the cell wall is a mixed polymer, known as *murein* or *peptidoglycan*. The peptidoglycan is made of long polysaccharide chains, which are cross-linked by short interconnecting peptides. The polysaccharide chains, called *glycan strands*, are composed of alternating units of two amino sugars, N-acetylglucosamine and N-acetylmuramic acid. A tetrapeptide (composed of L-alanine, D-glutamic acid, L-lysine, and D-alanine in *Staphylococcus aureus*) is attached to each N-acetylmuramic acid unit, forming side branches to the glycan strands. Many of these tetrapeptides are cross-linked to one another either directly or via short peptide chains. In *Staph. aureus*, the L-lysine of one tetrapeptide is linked via a pentaglycine to the D-alanine of another (Fig. 42-2). The resulting structure endows the wall with rigidity and the bacterium with its shape. The peptidoglycan layer of gram-negative bacteria is thinner than that of gram-positive bacteria and has fewer cross-links.

Inhibition of Cell Wall Synthesis

Peptidoglycan synthesis can be divided into three stages according to where the reactions take place. The first-stage reactions take place in the cytoplasm and result in the production of the precursor unit, uridinediphospho-N-acetylmuramyl pentapeptide. Cycloserine, an antibiotic which is used occasionally

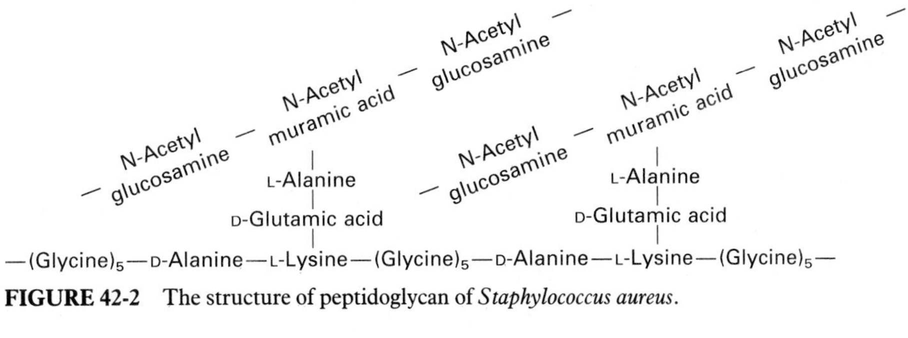

Site of Action

The cell wall, a structure unique to bacteria, has no counterpart in mammalian cells. It forms a rather rigid skeleton on the outer surface of the cytoplasmic membrane. The bacterial cytoplasmic membrane encases a

FIGURE 42-2 The structure of peptidoglycan of *Staphylococcus aureus*.

for the treatment of tuberculosis (Chap. 44), blocks cell-wall synthesis by competitive inhibition of alanine incorporation into the pentapeptide.

The second-stage reactions take place while the precursor unit is translocated across the cytoplasmic membrane. In the first reaction, *N*-acetylmuramyl pentapeptide moiety becomes attached (by a pyrophosphate bridge) to a carrier phospholipid bound to the cytoplasmic membrane. *N*-acetylglucosamine is then added to form a disaccharide-pentapeptide-*P-P*-phospholipid. Further modifications of the pentapeptide chain, such as the addition of pentaglycine in *Staph. aureus*, are then made. The modified disaccharide is subsequently cleaved from the membrane-bound phospholipid and is bonded to the growing point of the preexisting peptidoglycan, a reaction which is mediated by the enzyme *peptidoglycan synthetase*. The basic repeating units of peptidoglycan are thus put together to form linear glycopeptide polymers. Vancomycin (Chap. 43) inhibits cell-wall synthesis by inhibiting peptidoglycan synthetase.

The third and final stage of cell-wall synthesis takes place outside the cytoplasmic membrane. During this process, the linear glycopeptide polymers become cross-linked to each other by means of a transpeptidation reaction. The transpeptidase enzyme, which is membrane-bound, links the pentapeptide side chains by displacing a terminal D-alanine. Beta-lactam antibiotics inhibit the transpeptidation reaction. This initiates events that eventually lead to bacterial cell death.

Since beta-lactam antibiotics interfere with peptidoglycan biosynthesis and such synthesis does not occur in the cells of humans and other mammals, these agents are relatively nontoxic for human cells.

Autolytic Enzyme Activity

The fact that beta-lactam antibiotics inhibit cell-wall synthesis does not account for their rapid lethal action on bacteria. Important mediators of cell death after exposure to beta-lactam antibiotics are *autolysins* (murein hydrolases). Autolysins may be required to make nicks in the peptidoglycan lattice to enable new units to be inserted during growth, or they may be necessary to separate two daughter cells from one another during division. It has been suggested that the inhibition of cell wall synthesis "triggers" autolytic enzymes by deinhibiting their activity in some as yet undefined way. The uninhibited enzymes can then disrupt covalent bonds in the cell wall and cause bacterial death.

Certain bacterial strains that are "autolysin-deficient" have been identified. These organisms do not lyse in the presence of beta-lactam antibiotics, although their growth is inhibited. The term *tolerance* has been used to describe the dissociation between inhibition and killing of bacteria by agents that inhibit peptidoglycan synthesis. Tolerant organisms differ from those which are resistant in that they are still susceptible to the growth-inhibiting effect of the antibiotic but are tolerant with respect to the lytic action.

Penicillin-Binding Proteins

Beta-lactam antibiotics bind specifically to a number of proteins bound to the cytoplasmic membrane, known as *penicillin-binding proteins* (PBPs). These proteins are enzymes that are involved in transpeptidation reactions and in reshaping the cell wall during growth and division. The PBPs of a given organism are numbered in order of decreasing molecular weight. The PBP numbering system of gram-positive bacteria bears no relation to the PBP numbering of gram-negative bacteria. *Escherichia coli* have six PBPs. PBP-1a and PBP-1b are transpeptidases involved in peptidoglycan synthesis associated with cell elongation. Inhibition of these enzymes results in spheroplast formation and rapid lysis. PBP-2 is required for maintenance of the "rod" shape of the bacterium. Selective inhibition of this enzyme causes the production of osmotically stable, large round forms which eventually lyse. PBP-3 is required for septum formation during division. Selective inhibition of this enzyme results in formation of filamentous forms containing multiple rod-shaped units that cannot separate from each other. Different beta-lactam antibiotics have selective affinities for one or more PBPs. The inactivation of high-molecular-weight PBPs (PBP-1a, 1b, 2, or 3) causes bacterial cell death. In contrast, low-molecular-weight PBPs (PBP-4, 5, and 6) are not essential for bacterial viability, and their inactivation by beta-lactam molecules is not lethal to the bacteria.

MECHANISMS OF RESISTANCE

Bacterial resistance to beta-lactam antibiotics may be due to one or more of the following mechanisms: (1) inability of the drug to penetrate to the target site of its action, (2) alteration of PBPs resulting in reduced affinity for the drug, and (3) inactivation of the drug by bacterial enzymes.

Permeability Barrier

The beta-lactam antibiotics must penetrate through the outer cell envelope to reach their PBP targets on the cytoplasmic membrane. In gram-positive bacteria, the cell wall is usually the only layer external to the cytoplasmic membrane. In some species, there is a polysaccharide capsule exterior to the cell wall. Neither of these structures presents a barrier to the passage of small molecules like the beta-lactams. Therefore, inability to reach the PBP targets is unlikely to be a mechanism of resistance in gram-positive species.

Gram-negative bacteria have a more complex surface structure. A peptidoglycan layer again is external to the cytoplasmic membrane. Exterior to this layer, there is an outer membrane usually covered with a polysaccharide capsule. The outer membrane, which is composed of lipopolysaccharide and lipoprotein, constitutes a barrier to the passage of hydrophilic molecules. Penetration through this membrane is made possible by transmembrane channels, formed by proteins called *porins*, which allow diffusion of solutes into the interior of the bacterium. The ease with which beta-lactam antibiotics diffuse through the porin channels varies according to their size, charge, and hydrophilic properties.

Altered PBP Targets

A second mechanism of resistance to beta-lactam antibiotics is an alteration of PBP target resulting in reduced affinity for the beta-lactam molecule. Alterations in the binding characteristics of PBPs for beta-lactam compounds are responsible for the development of resistance in some organisms that are usually sensitive to these agents.

Beta-Lactamase Production

The most important mechanism of resistance to beta-lactam antibiotics is bacterial production of beta-lactamases. The beta-lactamases cleave the C—N bond in the beta-lactam ring of the antibiotic. Since an intact beta-lactam ring is an absolute requirement for interaction with the PBPs, cleavage of the ring destroys antibacterial activity.

There are many beta-lactamases, which can be distinguished on the basis of substrate profiles, gene location (chromosome or plasmid), and inducibility. Some of these enzymes primarily hydrolyze penicillins (penicillinase). Some hydrolyze mainly cephalosporins (cephalosporinase), and others have a broad substrate range. Some bacteria possess inducible beta-lactamases. The synthesis of these enzymes, which is normally repressed, is induced by the presence of a few beta-lactam antibiotics.

In gram-positive bacteria of clinical importance such as staphylococci, beta-lactamase production is plasmid-mediated with activity directed principally against penicillins and only slightly against cephalosporins. The enzyme is inducible and released in large amounts into the surrounding medium, where it carries out its protective role by destroying the penicillins in the environment. In aerobic gram-negative bacteria, beta-lactamases are produced in smaller amounts and retained in the periplasmic space, which lies between the cytoplasmic and the outer membranes of these organisms. Thus the enzyme is strategically located to destroy the beta-lactam compound before it reaches the cytoplasmic-membrane-bound PBP targets. These beta-lactamases may be either chromosomally or plasmid mediated, inducible or constitutively produced, and with an affinity for penicillins or cephalosporins or both. Some gram-negative anaerobes, particularly *Bacteroides fragilis*, produce beta-lactamase, which is retained in the periplasmic space and is usually chromosomally determined, although plasmid-mediated enzymes have been identified.

PENICILLINS

Penicillin G was discovered in 1928, when Alexander Fleming noted that a mold contaminating one of his cultures caused the bacteria in its vicinity to undergo lysis. Because the mold belonged to the genus *Penicillium*, he named the antibacterial substance *penicillin*.

Almost a decade later, a group of investigators at Oxford University isolated a crude preparation of penicillin, which was introduced for clinical trials in 1941. Early penicillin was a mixture of several penicillin compounds designated as F, G, X, and K. Penicillin G (benzylpenicillin), the most active of these, was purified and introduced into clinical medicine.

Major progress in the development of penicillins occurred in 1959, when the penicillin nucleus,

6-aminopenicillanic acid, was isolated from cultures of *Penicillium chrysogenum* that were depleted of side-chain precursors. Addition of various side chains to the nucleus led to the development of semisynthetic penicillins.

Chemistry

The basic penicillin structure is composed of a beta-lactam ring attached to a five-membered thiazolidine ring and a side chain (Fig. 42-3). Modifications of the penicillin molecule take place only on the acyl side chain (R). The side chain determines the antimicrobial spectrum, susceptibility to beta-lactamases, and the pharmacokinetic properties of a particular penicillin. All penicillins currently in use are available as either sodium or potassium salts.

Classification

Penicillins can be divided into four groups on the basis of their antimicrobial spectrum (Table 42-1). Differences within a group are usually of a pharmacologic nature, although one compound in a group may be more active than another against some organisms.

Penicillin G has a narrow antimicrobial spectrum. It is active against gram-positive bacteria and *Neisseria* species, but gram-negative bacilli are generally resistant. Penicillin G is degraded by gastric acid and destroyed by staphylococcal penicillinase. *Penicillin V*, another natural penicillin, is acid-resistant and used for oral administration.

Penicillinase-resistant penicillins (methicillin, nafcillin, oxacillin, cloxacillin, dicloxacillin) are active against penicillin G-resistant staphylococci. Their antimicrobial spectrum is limited to gram-positive organisms.

The antimicrobial spectrum of *aminopenicillins* (ampicillin, amoxicillin) resembles that of penicillin G except that it includes a limited number of gram-negative species. The *extended-spectrum penicillins* (carbenicillin, ticarcillin, mezlocillin, azlocillin, and piperacillin) are active against a much broader spectrum of gram-negative organisms. Both aminopenicillins and extended-spectrum penicillins are destroyed by staphylococcal penicillinase.

The addition of a *beta-lactamase inhibitor* (clavulanic acid or sulbactam) to an aminopenicillin or an extended-spectrum penicillin broadens the antimicrobial spectrum to include penicillin G-resistant staphylococci and many beta-lactamase-producing gram-negative bacilli.

Pharmacokinetics

There are marked differences in the oral absorption of various penicillins (Table 42-1). Penicillin G is acid-labile. Other penicillins available for oral administration are acid-stable. Peak serum levels are obtained 1 to 2 h after ingestion. When ingested with food, absorption is delayed to yield peak serum levels in 2 to 3 h.

Penicillins are bound to proteins (primarily albumin) in varying degrees, ranging from 20 percent for ampicillin to 97 percent for dicloxacillin. Only the free (unbound) drug exerts antibacterial activity, since the bound drug cannot reach the PBP target within the bacteria. Protein binding, however, is loose and rapidly reversible. An equilibrium exists between the antibiotic-protein complex and the free drug, not only in the serum but also in the interstitial fluid. Thus, although protein-bound penicillin is essentially inactive and relatively nondiffusible between these compartments, it serves as a constant reservoir, which releases more drug as the free drug is excreted or metabolized.

Penicillins diffuse quite readily into all body tissues and fluids except for brain, cerebrospinal fluid (CSF), eye, and prostate. In the presence of inflammation, therapeutic concentrations are attained in the brain and the CSF.

Penicillins are rapidly eliminated from the body with half-lives ranging from 30 to 70 min. Most penicillins are excreted mainly by the kidneys in the active unchanged form. Excretion occurs by glomerular filtration and by tubular secretion, which can be blocked with probenecid. Metabolism plays a major role in the elimination of nafcillin, oxacillin, cloxacillin, and dicloxacillin. Biliary excretion is important only for nafcillin (8 percent) and for mezlocillin, azlocillin, and piperacillin (20 to 30 percent)

Adverse Effects

Allergic reactions are the main adverse effects encountered with the use of the penicillins. Sensitization is usually the result of previous treatment with a penicillin. The penicillin molecule or its breakdown products may evoke allergy by acting as haptens combining

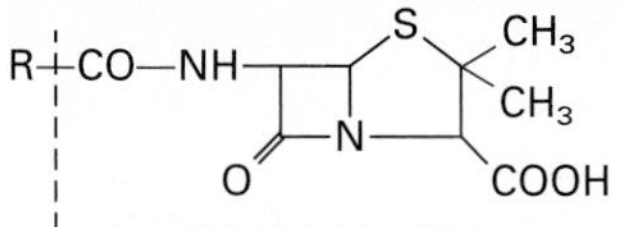

BASIC STRUCTURE

R Side chain	Generic name	Trade name(s)
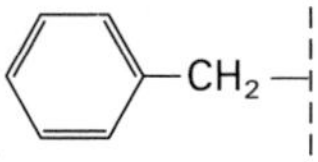	Penicillin G	—
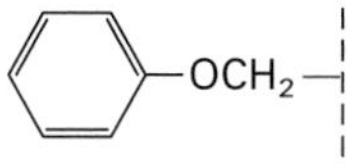	Penicillin V	—
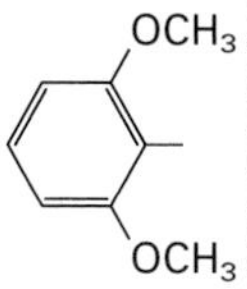	Methicillin	(Staphcillin)
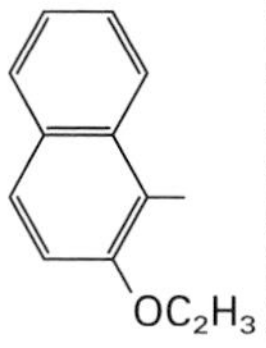	Nafcillin	(Unipen, Nafcil, others)
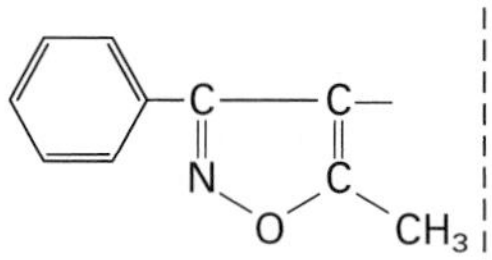	Oxacillin	(Bactocill, Prostaphin)
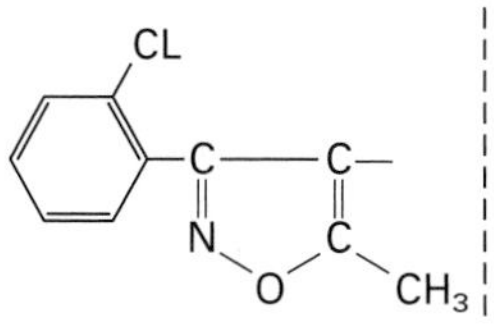	Cloxacillin	(Tegopen)
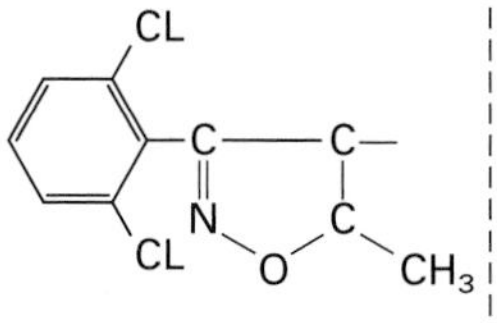	Dicloxacillin	(Dynapen, others)
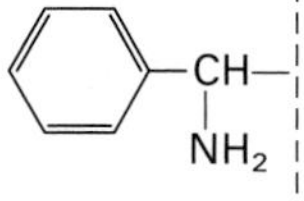	Ampicillin	(Omnipen, Polycillin, others)
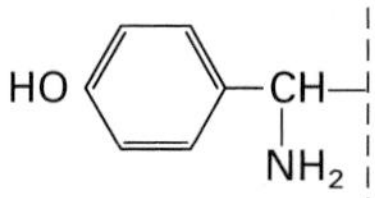	Amoxicillin	(Amoxil, Trimox, others)
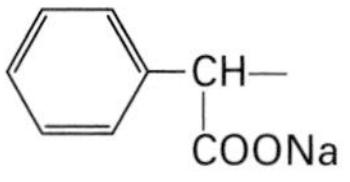	Carbenicillin	(Geocillin, Geopen, others)
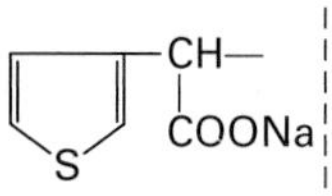	Ticarcillin	(Ticar)
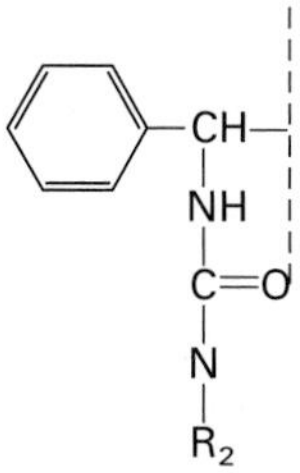	Azlocillin Mezlocillin Piperacillin	(Azlin) (Mezlin) (Pipracil)

FIGURE 42-3 Chemical structures of penicillins.

TABLE 42-1   Classification and pharmacokinetic properties of penicillins

Generic name	Oral absorption, %	Protein binding, %	Elimination half-life, h	Elimination half-life, h, anuria
Natural penicillins				
Penicillin G	20	55	0.5	4.0
Penicillin V	30	80	0.5	2.0
Penicillinase-resistant				
Methicillin	—	35	0.5	4.0
Nafcillin	10–20	88	0.5	1.0
Oxacillin	30	92	0.5	1.0
Cloxacillin	50	94	0.6	1.5
Dicloxacillin	70	97	0.7	2.2
Aminopenicillins				
Ampicillin	40	20	1.0	8.0
Amoxicillin	75	20	1.0	8.0
Extended spectrum				
Carbenicillin		50	1.1	15
Ticarcillin	—	50	1.2	15
Mezlocillin	—	30	1.0	3.6
Azlocillin	—	30	1.0	5.2
Piperacillin	—	30	1.0	4.0

with body proteins to form antigenic compounds. It is difficult to estimate the degree of cross allergy from one penicillin derivative to another, but allergy to one should be considered as allergy to all penicillins.

Immediate reactions include anaphylaxis (fatal in 10 percent), urticaria, bronchospasm, and angioedema. These are mediated by IgE antibodies and occur minutes to hours after administration of the penicillin. Late or delayed hypersensitivity reactions occur in 1 to 10 percent of patients receiving these drugs. Maculopapular skin rashes are the most common reactions and occur more frequently with ampicillin. These can be treated symptomatically and may subside despite continuation of the drug. Serum sickness, Stevens-Johnson syndrome, and exfoliative dermatitis are rare forms of allergic reactions that require discontinuation of the compound. Drug fever can occur with or without eosinophilia; it usually is low-grade but may be high with shaking chills. Eosinophilia may develop and is usually asymptomatic.

Penicillins are not nephrotoxic; however, allergic interstitial nephritis may occur, particularly with methicillin. It manifests itself by fever, occasional rashes, eosinophilia, the presence of eosinophils in the urine, and a rise in creatinine. Discontinuation of the penicillin will result in the return of renal function to normal in the majority of situations.

Hematologic reactions caused by penicillins are rare. Coombs-positive hemolytic anemia, immune thrombocytopenia, leukopenia, or neutropenia may occur. The white blood cell counts return to normal rapidly if the offending agent is discontinued. Neutropenia has been reported more frequently with nafcillin and oxacillin than with other penicillins. All penicillins at high concentrations, particularly carbenicillin and ticarcillin, impair platelet function, resulting in prolongation of the bleeding time but, rarely, a clinically significant bleeding.

Myoclonic jerks and seizures may develop when high doses of penicillins are given in the presence of renal insufficiency. The sodium content of ticarcillin (5.1 meq/g) and carbenicillin (4.7 meq/g) obligates the patient to receive 90 to 170 meq of sodium per day. The sodium overload can exacerbate congestive heart failure. Ureido penicillins (mezlocillin, azlocillin, piperacillin) contain less sodium (approximately 2 meq/g).

Administration of large doses of any penicillin, but most often carbenicillin and ticarcillin, may result in hypokalemia due to the large quantity of nonreabsorbable anions presented to the distal renal tubules.

Diarrhea may occur in 1 to 5 percent of patients taking penicillin; it is more common with oral ampicillin. *Clostridium difficile* colitis can develop with any of these agents. Transient elevations of transaminases may occur with most penicillins, especially oxacillin and carbenicillin. They are benign and reversible.

All the penicillins used at high doses for prolonged periods will abolish normal bacterial flora with resulting colonization with resistant gram-negative bacilli and/or fungi, followed occasionally by superinfection with these organisms.

Jarisch-Herxheimer reaction may occur when patients with syphilis are treated with penicillin G. It consists of fever, headache, myalgia, and malaise, which start abruptly, a few hours after therapy, and last up to 24 h. Herxheimer reaction occurs in 50 to 70 percent of patients with early syphilis and a small proportion of those with later stages of syphilis. Its pathogenesis is unclear.

Natural Penicillins

Natural penicillins, produced biosynthetically, include penicillin G (benzylpenicillin) and penicillin V (phenoxymethylpenicillin). The structural formulas of these compounds are shown in Fig. 42-3.

Antimicrobial Spectrum Penicillin G is highly active against nonenterococcal streptococci, including pneumococcus. Occasional strains are autolysin-deficient and therefore tolerant to the bactericidal action of the drug. Approximately 3 percent of clinically significant isolates of *Strep. pneumoniae* are relatively resistant to penicillin G (minimum inhibitory concentrations of 0.1 to 1.0 μg/mL). These strains require 5 to 100 times higher concentrations for inhibition than do sensitive strains. Although this level of resistance can be overcome by readily achievable serum or tissue concentrations, it is difficult to achieve CSF levels adequate to treat meningitis due to these organisms. Strains of pneumococci with high-level penicillin resistance have been detected but are very rare in the United States.

Enterococci (*Enterococcus faecalis, Enterococcus faecium,* and *Enterococcus durans*) are much less sensitive to penicillin G than are other streptococci. This is due to the presence of PBPs, which have low affinity for the drug. These organisms are also tolerant to the bactericidal action of penicillin G. Combinations of penicillin G and aminoglycosides (Chap. 43) usually have synergistic bactericidal effect against enterococci.

When penicillin G was first introduced, staphylococci were mostly sensitive. Within a few years, penicillin-resistant strains were encountered with increasing frequency, particularly among the hospital isolates. Today most strains of *Staph. aureus* and coagulase-negative staphylococci are resistant to penicillin G. Resistance is due to the production of penicillinase (a beta-lactamase), which is plasmid-mediated.

Penicillin G is active against most aerobic gram-positive bacilli, including *Listeria monocytogenes, Corynebacterium diphtheriae,* and *Bacillus anthracis.* However, *Nocardia* species and diphtheroids are resistant.

Neisseria meningitidis is highly sensitive to penicillin G. *Neisseria gonorrhoeae* is also susceptible, but its continued exposure to the antibiotic has led to a gradual decrease in sensitivity. This appears to be due to the additive effects of mutations affecting the binding affinity of PBPs and/or the permeability of the outer membrane. Strains of *N. gonorrhoeae* that do not produce penicillinase but are completely resistant to penicillin G have been detected in recent years. However, most resistant strains produce penicillinase, which is plasmid-mediated. Penicillinase-producing *N. gonorrhoeae* account for a significant proportion of isolates in some parts of the United States.

Penicillin G is moderately active against beta-lactamase-negative *Haemophilus influenzae.* All Enterobacteriaceae and *Pseudomonas* species are resistant to the drug. Penicillin G is active against *Pasteurella multocida,* a common cause of infection in animal-bite wounds; *Eikenella corrodens,* a common cause of infection in human bites; and *Streptobacillus moniliformis,* a cause of rat-bite fever.

Penicillin G is active against anaerobic bacteria, including peptococci, peptostreptococci, clostridia, *Actinomyces* species, *Fusobacterium,* and non-beta-lactamase-producing strains of *Bacteroides. Bacteroides fragilis* is resistant to penicillin G.

Treponema pallidum, leptospira, *Spirillum minor,* and *Borrelia* species are consistently sensitive to penicillin G. Penicillin G is ineffective against mycobacteria, *Chlamydia, Rickettsiae, Mycoplasma,* fungi, and protozoa.

The antibacterial spectrum of penicillin V is generally similar to that of penicillin G. It is, however, less active against meningococci and gonococci.

Pharmacokinectics   Penicillin G is destroyed by acid in the stomach; absorption after oral administration is irregular and variable. In order to achieve adequate absorption, it should be given 1 h before or 2 to 3 h after a meal. Penicillin V is acid-stable and is preferred for oral use. The absorption of penicillin V is subject to less variability and is not readily affected by proximity to meals.

Penicillin G is 55 percent bound to serum proteins. It is widely distributed throughout the body but does not enter the CSF when the meninges are normal. In the presence of meningeal inflammation, the concentrations attained in the CSF are approximately 5 percent of those in plasma.

Over 70 percent of a parenterally administered dose of penicillin G is excreted unchanged by the kidneys, predominantly via tubular secretion. Approximately 25 percent is metabolized in the liver, and a small amount is secreted into the bile in the unchanged form. The elimination half-life of penicillin G, which is 30 min with normal renal function, increases to 4.0 h in anuric patients.

Crystalline penicillin G is available as the potassium or sodium salt and may be given either intravenously or intramuscularly. The sodium salt is much more expensive than the potassium salt, and it rarely needs to be used. Administration of 4 million units (2.5 g) of crystalline penicillin G intravenously every 4 h results in a mean serum concentration of 20 units per milliliter. One unit of activity is equivalent to 0.625 mg of pure potassium penicillin G. Each million units contains 1.7 meq of potassium.

Given intramuscularly as an aqueous solution, penicillin G is very rapidly cleared from the body, and it is preferable to use a repository form. Repository penicillins provide tissue depots from which the drug is absorbed over hours in the case of procaine penicillin G or over days in the case of benzathine penicillin G. Repository penicillins are for intramuscular use and cannot be used intravenously or subcutaneously. After intramuscular injection of 600,000 units of procaine penicillin, the peak serum level is reached in about 2 h and detectable levels are maintained for 24 h. An intramuscular injection of 1.2 million units of benzathine penicillin G provides detectable serum levels for at least 15 days.

Clinical Use   In the nonallergic person, penicillin G is the drug of choice for infections caused by susceptible organisms. These include infections due to streptococci (except enterococci), gonococci, meningococci, non-beta-lactamase-producing anaerobes, *Pasteurella multocida* and *Eikenella corrodens*, syphilis, diphtheria, rat-bite fever, and anthrax. Penicillin V can be substituted for penicillin G in situations in which oral administration is suitable. Benzathine penicillin G (one monthly injection) is the most effective regimen for prevention of recurrent attacks of rheumatic fever. Penicillin V is used most commonly for group A streptococcal pharyngitis.

Penicillinase-Resistant Penicillins

Methicillin was the first penicillinase-resistant semisynthetic penicillin to be derived from the penicillin nucleus, 6-aminopenicillanic acid. Subsequently nafcillin and isoxazolyl penicillins (oxacillin, cloxacillin, and dicloxacillin) were developed (Fig. 42-3). These agents are of interest mainly because of their activity against staphylococci which are resistant to penicillin G.

Antimicobial Spectrum   Penicillinase-resistant penicillins are highly active against both penicillin G-sensitive and penicillin G-resistant *Staph. aureus* and coagulase-negative staphylococci. In vitro, methicillin is four- to eightfold less active than nafcillin and isoxazolyl penicillins; the activities of the latter agents are comparable. Occasional strains are autolysin-deficient and therefore tolerant to the bactericidal action of these agents. Combinations of penicillinase-resistant penicillins and aminoglycosides exhibit synergy against staphylococci.

Some strains of *Staph. aureus* and most coagulase-negative staphylococci are resistant to penicillinase-resistant penicillins. These strains are referred to as *methicillin-resistant*, although they are also oxacillin-, nafcillin-, and cephalosporin-resistant. The resistance is due to altered PBPs which have low affinity for beta-lactam compounds. Methicillin-resistant *Staph. aureus* has become an important cause of nosocomial infections in some parts of the United States.

Penicillinase-resistant penicillins are active against all streptococci with the exception of *Enterococcus* species. They are, however, less active than penicillin G against these organisms. Anaerobic gram-positive species, including peptococci, peptostreptococci, and clostridia, are also sensitive. These agents are inactive against gonococci, meningococci, and gram-negative bacilli (aerobic, anaerobic).

Pharmacokinetics Methicillin is acid-labile and therefore not useful for oral administration. Nafcillin is poorly and inconsistently absorbed from the gastrointestinal tract. Isoxazolyl penicillins are acid-stable and absorbed when administered orally. The presence of food in the stomach delays and decreases the absorption. After oral administration of equivalent doses, the serum concentrations of cloxacillin are twice those of oxacillin, and the serum levels of dicloxacillin are twice those of cloxacillin. These variations in serum levels are due to differences not only in absorption but also in clearance of these drugs.

With the exception of methicillin, which is 35 percent bound to serum proteins, penicillinase-resistant penicillins are highly protein-bound: nafcillin 88 percent, oxacillin 92 percent, cloxacillin 94 percent, and dicloxacillin 97 percent. Methicillin is excreted primarily into the urine in active unchanged form. Metabolism and biliary secretion play important roles in the excretion of nafcillin and isoxazolyl penicillins. Approximately 60 percent of an administered dose of nafcillin is inactivated in the liver. The elimination half-lives of nafcillin and oxacillin, which are 30 min with normal renal function, increase to 1.0 h in anuric patients. Dosage adjustments are therefore not necessary for either of these agents in patients with renal failure.

Clinical Use Penicillinase-resistant penicillins are the drugs of choice for infections due to penicillin G-resistant *Staph. aureus* or coagulase-negative staphylococci. Although indicated only for those infections, they are also effective in infections caused by nonenterococcal *Streptococcus* species, including groups A, B, C, and G streptococci and pneumococci. These agents, alone or combined with aminoglycosides, are ineffective in enterococcal infections.

Cloxacillin and dicloxacillin are available only for oral use and are the preferred agents for administration by this route. Oxacillin and nafcillin are available for both oral and parenteral use. Because of poor absorption, nafcillin is not recommended for oral administration. Methicillin is available only for parenteral administration. Because of a higher incidence of adverse effects (i.e., interstitial nephritis) and lower in vitro activity, methicillin is seldom used today.

Aminopenicillins

Ampicillin (2-aminobenzyl penicillin) differs from penicillin G by the presence of an amino group on the acyl side chain (Fig. 42-3). Bacampicillin is an ester of ampicillin. Amoxicillin differs from ampicillin by the presence of a hydroxyl group in the para position of the benzyl side chain.

Antimicrobial Spectrum The antibacterial activities of ampicillin and amoxicillin are similar. Bacampicillin has no antimicrobial activity; it is a prodrug that is rapidly hydrolyzed to ampicillin after absorption from the intestine. Like penicillin G, aminopenicillins are destroyed by staphylococcal penicillinase and are therefore ineffective against most *Staph. aureus* and coagulase-negative staphylococci. The activity of these agents against streptococci, gram-positive bacilli, and *Neisseria* species is equal to that of penicillin G, except that they are more potent against enterococci and *L. monocytogenes*.

Aminopenicillins are active against a few gram-negative species which are resistant to penicillin G. *H. influenzae* is susceptible except for strains that produce beta-lactamase. These strains account for 10 to 25 percent of isolates in many parts of the United States. Beta-lactamase production is plasmid-mediated. Approximately 80 percent of *E. coli* strains isolated from community-acquired infections are sensitive to aminopenicillins. Resistance is plasmid-mediated and is more common in hospital isolates. *Proteus mirabilis* is almost always sensitive to these agents. Most *Salmonella* and some *Shigella* strains are also susceptible, but other aerobic gram-negative species are resistant.

The activity of aminopenicillins against anaerobes is comparable to that of penicillin G.

Pharmacokinetics Ampicillin is 40 percent absorbed after oral administration; peak serum levels are delayed and lower if the drug is ingested with food. Amoxicillin is significantly better absorbed; the serum concentrations are approximately twice those achieved with a similar oral dose of ampicillin. The presence of food in the stomach does not alter absorption of amoxicillin. Bacampicillin is absorbed rapidly after oral administration and hydrolyzed immediately to ampicillin. The serum levels of ampicillin after an oral dose of bacampicillin are twice those attained with an equimolar dose of ampicillin. The presence of food in the stomach does not decrease or delay absorption of bacampicillin.

Ampicillin and amoxicillin are the least protein-bound (20 percent) penicillins. Both are excreted primarily (75 to 80 percent) by the kidneys in active unchanged form. A small fraction is inactivated, chiefly in the liver, and 2 to 3 percent is excreted unchanged into the bile. The elimination half-life of ampicillin, which is 1.0 h with normal renal function, increases to 8.0 h in anuric patients.

Clinical Use   Ampicillin is effective in a variety of infections caused by susceptible organisms. It is the drug of choice for infections caused by beta-lactamase-negative strains of *H. influenzae, L. monocytogenes,* and enterococci. For enterococcal endocarditis it is given in combination with an aminoglycoside in order to provide bactericidal activity against the organism.

Because of better absorption and a lower incidence of side effects (i.e., diarrhea), amoxicillin is preferred to ampicillin for oral administration. Bacampicillin is significantly more expensive than ampicillin. On a molar basis 400 mg of bacampicillin is equivalent to 278 mg of ampicillin.

Extended-Spectrum Penicillins

These agents, which include the carboxy penicillins (carbenicillin, ticarcillin) and the ureido penicillins (mezlocillin, azlocillin, piperacillin), have a broad spectrum of activity against aerobic gram-negative bacilli, including *Pseudomonas aeruginosa,* and anaerobic bacteria. Carbenicillin and ticarcillin have a carboxy group on the acyl side chain (Fig. 42-3). Mezlocillin, azlocillin, and piperacillin, all derivatives of ampicillin, have a ureido group ($-NH-CO-N-R_2$), in place of the amino group ($-NH_2$) of ampicillin, on the acyl side chain. The presence of a carboxy group or a ureido group on the acyl side chain leads to increased activity against gram-negative species primarily because of greater penetration through the outer membrane.

Antimicrobial Spectrum   All extended-spectrum penicillins are susceptible to staphylococcal penicillinase and thus inactive against penicillin G-resistant staphylococci. Carbenicillin and ticarcillin are ineffective against enterococci and less active than ampicillin against other streptococci and gram-positive bacilli.

The activity of ureido penicillins against these organisms, including enterococci, is comparable to that of ampicillin.

Extended-spectrum penicillins have a broad spectrum of activity against aerobic gram-negative bacilli. These include all organisms that are sensitive to ampicillin and most strains of *Enterobacter, Proteus vulgaris, Providencia, Morganella, Serratia marcescens, Acinetobacter,* and *Ps. aeruginosa.* There are some differences in the pattern of activity of these agents against gram-negative species. Ticarcillin is two- or fourfold more active than carbenicillin against *Ps. aeruginosa.* Mezlocillin has the same activity against *Ps. aeruginosa* as does ticarcillin, whereas azlocillin and piperacillin are two- to fourfold more active. *Klebsiella* species are uniformly resistant to carbenicillin and ticarcillin, whereas 50 to 80 percent of strains are susceptible to ureido penicillins. The activities of mezlocillin and piperacillin against enteric gram-negative bacilli are slightly superior to those of carbenicillin, ticarcillin, and azlocillin. Ureido penicillins are more active than carboxy penicillins against *H. influenzae,* but none is active against ampicillin-resistant isolates.

Extended-spectrum penicillins combined with an aminoglycoside show synergistic activity against many isolates of *Ps. aeruginosa* and against some strains of enteric gram-negative species.

Extended-spectrum penicillins have substantial activity against anaerobes, including the *Bacteroides fragilis* group. Approximately 80 percent of *B. fragilis* isolates are susceptible to these agents.

Pharmacokinetics   The extended-spectrum penicillins are not absorbed from the gastrointestinal tract and, therefore, must be given parenterally. Mezlocillin, azlocillin, and piperacillin are 30 percent protein-bound, whereas carbenicillin and ticarcillin are 50 percent bound to serum proteins.

Ninety-five percent of carbenicillin and 80 percent of ticarcillin administered intravenously are excreted in active unchanged form into the urine. Some ticarcillin (10 to 15 percent) is inactivated in the body, chiefly in the liver. The elimination half-lives of these agents, which are 1.1 h with normal renal function, increase to 15 h in anuric patients.

Mezlocillin, azlocillin, and piperacillin are also excreted primarily (55 to 70 percent) by the kidneys in active unchanged form. However 20 to 30 percent of the administered dose is excreted unchanged into the bile, and small fractions are inactivated in the body. The elimination half-lives of mezlocillin, piperacillin, and azlocillin, which are 1.0 h with normal renal function, increase to 3.6, 4.0, and 5.0 h, respectively, in anuric patients.

Clinical Use The extended-spectrum penicillins are most useful for infections caused by aerobic gram-negative bacilli and anaerobes. Because of the potential for the emergence of resistance during therapy, these agents should be combined with an aminoglycoside for the therapy of serious *Pseudomonas* infections. In compromised hosts, especially those with neutropenia, and in patients with intra-abdominal infections, pelvic infections, or nosocomial aspiration pneumonia, these agents are usually used in combination with an aminoglycoside.

Carbenicillin indanyl sodium is an α-carboxy ester of carbenicillin. It has no intrinsic activity of its own, but it is acid-stable and relatively well absorbed from the gastrointestinal tract. After absorption, the ester is rapidly hydrolyzed to free carbenicillin. Indanyl carbenicillin does not provide adequate serum or tissue levels for systemic infections; it is useful only for treatment of urinary tract infections, particularly those caused by *Ps. aeruginosa*.

Combinations with Beta-Lactamase Inhibitors

Beta-lactamases are responsible for the resistance of many bacteria to beta-lactam antibiotics. To overcome this type of resistance, a beta-lactam antibiotic may be combined with a beta-lactamase inhibitor, clavulanic acid or sulbactam. Clavulanic acid is a naturally occurring beta-lactamase inhibitor, which was isolated from *Streptomyces clavuligerus*. Sulbactam is a semisynthetic compound derived from 6-aminopenicillanic acid. Both agents function as a "suicide" rather than competitive inhibitor. By forming a complex with the beta-lactamase, they render the enzyme inactive so that a beta-lactam antibiotic can destroy the organism. Both clavulanic acid and sulbactam contain a beta-lactam ring but exhibit poor antibacterial activity. They readily cross the outer membrane of most enteric gram-negative bacilli to interact with beta-lactamses in periplasmic space. Both compounds inhibit approximately the same range of beta-lactamases.

Clavulanic acid   Sulbactam

Clavulanic acid is available in combination with amoxicillin (Augmentin) for oral use and in combination with ticarcillin (Timentin) for intravenous administration. Sulbactam is available in combination with ampicillin (Unasyn) for parenteral use.

Antimicrobial Spectrum Clavulanic acid and sulbactam do not influence the activity of the penicillin component of the combination against susceptible organisms. They do, however, broaden its antimicrobial spectrum to include beta-lactamase-producing strains of *Staph. aureus*, coagulase-negative staphylococci, *H. influenzae*, *Haemophilis ducreyi*, *N. gonorrhoeae*, *Branhamella catarrhalis*, and *Bacteroides*. All anaerobes including 100 percent of *B. fragilis* strains are sensitive to these combinations. The antibacterial spectra of the combinations also include beta-lactamase-producing strains of *E. coli*, *Proteus*, *Klebsiella*, and a few other enteric gram-negative species. No increased activity is provided against *Ps. aeruginosa*.

Pharmacokinetics The bioavailability of clavulanic acid after oral administration averages 60 percent of the administered dose. Fifty percent of an intravenously administered dose appears in the urine in the active unchanged form, and 50 percent is inactivated in the body. The elimination half-life of clavulanic acid is 1.1 h. The drug is 30 percent bound to serum proteins.

Approximately 50 percent of intravenously administered sulbactam is excreted unchanged in the urine. A small fraction is excreted into the bile, and the remainder is inactivated in the body. The elimination half-life of sulbactam is 1.0 h. The drug is 40 percent bound to serum proteins.

Clinical Use Amoxicillin–clavulanic acid is useful for treatment of infections caused by susceptible beta-lactamase-producing organisms. It is the oral drug of choice for human-bite or animal-bite infections in which staphylococci, streptococci, anaerobes, *Pasteurella multocida* (animal bite), and *Eikenella corrodens* (human bite) are the potential etiologic agents. The drug is available in tablets that contain 250 and 500 mg of amoxicillin, each with 125 mg of clavulanic acid. Two 250-mg tablets are *not* equivalent to a 500-mg tablet, because the amounts of clavulanic acid in the two tablets are higher and may increase gastrointestinal side effects.

Ticarcillin–clavulanic acid is useful for mixed infections in which *Staph. aureus* or beta-lactamase-producing anaerobes (especially *B. fragilis*) may be present. The combination is available in two forms: 3.1-g vials containing 3 g of ticarcillin with 0.1 g of clavulanic acid for systemic infections, and 3.2-g vials containing 3 g of ticarcillin with 0.2 g of clavulanic acid for urinary tract infections.

Ampicillin-sulbactam is effective in infections caused by susceptible beta-lactamase-producing organisms. It is particularly useful for mixed infections involving *Staph. aureus*, enterococcus, enteric bacilli, and/or anaerobes. The drug is available in 3-g vials containing 2 g of ampicillin with 1 g of sulbactam.

Amdinocillin

Amdinocillin, previously known as mecillinam, is a semisynthetic penicillin that binds specifically to PBP-2, in contrast to other penicillins and cephalosporins which bind primarily to PBP-1 and PBP-3. This agent is active only against enteric gram-negative bacilli and may be used to treat urinary tract infections. It acts synergistically with other penicillins and with cephalosporins against susceptible bacteria; however, its clinical role is unclear.

CEPHALOSPORINS

The first cephalosporin, known as *cephalosporin C*, was insolated from the fermentation products of a fungus, *Cephalosporium acremonium*. Hydrolysis of this compound produced 7-aminocephalosporanic acid, which was subsequently modified with different side chains to create an entire family of cephalosporin antibiotics.

Chemistry

The cephalosporin nucleus consists of a beta-lactam ring fused to a six-membered dihydrothiazine ring (Fig. 42-4). In contrast to the penicillin nucleus, the

First generation

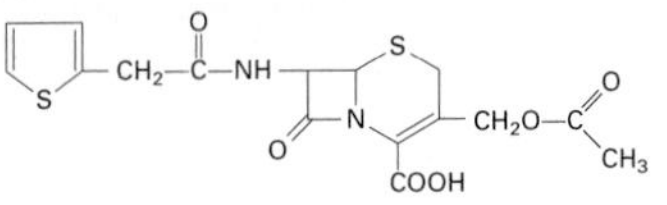

Cephalothin
(Keflin, Seffin)

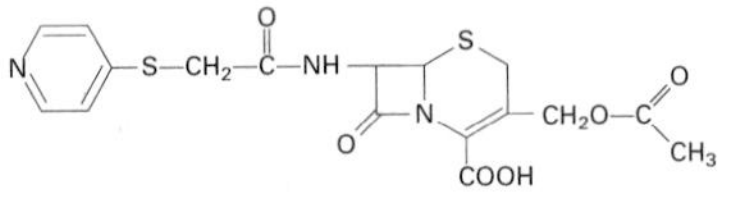

Cephapirin
(Cefadyl)

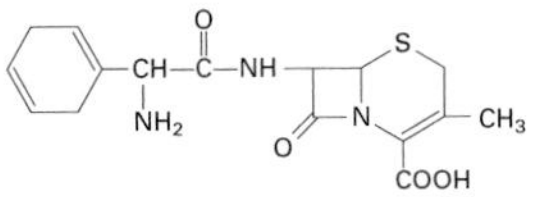

Cephradine
(Anspor, Velosef)

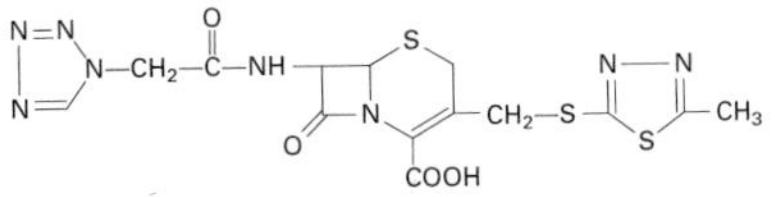

Cefazolin
(Ancef, Kefzol)

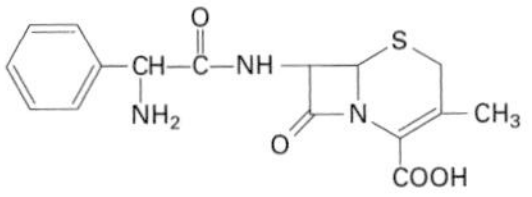

Cephalexin
(Keflex)

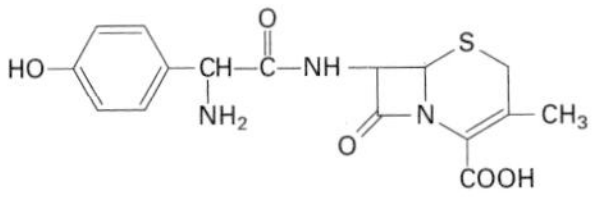

Cefadroxil
(Duricef, Ultracef)

FIGURE 42-4 Chemical structures of cephalosporins.

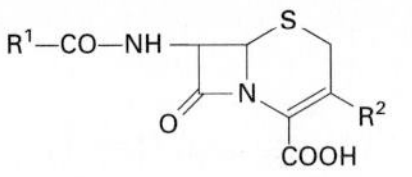

BASIC STRUCTURE

Second generation	Third generation
Cefuroxime (Ceftin, Zinacef)	Cefotaxime (Claforan)
Cefamandole (Mandol)	Ceftizoxime (Cefizox)
Cefonicid (Monocid)	Ceftriaxone (Rocephin)
Ceforanide (Precef)	Ceftazidime (Fortaz, Tazidime)
Cefoxitin (Mefoxin)	Moxalactam (Moxam)
Cefotetan (Cefotan)	Cefoperazone (Cefobid)
Cefaclor (Ceclor)	

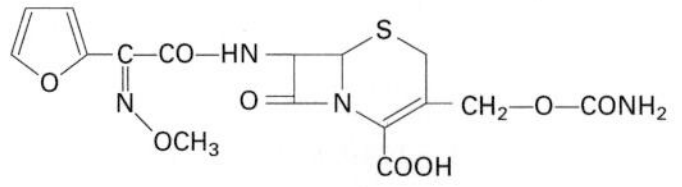

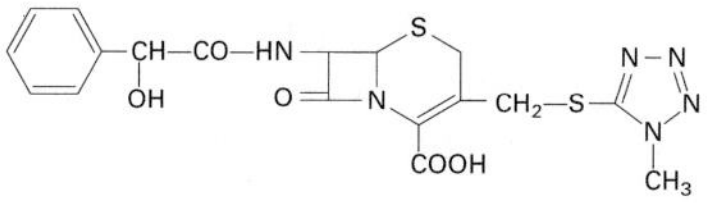

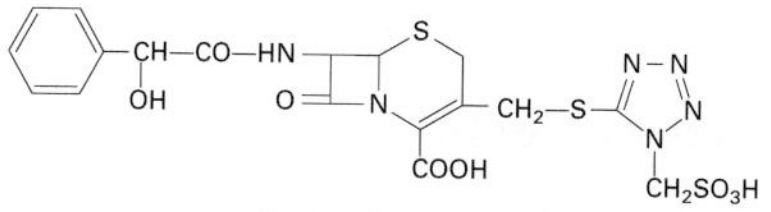

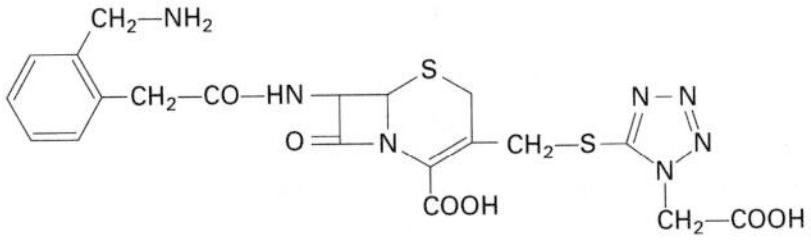

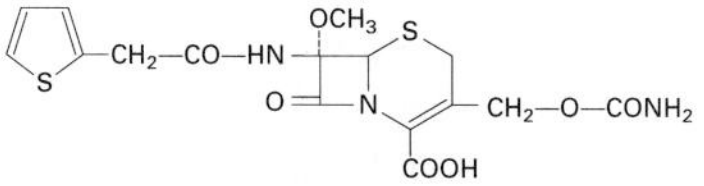

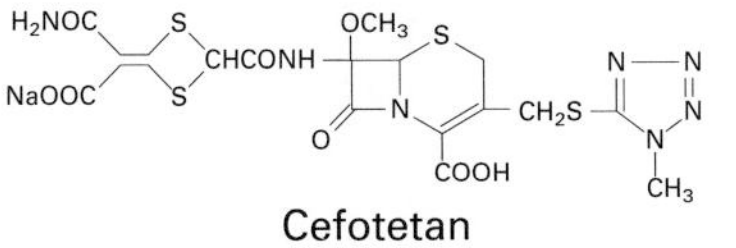

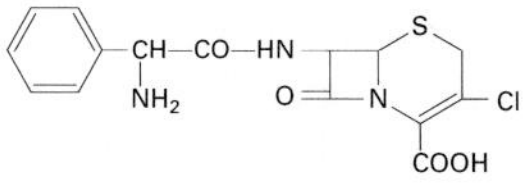

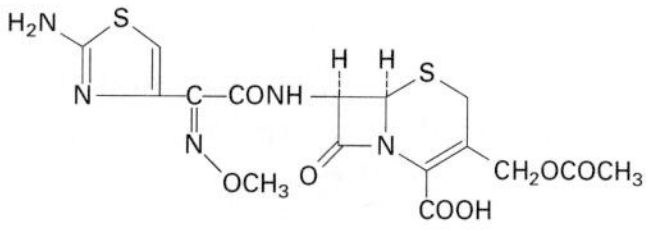

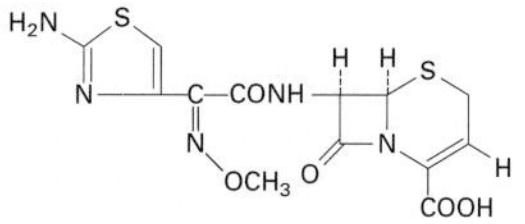

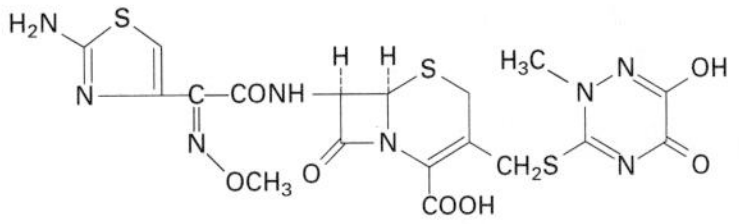

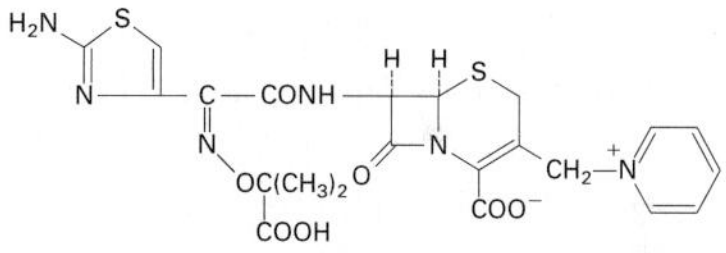

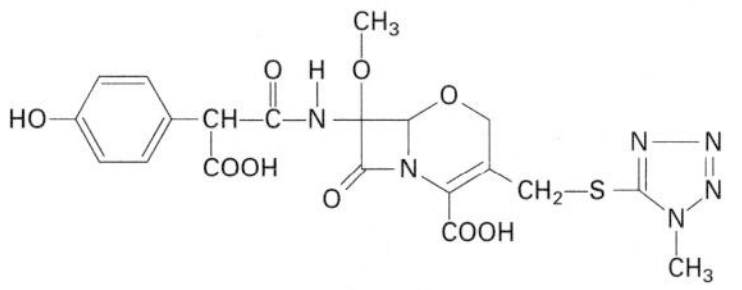

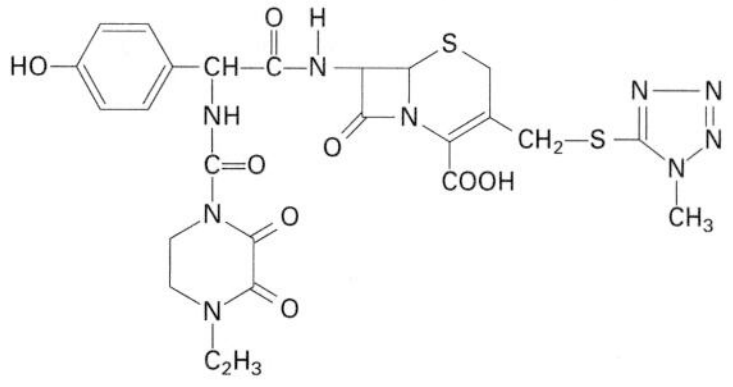

FIGURE 42-4 (*continued*)

cephalosporin nucleus is inherently more resistant to beta-lactamases. It also provides more sites for potential manipulation. Modifications of the acyl side chain at position R^1 alter antimicrobial activity, whereas substitutions at position R^2 are associated with changes in pharmacokinetics and metabolic parameters of the drug. Substitution of an acetoxy group ($—CH_2—O—CO—CH_3$) for R^2 (cephalothin, cephapirin, cefotaxime) is associated with significant metabolism to desacetyl derivative. The presence of a methylthiotetrazole group at this position (cefamandole, cefotetan, cefoperazone, and moxalactam) is associated with disulfiram-like reactions and hypoprothrombinemia. The presence of a methoxy group at α-7 position (cefoxitin and cefotetan), which, strictly speaking, identifies the compound as cephamycin rather than cephalosporin, confers resistance to gram-negative beta-lactamases.

Classification

Cephalosporins are classified into three groups, or *generations*, on the basis of their spectrum of activity against gram-negative bacilli (Table 42-2). Compounds within a generation differ from one another primarily in pharmacokinetic properties, although there may be significant difference in activity against certain organisms. The first-generation cephalosporins (cephalothin, cefazolin, cephapirin, cephradine, cephalexin, and cefadroxil) are hydrolyzed by many beta-lactamases produced by gram-negative organisms and therefore have a relatively narrow gram-negative spectrum. The second-generation compounds (cefuroxime, cefamandole, cefonicid, ceforanide, cefoxitin, and cefotetan) have greater beta-lactamase stability and a broader spectrum of activity against gram-negative organisms. The third-generation cephalosporins (cefotaxime, ceftizoxime, moxalactam, cefoperazone, ceftriaxone, and ceftazidime) are relatively resistant to hydrolysis by beta-lactamases and have the broadest gram-negative spectrum.

Pharmacokinetics

Three first-generation (cephalexin, cephradine, and cefadroxil) and two second-generation (cefaclor and cefuroxime axetil) cephalosporins are acid-stable and absorbed after oral administration. The other cephalo-sporins, including all third-generation compounds, are suitable only for parenteral administration.

The cephalosporins penetrate well into most body tissues and fluids. The first- and second-generation cephalosporins, with the exception of cefuroxime, do not penetrate the central nervous system (CNS) in high enough concentrations to treat meningitis. By contrast, the third-generation cephalosporins produce therapeutic levels in CSF when the meninges are inflammed.

Most cephalosporins are excreted unchanged into the urine by glomerular filtration and/or tubular secretion. Cephalothin, cephapirin, and cefotaxime are 20 to 30 percent metabolized, and the desacetyl metabolites are excreted into the urine. Cefoperazone and ceftriaxone are excreted chiefly into the bile in active unchanged form.

Adverse Effects

The adverse effects of cephalosporins are generally similar to those of penicillins. Allergic reactions described with penicillins may also occur with cephalosporins. Approximately 5 to 10 percent of patients allergic to penicillins will also prove allergic to cephalosporins. Cephalosporins should not be used in patients who have a history of immediate or accelerated reactions to penicillins or in patients with skin-test reactivity to antigens of penicillin metabolites (penicilloyl polylysine).

Hypoprothrombinemia may occur with cefamandole, cefoperazone, moxalactam, and cefotetan; it is related to the presence of a methylthiotetrazole side chain. Cefotetan has been less frequently associated with this complication. Moxalactam may also interfere with platelet aggregation and has been implicated more often than other cephalosporins in clinically significant bleeding. Therefore, it is not recommended for clinical use. Granulocytopenia or thrombocytopenia are rare complications of therapy with cephalosporins.

Diarrhea may occur with any of the cephalosporins, but it is more common with cefoperazone and ceftriaxone, which are predominantly excreted into the bile. *Clostridium difficile* colitis, manifested occasionally as pseudomembraneous colitis, has been reported with all cephalosporins. A disulfiram-like reaction may occur in patients who ingest alcohol while receiving moxalactam, cefoperazone, cefamandole, or cefotetan.

TABLE 42-2   **Classification and pharmacokinetic properties of cephalosporins**

Generic name	Protein binding, %	Elimination half-life, h	Elimination half-life, h, anuria
First generation			
For parenteral use			
Cefazolin	80	1.6	24
Cephalothin	60	0.6	3
Cephapirin	60	0.6	2
Cephradine	15	1.0	15
For oral use			
Cephalexin	15	1.0	20
Cefadroxil	20	1.5	20
Cephradine	15	1.0	15
Second generation			
For parenteral use			
Cefuroxime	50	1.5	21
Cefamandole	70	0.6	11
Cefonicid	95	4.5	65
Ceforanide	80	3.0	15
Cefoxitin	60	0.9	15
Cefotetan	88	3.5	35
For oral use			
Cefaclor	50	0.7	3
Cefuroxime axetil	50	1.5	21
Third generation			
For parenteral use			
Cefotaxime	30	1.0	2.6
Ceftizoxime	30	1.7	20
Cefoperazone	90	2.0	2.2
Ceftriaxone	90	8.0	12
Ceftazidime	15	1.8	24
Moxalactam	50	2.2	20

Beta-lactamase-stable cephalosporins, especially cefoxitin and the third-generation compounds, are potent inducers of chromosomally mediated beta-lactamases. A number of enteric species, notably *Enterobacter cloacae*, possess inducible beta-lactamases. Enzyme production, which is normally repressed, is markedly increased (i.e., derepressed) in the presence of the inducer. As a consequence, the organism becomes resistant to a broad range of beta-lactam antibiotics, including extended-spectrum penicillins and third-generation cephalosporins. The beta-lactamase-stable cephalosporins should be avoided in situations in which a first-generation cephalosporin would provide effective therapy or prophylaxis.

Superinfection with resistant organisms may occur during therapy with third-generation cephalosporins. These include enterococci, *Acinetobacter*, *Pseudomonas*, *Enterobacter*, and *Candida* species.

First-Generation Cephalosporins

Currently available first-generation cephalosporins for parenteral use include cefazolin, cephalothin, cephapirin, and cephradine (Fig. 42-4). The last agent is also available for oral administration. Cephalexin and cefadroxil are available only for oral use.

Antimicrobial Spectrum   The activity of the first-generation cephalosporins against gram-positive bacteria is almost identical to that of penicillinase-resistant penicillins. These agents are active against *Staph. aureus* and coagulase-negative staphylococci including strains that produce penicillinase. Methicillin-resistant strains, however, are uniformly resistant. The first-generation cephalosporins are active against nonenterococcal *Streptococcus* species including pneumococcus. They are, however, less potent than penicillin G against these organisms. *Enterococcus* species and *L. monocytogenes* are uniformly resistant to all cephalosporins.

The first-generation cephalosporins have a narrow spectrum of activity against gram-negative organisms. Most strains of *E. coli, Klebsiella, P. mirabilis,* and *Citrobacter diversus* are susceptible. Other gram-negative species, including *H. influenzae*, are resistant. These agents do not have clinically useful activity against gonococci and meningococci.

The first-generation cephalosporins are active against anaerobic bacteria with the exception of *B. fragilis*. Their activity against these organisms, however, is inferior to that of penicillin G.

Although the first-generation cephalosporins have identical antimicrobial spectra, these are some differences in their in vitro potencies. Cefazolin, cephalothin, and cephapirin are virtually identical, whereas cephradine, cephalexin, and cefadroxil are two- to fourfold less potent against most bacterial species. The in vitro potencies of the latter three agents are comparable.

Pharmacokinetics   Cephalexin, cephradine, and cefadroxil are almost completely absorbed after oral administration. Food delays absorption, resulting in lower peaks and more prolonged levels. All these agents are excreted into the urine in active unchanged form. Cefadroxil is eliminated more slowly than others; it can therefore be administered at less frequent intervals.

The pharmacokinetics of cephalothin and cephapirin are similar. Approximately 70 percent of the administered dose is excreted unchanged into the urine. The remainder is metabolized to desacetyl derivatives.

Because of metabolism, the half-lives of these agents are only modestly increased in anuric patients. Cefazolin and cephradine are excreted totally by the kidneys in active unchanged form. Their elimination half-lives (1.6 and 1.0 h, respectively) are longer than the elimination half-life of cephalothin or cephapirin (0.6 h) and increase substantially in anuric patients.

Clinical Use   The first-generation cephalosporins are alternatives to penicillins for treating staphylococcal and nonenterococcal streptococcal infections in patients who cannot tolerate penicillins. They are also effective in infections caused by susceptible strains of *E. coli, Klebsiella,* or *P. mirabilis.* Cefazolin is usually the preferred first-generation cephalosporin because it can be administered less frequently and it is relatively well tolerated after intramuscular injection.

The first-generation cephalosporins, especially cefazolin, are widely used for porphylaxis in cardiovascular, orthopedic, biliary, pelvic, and gastric surgeries. In this regard, they are preferable to second-generation cephalosporins because they are effective, they cost less, and they have a narrower spectrum.

Second-Generation Cephalosporins

The currently available second-generation cephalosporins for parenteral use include cefuroxime, cefamandole, cefonicid, ceforanide, cefoxitin, and cefotetan (Fig. 42-4). The latter two agents are 7-α-methoxy cephalosporins and, strictly speaking, cephamycins. Cefaclor and cefuroxime axetil are the second-generation cephalosporins available for oral administration.

Antimicrobial Spectrum   The gram-positive spectrum of second-generation cephalosporins is similar to that of first-generation compounds; it includes *Staphylococcus* species and nonenterococcal *Streptococcus* species. Against these organisms, the activities of cefuroxime and cefamandole are comparable to the activity of cefazolin, but other second-generation cephalosporins are significantly less active.

The second-generation cephalosporins are active against *N. meningitidis, N. gonorrhoeae,* and *Branhamella catarrhalis*, including strains that produce beta-lactamase. Cefuroxime is the most active member of the group against these organisms, whereas ceforanide has the least activity.

Cefuroxime and cefonicid are highly active against *H. influenzae*, including strains that produce beta-lactamase. Cefoxitin, cefotetan, and ceforanide are significantly less active. Cefamandole is relatively inactive against beta-lactamase-producing strains. The major difference between cefaclor and the oral first-generation cephalosporins is that cefaclor is active against *H. influenzae*, including strains that produce beta-lactamase.

The second-generation cephalosporins are more potent than first-generation agents against gram-negative species that are sensitive to the latter (i.e., *E. coli*, *Klebsiella*, and *P. mirabilis*). A variable percentage of strains of *Proteus vulgaris*, *Morganella morganii*, *Providencia*, and *Enterobacter* species are also susceptible to the second-generation cephalosporins. There are differences in the susceptibility of these organisms to the individual compounds, however; cefotetan is generally more active than others against these species.

Cefoxitin and cefotetan are the most active cephalosporins against anaerobes, especially *B. fragilis*. Approximately 80 to 90 percent of strains of *B. fragilis* are susceptible. The activities of other second-generation cephalosporins against anaerobic bacteria are comparable to those of the first-generation agents.

Pharmacokinetics Cefaclor is rapidly absorbed after oral administration; food intake significantly reduces its absorption. Cefuroxime axetil, an ester of cefuroxime, does not have antimicrobial activity. It is a prodrug that is rapidly hydrolyzed to cefuroxime after absorption.

Except for cefaclor, which undergoes some metabolism, all second-generation cephalosporins are excreted unchanged in the urine. There are significant differences in the rate of elimination of these agents. Cefamandole and cefoxitin are excreted rapidly with elimination half-lives of 0.6 and 0.9 h, respectively. Cefuroxime has an intermediate half-life (1.5 h), whereas ceforanide, cefotetan, and cefonicid have relatively long half-lives (3.0, 3.5, and 4.5 h, respectively), allowing less frequent administrations.

Among the second-generation cephalosporins, only cefuroxime penetrates into the CSF in concentrations adequate to treat meningitis.

Clinical Use Cefuroxime is commonly used for the treatment of community-acquired pneumonia. The potential pathogens, including pneumococcus and

H. influenzae, are all sensitive to the drug. Cefuroxime is an effective agent for the empiric therapy of bacterial meningitis in children.

Cefoxitin and cefotetan are valuable for treatment of mixed aerobic-anaerobic infections, including intra-abdominal infections, pelvic infections, nosocomial aspiration pneumonia, and foot infections in patients with diabetes. Cefonicid, because of its long half-life, is used in a once-daily regimen to treat a variety of mild to moderate infections. With the availability of cefuroxime and cefonicid, which possess distinct advantages over cefamandole and ceforanide, respectively, in terms of both pharmacokinetics and antimicrobial activity, the clinical use of the latter compounds is uncertain.

Third-Generation Cephalosporins

Currently available third-generation cephalosporins include cefotaxime, ceftizoxime, ceftriaxone, cefoperazone, ceftazidime, and moxalactam (Fig. 42-4). All are available for parenteral use only. Moxalactam is an oxa-beta-lactam agent, not a true cephalosporin, since it has an oxygen atom rather than a sulfur atom in the six-membered ring. However, its antimicrobial spectrum and pharmacokinetic properties are similar to those of third-generation cephalosporins.

The third-generation cephalosporins differ from each other primarily in pharmacokinetic properties. There are also some differences in their antimicrobial activity, especially with respect to *Ps. aeruginosa* and *Staph. aureus*.

Antimicrobial Spectrum Cefotaxime and ceftizoxime are active but approximately fourfold less potent than the first-generation cephalosporins against *Staph. aureus*. Ceftriaxone and cefoperazone are slightly less active. Ceftazidime and moxalactam have poor antistaphylococcal activity. The third-generation cephalosporins, except for moxalactam, are approximately as potent against nonenterococcal *Streptococcus* species as are the first-generation compounds.

The third-generation cephalosporins are highly active against *N. meningitidis*, *N. gonorrhoeae*, *Branhamella catarrhalis*, and *H. influenzae*, including strains that produce beta-lactamase. Ceftriaxone is the most active agent against *N. gonorrhoeae*.

Because of resistance to beta-lactamases, the third-generation cephalosporins provide a potent broad spectrum of activity against aerobic gram-negative bacteria that is markedly greater than that provided by the second-generation compounds. Most gram-negative species, including *E. coli*, *Klebsiella*, *Proteus*, *Providencia*, *Morganella morganii*, *Serratia marcescens*, and *Citrobacter*, are highly susceptible to these agents. Strains of *Enterobacter* show variable sensitivity. With the exception of cefoperazone, which is slightly less active in vitro, other third-generation agents have comparable activity against these organisms.

Ceftazidime is the most active third-generation cephalosporin against *Ps. aeruginosa*. Cefoperazone exhibits moderate activity against this organism; other third-generation compounds do not have significant anti-pseudomonal activity. *Pseudomonas maltophila*, *Pseudomonas cepacia*, and *Acinetobacter* species are resistant to the third-generation cephalosporins.

The third-generation cephalosporins are active against anaerobes; however, 20 to 60 percent of the strains of *B. fragilis* are resistant. Ceftizoxime and moxalactam are more active than others against this organism.

Pharmacokinetics The third-generation cephalosporins penetrate well into the CNS. The CSF concentrations in patients with meningitis are in the therapeutic range for susceptible organisms.

Ceftizoxime, ceftazidime, and moxalactam are excreted almost entirely by the kidneys in active unchanged form. Therefore, significant adjustments in dosage are required in patients with renal failure. Metabolism and biliary excretion play important roles in the elimination of other third-generation agents. Twenty to thirty percent of administered cefotaxime is metabolized to a desacetyl derivative that has antimicrobial activity; the remainder is excreted unchanged in the urine. Approximately 40 percent of ceftriaxone and 70 percent of cefoperazone administered parenterally are excreted into the bile in active unchanged form. Neither of these two agents requires dosage adjustment in patients with renal failure.

The elimination half-lives of the third-generation cephalosporins vary widely. Cefotaxime has a relatively short half-life (1.0 h), whereas ceftriaxone has a long half-life (8.0 h), allowing once-a-day administration. Ceftizoxime, ceftazidime, cefoperazone, and moxalactam have intermediate half-lives, ranging from 1.7 to 2.2 h (Table 42.2).

Clinical Use Infections caused by multiply resistant gram-negative bacilli are the main indication for the use of third-generation cephalosporins. For infections involving *Ps. aeruginosa*, ceftazidime is the third-generation agent of choice.

The third-generation cephalosporins are useful agents for the treatment of meningitis caused by susceptible bacteria. Ceftriaxone (or cefotaxime) is now considered the drug of choice for empiric therapy of bacterial meningitis in children and for *H. influenzae* meningitis. A combination of ceftriaxone and ampicillin is as effective as the conventional ampicillin-gentamicin regimen in neonatal meningitis. The third-generation cephalosporins are also the drug of choice for gram-negative bacillary meningitis.

Ceftazidime is effective monotherapy for the empiric treatment of febrile neutropenic patients. Because of increasing prevalence of penicillin-resistant *N. gonorrhoeae*, ceftriaxone has become the drug of choice for gonorrhea in most parts of the United States.

CARBAPENEMS

The term carbapenem denotes similarity with the 4:5 fused ring structure of penicillins, the substitution of carbon for sulfur, and the presence of unsaturation in the five-membered ring. Imipenem (*N*-formimidoyl thienamycin) is the only carbapenem currently available for clinical use. It is derived from thienamycin, which was isolated form *Streptomyces cattleya*.

In contrast with penicillins and cephalosporins, which have an acyl amino side chain attached to the beta-lactam ring, imipenem has a hydroxyethyl side chain. Marked resistance to hydrolysis by beta-lactamases is provided by the trans configuration of the side chain which contrasts with the cis configuration of the penicillins and cephalosporins.

Imipenem binds primarily to PBP-2 and PBP-1b. Its high affinity for PBP-2 contrasts with other beta-lactam antibiotics. Bacteria exposed to imipenem assume a spherical shape which is rapidly followed by lysis.

Imipenem is a potent inducer of chromosomally mediated beta-lactamases that can cleave other beta-lactam antibiotics. The organisms, however, remain susceptible to imipenem owing to the drug's exceptional resistance to beta-lactamases.

Imipenem

Cilastatin

Imipenem undergoes enzymatic inactivation in the kidneys resulting in low and variable urinary concentrations of the active antibiotic. To overcome this problem and make the drug useful for urinary tract infections, it is combined with cilastatin, a compound that inhibits renal metabolism of the drug. Imipenem is available only in a fixed 1:1 combination with cilastatin (Primaxin) for parenteral use.

Antimicrobial Spectrum Imipenem is highly active against *Staph. aureus* and coagulase-negative staphylococci. Its level of activity against *Staph. aureus* is superior to that displayed by penicillinase-resistant penicillins. Many strains of methicillin-resistant *Staph. aureus* and methicillin-resistant coagulase-negative staphylococci are resistant to imipenem.

Imipenem is highly active against nonenterococcal *Streptococcus* species. Enterococci exhibit variable susceptibility, depending on the species. *Enterococcus faecalis* is usually sensitive, whereas *Enterococcus faecium* is commonly resistant. Like penicillin G and ampicillin, the susceptible enterococci exhibit tolerance to the bactericidal action of imipenem. The combination of imipenem and aminoglycosides has synergistic activity against these organisms. Imipenem is active against *L. monocytogenes* and *Nocardia* species; diphtheroids are usually resistant.

Imipenem is highly active against *N. meningitidis*, *N. gonorrhoeae* (including strains that produce beta-lactamase), and *H. influenzae*. Gram-negative enteric species are generally susceptible to imipenem, although occasional resistant strains are encountered. With few exceptions, the level of activity of imipenem against these organisms is comparable to that of third-generation cephalosporins. The third-generation cephalosporins are substantially more active than imipenem against *Proteus*, *Providencia*, and *Morganella*. However, *Enterobacter* strains are more frequently sensitive to imipenem. In contrast to cephalosporins, imipenem is highly active against *Acinetobacter* species. Since imipenem has remarkable stability to beta-

lactamase attack, there is little cross-resistance between penicillins or cephalosporins and imipenem.

One important feature of imipenem is its activity against *Ps. aeruginosa*. Its level of activity against this organism is comparable to ceftazidime. *Ps. maltophila* and *Ps. cepacia* are usually resistant to imipenem.

Imipenem is highly active against anaerobes, including *B. fragilis*. It is the most potent beta-lactam antibiotic against *B. fragilis* and other penicillin G-resistant anaerobes. Occasional strains of *Fusobacterium* are resistant to imipenem.

Pharmacokinetics Imipenem is only 20 percent bound to serum proteins. It penetrates into all body tissues and fluids, including CSF, if the meninges are inflamed.

Approximately 75 percent of administered imipenem is excreted unchanged by the kidneys via glomerular filtration and tubular secretion. A renal dipeptidase enzyme (dehydropeptidase I), located in the luminal brush border of the proximal tubular epithelium, inactivates the drug after it is cleared from the plasma. Cilastatin, a competitive inhibitor of this enzyme, protects imipenem from renal degradation, thereby assuring high levels of unchanged antibiotic in the urine. Cilastatin is devoid of antimicrobial activity and does not affect the activity of imipenem. Approximately 25 percent of administered imipenem is metabolized outside the kidneys.

The elimination half-lives of both imipenem and cilastatin are 1.0 h. In anuric patients, the half-life of imipenem increases to 3.0 h and that of cilastatin to 13 h.

Clinical Use Infections caused by multiply resistant gram-negative species (mostly nosocomial) and mixed infections involving *Staph. aureus*, gram-negative bacilli, and anaerobes are the main indications for imipenem. Because of its potent activity against anaerobes, imipenem is effective monotherapy for intra-abdominal infections. Similar to ceftazidime, imipenem is effective monotherapy for the empiric treatment of febrile neutropenic patients. For *Ps. aeruginosa* infections, imipenem should be used in combination with an aminoglycoside in order to reduce the development of resistance.

Adverse Effects Allergic reactions described with penicillins may occur with imipenem. Cross-allergy with other beta-lactam antibiotics may occur, and imipenem should not be used in patients who have a history of Ig E-mediated reactions to penicillins or cephalosporins.

Nausea and vomiting occur more commonly with imipenem than with other parenteral beta-lactam antibiotics. Seizures have been reported in 1.5 percent of patients receiving imipenem. These generally occur in the elderly and in patients with predisposing factors such as head trauma, antecedent CNS disorder, and renal functional impairment. Superinfection with resistant organisms (mainly *Candida* and resistant *Pseudomonas* species) may occur during therapy with imipenem.

MONOBACTAMS

Aztreonam is the first monocyclic beta-lactam, known as *monobactam*, to be available for parenteral use. It is a totally synthetic compound. The alpha-methyl group at position 4 enhances the stability of the ring to beta-lactamase attack. The amino acyl side chain, identical to that of ceftazidime, is responsible for the potent activity of the drug against aerobic gram-negative bacteria. Aztreonam binds primarily to PBP-3, resulting in the formation of filaments and ultimately lysis of bacteria.

Aztreonam

Aztreonam is highly resistant to hydrolysis by most bacterial beta-lactamases. Despite this stability, it does not induce the production of chromosomally mediated beta-lactamases, as do the cephalosporins and imipenem.

Antimicrobial Spectrum Aztreonam has no activity against gram-positive organisms and anaerobes. Its antimicrobial spectrum is limited to aerobic gram-negative species.

Aztreonam is active against *N. meningitidis*, *N. gonorrhoeae*, *H. influenzae*, and enteric gram-negative species, including *E. coli*, *Klebsiella*, *Proteus*, *Morganella*, *Providencia*, *Serratia marcescens*, *Enterobacter*, and *Citrobacter*. Its potency against these organisms is comparable to that of third-generation cephalosporins. Aztreonam is active against *Ps. aeruginosa*, but its potency against this organism is less than that of ceftazidime. In vitro synergy with aminoglycosides occurs in 30 to 60 percent of susceptible strains. *Acinetobacter*, *Ps. maltophila*, and *Ps. cepacia* are usually resistant to aztreonam.

Pharmacokinetics Aztreonam is not absorbed after oral administration. It is 55 percent bound to serum proteins and penetrates into all body tissues and fluids, including CSF if the meninges are inflamed.

Approximately 70 percent of administered aztreonam is excreted unchanged by the kidneys via glomerular filteration and tubular secretion. A small fraction is excreted unchanged into the bile, and 25 to 30 percent is inactivated in the body. The elimination half-life of aztreonam, which is 1.7 h with normal renal function, increases to 6.0 h in anuric patients.

Clinical Use Aztreonam is a useful agent for infections caused by aerobic gram-negative bacilli. In patients with documented or suspected mixed infections, it should be used in combination with other agents such as clindamycin, metronidazole, nafcillin, or vancomycin. Aztreonam has a very similar antimicrobial spectrum to aminoglycoside and is a potential substitute for these agents in most instances.

Adverse Effects Allergic skin reactions occur in 1.5 percent of patients treated with aztreonam. There is very little cross-reactivity between aztreonam and other beta-lactam antibiotics; therefore, it can be used in patients allergic to penicillins or cephalosporins. Diarrhea occurs infrequently, and *Clostridium difficile* colitis is less commonly reported with aztreonam than with other beta-lactam antibiotics.

BIBLIOGRAPHY

Adkinson, N. F., Jr., A. Saxon, M. R. Spence, and E. A. Swabb: "Cross Allergenicity and Immunogenicity of Aztreonam," *Rev. Infect. Dis.*, 7 (**Suppl. 4**):S613–S621 (1985).

Barriere, S. L., and J. F. Flaherty: "Third-Generation Cephalosporins: A Critical Evaluation," *Clin. Pharmacy*, 3:351–373 (1984).

Barza, M: "Imipenem: First of a New Class of Beta-Lactam Antibiotics," 103:552–560 (1985).

Bauernfeind, A: "Classification of Beta-Lactamases," *Rev. Infect. Dis.*, 8 (**Suppl. 3**):S470–S481 (1986).

Beam, T. R., Jr.: "Ceftriaxone: A Beta-Lactamase-Stable, Broad-Spectrum Cephalosporin with an Extended Half-Life," *Pharmacotherapy*, 5:237–253 (1985).

Childs, S. J., and G. P. Bodey: "Aztreonam," *Pharmacotherapy*, 6:138–152 (1986).

Creeland, R, and E. Squires: "Antimicrobial Activity of Ceftriaxone: A Review," *Am. J. Med.*, 77 (**Suppl. 4C**):3–11 (1984).

Donowtiz, G. R., and G. L. Mandell: "Beta-Lactam Antibiotics," *N. Engl. J. Med.*, 318:419–426, 490–500 (1988).

Drusano, G. L., S. G. Schimpff, and W. L. Hewitt: "The Acylampicillins: Mezlocillin, Piperacillin, and Azlocillin," *Rev. Infect. Dis.*, 6:13–32 (1984).

Eliopoulos, G. M., and R. C. Moellering, Jr.: "Azlocillin, Mezlocillin, and Piperacillin: New Broad-Spectrum Penicillins," *Ann. Intern. Med.*, 97:755–760 (1982).

Gentry, L. O.: "Antimicrobial Activity, Pharmacokinetics, Therapeutic Indications and Adverse Reactions of Ceftazidime," *Pharmacotherapy*, 5:254–267 (1985).

Greenwood, D: "An Overview of the Response of Bacteria to Beta-Lactam Antibiotics," *Rev. Infect. Dis.*, 8 (**Suppl. 5**):S487–S495 (1986).

Kropp, H, L Gercken, J. G. Sundelof, and F. M. Kahan: "Antibacterial Activity of Imipenem: The First Thienamycin Antibiotic," *Rev. Infect. Dis.*, 7 (**Suppl. 3**):S389–S410 (1985).

Kucers, A, and N. M. Bennett: *The Use of Antibiotics*, J. B. Lippincott, Philadelphia; 1987, pp. 3–584.

LeFrock, J. L., R. A. Prince, and R. D. Leff: "Mechanism of Action, Antimicrobial Activity, Pharmacology, Adverse Effects, and Clinical Efficacy of Cefotaxime," *Pharmacotherapy*, 2:174–183 (1982).

McCloskey, R. V., J. L. LeFrock, B. R. Smith, and G. R. Aronoff: "Microbiology, Pharmacology, and Clinical Use of Mezlocillin Sodium," *Pharmacotherapy*, 2:300–310 (1982).

Molavi, A, and J. L. LeFrock: "Antistaphylococcal Penicillins," in B. A. Cunha and A. M. Ristuccia (eds.), *Antimicrobial Therapy*, Raven Press, New York, 1984, pp. 183–195.

Neu, H. C.: "Ceftizoxime: A Beta-Lactamase-Stable, Broad-Spectrum Cephalosporin. Pharmacokinetics, Adverse Effects and Clinical Use," *Pharmacotherapy*, 4:47–58 (1984).

Neu, H. C.: "Contribution of Beta-Lactamases to Bacterial Resistance and Mechanisms to Inhibit Beta-Lactamases," *Am. J. Med.*, 79 (**Suppl. 5B**):2–12 (1985).

Neu, H. C.: "Beta-Lactam Antibiotics: Structural Relationships Affecting in Vitro Activity and Pharmacologic Properties," *Rev. Infect. Dis.*, 8 (**Suppl. 3**):S237–S259 (1986).

Neu, H. C.: "Aztreonam: The First Monobactam," *Med. Clin. North Am.*, 72:555–566 (1988).

Patel, I. H., and S. A. Kaplan: "Pharmacokinetic Profile of Ceftriaxone in Man," *Am. J. Med.*, 77 (**Suppl. 4C**):17–25 (1984).

Sher, TH: "Penicilin Hypersensitivity—A Review," *Pediat. Clin. North Am.*, 30:161–176 (1983).

Sutherland, R., A. S. Beale, R. J. Boon, K. E. Griffin, et al.: "Antibacterial Activity of Ticarcillin in the Presence of Clavulanate Potassium," *Am. J. Med.*, 79 (**Suppl. 53**):13–24 (1985).

Swabb, E. A.: "Review of the Clinical Pharmacology of the Monobactam Antibiotic Aztreonam," *Am. J. Med.*, 78 (**Suppl. 2A**):11–18 (1985).

Sykes, R. B., and D. R. Bonner: "Discovery and Development of the Monobactams," *Rev. Infect. Dis.*, 7 (**Suppl. 4**):S579–S593 (1985).

Tomasz, A: "Penicillin-Binding Proteins and the Antibacterial Effectiveness of Beta-Lactam Antibiotics," *Rev. Infect. Dis.*, 8 (**Suppl. 3**):S260–S278 (1986).

Antimicrobials II: Erythromycin, Clindamycin, Vancomycin, Metronidazole, Aminoglycosides, Quinolones, Chloramphenicol, and Tetracyclines

Abdolghader Molavi

The antimicrobials discussed in this chapter include some which are sometimes called *broad spectrum*. This designation may be misleading, since all antimicrobials have limitations to their antimicrobial spectra. Even an agent with a spectrum as broad as that of chloramphenicol is often ineffective against *Enterobacter, Proteus vulgaris, Pseudomonas,* and some strains of *Staphylococcus aureus.*

These antimicrobials may be grouped into the following categories: (1) agents used primarily in the therapy of infections caused by gram-positive bacteria (erythromycin and vancomycin); (2) agents used primarily in the treatment of infections caused by anaerobes (clindamycin and metronidazole); (3) agents used primarily in the treatment of infections caused by gram-negative bacteria (aminoglycosides and quinolones); and (4) broad-spectrum antimicrobials (chloramphenicol and tetracyclines).

AGENTS USED PRIMARILY AGAINST GRAM-POSITIVE ORGANISMS

Erythromycin

Erythromycin was isolated in 1952 from a strain of *Streptomyces erythreus.* It belongs to a group of antibiotics known as *macrolides,* so named because they con-

tain a macrocyclic lactone ring (14-membered in erythromycin) to which one or more deoxy sugars are attached.

Mechanism of Action Erythromycin and most other antibiotics discussed in this chapter inhibit bacterial protein synthesis. The basic mechanisms of protein synthesis in bacteria and in man are similar. There are, however, sufficient differences to allow certain antibiotics to be selectively toxic to bacteria.

The initial step in protein synthesis is the transcription of the genetic code from the DNA onto the messenger RNA (mRNA), a process catalyzed by DNA-dependent RNA polymerase (transcriptase). The sequence of nucleotides in mRNA reflects the nucleotide order in DNA and thus contains the information determining the sequence in which amino acids will be joined to form a specific protein.

Protein synthesis occurs on the ribosomes, which can be considered as the "workbench" upon which various amino acids are joined to form polypeptide chains. Bacteria contain 70-S ribosomes which are made of two unequal portions: a larger 50-S subunit and a smaller 30-S subunit. The two subunits have different functions. Messenger RNA binds to the 30-S subunit, while the 50-S subunit is a site for the attachment of amino acids and a site for holding the growing peptide chains. These sites, known as the acceptor (A) site and the donor (P) site, respectively, are in close proximity to each other.

Amino acids are brought to the ribosome-mRNA complex by transfer RNA (tRNA). For each amino acid to be incorporated into a protein molecule, there is a specific tRNA. Each tRNA is also specific for one nucleotide sequence (nucleotide triplet or codon) in the mRNA. The tRNA is thus a two-ended molecule in which one end is specific for an amino acid and the other end specific for a region of three nucleotides in the mRNA. The aminoacyl-tRNA binds to the A site on the 50-S subunit.

Growth of peptide chains is achieved by the transfer and binding of a peptide chain from the P site onto the amino acid at the A site, a process catalyzed by peptidyl transferase. After the formation of the peptide bond, a complicated "translocation" takes place. The tRNA with the newly elongated peptide chain moves from the A site to the P site, and the 30-S subunit moves one codon along the mRNA. The A site is now unoccupied and ready to receive another aminoacyl-tRNA directed by the next code triplet on the mRNA. The process of elongation continues until the protein chain is complete.

Erythromycin inhibits protein synthesis by binding in a reversible manner to the 50-S ribosomal subunit and interferes with the translocation. Erythromycin binds to and blocks the P site, thereby preventing the proper association of the peptidyl-tRNA with its binding site after formation of the peptide bond.

Erythromycin is classified as a bacteriostatic antibiotic. It may, however, have a bactericidal action against some microbial species at achievable serum concentrations.

Antimicrobial Spectrum

Gram-Positive Aerobic Bacteria Erythromycin is highly active against nonenterococcal *Streptococcus* species (including groups A, B, C, and G streptococci, *Strep. viridans*, and *Strep. pneumoniae*), although occasional resistant clinical isolates are encountered. Enterococci (*Enterococcus faecalis* and *Enterococcus faecium*) are usually resistant. Most clinical isolates of *Staph. aureus* are sensitive to erythromycin, but resistant strains are encountered, particularly in hospitals (7 to 14 percent of isolates). Coagulase-negative staphylococci are frequently resistant. A majority of strains of *Corynebacterium diphtheriae*, *Bacillus anthracis*, and *Listeria monocytogenes* are sensitive to erythromycin.

Gram-Negative Aerobic Bacteria Erythromycin is active against *Neisseria* species, *Bordetella pertussis*, *Branhamella catarrhalis*, *Legionella* species, *Campylobacter jejuni*, *Haemophilus ducreyi*, and some *Haemophilus influenzae* strains. *Enterobacteriaceae* and other gram-negative bacilli are invariably resistant.

Anaerobic Bacteria Erythromycin has a wide range of activity against gram-positive anaerobic bacteria, including *Peptococcus*, *Peptostreptococcus*, *Clostridium*, *Propionibacterium*, and *Actinomyces*. Its activity against gram-negative anaerobes is variable. *Bacteroides fragilis* group and *Fusobacterium* species are usually resistant, but other *Bacteroides* species are susceptible.

Other Organisms Erythromycin is active against *Mycoplasma pneumoniae*, *Ureaplasma urealyticum*, *Chlamydia trachomatis*, *Rickettsia*, *Treponema pallidum*, and some atypical myobacteria.

Mechanisms of Resistance Bacterial resistance to erythromycin may be due to one of the following mechanisms: (1) Inability to penetrate through the cell envelope. This is responsible for the resistance of organisms, such as *Enterobacteriaceae*, which are innately resistant to erythromycin. (2) Methylation of adenine in the 23-S ribosomal RNA of the 50-S subunit, resulting in decreased binding affinity of erythromycin for its target. This is mediated by a plasmid that contains the gene for the methylating enzyme and is the usual mechanism of resistance in gram-positive species. The resistance may be constitutive or inducible by subinhibitory concentrations of erythromycin.

Pharmacokinetics Erythromycin base is very bitter, insoluble in water, and inactivated by gastric acid. To improve absorption, the preparations of erythromycin base are made with an acid-resistant coating, which delays drug dissolution until it reaches the small bowel (enteric-coated tablets, enteric-coated granules in capsules, "film"-coated tablets). Several salts and esters of erythromycin have also been prepared with the aims of eliminating the bitterness (important in pediatric preparations) and improving the absorption. These include erythromycin stearate (a salt), erythromycin ethyl succinate (an ester), and erythromycin estolate (lauryl sulfate salt of the propionyl ester of erythromycin). The stearate salt dissociates in the intestine, and the drug is absorbed as the base. The ester derivatives are absorbed intact and partially hydrolyzed to the free base in the blood; the esters do not have significant antibacterial activity. The serum concentrations of bioactive erythromycin after oral administration of various enteric-coated preparations, salts or esters of the drugs are approximately the same.

Erythromycin gluceptate and erythromycin lactobionate are soluble salts of erythromycin that can be administered intravenously. The serum concentrations after intravenous administration of these compounds are substantially higher than those achieved with the oral preparations.

Erythromycin is 65 percent bound to plasma proteins. It is widely distributed in the tissues (including prostate) and body fluids. It does not diffuse across the normal meninges, but low levels are detectable in the cerebrospinal fluid (CSF) when the meninges are inflamed. Erythromycin is actively concentrated intracellularly by polymorphonuclear leukocytes and alevolar macrophages.

Approximately 2.5 percent of an orally administered dose and 15 percent of a parenterally administered dose are excreted unchanged in the urine. A smaller proportion is excreted into the bile in active form. Most of the administered dose is inactivated in the body, probably in the liver.

The elimination half-life of erythromycin in persons with normal renal function is 1.4 h, increasing to about 5.0 h in anuric patients. Only minor, if any, dosage reduction is necessary in patients with end-stage renal disease. However, in patients with severe hepatic disease the drug may accumulate and dosage reduction may be necessary. Erythromycin is not removed by either peritoneal dialysis or hemodialysis.

Adverse Effects Erythromycin is one of the safest antibiotics ever developed. Allergic reactions (skin rash, fever, and eosinophilia) occur rarely. The most common adverse effect with oral therapy is epigastric pain and nausea, which may also occur with intravenous administration.

Erythromycin should not be administered intramuscularly because it causes severe local pain. Thrombophlebitis occurs relatively frequently when the drug is administered through peripheral veins.

The most serious adverse effect of erythromycin is cholestatic hepatitis, which occurs primarily with erythromycin estolate. The syndrome is probably a hypersensitivity reaction to the specific structure of the estolate compound. Since administration of erythromycin estolate does not yield higher serum levels of the bioactive erythromycin and since the estolate is almost uniquely associated with cholestatic hepatitis, its use is not recommended.

Transient hearing loss is a rare complication of therapy with erythromycin; it occurs most often in association with intravenous administration of high doses. The hearing loss disappears promptly after therapy is discontinued.

Clostridium difficile colitis is rarely associated with the use of erythromycin.

Clinical Use Erythromycin is an alternative to penicillin for the treatment of infections caused by susceptible organism. It is the drug of choice for *Mycoplasma* pneumonia, *Legionella* pneumonia, pertussis, diphtheria, chancroid, *Campylobacter* enteritis, chronic prostatitis due to *Chlamydia*, and *Chlamydia trachomatis* infections during pregnancy and childhood.

Vancomycin

Vancomycin was isolated in 1956 from *Streptomyces orientalis* (currently designated as *Nocardia orientalis*). Based on its carbohydrate and peptide content, vancomycin is classified as a glycopeptide antibiotic. It has a molecular weight of 1449, considerably higher than that of any other antibiotic.

When vancomycin was first introduced for clinical use, the commercial preparations contained more than 20 percent impurities. Current formulations contain less than 10 percent impurities and are associated with a significantly reduced adverse effects.

Mechanism of Action   Vancomycin is a bactericidal agent which inhibits cell wall synthesis. In contrast to beta-lactam antibiotics, which inhibit the third stage of peptidoglycan synthesis, vancomycin interferes with the second stage. It inhibits the reaction in which the repeating unit of the cell wall is separated from the cytoplasmic membrane-bound phospholipid and linked to the preexisting peptidoglycan. As with beta-lactam antibiotics, autolysins mediate the lethal action of vancomycin after inhibition of peptidoglycan synthesis.

Antimicrobial Spectrum   Virtually all gram-positive bacteria are sensitive to vancomycin; however, the drug has no significant activity against gram-negative organisms.

Vancomycin is active against both methicillin-susceptible and methicillin-resistant strains of *Staph. aureus* and coagulase-negative *Staphylococcus* species; resistance in these organisms is extremely rare. Some strains are deficient in autolysins and exhibit tolerance to the bactericidal action of vancomycin. All *Streptococcus* species (including groups A, B, C, and G streptococci, *Strep. viridans*, and *Strep. pneumoniae*) are sensitive to vancomycin; occasional strains are tolerant. Vancomycin has marked inhibitory activity against *Enterococcus* species, but it is usually not bactericidal in concentrations which are attained clinically. A synergistic bactericidal effect is obtained when vancomycin is combined with an aminoglycoside. Diphtheroids, *Bacillus anthracis*, and *Listeria monocytogenes* are sensitive to vancomycin.

Anaerobic gram-positive bacteria including *Peptococcus*, *Peptostreptococcus*, *Clostridium* species (including *C. difficile*), and *Actinomyces* are sensitive to vancomycin. *Bacteroides fragilis* and a significant proportion of other *Bacteroides* and *Fusobacterium* strains are resistant.

Mechanisms of Resistance   Resistance of gram-negative organisms to vancomycin is due to the permeability barrier provided by the outer membrane. Resistance among gram-positive species is rare and probably due to altered target site. There is no cross-resistance between vancomycin and other antibiotics.

Pharmacokinetics   Vancomycin is absorbed poorly from the gastrointestinal tract. Intramuscular injections are very painful, so it is administered intravenously.

Vancomycin is 55 percent bound to plasma proteins. It diffuses readily into most body fluids and tissues. Penetration into the CSF is poor when the meninges are intact. With meningeal inflammation, CSF concentrations of 4 to 10 percent of the concurrent serum levels are attained. Biliary concentrations are generally low and in the subtherapeutic range.

Virtually all of the administered vancomycin is excreted unchanged by the kidneys, primarily by glomerular filtration. The elimination half-life of vancomycin in persons with normal renal function is 7 to 8 h; in functionally anephric patients it is extended to several days. There is great variability in the half-life values in patients with impaired renal function; hence maintenance doses of the drug should be guided by serum levels. Vancomycin is not cleared by either peritoneal dialysis or hemodialysis.

Adverse Effects   With the purified preparations now available, adverse reactions are less frequent than when vancomycin was first introduced. Allergic reactions are uncommon. Phlebitis at the site of the infusion may occur if the drug is administered through a peripheral vein.

Rapid intravenous infusion of vancomycin may cause tingling, erythema, or flushing of the face, neck, and thorax, occasionally associated with hypotension. This reaction (the "red-neck syndrome") occurs during or shortly after administration of the drug and appears to be due to histamine release. It is recommended that vancomycin be administered by slow intravenous infusion over a period of 60 min.

The most important, though infrequent, adverse effect of vancomycin is ototoxicity. Tinnitus and dizziness may occur and are usually reversible. High-frequency hearing loss or deafness may also result, which is often irreversible. Ototoxicity is more frequent in the elderly and in patients with impaired renal function; it correlates with high serum concentrations. Vancomycin levels should be monitored during therapy particularly in the elderly and those with diminished renal function.

Nephrotoxicity was relatively common with early impure preparations of vancomycin and was usually reversible. With current preparations, nephrotoxicity is uncommon. Renal function should be monitored during therapy with vancomycin.

Clinical Use   Vancomycin is the drug of choice for (1) infections caused by methicillin-resistant strains of *Staph. aureus, Staph. epidermidis* and other coagulase-negative staphylococci, (2) endocarditis caused by *Staphylococcus* species or streptococci in patients allergic to penicillins and cephalosporins, (3) enterococcal infections in penicillin-allergic patients, (4) diphtheroid infections, and (5) seriously ill patients with *Clostridium difficile* colitis (administered orally).

In patients with end-stage renal disease vancomycin is given once every 5 to 7 days and is often the preferred agent for the treatment of infections caused by susceptible bacteria.

AGENTS USED PRIMARILY AGAINST ANAEROBES

Clindamycin

Lincomycin, the first lincosamide available for clinical use, was isolated in 1962 from *Streptomyces linconensis*. Clindamycin is the 7(*S*)-chloro-7-deoxy derivative of lincomycin. It is superior to the parent compound in all desirable properties, including gastrointestinal absorption, antibacterial activity, and antimicrobial spectrum.

Clindamycin

Mechanism of Action   Clindamycin binds to the 50-S ribosomal subunits of bacteria and inhibits protein synthesis. The presence of clindamycin on the ribosome inhibits the peptidyl transferase reaction by interfering primarily with the binding of the aminoacyl-tRNA to the A site.

Clindamycin is a bacteriostatic antibiotic. It may, however, have bactericidal action against some bacteria at achievable serum concentrations.

Antimicrobial Spectrum

Aerobic Bacteria   Clindamycin is active against non-enterococcal *Streptococcus* species, including groups A, B, C, and G streptococci, *Strep. viridans*, and *Strep. pneumoniae*; however, enterococci are invariably resistant. Most strains of *Staph. aureus* are sensitive to clindamycin; methicillin-resistant isolates are frequently resistant. The in vitro potency of clindamycin against *Staph. aureus* is comparable to that of erythromycin. The activity of clindamycin against coagulase-negative staphylococci is variable; up to 60 percent of strains may be resistant. *Corynebacterium diphtheriae* and *bacillus anthracis* are sensitive to clindamycin.

Practically all the aerobic gram-negative bacilli are resistant to clindamycin. Unlike erythromycin, clindamycin is not active against *Mycoplasma pneumonia*.

Anaerobic Bacteria   Clindamycin is highly active against anaerobes. *Peptococcus, Peptostreptococcus, Actinomyces, Propionibacterium*, and *Clostridium perfringens* are usually sensitive. Approximately 10 percent of *Peptococcus* strains and 10 to 20 percent of clostridial strains other than *C. perfringens* are resistant to clindamycin.

Bacteroides species, including *B. fragilis*, and *Fusobacterium* species are usually sensitive to clindamycin; about 4 to 10 percent of *B. fragilis* strains are resistant.

Mechanisms of Resistance   Bacterial resistance to clindamycin may be due to (1) inability to penetrate the cell envelope (*Enterobacteriaceae*) or (2) an alteration in the ribosomal binding site. The latter is brought about by methylation of the 23-S ribosomal RNA of the 50-S ribosomal subunit and is plasmid-mediated.

Pharmacokinetics   Clindamycin hydrochloride is rapidly and virtually completely (90 percent) absorbed from the gastrointestinal tract. The presence of food in the stomach does not significantly affect absorption.

Clindamycin hydrochloride is poorly soluble in water. For children and elderly patients unable to swallow capsules, clindamycin palmitate (a water-soluble ester) is available as oral solution. This ester has no antibacterial activity but is rapidly hydrolyzed in the blood to active drug. Another water-soluble ester of clindamycin, clindamycin-2-phosphate, is available for parenteral administration. It also has no antimicrobial activity but is hydrolyzed rapidly in the blood to active parent compound.

Clindamycin is 60 percent bound to plasma proteins. It is widely distributed in the tissues and body fluids. High levels are achieved in bone and synovial fluid, but passage into the CSF is very poor even when the meninges are inflamed. Like erythromycin, clindamycin is actively transported into polymorphonuclear leukocytes and macrophages.

About 10 percent of administered clindamycin is excreted unchanged in the urine, and a fraction is eliminated unchanged into the bile. Most of the drug is metabolized, mainly in the liver, to products with variable antibacterial activity which are excreted into the urine and bile.

The elimination half-life of clindamycin in persons with normal renal function is 2.4 h, increasing to about 6.0 h in anuric patients. Dosage adjustment is usually not necessary in functionally anephretic patients if hepatic function is normal. In patients with severe hepatic disease, the elimination half-life of clindamycin is prolonged significantly and dosage adjustment is necessary. Neither hemodialysis nor peritoneal dialysis removes significant amounts of clindamycin.

Adverse Effects   The most frequent adverse effects of clindamycin are gastrointestinal reactions. Nausea, vomiting, and epigastric pain may occur with either oral or parenteral administration. Diarrhea occurs in 5 to 15 percent of patients; it is more common with oral administration. The diarrhea is occasionally due to *Clostridium difficile*, which is resistant to clindamycin and produces a toxin that causes colitis. The latter may present as pseudomembraneous colitis manifested by fever, abdominal cramps, and diarrhea, which may be bloody.

Allergic reactions, including skin rashes and fever, are rare with clindamycin. Reversible elevations of transaminases (serum glutamic oxaloacetic transaminase, SGOT; serum glutamic pyruvic transaminase, SGPT) may occur and are usually due to interference by clindamycin with the colorimetric method of enzymatic measurements. However, rare cases of hepatotoxicity have been reported.

Clinical Use   Clindamycin is used most commonly for the treatment of anaerobic infections, especially those involving *B. fragilis*, such as intra-abdominal infection and female pelvic infection. Most of these infections are polymicrobial, involving gram-negative aerobes as well as anaerobes. Therefore clindamycin is frequently administered in combination with an aminoglycoside or aztreonam. Clindamycin is a satisfactory alternative to penicillin G for the treatment of actinomycosis in penicillin-allergic patients.

Clindamycin is a useful alternative to beta-lactam antibiotics for the treatment of infections due to *Staph. aureus* or streptococci. It is particularly useful for osteomyelitis and septic arthritis because of the high concentrations which are achieved in the bone.

Metronidazole

Metronidazole is a synthetic antimicrobial agent that was initially introduced into clinical medicine in 1960 for the treatment of vaginal trichomoniasis. It is a nitroimidazole compound and has a low molecular weight (170).

Metronidazole

Mechanism of Action   Metronidazole has a bactericidal action that is specific for obligate anaerobes and occurs in the following sequence: (1) penetration into the bacterial cell, (2) reductive activation, and (3) toxic effect of the reduced intermediate product(s).

Metronidazole diffuses readily into both aerobic and anaerobic bacteria. Activation of the drug requires a reduction process that occurs only in anaerobic organisms and in facultative bacteria under anaerobic conditions. Reduction occurs at the nitro group of the drug by the low-redox-potential electron-transport proteins. This biochemical reaction decreases the concentration of unchanged metronidazole and maintains a gradient that enables more of the drug to enter the bacterium. An unstable, and as yet unidentified, intermediate product of metronidazole reduction interacts with bacterial DNA and produces cell death.

Antimicrobial Activity   Metronidazole is highly active and bactericidal against the majority of obligate anaerobes, but it has no activity against aerobic organisms.

Anaerobic Bacteria Metronidazole is highly active against *Peptococcus, Peptostreptococcus, Clostridium, Bacteroides* (including *B. fragilis*), and *Fusobacterium;* resistant strains are extremely rare. The activity of metronidazole against non-spore-forming gram-positive bacilli *(Actinomyces, Eubacterium, Bifidobacterium,* and *Propionibacterium)* is variable; 40 to 60 percent of strains are resistant.

Anaerobic Protozoa Metronidazole is highly active against anaerobic protozoa, including *Trichomonas vaginalis, Entamoeba histolytica, Giardia lamblia,* and *Balantidium coli.* Occasional strains of *T. vaginalis* may be resistant (see Chap. 46).

Mechanisms of Resistance The mechanism of metronidazole resistance is unclear. Resistant strains appear less able to reduce the drug to active intermediate compounds and, therefore, are less likely to accumulate the drug within the cell.

Pharmacokinetics Metronidazole is well absorbed (85 percent) after oral administration. The presence of food in the stomach delays absorption, but the bioavailability remains unchanged.

Metronidazole is 10 percent bound to plasma proteins. The small size of the molecule, lipid solubility, and the low protein binding account for its wide distribution in tissues and body fluids. Metronidazole penetrates well into the CSF even when the meninges are normal. In patients with meningitis, the concentrations in the CSF are equal to those in the serum.

Approximately 10 to 15 percent of administered metronidazole is excreted unchanged in the urine. Most of the drug is metabolized in the liver; the metabolites are excreted in the urine. The elimination half-life of metronidazole in persons with normal renal function is 7.0 h.

In anuric patients, the elimination half-life of metronidazole is only slightly extended (10 h), but accumulation of metabolites does occur. Since the metabolites are removed by dialysis, no dosage adjustment is necessary in anuric patients on dialysis. Metronidazole metabolites have not been definitely associated with adverse effects. In patients with severe liver disease, the plasma clearance of metronidazole is decreased, and the dosage regimen should be adjusted to avoid toxicity.

Adverse Effects The incidence of untoward effects associated with the use of metronidazole is low. An unpleasant metallic taste, anorexia, nausea, and vomiting are occasionally experienced. Neurotoxicity manifested by sensory neuropathy, ataxia, and rarely encephalopathy and seizures are rare complications which may occur after prolonged treatment with high doses.

Metronidazole may produce a disulfiram-like reaction; alcohol ingestion is therefore contraindicated in patients taking the drug. Metronidazole increases the hypoprothrombinemic effect of racemic sodium warfarin by inhibiting its hepatic metabolism.

Clinical Use Metronidazole is effective in the therapy of a wide variety of anaerobic infections, including those involving *B. fragilis,* such as intra-abdominal and female pelvic infections. Since most of these infections are mixed, involving both aerobes and anaerobes, it is often necessary to combine metronidazole with another antimicrobial agent active against aerobic bacteria.

Because of its excellent CNS penetration, metronidazole is usually included in regimens used to treat brain abscess. Metronidazole is the drug of choice for nonspecific vaginitis. It is an alternative to vancomycin (oral) for the therapy of *C. difficile* colitis in patients who are not severely ill.

Metronidazole is the drug of choice for amebiasis, giardiasis, and vaginal trichomoniasis (see Chap. 46).

AGENTS USED PRIMARILY AGAINST GRAM-NEGATIVE ORGANISMS

Aminoglycosides

Aminoglycosides are compounds which contain two or more aminosugars linked by glycosidic bonds to an aminocyclitol ring. The six-membered aminocyclitol ring is either streptidine (as in streptomycin) or 2-deoxystreptamine (as in other aminoglycosides).

Of the eight aminoglycosides currently available in the United States, five are derived from *Streptomyces* species: streptomycin (isolated in 1943 from *Streptomyces griseus*), neomycin (isolated in 1949 from *Strep. fradiae*), paromomycin (isolated in 1956 from *Strep.*

rimosus), kanamycin (isolated in 1957 from *Strep. kanamyceticus*), and tobramycin (isolated in 1967 from *Strep. tenebrarius*). Gentamicin was isolated in 1963 from *Micromonospora purpurea*. Amikacin and netilmicin are both semisynthetic. Amikacin is produced through chemical modification of kanamycin; netilmicin is a semisynthetic derivative of sisomicin, an investigational aminoglycoside isolated from *Micromonospora inyoensis*. The spelling of gentamicin and netilmicin with *micin* rather than *mycin* denotes origin from *Micromonospora* rather than *Streptomyces* species.

Neomycin and paromomycin are too toxic for parenteral administration. Kanamycin, the most commonly used aminoglycoside in the 1960s, is seldom employed today. The discussion that follows focuses on streptomycin, gentamicin, tobramycin, amikacin, and netilmicin. Gentamicin consists of a mixture of roughly equal amounts of three individual components: gentamicin C_1, C_{1a}, and C_2 (see Fig. 43-1).

Mechanism of Action   The aminoglycoside antibiotics are rapidly bactericidal. These agents inhibit protein synthesis and produce misreading of the genetic code.

An essential element in the process leading to lethality is the active transport of the aminoglycoside from external milieu into the bacterial cell. The transport mechanism results in the accumulation of aminoglycosides inside bacterial cells to concentrations far in excess of the external concentrations.

Aminoglycosides diffuse readily through the porin channels in the outer membrane of gram-negative bacteria and enter the periplasmic space. Transport across the cytoplasmic (inner) membrane is energy-dependent and occurs in two phases. In the first phase (termed *energy-dependent phase I*), the strongly cationic aminoglycoside binds to anionic transporters and is driven across the cytoplasmic membrane by the membrane potential which is negative on the interior. A faster rate of aminoglycoside uptake (termed *energy-dependent phase II*) starts after the aminoglycoside interacts with the ribosome. The energy-dependent uptake of the aminoglycosides is inhibited by both a reduction in pH and anaerobiosis, which impair the ability of bacteria to maintain membrane potential necessary for transport.

The primary intracellular site of action of aminogly-cosides is the bacterial ribosome. There appears to be at least two different types of ribosomal binding: one unique to streptomycin and one shared by other aminoglycosides. Streptomycin binds to the 30-S ribosomal subunit. Other aminoglycosides bind to multiple sites on both 30-S and 50-S ribosomal subunits and fail to compete with streptomycin binding to the 30-S ribosome.

The binding of aminoglycosides to the ribosome results in (1) inhibition of protein synthesis and (2) misreading of the genetic code of the mRNA template with resultant incorporation of incorrect amino acids into the growing polypeptide chains. However, neither of these effects explains the bactericidal effect of aminoglycosides. Some other antibiotics inhibit protein synthesis as effectively as do the aminoglycosides and yet fail to cause a lethal event, that is, produce only bacteriostasis. The mechanism of rapid lethal action of aminoglycosides remains unclear.

Antimicrobial Spectrum   The antimicrobial spectrum of aminoglycosides includes aerobic and facultative gram-negative bacilli, *Staph. aureus*, and myobacteria. These antibiotics have no activity against anaerobic microorganisms, chlamydiae, or rickettsiae.

Gram-Positive Aerobic Bacteria   *Staph. aureus* and *Staph. epidermidis* are usually quite susceptible, especially to the 2-deoxystreptamine-containing aminoglycosides (gentamicin, tobramycin, netilmicin, and amikacin). *Streptococci* and *Listeria monocytogenes* are generally resistant to clinically achievable concentrations. In the case of enterococci, resistance is related to decreased intracellular transport, although some strains also have ribosomal resistance, especially to streptomycin. Such strains exhibit high-level resistance with minimum inhibitory concentrations (MICs) greater than 1000 μg/mL. The combination of an aminoglycoside and penicillin G (or vancomycin) has synergistic bactericidal action against enterococci, except for strains that exhibit high-level resistance.

Gram-Negative Aerobic Bacteria   Gentamicin, tobramycin, netilmicin, and amikacin are active against aerobic and facultative gram-negative bacteria, including *E. coli*, *Klebsiella*, *Proteus*, *Providencia*, *Morganella*, *Enterobacter*, *Serratia*, *Citrobacter*, *Francisella tularensis*, *Yersinia pestis*, *H. influenzae*,

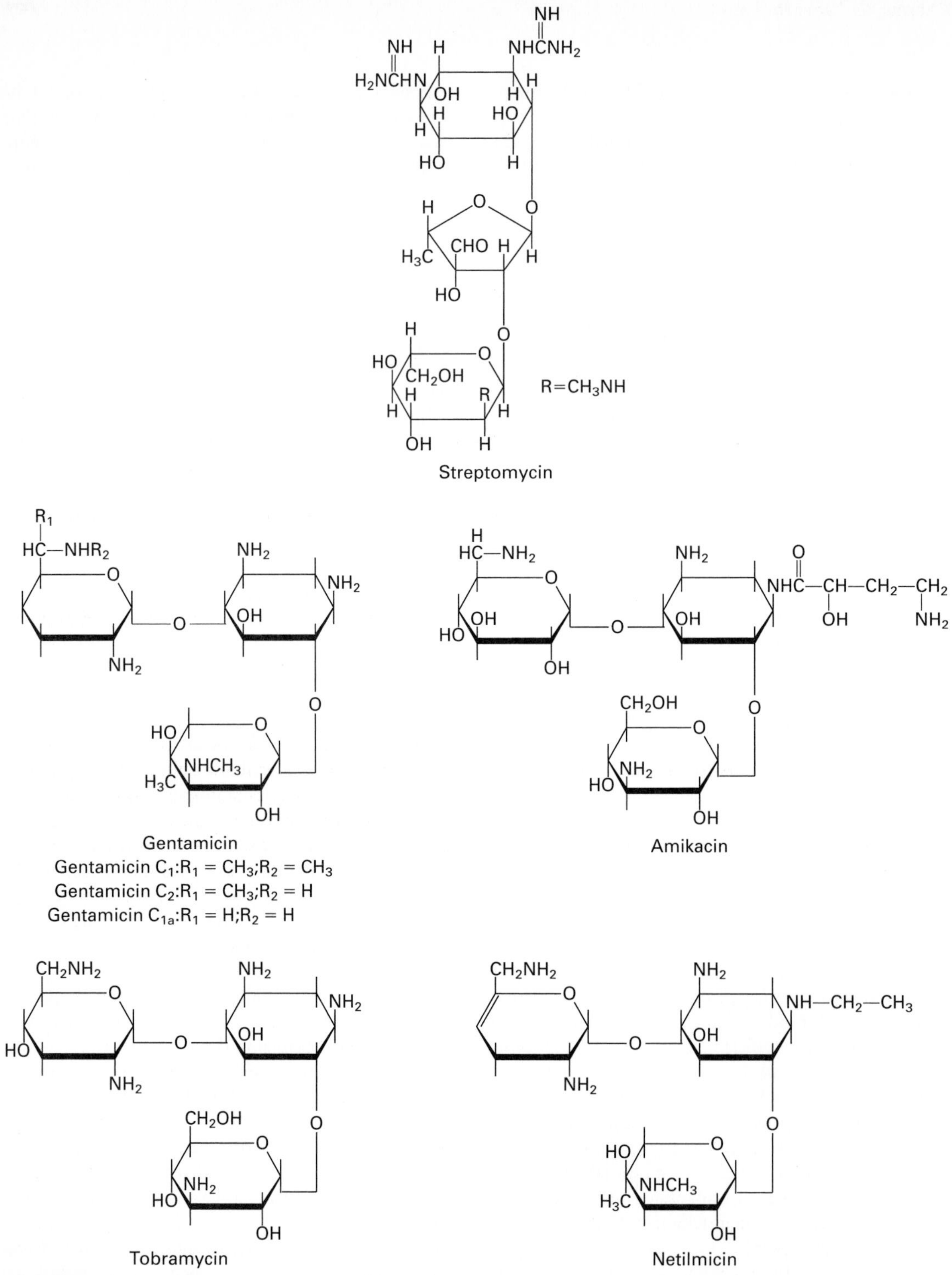

FIGURE 43-1   Structural formulas of aminoglycosides.

N. menigitidis, N. gonorrhoeae, Brucella, Acinetobacter, Ps. aeruginosa, and other *Pseudomonas* species. Gentamicin and tobramycin share very similar in vitro profiles; gentamicin is somewhat more potent against *Serratia marcescens,* and tobramycin is 2 to 4 times more potent against *Ps. aeruginosa.* The susceptibility of other organisms to these two aminoglycosides is virtually identical. Netilmicin shares the spectrum of gentamicin and tobramycin, but some *E. coli, Klebsiella, Enterobacter,* and *Citrobacter* strains that are gentamicin-resistant are susceptible to netilmicin. Amikacin is active against many strains of gram-negative species that are resistant to other aminoglycosides. The gram-negative spectrum of streptomycin is similar to other aminoglycosides; however, resistant strains are common, and *Pseudomonas* species are usually resistant.

Mycobacteria Streptomycin is the most active aminoglycoside against *Mycobacterium tuberculosis.* Amikacin possesses significant activity against *Mycobacterium fortuitum.* The antimycobacterial activities of gentamicin, tobramycin, and netilmicin are not significant clinically.

Mechanisms of Resistance Bacterial resistance to aminoglycosides can occur by one of the following mechanisms: (1) altered ribosomal binding site, (2) impaired intracellular transport, and (3) inactivation of the drug by microbial enzymes.

Streptomycin binds to a specific protein (S_{12}) on the 30-S subunit of the ribosome. Alteration of this protein by mutation renders ribosomes unable to bind streptomycin and makes the organism totally resistant. Mutational resistance to streptomycin occurs with relatively high frequency; the mutants exhibit high-level resistance to the drug. Gentamicin, tobramycin, netilmicin, and amikacin bind to multiple sites on both ribosomal subunits. Due to the requirement for multiple mutational events, mutational resistance to these agents is exceedingly uncommon.

A second mechanism of resistance is impaired intracellular transport which leads to resistance to all aminoglycosides. This type of resistance is uncommon among gram-negative aerobic or facultative bacilli. Since the transport of aminoglycosides across the cytoplasmic membrane is an oxygen-dependent active process, strictly anaerobic bacteria are invariably resistant to these agents.

The most significant mechanism of resistance in clinical isolates is the plasmid-mediated production of enzymes that phosphorylate, adenylate, or acetylate specific hydroxyl or specific amino groups on the aminoglycoside molecule. The aminoglycoside-modifying enzymes are not secreted extracellularly. Instead, they are found in the periplasmic space. As the drug penetrates the outer membrane and reaches the periplasmic space, it is altered by the enzyme. The modified drug competes with the unaltered drug for intracellular transport but fails to bind to ribosomes. As a consequence, the second energy-dependent phase of aminoglycoside uptake is inhibited. Many of these enzymes (over 20) have been identified. Aminoglycosides vary in their ability to resist enzymatic inactivation. Gentamicin and tobramycin are both susceptible to the same enzymes; netilmicin is more resistant to such modifications. Amikacin is least vulnerable to the enzymes that are currently prevalent.

Pharmacokinetics Aminoglycosides are very poorly absorbed from the intestinal tract (less than 1 percent) and must be given parenterally. Streptomycin is 35 percent bound to plasma proteins; other aminoglycosides have negligible protein binding (0 to 10 percent). The aminoglycosides penetrate into various tissues, except for the brain and the prostate. High concentrations are found in the renal cortex and in the endolymph and perilymph of the inner ear. Penetration into bronchial secretions is poor, and the biliary concentrations are lower than the concurrent serum levels. Penetration into the CSF and occular fluids is poor even in the presence of inflammation. The CSF concentrations approach 20 percent of the serum levels when the meninges are inflamed. Higher levels are obtained in the neonates, perhaps because of immaturity of the blood-brain barrier.

The aminoglycosides are excreted entirely by kidneys in active unchanged form. Less than 1 percent of a parenterally administered dose appears in feces. The elimination half-lives of gentamicin, tobramycin, netilmicin, amikacin, and streptomycin in persons with normal renal functions are identical, 2.0 to 2.5 h. In functionally anephritic patients, the half-lives are prolonged to 40 to 60 h. Dosage adjustment is essential with any degree of renal impairment. The aminoglycosides are removed from the body by either hemodialysis or peritoneal dialysis.

Adverse Effects   The incidence of allergic reactions to aminoglycosides is very low. The principal toxicities are ototoxicity, nephrotoxicity, and neuromuscular blockade.

Ototoxicity   All aminoglycosides are capable of causing ototoxicity. Their toxic effect on the neuroepithelial cells of the inner ear may produce either cochlear damage or vestibular impairment or both. Although relatively uncommon, ototoxicity is especially worrisome because of its frequent irreversibility, its occurrence even after discontinuation of the drug, and its cumulative nature with repeated courses of aminoglycosides.

The auditory toxicity of aminoglycosides is manifest clinically as neurosensory hearing loss. The initial manifestations are tinnitus and/or high-frequency hearing loss (usually bilateral). Since the latter is outside the conversational range, it can only be detected by audiometry. Loss of low-tone hearing occurs if exposure is continued. Vestibular toxicity is manifest clinically by vertigo, dizziness, and/or ataxia. The occurrence and the severity of both auditory toxicity and vestibular toxicity correlate with high serum levels and prolonged therapy with aminoglycosides.

The auditory toxicity of aminoglycosides is due to selective destruction of the hair cells of the organ of Corti. The hair cells located in the basal turn of the cochlea are affected first, with destruction progressing toward the apex. The progression is consistent with clinical experience, since the basal region responds to high-frequency and the apex to low-frequency tones. The vestibular system is affected primarily by damage to type I hair cells of the summit of the ampullar cristae. Neither cochlear nor ampullar cells can regenerate once they have been destroyed, thus accounting for irreversibility.

The cellular damage in the inner ear is due to the high concentrations of aminoglycosides in the perilymph and endolymph that bathe the cells. Aminoglycosides enter the perilymph and the endolymph when concentrations in plasma are high. Diffusion back into the blood stream is slow, and their half-lives in these fluids (10 to 12 h) are much longer than their plasma half-lives.

The incidence of aminoglycoside-induced auditory and vestibular toxicity is low if clinically detectable hearing loss or vestibular dysfunction is required, but it is higher if more sensitive measures of auditory or vestibular function are used.

Nephrotoxicity   All aminoglycosides are capable of causing nephrotoxicity. The toxicity is due to marked accumulation and avid retention of these drugs in the renal cortex by the proximal tubular cells.

Nephrotoxicity manifests itself initially by proteinuria, cylindruria, and inability to concentrate the urine. This is followed by a reduction in glomerular filtration rate with a rise in serum creatinine and blood urea nitrogen. The impairment in renal function is almost always reversible, since the proximal tubular cells have the capacity to regenerate.

Streptomycin does not concentrate much in the renal cortex; it is the least nephrotoxic aminoglycoside. The nephrotoxic potentials of gentamicin, amikacin, and netilmicin are similar. Tobramycin may be less nephrotoxic, but this is controversial.

Risk factors for development of nephrotoxicity from aminoglycosides include advanced age, preexisting renal disease, and concurrent use of vancomycin, amphotericin B, cephalothin, cisplatin, and cyclosporin.

Neuromuscular Blockade   All aminoglycosides are capable of producing neuromuscular blockade resulting in respiratory paralysis. This effect is associated with very high concentrations, which is usually achieved by rapid intravenous administration of large boluses.

The mechanism responsible for aminoglycoside-induced neuromuscular blockade involves both an inhibition of the presynaptic release of acetylcholine and a reduction in sensitivity of the postsynaptic receptor for acetylcholine. Calcium overcomes the effect of the aminoglycoside at the neuromuscular junction, and the intravenous administration of a calcium salt is the preferred treatment of this toxicity.

Clinical Use   Gentamicin, tobramycin, amikacin, and netilmicin are useful and effective agents for the treatment of infections involving aerobic or facultative gram-negative bacilli. For serious infections caused by *Ps. aeruginosa*, these agents are used in combination with an extended-spectrum penicillin, ceftazidime, imipenem, or aztreonam.

Streptomycin is the drug of choice for the treatment of tularemia (*Francisella tularensis*), plague (*Yersinia pestis*), and brucellosis (in combination with tetracycline). It is not used for other gram-negative bacillary infections because high-level resistance may develop during therapy due to a single-step mutation.

Streptomycin or gentamicin in combination with penicillin G is the treatment of choice for enterococcal endocarditis.

Spectinomycin Spectinomycin, isolated from *Streptomyces spectabilis*, is an aminocyclitol antibiotic but not an aminoglycoside, since it contains neither an amino sugar nor a glycosidic bond.

Similar to streptomycin, spectinomycin binds to the 30-S ribosomal subunit and inhibits protein synthesis. However, misreading of the genetic code does not occur.

Although spectinomycin has a wide spectrum of activity, it is used only for gonococcal infections. Other gram-negative bacteria develop resistance during therapy. Resistance to spectinomycin is rarely seen in *N. gonorrhoeae*.

Spectinomycin does not enter saliva and is not effective in gonococcal pharyngitis. It is completely excreted into the urine as unchanged drug, and its half-life is about 1 h.

Spectinomycin is neither ototoxic nor nephrotoxic. It is used for the treatment of penicillinase-producing gonococcal infections. Spectinomycin is administered only by intramuscular injection.

Quinolones

Nalidixic acid was the first of a new class of antimicrobial agents, the quinolones, that was synthesized in 1962 and introduced for the treatment of urinary tract infections. A number of chemically related compounds were synthesized in the subsequent years, but all had suboptimal pharmacokinetic profile, narrow antimicrobial spectrum, and microbial resistance problems. Major progress came with the synthesis of fluoroquinolones in the 1980s. These agents differ from the older compounds in that they have a fluorine at the C-6 position and a piperazinyl moiety at the C-7 position of the quinolone nucleus. The 6-fluoro modification increases potency against gram-negative bacteria and broadens the spectrum to include gram-positive organisms. The 7-piperazinyl group provides activity against *Pseudomonas aeruginosa*. Substituents at the N-1 position of the quinolone and the para position of the piperazine ring vary from agent to agent. The fluoroquinolones currently available in the United States include norfloxacin and ciprofloxacin, both supplied in oral form. Intravenous ciprofloxacin and many other fluoroquinolones are currently under investigation.

Mechanism of Action The fluoroquinolones are potent bactericidal agents that alter the structure and function of bacterial DNA by interfering with the activities of the enzyme DNA gyrase (topoisomerase II). This enzyme is responsible for (1) the insertion of negative superhelical twists (negative supercoils) into covalently closed circular DNA, and (2) breaking and rejoining (catenation, decatenation) of DNA circles interlocked like links in a chain. DNA gyrase is essential to accommodate the bacterial DNA, approxi-

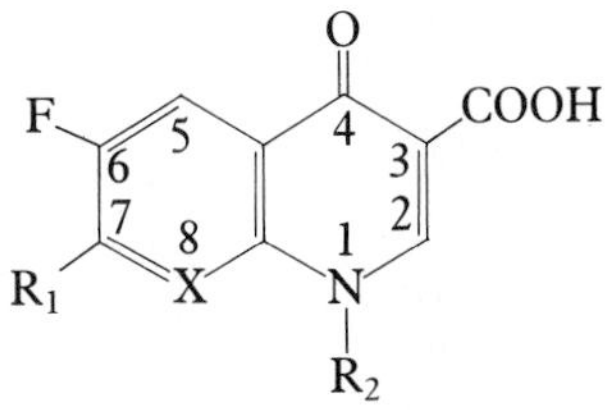

X Carbon or nitrogen

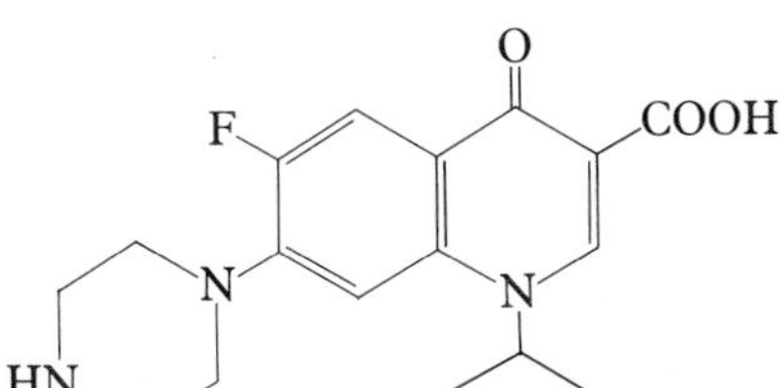

Ciprofloxacin

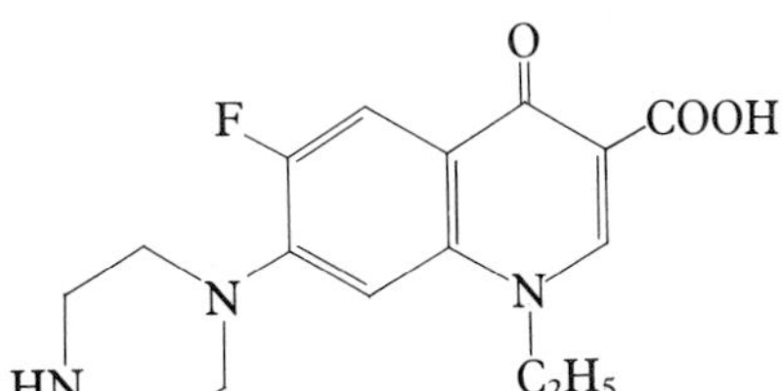

Norfloxacin

mately 1300 μm in *E. coli*, within a cell which is only 2 to 3 μm in length. This enzyme is required for DNA replication, DNA repair, recombination, transposition, and transcription of certain operons. DNA gyrase is composed of two A subunits and two B subunits; quinolones interfere primarily with the action of the A subunit.

Antimicrobial Spectrum   Ciprofloxacin and norfloxacin have a similar antimicrobial spectrum. However, depending on the organism, norfloxacin is two- to eightfold less active.

Gram-Negative Bacteria   Ciprofloxacin is highly active against aerobic gram-negative bacteria. *Escherichia coli, Klebsiella, Enterobacter, Serratia marcescens, Proteus, Morganella, Providenica, Citrobacter, Acinetobacter, Eikenella corrodens, Pasteurella multocida, Aeromonas hydrophila, Salmonella, Shigella, Campylobacter jejuni, Yersinia enterocolitica*, and *Vibrio* are highly sensitive. The in vitro potency of ciprofloxacin against these organisms is greater than that of third-generation cephalosporins, imipenem, aztreonam, or aminoglycosides. *Pseudomonas aeruginosa* is sensitive to ciprofloxacin; however, most strains of *Ps. cepacia* and *Ps. maltophila* are resistant.

Ciprofloxacin is highly active against *Haemophilus influenzae, Haemophilus ducreyi, Branhamella catarrhalis, Neisseria gonorrhoeae* (including beta-lactamase-producing strains), and *Neisseria meningitidis;* its activity against these organisms is comparable to those of third-generation cephalosporins.

Gram-Positive Bacteria   Ciprofloxacin is active against both methicillin-susceptible and methicillin-resistant strains of *Staph. aureus, Staph. epidermidis*, and other coagulase-negative staphylococci. *Streptococcus* species (including groups A, B, C, D, and G streptococci and *Strep. pneumoniae*) and *Corynebacterium* species are only marginally susceptible to ciprofloxacin.

Other Organisms   The activity of ciprofloxacin against anaerobic bacteria is poor. The drug is active against *Mycobacterium tuberculosis, Mycobacterium kansasii*, and *Mycobacterium fortuitum* at concentrations which are therapeutically achievable.

Mechanisms of Resistance   Two mechanisms of bacterial resistance to fluoroquinolones have been identified: (1) alteration of the A subunit of DNA gyrase and (2) decreased outer membrane permeability. Resistance is chromosomally mediated; no plasmid-mediated resistance has been demonstrated. Spontaneous single-step mutations to fluoroquinolone resistance occur at a very low frequency. Development of resistance during therapy is rare and occurs most often in *Ps. aeruginosa* isolates from patients with cystic fibrosis.

Pharmacokinetics   Fluoroquinolones are absorbed from the gastrointestinal tract to varying degrees; nofloxacin is less absorbed than ciprofloxacin. Food delays absorption but does not affect other pharmacokinetic parameters. Concurrent administration of antacids containing magnesium hydroxide or aluminum hydroxide interferes with the gastrointestinal absorption. The bioavailability of orally administered ciprofloxacin is approximately 70 percent.

Ciprofloxacin is 35 percent bound to plasma proteins. It penetrates well in various tissues (including prostate), body fluids (including salivary secretions), and human cells (including macrophages and neutrophils). Penetration into the CSF is poor when the meninges are normal; higher levels are achieved in the presence of meningeal inflammation. The tissue concentrations of norfloxacin are lower than those of ciprofloxacin, however, substantial levels are attained in the kidney and prostatic tissues.

Fluoroquinolones are eliminated through renal excretion and metabolism. Renal excretion occurs by both glomerular filtration and tubular secretion. Approximately 40 to 45 percent of an orally administered ciprofloxacin is excreted unchanged into the urine, and 15 to 20 percent is metabolized. Renal excretion accounts for 30 percent of administered norfloxacin; 10 to 15 percent is metabolized. Biliary excretion of these compounds is not significant.

The elimination half-lives of ciprofloxacin and of norfloxacin in persons with normal renal function are 4.0 h, increasing to 9.0 h in anuric patients.

Adverse Effects   Adverse effects associated with the fluoroquinolones are infrequent. These include gastrointestinal disturbance (nausea, vomiting, or diarrhea), CNS disturbance (headache, restlessness, dizziness, tremors, and very rarely seizure), skin reactions (rashes, pruritus, photosensitivity), and transient elevations of serum transaminases, lactate dehydrogenase, and alkaline phosphatase.

Ciprofloxacin inhibits theophylline metabolism, thereby elevating its serum concentrations. In patients receiving both drugs, serum theophylline levels should be monitored and dosage adjustments made.

Clinical Use   Norfloxacin and ciprofloxacin are both effective for the treatment of urinary tract infections. Ciprofloxacin is also effective in bacterial prostatitis, uncomplicated gonorrhea (including those caused by penicillinase-producing *N. gonorrhoeae*), and osteomyelitis and pulmonary infections caused by susceptible organisms. It is efficacious in the treatment of most acute infectious diarrheas, including travelers' diarrhea, shigellosis, and *Campylobacter* enteritis.

BROAD-SPECTRUM ANTIMICROBIALS

Chloramphenicol

Chloramphenicol was originally isolated in 1947 from *Streptomyces venezuelae;* however, it is now manufactured synthetically.

$$O_2N - \text{(ring)} - \underset{|}{\overset{OH}{CH}}\underset{|}{\overset{CH_2OH}{CH}} - NH - \overset{O}{\overset{||}{C}} - CHCl_2$$

Chloramphenicol

Mechanism of Action   Chloramphenicol inhibits protein synthesis in bacteria and, to a lesser extent, in eukaryotic cells. The drug diffuses well into bacterial cells, where it binds reversibly to the 50-S ribosomal subunit. This prevents the attachment of the amino acid–containing end of the tRNA to its binding site on the 50-S ribosome. The binding of the aminoacyl-tRNA to the 30-S subunit is not affected. In the presence of chloramphenicol, the association of the amino acid substrate with peptidyl transferase does not occur and peptide bond formation is prevented.

Chloramphenicol has a bacteriostatic action against susceptible organisms. It has, however, "cidal" activity against *H. influenzae*, *Strep. pneumoniae*, and *N. meningitidis* at clinically achievable concentrations.

Mammalian cells contain 80-S ribosomes, and the protein synthesis in these, unlike that in bacterial 70-S ribosomes, is unaffected by chloramphenicol. The drug, however, inhibits mitochondrial protein synthesis in mammalian cells, perhaps because mitochondrial ribosomes resemble bacterial ribosomes; both are 70-S.

Antimicrobial Spectrum   Chloramphenicol has a broad spectrum of antimicrobial activity that includes gram-positive and gram-negative aerobic and anaerobic bacteria, spirochetes, mycoplasma, chlamydiae, and rickettsiae.

Aerobic Bacteria   Chloramphenicol is highly active against methicillin-sensitive *Staph. aureus*, nonenterococcal *Streptococcus* species (including *Strep. pneumoniae*), and *Listeria monocytogenes*. Enterococci and methicillin-resistant staphylococci are usually resistant.

Chloramphenicol is highly active against *N. meningitidis*, *N. gonorrhoeae*, *H. influenzae*, *Bordetella pertussis*, *Salmonella*, and *Brucella;* occasional strains may be resistant. The activity of the drug against other gram-negative bacteria is variable. Most strains of *E. coli*, *Proteus mirabilis*, *Klebsiella*, and *Shigella* are sensitive; resistance among other enteric species is more frequent. *Ps. aeruginosa* is invariably resistant to chloramphenicol.

Anaerobic Bacteria   Chloramphenicol is one of the most active antimicrobials against anaerobic bacteria. *Peptococcus*, *Peptostreptococcus*, *Clostridium*, *Actinomyces*, *Bacteroides* (including *B. fragilis*), *Fusobacterium*, and other anaerobic bacteria are all susceptible to chloramphenicol.

Other Organisms   Chloramphenicol is active against spirochetes, *Mycoplasma* species, *Chlamydia*, and *Rickettsia*.

Mechanisms of Resistance   Resistance to chloramphenicol is usually due to the presence of a plasmid that determines the production of chloramphenicol acetyltransferase. This enzyme acetylates the drug, a modification that renders it unable to bind to the 50-S subunit of the bacterial ribosome. Three distinct acetyltransferases are determined by plasmids in gram-negative bacteria; staphylococcal plasmids specify four closely related variants that are inducible. The resistance plasmids in gram-negative bacilli frequently carry determinants for multiple-drug resistance and can be transferred from one organism to another by conjugation.

Although chloramphenicol resistance is usually due to plasmid-mediated acetyltransferase production, impaired outer membrane permeability and mutations to ribosomal insensitivity have also been described.

Pharmacokinetics Chloramphenicol administered orally in capsules is rapidly and completely absorbed from the intestinal tract. Since the drug is exceedingly bitter, a suspension of tasteless chloramphenicol palmitate (an ester) is available for children. The ester is a prodrug which has no antimicrobial activity. It is hydrolyzed rapidly in the intestine to active chloramphenicol which is then absorbed. The bioavailability of chloramphenicol palmitate is the same as the chloramphenicol capsules.

Chloramphenicol is poorly soluble in water. A soluble ester of the drug, chloramphenicol succinate, is available for parenteral administration. The ester has no antimicrobial activity, but it is rapidly hydrolyzed in the body to active drug. The serum levels of active chloramphenicol following intravenous administration of the succinate ester are in the same range as those obtained with comparable doses of oral chloramphenicol. Absorption after intramuscular injection is unpredictable, and this route is not recommended.

Chloramphenicol is 45 percent bound to plasma proteins. It is lipid-soluble and diffuses well into tissues and body fluids, and it also crosses the placenta. The CSF concentrations are 50 to 65 percent of the concurrent serum levels in the presence or absence of meningeal inflammation.

About 10 percent of orally administered chloramphenicol is excreted unchanged in the urine. The remaining 90 percent is metabolized to a glucuronide conjugate which has no antibacterial activity and is excreted into the urine.

A variable percentage of intravenously administered chloramphenicol succinate is excreted into the urine in unchanged ester form. The remainder of the dose is hydrolyzed to active chloramphenicol, which is eliminated by hepatic metabolism and renal excretion.

The elimination half-life of chloramphenicol in persons with normal renal and hepatic function is 4.0 h. In anuric patients, the half-life is not altered signifi-

cantly and dosage adjustment is not necessary. Inactive metabolites accumulate in these patients, but they are not associated with adverse effects. In patients with hepatic failure, the dose of chloramphenicol should be reduced.

Adverse Effects Hematologic toxicity is by far the most important adverse effect of chloramphenicol. This can be divided into two types. The first is a reversible bone marrow depression due to a direct pharmacologic effect of the antibiotic as a result of inhibition of mitochondrial protein synthesis. It is manifest by reticulocytopenia and anemia with or without leukopenia and/or thrombocytopenia. This type of toxicity is common, occurs during the course of therapy, and is dose-related. It is more likely to occur when serum levels exceed 25 μg/mL and is reversible when the antibiotic is discontinued.

The second type of toxicity is a rare but generally fatal aplastic anemia, which occurs in one of 25,000 to 40,000 patients who receive chloramphenicol. Aplastic anemia usually develops weeks to months after administration of the drug but may occur during the course of therapy. The incidence is not related to the dose; however, it seems to occur more commonly in individuals who undergo prolonged therapy and especially in those who are exposed to the drug on more than one occasion. The pathogenesis of this idiosyncratic reaction is unknown.

Complete blood count should be obtained twice weekly on all patients receiving chloramphenicol. If the white blood cell count decreases below 2500 per mm^3, the antibiotic should be discontinued if the clinical condition allows.

Chloramphenicol can produce a potentially fatal toxic reaction, called *gray syndrome*, in newborn infants, especially premature babies. It is characterized by abdominal distension, vomiting, cyanosis, circulatory collapse, and death. Gray syndrome is due to diminished ability of neonates to conjugate chloramphenicol, resulting in high serum concentrations.

Allergic reactions including skin rash and drug fever are very rare with chloramphenicol. Nausea, vomiting, and diarrhea may occur but are uncommon. Hemolytic anemia may develop in persons with severe glucose-6-phosphate dehydrogenase deficiency (Mediterranean type) who are treated with chloramphenicol.

Chloramphenicol inhibits the activity of certain hepatic microsomal enzymes and interferes with the metabolism of warfarin, phenytoin, tolbutamide, and chlorpropamide. Toxicity due to these drugs may occur if they are administered in usual doses to a patient who is also receiving chloramphenicol.

Clinical Use Chloramphenicol is a potentially toxic agent that has very few clinical indications. It is a drug of first choice for the treatment of typhoid fever and is often included in regimens used to treat brain abscess. Until recently, chloramphenicol was the drug of choice for the empiric therapy of bacterial meningitis in children (in combination with ampicillin) and for ampicillin-resistant *H. influenzae* meningitis. The third-generation cephalosporins are now preferred in these conditions.

Chloramphenicol is an effective alternative in a number of infections when the drug of first choice cannot be used. These include rickettsial infections, brucellosis, and meningitis caused by *Strep. pneumoniae, N. meningitidis,* or *H. influenzae.*

The risk of aplastic anemia does not contraindicate the use of chloramphenicol in situations in which it is necessary. However, the drug should never be employed in infections which can be safely and effectively treated with other antimicrobial agents. Chloramphenicol should never be used for prophylaxis or for treatment of minor infections. Prolonged use and repeated exposure should be avoided.

Tetracyclines

The tetracyclines are a family of chemically related compounds that share in common a four-benzene-ring structure. The first of these compounds, chlortetracycline (isolated from *Streptomyces aureofaciens*), was introduced in 1948. Subsequently six congeners were introduced which are currently available in the United States. Oxytetracycline (isolated from *Streptomyces rimosus*) became available in 1950, tetracycline (semisynthetic) in 1952, demeclocycline (isolated from a mutant strain of *Streptomyces aureofaciens*) in 1959, methacycline (semisynthetic) in 1961, doxycycline (semisynthetic) in 1966, and minocycline (semisynthetic) in 1972. Although there are some differences among these agents in terms of pharmacokinetic properties and antimicrobial activity, they are very much alike.

Tetracycline

Congener	Substituent(s)	Position(s)
Oxytetracycline	—OH,—H	(5)
Demeclocycline	—OH,—H; —Cl	(6; 7)
Methacycline	—OH,—H; =CH$_2$	(5; 6)
Doxycycline	—OH,—H; —CH$_3$,—H	(5; 6)
Minocycline	—H,—H; —N(CH$_3$)$_2$	(6; 7)

Mechanism of Action The tetracyclines bind to the 30-S ribosomal subunit of bacteria and inhibit protein synthesis. An essential element in this process is the active transport of the drug across the cytoplasmic membrane. This energy-dependent transport mechanism results in the accumulation of the antibiotic inside the bacterial cell. Once within the cell, the tetracyclines bind reversibly to the 30-S ribosomal subunit. This blocks the attachment of the aminoacyl-tRNA to the mRNA–30-S ribosome and results in inhibition of protein synthesis. Tetracyclines have a bacteriostatic action against susceptible organisms.

The selective toxicity of tetracyclines resides in their differential entry into bacterial cells; mammalian cells lack the active transport system found in bacteria.

Antimicrobial Spectrum The antimicrobial spectra of all the tetracyclines are almost identical. Some differences, however, in the degree of activity against various organisms do exist among the congeners.

Gram-Positive Aerobic Bacteria The activity of tetracyclines against *Staph. aureus* and coagulase-negative staphylococci is variable, and the prevalence of resistant strains varies considerably. *Streptococcus pneumoniae* and *Strep. pyogenes* are usually sensitive, but 10 to 30 percent of the strains may be resistant.

Resistance is more frequent in other *Streptococcus* species; enterococci are usually resistant. Minocycline is the most active tetracycline against *Staph. aureus* and streptococci, closely followed by vibramycin. Both are active against a proportion of strains which are resistant to other tetracyclines.

Gram-Negative Aerobic Bacteria   Tetracyclines are active against *N. gonorrhoeae, N. meningitidis, H. influenzae, Branhamella catarrhalis, Legionella, Brucella, Vibrio cholerae, Vibrio vulnificus, Yersinia pestis, Yersinia enterocolitica, Francisella tularensis,* and *Pasteurella multocida.* Enteric gram-negative species, except for a small proportion of *E. coli* and *Enterobacter* strains, are resistant.

Anaerobes   Tetracyclines are active against many anaerobic bacteria; their activity against *Actinomyces* is particularly relevant clinically. Most strains of the various anaerobic species (75 percent of *B. fragilis* strains) are sensitive to doxycycline, the most active congener against these organisms.

Other Organisms   Tetracyclines are active against *Mycoplasma, Ureaplasma urealyticum, Chlamydia trachomatis, Chlamydia psittaci (psittacosis), Rickettsia, Treponema pallidum, Borrelia recurrentis* (relapsing fever), *Borrelia burgdorferi* (Lyme disease), *Leptospira,* and *Spirillum minor* (rat-bite fever). Doxycycline is active against *Mycobacterium fortuitum.*

Mechanisms of Resistance   Tetracycline resistance in clinical isolates is associated with a decreased ability to accumulate the antibiotic within the cell. It is mediated by plasmids and is inducible. The resistance plasmids contain genetic information for a number of proteins that appear to decrease influx of the drug into the cell or provide an efflux system that actively transports the drug out of the cell. Resistance to one tetracycline usually implies resistance to all, except for *Staph. aureus,* which is more sensitive to minocycline, and *B. fragilis,* which is more sensitive to vibramycin.

Pharmacokinetics   The tetracyclines are absorbed from the stomach and upper small intestine. The percentage of an oral dose that is absorbed varies from 60 percent for oxytetracycline to 95 percent for minocycline (Table 43-1). The presence of food in the stomach does not affect the absorption of doxycycline or minocycline, but it reduces the absorption of other tetracyclines. All the tetracyclines from stable chelates with divalent or trivalent cations. Absorption is markedly decreased when these drugs are administered simultaneously with milk (which contains calcium), antacids (which contain magnesium or aluminum), or iron preparations.

The tetracyclines bind to plasma proteins to various extents and diffuse into most tissues and body fluids. Penetration into the CSF is highest for minocycline, followed by vibramycin, and correlates with lipid solubility. The CSF levels are approximately 10 to 20 percent of the concurrent serum concentrations. Penetration into prostatic tissue is also highest for these two compounds. Minocycline penetrates well into salivary secretions; this accounts for its efficacy as a prophylactic agent in meningococcal carriers. All tetracyclines cross the placental barrier and are excreted in breast milk in concentrations that are usually a fraction of maternal serum levels.

TABLE 43-1   Pharmacokinetic features of the tetracyclines

Drug	Absorption, %	Protein binding, %	Elimination half-life, h	Excreted unchanged in urine, %
Tetracycline	75	65	8	60
Oxytetracycline	60	35	8	60
Demeclocycline	65	80	14	40
Methacycline	60	80	14	50
Doxycycline	95	90	16	35
Minocycline	95	80	16	10

Tetracyclines, with the exception of minocycline, are excreted in the urine (unchanged) and the feces. The proportion of the dose which is excreted in the urine varies with the individual compound (Table 43-1). The remainder of the dose is eliminated in the feces as a result of drug secretion into the intestinal tract, unabsorbed drug (oral administration), and biliary excretion (a small fraction). Cationic chelation in the intestine prevents reabsorption in the lower intestine. Less than 30 percent of administered minocycline is recovered in the urine and the feces, suggesting that most of the drug is metabolized. Metabolism does not play a significant role in the elimination of other tetracyclines. The elimination half-lives of tetracyclines range from 8 h (tetracycline and oxytetracycline) to 16 h (doxycline and minocycline).

In anuric patients the elimination half-life of doxycycline remains unchanged due to increased excretion in the feces, and dosage adjustment is not necessary. This drug is the tetracycline of choice in patients with renal failure. The tetracyclines are not removed by peritoneal dialysis or hemodialysis.

Adverse Effects   Allergic reactions including skin rash and drug fever are infrequent with tetracyclines. Photosensitivity reactions are more common in patients receiving demeclocycline, but they occur with all tetracyclines.

Epigastric pain, nausea, and vomiting are relatively common with tetracyclines. Diarrhea may occur and can be due to *Clositridium difficile* colitis.

Tetracyclines may be deposited in the deciduous teeth of children if they receive these drugs early in life, or if their mother is treated by tetracyclines during the second and third trimesters of pregnancy. This causes a yellow-brown discoloration of the teeth. These drugs may also produce a lifelong discoloration of the permanent teeth if they are administered to children under 8 years of age. Tetracyclines should not be administered to pregnant women and to children under 8 years of age.

Patients receiving minocycline, but not other tetracyclines, may experience vestibular toxicity, manifested by dizziness, tinnitus, vertigo, and ataxia. The symptoms are reversible within several days after discontinuation of the drug. Vestibular toxicity has significantly limited the use of minocycline.

Other side effects associated with tetracyclines include hepatic toxicity (with high doses especially in pregnant women), aggravation of preexisting renal failure (least common with doxycycline), and superinfection with *Candida* and resistant bacteria.

Clinical Use   Tetracyclines are the drug of choice for a wide variety of infections, including chlamydial infections (urethritis, pelvic inflammatory disease, lymphogranuloma venereum, psittacosis), rickettsial infections (Rocky Mountain spotted fever, Q fever, etc.), Lyme disease, leptospirosis, relapsing fever, brucellosis (in combination with streptomycin), mycoplasma pneumonia (many prefer erythromycin), plague, cholera, vibrio vulnificus infections, and granuloma inguinale (*Calymmatobacterium granulomatis*) and infections caused by *Mycobacterium fortuitum* (only doxycline). In addition, they are effective alternatives in a number of infections when the drug of first choice cannot be used. These include actinomycosis, rat-bite fever, syphilis, tularemia, and *Yersinia enterocolitica* enteritis. Long-term low-dose tetracycline therapy is frequently used to control severe acne.

BIBLIOGRAPHY

Craig, W. A., J. Gudmundsoon, and R. M. Reich: "Netilmicin Sulfate: A Comparative Evaluation of Antimicrobial Activity, Pharmacokinetics, Adverse Reactions and Clinical Efficacy," *Pharmacotherapy*, **3**:305–315 (1983).

Dhawan, V. K., and H. Thadepalli: "Clindamycin: A Review of Fifteen Years of Experience," *Rev. Infect. Dis.*, **4**:1133–1153 (1982).

Francke, E. L., and H. C. Neu: "Chloramphenicol and Tetracyclines," *Med. Clin. North Am.*, **71**:1155–1168 (1987).

Goldman, P: "Metronidazole," *N. Engl. J. Med.*, **303**:1212–1218 (1980).

Hooper, D. C., and J. S. Wolfson: "The Fluoroquinolones: Pharmacology, Clinical Uses, and Toxicities in Humans," *Antimicrob. Agents Chemother.*, **28**:716–721 (1985).

LeBel, M.: "Ciprofloxacin. Chemistry, Mechanism of Action, Resistance, Antimicrobial Spectrum, Pharmacokinetics, Clinical Trials, and Adverse Reactions," *Pharmacotherapy*, **8**:3–30 (1988).

Leitman, P. S., and C. R. Smith: "Aminoglycoside Nephrotoxicity in Humans," *Rev. Infect. Dis.*, **5 (Suppl. 2)**:S284–S293 (1983).

Moore, R. D., C. R. Smith, J. J. Lipsky, E. D. Mellits, et al.: "Risk Factors for Nephrotoxicity in Patients Treated with Aminoglycosides," *Ann. Intern. Med.*, **100**:352–357 (1984).

Neu, H. C.: "Quinolones. A New Class of Antimicrobial Agents with Wide Potential Uses," *Med. Clin. North Am.*, **72:**623–636 (1988).

Pancoast, S. J.: "Aminoglycoside Antibiotics in Clinical Use," *Med. Clin. North Am.*, **72:**581–611 (1988).

Tally, F. P., and E. Sullivan: "Metronidazole: In Vitro Activity, Pharmacology and Efficacy in Anaerobic Bacterial Infections," *Pharmacotherapy*, **1:**28–38 (1981).

Tadepalli, H., M. B. Bansal, B. Rao, R. See, et al.: "Ciprofloxacin: In Vitro, Experimental and Clinical Evaluation," *Rev. Infect. Dis.*, **10:**505–515 (1988).

Wolfson, J. S., and D. C. Hooper: "Norfloxacin: A New Targeted fluoroquinolone Antimicrobial Agent," *Ann. Intern. Med.*, **108:**238–251 (1988).

C H A P T E R **44**

Antimicrobials III: Sulfonamides, Trimethoprim, and Antimycobacterial Agents

Abdolghader Molavi

SULFONAMIDES

Sulfonamides are synthetic antimicrobial agents derived from sulfanilamide (*para*-aminobenzenesulfonamide). They are structural analogs of *para*-aminobenzoic acid (PABA), a factor required by bacteria for folic acid synthesis (Table 44-1). The nature of substitutions at the sulfonyl radical (SO_2) determines the antimicrobial potency and the pharmacokinetic properties of the individual compound.

The sulfonamides currently available include sulfisoxazole, sulfamethoxazole, sulfadiazine, sulfamethizole, and trisulfapyrimidines (a mixture of sulfamerazine, sulfamethazine, and sulfadiazine); the first two are most commonly used. A long-lasting sulfonamide, sulfadoxine, is available only in fixed combination with pyrimethamine for prophylaxis and treatment of falciparum malaria.

Mechanism of Action

The sulfonamides are bacteriostatic compounds that inhibit bacterial growth via interference with microbial folic acid synthesis. More specifically, sulfonamides inhibit competitively the conversion of PABA to folic acid mediated by the enzyme dihydropteroate synthetase (Fig. 44-1).

Folic acid is essential for purine and ultimately DNA synthesis in both bacterial and mammalian cells. Because animal cells are unable to synthesize folic acid, this compound must be supplied in the diet. Folic acid enters mammalian cells by an active transport mechanism. Since it does not enter most bacterial cells, bacteria must synthesize the compound. This difference between the bacterial and mammalian cells is the basis for selective toxicity of sulfonamides.

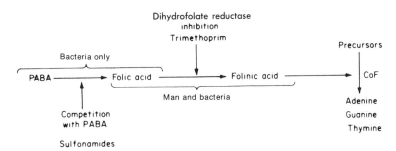

FIGURE 44-1 The diagram shows the site of action of competitors of PABA in contrast to inhibitors of dihydrofolate reductase in the chain of synthesis and utilization of folic acid by bacteria and humans.

TABLE 44-1   Chemical formulas and pharmacokinetic properties of selected sulfonamides

$$NH_2 - \underset{\text{(benzene ring)}}{\bigcirc} - SO_2 - NH - R_1$$

Drug	Structural formula of R_1	Route of administration	Protein binding	Elimination half-life, h	Percent excreted unchanged
Sulfisoxazole		Oral	85	6	40–70
Sulfadiazine		Oral	40	10	65
Sulfamethoxazole		Oral	65	10	30
Sulfamerazine		Oral	75	10	
Sulfamethazine		Oral	80	10	20–40
Sulfamethizole		Oral	90	1–2	95
Sulfameter		Oral	80	34–37	70–80

Antimicrobial Spectrum

The sulfonamides have a wide range of antimicrobial activity that includes *Staphylococcus aureus*, nonenterococcal *Streptococcus* species, *Listeria monocytogenes*, *Nocardia* (particularly relevant clinically), *Neisseria*, *Haemophilus influenzae*, enteric gram-negative species (especially *Escherichia coli* and *Proteus mirabilis*), and some anaerobic bacteria. Resistance, however, is widespread, being found in 10 to 50 percent of strains of various species.

Sulfonamides, particularly when combined with pyrimethamine or trimethoprim, are active against some protozoa, including *Toxoplasma*, *Plasmodium falciparum*, and *Pneumocystis carinii*.

Mechanisms of Resistance

Bacterial resistance to sulfonamides may develop by mutation, resulting in either microbial overproduction of PABA or an altered dihydropteroate synthetase less readily inhibited by the drug. Resistance also may be mediated by plasmids that code for the production of drug-resistant dihydropteroate synthetase or result in decreased permeability of the cell envelope to sulfonamides.

Pharmacokinetics

The sulfonamides are rapidly and almost completely absorbed from the gastrointestinal tract. These drugs bind to plasma proteins to various extents and readily diffuse into various tissues and body fluids. The sulfonamides penetrate into the cerebrospinal fluid (CSF), even in the absence of meningeal inflammation, but the levels achieved vary somewhat with each drug. Sulfadiazine achieves the highest CSF levels, approximately 60 percent of the concurrent serum concentrations when the meninges are inflamed. High levels also occur in saliva and breast milk. Sulfonamides readily cross the placenta and enter the fetal circulation.

The sulfonamides are metabolized to various degrees, primarily in the liver, by acetylation on the *para*-amino moiety. The acetylated metabolites have no antibacterial activity and yet remain the toxic potentialities of the parent compound.

The sulfonamides are excreted into the urine as unchanged drug and the acetylated metabolites. Biliary excretion is not significant. The elimination half-lives of sulfonamides vary widely, ranging from 6 h (sulfisoxazole) to 6 to 8 days (sulfadoxine).

Adverse Effects

Nausea, vomiting, and diarrhea may occur but are uncommon. Allergic reactions, particularly rashes, occur in about 3 percent of patients receiving sulfisoxazole or sulfamethoxazole, the two preparations most commonly used in the United States. In addition to a variety of rashes, sulfonamides can cause drug fever, erythema multiforme (including Stevens-Johnson syndrome), erythema nodosum, vasculitis resembling periarteritis nodosa, and a serum sickness-like syndrome.

Crystalluria, particularly in acid urine, may occur and tubular deposits of sulfonamide crystals can result in renal damage. This complication occurs rarely, if at all, with sulfisoxazole, which is highly soluble in urine. Sulfamethoxazole is slightly less soluble. Sulfadiazine has a lower solubility than the above drugs, and therefore it is important to maintain a high fluid intake when this drug is used. Alkalinization of the urine may also be desirable, since the solubility increases greatly with slight elevations of pH. Since the solubility of one agent is independent of another, while the antibacterial activity is additive, trisulfapyrimidine (a mixture of sulfadiazine, sulfamerazine, and sulfamethazine) is associated with a lower incidence of crystalluria than are the individual components.

Leukopenia, agranulocytosis (reversible), and acute hemolytic anemia (sometimes related to a glucose-6-phosphate dehydrogenase deficiency) are among the serious complications of sulfonamide therapy.

Sulfonamides should not be administered during the last month of pregnancy because they compete for bilirubin-binding sites on plasma ablumin and increase fetal levels of unconjugated bilirubin, increasing the risk of kernicterus.

Sulfonamides inhibit the metabolism of sodium warfarin, phenytoin, tolbutamide, and chlorpropamide. Dosage adjustment may be necessary when a sulfonamide is given concurrently.

Clinical Use

Sulfonamides are primarily used for the treatment of uncomplicated urinary-tract infections. A vast majority of organisms (*E. coli* and *Proteus mirabilis*) responsible for acute urinary-tract infections acquired in the community are sensitive to these agents.

Sulfonamides are quite effective in the therapy of *Nocaria asteroides* infections; trimethoprim-sulfamethoxazole, however, is the drug of choice.

Sulfonamides are effective in preventing streptococcal pharyngitis and recurrence of rheumatic fever (used in penicillin-allergic patients). They are effective in preventing meningococcal disease in close contacts if the infective organism is known to be sensitive.

Sulfadiazine combined with pyrimethamine is the regimen of choice for the treatment of toxoplasmosis. Sulfadoxine-pyrimethamine (Fansidar) is effective for treatment (in combination with quinine) and for prevention of chloroquine-resistant falciparum malaria.

TRIMETHOPRIM AND TRIMETHOPRIM-SULFAMETHOXAZOLE

Trimethoprim is a synthetic antimicrobial compound which is available as a single agent and in a fixed combination with sulfamethoxazole, trimethoprim-sulfamethoxazole (TMP-SMX). The structural formula of trimethoprim is as follows:

Trimethoprim

MECHANISM OF ACTION

Trimethoprim interferes with the action of dihydrofolate reductase, the enzyme that reduces dihydrofolic to tetrahydrofolic acid, an essential step in purine and, ultimately, DNA synthesis (Fig. 44-1). The sulfonamides inhibit an earlier reaction in the same biosynthetic pathway (i.e., the incorporation of *para*-aminobenzoic acid into dihydrofolic acid). The sequential blockade of the same biosynthetic pathway by these agents results in a high degree of synergistic activity against a wide spectrum of microorganisms.

The reduction of dihydrofolic to tetrahydrofolic acid in humans is also catalyzed by dihydrofolate reductase. However, trimethoprim has at least 10,000 times more inhibitory effect on the bacterial enzyme than on the corresponding mammalian enzyme. This difference in intrinsic sensitivity of the enzyme is the primary basis for the selective toxicity of trimethoprim.

Trimethoprim has a bacteriostatic action on susceptible bacteria. In combination with sulfamethoxazole, a bactericidal effect is obtained against many organisms.

Antimicrobial Spectrum

Trimethoprim has a wide range of antimicrobial activity. It is 20 to 100 times more potent than sulfamethoxazole against most bacterial species. The combination of trimethoprim and sulfamethoxazole exhibits synergism against susceptible organisms. Although the optimal concentration ratio of these agents for synergism varies for different bacteria, the most effective ratio for the greatest number of organisms is 20 parts of sulfamethoxazole to one part of trimethoprim. Synergism, however, occurs over a wide ratio of drug concentrations, with trimethoprim susceptibility being the most important predictor of susceptibility to the drug combination.

Gram-Positive Aerobic Bacteria   Trimethoprim is active against *Staph. aureus* (including penicillin-resistant and some methicillin-resistant strains), *Staph. epidermidis*, *Streptococcus* species, and *Listeria monocytogenes*. The susceptibility of enterococci is variable and depends on the medium used for sensitivity determination. The activity of trimethoprim against *Nocardia* is inferior to that of sulfonamides.

Gram-Negative Aerobic Bacteria   Most strains of enteric gram-negative bacilli including *E. coli*, *Enterobacter*, *Proteus*, *Klebsiella*, *Providencia*, *Morganella*, *Serratia marcescens*, *Citrobacter*, *Salmonella*, *Shigella*, and *Yersinia enterocolitica* are sensitive to trimethoprim. Trimethoprim is quite active against *Legionella*, *Acinetobacter*, *Vibrio*, *Aeromonas*, *Ps. maltophila*, and *Ps. cepacia*, but *Ps. aeruginosa* is invariably resistant.

H. influenzae (including ampicillin-resistant strains) and *H. ducreyi* are susceptible to trimethoprim. Pathogenic *Neisseria* (meningococci and gonococci) and *Branhamella catarrhalis* are moderately resistant to trimethoprim but often sensitive to TMP-SMX.

Other Organisms Anaerobic bacteria are generally resistant to trimethoprim. The activity of TMP-SMX against these organisms is due to the sulfamethoxazole component. *Pneumocystis carinii* is sensitive to TMP-SMX.

Mechanisms of Resistance

Bacterial resistance to trimethoprim may be due to any of the following mechanisms: (1) inability of the drug to penetrate through the cell envelope (*Ps. aeruginosa*), (2) the presence of a dihydrofolate reductase that is not susceptible to trimethoprim inhibition, (3) overproduction of dihydrofolate reductase, and (4) mutation resulting in thymine dependence, whereby the organism requires exogenous thymine (found in purulent material) for DNA synthesis, thus bypassing the metabolic blockade produced by trimethoprim.

Trimethoprim-resistant bacteria may arise by mutation. However, resistance in gram-negative organisms is often associated with the acquisition of a plasmid that codes for an altered dihydrofolate reductase.

The frequency of development of bacterial resistance to TMP-SMX is lower than it is to either of the agents alone.

Pharmacokinetics

Trimethoprim is absorbed almost completely from the gastrointestinal tract. The administration of sulfamethoxazole does not affect the rate of absorption of trimethoprim.

Trimethoprim is 45 percent bound to plasma proteins. It is lipid-soluble and penetrates readily into tissues (including prostate) and body fluids. The volume of distribution of trimethoprim is significantly larger than that of sulfamethoxazole. The ratio of trimethoprim to sulfamethoxazole in the available oral and intravenous preparations of TMP-SMX is 1:5. After the components have been distributed throughout the body, the concentration ratio of the bioactive forms in blood and tissues is about 1:20, which is optimal for synergy.

Trimethoprim penetrates well into the CSF. With normal meninges, the CSF levels are approximately 20 percent of the concurrent serum concentrations; this increases to 40 percent when the meninges are inflamed. Sulfamethoxazole also penetrates well into the CSF, achieving levels which are 12 percent of the concurrent serum concentrations; this increases to 25 percent when the meninges are inflamed.

Approximately 60 to 80 percent of administered trimethoprim is excreted unchanged into the urine. The remainder is inactivated in the liver and the metabolites are excreted by the kidney. The elimination half-life of trimethoprim in persons with normal renal function is 10 h. In functionally anephric patients it is extended to 24 to 30 h.

Approximately 30 percent of administered sulfamethoxazole is excreted unchanged in the urine; the remainder is inactivated in the liver, and the metabolites are excreted by the kidney. The elimination half-life of sulfamethoxazole in persons with normal renal function is 10 h. In anuric patients it is extended to 24 to 30 h.

Both trimethoprim and sulfamethoxazole are removed by hemodialysis.

Adverse Effects

Nausea, diarrhea, and hypersensitivity reactions are the most frequent adverse effects of trimethoprim. Trimethoprim can interfere with human folate metabolism if large doses are given over prolonged periods. In persons with suboptimal folate nutrition, megaloblastosis, granulocytopenia, and thrombocytopenia may occur. The administration of folinic acid (tetrahydrofolic acid) usually prevents or treats effectively the antifolate effects of trimethoprim, without affecting its antibacterial efficacy except possibly against enterococci.

The side effects of TMP-SMX are a summation of those due to the sulfonamide component and those caused by trimethoprim; most are caused by the former. Rash is quite common in patients with acquired immunodeficiency syndrome (AIDS) when TMP-SMX is administered to treat *Pneumocystis carinii* pneumonia.

Clinical Use

Although trimethoprim is available as a single agent, it is most commonly used in combination with sulfamethoxazole.

TMP-SMX is effective in the therapy of urinary-tract infections, prostatitis, epididymo-orchitis, and other infections caused by susceptible organisms. It is the drug of choice for *Nocardia asteroides* infection and for *Pneumocystis carinii* pneumonia.

TMP-SMX is a drug of choice for shigellosis, travelers' diarrhea, and *Yersinia enterocolitica* enteritis. It is a second-line drug for *Listeria* meningitis, *Legionella* infection, and typhoid fever.

TMP-SMX is effective in meningitis due to susceptible gram-negative bacteria. It is most useful when meningitis is caused by *Acinetobacter*, *Ps. maltophila*, and *Enterobacter*, organisms which are frequently resistant to the third-generation cephalosporins.

ANTITUBERCULOSIS DRUGS

The drugs used for the chemotherapy of tuberculosis are divided into two groups. The "first-line" agents combine the greatest level of efficacy with relatively low toxicity. These include isoniazid, rifampin, ethambutol, pyrazinamide, and streptomycin. A great majority of patients with tuberculosis can be successfully treated with the first-line drugs. Occasionally, because of microbial resistance and/or patient-related factors, it may be necessary to use the "second-line" drugs. These agents, which include ethionamide, cycloserine, capreomycin, kanamycin, and *para*-aminosalicylic acid, have important limitations that interfere with their usefulness in treating tuberculosis.

Chemotherapy of tuberculosis must include simultaneous administration of two or more effective drugs to prevent multiplication of drug-resistant mutants. With monotherapy, resistant organisms are readily selected. Treatment should be continued long enough to eradicate persisters (slowly growing intracellular organisms) in order to prevent relapse.

Isoniazid

Isoniazid, isonicotinic acid hydrazide (INH), is a synthetic compound which was introduced in 1953 for the treatment of tuberculosis. Its structural formula is

$$\text{N} \diagup \!\!\!\!\!\!\bigcirc\!\!\!\!\!\!\diagdown \text{C}-\text{NH}-\text{NH}_2$$
$$\text{O}$$

Isoniazid

Mechanism of Action Isoniazid has a bactericidal action on *Mycobacterium tuberculosis*. It inhibits the synthesis of mycolic acids, important constituents of the mycobacterial cell wall. Mycolic acids are unique to mycobacteria, and this action accounts for the selective toxicity of the drug for these organisms.

Antimicrobial Activity Isoniazid is highly active against rapidly multiplying *M. tuberculosis*, which resides in cavitary pulmonary lesions; it is less effective against slowly multiplying intracellular organisms. Atypical mycobacteria, except for *Mycobacterium kansasii* and *Mycobacterium xenopi*, are usually resistant to the drug.

Mechanisms of Resistance Naturally occurring isoniazid-resistant mutants occur at random and spontaneously in growing populations of tubercle bacilli at a rate of one per 10^5 to 10^6 organisms. These mutants exhibit decreased isoniazid uptake. Large populations of the organism, like the 10^9 to 10^{10} bacilli in open pulmonary cavities, contain significant numbers of resistant mutants. If isoniazid is used singly for treatment of tuberculosis, the sensitive organisms are killed while the resistant mutants multiply and eventually emerge as the dominant phenotype. The shift from primarily sensitive to mainly insensitive microorganisms during therapy is termed *secondary* (or acquired) *resistance;* it occurs within a few weeks.

Strains of *M. tuberculosis* resistant to isoniazid may be isolated from patients who have not received previous treatment with this drug (primary resistance). The primary isoniazid resistance occurs with an average frequency of 4.4 percent in the United States. The incidence is higher in certain populations, including Asians and Hispanics.

Pharmacokinetics Isoniazid is well absorbed when given by mouth and also may be administered parenterally. Both food and antacids reduce its bioavailability.

Isoniazid is less than 10 percent bound to plasma proteins. It is widely distributed throughout the body, including the central nervous system (CNS), and enters readily into macrophages. Concentrations in the CSF are about 20 percent of those in the serum in the presence or absence of meningeal inflammation. Isoniazid passes readily across the placenta and enters fetal circulation.

Most of the administered isoniazid is metabolized in the liver to inactive products which are excreted in the urine. Inactivation occurs primarily via acetylation by the hepatic enzyme N-acetyl transferase, which converts isoniazid to acetyl isoniazid. The rate at which humans acetylate isoniazid is genetically determined. There is bimodal distribution of slow and rapid inactivators of the drug due to differences in the activity of the enzyme acetyl transferase. Slow inactivators are autosomal homozygous recessives; rapid inactivators are either heterozygous or homozygous dominants. The frequency of the two phenotypes varies in populations of different racial origin. In the United States, 58 percent of Caucasians are slow inactivators. The mean elimination half-life of isoniazid in rapid inactivators is about 80 min, whereas it is 180 min in slow inactivators. The average serum concentration of active isoniazid in rapid inactivators is 30 to 50 percent of that present in slow inactivators. There is, however, no evidence of a difference in therapeutic efficacy related to the rate of acetylation of isoniazid in patients receiving the drug every day.

Some unchanged active isoniazid is excreted in the urine; the amount depends on the rate of acetylation. Rapid inactivators excrete about 3 percent of the dose unchanged in the urine. The fraction excreted this way is several times higher in slow inactivators.

Adverse Effects Peripheral neuropathy is a relatively common adverse effect of isoniazid. It is manifest by paresthesias in the "stocking-glove" distribution and occurs more frequently if high doses of the drug are used. Peripheral neuropathy is due to the effects of isoniazid on pyridoxine metabolism and can be prevented by prophylactic administration of pyridoxine.

Asymptomatic transaminase elevation occurs in 10 to 20 percent of patients receiving isoniazid. Severe hepatitis is much less frequent. Age appears to be the most important factor in determining the risk of hepatotoxicity. Hepatitis is rare in persons less than 20 years old, but it occurs in 0.3 percent of those 20 to

34 years old. The incidence increases to 1.2 percent in persons 35 to 49 years old and 2.3 percent in those 50 to 65 years old. Hepatitis can occur at any time during treatment, but it is more common in the first 2 months. Routine monitoring of serum transaminases is not necessary during isoniazid therapy. However, the patient should be monitored clinically, and if symptoms suggesting hepatitis occur, appropriate laboratory tests should be performed.

Other adverse effects of isoniazid include hypersensitivity reactions, drug fever, and agranulocytosis. Isoniazid inhibits metabolism of phenytoin and carbamazepine; toxicity due to these agents may occur if they are coadministered with isoniazid.

Clinical Use Isoniazid is the most important drug for the treatment of both pulmonary and extrapulmonary tuberculosis. It is active against both extracellular and intracellular organisms. To prevent secondary resistance, isoniazid must be used with another effective drug (usually rifampin) for the chemotherapy of tuberculosis. A 9-month regimen consisting of isoniazid and rifampin is highly effective.

Isoniazid, administered singly, is the drug of choice for chemoprophylaxis in persons at risk of developing tuberculosis such as household contacts of persons with active disease, persons known to have become infected within the preceding year, and tuberculin skin-test reactors under 35 years of age.

Pyridoxine should be administered with isoniazid to prevent peripheral neuropathy, especially in malnourished patients, the elderly, pregnant women, alcoholics, and patients with end-stage renal disease.

Rifampin

Rifampin is a semisynthetic derivative of rifamycin B, a macrocyclic compound produced by *Streptomyces mediterranei* (currently designated *Nocardia mediterranei*). It was introduced for clinical use in 1968. The structural formula of rifampin is shown on page 628.

Mechanism of Action Rifampin exerts a bactericidal effect by inhibition of RNA synthesis. The drug inhibits DNA-dependent RNA polymerase, preventing chain initiation but not elongation.

Rifampin does not bind to nuclear RNA polymerase in mammalian cells and does not affect the corre-

Rifampin

sponding RNA synthesis. It can inhibit mitochondrial RNA synthesis; however, the concentration required is several hundred times that which inhibits bacterial RNA synthesis.

Antimicrobial Activity   Rifampin is highly active against *M. tuberculosis.* Among atypical mycobacteria, *Mycobacterium kansasii, Mycobacterium marinum,* and most strains of *Mycobacterium scrofulaceum* and *Mycobacterium xenopi* are sensitive; the susceptibility of others is variable. Rifampin is rapidly bactericidal against *Mycobacterium leprae.*

In addition to mycobacteria, rifampin exhibits bactericidal activity against a wide range of organisms. It is extremely active against *Staph. aureus* and coagulase-negative staphylococci, including methicillin-resistant strains, and is also effective against nonenterococcal *Streptococcus* species and *Listeria monocytogenes.* Among the gram-negative species, *Neisseria meningitidis, Haemophilus influenzae* (including ampicillin-resistant strains), and *Legionella* sp. are highly sensitive. Others, except for *Brucella* and some strains of *E. coli* and *Proteus mirabilis,* are resistant. Anaerobic cocci, *Clostridium* sp., and *Bacteroides* sp. are frequently susceptible to rifampin.

Mechanisms of Resistance   Naturally occurring rifampin-resistant mutants can be detected both in vitro and in vivo among bacteria sensitive to the drug. Resistance is due to an alteration of the DNA-dependent RNA polymerase which is produced by a single-step mutation. Approximately one of every 10^7 to 10^8 organisms is resistant to the drug. When

rifampin is used singly for the treatment of tuberculosis or other infections, the sensitive organisms are killed while the resistant mutants multiply and emerge as the dominant phenotype. Secondary resistance can be prevented if rifampin is used with another effective chemotherapeutic agent.

Primary resistance to rifampin occurs with a frequency of less than 1 percent in the United States. The incidence is significantly higher in developing countries.

RNA polymerases of gram-negative and gram-positive bacteria are equally sensitive to rifampin; resistance of gram-negative species is due to impaired penetration of the drug through the outer membrane.

Pharmacokinetics   Rifampin is well absorbed from the gastrointestinal tract. Serum levels are slightly lower if the drug is taken immediately after food.

Rifampin is 80 percent bound to plasma proteins. It penetrates readily into tissues and body fluids, including CSF and saliva. The CSF concentrations are approximately 50 percent of the concurrent serum levels when the meninges are inflamed. Rifampin is lipid-soluble and penetrates well into leukocytes, macrophages, and peripheral nerves. It passes readily across the placenta and enters fetal circulation.

Rifampin is metabolized in the liver by deacetylation to desacetylrifampin, which is also biologically active but less so than the parent compound. Both the unaltered drug and the deacetylated metabolite are excreted in the bile. Unaltered drug is reabsorbed from the intestine in an enterohepatic cycle, but the metabolite is very poorly reabsorbed. Eventually, most of the administered dose is eliminated in the feces.

A small fraction (10 to 20 percent) of the dose is excreted in the urine, mostly in the form of desacetylrifampin. The dosage of rifampin does not have to be modified in the presence of renal failure. However, when hepatic function is impaired, the dosage should be adjusted.

The elimination half-life of rifampin shortens progressively during the first 7 to 10 days of therapy. The drug induces hepatic microsomal enzymes which increase its own rate of metabolism. The half-life of rifampin, which is 3.5 h at the onset of therapy, decreases to 2.0 h after daily administration for 1 to 2 weeks and remains constant thereafter.

Adverse Effects   In general, rifampin is a well-tolerated drug. Nausea, vomiting, and abdominal pain are uncommon. Asymptomatic transaminase elevation may occur during the first few weeks of therapy; however, the incidence of overt hepatitis is less than 1 percent.

Other adverse effects of rifampin include allergic reactions, drug fever, and rare instances of thrombocytopenia, leukopenia, hemolytic anemia, and acute renal failure.

Because rifampin induces hepatic microsomal enzymes, it may accelerate clearance of drugs metabolized by the liver. These include methadone, warfarin, glucocorticoids, estrogens, propranolol, quinidine, cardiac glycosides, cyclosporin, and the sulfonylureas. By accelerating estrogen metabolism, rifampin may interfere with the effectiveness of oral contraceptives.

Rifampin and its metabolite give a red-orange color to urine, saliva, sweat, and tears. Patients should be warned of this and of possible permanent discoloration of soft contact lenses.

Clinical Use   Rifampin is a most effective drug for treatment of both pulmonary and extrapulmonary tuberculosis, including tuberculous meningitis. Like isoniazid, rifampin should never be used alone for the treatment of tuberculosis. Rifampin is also included in chemotherapeutic regimens of various forms of leprosy.

Rifampin is effective in eliminating meningococci and *H. influenzae* from the pharynx. It is the drug of choice for chemoprophylaxis of meningococcal disease and *H. influenzae* meningitis. Short-term chemoprophylaxis is usually associated with very few side effects except for red discoloration of urine and permanent staining of soft contact lenses.

Rifampin combined with nafcillin or vancomycin is the treatment of choice for prosthetic valve endocarditis due to *Staph. epidermidis*. In patients with *Staph. aureus* endocarditis, rifampin may be a useful addition to nafcillin or vancomycin if there are myocardial, splenic, or brain abscesses.

Ethambutol

Ethambutol was discovered in 1961 while randomly selected synthetic compounds were being screened for antimycobacterial activity. Its structural formula is

$$\text{H—}\underset{\underset{C_2H_5}{|}}{\overset{\overset{CH_2OH}{|}}{C}}\text{—NH—CH}_2\text{—CH}_2\text{—HN—}\underset{\underset{CH_2OH}{|}}{\overset{\overset{C_2H_5}{|}}{C}}\text{—H}$$

Ethambutol

Mechanism of Action   Ethambutol has a bacteriostatic action against *M. tuberculosis*, but the precise mechanism is not known. The drug inhibits the transfer of mycotic acids into the cell wall of *Mycobacterium smegmatis*. This effect is rapid and occurs at low concentrations. An effect on the transfer of mycolic acid to the cell wall would explain the selective toxicity of ethambutol for mycobacteria.

Antimicrobial Activity   Ethambutol is only active against mycobacteria; all other bacteria are completely resistant. It is active against *M. tuberculosis*, *M. kansasii*, and most strains of *M. scrofulaceum*. The sensitivity of other atypical mycobacteria is variable.

Mechanism of Resistance   The incidence of primary resistance to ethambutol is less than 1 percent in the United States. Secondary resistance develops when the drug is used without another effective agent for the treatment of tuberculosis. The mechanism of resistance to ethambutol is not known.

Pharmacokinetics   Approximately 80 percent of orally administered ethambutol is absorbed from the gastrointestinal tract.

Ethambutol is 20 to 30 percent bound to plasma proteins. It is widely distributed throughout the body and enters into macrophages. Penetration through noninflamed meninges is poor, but therapeutic concentrations are attained in the CSF when the meninges are inflamed. The drug penetrates into pulmonary parenchyma and caseous tuberculous lesions, where the levels achieved are 5 to 10 times and 3 times the simultaneous serum concentrations, respectively. Ethambutol readily passes across the placenta and enters fetal circulation.

Most of the absorbed ethambutol is excreted unchanged in the urine. Up to 15 percent is converted into various inactive metabolites which are also excreted in the urine. The elimination half-life of ethambutol is 4.0 h; it is prolonged to 7.0 h in patients with renal failure.

Adverse Effects   Ethambutol is generally well tolerated and produces very few adverse reactions. Retrobulbar neuritis is the most important untoward effect. Symptoms include decreased visual acuity, central scotoma, and color blindness, but sometimes the only change is constriction of visual fields. Vision may be unilaterally or bilaterally affected, and the degree of impairment is related to the duration of therapy after the symptoms first become apparent. Retrobulbar neuritis is completely reversible if ethambutol is promptly withdrawn; permanent impairment of vision may result if the drug is continued long after the onset of symptoms. Visual toxicity of ethambutol is dose related; the incidence is 1 to 2 percent with the currently recommended doses. Patients receiving ethambutol should be instructed to report any visual disturbances. Testing of visual acuity, visual fields, and color discrimination is recommended every 4 to 6 weeks.

Other adverse effects of ethambutol include allergic reactions, drug fever, gastrointestinal upset, hyperuricemia, arthralgia, and peripheral neuritis. The latter manifests itself by numbness and tingling in extremities, which disappear when the drug is withdrawn.

Clinical Use   Ethambutol is an effective drug for the treatment of tuberculosis. It is used mainly as a "companion" drug with either isoniazid or rifampin to prevent emergence of resistance. If isoniazid resistance is suspected, ethambutol is added to the currently recommended initial regimen (isoniazid-rifampin or isoniazid-rifampin-pyrazinamide) until susceptibility tests are completed. If the isolate is sensitive to isoniazid and rifampin, ethambutol is discontinued.

Pyrazinamide

Pyrazinamide, a derivative of nicotinamide, was synthesized in 1952. Its structural formula is

Pyrazinamide

Pyrazinamide has a bacterial action against tubercle bacilli in vitro when the pH of the growth medium is slightly acidic (pH 5.0 to 5.5); it has little or no activity at neutral pH. The drug is active against organisms in macrophages, due to the acidic environment within the phagosomes. It has no activity against organisms which reside in cavitary pulmonary lesions and multiply rapidly at a neutral pH. The precise mechanism of action of pyrazinamide is not known.

Pyrazinamide is completely absorbed from the gastrointestinal tract. It is widely distributed throughout the body and readily penetrates into macrophages. Pyrazinamide enters into the CSF, at least in patients with tuberculous meningitis.

Most of the absorbed pyrazinamide is metabolized in the liver, and the metabolites are excreted in the urine. Only 3 to 4 percent of the dose is excreted unchanged in the urine. The elimination half-life of pyrazinamide is 9.0 h.

Hepatotoxicity is the most serious adverse effect of pyrazinamide. Asymptomatic elevations of transaminases are relatively common, but overt hepatitis is infrequent. Hepatotoxicity of pyrazinamide is dose-related. With the currently recommended doses it is quite uncommon.

The other main side effect of pyrazinamide is arthralgia associated with raised serum uric acid. This is due to the interference of pyrazinoic acid (a metabolite of pyrazinamide) with the tubular secretion of uric acid.

Because of the high incidence of hepatotoxicity associated with higher than the currently recommended doses, pyrazinamide was previously regarded as a "reserve drug." In recent years, it has emerged as a first-line drug for the treatment of tuberculosis, particularly in short-course regimens. A 6-month regimen consisting of isoniazid, rifampin, and pyrazinamide given for 2 months followed by isoniazid and rifampin for 4 months is as effective as a 9-month regimen consisting of isoniazid and rifampin. Continuing pyrazinamide beyond the initial 2 months does not seem to improve the outcome. In contrast to other first-line drugs, pyrazinamide has little ability to prevent emergence of drug resistance.

Streptomycin

Streptomycin was the first clinically effective drug to become available for the treatment of tuberculosis. It is an aminoglycoside antibiotic discussed in Chap. 43. The following brief comments pertain to its antimycobacterial activity and its role in the treatment of tuberculosis.

Streptomycin is active against *M. tuberculosis* and *M. kansasii;* other atypical mycobacteria are only occasionally susceptible. It has a bactericidal effect against extracellular organisms, but it does not enter macrophages and, therefore, has no effect against intracellular mycobacteria.

There are naturally occurring mutants in any large population of tubercle bacilli that are resistant to streptomycin. Such resistant mutants occur with a frequency of one in 10^6 to 10^7 organisms. Use of streptomycin singly for the treatment of tuberculosis leads to development of secondary resistance. Primary resistance to streptomycin is found in 2 to 3 percent of isolates of *M. tuberculosis* in the United States.

The most common serious adverse effect of streptomycin is ototoxicity. This usually results in vertigo and ataxia, but hearing loss may also occur. Streptomycin is significantly less nephrotoxic than other aminoglycosides. The risks of ototoxicity and nephrotoxicity are related both to the cumulative dose and to serum concentrations.

Streptomycin is used primarily for infections caused by isoniazid- or rifampin-resistant organisms. It should be used with extreme caution in the elderly and in patients with renal insufficiency.

Second-Line Drugs

Ethionamide   Ethionamide is a derivative of isonicotinic acid. It is active against *M. tuberculosis* and *M. leprae*. Ethionamide is well absorbed from the gastrointestinal tract. It is metabolized by the liver with metabolites excreted mainly in the urine. Ethionamide causes a high frequency of gastrointestinal side effects (nausea, vomiting, and abdominal pain), often necessitating discontinuation of the drug. Other adverse effects include hepatotoxicity, which occurs in 5 percent of patients, and neurotoxicity (mental disturbances, peripheral neuropathy).

Cycloserine   Cycloserine is an antibiotic isolated from *Streptomyces orchidaceus*. It interferes with the first stage of cell wall synthesis (Chap. 42). Cycloserine is readily absorbed when administered orally. Approximately two-thirds of the drug is excreted unchanged in the urine, and the remainder is metabolized to inactive forms. Cycloserine causes behavioral disturbances in a large number of patients to whom it is administered; seizures and peripheral neuropathy may also occur.

Capreomycin   Capreomycin is a polypeptide antibiotic isolated from *Streptomyces capreolus*. It is active only against mycobacteria. Capreomycin is not absorbed after oral administration and must be administered intramuscularly. About 50 to 60 percent of an administered dose is excreted unchanged in the urine; the remainder is inactivated in the body. Nephrotoxicity and ototoxicity (vertigo, tinnitus, and deafness) are the most serious adverse effects of capreomycin.

Kanamycin   Kanamycin is an aminoglycoside antibiotic isolated from *Streptomyces kanamyceticus*. Ototoxicity and nephrotoxicity are the main adverse effects.

Para-Aminosalicylic Acid (PAS)   PAS has weak bacteriostatic activity against *M. tuberculosis*. It is 85 percent absorbed from the gastrointestinal tract. PAS is excreted in unchanged active form (20 percent) and as metabolites (80 percent) in the urine. The usual dose of the drug (10 to 12 g daily) is associated with a high frequency of gastrointestinal intolerance, which often causes poor patient compliance. In addition, hypersensitivity reactions occur in 5 to 10 percent of patients.

DRUGS FOR TREATMENT OF LEPROSY

Chemotherapy of leprosy, until 1982, consisted of dapsone, which produced gratifying clinical results. With the emergence of both primary and secondary resistance to dapsone as a consequence of its long-term use as monotherapy, it has now become imperative that multidrug regimens be administered to all patients with leprosy. Drugs currently used include dapsone, rifampin, and clofazimine. Ethionamide, a second-line drug for tuberculosis, is active against *Mycobacterium leprae*, but it is not a drug of first choice for inclusion in chemotherapeutic regimens.

Dapsone

Dapsone (4,4-diaminodiphenylsulfone, DDS) is a sulfone which was first introduced for the therapy of leprosy in 1941. Its structural formula is

$$NH_2 - \text{<benzene ring>} - SO_2 - \text{<benzene ring>} - NH_2$$

Dapsone

Dapsone is a structural analog of para-aminobenzoic acid. Its mechanism of action involves competitive inhibition of the enzyme dihydropteroate synthetase, thereby blocking the synthesis of folic acid. Dapsone is weakly bactericidal for *M. leprae*. Secondary resistance may develop years after commencing therapy, mainly in multibacillary leprosy. Primary dapsone resistance occurs with a frequency of 2.5 to 4.0 percent, depending on geographic location.

Dapsone is slowly and nearly completely absorbed from the gastrointestinal tract. It is 70 percent bound to plasma proteins and penetrates readily into tissues and body fluids. Dapsone is acetylated by the same polymorphic *N*-acetyl transferase that acetylates isoniazid. Although the concentration of dapsone is higher in slow acetylators than it is in rapid acetylators, the acetylation phenotype does not affect the overall half-life of the drug. Dapsone is ultimately excreted in the urine, predominantly as glucuronide and sulfate conjugates. Its elimination half-life is 25 to 27 h, but there is wide variation between different individuals (13 to 53 h).

The most common adverse reactions to dapsone are hemolytic anemia and methemoglobinemia. Hemolysis is a dose-related effect and occurs more commonly in persons with glucose-6-phosphate dehydrogenase deficiency. The most serious hematologic side effect is marrow suppression, which is rare, but deaths due to agranulocytosis and aplastic anemia have been reported.

Other adverse effects of dapsone include allergic reactions, drug fever, nausea, vomiting, vertigo, tinnitus, blurred vision, and peripheral neuropathy (predominantly motor). Patients with lepromatous leprosy may develop erythema nodosum leprosum during the first year of therapy. The reaction is characterized by fever and tender erythematous skin nodules, sometimes accompanied by malaise, joint swelling, and immune complex glomerulonephritis.

The only major indication for dapsone continues to be leprosy. For treatment of multibacillary forms of leprosy a triple drug combination of dapsone, rifampin, and clofazimine is recommended. For the paucibacillary forms dapsone combined with rifampin is employed. The combination of dapsone and trimethoprim is effective in the treatment of *Pneumocystis carinii* pneumonia.

Clofazimine

Clofazimine is a substituted iminophenazine that was first shown to be useful for the treatment of leprosy in 1962. It was reserved mainly for the treatment of dapsone-resistant leprosy until 1982, when it was recommended by the World Health Organization as part of the three-drug combination (dapsone, clofazimine, and rifampin) for all multibacillary forms of leprosy. Its structural formula is

Clofazimine

Clofazimine is weakly bactericidal for *M. leprase*. In addition, it is active against *Mycobacterium avium-intracellulare*. Although its mechanism of action is not well understood, there is some evidence that it may act by inhibiting template formation of DNA.

The pharmacokinetics of clofazimine are complex. The rate of absorption from the gastrointestinal tract ranges from 45 to 62 percent. Clofazimine is widely distributed in the body and retained for a long time. It is highly lipophilic and tends to be deposited predominantly in fatty tissue, skin, cells of the reticuloendothelial system, and the distal small intestine at the site of absorption. It is taken up by macrophages throughout the body. Clofazimine is not excreted in the urine or metabolized to any significant extent, biliary excretion appears to be the major route of disposition. The elimination half-life of clofazimine is 70 days. A dose of 100 mg daily has been calculated to eventually result in total accumulation of at least 10 g of the drug in the tissues.

At recommended doses, clofazimine is well tolerated. It causes a red-brown pigmentation of the skin within a few weeks of treatment; this clears gradually over months after withdrawal of the drug. Clofazimine also imparts a red color to urine, sputum, and sweat.

Clofazimine is used in a triple-drug combination (dapsone-rifampin-clofazimine) for the treatment of multibacillary forms of leprosy. It is also recommended, as part of a multidrug regimen, for *M. avium-intracellulare* infections in patients with acquired immunodeficiency syndrome.

BIBLIOGRAPHY

Acocella, G., and R. Conti: "Interaction of Rifampicin with Other Drugs," *Tubercle*, **61**:171–177 (1980).

Alexander, M. R., S. G. Louie, and B. G. Guernsey: "Isoniazid-Associated Hepatitis," *Clin. Pharmacol.*, **1**:148–153 (1982).

Bass, J. B., Jr., L. S. Farer, P. C. Hopewell, and R. F. Jacobs: "Treatment of Tuberculosis and Tuberculosis Infection in Adults and Children," *Am. Rev. Resp. Dis.*, **134**:355–363 (1986).

Foltzer, M. A., and R. E. Reese: "Trimethoprim-Sulfamethoxazole and Other Sulfonamides," *Med. Clin. North Am.*, **71**:1155–1168 (1988).

Grosset, J.: "Bacteriologic Basis of Short-Course Chemotherapy for Tuberculosis," *Clin. Chest Med.*, **1**:231–241 (1980).

Hastings, R. C., and S. G. Franzblau: "Chemotherapy of Leprosy," *Ann. Rev. Pharmacol. Toxicol.*, **28**:231–245 (1988).

Reed, M. D., and J. L. Blumer: "Clinical Pharmacology of Antitubercular Drugs," *Ped. Clin. North Am.*, **30**:177–183 (1983).

Salter, A. J.: "Trimethoprim-Sulfamethoxazole: An Assessment of More Than 12 Years of Use," *Rev. Infect. Dis.*, **4**:196–236 (1982).

Stratton, M. A., and M. T. Reed: "Short-Course Drug Therapy for Tuberculosis," *Clin. Pharm.*, **5**:977–987 (1986).

C H A P T E R 45

Antimycotic and Antiviral Drugs

Gerald H. Sterling

ANTIMYCOTIC AGENTS

For therapeutic purposes, fungal infections are divided into three categories: dermatophytic, mucocutaneous, and systemic. Dermatophytic fungal infections are the most common and involve the skin, hair, and nails; common infections include athlete's foot, ringworm, and *Tinea cruris*. Most infections can be treated with over-the-counter or prescription topical agents such as tolnaftate, undecylenic acid, haloprogin, clotrimazole, and miconazole. For deep infection, particularly of the nail beds, griseofulvin administered orally is the drug of choice. Ketoconazole, an imidazole derivative is being investigated for chronic oral treatment of dermatophytes.

Mucocutaneous infections, mostly *Candida albicans*, involve the moist skin and mucous membranes (e.g., gastrointestinal tract, perianal and vulvovaginal areas). Agents used topically include amphotericin B, miconazole, clotrimazole, and nystatin. Ketoconazole, administered orally, is safe and effective for treatment of chronic infections.

Systemic fungal infections occur much less frequently, but they are a serious problem because they are usually chronic in nature and difficult to diagnose. Also, any drug given systemically has the possibility of more severe adverse effects. Amphotericin B is a reliable drug for most infections, despite its toxicity. It is commonly used in combination with flucytosine. Ketoconazole is most useful for chronic infections, since it is both effective and well tolerated. Potassium iodide is available specifically for treatment of *Sporothrix schenckii*.

Amphotericin B

Amphotericin B is a large polyene antibiotic derived from *Streptomyces nodosus*. The compound has a broad spectrum of antifungal activity, including *Candida albicans*, *Leishmania brasiliensis*, *Mycobacterium leprae*, *Histoplasma capsulatum*, *Blastomyces dermatitidus*, and *Coccidioides immitis*. It has both fungistatic and fungicidal activity, dependent on the dose used. Its chemical structure is shown in Fig. 45-1.

Mechanism of Action The antifungal activity of amphotericin B is due to its binding to sterols, particularly ergosterol, in the cell membrane of sensitive fungi (see Table 45-1). This interaction creates pores in the membrane and increases membrane permeability to small molecules, thus reducing the function of the membrane as an osmotic barrier and making the cell more susceptible to destruction. Amphotericin B is active in growing and resting cells. The compound, however, is not highly selective and will interfere with membrane function of the mammalian host cell.

Pharmacokinetics Amphotericin B is poorly absorbed from the gastrointestinal tract due to its large, bulky structure. When given by intravenous infusion, peak plasma levels are attained very rapidly. The plasma half-life is 24 h, though active drug can be detected in the plasma for up to 7 weeks after the last administered dose. The persistence of the drug in the body is consistent with its uptake into tissue reservoirs from which the drug is later slowly released.

Only 2 to 5 percent of the drug is excreted in the

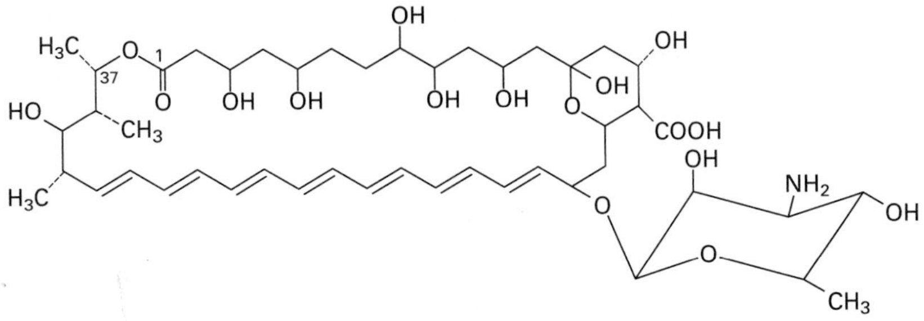

Amphotericin B

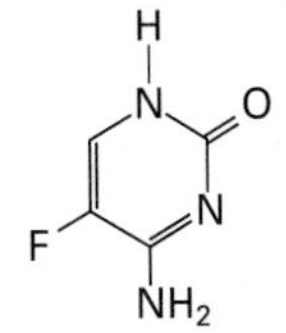

Flucytosine

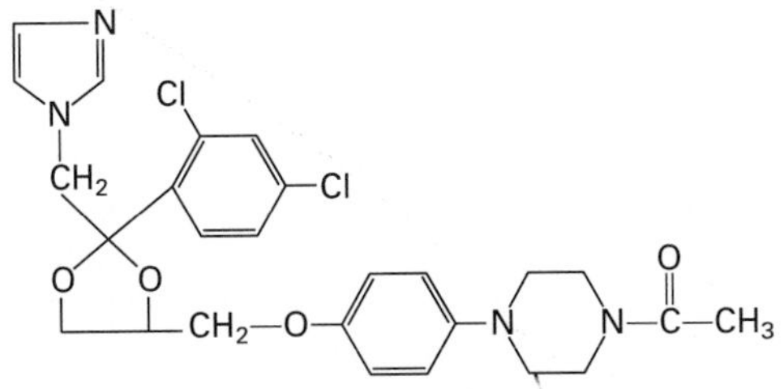

Ketoconazole

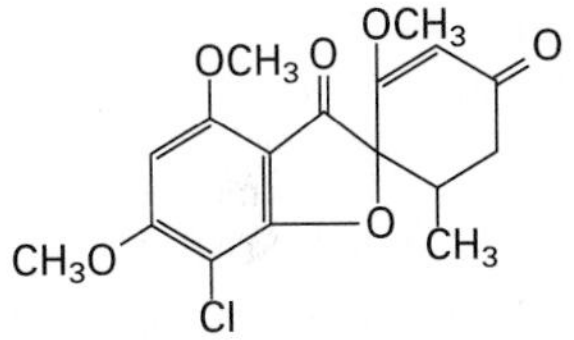

Griseofulvin

FIGURE 45-1 Structures of common antimycotic agents.

TABLE 45-1 Mechanisms of antifungal agents

Drugs	Mechanism of action
Polyene antimycotics Amphotericin B Nystatin	Bind to sterols (e.g., ergosterol) in cell membranes, forming pores or channels which increase membrane permeability, making the cell more susceptible to destruction.
Flucytosine	Converted to 5-fluorouracil and 5-fluorodeoxyuridylic acid in sensitive fungi. 5-Fluorodeoxyuridylic acid inhibits thymidylate synthetase. Triphosphate of 5-fluorouracil is incorporated into RNA.
Griseofulvin	Inhibits fungal cell mitosis by disrupting the mitotic spindle.
Imidazole antimycotics Ketoconazole Miconazole Clotrimazole Econazole Butoconazole	Inhibit ergosterol biosynthesis to destabilize the membrane.

urine unchanged. The distribution of amphotericin B is limited; it crosses the blood-brain barrier poorly, though this may increase in the presence of inflammation. Thus the drug may have to be administered by intrathecal or intraventricular routes for fungal meningitis. It is also available for topical administration.

Adverse Reactions Most patients receiving intravenous amphotericin B exhibit the side effects associated with this form of administration. Within 3 h after infusion is begun, an acute hypersensitivity reaction may occur. Symptoms include fever, chills, headache, nausea, vomiting, abdominal pain, hypotension, flushing, sweating, and delirium. Hydrocortisone, added to the infusion, may reduce this reaction. Renal impairment is probably the most prevalent adverse reaction in patients receiving amphotericin B. This effect is time- and dose-dependent; it is reversible if recognized early enough and the dose of the drug reduced. Other adverse reactions may include fatigue, enteritis, thrombocytopenia, hypokalemia, and phlebitis at the injection site. Intrathecal administration may also produce paresthesias and nerve palsies.

Therapeutic Uses Despite its many adverse reactions, amphotericin B remains the primary drug for therapy of acute, severe, systemic fungal infections. It is useful topically for local dermatophytic and mucocutaneous infections. Despite its poor absorption from the gastrointestinal tract, amphotericin B is available for oral administration in combination with tetracycline, but only for its local effects.

Nystatin

Nystatin was isolated in 1949 from *Streptomyces* and was the first antimycotic antibiotic to be discovered. It is a polyene antibiotic, structurally similar to amphotericin B. Nystatin has a fairly broad spectrum of activity including yeast and various fungi. The mechanism of nystatin's antifungal activity is similar to that of amphotericin B in that it binds to sterols in fungal cell membranes (Table 45-1). This increases membrane permeability, making the cell more susceptible to destruction.

Nystatin is available for topical or oral administration. When used topically, the drug does not cross the skin or mucous membranes. Absorption from the gastrointestinal tract is negligible following oral adminis-

tration. Therefore, nystatin has few adverse reactions when given by either route. Used topically, the only potential problem is local burning and itching. Large doses, administered orally, can produce gastrointestinal upset, including nausea, vomiting, and diarrhea. Nystatin is not available for systemic administration due to its renal toxicity. Therapy with nystatin is limited to the prevention and topical treatment of superficial candidal infections of the skin and mucous membranes including gums, gastrointestinal tract, rectum, and vagina.

Flucytosine

Flucytosine is a fluorinated pyrimidine derivative (see Fig. 45-1). Its spectrum of activity is narrower than that of amphotericin B; it includes *Candidiasis*, *Cryptococcosis*, and *Chromomycosis*. Clinical use has been disappointing due to a high incidence of resistance. It does, however, have a synergistic effect when used in combination with amphotericin B.

Mechanism of Action (Table 45-1) Flucytosine is converted in sensitive fungi to 5-fluorouracil. This compound is further biotransformed to 5-fluorodeoxyuridylic acid, an inhibitor of thymidylate synthetase and thus DNA synthesis. The triphosphate of 5-fluorouracil can also be incorporated into and produce defective RNA. This mechanism is fairly selective, since mammalian cells do not convert large amounts of flucytosine to 5-fluorouracil.

Pharmacokinetics Flucytosine is well absorbed from the gastrointestinal tract and is therefore used by the oral route. It is well distributed throughout the body. The plasma half-life is 3 to 6 h. Approximately 80 percent of the drug is excreted in the urine unchanged. Therefore the drug must be used with extreme caution in patients with renal impairment. The physician should also be aware that amphotericin B, which can reduce renal function, may increase the toxicity of flucytosine when they are used in combination.

Adverse Reactions The most common adverse reactions of flucytosine include nausea, vomiting, diarrhea, and rash. Anemia, leukopenia, thrombocytopenia, and elevation of hepatic enzymes, BUN, and creatinine have been reported. Therefore frequent monitoring of hepatic function and hematologic status is indicated during therapy. Less common reactions include sedation, vertigo, headache, and confusion.

Therapeutic Use Flucytosine is primarily used in combination with amphotericin B for treatment of selected systemic fungal infections. The agent is rarely used alone.

Griseofulvin

The spectrum of antimycotic activity of griseofulvin includes dermatophytic infections of the skin, nails, and scalp. It is fungistatic. The compound is inactive against yeast, bacteria, and fungi causing deep, systemic mycotic infections. Resistance to its effectiveness can develop.

Mechanism of Action The mechanism of griseofulvin's antimycotic activity appears to be its ability to inhibit fungal cell mitosis, thus producing multinucleated defective cells (Table 45-1). It acts by binding to microtubules, disrupting the mitotic spindle.

Pharmacokinetics Griseofulvin, administered orally, undergoes variable absorption from the gastrointestinal tract. Due to its lipid solubility, absorption is enhanced when taken with a fatty meal. Its plasma half-life is approximately 24 h. The drug distributes to growing nails and skin, binding to keratin and making the cells resistant to fungal infection. Therefore, only new growth is protected against the fungal infection. The drug is biotransformed in the liver, mostly to 6-methyl-griseofulvin, which is slowly excreted in the urine.

Adverse Reactions Serious adverse reactions to griseofulvin are rare. Common side effects include headache, lethargy, fatigue, blurred vision, insomnia, and gastrointestinal upset. Hepatotoxicity has been reported. Griseofulvin reduces the effectiveness of oral anticoagulants by enhancing their metabolism. Concomitant use of barbiturates enhances the metabolism of griseofulvin and may require an increase in dose.

Therapeutic Use Griseofulvin is administered orally for treatment of dermatophytic fungal infections. Since it does not destroy the fungal cells, but only inhibits new growth, the compound must be given for prolonged periods, usually several months.

Imidazoles

Several imidazole analogs are available for treatment of fungal infections. Those agents used for systemic administration include ketoconazole and miconazole; those used topically include miconazole, clotrimazole, econazole, and butoconazole.

Mechanism of Action The imidazoles' antifungal activity is due to their ability to selectively increase fungal cell membrane permeability by interfering with the biosynthesis of sterols, particularly ergosterol (Table 45-1). They are therefore, unlike amphotericin B, only effective in growing cells. Host cells are not affected by this action, since humans use exogenous preformed sterols.

Ketoconazole

Ketoconazole has broad antifungal activity including many candidal infections. The chemical structure is shown in Fig. 45-1.

Pharmacokinetics Ketoconazole is readily absorbed from the gastrointestinal tract under acidic conditions. Agents that reduce gastric acidity (e.g., anticholinergics, H_2 blockers, antacids) reduce absorption and decrease its therapeutic effectiveness. Peak plasma levels occur approximately 2 h after oral administration. The drug is biotransformed in the liver, metabolites being excreted in the urine. Ketoconazole does not penetrate well into the cerebrospinal fluid which limits its effectiveness in treatment of central nervous system infections.

Adverse Reactions The most frequent side effects of ketoconazole are nausea, vomiting, and diarrhea. Other effects include rash, itching, dizziness, constipation, fever, chills, and headache. Ketoconazole also has antiandrogenic effects by reducing testosterone synthesis. Gynecomastia and impotence have been reported. Hepatocellular toxicity, including fatalities, has been associated with ketoconazole. Hepatic function should be monitored during drug therapy.

Therapeutic Uses Ketoconazole has been shown to be most effective in chronic suppressive therapy. It is very effective in treatment of chronic mucocutaneous candidiasis and is under investigation for dermatophytic infections, administered by the oral route. Therapy may be for up to 1 year. Slow improvement makes ketoconazole less useful for acute, severe systemic mycoses.

Miconazole

Miconazole is another synthetic antimycotic imidazole derivative designed initially for topical treatment of candidal and dermatophytic infections of the skin and for vaginal candidiasis. Its primary use is still topical. Miconazole, administered intravenously, is highly toxic and therefore only used for severe systemic fungal infections in which patients do not respond or cannot tolerate amphotericin B. All other systemic use has been taken over by ketoconazole. Adverse reactions to topically administered miconazole include local burning, itching, and rash. Intravenous administration can cause nausea, vomiting, and anemia. Anaphylactoid reactions, central nervous system toxicity, hyponatremia, and phlebitis have been reported.

Clotrimazole

Clotrimazole is closely related to miconazole. It has broad antifungal activity and is very effective when applied topically to the skin and vaginal mucosa. Clinical improvement from vulvovaginal candidiasis usually occurs within 1 week. Other dermatophytes may take longer. Clotrimazole is also available as a topical oral form (troche) for treatment of oropharyngeal candidiasis. Adverse reactions from topical administration are local and include erythema, blistering, edema, pruritus, and urticaria. Used topically, less than 0.5 percent is absorbed through the intact skin, 5 to 10 percent from the vagina.

Econazole

Econazole is a derivative of miconazole, useful topically for the treatment of tinea pedis, tinea cruris, tinea corporus, tinea versicolor, and cutaneous candidasis. When applied topically, less than 1 percent is absorbed systemically. Therefore, adverse reactions are local, consisting of burning, itching, and rash.

Butoconazole

Butoconazole is an imidazole derivative particularly effective against vaginal infections produced by *Candida albicans* and *Candida tropicalis*. It is only used topically, and therefore only local adverse reactions have been reported.

Additional Antimycotic Compounds: Topically Applied Agents

Though orally administered griseofulvin is very useful in the treatment of dermatophytic infections, many mild or superficial infections can be treated effectively with topical agents, thus causing less adverse reactions. Such compounds shown to be effective include undecylenic acid, tolnaftate, haloprogin, and ciclopirox olamine in addition to miconazole and clotrimazole, which have previously been mentioned.

Preparations

Amphotericin B (Fungizone) is available in a vial containing 50 mg, which must be dissolved for intravenous administration; and in a cream, lotion, and ointment containing 3% amphotericin B.

Butoconazole (Femstat) is available as a 2% vaginal cream.

Econazole (Spectazide) is available as a 1% cream.

Clotrimazole (Lotrimin, Mycelex) is supplied as a 1% cream, lotion, or solution, 100-mg vaginal tablets, and 10-mg troches.

Flucytosine (Ancobon) is available in capsules containing 250 and 500 mg.

Griseofulvin (Fulvicin U/F and P/G, Grifulvin V, Grisactin) is available in capsules containing 125 or 250 mg, in tablets containing 250 or 500 mg, in tablets (microsized) containing 125 to 330 mg, and in a suspension containing 125 mg per 5 mL.

Haloprogin (Halotex) is available as a 1% cream or solution.

Ketoconazole (Nizoral) is supplied in 200-mg tablets for oral administration.

Miconazole (Monistat, Micatin) is available as a nitrate salt in a topical cream (2%), spray, powder, or lotion. It is also supplied as a 2% vaginal cream and vaginal suppositories (100 and 200 mg). Miconazole is available as a solution (10 mg/mL) for infusion.

Nystatin (Mycostatin, Nilstat) is available in an oral suspension containing 100,000 units/mL, in oral tablets containing 500,000 units, in topical cream, lotion, ointment, and powder containing 100,000 units/g, and in vaginal tablets containing 100,000 units each.

Tolnaftate (Aftate, Tinactin) is available as a 1% cream, gel, powder, aerosol powder, topical solution, or topical aerosol.

Undecylenic acid (Desenex) is available as a cream, foam, ointment, powder, soap, and solution.

ANTIVIRAL AGENTS

The chemotherapy of viral infections has been approached by three different modalities. These include (1) prophylactic immunization, (2) use of an endogenous antiviral substance (i.e., interferon), and (3) antiviral drugs. Immunization has made great strides in the prevention of many viral infections; among those for which vaccines have been produced include measles, mumps, polio, rubella, smallpox, and specific types of influenza. Interferons are a group of endogenous antiviral substances produced by lymphocytes and viral-infected cells. Interferons and inducers of endogenous synthesis are currently being evaluated. Though clinical studies have demonstrated effectiveness in specific instances, the ultimate use of interferons has not yet been determined. Interferons are discussed in more detail in Chap. 41.

Progress in the development of clinically useful antiviral agents has only recently made significant strides in the treatment of herpes simplex virus and, more recently, of acquired immunodeficiency syndrome (AIDS). These drugs act by inhibiting viral cell multiplication.

There are three stages to multiplication of viruses: (1) adsorption, penetration, and uncoating as the virus enters the host cell and sheds its protective coat; (2) synthesis of viral components; and (3) assembly and release of the virus which can destroy or permanently change the cell (Fig. 45-2). The antiviral drugs currently available which effectively interfere with viral multiplication are amantadine, vidarabine, trifluridine, idoxuridine, acyclovir, ribavirin, and zidovudine.

Amantadine

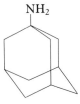

Amantadine

Amantadine is a synthetic stable amine with an unusual structure. The compound has a very narrow spectrum of antiviral activity and is only indicated in the treatment or prophylaxis of influenza A virus. The prophylactic use of amantadine is considered in high-risk patients, such as elderly persons in nursing homes, during influenza A epidemics. It is also used for treatment of Parkinson's disease.

Mechanism of Action The exact mechanism of amantadine's antiviral activity is not fully understood. Amantadine is thought to inhibit the adsorption of viral particles to host cells, resulting in delayed penetration of the virus into the cell and/or inhibition of uncoating (Fig. 45-2). Recent studies have demonstrated that the drug may also inhibit virus assembly.

Pharmacokinetics Amantadine is rapidly and completely absorbed following oral administration. The elimination half-life is 12 to 36 h, with peak levels occurring within 2 to 4 h. Amantadine is not significantly biotransformed; approximately 90 percent is eliminated unchanged in the urine.

Adverse Reactions Amantadine is fairly well tolerated. The major adverse reactions when used as an antiviral drug primarily involve the central nervous system. The reactions include confusion, ataxia, sleep disorders, tumors, and hallucinations. Anticholinergic effects have also been reported. Anorexia, nausea, vomiting, and orthostatic hypotension may also occur. Occasionally, amantadine may cause livedo reticularis, edema, and slurred speech. Generally, the adverse reactions are dose-related and reversible. The drug increases susceptibility to rubella and is therefore contraindicated in patients exposed to rubella. It is excreted in breast milk and thus should not be given to nursing mothers. Animal studies have demonstrated teratogenic effects.

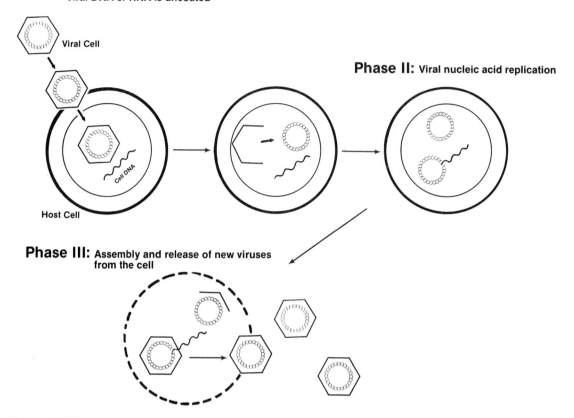

Phase I: Virus Adsorbs to and penetrates the cell
Viral DNA or RNA is uncoated

Viral Cell

Phase II: Viral nucleic acid replication

Cell DNA

Host Cell

Phase III: Assembly and release of new viruses
from the cell

Phase I inhibitor	
Amantadine	Blocks adsorption and penetration.
Phase II inhibitors	
Acyclovir	Triphosphate (acyclo GTP) competitively inhibits viral DNA polymerase. It also incorporates into DNA, acting as a chain terminator.
Vidarabine	Triphosphate inhibits viral DNA polymerase.
Trifluoridine	Triphosphate inhibits viral DNA polymerase.
Idoxuridine	Triphosphate inhibits viral DNA polymerase and incorporates into DNA viruses.
Ribaviron	Reduces nucleic acid synthesis. Exact mechanism is unknown.
Zidovudine	Interferes with replication. Exact mechanism is unknown.

FIGURE 45-2   Viral cell multiplication.

Acyclovir

Acyclovir [acycloguanosine, 9-(2-hydroxyethoxy-methyl)guanine] is a nucleoside analog of the pyrimidine, guanosine. It has the following chemical structure, which includes a linear (acyclic) side chain instead of a cyclic sugar:

Acyclovir

Mechanism of Action The mechanism of acyclovir's antiviral activity involves its conversion to the triphosphate and subsequent inhibition of viral DNA synthesis; its activity is highly selective (Fig. 45-2). The compound enters herpes virus–infected cells and is phosphorylated to the monophosphate by herpes virus–induced thymidine kinase; uninfected cells do not use acyclovir as a substrate. The monophosphate is further converted into the diphosphate and to the triphosphate (acyclo GTP). Acyclo GTP is a competitive inhibitor of herpes viral DNA polymerase and is also incorporated into viral DNA, where it functions as a chain terminator, thus preventing the further elongation of the DNA molecule and therefore viral replication. Other antiviral mechanisms may be involved against cytomegalovirus and Epstein-Barr virus.

Pharmacokinetics Acyclovir is available for topical, oral, and intravenous administration. Transcutaneous absorption is limited; therefore, no drug is detectable in blood or urine following topical use. Absorption of acyclovir from the gastrointestinal tract following oral administration is limited (15 to 30 percent); the concentration of drug in the blood is much lower than following intravenous administration. Acyclovir is widely distributed in tissues and body fluids; concentration in cerebrospinal fluid is approximately 50 percent of plasma values. Plasma protein binding is relatively low. The major route of elimination of acyclovir is renal excretion of unchanged drug by glomerular filtration and tubular secretion; this accounts for 60 to 90 percent of the intravenous dose. Therefore, plasma half-life and total body clearance are dependent on renal function. The only major urinary metabolite is 9-carboxymethoxymethylguanine, which may account for up to 14 percent of the dose. Plasma half-life in a patient with normal renal function is 2.5 to 3.5 h. Probenecid, which alters the tubular secretion of acyclovir, reduces its urinary excretion and thus increases its plasma half-life.

Therapeutic Use In vitro, acyclovir has been shown to be effective against herpes simplex, varicella zoster, Epstein-Barr virus, and, to a lesser extent, cytomegalovirus. It has proven effective in the treatment of mucocutaneous herpes and genital and disseminated adult herpes simplex. Though not yet approved, it has been shown to be effective in therapy of herpes encephalitis, neonatal herpes, varicella zoster, and as an ophthalmic solution in herpes keratitis.

Acyclovir ointment is indicated in the management of initial herpes genitalis and in limited non-life-threatening cutaneous herpes simplex virus infections in immunocompromised patients. The compound produces a decrease in healing time and duration of viral shedding and pain. There is no evidence of clinical benefit in patients with recurrent herpes genitalis or herpes labialis.

Oral acyclovir is indicated in the treatment of initial episodes and treatment or suppression of recurrent episodes of genital herpes infection and in varicella zoster. Intravenous administration is indicated for the treatment of initial and recurrent mucosal and cutaneous herpes simplex infections in immunocompromised adults and children. It is also indicated for severe initial clinical episodes of herpes genitalis in patients who are not immunocompromised.

Adverse Reactions Only local adverse reactions occur with acyclovir ointment. These include mild pain, transient burning and stinging, pruritus, and rash. The most common adverse reactions to oral administration of the drug are nausea, vomiting, and headache. Less frequent reactions include diarrhea, dizziness, anorexia, fatigue, edema, skin rash, leg pain, adenopathy, and sore throat. Acyclovir may also cause fever, palpitations, acne, and depression.

The most frequent adverse reactions to intravenous acyclovir are inflammation or phlebitis at the injection site, transient elevation of serum creatinine, and rash or hives. Less frequent reactions include diaphoresis, hematuria, hypotension, headache, and nausea. Administered systemically, the drug is well tolerated.

Vidarabine

Chemically, vidarabine (adenine arabinoside) is a stereoisomer of adenosine. Its chemical structure includes an arabinoside rather than a ribose sugar (see top of page 642).

Vidarabine, like acyclovir, is converted to the mono-, di-, and triphosphate in virus-infected cells. Vidarabine triphosphate inhibits DNA polymerase, thus reducing DNA synthesis (Fig. 45-2). It is fairly selective for viral DNA polymerase.

Vidarabine is administered either intravenously or topically. It cannot be given by subcutaneous or intra-

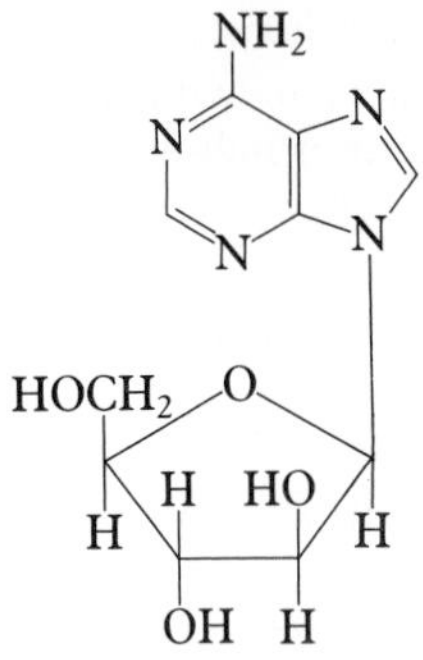

NH$_2$

Vidarabine

muscular routes due to its low solubility and poor absorption. When given intravenously, the drug is infused for 12 to 24 h; plasma half-life is approximately 4 h. The compound is deaminated to arabinosylhypoxanthine, which is primarily excreted into the urine; only 1 to 3 percent appears in the urine as parent compound.

Vidarabine is useful as an ophthalmic preparation for topical treatment of herpes simplex keratitis. It is not used for treatment of herpes simplex infection of the skin or mucous membranes. It is also available for intravenous administration in the treatment of herpes simplex encephalitis, other severe systemic herpes infections, and varicella zoster. Recently acyclovir has replaced vidarabine as the drug of choice in treatment of herpes simplex encephalitis and may be preferred in patients with varicella zoster.

Used systemically, the most common adverse reactions include anorexia, nausea, vomiting, and diarrhea. Occasionally, the drug may cause tremors, dizziness, hallucinations, confusion, psychosis, and ataxia. The drug may also decrease the hemoglobin and hematocrit, the white blood count, and the platelet count. Elevation in serum glutamic oxaloacetic transaminase (SGOT) has also been observed. In addition, the drug may cause weight loss, pruritus, rash, and hematemesis. Major adverse reactions of vidarabine when applied to the eye are rare. Some localized burning and itching may occur.

The drug is contraindicated in patients who develop hypersensitivity reactions. The drug should not be given to patients susceptible to fluid overloading, cerebral edema, or with impaired renal function. Those patients with reduced renal function may require a lower dose of the drug.

Trifluridine

Trifluridine (trifluorothymidine) is a halogenated thymidine derivative used as an ophthalmic solution for herpes simplex–induced keratoconjunctivitis. Its mechanism of action is similar to acyclovir and vidarabine (Fig. 45-2). It is converted to the triphosphate, which inhibits DNA polymerase. Adverse reactions include local burning or stinging; no systemic effects have been reported following topical use. The drug appears to be as effective, yet better tolerated, as idoxuridine.

Idoxuridine

Idoxuridine is a halogenated derivative of deoxyuridine. Its structure is as follows:

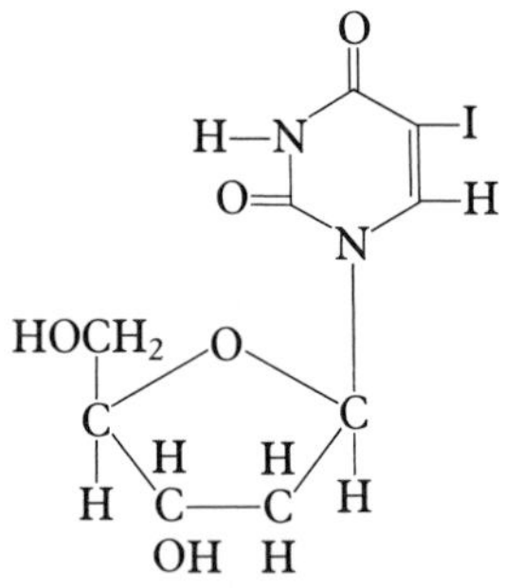

Idoxuridine

The major action of idoxuridine is on DNA viruses; it has little or no effect on RNA viruses. The primary action of idoxuridine is the inhibition of the replication of DNA viruses by its incorporation into the virus.

The major use of the drug is in the treatment of herpes simplex keratitis. It is used topically on the eye. Because of its severe adverse reactions, the drug is not given systemically.

When applied topically to the eye, idoxuridine may cause the following adverse reactions: inflammatory edema of the eyelids, photophobia, lacrimal duct occlusion, and contact dermatitis.

Ribavirin

Ribavirin is a synthetic nucleoside analog. Its chemical structure is shown on page 643.

In vitro, ribavirin is effective against several DNA and RNA viruses, including respiratory syncytial

$$H_2NC \overset{\displaystyle O}{\underset{}{\parallel}}$$

Ribavirin

virus (RSV), herpes simplex, and influenza A and B viruses. It is approved for aerosol treatment of infants and young children with severe RSV infections. The compound acts by interfering with guanidine monophosphate. Thus nucleic acid synthesis is reduced. Adverse reactions may include rash, headache, and fatigue. The drug may precipitate on the valves and tubing of a mechanical respirator, causing malfunctions. This may limit its use in those individuals who would most benefit from it. The drug has been used experimentally in AIDS patients, with mixed results.

Zidovudine

Zidovudine (formerly azidothymidine or AZT) has recently been approved for the treatment of AIDS patients with *Pneumocystis carinii* pneumonia or advanced AIDS-related complex. The drug interferes with HIV (human T-cell lymphotropic virus, HTLV-III) replication. Zidovudine prolongs patients' lives, but it has many toxic effects. Adverse reactions include insomnia, myalgia, nausea, severe headache, anemia, and neutropenia. Many other agents, including ribavirin, ampligen, dideoxycytidine, and foscarnet, are currently being investigated in the therapy of AIDS.

Current Use of Antiviral Agents

The development of effective, clinically useful antiviral agents has been difficult, since drugs inhibiting viral replication would also have effects on the host cells. However, over the past few years several effective agents have been placed on the market. A summary of drugs effective in treatment of various viral infections is presented in Table 45-2.

TABLE 45-2   Summary of treatment of viral infections

Viral infection	Drugs available
Herpes simplex	
Keratitis	Trifluridine*, vidarabine Idoxuridine
Genital	Acyclovir
Encephalitis	Acyclovir[†], vidarabine
Neonatal	Acyclovir[†], vidarabine
Disseminated, adult	Acyclovir*, vidarabine
Influenza A	Amantadine
Varicella zoster	Vidarabine, acyclovir[†]
Respiratory syncytial virus	Ribavirin
Acquired immunodeficiency syndrome	Zidovudine

*Currently accepted drug of choice.
†Not yet approved for this use by FDA.

Acyclovir has been a major advancement in the therapy of herpes simplex and is useful by topical and systemic administration. It is also considered useful in treating varicella zoster infections. Vidarabine is approved for treating herpes simplex encephalitis, shingles, and chicken pox in immunocompromised patients and neonatal herpes. It is useful in treating acyclovir-resistant strains of herpes simplex virus. Trifluridine is used topically for treatment of herpes simplex keratitis. Amantadine has very specific use in prophylaxis and treatment of influenza A virus. Ribavirin is used in a hospital setting for treatment of RSV infection in specific patients.

Zidovudine is currently the only drug approved for the treatment of HIV infections responsible for AIDS. However, currently numerous agents are in clinical trials, and much research is being conducted for a more effective agent in treatment of AIDS.

Preparations

Acyclovir (Zovirax) is available as an ointment (5%) for topical administration, 200-mg capsules for oral administration, and as a sterile powder equivalent to 500 mg in 10-mL containers for intravenous administration.

Amantadine (Symmetrel) is available in 100-mg capsules and in a syrup containing 50 mg in 5 mL.

Idoxuridine (Dendrid, Herplex, Stoxil) is available as a 0.5% ointment and a 0.1% solution for use in the eye.

Ribavirin (Virazole) is supplied in 100-mL glass vials with 6 g of drug to be reconstituted in 300 mL of water for use as an aerosol.

Trifluridine (Viroptic) is available as a 1% sterile ophthalmic solution (10 mg/mL) in a 7.5-mL bottle.

Vidarabine (Vira-A) is supplied as a 3% ophthalmic ointment and a sterile suspension containing 200 mg of the monohydrate per milliliter in a 5-mL vial.

Zidovudine (Retrovir) is available in 100-mg capsules for oral administration.

BIBLIOGRAPHY

Appel, G. B., and H. C. Neu: "The Nephrotoxicity of Antimicrobial Agents," *N. Engl. J. Med.*, **296**:784–787 (1977).

"Antifungal Agents for Systemic Mycoses," in *AMA Drug Evaluations*, 6th ed., 1986, pp. 1553–1564.

"Antiviral Agents," in *AMA Drug Evaluations*, 6th ed., 1986, pp. 1615–1631.

Bean, B., and D. Aeppli: "Adverse Effects of High-Dose Intravenous Acyclovir in Ambulatory Patients with Acute Herpes Zoster," *J. Infect. Dis.*, **151**:362 (1985).

Bennet, J. E.: "Chemotherapy of Systemic Mycoses," *N. Engl. J. Med.*, **290**:30–32, 320–323 (1974).

Bryson, Y. J., et al.: "Treatment of First Episodes of Genital Herpes Simplex Virus Infection with Oral Acyclovir," *N. Engl. J. Med.*, **308**:916 (1983).

Dismukes, W. E., et al.: "Treatment of Systemic Mycoses with Ketoconazole: Emphasis on Toxicity and Clinical Response in 52 Patients," *Ann. Intern. Med.*, **98**:13 (1983).

Galasso, G. J., T. C. Merigan, and R. A. Buchanan (eds.): *Antiviral Agents, and Viral Diseases of Man*, Raven Press, New York, 1979.

Gnann, J. W., Jr., and R. J. Whitley: "Current Status of Antiviral Chemotherapy," *Intern. Med.*, **4**:49–61 (1983).

Hirsch, M. S., and M. N. Swartz: "Antiviral Agents," *N. Engl. J. Med.*, **302**:903–907, 949–953 (1980).

Hirsch, M. S., and R. T. Schooley: "Treatment of Herpes Virus Infections" (J. Koch-Weser, ed.), *N. Engl. J. Med.*, **309**:963–970 (1983).

Hirsch, M. A., and R. T. Schooley: Part II, *N. Engl. J. Med.*, **309**:1034–1039 (1983).

King, K.: "Antifungal Chemotherapy," *Med. J. Australia*, **143**:287–290 (1985).

Knight, V., and B. E. Gilbert: "Biochemistry and Clinical Applications of Ribavirin," in *Antimicrob. Agents Chemother.*, **30**:201–205 (1986).

Kucers, A., and N. McK, Bennett: *The Use of Antibiotics*, 2d ed., Lippincott, Philadelphia, 1975, pp. 561–603, 609–636.

Hoeprich, P. D.: "Chemotherapy of Systemic Fungal Diseases," *Ann. Rev. Pharmacol. Toxicol.*, **18**:205–231 (1978).

Medoff, G., and G. S. Kobayashi: "Strategies in the Treatment of Systemic Fungal Infections," *N. Engl. J. Med.*, **302**:145–155 (1980).

Newberry, W. M.: "Drug Treatment of the Systemic Mycoses," *Semin. Drug Treat.*, **2**:313–329 (1979).

Pratt, W. B.: *Chemotherapy of Infection*, Oxford, New York, 1977, pp. 265–303, 409–448.

Scholer, H. J.: "Flucytosine," in D. C. E. Speller (ed.), *Antifungal Chemotherapy*, Wiley, New York, 1979, chap. 4.

Shepp, D. H., et al.: "Treatment of Varicella-Zoster Virus Infection in Severely Immunocompromised Patients: Randomized Comparison of Acyclovir and Vidarabine," *N. Engl. J. Med.*, **314**:208–212 (1986).

Smego, R. A., Jr.: "Combined Therapy with Amphotericin B and Flucytosine for *Candida Menigitis*," *Rev. Infect. Dis.*, **6**:791 (1984).

Smith, R. A., R. W. Sidwell, and R. K. Robins: "Antiviral Mechanisms of Action," *Ann. Rev. Pharmacol. Toxicol.*, **20**:259–284 (1980).

Stevens, D. A.: "Drugs for Systemic Fungal Infections," *Ration. Drug Ther.*, **13:**1–7 (1979).

Streissle, G., et al.: "New Antiviral Compounds," *Adv. Virus Res.*, **30:**83–138 (1985).

Whitley, R. J., et al.: "Herpes Simplex Encephalitis: Vidarabine Therapy and Diagnostic Problems," *N. Engl. J. Med.*, **304:**313 (1981).

Whitley, R. J., et al.: "Vidarabine versus Acyclovir Therapy for Mucocutaneous Herpes Simplex Encephalitis," *N. Engl. J. Med.*, **314:**144–149 (1986).

Young, L. S.: "Current Needs in Chemotherapy for Bacterial and Fungal Infections," *Rev. Infect. Dis.*, **7:**S380–S388 (1985).

C H A P T E R   **46**

Drugs Used in Protozoan Infections

Joseph R. DiPalma

The most common protozoan infections in the United States are trichomoniasis, amebiasis, giardiasis, and toxoplasmosis. Malaria, leishmaniasis, and trypanosomiasis are more prevalent in subtropical and tropical zones (Table 46-1). Because of immigration, returning soldiers, and widespread travel, all protozoan diseases are of economic, medical, and societal importance worldwide.

Protozoa are unicellular organisms with a much more versatile and adaptable metabolism than bacteria. They have complex life cycles and thus exist in several different forms which may require different chemotherapeutic approaches. In addition, some have insect vectors and animal reservoirs which may require chemical measures to eliminate this source of infection. It is, therefore, not surprising that numerous chemotherapeutic agents have been and are being employed to combat these parasites (Table 46-1).

This chapter discusses the chemotherapy of malaria in some detail as the prime example of antiprotozoan chemotherapy. Then the other agents useful today in the therapy of other protozoan infections are discussed mainly from the viewpoint of their pharmacologic properties and usefulness in other protozoan diseases.

ANTIMALARIAL AGENTS

Although now uncommon in most parts of the world, malaria remains the most devastating disease in many tropical "third world" countries (see Table 46-1). This disease is particularly fatal to young children, who typically experience mortality in excess of 15 percent.

Many factors contribute to the success of the malaria parasite despite significant efforts to remove the *Anopheles* mosquito, which carries the parasite, and to treat infected populations. War and poverty in areas where malaria is endemic, e.g., Vietnam, have favored a recrudescense of the disease. An increase in air travel has also caused its reintroduction into areas previously freed. Constant vigilance is necessary even in temperate zone countries because the *Anopheles* mosquito is ubiquitous.

LIFE CYCLE OF THE MALARIA PARASITE

Malaria is the result of infestation with protozoa belonging to the genus *Plasmodium*. Of the many species which exist, only four infect humans: *Plasmodium falciparum*, *Plasmodium vivax*, *Plasmodium malariae*, and *Plasmodium ovale*. Infestation by the first two organisms is far more common, and *P. falciparum*, because some of its many strains have acquired resistance to antimalarial drugs, is the most problematic species from a therapeutic standpoint. A proper understanding of the chemotherapy of malaria can best be achieved by examining the life cycle of the parasite in the female *Anopheles* mosquito and in humans. This is shown in Fig. 46-1. The female *Anopheles* mosquito requires a blood meal prior to laying her eggs. When the female bites an infected host (whose blood contains male and female sexual forms of the malarial parasite) fertilization occurs in the stomach of the mosquito. The resulting zygote penetrates the stomach wall and

TABLE 46-1   The most common protozoan infections and the indicated drug therapy

Disease	Worldwide distribution	Drugs
Malaria	USA: 1000–2000 cases/year Tropical regions: at least 200 million infected, 1 million deaths annually	Quinine, mefloquine Chloroquine Primaquine Proguanil Pyrimethamine Trimethoprim Sulfonamides Qinghaosu, artemisinine
Amebiasis	USA: 3–5% of population infected Tropical regions: 10% of population infected	Diloxamide furvate Metronidazole Tinidazole Emetine Dehydroemetine Iodoquinol Paromomycin Carbarsone Chloroquine
Leishmaniasis	USA: uncommon Tropical regions: 12 million new cases/year	Sodium stibogluconate Amphotericin B Metronidazole Allopurinol Nifurtimox
Trypanosomiasis	USA: uncommon South American and Caribbean: 10 million cases (Chagas disease) Africa: many millions in tropical belt	Pentamidine Melarsoprol Nifurtimox Suramin
Giardiasis	USA: 2–10% of population, mainly nonsymptomatic Worldwide: very common	Metronidazole Quinacrine Furazolidone
Trichomoniasis	Worldwide: pandemic proportions	Metronidazole
Toxoplasmosis	Worldwide: serological evidence of infection in 50% population	Pyrimethamine-sulfadiazine
Pneumonia caused by *P. carinii*	Worldwide: high incidence in immunodeficiency states such as AIDS	Trimethoprim-sulfamethoxazole Pentamidine

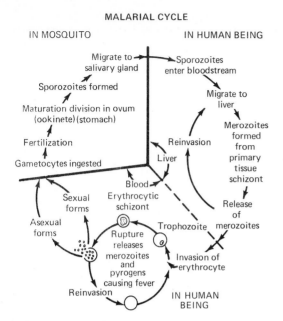

FIGURE 46-1   Life cycle of the malarial parasite. (Schematic diagram after W. B. Pratt, *Fundamentals of Chemotherapy*, Oxford, New York, 1973.)

forms a cyst on its outer surface. After many cell divisions, this oocyst bursts, releasing thousands of sporozoites into the body cavity. Sporozoites migrate to the salivary glands and are injected when the mosquito bites a suitable host. Once injected, these sporozoites disappear rapidly from the blood and appear within liver parenchymal cells and elsewhere. In the liver the sporozoites divide asexually and mature to form a hepatic (exoerythrocytic) schizont containing many merozoites. When this schizont ruptures, merozoites are released into the blood and may reinvade parenchymal cells to form secondary hepatic schizonts or may invade red blood cells where they multiply asexually to form erythrocytic schizonts. At this point, the patient is asymptomatic and will remain so until these erythrocytic schizonts rupture, releasing merozoites and pyrogens into the blood. Clinically this event is marked by the first in a series of febrile episodes. Some of the merozoites released will reinvade red blood cells to form new (secondary erythrocytic) schizonts, others will undergo sexual division and become male and female gametocytes. These sexual forms are ingested

when a new female *Anopheles* bites the infected host, and the process begins again.

Based on the complex life cycle of the malarial parasite in humans, there are certain terms describing more accurately the goals and purposes of chemotherapy. These are defined in Table 46-2. *Suppressive therapy* only affects the asexual, erythrocytic forms. This type of therapy will ensure that clinical symptoms do not appear, but it does not affect the infectivity of the host for the mosquito, nor does it ensure that a relapse will not occur when chemotherapy is terminated. Therapy with a *radical curative agent* will eliminate secondary-tissue schizonts and thus ensure that no relapse can occur at a later date. *Causal prophylaxis* refers to action on primary-tissue schizonts, which may be achieved by some drugs which attack both erythrocytic and primary-tissue (exoerythrocytic) schizonts. *Plasmodium falciparum* does not form secondary-tissue schizonts; thus causal prophylaxis achieves a radical cure in this case, but not for the other plasmodia which infect humans.

CHEMOTHERAPEUTIC AGENTS

The chemotherapy of malaria is designed to interfere with specific stages of the parasite's life cycle. The drugs presented here are divided into three groups: those that affect the erythrocytic stage of the life cycle, those that disrupt the exoerythrocytic (or hepatic) stage, and those that attack both stages simultaneously.

Drugs Effective against Erythrocytic Stages of Plasmodium Infestation

Two classes of drugs are particularly useful in the erythrocytic stage of malarial infections: these are the 4-aminoquinolines and quinoline methanols.

4-Aminoquinolines

The 4-aminoquinolines (chloroquine, amodiaquine, and hydroxychloroquine) are synthetic compounds. The substitution of an amino group at position 4 of the quinoline ring is the most important structural characteristic. The composition of the side chain may vary, but this is not as critical as the presence of a chlorine atom at the 7 position of the ring. Amodiaquine, ex-

TABLE 46-2   Major antimalarial drugs classified in relation to the different stages of the malarial parasite

Stage	Type of therapy	Effective drugs	Purpose
Sporozoites	True causal prophylaxis	None	If effective drugs were available to destroy sporozoites, malarial infection could be prevented. A vaccine is being developed which may be effective.
Exoerythrocytic (primary)	Causal prophylaxis	Chloroguanide†	Drugs are effective against primary tissue schizonts. Therapy prevents erythrocytic infection.
Exoerythrocytic (secondary)	Radical (antirelapse therapy)	Primaquine	Only this drug is active against the secondary tissue schizonts, and thus it eliminates the source of recurrent invasion of the blood cells.
Erythrocytic	Suppressive* (schizontocidal)	Quinine Chloroquine Hydroxychloroquine Mefloquine Amodiaquine† Chloroguanide† Pyrimethamine	Used for the temporary prevention of clinical symptoms. The tissue schizonts are not destroyed, and upon arrest of the therapy relapse frequently occurs.
Sexual	Gametocidal	Primaquine	Used to prevent the spread of infection from man to the mosquito and thus back to the animal reservoir. Important only in endemic and epidemic areas.
Mosquito	Sporontocidal (antisporogonic, gametostatic)	Pyrimethamine Primaquine	At best gametocytes are resistant, and those escaping destruction in the host may still be inhibited from developing in the mosquito by therapy of the host.

*Other terms which apply are *clinical cure* and *clinical prophylaxis*.
†Not available in the United States.

tensively used abroad, is not available in the United States.

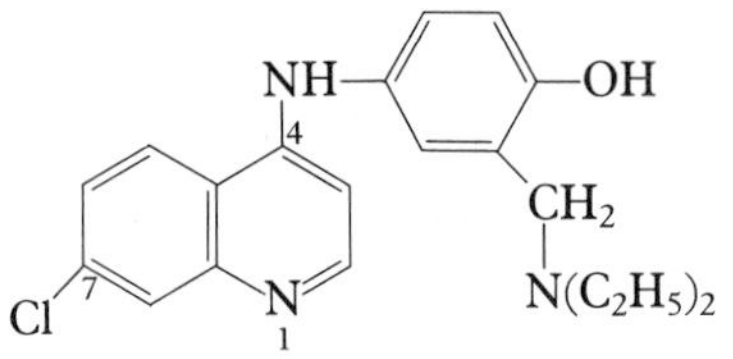

Amodiaquine

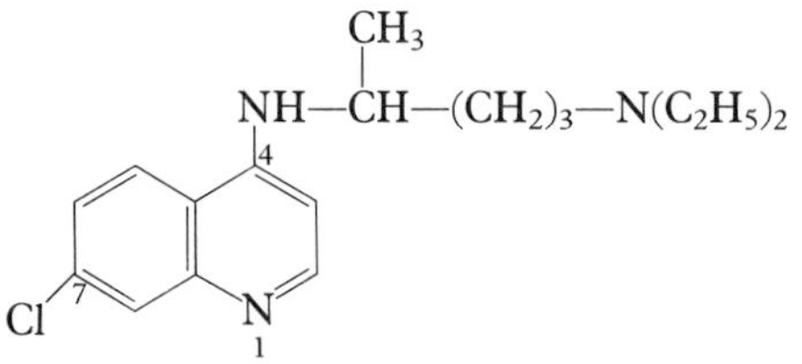

Chloroquine

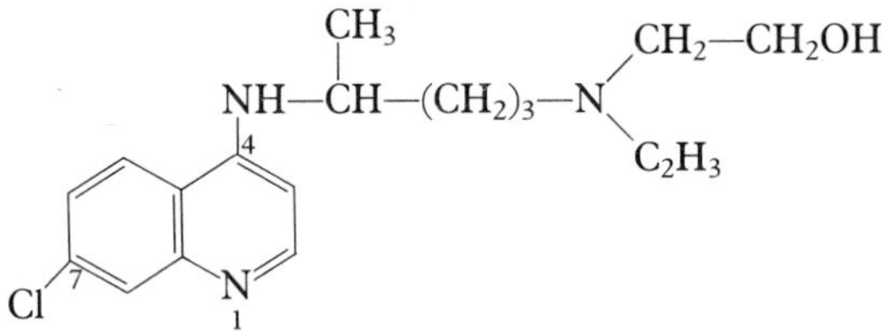

Hydroxychloroquine

The prototype compound in this group is chloroquine, and its pharmacology will be considered representative of the entire group.

Mechanism of Action Chloroquine and its congeners inhibit nucleic acid synthesis by interfering with the template function of DNA. This is accomplished by a preferential hydrogen bonding with purine molecules and a subsequent intercalation of the chloroquine molecule between stacked base pairs in the DNA helix. In this way, chloroquine prevents transcription and translation, reducing DNA and RNA synthesis. The selective toxicity of chloroquine is attributed to the ability of parasitized red blood cells to concentrate this drug at levels many times that found in plasma and about 25 times that found in normal erythrocytes. Red blood cells parasitized by strains of malaria which have developed resistance to chloroquine, e.g., *P. falciparum*, have a reduced ability to concentrate this drug.

A recent finding is that aggregates of ferriprotoporphyrin IX which are released by the plasmodium into red blood cells serve as receptors for chloroquine and related compounds. This explains the accumulation of the drug in parasitized red blood cells. The ability of *P. falciparum* to acquire resistance to chloroquine may reside in altered production of ferriprotoporphrin IX.

There is also an acid-vesicle hypothesis. Chloroquine has a high tissue affinity and is concentrated in the cytoplasm of the parasite. As a weak base it raises the pH of the intracellular lysosomes and endosomes. Acidification of these organelles is necessary for the parasitic invasion of mammalian cells. Consequently the parasite growth and development are inhibited.

Pharmacokinetics The oral bioavailability of chloroquine is in the range of 90 percent. After an oral dose, maximum blood levels are achieved in 6 h. Approximately 55 percent of the total plasma concentration is bound to plasma proteins. Extensive tissue binding, however, contributes to a large apparent volume of distribution. Normal red blood cells concentrate this drug at levels twice that found in plasma; liver, lung, kidney, and heart concentrate it at 10 times plasma levels. The half-life is 5 days. Twenty-five percent appears unchanged in the urine, the rest as the *N*-desethyl derivative. The parent compound appears in greater concentration in acidic urine.

Pharmacodynamics Chloroquine has a slight quinidine-like effect on the heart and depresses cardiac function in higher doses, especially when administered parenterally.

In larger doses chloroquine has unique actions apart from its antimalarial activity. It has distinct anti-inflammatory capability, especially against inflammatory diseases such as rheumatoid arthritis and chronic discoid lupus erythematosus. This action is believed to be due to the suppression of the immune process. At such doses, however, toxicity is greatly increased and may outweigh clinical benefit.

Other actions include enzyme inhibition; binding of melanin, porphyrin, and nucleic acids; and antihistaminic effects.

Therapeutic Uses Treatment of malaria in adults requires 600 mg of the base initially, followed by 300 mg in 6 h, then 300 mg daily for 2 more days. For prophylaxis, 300 mg is required once weekly. Treatment should start 2 weeks before entering the endemic area and continue for 8 weeks after returning. To prevent malaria, primaquine should be added immediately after an individual has left an endemic area, especially if the predominant plasmodium is other than *P. falciparum*.

A level of 10 ng/mL clears the blood of parasites, but a plasma concentration of 250 to 280 ng/mL is required to achieve therapeutic results in rheumatoid arthritis. Consequently, much larger doses must be employed in rheumatoid arthritis and discoid lupus. These are on the order of 150 mg of the base daily for 6 to 12 weeks.

The therapy of amebic abscess of the liver may also include chloroquine; 300 mg of the base daily for 10 weeks is the regimen commonly used.

Adverse Reactions   Other than mild gastrointestinal complaints, side actions are almost unknown with doses of chloroquine used to treat malaria. However, the high doses required as anti-inflammatory medication lead to a variety of severe reactions. Generalized loss of hair pigment and a blue-black pigmentation of the skin and mucous membranes may occur. More important are the keratopathy and retinopathy resulting in constriction of the visual fields and loss of central vision. Early changes are reversible, but later the visual changes become permanent. Prolonged therapy should be attended by periodic ophthalmologic examinations. Mothers receiving high doses during pregnancy may give birth to children with sensorineural deafness. Lichen planus skin eruption and even exfoliative dermatitis have occurred. Intravenous doses, especially in children, may cause fatal cardiorespiratory collapse. Deaths have been associated with blood levels as low as 1 μg/mL.

Drug Interactions   Chlorpromazine blocks the melanin binding of chloroquine, and as a consequence has been suggested as a preventative of retinopathy; this combination, however, cannot be recommended at the present time. Simultaneous use of gold salts and phenylbutazone (for rheumatoid arthritis) may enhance the likelihood of exfoliative dermatitis. Intestinal absorption of chloroquine may be decreased by the presence of kaolin or antacids.

Quinoline Methanols

Source and Chemistry   The second group of drugs useful against the erythrocytic stages of malarial infection is the quinoline methanols. This group includes the cinchona alkaloids, among which only quinine is still used in the therapy of malaria. Quinine is obtained from the bark of the cinchona tree, which grows in South America and in the plantations of the East Indies. Quinine is the levorotatory isomer of quinidine and consists of a quinoline ring substituted in the 4 position with a methylene bridge to a quinuclidine ring structure. There are two groups, a methoxy group on the 6 position of the quinoline ring and a vinyl group on the quinuclidine ring, which enhance activity but are not absolutely necessary.

l-Quinine
d-Quinidine

Quinine possesses other physical properties of importance. It fluoresces easily, polarizes light, and screens out ultraviolet light. Its bitter taste gives it the property of a stomachic, and it finds use in proprietary products such as quinine water.

Mechanism of Action   Quinine attaches to plasmodial DNA in a manner similar to chloroquine, interfering with nucleic acid synthesis by preventing replication and transcription. Quinine also depresses a great number of enzyme systems and has been characterized as a generalized protoplasmic poison. This fact correlates well with quinine's membrane actions, local anesthetic effect, and cardiac-depressant effect.

Pharmacodynamics   Quinine has analgesic and antipyretic properties similar to the salicylates. When applied locally, quinine has a local anesthetic action in which it briefly stimulates and then paralyzes sensory neurons. Because of its nature as a protoplasmic poison, local tissue destruction often results, which prolongs its action for weeks or months.

Quinine causes a quinidine-like depression of myocardial excitability and conduction velocity. Intravenous injection of quinine, particularly when administered rapidly, has a direct relaxant effect on vascular smooth muscle, causing a profound fall in blood pressure, which may reach the proportions of circulatory collapse. This effect may be combatted with norepinephrine or other suitable vasopressors.

Quinine inhibits cholinesterase, and it has a distinct but weak curare-like action. Because of this latter effect, quinine will aggravate the clinical syndrome of myasthenia gravis. On the other hand, quinine is quite useful in relieving the excessive tone of muscle in myotonia congenita and in the night cramps of peripheral vascular disease.

In usual therapeutic doses quinine contracts the pregnant uterus. This action, now obsolete in clinical practice, has been used to precipitate labor; it is generally used with other agents such as castor oil. As an abortifacient, quinine must be used in toxic doses and is seldom successful.

Pharmacokinetics Quinine is rapidly and completely absorbed from the gastrointestinal tract, reaching a maximum plasma concentration in 1 to 2 h. This drug is widely distributed, achieving its highest concentrations in the liver, lung, kidney, and spleen. Leukocytes concentrate quinine, but erythrocytes contain less of the compound than does the plasma. Plasma protein binding is approximately 70 percent. Biotransformation occurs by hydroxylation at position 2 of the quinoline ring in the liver drug-metabolizing microsomal system. About 10 percent is found unchanged in the urine. The plasma level falls rapidly to negligible levels in 6 to 8 h, and hence daily doses are required.

Therapeutic Uses Administered by the oral route, quinine is effectively combined with pyrimethamine, sulfadiazine, and/or tetracycline in treating an uncomplicated attack of chloroquine-resistant *P. falciparum*. Quinine administered by intravenous drip is the therapy of choice for an acute attack of chloroquine-resistant *P. falciparum*. Because of adverse reactions, its use is fairly limited. The only indication for quinine is malaria, and only when there is a synthetic drug-resistant strain. It is, however, occasionally prescribed for night cramps.

Adverse Reactions Quinine has many toxicities and side actions because of its complex pharmacology. The acute oral fatal dose is estimated to be in excess of 8 g. All persons who must take quinine chronically eventually suffer from *cinchonism,* a syndrome similar to salicylism. In mild cases it consists of ringing in the ears, headache, nausea, and disturbances of vision. More advanced cases show color-vision changes, photophobia, constriction of visual fields, and scotomas. In fact, *quinine amblyopia* is a term applied to severe cases. Confusion, excitement, and delirium may eventually result.

Skin reactions do occasionally occur. These usually consist of a scarlatiniform rash. More often it is urticarial in nature. Angioneurotic edema and asthmatic attacks which respond to epinephrine also occur. Purpura is not uncommon and is caused by thrombocytopenia. Recovery is rapid as soon as the drug is stopped.

Intravenous therapy with quinine requires great care to avoid severe reactions. It must be injected slowly and in very dilute solutions.

Another phenomenon associated with quinine toxicity is blackwater fever, a syndrome characterized by excessive intravascular hemolysis, hemoglobinuria, azotemia, and renal failure and resulting in a mortality of 20 to 30 percent. This reaction has been associated particularly, if not exclusively, with *P. falciparum* infection. It was originally believed that only patients treated with quinine could display this disorder, which was attributed to a drug-induced autoimmune state. It is now known, however, that patients receiving no medication at all can experience blackwater fever. Its exact cause remains an enigma.

Mefloquine This is an antimalarial developed for treatment and prevention of chloroquine-resistant strains of *P. falciparum* malaria. Chemically, mefloquine is an analog of quinine. It differs from quinine in that the side chain is a piperidyl ring rather

Mefloquine

than quinuclidine. In addition there is the substitution of fluoromethyl groups at positions 2 and 8 of the quinoline ring. The 2-position fluoromethyl group blocks ring hydroxylation at this point, which, it will be recalled, is a major site of biotransformation for quinine.

As might be expected, mefloquine shows similarities to quinine both in its pharmacology and therapeutic spectrum. Studies have shown the same predilection for blood pressure reduction and depression of cardiac function when mefloquine is injected intravenously in a dose of 2 to 3 mg/kg/min.

In human phase I studies single oral doses of up to 2 g were well tolerated. There was some dizziness and nausea, but this was not associated with any neurological signs. Human trials showed mefloquine to be both a good prophylactic and therapeutic drug for malarial infections, and many investigators believe this drug to be the most effective single-dose agent for chloroquine-resistant *P. falciparum*. Doses of 500 mg/week proved to be an effective suppressive dose not only for *P. falciparum but also for P. vivax*. Naturally acquired *P. falciparum* infections responded to single oral doses of 1.5 g.

At the present time mefloquine is an investigational drug and is not available for wide distribution. Some strains of *P. falciparum* resistant to mefloquine have already been reported. It is likely that mefloquine will be used for prophylaxis combined with pyrimethamine-sulfadoxine.

Qinghaosu, Artemisinine What is amazing is the variety of substances which have chemotherapeutic action against malarial parasites. A recent discovery is a heterocyclic compound lacking nitrogen and, therefore not an alkaloid, extracted from a Chinese herbal medicine. Actually the plant *Artemisia amma* also grows in the United States. The chemical structure is

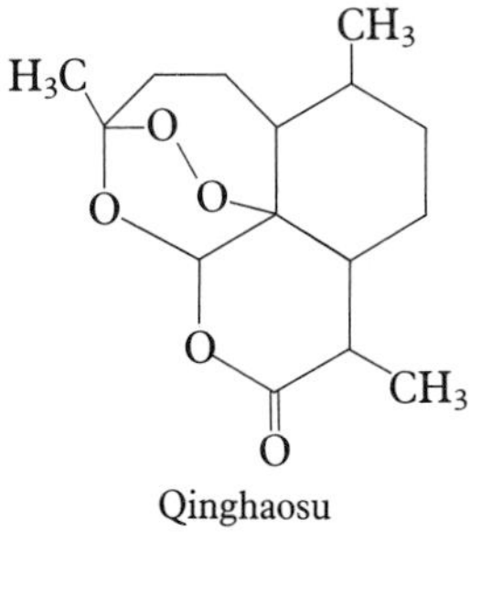

Qinghaosu

Extremely insoluble qinghaosu is given either orally or intramuscularly. Its activity resembles that of quinine in that it works rapidly against the erythrocytic stage of malaria. It has no effect on the hepatic forms. The main interest in qinghaosu is its effectiveness against chloroquine-resistant *P. falciparum* malaria. Indeed it has been effective even in the cerebral form of this infection. Unfortunately, when qinghaosu is used alone there is a high relapse rate.

Drugs Effective against the Hepatic (Exoerythrocytic) Forms of Plasmodium Infestation

8-Aminoquinolines

Source and Chemistry These are synthetic compounds first introduced in Germany in 1926. After World War II, further investigation in the United States led to the development of a compound with a good therapeutic index. This drug is known as primaquine, and its structure is shown below:

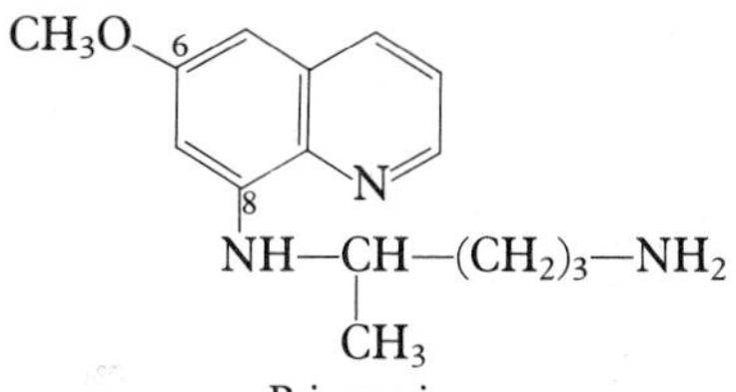

Primaquine

The shift of the side chain from the 4 position of the quinoline nucleus to the 8 position completely changes the spectrum of primaquine's activity. In contrast to the 4-aminoquinolines, primaquine has virtually no effect on erythrocytic forms of the malarial parasite: its activity is restricted to the tissue forms of the parasite in humans and in the mosquito (Table 46-2). This makes primaquine an extremely valuable aid because it permits a radical cure and causal prophylaxis which cannot be achieved with the other purely erythrocytic drugs.

Mechanism of Action The site of action of primaquine is within the mitochondria of the malaria parasite. Here primaquine is believed to interfere with electron transport, causing oxidative damage to mitochondrial enzyme systems. This results in swelling and vacuolation of the parasite's mitochondria. Host mitochondria are not affected. In addition, primaquine attacks the sexual forms of the parasite in human blood and renders them incapable of maturation division in the mosquito. This is probably accomplished by causing oxidative damage to electron-rich nucleic acids within the gametocytes. Primaquine, therefore, can be used to prevent the spread of malaria in endemic areas.

Pharmacokinetics   Primaquine is rapidly and completely absorbed from the gastrointestinal tract, achieving maximum plasma concentrations within 2 h of an oral dose. Primaquine is not as extensively tissue-bound as are the 4-aminoquinolines but is somewhat concentrated in the liver and, in descending order, the lung, brain, heart, and skeletal muscle.

Primaquine is rapidly biotransformed in the liver to active quinoline products which are potent oxidizing agents. After 8 to 10 h, following an oral dose, the plasma level of the parent compound is very small; only 1 percent of the original dose is excreted unchanged in the urine. One of the major biotransformation products, the 6-hydroxyl derivative, undergoes conjugation prior to urinary excretion.

Pharmacodynamics   In the usual therapeutic doses primaquine has only minor actions. In some respects, it is similar to quinine because in concentrations of 2 to 4 μg/mL the isolated mammalian uterus contracts, and when the concentration is raised to 10 μg/mL, the uterus relaxes. Because intravenous injection may produce a fall in blood pressure, cardiac arrhythmias, and electrocardiographic changes, its use by this route is not recommended.

Therapeutic Uses   Primaquine's only use is the radical cure or causal prophylaxis of malaria. In adults 15 mg of the base are given daily for 14 days concomitantly or consecutively with chloroquine. For prophylaxis, after an individual has left a malarious area, 15 mg (base) are used daily for 14 days. In some cases, when the organism is *P. vivax*, 30 mg (base) daily for 14 days might be necessary.

Adverse Reactions   Much is now known about the phenomenon called *primaquine sensitivity*, a form of intravascular hemolysis accompanied by the formation of methemoglobin. The mechanism by which this sensitivity arises is common to a number of drugs which are capable of acting as oxidants and is believed to be intimately related to the mechanism by which primaquine exerts its schizontocidal and gametocidal actions.

Red blood cells contain many components which are particularly sensitive to oxidative damage, notably, hemoglobin and the cell membrane. Normal erythrocytes which are exposed to oxidants, e.g., primaquine, neutralize these offensive agents via reduced cofactors (NADH and NADPH), which permit the reduction of oxidized glutathione (GSSG) to reduced glutathione (GSH). Reduced glutathione in turn gives up its electrons to the oxidant, neutralizing it, and in this process is, itself, oxidized to GSSG. As long as reduced cofactors are available, this protective cycle continues (see Fig. 46-2). The hexose monophosphate shunt serves a homeostatic role by producing reduced cofactors in direct response to the levels of oxidized glutathione (GSSG) present in the erythrocyte, using the enzyme glucose-6-phosphate dehydrogenase (G6PD).

Primaquine and certain other drugs, including sulfones, menadiol, and sulfonamides, are converted to oxidant products in the blood. These metabolites consume electrons and, in the absence of protective GSH, do oxidative damage to hemoglobin, forming methemoglobin, and to the red blood cell membrane, causing hemolysis.

Primaquine sensitivity is most common in persons who belong to ethnic groups originating in the Mediterranean basin and is linked closely to a genetic defect: a deficiency of G6PD, which leads to increased fragility of the red blood cells. Actually, old cells are affected first, and the hemolysis is dose-dependent. Using small doses of primaquine (15 mg of base once a week), few individuals experience hemolysis. With larger doses hemolysis is apt to occur in sensitive individuals. Because the resulting hemolysis can be severe and because the procedure is easily accomplished, it is worthwhile to screen patients for G6PD deficiency prior to the initiation of primaquine therapy.

Primaquine may also cause abdominal discomfort, nausea, headache, changes in visual accommodation, and pruritus. The predisposition for intravascular hemolysis in susceptible individuals is its principal side effect. Some methemoglobinemia is frequently attendant with its use but rarely requires cessation of the 14-day course of therapy. Drug interactions are generally not a problem.

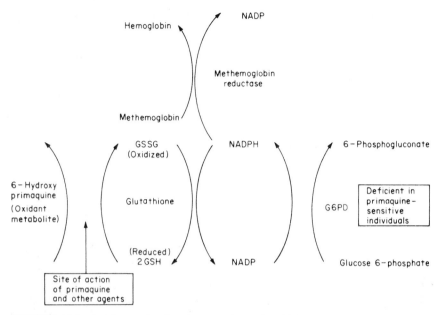

FIGURE 46-2 A schema showing the complex cycle which renders the red blood cell susceptible to hemolysis in primaquine-sensitive individuals. The deficiency in G6PD makes it possible for primaquine to oxidize glutathione because of inadequate production of NADPH. An added complication is failure of conversion of methemoglobin to hemoglobin, which also requires NADPH.

Drugs Effective against Erythrocytic and Hepatic Forms of Plasmodium Infestation

Folate Metabolism Inhibitors: Biguanides and Diaminopyrimadines Early studies showed that sulfones and sulfonamides had some curative value in malarial infections. However, it was not until such compounds as chloroguanide and pyrimethamine became available that a new class of drugs with a different mechanism of action in malaria were discovered. Experimental studies showed a marked synergism between sulfonamides and pyrimethamine. In field studies it was shown that either biguanides or diaminopyrimidines alone were prophylactic and curative in malarial infections. It was later discovered that all strong inhibitors of dihydrofolate reductase such as trimethoprim could destroy the malarial parasite with relatively little damage to the human host. The scheme shown in Fig. 44-1 serves to illustrate the synergistic relationship between sulfonamides, which compete for *para*-aminobenzoic acid (PABA), and the inhibitors of dihydrofolate reductase.

Source and Chemistry Chloroguanide was introduced in England in 1945, the result of work on a long series of biguanide compounds. A few years later pyrimethamine was discovered as the culmination of intensive study of antimetabolites of folic acid. Trimethoprim was a still later development. The close structural resemblance of these compounds is shown in Fig. 46-3. One may also perceive similarities between the pteridine ring of folic acid and the diaminopyrimidine structure of pyrimethamine. Undoubtedly this contributes to the affinity of these compounds for a receptor site of dihydrofolate reductase (DHFR).

Mechanism of Action All these compounds are inhibitors of DHFR in bacteria, plasmodia, and humans. Fortunately, they have a high relative affinity for bacterial and protozoal DHFR: pyrimethamine, for example, inhibits parasitic DHFR at a level several hundred times lower than that required to inhibit human DHFR. This serves as a basis for a selective toxicity which favors the host against the parasite.

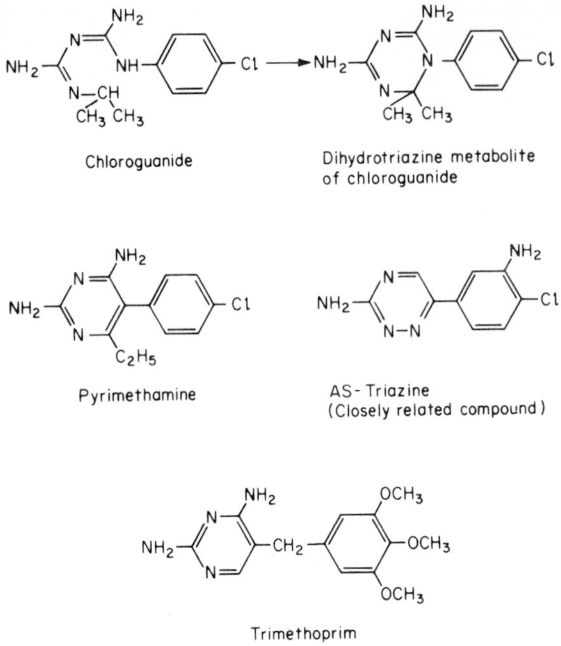

Chloroguanide → Dihydrotriazine metabolite of chloroguanide

Pyrimethamine

AS-Triazine (Closely related compound)

Trimethoprim

FIGURE 46-3 Drugs classified as biguanides and diaminopyrimidines. Note that chloroguanide is shown in the folded form to indicate its close relationship to pyrimethamine and to its dihydrotriazine metabolite.

This selective toxicity can be enhanced by providing the host with folinic acid, which the parasite cannot utilize.

Chloroguanide is inactive in vitro. In the body it is converted to a dihydrotriazine compound, which is active. This represents one of the unique examples of a conversion of an inactive drug to an active one by a biotransformation mechanism (see Fig. 46-3).

The biguanides and diaminopyrimidines are active against both the exoerythrocytic and the erythrocytic forms of plasmodia. They are most useful in suppressive therapy, but a causal cure may be obtained when treating *P. falciparum* infections. They also have an effect on gametocytes such that they are unable to undergo maturation, thus preventing sporogony in the mosquito's gut sporozoite formation. The major disadvantage of these drugs is the rapidity with which the parasite develops resistance to them. This includes *P. falciparum* and *P. vivax* as well as many experimental strains.

Pharmacokinetics Chloroguanide is slowly absorbed from the gastrointestinal tract. However, 60 to 70 percent of a given dose is eventually absorbed. Peak serum levels occur in 2 to 4 h and decline gradually over 24 h. Approximately 25 percent is bound to plasma proteins. On chronic administration there is little or no accumulation. In humans 40 to 60 percent of the chloroguanide absorbed is excreted in the urine, while 10 percent is secreted into the intestinal tract and lost with the feces. As mentioned before, chloroguanide itself is inactive and must be converted to the triazine (closed ring) compound to be effective (Fig. 41-4).

Pyrimethamine and trimethoprim are rapidly absorbed in the gastrointestinal tract. Peak plasma levels occur in 2 to 4 h, and some is found in the blood after 24 h. Tissue concentrations are high; even the cerebrospinal fluid has significant levels. Pyrimethamine is secreted in mother's milk at concentrations high enough to provide chemosuppression of malaria in a breast-fed infant. Several unidentified products of biotransformation of pyrimethamine and 4-hydroxylated products of trimethoprim are found in the urine.

Pharmacodynamics As might be expected, this group of drugs exhibits no special organ effects. Their action is restricted to those metabolic systems affected by folate metabolism, including the reticuloendothelial system and gastrointestinal tract (see "Adverse Reactions," below).

Therapeutic Use Chloroguanide is used in the prophylaxis of malaria. It has a low incidence of side effects and is useful in chloroquine-resistant *P. falciparum* infection. Therapy is begun 2 weeks before entering the malarious area and continued for 8 weeks after the return. It will not prevent malaria unless primaquine is added to the regimen after the patient has left the endemic area.

Pyrimethamine or trimethoprim administered alone may be used like chloroguanide for the prophylaxis of malaria. However, used alone, these drugs are not very effective in the treatment of a primary attack of malaria. When they are combined with a sulfonamide or a sulfone (Fansidar) they have been used successfully in treating chloroquine-resistant *P. falciparum* malaria, providing a 95 to 98 percent cure with only minor host toxicities. Combination therapy also significantly reduces the dosage required and the development of resistance.

Combined with triple sulfonamides given simultaneously, pyrimethamine has had considerable use in the therapy of *toxoplasmosis*, another parasitic infection. In this application, it is usually advisable to supplement with folinic acid.

Adverse Reactions The toxicity of these drugs resides in their dihydrofolate reductase-inhibiting ability. The usual doses either for the prophylaxis or for the therapy of malaria do not have appreciable effects. However, larger doses and use for prolonged periods can cause the symptoms of folic acid deficiency. These include bone marrow depression and megaloblastosis, and they are readily reversible by the administration of folinic acid or by cessation of treatment. In endemic areas, where continual use is expected, the simultaneous administration of folinic acid is recommended. Because of its membrane-penetrating ability, the use of these drugs in pregnant women is not advisable.

Of course, the sulfonamides and sulfones used with these drugs have their own toxicity (see Chap. 44). Skin rashes which occur may be due to either ingredient, but the sulfonamides are more culpable.

Miscellaneous Drugs

As mentioned previously, the malarial parasite is susceptible to many different drug groups. The main problem is the development of resistance, especially in the case of *P. falciparum* infections. As a consequence, different drugs are used in combination as the occasion requires.

Quinacrine Quinacrine is an acridine derivative closely related to the 4-aminoquinolines chemically and in clinical use. It was the main drug for prophylaxis and therapy during World War II. It is now rarely used as an antimalarial, but it finds use in amebiasis and giardiasis. It is also used as a sclerosing agent intrapleurally for the prevention of recurrence of pneumothorax.

Tetracycline This antibiotic (described in Chap. 43) is quite active in most malarial species. Seldom used as the sole agent, it is an alternative drug most

often combined with another agent such as pyrimethamine, sulfonamides, or sulfone in cases of resistant strains. Doxycycline is the preparation most frequently used.

Dapsone Dapsone is 4,4-diaminodiphenylsulfone and is also known as DDS. As a sulfone it has much the same characteristics as sulfonamides with somewhat greater toxicity. Dapsone has been widely used for the therapy of leprosy. It also finds utility in the prophylaxis of malaria. Because of the easy development of resistance, it is combined with pyrimethamine.

Preparations

Amodiaquine (Camoquin) is not available in the United States.

Chloroguanide (Paludrine) is not available in the United States.

Chloroquine (Aralen) is available in tablets containing 500 mg (equivalent to 300 mg of base) and for injection in solutions containing 50 mg/mL (equivalent to 40 mg of base) in 5-mL ampuls.

Hydroxychloroquine (Plaquenil) is available in tablets containing 200 mg (equivalent to 155 mg of base).

Primaquine phosphate is available in tablets containing 25.3 mg (equivalent to 15 mg of base).

Pyrimethamine (Daraprim) is available in tablets containing 25 mg.

Quinacrine (Atabrine) is available in tablets containing 200 mg.

Quinine is available as the sulfate salt in capsules containing 130, 195, 200, 260, 300, and 325 mg. As the hydrochloride salt it is available as powder for dilution for intravenous injection from the Centers for Disease Control. In an emergency quinidine sulfate can be substituted.

Mixtures *Chloroquine-primaquine* is available as tablets containing chloraquine 500 mg and primaquine 79 mg.

Pyrimethamine-sulfadoxine (Fansidar) is available as tablets containing 500 mg of sulfadoxine and 25 mg of pyrimethamine.

AMEBIASIS

Entamoeba histolytica, the causative agent of amebiasis, has a very complicated life cycle in its human host.

It may exist as an asymptomatic infection, as a mild to moderate intestinal infection (nondysenteric colitis), much more severe intestinal infection causing dysentery and invasion of the wall of the intestine, and finally as a systemic stage with abscesses usually in the liver but also in late stages appearing in other parts of the body, such as the brain. As shown in Table 46-1, many drugs are utilized to treat amebiasis in its various stages. None are completely effective because the cystic form of the organism is extremely resistant to chemotherapy. In addition, chemotherapeutic agents cannot penetrate the heavily walled abscesses, which in most cases must be surgically drained and removed.

Metronidazole

Originally introduced about 30 years ago for the treatment of trichomoniasis, metronidazole has proven to be a remarkably effective chemotherapeutic agent not only for amebiasis but also for leishmaniasis, trichomoniasis, and giardiasis. It is also effective in bacterial anaerobic infections.

Metronidazole is amebicidal for *Entamoeba histolytica* in both the intestinal (luminal) and tissue stages. At the present time it is the preferred drug for amebiasis except for asymptomatic cyst carriers. Since oral doses are completely absorbed, another luminal amebicide must be given, usually iodoquinol, to eradicate intestinal ameba and thus prevent relapse. The complete pharmacology, including chemistry, is described in Chap. 44.

Diloxanide Furoate

Since the late 1950s, diloxanide furoate has been used mainly outside the United States to treat the intestinal phase of amebiasis. Although not clearly more effective than luminal amebosides, it has fewer side effects.

Diloxanide furoate

Diloxanide is a dichloroacetamide derivative that is insoluble in water and must be protected from light. There are no pharmacologic effects from ordinary doses. Diloxanide is rapidly absorbed in the intestine, reaching a peak blood level in about 1 h. After conjugation to the glucuronide, it is excreted in the urine in about 6 h.

Used alone, diloxanide is effective in the asymptomatic early stage of amebiasis infection. Combined with metronidazole, it is usually curative in the purely luminal stage of amebiasis. It has no effect on the cystic form of the ameba. Except for the gastrointestinal (GI) complaints, there are few or no adverse reactions. It should not be used in children under 2 years of age or in pregnant females.

Diloxanide is available as 500-mg tablets from the Centers for Disease Control. The usual dose in adults is 500 mg three times daily with meals for 10 days.

Emetine

Traditionally and historically, emetine, an alkaloid extracted from ipecac (Brazil root), has been a major drug in the therapy of amebiasis. A very toxic alkaloid, it has been largely replaced by metronidazole. Its use is restricted to severe cases of bowel wall infestation by the ameba resistant to other amebicides. For this purpose it and a close relative, dehydroemetine, are used subcutaneously and intramuscularly. By these routes emetine has no effect on intraluminal parasites, although it is effective as a direct agent. However, it is no longer used as an oral drug.

Emetine is thought to act by inhibiting polypeptide chain elongation; hence protein synthesis in parasites and mammalian cells is arrested. As a general irritant and protoplasmic poison, emetine has actions on the GI tract, cardiovascular, neuromuscular, and central nervous systems, which are generally considered adverse effects and often preclude use of the drug. When necessary to resort to emetine, it is best to closely watch the patient in a hospital setting.

Idoquinol

This agent is useful in amebal intraluminal infections only. As such it is indicated in mild infections. The mechanism of action is unknown. Its chemistry is as follows:

Iodoquinol

Absorption is poor in the GI tract, and this is advantageous because it is the locus of action of the drug. Some is absorbed, however, and metabolic studies indicate a half-life of 11 to 14 h. Thyroid function tests are unreliable in patients taking iodoquinol. Adverse reactions consist of rashes (acneform, popular and pustular iododerma), GI disturbances, fever, and enlargement of the thyroid. Iodoquinol in large doses over a long period can also cause optic neuritis, atrophy, and peripheral neuropathy.

Iodoquinol is also used as a powder which is insufflated intravaginally for trichomonas infections. By this route it is generally a safer drug because absorption is minimized.

Paromomycin

As an aminoglycoside antibiotic, paromomycin is a close relative of neomycin and streptomycin. It is active against the intestinal stage of amebiasis. It is also effective against enteric bacteria *Salmonella* and *Shigella*.

Only a very small portion of orally administered paromomycin is absorbed. Nearly 100 percent of the drug is recovered in the stool. As a result, paromomycin is effective only in the intraluminal stage of amebiasis.

The side effects are usually restricted to nausea and vomiting and sometimes cramps and diarrhea. In an ulcerated bowel considerable absorption can occur, which may result in renal toxicity and ototoxicity commonly associated with the aminoglycosides. Superinfection is another complication which requires vigilance.

Paromomycin (Humatin) is available in 250-mg capsules. The dose is 25 to 35 mg/kg daily in three divided doses.

Arsenicals

The use of pentavalent arsenicals to treat amebiasis is now obsolete. However, carbarsone, a pentavalent organic arsenical, is still available. It contains 29 percent arsenic, which is the active agent. As a heavy metal it combines with sulfhydryl (SH) groups in essential enzyme systems of the parasites. Unfortunately, arsenic is also toxic to the host (see Chap. 48). Carbarsone is not active against cystic forms of the ameba and should not be used in systemic infections. If used early enough, it does prevent cyst formation by killing trophozoites.

Chloroquine

This antimalarial drug is also very useful in amebiasis. It is effective against the trophozoite stage and does prevent and eradicate liver abscess. Chloroquine is not used and is ineffective in the luminal stage of amebiasis. Chloroquine is the drug of choice in a later stage, when ulceration of the mucosa is present and the danger of invasion of the intestinal wall and metastatic liver abscess is probable. While the ideal dose of chloroquine for this purpose is unsettled, it lies above that used in malaria and certainly below that used in rheumatoid arthritis (see Chap. 23). At this dosage level the toxicity of chloroquine is certainly acceptable. (See under "Malaria" for complete description of chloroquine.)

LEISHMANIASIS

A group of trypanosome protozoal parasites of the genus *Leishmania* cause a variety of diseases which are known generally as leishmaniasis. The insect vector is a biting sandfly, which transmits the infection from human to human or from rodents and canines to humans. Kala azar in India is caused by *L. donovani*. This is a serious chronic systemic disease with spleenomegaly and hepatomegaly with dysentery, which if untreated is usually fatal. *L. tropica* and *L. mexicana* cause only a cutaneous lesion, and spontaneous recovery is the rule. *L. braziliensis* infection results in destructive ulcers of mucous membranes, which require treatment for recovery.

Sodium Stibogluconate

Antimony trivalent organic salts have been the traditional and effective therapy for kala azar or visceral leishmaniasis. More recently a pentavalent compound, sodium stibogluconate, has been found to be more convenient to use. Its chemistry is as follows:

Sodium stibogluconate

In the body sodium stibogluconate is probably converted to the trivalent form of antimony. Although the mechanism of action is unknown, antimony, like other metals, is known to react with sulfhydryl groups. Intestinal absorption is poor, and the drug must be given intramuscularly or intravenously. Excretion is 80 to 90 percent complete via the kidneys in 6 h. A course of treatment is usually 6 daily administrations of 600 mg of pentavalent antimony. Sodium stibogluconate is available in the United States only from the Centers for Disease Control.

Other drugs have been used successfully in various forms of leishmaniasis. These include amphotericin B (Fungizone) for the visceral form resistant to antimony. Metronidazole has been used in the Mexican cutaneous form. A promising approach is the use of allopurinol in kala azar. This relatively nontoxic drug in humans is converted to toxic metabolites only in the parasites (see Chap. 23 for pharmacology).

TRYPANOSOMIASIS

In Africa trypanosomiasis is transmitted by the tsetse fly and is commonly known as sleeping sickness. The parasites *T. brucai* exist in two subspecies, *rhodesiense* and *gambiense*. The former causes a progressive fatal form of the disease with early CNS involvement. The latter has late CNS invasion, which gives rise to the symptoms of sleeping sickness.

American trypanosomiasis (Chagas disease) is common in South America. It is transmitted by bloodsucking triatomid insects. The main pathology is cardiomyopathy, hypertrophy of the esophagus and colon, which is eventually fatal.

Pentamidine

Fortunately, the diamidine group of drugs active against trypanosomes was discovered. Of this group pentamidine is the most stable and most widely used. Its chemistry is as follows:

Pentamidine

Pentamidine has a selective spectrum of activity against trypanosomes. It is particularly effective against *T. gambiense* infections both for prevention and treatment. Pentamidine is less effective but still useful in *T. rhodesiense* infections. Other trypanosomes which are susceptible are *L. donovani* and *P. carinii*.

There are several possible chemotherapeutic actions. Uptake by the parasite is energy dependent and in susceptible organisms is very rapid. Pentamidine is highly positively charged and may react with DNA or nucleotides. Pentamidine's activity is antagonized by glucose, and thus it may interfere with glycolysis.

Adverse reactions include initial respiratory stimulation followed by depression, fall in blood pressure, tachycardia, dizziness, headache, and GI symptoms. Diamidines can be nephrotoxic and also cause sometimes fatal CNS symptoms (ataxia, seizures).

Available as the isethionate salt (Pentam) in 300-mg single-dose vials; it is given IM or IV after dilution. The dose is 4 (mg/kg)/day for 14 days.

Clinical use of pentamidine in the United States is for *P. carinii* infections resistant to other agents. Pentamidine's use in trypanosomiasis is mainly preventive and is also used for the early stages without CNS involvement.

Melarsoprol

The later stages of trypanosomiasis (CNS) are treated with melarsoprol, an organic arsenical. Chemically it is a condensation product of melarsen oxide with dimercaprol, an arsenical antagonist. The chemical structure is as follows:

Melarsoprol

This arrangement lowers the toxicity of the arsenic while retaining its trypanosomicidal activity. The mechanism of action is probably due to the action of arsenic in reacting with sulfhydryl groups. It is given only intravenously as slowly as possible to avoid GI symptoms. A severe adverse reaction is a reactive encephalopathy, which occurs at the end of the first week of therapy. Unfortunately, the more severe the CNS disease, the more likely is the encephalopathy to occur. Melarsoprol is available only from the Centers for Disease Control.

Other Trypanosomicidal Drugs

Suramin Sodium An older drug, suramin is interesting because it is derived from the observation that certain dyes (trypan red and blue and afridol violet) had trypanosomicidal activity. Chemically suramin consists of two large organic dye molecules which are joined by a urea linkage. Now less used than previously, it is still a drug of choice in the early stages of African trypanosomiasis. It is given intravenously, and the patient must be watched for adverse reactions such as shock and loss of consciousness, colic, and acute urticaria. Late toxicity may consist of albuminuria and peripheral neuritis.

Suramin is of no value in South American trypanosomiasis. It is, however, the drug of choice in the filarial infection *onchocerciasis*.

Nifurtimox (Lampit) In acute Chagas infection with *T. cruzi*, nifurtimox is a drug of choice. A nitrofurazone derivative, its structural formula is as follows:

$$O_2N \overset{\displaystyle O}{\diagdown} CH{=}N{-}N \overset{\displaystyle }{\diagdown} SO_2$$

$$H_3C$$

Nifurtimox

It apparently is capable of forming chemically reactive radicals (superoxide, hydrogen peroxide, hydroxyl) in the parasite. The parasite *T. cruzi* lacks catalase and glutathione peroxidase, thus increasing the susceptibility of the organism to hydrogen peroxide. The drug can cause serious GI disturbances, allergic reactions, and neurologic syndromes, so its use in the chronic form of Chagas disease is impractical. It is obtainable from the Centers for Disease Control.

OTHER PROTOZOAL DISEASES

Giardiasis

This protozoan intestinal disease is quite common and has occurred in endemic form in the United States. Often asymptomatic, it can invade the intestinal wall, causing ulceration and severe foul diarrhea. The cystic form is very resistant to therapy and may cause abscesses in the liver and other organs.

Quinacrine (Atabrine) has been the main therapy, but metronidazole, with much lower toxicity, is probably just as active and is replacing the former drug. In especially resistant cases the two drugs may be used together.

Furazolidone (Furoxone), a broad-spectrum antibacterial antinfective, is also active against *Giardia lamblia*. Since it is relatively less toxic than metronidazole, it has been recommended for use in children.

Other protozoal diseases are toxoplasmosis and trichomoniasis and pneumonia caused by *P. carinii*. The last is of particular importance because it is a frequent complication of AIDS. (See Table 46-1 and Chap. 43 for therapy.)

BIBLIOGRAPHY

Barrett-Connor, E.: "Drugs for the Treatment of Parasitic Infection," *Med. Clin. North Am.*, **66**:245 (1982).

Bushby, S. R. M., and G. H. Hitchings: "Trimethoprim, a Sulphonamide Potentiator," *Br. J. Pharmacol.*, **33**:72 (1968).

Cox, F. E.: "Malaria Vaccines. The Shape of Things to Come," *Nature*, **333**:702 (1988).

"Drugs for Parasitic Infections," *Med. Lett. Drugs Ther.*, **26**:27 (1984).

Goldman, P.: "Metronidazole," *N. Engl. J. Med.*, **303**:1212 (1980).

Jiang, J. B., et al.: "Antimalarial Activity of Mefloquine and Qinghaosu," *Lancet*, **2**:285 (1982).

Krogstad, D. J., H. C. Spencer, Jr., and G. R. Healy: "Amebiasis," *N. Engl. J. Med.*, **298**:262 (1978).

LeFrock, J. L.: "Drugs for Protozoan Infections," *Am. Fam. Physician*, **35**:247–251 (1987).

Lerman, S. J., and R. A. Walker: "Treatment of Giardiasis. Literature Review and Recommendation," *Clin. Pediatr.*, **21**:409 (1982).

Lister, G. D.: "Delayed Myocardial Intoxication following the Administration of Dehydroemetine Hydrochloride," *J. Trop. Med. Hyg.*, **71**:219 (1986).

Lossick, J. G.: "Treatment of *Trichomonas vaginalis* Infection," *Rev. Infect. Dis.*, **4**(Suppl.):S801 (1982).

Marsden, P. D.: "Current Concepts in Parasitology Leishmaniasis," *N. Engl. Med.*, **300**:350 (1979).

Phillips, R. E., et al: "Intravenous Quinidine for the Treatment of Severe *Falciparum malaria*: Clinical and Pharmacokinetic Studies," *N. Engl. J. Med.*, **312**:1273 (1985).

"Recommendations for the Prevention of Malaria in Travelers," *MMWR* **6**:37:277–284 (1988).

Wolfe, M. S.: "The Treatment of Intestinal Protozoan Infections," *Med. Clin. North Am.*, **66**:707 (1982).

Wyler, D. J.: "The Ascent and Decline of Chloroquine," *JAMA*, **251**:2420 (1984).

Chemotherapy of Helminthiases

Benjamin Z. Ngwenya

Helminthic infections represent a major problem to the health of millions of people throughout the world, especially in the subtropics and the tropics. The anthelmintic drugs are utilized to eradicate and control human intestinal helminthiases and may improve the health of the individual by alleviating the parasite-related suffering. The anthelmintic drugs covered in this chapter are listed alphabetically in Table 47-1. Most of the anthelmintics listed are active against specific helminths, and some are known to be toxic. It is advisable that before a drug is prescribed, a diagnosis and identification of the parasite must be made. This can be accomplished by finding the adult parasites and their characteristic eggs or larvae in feces, urine, sputum, blood, and tissues of the infected host. The anthelmintic of choice (Table 47-1) for the treatment of parasitic infection is usually the most active agent against the pathogenic parasite or the least toxic alternative among relatively effective anthelmintics.

This chapter provides some basic information for effective and safe anthelmintic drug treatment required by the prescriber to understand the essential pharmacology of the drugs used. The main intention is to provide information on chemistry, mechanism of action (if known), pharmacokinetics, clinical uses, adverse effects, and dose schedule of anthelmintic drugs.

ALBENDAZOLE

Chemistry

Albendazole, a synthetic benzimidazole carbamate derivative, is a broad-spectrum derivative, anthelmintic agent. It is practically insoluble in water and slightly soluble in most organic solvents. Its structure is as follows:

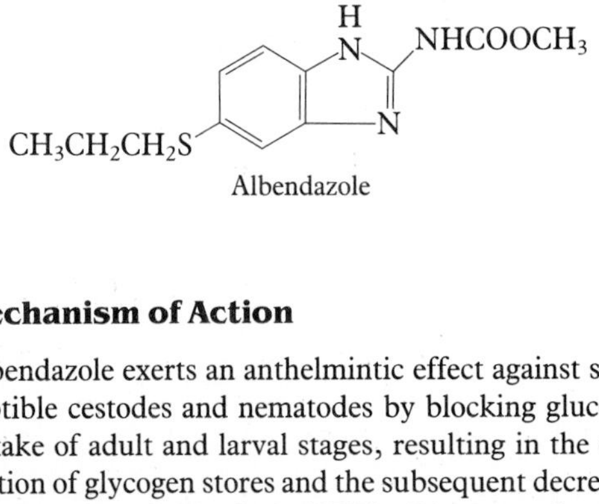

Albendazole

Mechanism of Action

Albendazole exerts an anthelmintic effect against susceptible cestodes and nematodes by blocking glucose uptake of adult and larval stages, resulting in the depletion of glycogen stores and the subsequent decrease of adenosine triphosphate (ATP). Consequently, the parasites are immobilized and die. The drug is ovicidal against *Ascaris lumbricoides, Ancylostoma duodenale, Necator americanus,* and *Trichuris trichiura* and larvicidal against *Necator americanus.*

TABLE 47-1   The choice of drugs for the treatment of helminthic infections

Infecting agent disease	Anthelmintic of choice	Alternative anthelmintics
Cestodes (tapeworms)		
Cysticercus cellulosae (pork tapeworm larval stage) Cysticercosis	Praziquantel	Surgery
Diphyllobothrium latum (fish tapeworm) Diphyllobothriasis	Niclosamide	Praziquantel or paromomycin
Dipylidium caninum (dog tapeworm) Dipylidiasis	Niclosamide	Praziquantel
Echinococcus granulosus (hydatid worm) Echinococcosis	Surgery or mebendazole	Albendazole
Echinococcus multilocularis (hydatid worm) Echinococcosis	Surgery or mebendazole	Albendazole
Hymenolepis diminuta (rat tapeworm) Hymenolepiasis	Niclosamide	Praziquantel
Hymenolepis nana (dwarf tapeworm) Hymenolepiasis	Praziquantel	Niclosamide or paromomycin
Taenia saginata (beef tapeworm) Taeniasis	Niclosamide	Praziquantel, paromomycin
Taenia solium (pork tapeworm) Taeniasis	Niclosamide	Praziquantel, paromomycin, or mebendazole
Nematodes (roundworms)		
Acanthocheilonema perstans Acanthocheilonemiasis	Diethylcarbamazine	None
Ancylostoma braziliense (dog and cat hookworm) Ancylostomiasis (cutaneous larva migrans, creeping eruption)	Thiabendazole or albendazole	Diethylcarbamazine

TABLE 47-1 (*continued*)   **The choice of drugs for the treatment of helminthic infections**

Infecting agent disease	Anthelmintic of choice	Alternative anthelmintics
Nematodes (roundworms) (*continued*)		
Ancylostoma caninum (dog hookworm) Ancylostomiasis (cutaneous larva migrans, creeping eruption)	Thiabendazole or albendazole	Diethylcarbamazine
Ancylostoma duodenale (human hookworm) Ancylostomiasis	Mebendazole or pyrantel pamoate	Tetrachloroethylene, levamisole, or bephenium
Angiostrongylus cantonensis Angiostrongyliasis	Levamisole or thiabendazole	None
Anisakis sp. Anisakiasis	Surgical removal	Thiabendazole
Ascaris lumbricoides (roundworm) Ascariasis	Pyrantel pamoate or mebendazole	Piperazine citrate, levamisole
Brugia malayi (Malayan filarial worm) Malayan filariasis	Diethylcarbamazine	None
Dracunculus medinensis (guinea worm) Dracunculiasis	Niridazole or metronidazole	Thiabendazole, mebendazole
Enterobius vermicularis (pinworm) Enterobiasis	Pyrantel pamoate or mebendazole	Pyrvinium pamoate or albendazole
Combined infection with human hookworm and *Ascaris*	Mebendazole or pyrantel pamoate	Bephenium or albendazole
Multiple infection with human hookworm, ascariasis, and trichuriasis	Mebendazole or pyrantel pamoate	Albendazole
Intestinal capillariasis	Mebendazole	Thiabendazole
Loa loa (eyeworm) Loiasis	Diethylcarbamazine	None

TABLE 47-1 (*continued*)   **The choice of drugs for the treatment of helminthic infections**

Infecting agent disease	Anthelmintic of choice	Alternative anthelmintics
Nematodes (roundworms) (*continued*)		
Necator americanus (human hookworm) Necatoriasis	Mebendazole or tetrachloroethylene, pyrantel pamoate	Levamisole or bephenium
Onchocerca volvulus (filarial worm) Onchocerciasis	Diethylcarbamazine followed by suramin	Mebendazole, ivermectin
Strongyloides stercoralis (threadworm) Strongyloidiasis	Thiabendazole	Mebendazole, albendazole
Toxocara canis (dog ascarid) Toxocariasis (Viceral larva migrans)	Diethylcarbamazine or thiabendazole	Mebendazole
Toxocara cati (cat ascarid) Toxocariasis (Visceral larva migrans)	Diethylcarbamazine or thiabendazole	Mebendazole
Trichinella spiralis Trichinosis	Steroids for severe symptoms plus thiabendazole	Mebendazole
Trichostrongylus species Trichostrongyliasis	Pyrantel pamoate or mebendazole	Levamisole or bephenium
Trichuris trichiura (whipworm) Trichuriasis	Mebendazole	Pyrantel pamoate or albendazole
Tropical eosinophilia	Diethylcarbamazine	None
Wuchereria bancrofti (filarial worm) Bancroft's filariasis	Diethylcarbamazine	None
Trematodes (flukes)		
Clonorchis sinensis (liver fluke) Clonorchiasis	Praziquantel	Mebendazole or albendazole

TABLE 47-1 *(continued)*   **The choice of drugs for the treatment of helminthic infections**

Infecting agent disease	Anthelmintic of choice	Alternative anthelmintics
Trematodes (flukes) *(continued)*		
Fasciola hepatica (sheep liver fluke) Fascioliasis	Bithionol	Praziquantel, emetine, or dehydroemetine
Fasciolopsis buski (large intestinal fluke) Fasciolopsiasis	Praziquantel or niclosamide	Tetrachloroethylene, dichlorophen, or bephenium
Heterophyes heterophyes Heterophyiasis	Praziquantel or niclosamide	Tetrachloroethylene, bephenium
Metagonimus yokogawai (Yokogawa's fluke) Metagonimiasis	Praziquantel or niclosamide	Tetrachloroethylene, bephenium
Opisthorchis species (liver fluke) Opisthorchiasis	Praziquantel	Mebendazole or albendazole
Paragonimus westermani (lung fluke) Paragonimiasis	Praziquantel	Bithionol
Schistosoma haematobium (vesical blood fluke) Vesical schistosomiasis Urinary bilharziasis	Praziquantel	Metrifonate
Schistosoma japonicum (Oriental blood fluke) Oriental schistosomiasis Katayama disease	Praziquantel	Niridazole
Schistosoma mansoni (Manson's blood fluke) Schistosomal dysentery Intestinal bilharziasis	Praziquantel	Oxamniquine
Trematodes (roundworms)		
Schistosoma mekongi (Mekong schistosome)	Praziquantel	

Pharmacokinetics

Orally administered albendazole is rapidly absorbed from the gastrointestinal tract and is metabolized to yield mainly albendazole sulfoxide and other metabolites. Large amounts of the metabolites formed by hydroxylation and hydrolysis of albendazole sulfoxide are mainly excreted in the urine, and only a trace amount is excreted in the feces. The plasma elimination half-life of the sulfoxide is about 8 to 9 h.

Pharmacodynamics

Albendazole itself is not detected in plasma due to its rapid metabolism. The sulfoxide metabolite appears to mediate most of the anthelmintic effect of albendazole. Based on animal model and limited human studies, albendazole has no pharmacologic effects at therapeutic oral doses of 5 mg/kg. However, intravenous administration of higher doses causes cardiovascular depression in animal studies. In long-term (30 days) studies in dogs and rats, elevation of alkaline phosphotase, diarrhea, leukopenia, and anemia were noted in few animals at dose level of 48 mg/kg/day. Teratogenecity and embryotoxicity have been reported in pregnant rats and rabbits treated with 30 mg/kg/day.

Adverse Effects

When used at recommended dosage for 1 to 3 days, albendazole appears to be practically free of adverse effects. However, mild transient headache, nausea, diarrhea, epigastric distress, lassitude, insomnia, and dizziness have been reported in about 6 percent of the patients. Placebo-controlled experiments suggest that the incidence of side effects attributed to the drug was similar to that in the control group. A few cases of transient abdominal pain, low-grade transaminase elevations, mild transient neutropenia, and fever have been reported during albendazole treatment. Further evaluation of the type and severity of the side effects of the drug after both single and repeated treatment is warranted.

Clinical Uses

Administration of albendazole has been used effectively against *A. lumbricoides*, *A. duodenale*, *N. americanus*, *T. trichiura*, and *Enterobius vermicularis*. A sin-gle dose of orally administered albendazole to 1455 patients resulted in cure rates of 70, 80, 88, and 100 percent for trichuriasis, ascariasis, necatoriasis, and enterobiasis, respectively. To attain a satisfactory reduction in worm burden in patients with heavy trichuriasis and nectoriasis and high cure rates in ascariasis may require a higher initial single dose or repeated treatment for several days (2 to 3 days). The cure rates of the drug in patients who attain low-plasma concentration levels of the sulfoxide metabolite remains to be elucidated.

Contraindications

Albendazole has been shown to be teratogenic and embryotoxic in some experimental animals. Therefore, it is not recommended during pregnancy and lactation. Its safety has not been established in children under 2 years of age. The drug should be used with caution in patients with history of hematologic and liver diseases.

BEPHENIUM HYDROXYNAPHTHOATE

Chemistry

Bephenium, a quaternary ammonium compound of bephenium hydroxynaphthoate, is an anthelmintic agent. The drug is sensitive to light and therefore should be protected. It is practically insoluble in water. Its structure is as follows:

$$C_6H_5OCH_2CH_2-\overset{\overset{\displaystyle CH_3}{|}}{\underset{\underset{\displaystyle CH_2C_6H_5}{|}}{N^+}}-CH_3 \cdot \text{anion}$$

Bephenium hydroxynaphthoate

Mechanism of Action

Bephenium exerts its anthelmintic effects by acting as a cholinergic agonist, inducing initial excitation and the subsequent paralysis of the parasite.

Pharmacokinetics

Bephenium is insoluble in water. After ingestion, absorption from the gastrointestinal mucosa is minimal. Studies show that less than 0.5 percent of the prescribed dose is excreted in the urine 24 h posttreatment. Specific analytical methods for determination of this drug are not available.

Adverse Effects

Bephenium has a bitter taste. This minor problem can be alleviated by giving the drug with a sweet drink. Adverse effects such as nausea, vomiting, and headache have been observed soon after drug ingestion. Vertigo has been reported in a few cases.

There are no reports concerning teratogenicity and embryotoxicity. Long-term toxicity studies are not available.

Clinical Uses

In several studies, a single dose of bephenium resulted in cure rates of 80 to 100 percent of patients with ancylostomiasis (*Ancylostoma duodenale*). However, the drug is less effective against *N. americanus*. In ascariasis, success rates with a single-dose treatment are about 50 to 70 percent. More effective alternative drugs are available.

Contraindications

Patients with inflammatory bowel diseases should not be given this drug. There are no untoward reactions to the pregnant women that have been reported. Nevertheless, superior alternative drugs should be considered for use first.

BITHIONOL

Chemistry

Bithionol is a dichlorophenol structurally similar to hexachlorophene. It is the anthelmintic of choice for the treatment of human infection by *Fasciola hepatica* (sheep liver fluke) and is an alternative to the drug praziquantel for the treatment of pulmonary paragonimiasis (lung fluke) and acute cerebral paragonimiasis. This drug is not marketed in the United States. It is distributed by the Centers for Disease Control (CDC),

Atlanta, Georgia. Bithionol is practically insoluble in water. Information on storage and stability of the drug is not available. Its structure is as follows:

Bithionol

Mechanism of Action

Although the exact mechanism of anthelmintic action of bithionol has not been fully elucidated, the drug appears to inhibit oxidative phosphorylation in *Paragonimus westermani*. Morphological alteration in *F. hepatica* has been attributed to the drug.

Pharmacokinetics

Although no specific analytical method for assaying the metabolic fate of bithionol exists, the drug is readily absorbed from the gastrointestinal tract and glucuronidated in the liver. The drug excretion appears to be mainly through the kidney.

Pharmacodynamics

Anorexia, nausea, vomiting, and diarrhea have been observed in few patients and are probably due to effects of the drug. Urticaria or skin rashes together with pruritus have been reported. There are insufficient data on bithionol treatment during pregnancy and lactation to recommend its use in such patients.

Adverse Effects

Side effects have been reported in about one-third of the patients. Usually the effects are mild and transient. The most common side effects are abdominal cramps and diarrhea. Diarrhea in these patients may be accompanied by anorexia, nausea, and vomiting. Some patients receiving long-term therapy may develop pruritic, urticaria, or papular skin rashes. Since the onset of skin rashes occurs after a latent period of a week or more of therapy, they could be due to allergic reactions resulting from massive release of antigens from the dying parasites. Other infrequent side effects are leukopenia and proteinuria.

Clinical Uses

Bithionol is the anthelmintic of choice for the treatment of fascioliasis (sheep liver fluke) and as an alternative to praziquantel for the treatment of human infections by *Paragonimus* species. A treatment regimen with 10 to 50 mg/kg on alternate days for a total of 15 doses resulted in a cure rate of 91 to 97 percent in patients with pulmonary paragonimiasis. However, in patients with combined pulmonary and cerebral paragonimiasis, the results were less satisfactory. In patients with acute cerebral paragonimiasis, bithionol effectiveness may be enhanced by administering more than one course of treatment. The drug effectiveness is minimal in patients with long-term cerebral paragonimiasis.

Although meager information is available on the efficacy of bithionol in fascioliasis, it should be tried first as the drug of choice for treatment of human infection by *F. hepatica*, because praziquantel is ineffective and dihydroemetine is more toxic.

Contraindications

There is limited experience with bithionol treatment during pregnancy and lactation. Therefore, its use in such patients is not recommended. In children under 8 years of age, the efficacy and safety of bithionol have not been established, and it should be used with caution. The development of toxic hepatitis and leukopenia should be evaluated by liver function and hematologic test, respectively. It appears that the drug does not worsen the neurologic condition of patients with cerebral paragonimiasis, but the evidence is inconclusive.

DIETHYLCARBAMAZINE

Chemistry

Diethylcarbamazine, a piperazine derivative, is an effective drug for the treatment of filariasis. It is available as the citrate salt containing 51 percent of the active base. The drug is highly soluble in water. It should be stored in airtight containers and protected from light. Its structure is as follows:

Diethylcarbamazine

Mechanism of Action

The exact mechanism of antimicrofilarial activity of diethylcarbamazine has not been fully elucidated. The drug causes rapid sensitization of the microfilariae, and they become trapped in the reticuloendothelial system. The drug also causes a rapid disappearance of microfilariae of *Brugia malayi, Loa loa, and Wuchereria bancrofti* from the circulatory system.

Pharmacokinetics

Orally administered diethylcarbamazine is rapidly absorbed from the gastrointestinal tract. A single dose produces a peak plasma level of 1.5 μg/mL within 1 to 3 h. The minimum effective plasma level is about 1 mg/mL. The drug is rapidly distributed and equilibrated with all tissues, except fat. Its half-life is about 2 to 3 h and 10 h in the presence of acidic and alkaline urine, respectively. Diethylcarbamazine is excreted primarily in the urine within 30 h, either as unchanged drug or as *N*-oxide. Less than 10 percent of the drug is excreted in feces.

Adverse Effects

At therapeutic levels, diethylcarbamazine is relatively safe. However, mild transient malaise, headache, joint pains, anorexia, nausea, and vomiting occur in 2 to 4 h posttreatment. There are specific adverse effects seen only in filarial-infected patients.

Parasite-Induced Reactions These reactions are assumed to be caused by the release of foreign proteins (antigens) from dying microfilariae or adult worms in sensitized patients. Usually the reactions are associated with intensified eosinophilia and leukocytosis. In lymphatic filariasis, the reactions may be very severe in heavy infections, producing a syndrome known as the *Mazzotti reaction*. It is characterized by generalized pruritus, rash, edema of the skin, erythema, lymphangitis, chills, conjunctiva, tearing, photophobia, and sweating. Respiratory distress, tachycardia, and hyperpyrexia have also been reported. The severity of the Mazzotti reaction is directly related to the microfilarial burden in the skin. Treating the patient with antiserotonins, antihistamines, or antiprostaglandins will not diminish the Mazzotti reaction. However, the severity of the Mazzotti reaction may be alleviated by systemic administration of corticosteroids, but this reduces the efficacy of diethylcarbamazine. In loiasis, treatment may aggravate ocular lesions and result in blindness due to reaction against the dying microfilariae.

Clinical Uses

Diethylcarbamazine is indicated for the treatment of *W. bancrofti*, *B. malayi*, *L. loa*, and *Onchocerca volvulus*. The drug has a high therapeutic efficacy against these parasites. It is also used in *Mansonella streptocerca* infections and in tropical eosinophilia. Diethylcarbamazine has been used for mass treatment to reduce transmission of *W. bancrofti*. The drug may be given in low doses as a medicated salt, which is stable in cooking and seems to be free of adverse effects but still active against the microfilariae. The drug has also been recommended for prophylactic measures against *L. loa*, *W. bancrofti*, and *B. malayi* infections.

Contraindications and Precautions

Although there are no absolute adverse effects, diethylcarbamazine should be used with caution in patients with hypertension and renal disease. Dosage should be adjusted in patients with high urinary pH, because renal function and pH are critical factors associated with the excretion of the drug. In patients with onchocerciasis or mixed filariasis, dosage of diethylcarbamazine should be increased gradually.

LEVAMISOLE

Chemistry

Levamisole hydrochloride, an imidazothiazole derivative, is the L isomer of DL-tetramisole. The drug is highly effective against *A. lumbricoides*, *A. duodenale*,

and *Trichostrongylus* spp., and it has moderate effects against *Strongyloides stercoralis*. Levamisole is not marketed in the United States. Its structure is as follows:

Levamisole

Mechanism of Action

Levamisole appears to have ganglion-stimulating effects on parasite tissue at both parasympathetic and sympathetic sites. This may contribute to the drug's anthelmintic effect. Its mechanism of action as an immunomodulating agent is still under investigation. The available data suggest that the drug affects host defenses by augmenting the cell-mediated immunity.

The drug seems to be useful only when the patient has depressed cell-mediated immunity, and it has insignificant effect on normal immune mechanism at therapeutic dosage. At higher doses, the drug acts as an immunomodulator for cell-mediated immunity.

Pharmacokinetics

Levamisole is soluble in water. Following oral administration, levamisole is rapidly and extensively absorbed from the gastrointestinal tract. A single oral dose of 2.5 mg/kg produces peak plasma levels of 0.5 to 0.7 mg/mL within 2 to 4 h. The drug is extensively metabolized in the liver and is widely distributed to the tissues with highest concentration attained in about 4 h. The elimination of the drug is almost complete in 48 h. One of the metabolites, hydroxylevamisole, is excreted in urine, and about 5 percent of the administered dose is excreted unchanged in the urine. About 4 percent of the drug is excreted in feces and 70 percent is excreted in urine within 72 h.

Pharmacodynamics

Levamisole is reported to have a reversible ganglion-stimulating activity on mammalian tissues at parasympathetic and sympathetic sites. The resultant drug stimulation of skeletal, central, and autonomic nervous system produces mood-elevating effects in patients. In helminths, levamisole stimulates ganglion-like structures, inducing muscle contractions and neuromuscular paralysis. This results in the expulsion of the worms by normal peristalsis. The drug has also been reported to restore cell-mediated immune response in immunologically depressed patients.

Adverse Effects

When levamisole is administered as a single dose for treatment of nematode infections, adverse effects are mild and transient. They include headache, nausea, vomiting, abdominal pain, weakness, dizziness, and skin rash.

Clinical Uses

In several studies, a single dose of 15 to 150 mg levamisole cured 90 percent of patients with ascariasis. In *A. duodenale* infections, a single oral dose of 150 mg has been reported to produce cure rates of 90 to 100 percent. However, the drug is not as effective when used for the treatment of *N. americanus* infection.

Contraindications

There are no known contraindications in the use of levamisole for the treatment of nematodiasis.

MEBENDAZOLE

Chemistry

Mebendazole is a synthetic benzimidazole derivative. It is a broad-spectrum anthelmintic agent. The drug occurs as a white-yellowish powder and is nearly insoluble in alcohol and water. Tablets should be stored in tightly closed containers and have an expiration date of 3 years. Its structure is as follows:

Mebendazole

Mechanism of Action

The exact mechanism of anthelmintic action of mebendazole has not been completely elucidated. The drug selectively and irreversibly inhibits glucose up-

take by the parasites, resulting in glycogen depletion which leads to the ultimate death of the parasites. Mebendazole does not affect blood glucose concentrations in humans.

Pharmacokinetics

Orally administered mebendazole is minimally absorbed from the gastrointestinal tract. It is indicated that about 2 to 10 percent of an oral dose is absorbed, and peak plasma concentration of the drug occurs about 0.5 to 7 h postadministration. The drug is rapidly metabolized via decarboxylation to 2-amino-5(6)-benzimidazolyl phenylketone. The excretion half-life of mebendazole is about 3 to 9 h, and the drug is eliminated in the urine either unchanged or as a decarboxylated derivative over a 24 to 48 h period. The drug may also be excreted via the bile into feces.

Pharmacodynamics

Mebendazole appears to be almost inert in humans. Studies in pregnant rats indicate that the drug has teratogenic and embryotoxic activity. In human studies, no teratogenic risk was associated with mebendazole therapy in 170 full-term deliveries.

Adverse Effects

At recommended dosage for a short-term (1 to 3 days) usage, mebendazole appears to be remarkably free of adverse effects. Few cases of transient nausea, vomiting, abdominal pain, and diarrhea have been reported in patients with massive infections. Higher or massive doses of mebendazole have been shown to induce bone marrow toxicity.

Clinical Uses

Mebendazole is indicated for the treatment of tricuriasis, ascariasis, trichostrongylosis, and ancylostomiasis. A dose of 100 mg twice daily for 3 days produces 90 to 100 percent cure rates for ascariasis and trichostrongyliasis. In trichuriasis and hookworm infections, cure rates of 60 to 90 percent and 70 to 95 percent are obtained, respectively. Mebendazole studies show cure rates of 90 to 100 percent for *E. vermicularis* (pinworm). The cure rates of mebendazole compare favorably with dose regimen of pyrantel pamoate and pyrvinium pamoate. However, mebendazole has the added advantage of fewer adverse effects. Mebendazole is also used as the drug of choice in patients who have capillariasis. The drug is an effective alternative to thiabendazole for the treatment of toxocariasis (dog and cat ascarid).

Contraindications

Mebendazole is contraindicated in patients who are pregnant or hypersensitive to the drug. Mebendazole should be used with caution in patients with severe hepatic parenchymal disease because the drug is poorly detoxified in such patients. The safety of mebendazole in children under 2 years of age has not been established. It should be used in children with caution.

NICLOSAMIDE

Chemistry

Niclosamide, a salicylamide derivative, is an effective anthelmintic agent. It is available as a cream-colored or yellowish-white powder or pale yellow crystals. The drug is slightly soluble in alcohol and practically insoluble in water. Niclosamide tablets should be stored below 30°C and avoid freezing and exposure to light. Its structure is as follows:

Niclosamide

Mechanism of Action

Niclosamide, an anthelmintic agent, exerts its effect against cestodes via the inhibition of mitochondrial oxidative phosphorylation in the parasites. The mechanism of niclosamide action is also related to its inhibition of glucose and oxygen uptake in the parasite. The drug-induced alteration of the parasite integument may render the cestodes susceptible to digestion by the host intestinal proteolytic enzymes. At therapeutic doses, the drug appears to have no pharmacologic effect on human cells.

Pharmacokinetics

Orally administered niclosamide is minimally absorbed from the gastrointestinal tract. Therefore, only trace amounts of an oral dose of niclosamide reach the circulatory system. Although the exact metabolic fate of the drug has not been elucidated, limited evidence indicate that the drug is metabolized in the gastrointestinal tract and excreted in feces.

Pharmacodynamics

Limited evidence suggest that orally administered niclosamide in animals and humans has not been associated with hematologic, hepatic, or renal abnormalities. However, extensive pharmacologic evaluation of niclosamide in humans has not been reported.

Adverse Effects

Niclosamide is generally well tolerated at recommended dosage (2 g). Niclosamide therapy may be associated with transient and mild to severe side effects. The infrequent adverse effects are abdominal discomfort, nausea, vomiting, and diarrhea; rarely reported adverse effects associated with niclosamide treatment include fever, headache, pruritus ani, skin rash, and urticaria, some of which may be attributed to a hypersensitivity reaction to massive antigens absorbed from disintegrating tapeworms.

Clinical Uses

Niclosamide is effective against adult intestinal cestodes such as *Diphyllobothrium latum* (fish tapeworm), *Taenia saginata* (beef tapeworm), *Taenia solium* (pork tapeworm), *Dipylidium caninum* (cat and dog tapeworm), *Hymenolepis diminuta* (rat tapeworm), and *Hymenolepis nana* (dwarf tapeworm).

A single 2-g oral dose of the drug results in cure rates of 85 and 95 percent for adult *D. latum* and *T. saginata* or *T. solium*, respectively. The drug is ineffective for the treatment of cysticercosis (an invasive larval disease) acquired by humans via the ingestion of the eggs of *T. solium*. Niclosamide is effective against the adult *H. nana* tapeworms but not against tissue-embedded cysticercoides. The cure rate for *H. nana* is about 75 percent for a treatment regimen of 5 to 7 days. Promising results have been reported in patients treated for *D. caninum* and *H. diminuta* infections. Niclosamide is also considered the drug of choice for the treatment of intestinal fluke (*Fasciolopsis buski*) infection.

Contraindications

Niclosamide exerts its effect against intestinal cestodes and should not be used in the treatment of invasive larval disease (cysticercosis). It is advisable not to use niclosamide for the treatment of *T. solium*, because the drug causes disintegration of proglottids (worm segments) and release of infective eggs. The presence of the eggs in the intestinal tract is correlated with a serious theoretical risk of the development of cysticercosis. To avoid this possibility, some clinicians consider praziquantel the drug of choice for the treatment of *T. solium*.

Consumption of alcohol is contraindicated on the day of treatment and for 1 day past treatment. The drug is also contraindicated in patients who are hypersensitive to the drug. Niclosamide safety in children under 2 years of age has not been established.

NIRIDAZOLE

Chemistry

Niridazole is a nitrothiazole derivative and has schistosomicidal and amebicidal action. Its structure is as follows:

Niridazole

Mechanism of Action

The mechanism of action of niridazole is not clear. In animals infected with *Schistosoma mansoni*, niridazole induces a "liver shift" of adult schistosomes, which results in their death. The drug is also rapidly concentrated in the parasites, causing inhibition of phosphorylase activation that results in glycogen depletion of the adult worms. The drug has been reported to cause inhibition of oogenesis and spermatogenesis, and reduction in the size of the parasite and interruption of egg production.

Pharmacokinetics

After oral administration, niridazole is absorbed slowly over a period of 10 to 15 h. The drug is extensively metabolized to 4-hydroxyniridazole and 4-ketoniridazole. Peak plasma concentration is reached in 6 h. The drug has a half-life of only a few hours. However, the drug metabolites are bound to serum proteins and have a half-life of approximately 40 h. Niridazole is mostly excreted as metabolites equally in the urine and feces.

Pharmacodynamics

Niridazole produces reduced glycogen levels in animal muscles. This glycogen depletion may account for some of the drug's adverse effects in humans. The drug also causes temporary inhibition of spermatogenesis. Furthermore, niridazole has anti-inflammatory properties, suppresses cell-mediated immunity, and has antibacterial effect. No reports are available on its effects on human peripheral blood counts or bone marrow.

Adverse Effects

Adverse effects of niridazole are transient and occur in about 70 percent of patients. The most frequent include nausea, vomiting, abdominal pain, anorexia, headache, fatigue, diarrhea, muscle ache, dizziness, sweating, palpitation, and skin rash. These adverse effects appear about 3 to 4 days after treatment and disappear days after therapy. Niridazole may cause hemolysis in patients with glucose-6-phosphate dehydrogenase deficiency. Gastrointestinal hemorrhage and Stevens-Johnson syndrome have rarely been associated with the drug.

Blood counts and liver function tests should be monitored during the course of therapy. The drug and its metabolites have been reported to have carcinogenic and mutagenic properties.

Clinical Uses

Niridazole is indicated for the treatment of *Dracunculus medinensis*. The drug reduces swelling and pain during treatment and facilitates spontaneous expulsion of the worms. In *Schistosoma japonicum* infections, niridazole is used as an alternative drug and in

Schistosoma haematobium and *S. mansoni* infections, it should be considered a tertiary drug, to be used only if the drug of choice is not available.

Contraindications

Niridazole should always be administered under strict daily medical supervision. Niridazole is contraindicated for patients with impaired liver function, glucose-6-phosphate dehydrogenase, history of liver disease, cardiac or renal disease, hepatosplenic disease caused by schistosomiasis, hypertension, history of psychiatric disorder, epilepsy, and gastrointestinal ulcer. Patients with debilitating conditions such as anemia, malnutrition, and infections should have these conditions corrected prior to therapy.

PIPERAZINE

Chemistry

Piperazine is available as a variety of salts: tartrate, citrate, adipate, phosphate, and also as a hexahydrate containing 40 percent of the base. The drug is relatively soluble in water. Its structure is as follows:

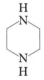

Piperazine

Mechanism of Action

Piperazine is used to treat enterobiasis and ascariasis. The drug causes a paralysis of the nematodes by blocking acetylcholine possibly at the myoneural junction. This causes the parasites to detach from the intestinal wall, and they are expelled live by normal bowel peristalsis.

Pharmacokinetics

Piperazine is readily absorbed from the intestinal tract. Peak plasma levels are attained in 2 to 4 h. The drug appears to be excreted mainly unchanged in the urine 2 to 6 h after the drug intake. The drug excretion in urine varies among patients from 15 to 70 percent of the original dose.

Pharmacodynamics

Piperazine appears to be almost free of pharmacologic effects in humans. However, a potentially carcinogenic nitrosamine derivative (mononitrosopiperazine) has been reported in urine and gastric fluids of volunteers administered therapeutic doses of the drug.

Adverse Effects

Mild and transient side effects occur occasionally. These include nausea, vomiting, abdominal cramps, diarrhea, and rare neurologic side effects such as incoordination, vertigo, tremors, lethargy, hyporeflexia, muscular weakness, and blurring of vision.

Clinical Uses

Piperazine is indicated as an alternative drug for treating ascariasis and enterobiasis. For ascariasis, a dose of 75 mg/kg once daily for 2 days gives cure rates of over 90 percent. In enterobiasis, it requires a 7-day course of treatment to effect cure.

Contraindications

The drug should not be administered to patients with a history of impaired hepatic or renal function, epilepsy, or chronic neurologic disease. Piperazine should be administered with caution in patients with anemia or severe malnutrition. The teratogenic potential of the drug has not been fully elucidated.

PRAZIQUANTEL

Chemistry

Praziquantel, a synthetic pyrazinoisoquinoline derivative, is a broad-spectrum anthelmintic agent. It is structurally unrelated to other anthelmintic agents currently available. The drug occurs as a hygroscopic, crystalline, colorless powder and has a distinctly bitter taste. It is slightly soluble in water and is soluble in alcohol.

Praziquantel tablets should be stored in tightly closed containers at a temperature below 30°C. Its structure is as follows:

Praziquantel

Mechanism of Action

The precise mechanism of action of praziquantel has not been fully elucidated. Praziquantel appears to kill the adult schistosomes by increasing the permeability of the cell membrane of the parasite to calcium and consequent influx of calcium ions. This results in drug-induced massive contraction and subsequent paralysis of the parasite's muscles. This causes immobilization of their suckers, resulting in parasite detachment from their sites of residence in the mesenteric veins or vesical plexus. The worms are then carried to the liver, where they elicit tissue reaction with subsequent phagocytosis. The drug appears also to be active against the schistosomal infective stage (cercaria) for humans and animals.

Praziquantel has also been shown to cause irreversible focal vacuolization and subsequent disintegration of the trematodes and cestodes.

Pharmacokinetics

Praziquantel is well absorbed (about 80 percent) after oral administration. A small portion of the drug reaches the blood unchanged. Peak plasma drug concentration (1 mg/mL) is reached 1 to 2 h after a single oral administration of 50 mg/kg. The concentration of the drug in cerebrospinal fluid is reported to be 14 to 20 percent of the plasma concentration.

Praziquantel has a serum half-life of approximately 0.8 to 1.5 h in normal adults. The serum half-life of the metabolites is about 4 to 5 h. Although the precise metabolic fate of praziquantel is unclear, most of the drug is quickly and extensively metabolized in the liver via hydroxylation to monohydroxylated and polyhydroxylated metabolites.

The drug and its metabolites are mostly excreted in urine. Approximately 70 to 80 percent of orally administered dose is excreted in urine as metabolites within 24 h.

Pharmacodynamics

At recommended dosage, praziquantel has not produced major alterations in hematologic and biochemical tests. No reactions have been reported in patients with glucose-6-phosphate dehydrogenase deficiencies or hemoglobinopathies. No significant damage to vital organs has been observed.

In animal studies, signs of cerebral toxicity have been reported in animals receiving doses of about 100 times the therapeutic levels. Mutagenecity studies show no abnormalities. Tests for teratogenicity, embryotoxicity, and carcinogenecity have been reported to be negative.

Adverse Effects

At recommended dosage, praziquantel is generally well tolerated. The drug is associated with frequent occurrence of transient and mild to moderate side effects such as malaise, headache, abdominal pain, and dizziness, which occur in about 90 percent of patients. Diarrhea, anorexia, and vomiting have also been reported. Other side effects are pruritus, skin rashes, low-grade fever, and elevated eosinophilia. Heavily infected patients are associated with increased frequency of side effects. The intensity and frequency of the adverse effects appear to be dose-related. The drug has not been shown to produce carcinogenic or mutagenic effects.

Clinical Uses

Praziquantel is indicated for the treatment of all forms of human schistosomiasis. The drug is highly effective, has low toxicity, and is easily administered orally. Praziquantel is well tolerated by patients in the chronic stage (hepatosplenic stage) of advanced schistosomiasis. The drug produces cure rates of 75 to 95 percent and/or 80 to 98 percent egg reduction in infected patients. Praziquantel is the drug of choice in the treatment of *S. mansoni*, *S. haematobium*, and *S. japonicum*. The drug has also been shown to be effective against *S. intercalatum* or *S. mekongi*.

Praziquantel has also been used effectively in the treatment of other trematode infections caused by *Paragonimus westermani*, *Clonorchis sinensis*, *Metagonimus yokogawai*, *Heterophyes heterophyes*, and *Fasciolopsis buski* and is currently considered the drug of choice. Praziquantel is also effective against cestodes infection, including *T. solium*, *T. saginata*, *D. latum*, and *H. nana*. Some clinicians consider praziquantel the drug of choice for *T. solium* because paromomycin and niclosamide cause disintegration of proglottids and release of eggs which may produce *Cysticercus cellulosae* infection.

Contraindications

Praziquantel should not be administered in patients who are hypersensitive to the drug. Preferably the drug should not be taken during pregnancy. Patients should be advised not to drive because the drug causes dizziness and drowsiness on the day of and the day after therapy. Safety of the drug in children under 4 years of age has not been established.

PYRANTEL PAMOATE

Chemistry

Pyrantel pamoate, a pyrimidine derivative, is a highly effective anthelmintic agent. Each 100 mg of pyrantel base is equivalent to 290 mg pyrantel pamoate. The drug occurs as a yellow-to-tan solid and is insoluble in alcohol and in water. Pyrantel pamoate is available commercially as an oral suspension, and it should be stored in high-resistant container at a temperature below 30°C. Its structure is as follows:

Pyrantel pamoate

Mechanism of Action

Pyrantel pamoate exerts its anthelmintic effect via the inhibition of neuromuscular transmission. In susceptible worms, a spastic neuromuscular paralysis occurs, resulting in the expulsion of the worms from the intestinal tract of the host. Pyrantel also exerts its effect against parasites via release of acetylcholine and inhibition of cholinesterase.

Pharmacokinetics

Orally administered pyrantel pamoate is poorly absorbed from the gastrointestinal tract. Peak plasma concentrations (50 to 130 mg/mL) are attained in 1 to 3 h. The drug is partially metabolized in the liver, and about 7 percent is excreted in urine unchanged or as metabolites. About 50 percent of an oral dose of the drug is excreted unchanged in the feces.

Pyrantel does not appear to produce any clinically significant alterations in urinary values at therapeutic dosages. However, minimal transient increases in serum concentrations of SGOT have been reported in a few patients.

Adverse Effects

Adverse effects of pyrantel pamoate occur in 4 to 20 percent of patients and are usually infrequent, mild, and transient. They include abdominal cramps, nausea, diarrhea, vomiting, headache, insomnia, drowsiness, rash, fever, and weakness.

Clinical Uses

Pyrantel is administered orally. It is used for the treatment of ascariasis, enterobiasis, and hookworm disease. The drug has cure rates of 85 to 100 percent in patients infected with ascariasis and 90 to 100 percent in patients with enterobiasis. Pyrantel pamoate, like mebendazole, is currently considered a drug of choice for *E. vermicularis* and *A. lumbricoides*. Mebendazole is as effective as pyrantel. However, Mebendazole has been reported to produce fewer adverse effects than pyrantel. Pyrantel has also been used for the treatment of *A. duodenale* and *N. americanus*, producing cure rates of 92 to 96 percent and 48 to 93 percent, respectively.

Contraindications

There are no reports on contraindications to pyrantel pamoate, but it should be used with caution in patients with severe anemia and liver dysfunction, because minimal transient increase in serum concentration of SGOT have been reported in few patients.

THIABENDAZOLE

Chemistry

Thiabendazole is a benzimidazole derivative and a broad-spectrum anthelmintic agent. It is structurally related to mebendazole. Thiabendazole is a white, practically odorless powder, and it is tasteless, slightly soluble in alcohol, and insoluble in water. The drug is commerically available as an oral suspension with sorbic acid as a preservative. The oral suspension and tablets should be stored in tightly closed containers. Its structure is as follows:

Thiabendazole

Mechanism of Action

The exact mechanism of anthelmintic activity of thiabendazole is not clearly elucidated. The drug has been shown to inhibit the enzyme fumarate reductase, a helminth-specific enzyme. In animal studies, the drug has been shown to have analgesic, anti-inflammatory, and antipyretic effects.

Absorption, Metabolisms, and Secretion

Thiabendazole is administered topically or orally. The drug is rapidly absorbed from the gastrointestinal tract and through the skin. Following oral administration, peak plasma concentrations are achieved within 1 to 2 h. The drug is extensively metabolized in the liver to 5-hydroxythiabendazole and is conjugated with glucuronic or sulfuric acid. These metabolites are excreted in feces and urine. About 90 percent of an orally administered drug is eliminated in urine within 48 h as glucuronic or sulfate conjugates of 5-hydroxythia-

bendazole. Approximately 5 percent of an oral dose of thiabendazole is eliminated in feces over the first 24 h.

Pharmacodynamics

Thiabendazole does not appear to induce significant effects on respiratory and cardiovascular systems. The drug has anti-inflammatory properties and immuno-modulating effects on T-cell function. Thiabendazole has not been shown to be safe in pregnancy and lactation. No evidence of mutagenic and carcinogenic potential has been reported in several short- and long-term animal studies.

Adverse Effects

At the recommended dosage (25 mg/kg twice daily for 2 days), 7 to 50 percent of patients experience mild and transient side effects. The commonly observed side effects include headache, nausea, vomiting, abdominal pain, and dizziness. The side effects occur 3 to 4 h postadministration of thiabendazole and last up to 2 to 8 h. The incidence of these side effects increases with the administration of higher doses and length of treatment. Occasionally, epigastric distress, skin reaction, diarrhea, fatigue, and drowsiness may occur. Hypersensitivity reactions such as chills, fever, anaphylaxis, angioedema, and lymphadenopathy have been reported in thiabendazole-treated patients.

Clinical Uses

Thiabendazole is a broad-spectrum anthelmintic, active against most human intestinal nematode infections, including *Angiostrongylus cantonensis*, *Strongyloides stercoralis*, *Trichinella spiralis*, *Toxocara canis*, *Toxocara cati*, *Ancylostoma caninum*, *Ancylostoma braziliense*, *A. duodenale*, *Dracunculus medinensis*, *Capillaria philippinensis*, and *Anisakis* sp. The drug is both ovicidal and larvicidal.

Although, thiabendazole has been reported to be larvicidal against *T. spiralis* in animals and active against the intestinal phase in human infections, its activity against migrated and encysted larvae in human infections has not been established. The thiabendazole effect of the intestinal phase of trichinosis is limited. Its use will ameliorate the signs and symptoms without subsequent changes in laboratory finding. Clinical manifestations of trichinosis can also be controlled via the use of corticosteroids or ACTH in severe infections.

Thiabendazole is highly effective in the treatment of *S. stercoralis*, cutaneous larva migrans, and *A. cantonensis*. Its activity against other parasites is variable. Despite the fact that thiabendazole is a broad-spectrum drug, it is no longer recommended for treatment of many nematodes (hookworm, ascariasis, and pinworm) infections due to its potential toxicity.

Contraindications

Thiabendazole should be given with caution and careful monitoring to patients with a history of renal dysfunction and drug hypersensitivity. If hypersensitive reactions develop during treatment, the use of the drug should be discontinued immediately. Supportive therapy is indicated for dehydrated, malnourished, or anemic patients before administration of thiabendazole. Since the drug can induce adverse effects on the CNS, it should not be given during the day for patients requiring mental alertness, such as driving a motor vehicle and operating machinery. Ideally, such activities should be avoided.

PREPARATIONS

Zentel tablets 200 mg.

Alcopar sachet containing 5 g of bephenium hydroxynaphthoate.

Diethylcarbamazine citrate (Hetrazan, Banocide, Caricide) is available as 50-mg or 100-mg tablets or as a syrup containing 30 or 24 mg/mL. The dosage is expressed in milligrams of the base. A 50-mg base is equivalent to 100-mg citrate.

Levamisole (Ketrax, Solaskil) is available as levamisole hydrochloride: 188 mg is equivalent to a 100-mg levamisole base. It is marketed as tablets containing 50 to 150 mg base and as an oral solution containing 8-mg base/mL.

Mebendazole (Vermox) is prepared as tablets of 100 mg, and it is also available in some countries as an oral suspension containing 20 mg/mL. The tablets may be chewed, crushed and mixed with food, or swallowed whole. Some studies have shown that administration of the drug with food containing fat enhances absorption of the drug. This situation may be desirable in treatment of dracunculiasis, hydatid disease, and trichonosis, where high plasma concentration of the drug is required.

Thiabendazole (Mintezol) is available as an oral suspension containing 100 mg/mL and as chewable tablets containing 500 mg.

Niclosamide (Niclocide, Yomesan, Tredemine) is available as chewable tablets. Each tablet contains 500 mg of the drug.

Niridazole (Ambilhar) is available as tablets containing 100 and 500 mg.

Piperazine is available as various salts. Piperazine citrate (Antepar) is prepared as an oral solution containing 110 mg citrate, which is equivalent to 100 mg hexahydrate, or as tablets containing 500 mg piperazine hexahydrate. The therapeutic efficacy of the various piperazine salts appears to be the same.

Pyrantel pamoate (Antiminth, Cobantrin) is available as a suspension containing 50 mg pyrantel base/mL and as chewable tablets containing 125 mg base/mL. The drug may be given as a single dose with fruit juice or milk, if desired.

BIBLIOGRAPHY

Awadzi, K., et al.: "The Effects of Moderate Urine Alkalinisation on Low Dose Diethylcarbamazine Therapy in Patients with Onchocerciasis," *Br. J. Clin. Pharmacol.*, **21**:669 (1986).

Bruce, S. I.: "New Anthelmintics," in M. S. Howell (ed.), *Parasitology—Quo Vadis*, Proceedings of the Sixth International Congress of Parasitology, Australian Academy of Science, 1986, pp. 131–140.

Coleman, D. L., and M. Barry: "Relapse of *Paragonimus westermani* Lung Infection after Bithionol Therapy," *Am. J. Trop. Med. Hyg.*, **31**:71 (1982).

Farid, Z., et al.: "Comparative Single Dose Treatment of Hookworm and Roundworm Infections with Levamisole, Pyrantel and Bephenium," *J. Trop. Med. Hyg.*, **80**:107–108 (1977).

Gilling, P. C., and Heidelberger: "Effects of Praziquantel a New Antischistosomial Drug on the Mutation and Transformation of Mammalian Cells," *Cancer Res.*, **42**:2692 (1982).

Gustofsson, L. L., Beerman, and Y. A. Abdi: *Handbook of Drugs for Tropical Parasitic Infections*, Taylor and Francis, Inc., New York, 1987.

Johnson, R. J., et al.: "Paragonimiasis: Diagnosis and the Use of Praziquantel in Treatment," *Rev. Infect. Dis.*, **7**:200 (1985).

Kale, O. O., T. Elemile, and F. Enahoro: "Controlled Comparative Trial of Thiabendazole and Metronidazole in the Treatment of Dracontiasis," *Ann. Trop. Med. Parasitol.*, **77**:151 (1983).

Kammerer, W. S., and P. M. Schantz: "Long Term Followup of Human Hydatid Disease (Echinococcus Granulosus) Treated with a High-Dose Mebendazole Regimen," *Am. J. Trop. Med. Hyg.*, **33**:132 (1984).

Pearson, R. D., and E. L. Hewlett: "Niclosamide Therapy for Tapeworm Infections," *Ann. Intern. Med.*, **102**:550 (1985).

Renoux, G.: "The General Immunopharmacology of Levamisole," *Drugs*, **19**:89 (1980).

Wilson, K. H., and C. A. Kauffman: "Persistent *Strongyloides stercoralis* in a Blind Loop of Bowel: Successful Treatment with Mebendazole, *Arch. Intern. Med.*, **143**:357 (1983).

Toxicology|

SECTION EDITOR

Joseph R. DiPalma

C H A P T E R 48

Heavy Metals and Antagonists

Benjamin Calesnick

Since life began, heavy metals found in the environment produce a hazard to biologic organisms. Some diseases of humans can be traced to heavy-metal poisoning associated with the development of metal mining, refining, and use. Even with the present recognition of the hazards of heavy metals (see Table 48-1), the incidence of intoxication remains significant and the need for effective therapy remains high.

Heavy metals are not metabolized and therefore persist in the body and accumulate. Most often they combine with sulfhydryl groups. Since these are present in many enzymes, cell function is severely disrupted. Some metals such as iron, zinc, cobalt, copper, and a few trace elements perform vital cellular functions usually as cofactors or even as electron donors (hemoglobin, for example).

Since this is a vast subject and cannot be covered in depth in this book, the plan for this chapter is as follows: the toxicology of lead, mercury, gold, and arsenic as primary examples of heavy-metal toxicity is discussed in some detail. Next the main antagonists (chelating agents) which have proven to be useful in therapy are described. Finally, other metals such as zinc and aluminum are briefly described.

LEAD

Lead forms two well-defined series of compounds in which the metal is bivalent and tetravalent, respectively. Metallic lead is a soft metal having little tensile strength and is the heaviest of the common metals, with the exception of gold and mercury. In air which contains moisture and carbon dioxide, lead becomes oxidized on the surface, forming a protective layer which is both compact and adherent.

Lead is found in practically all foods as well as in the air, and can therefore be both ingested and inhaled. Industrial uses of lead, such as the manufacture of batteries, cables, automotive body paints, and ceramics, provide potential sources of lead exposure. Some paint pigments contain lead: white lead (basic lead carbonate) and red lead (lead oxide). Formerly, paints used for interior and exterior surfaces contained lead pigments. Even though this application of lead has largely been discontinued, the hazard still remains, especially in dilapidated dwellings where peeling of multicoated walls and woodwork constitutes the most important single source of lead poisoning in young children.

Absorption, Distribution, and Excretion

The average daily American dietary intake of lead may vary from 0.12 to 0.35 mg. About 0.04 mg of lead is inhaled daily. Of this amount, 30 to 50 percent is retained by the lung and readily absorbed. Only about 10 percent of ingested lead is absorbed in an adult. In contrast to this low absorption in adults, the absorption of dietary lead in normal infants and young children has been found to be approximately 50 percent. This fact makes lead ingestion more of a hazard to children than to adults. Inorganic lead does not readily penetrate intact skin; however, lipid-soluble forms

TABLE 48-1   Summary of heavy-metals toxicology

Metal	Chemical form absorbed	Distribution	Target organs	Normal concentration
Lead	Inorganic lead oxides and salts	Bone (90%), teeth, hair, blood (erythrocytes), liver, kidneys	Hematopoietic tissues and liver, CNS, kidneys, neuromuscular junction	Blood: 0–40 μg/dL Urine: 0–100 μg/24 h
	Organic (tetraethyl lead)	Liver	CNS	
Mercury	Elemental mercury	CNS (where it is trapped as Hg^{2+}), kidneys (following conversion of elemental Hg to Hg^{2+})	CNS (neuropsychiatric due to elemental Hg and its Hg^{2+} metabolite), kidneys (substantial due to conversion of elemental Hg to Hg^{2+})	Blood: 0–0.10 μg/mL Urine: 0–20 μg/L
	Inorganic: Hg^+ (less toxic): Hg^{2+} (more toxic)	Kidneys (predominant), blood, brain (minor)	Kidneys, GI	
	Organic: alkyl	Kidneys, brain, blood	CNS	
Arsenic	Inorganic arsenic salts	Red blood cells (95–99% bound to globin) (24 h); then to liver, lungs, kidneys, wall of GI tract, spleen, muscle, nerve tissues (2 weeks); then to skin, hair, and bone (years)	Increased vascular permeability leading to vasodilation and vascular collapse. Uncoupling of oxidative phosphorylation resulting in impaired cellular metabolism	Blood: 0–0.10 mg/L Urine: 0.0–20 μg/L
Zinc	Elemental zinc	Red blood cells and plasma proteins; prostate, liver, and choroid plexus intestine	Bone, brain, skeletal muscle, eye tissue	Blood: 50–160 μg/dL Urine: 110–600 μg/ 24 h
Aluminum	Inorganic aluminum oxides and salts	Intestine, liver, spleen	Brain	Blood: 0–6 mg/L Urine: 6–92 μg/24 h
Cadmium	Inorganic cadmium salts	GI tract, lungs	Lungs, kidneys, intestine	Blood: 0–10 μg/L Urine: 5 μg/L

TABLE 48-1 (*continued*)   **Summary of heavy-metals toxicology**

Metal	Chemical form absorbed	Distribution	Target organs	Normal concentration
Manganese	Inorganic manganese oxides and salts	Liver, kidneys, intestine, and pancreas	Basal ganglia, cerebellum	Blood: 0.1–1.0 μg/dL Urine: 10 μg/L
Gold	Gold salts	Liver, kidneys, spleen, pancreas, intestine	Skin, kidneys, and liver	Blood: 3–6 mg/L

such as tetraethyllead are significantly absorbed. Some of the absorbed lead is excreted via the bile into the gastrointestinal tract and passes out in the feces with the unabsorbed portion. Thus the fecal excretion of lead approximates that which is ingested with food. The remainder of the absorbed lead is excreted in the urine. Therefore, the daily intake of lead is equal to the daily output under normal conditions.

Lead is a bone-seeker. Over 90 percent of the human body burden of lead is found in bone. Of the soft tissues, liver, muscle, skin, dense connective tissues, and hair contain the largest amounts, in that order. Of major concern is the distribution of lead into the brain, kidney, and hematopoietic system, where it produces toxicologic effects.

Blood and urinary lead levels have been determined in people from all parts of the world. The worldwide "average" urinary and blood lead levels are 35 μg/L and 10 to 25 μg per 100 mL, respectively. The urinary level of lead indicative of a hazardous exposure is 150 μg per liter of urine, while 80 μg per 100 mL of blood indicates dangerous exposure. Recent reports have indicated that even very low levels of lead in the plasma may alter normal physiologic function.

Acute Lead Poisoning

Acute lead poisoning is rare; it may result from the massive inhalation of large quantities of finely divided lead or lead fumes. The symptoms include sweet metallic taste, salivation, vomiting, abdominal pain, intestinal colic, lowered body temperature, and cardiovascular collapse. Death may result in 1 or 2 days.

Chronic Lead Poisoning

The signs and symptoms of chronic lead poisoning can be divided into five categories: (1) hematologic, (2) neurologic, (3) renal, (4) gastrointestinal, and (5) other.

Hematologic Signs   A sign of lead intoxication may be the appearance of stippled cells in the peripheral blood. These juvenile forms of erythrocytes are not in themselves diagnostic since basophilic stippling can occur in a variety of blood dyscrasias. Furthermore, stippling is observed in only 60 percent of childhood lead intoxications. Basophilic stippling, however, is an indication that lead interferes with hemoglobin synthesis. An important chemical clue to the effects of lead on the hematopoietic system is the appearance of coproporphyrin III in the urine. Inconclusive evidence reveals lower activity of coprogenase with increasing blood lead levels (see Table 48-2). This finding alone may be misleading, since coproporphyrinuria occurs in a large variety of other diseases and poisonings. An excellent correlation exists, however, between the amount of lead in the urine and the appearance of urinary coproporphyrins.

Another consistent finding in lead poisoning is the appearance of δ-aminolevulinic acid in the urine. This results from an inhibition by lead of the enzyme aminolevulinic acid dehydratase, which converts δ-aminolevulinic acid to porphobilinogen (see Table 48-2). Aminolevulinic acid dehydratase has been shown to be inhibited with blood lead levels as low as 5 μg/mL. Urinary lead and coproporphyrin levels have been shown to correlate well with the appearance of δ-aminolevulinic acid. Evidence has been presented

**TABLE 48-2   Toxic effects of lead
on hemoglobin synthesis**

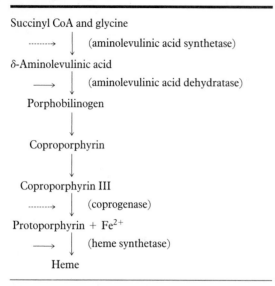

Key: ⟶, steps inhibited by lead; ┄┄➤, steps at which lead is
thought to act, but evidence is inconclusive.

that a raised urinary δ-aminolevulinic acid level provides an earlier sign of lead exposure than a raised coproporphyrin level. Less conclusive evidence reveals lower activity of aminolevulinic acid synthetase with increasing blood lead levels. The decrease in activity, however, might simply be due to product inhibition as δ-aminolevulinic acid levels rise.

Lead also interferes with the incorporation of iron into protoporphyrin by the activity of heme synthetase to form heme. Protoporphyrin levels rise in bone marrow and erythrocytes. The anemia associated with lead poisoning is of the hypochromic, normocytic type and is seldom severe. Hemoglobin values rarely fall below 60 percent or the red blood cell count below 4×10^6 per milliliter.

Neurologic Signs   The neurotoxic effects of lead at high doses have been well documented. The central nervous system manifestations of lead poisoning are termed *lead encephalopathy*. Today, these symptoms occur rarely in adults, and only after very high doses of lead; they are of more importance and of higher frequency in children. The early symptoms include irritability, headache, insomnia, restlessness, and ataxia.

Later, confusion, delirium, convulsions, and coma may develop. Morphologic changes appear as nonspecific lesions in the cerebrum and cerebellum. Accumulations of serous fluid which distort the normal architecture, and capillary damage and hemorrhages of the meninges, are evident. It is believed that these changes are secondary to increased cranial pressure due to edema.

Recent evidence has demonstrated that children with blood lead levels considered subclinical intoxication may have mild neurologic dysfunction, though no overt symptoms have been observed. Therefore permissible exposure levels of lead in children are being revised downward by the Centers for Disease Control. The reason has been the demonstration that lead at extremely low concentrations has an inhibitory effect in brain and aminolevulinic acid dehydratase, adenylcyclase, and on mitochondrial function. In addition, there are peripheral neurologic effects known as *lead palsy*. This peripheral neuropathy leads to muscle paralysis which involves primarily the extensor muscles of the wrist and foot. In advanced cases the antigravity muscles may atrophy. Contraction of the flexors produces a limb which is immovable and extremities with a clawlike appearance.

Renal Signs   The effects of lead on the kidney have only been observed at very high doses and occur in both adults and children. One effect is proximal tubular damage, which is readily reversible by chelation therapy. The second major effect involves reduced glomerular function associated with vascular damage and fibrosis. These effects occur at levels of lead above that affecting hemoglobin formation and brain function.

Gastrointestinal Signs   Lead stimulates the smooth muscle of the gut, giving rise to intestinal symptoms such as distention after meals, constipation, nausea, and vomiting. Appetite loss leads to loss of body weight and easy fatigability. Dull pains in various parts of the abdomen precede colic. Colic is important diagnostically, since it constitutes a symptom for which the patient seeks relief. Characteristically, the onset of lead colic is sudden and usually occurs at night with severe pain.

Other Signs   Another nonspecific sign of lead intoxication is the appearance of a lead line at the margin of the gums. Today, the lead line is infrequent because of better dental hygiene. A black or purplish line is formed when lead sulfide is precipitated at the gingival borders; sulfides produced by bacteria react with lead in the saliva. Other metals, for example, bismuth, mercury, tin, and arsenic, produce similar precipitates at the gingival border, illustrating the nonspecificity of the lead line in diagnosing lead intoxication.

Lead poisoning invariably produces changes in skin coloration known as *lead hue* or *lead pallor*. The patient takes on a pale or ashen-gray appearance.

A summary of the clinical signs and symptoms of lead intoxication in the order of their occurrence is given in Table 48-3.

TABLE 48-3   Lead intoxication

Reactions	Signs and symptoms
Subjective	Weakness
	Anorexia
	Fatigue
	Nervousness
	Tremor
	Nausea
	Loss of body weight
	Headache
	Gastrointestinal
	Constipation
	Gastric pain
	Colic
	Weakness of extensor muscles
	Impotence, amenorrhea
Objective	Pallor (constricted arterioles), loss of weight
	Increased δ-aminolevulinic aciduria
	Porphyrinuria (coproporphyrin III)
	Constipation
	Blood
	Increased lead content
	Possible slight increase in serum
	bilirubin and serum iron
	Anemia (basophilic stippling)
	Bone marrow
	Basophilic stippled erythroblasts
	Possible increase in erythropoiesis
	Lead line
	Weakness of extensor muscles
	Tremor

Tetraethyllead and Tetramethyllead

Tetraethyllead and tetramethyllead are oily lipid-soluble compounds used as antiknock additives in gasoline. Although they are absorbed through the skin, appreciable time is required to achieve a toxic level by this route. Organic lead compounds gain entry in the body mainly via the respiratory tract, usually in handling and during tank-cleaning operations. Because of close and skillful industrial hygienic supervision, intoxication by these compounds is rare.

Tetraethyllead produces symptoms which are referable predominantly to the CNS. The patient is irritable, suffers from insomnia, has wild nightmares, and is emotionally unstable. In later stages, the patient hallucinates, becomes hyperexcitable, and requires restraint. Also seen are gastrointestinal effects including anorexia, vomiting, and mild diarrhea. There is no effect on porphyrin metabolism. Blood lead levels remain near normal in tetraethyllead intoxication, whereas urine lead levels increase markedly, exceeding those found in inorganic lead poisoning.

Treatment of Lead Intoxication

The mainstay for treatment of lead poisoning in both adults and children is chelation therapy. The three drugs primarily used are calcium disodium edetate, dimercaprol, and penicillamine. Therapy in children usually involves intramuscular injections of calcium disodium edetate combined with dimercaprol, followed by penicillamine orally for several days. (The individual agents are discussed below.) Supportive measures include continuous intravenous infusion of 10 percent dextrose in water to increase urine flow before administration of the chelating agent.

MERCURY

Mercury exists in three states of oxidation: as the element, in a monovalent (mercurous) form, and in a divalent (mercuric) form. Divalent mercury can form covalent bonds with carbon atoms: mercury in this form is usually referred to as *organic* mercury. The organomercurial diuretics and many of the mercurial fungicides contain mercury covalently bound to carbon.

Elemental or metallic mercury is a highly toxic, somewhat volatile liquid. Human exposure to mercury vapor is mainly occupational and has been noted since antiquity. Mercurous chloride (calomel) is the best known of the mercurous compounds. It is still used in some skin creams as an antiseptic and was once frequently employed as a cathartic. The mercuric salts are the most irritating and acutely toxic forms of mercury. Mercuric salts have wide application in industry—as catalysts in the production of vinyl plastics and to suppress the growth of slime molds in the manufacturing of paper pulp. It has recently been observed that microorganisms in river water can synthesize methylmercury from the inorganic forms of mercury such as those discharged in industrial waste. Therefore, discharge of mercury into rivers from industries has led to problems of environmental pollution in Japan, Sweden, and the United States.

All the organomercurials in use today contain mercury having only one covalent link to a carbon atom. From a pharmacologic standpoint, they cannot be considered as a single group. The mercurial diuretics have the lowest toxicity of the organic mercury compounds. Next in order of increasing toxicity are the phenylmercury salts, used as fungicides in seed dressing. Phenylmercuric nitrate was used in some hemorrhoidal preparations and in a proprietary throat lozenge. Methoxyethylmercury chloride belongs to a new group of mercury fungicides whose toxicity is similar to that of the phenylmercury compounds. The alkylmercury salts are by far the most dangerous of all the compounds of mercury. The simple salts such as methylmercury chloride and ethylmercury chloride are sufficiently volatile to produce serious toxic effects by inhalation. Methylmercury dicyandiamide is less volatile. All the alkyl mercurials produce characteristic and usually irreversible damage to the CNS. They have had extensive use as fungicides.

Mechanism of Toxic Action

Mercury has a specific affinity for the sulfur atom in thiol groups of enzymes and other proteins, inactivating these substances. This uniquely high affinity for sulfur is ultimately responsible for the toxicity of all compounds of mercury. The organic moiety of the organomercurials and the dissociable anion in the mercuric salts undoubtedly account for the differences found between the compounds, such as the degree and type of toxic symptoms, and the differences in hazardous properties associated with volatility and solubility.

Absorption, Distribution, and Excretion

Mercury may be absorbed into the body via the respiratory and gastrointestinal tracts, and the skin. In general, most compounds of mercury, both organic and inorganic, are well absorbed except mercurous chloride (HgCl). Mercurous chloride is poorly absorbed from the gastrointestinal tract because of its low solubility; an equivalent dose of mercuric chloride would be lethal.

The pattern of deposition of mercury is an important consideration in the toxicology of this metal. Both organic and inorganic mercury compounds, if present at a sufficient concentration, will produce toxic effects in any cell with which they come in contact. Irrespective of the route of administration, mercury is distributed within a few hours to all organs of the body. The mercury in plasma is protein-bound, and the mercury present in red blood cells is bound to the cysteine residues of hemoglobin.

Mercury is excreted in the urine, bile, feces, sweat, and saliva. Urinary and fecal routes of excretion are the most important for elimination.

The biologic half-life in humans for methylmercury is close to 70 days, corresponding to an excretion of about 1 percent per day of the body burden. The decrease in blood mercury follows a similar time course. The half-life of clearance from the brain is about 20 percent longer than the clearance from the whole body.

Normal Levels of Mercury

For mercury, the intake rate roughly balances the total urinary and fecal excretion. A statistical analysis of over 800 samples from 15 countries indicates that 84 percent of the general population have urinary concentrations of less than 5 μg/L. A zero value, that is, less than 0.5 μg/L, was found in 79 percent of the samples. The 95 percent confidence limit indicates an upper limit for "normal" mercury in urine of 20 to 25 μg/L and for blood, 4 μg per 100 mL (see Table 48-1 for average values). Fecal excretion was reported in earlier studies to average 10 μg of mercury per day.

Chronic and Acute Poisoning from Inorganic Mercury

No clinical distinction has been made between symptoms associated with exposure to mercury vapor and to mercuric salts. The experimental findings of higher brain levels associated with the vapor suggest that central nervous system disturbances would be more pronounced following exposure to this form of mercury.

Symptoms involving the CNS are the most frequently seen, the principal features being tremor and psychologic disturbances (erethismus mercurialis). Proteinuria and progressing renal damage may occur. Symptoms related to the mouth such as gingivitis, stomatitis, and excessive salivation often occur. These symptoms may be connected with the secretion of mercury in the saliva. Dermatitis has been observed in some workmen exposed to mercury. Mercurialentis (a colored reflex from the lens) is seen in chronic exposure, but does not indicate intoxication. A number of nonspecific symptoms such as anorexia, weight loss, anemia, and muscular weakness are also associated with chronic exposure.

The symptoms associated with acute oral intake of inorganic mercury salts are acute gastroenteritis with abdominal pain, vomiting, and some bloody diarrhea. Anuria and uremia are associated with severe kidney damage and may appear a day or more after exposure and frequently precede a fatal outcome. The approximate lethal dose to humans of mercuric chloride is 1 g. Acute exposure to high concentrations of mercury vapor may give rise to a condition characterized by a metallic taste, nausea, abdominal pain, vomiting, diarrhea, headache, and sometimes albuminuria. A few days later the salivary glands swell, stomatitis and gingivitis develop, and a dark line of mercurous sulfide (HgS) forms on the inflamed gums. The teeth may loosen and ulcers may form on the lips and cheeks.

Chronic and Acute Poisoning from Organomercurial Compounds

The symptoms of chronic and acute exposure to organomercurial compounds are the same. Symptoms may appear weeks to months after an acute exposure, and include ataxia; slurring of speech; numbness and tingling of the lips, hands, and feet; concentric restriction of the visual fields; impairment of hearing; and emotional disturbances. The symptoms are irreversible in cases of severe poisoning.

Mothers ingesting large amounts of methylmercury give birth to babies suffering from palsy, convulsions, and mental retardation. Experimental work indicates that methylmercury compounds are potent inhibitors of cell division and chromosome segregation.

Evidence based on cases of industrial poisoning and ingestion of methylmercury in food indicates that symptoms are first observed at concentrations of 100 μg per 100 mL of whole blood. Fatalities are associated with brain levels of 10 μg per gram wet weight of tissue. It is likely that blood levels of 10 μg per 100 mL or less are not associated with toxic symptoms.

Treatment of Mercury Poisoning

The treatment of mercury poisoning aims at the removal of mercury from the gastrointestinal tract and the inactivation with subsequent excretion of mercury which has been absorbed. Though calcium disodium edetate, penicillamine, and dimercaprol all increase the excretion of mercury, dimercaprol has greater efficacy. Therefore it remains the drug routinely used in the treatment of acute mercury poisoning (see section on dimercaprol, below). Diaphoresis is a useful adjunctive measure.

ARSENIC

Arsenic is readily available in inorganic and organic forms. Inorganic arsenic is an active constituent in many fungicides, herbicides, and pesticides. It is used in the paint and dye industry and was at one time used extensively in cosmetics. Organic arsenicals are used today to treat protozoan infestations such as trypanosomiasis and amebiasis. Arsanilic acid is fed to poultry and livestock to enhance growth rate.

Arsenic exists in the elemental form, and in salts where it is trivalent or pentavalent. The arsenites, for example, potassium arsenite, $KAsO_2$, and salts of arsenous acid, $H_2As_2O_4^{2-}$, contain trivalent arsenic. The pentavalent oxidation state is found in the arsenates such as lead arsenate, $PbHAsO_4$. These are salts of arsenic acid, H_3AsO_4. The arsenites have a high affinity for thiol groups and are considerably more toxic than the arsenates. The latter have properties similar to those of phosphate and have no affinity for thiol groups.

The organic arsenicals contain arsenic linked to a carbon atom by a covalent bond, where arsenic exists in the trivalent or pentavalent state. Arsphenamine contains trivalent arsenic; sodium arsanilate contains the element in the pentavalent form. Their structures are given on page 690.

Arsphenamine

Sodium arsanilate

Arsine, AsH_3, is a colorless gas with a garliclike odor and is produced by the action of nascent hydrogen on the elemental form of arsenic. It produces toxic effects which are different from those of the other compounds of arsenic.

Biochemical Mechanism of Toxic Action

Trivalent arsenical compounds, both the inorganic arsenic salts and the monosubstituted organic arsenicals, possess a high affinity for vicinal thiol groups. Thus, reactions with thiol functional groups lead to the formation of stable five-membered rings.

It is likely that this affinity of trivalent arsenic for thiol groups of enzymes and other proteins in tissues is ultimately responsible for the toxicity of this class of arsenic compounds.

Absorption, Distribution, and Excretion

Systemic poisoning can be produced by absorption from the lungs, the gastrointestinal tract, and through the skin.

After acute exposure, arsenic is deposited in tissues such as the liver, kidney, intestine, spleen, and lungs, in that order. Arsenic appears in hair about 2 weeks after the first exposure, where it is bound to the sulfide linkages in keratin. Chronic exposure leads to accumulation in hair, bone, and skin. Arsenic may be found in high concentrations in the hair years after cessation of exposure and after most of the metal has been removed from the soft tissues.

Arsenic passes the blood-brain barrier slowly. Brain levels are among the lowest in the body. Arsenic read-ily crosses the placental barrier, and fetal damage has been reported.

The pathways and products of biotransformation of arsenic have not been well defined.

Excretion occurs by all physiologic routes—feces, urine, sweat, and milk. In general, the arsenite salts are lost mainly via the feces, and the arsenates via the urine. Arsenate excretion is more rapid than arsenite excretion and probably occurs via the phosphate excretory mechanisms.

Symptoms of Acute Toxicity

Acute arsenic poisoning occurs because arsenic, especially in the form of As_2O_3 (arsenic trioxide, arsenous acid) is readily available, practically tasteless, has the appearance of sugar, and is quickly absorbed from the gastrointestinal tract. Oral intake is followed by an asymptomatic period of about 30 min. The victim then experiences a tightness in the throat, difficulty in swallowing, and stomach pains. Projectile vomiting may ensue, which can be lifesaving. Other effects quickly follow, such as intensive diarrhea with watery feces containing shreds of mucus. Depressed urine flow is characteristic of acute arsenic intoxication. Symptoms of shock due to hypovolemia may develop. Death usually results in 1 to 3 days, with the victim in a state of collapse. Deaths which occur up to 14 days after poisoning are caused by nephritis. Ingestion of 100 μg of arsenous acid will cause severe poisoning; the minimal lethal dose in humans is quoted as 1 g.

Inhalation of arsine gas leads to rapid hemolysis, which gives rise to anemia, reduced red blood cell count, and hemoglobin in the urine. The released hemoglobin causes jaundice and may block the kidney tubules. Death usually results from anoxemia in 2 to 9 days after exposure. Some symptoms of typical arsenic poisoning may also appear.

Symptoms of Chronic Poisoning

Nausea, vomiting, and diarrhea occur but are less pronounced than in cases of acute poisoning. The mucous membranes are affected, giving rise to symptoms of the common cold. The horny layer of the skin is stimulated, leading to the appearance of dark brown scales. Peripheral neuritis similar to that associated with chronic alcoholism is observed in approximately 5 percent of the cases of chronic arsenic poisoning. The afferent motor nerves and sensory fibers are affected, especially in the legs. The ankle jerk disappears and the leg muscles atrophy. Tremors have been reported in 10 percent of the cases of chronic exposure. Renal cortical necrosis has also been reported.

Continued exposure to arsine gas generally results in symptoms similar to the picture of arsenic poisoning. Arsine binds to red blood cells, making them susceptible to hemolysis. This results in a steady level of anemia.

Skin keratoses result from prolonged exposure to arsenic, and may become malignant. Arsenic has been reported as an industrial carcinogen implicated in producing lung and skin carcinomas.

The Action of Arsenic on Capillaries

Arsenic produces dilatation of capillaries, and an increase in permeability of the capillary walls. This results in a fall in blood pressure and tissue edema leading to a state of stock.

Capillary damage is especially pronounced in the splenic area. The loss of plasma proteins into the intestinal areas causes blisters under the mucosal layer. Stimulated intestinal peristalsis leads to diarrhea and the shedding of epithelial cells.

Capillary and epithelial cell damage also occurs in the kidneys. Protein and red blood cells appear in the urine. The depression in urine flow results from both the vascular damage to kidney and the loss of fluid in the capillary beds.

Treatment of Arsenic Poisoning

Dimercaprol is the primary agent used in the treatment of chronic arsenic poisoning. When the urinary level of arsenic falls below 50 mg in 24 h, chelation therapy should be stopped. (See under "Dimercaprol," below.)

GOLD

At present, gold compounds have a therapeutic usefulness limited to the treatment of rheumatoid arthritis of the peripheral joints and of certain rare skin diseases such as discoid lupus. Colloidal radioactive gold, because of its distribution in the body and its short half-life, has been used as a radiation source in the treatment of cancer.

Absorption, Distribution, and Excretion

Gold compounds administered by intramuscular injection, either in an aqueous solution or as an oil suspension, are absorbed very slowly from the site of injection. They are carried in the blood plasma in a nondialyzable form, with little in the cells, and are distributed throughout the soft tissues of the body. Even after a single injection, gold appears in the blood and urine for months afterward. Of the gold that is absorbed, about 20 percent is rapidly excreted, mostly in the urine in the case of soluble compounds and in the feces in the case of insoluble compounds, and about 80 percent is fixed for long periods in the tissues. With therapeutic doses, the levels in plasma and urine in humans contain about 1 to 2 mg per 100 mL.

Use of Gold Compounds in Treatment of Rheumatoid Arthritis

The principal therapeutic use of gold compounds is in the treatment of adult or juvenile rheumatoid arthritis. Gold, certainly no miracle drug, nevertheless offers considerable benefit to many individuals subjected to a painful and prolonged disease. Gold compounds are most efficacious in the early stages of the arthritic disease, reducing the inflammatory process but without inducing any repair process in the joints. The mechanism of their anti-inflammatory action is unknown. There are two disadvantages associated with chrysotherapy (use of gold in treating disease). One is that patients who show improvement as a result of treatment may relapse after treatment is discontinued. The second disadvantage is the toxicity: gold compounds should be used with great caution, especially in aged individuals. The drug should only be used as part of a complete therapeutic course, not alone.

Adverse Reactions

The most frequent toxic reaction to gold is a dermatitis—an erythema urticaria, or rash—often with gastrointestinal disturbances. These reactions are usually preceded by pruritus, which is one of the best alarm signals. The skin lesions may last for some time but will eventually disappear after gold therapy has been discontinued. In some cases, severe exfoliative dermatitis results. Gold may be toxic to the kidney, producing a nephropathy or glomerulosis. Gastrointestinal damage (gastritis, colitis, or stomatitis) and hepatitis have been rarely observed. Blood dyscrasias, such as leukopenia, agranulocytosis, thrombopenia, or aplastic anemia, are rare but are very serious when they occur. Anaphylactoid or nitritoid-type reactions have been reported. Symptoms include flushing, fainting, dizziness, sweating, and gastrointestinal upset. Toxic effects may occur immediately or at any time during therapy.

Contraindications to the use of gold are impaired renal or hepatic function, skin lesions, or abnormalities of the hematopoietic system. The drugs should be used in pregnancy only when essential.

Treatment of Gold Toxicity

Treatment consists primarily of topical or systemic administration of corticosteroids. Severe cases of toxicity respond well to treatment with dimercaprol; penicillamine also increases urinary gold excretion.

Preparations

A variety of gold preparations are available for clinical use.

Parenteral *Gold sodium thiomalate* (Myochrysine) contains about 50 percent gold and is available in aqueous solution in 10-, 25-, 50-, or 100-mg/mL ampuls.

Aurothioglucose (Gold Thioglucose, Solganal) is supplied as a suspension in sesame oil containing 5 percent (50 mg/mL) aurothioglucose. A dose schedule commonly accepted is 10 to 20 mg weekly until a total of 200 to 300 mg is reached. Some clinicians use a maximum of 25 mg weekly. There are many variants of this schedule, but it seems clear that weekly doses greater than 50 mg increase the frequency of toxic reactions.

Oral *Auranofin* (Ridaura) capsules 3 mg.

HEAVY-METAL ANTAGONISTS

The basis for treatment of heavy-metal toxicity is chelation therapy. Heavy metals produce their toxic effects by binding with endogenous ligands, forming complexes which block or inhibit some physiologic or biochemical process. Chelating agents bind to the metal ions, thus competitively inhibiting the binding of the metals to the ligands. The chelates, being more water-soluble, are readily excreted in the urine. In some heavy-metal toxicity, such as that produced by cadmium and gold, present chelating agents are contraindicated, since these chemical complexes may increase the risk of renal toxicity.

Calcium Disodium Edetate

Chemistry Calcium disodium edetate is the calcium chelate of the disodium salt of ethylenediaminetetraacetic acid (EDTA). EDTA binds cations generally. Sodium and potassium are held most weakly. Calcium, magnesium, and barium are bound more tightly but can be displaced by cobalt, chromium, cadmium, copper, nickel, and lead, whose chelates have higher stability constants.

Ethylenediaminetetraacetic acid (EDTA)

Calcium disodium EDTA (calcium disodium edetate)

Mechanism of Action The therapeutic action of calcium disodium edetate in heavy-metal intoxication is due to the ability of the heavy metals such as lead to displace the sodium and calcium to form stable, soluble metal chelates. It is generally held that calcium disodium EDTA mobilizes lead from the soft tissues. Subsequently, the soft-tissue stores are replenished by the redistribution of lead from bone. The lead chelate formed by EDTA is represented structurally on page 693.

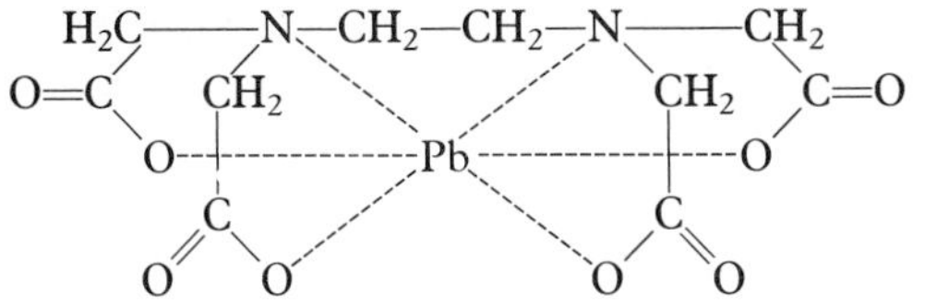

$$H_2C-N-CH_2-CH_2-N-CH_2$$

$$O=C \quad CH_2 \qquad\qquad CH_2 \quad C=O$$

$$O-\!\!\!-\!\!\!-\!\!\!-\!\!\!-\!\!\!-\!\!\!-Pb-\!\!\!-\!\!\!-\!\!\!-\!\!\!-\!\!\!-\!\!\!-O$$

$$C \qquad\qquad\qquad C$$

$$O \quad O \qquad\qquad O \quad O$$

Pharmacokinetics The absorption of calcium disodium EDTA from the gastrointestinal tract after oral administration is poor. Following parenteral administration, 50 percent of a dose is excreted unchanged in the urine within 1 h; almost 100 percent is excreted in the urine within 24 h. The drug is distributed exclusively in body fluids. In blood, all of the drug is found in the plasma.

Therapeutic Uses Calcium disodium EDTA is primarily used in the diagnosis and treatment of lead intoxication. It is ineffective in the treatment of arsenic and mercury toxicity and has questionable activity against other heavy metals.

Routes of Administration and Dosage As a diagnostic agent for plumbism, calcium disodium EDTA is given intramuscularly in 1.5 percent procaine hydrochloride at intervals of 8 h for 24 h. For the treatment of lead intoxication, the intravenous route of administration is preferred in adults. The therapeutic dosage is determined by the concentration of lead in the blood, the size of the patient, and reactions to the drug. The average dose for adults is 3 to 5 g/day for 3 to 5 days in two daily doses, each given in saline or 5 percent dextrose solution. For greater convenience and safety in treating children, the drug is usually administered intramuscularly at a dose of 50 mg/kg daily. In children with acute encephalopathy the mortality rate is reduced to about 25 percent when they are treated with calcium disodium edetate alone. However, administration of calcium disodium edetate alone to an individual with a relatively high concentration of lead (>60 μg per 100 mL) can intensify the toxic effects of lead. For this reason it is never given alone to children, but is given in combination with dimercaprol. Dimercaprol at 4 mg per kilogram of body weight is given intramuscularly initially, followed by the same dose of dimercaprol combined with 12.5 mg per kilogram of calcium disodium edetate. Calcium disodium edetate is also available for oral administration to enhance the absorption of lead from the gastrointestinal tract as well as promote its excretion in urine. However, this route may lead to a concomitant decrease in fecal lead excretion, making its beneficial effect questionable. Oral administration may be more effective in the treatment of poisoning from inorganic lead than from organic lead (tetraethyllead).

Adverse Reactions The most common adverse reactions are pain at the site of intramuscular injection and gastrointestinal irritation following oral administration. The principal toxic effect is renal tubular necrosis. An excessive chelation syndrome may be produced by large doses or prolonged administration. This is an acute febrile state with marked myalgia, headache, nasal congestion, nocturia, and chills. The symptoms subside upon removal of the drug. Deaths have been reported rarely. The drug is contraindicated in patients with severe renal disease. Precautions should also be taken in patients with active or inactive tuberculosis. Safety in pregnancy has not been established; therefore, the drug should not be used in women of childbearing age unless potential benefit outweighs the risk.

Dimercaprol

Dimercaprol has the following structure:

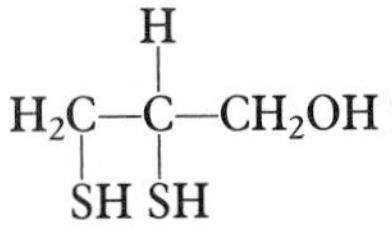

$$\overset{\displaystyle H}{H_2C-\underset{\underset{\displaystyle SH\ SH}{|}}{\overset{|}{C}}-CH_2OH}$$

2,3-Dimercaptopropanol

Mechanism of Action Dimercaprol forms stable chelates with arsenic, gold, and mercury, thus enhancing their excretion. In the case of mercury, the drug may form two different complexes:

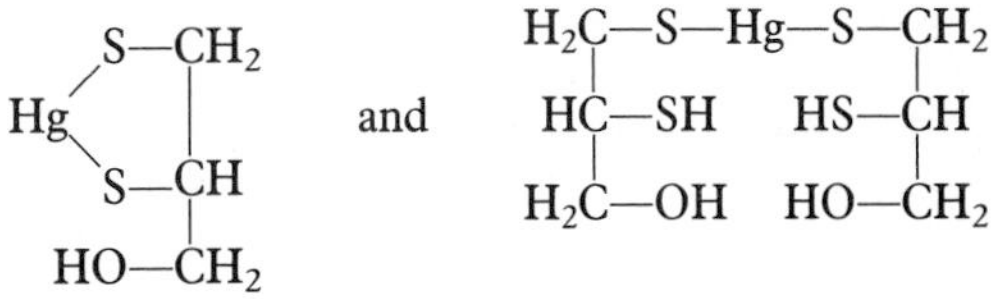

$$Hg\overset{\displaystyle S-CH_2}{\underset{\displaystyle HO-CH_2}{\overset{|}{\underset{\displaystyle S-CH}{}}}} \qquad \text{and} \qquad \begin{array}{c} H_2C-S-Hg-S-CH_2 \\ HC-SH \quad HS-CH \\ H_2C-OH \quad HO-CH_2 \end{array}$$

At a molar ratio of dimercaprol to Hg^{2+} of 1, a chelate is formed. When the molar ratio is 2, a complex forms containing two dimercaprol molecules to one atom of mercury. This compound is water-soluble at pH 7.5 and binds mercury more tightly than does the chelate. The drug prevents the inhibition of sulfhydryl enzymes by the heavy metal and also reactivates the enzymes.

Pharmacokinetics When administered intramuscularly as a 10 percent solution of dimercaprol in oil, the drug reaches a peak plasma level within 1 h. The drug is biotransformed very rapidly by the liver and almost completely excreted in the urine with 4 h.

Therapeutic Uses Dimercaprol is highly effective in the treatment of arsenic, gold, and mercury poisoning. It is effective in acute mercury poisoning when administered within 1 to 2 h following ingestion. It is not effective in treatment of chronic mercury poisoning. Dimercaprol is also used in combination with calcium disodium EDTA for use in lead poisoning in children.

Route of Administration and Dosage Dimercaprol is given only by deep intramuscular injection. For therapy of arsenic and gold intoxication, it is given for approximately 10 days as follows: 2.5 mg/kg, four times daily for 2 days, two times on the third day, and once on days 4 to 10. For acute mercury toxicity, the drug is given at 5 mg/kg initially, followed by 2.5 mg/kg once or twice on days 2 to 10. (For dosage in treatment of lead toxicity, see under "Calcium Disodium Edetate," above.)

Adverse Reactions At therapeutic doses, side effects to dimercaprol are generally mild. At larger doses, adverse reactions such as nausea and vomiting, headache, burning sensation in mouth and throat, salivation, lacrimation, and anxiety and restlessness have been reported. These are usually relieved by administration of an antihistamine. The most prominent toxic effect reported has been hypertension and tachycardia, the response being proportional to the dose administered. High doses can produce convulsions or coma. The drug is potentially nephrotoxic. Because the drug-metal complex breaks down easily under acid conditions, producing an alkaline urine protects the kidney during therapy. Iron should not be given to the patient taking dimercaprol because iron will complete

with the toxic metal for complexing. The safety of dimercaprol has not been established during pregnancy.

Penicillamine

Penicillamine is D-3-mercaptovaline.

$$HS-\underset{\underset{CH_3}{|}}{\overset{\overset{CH_3}{|}}{C}} - \underset{\underset{NH_2}{|}}{\overset{\overset{H}{|}}{C}} - COOH$$

Penicillamine

Mechanism of Action Penicillamine acts by binding to copper, iron, mercury, and lead, producing chelates which are readily excreted in the urine. It is superior to other heavy-metal antagonists in chelating copper and is used therapeutically to remove excess copper. It also interacts with cystine, increasing its excretion in cystinuria.

Pharmacokinetics Penicillamine is well absorbed from the gastrointestinal tract following oral administration. The drug is relatively stable to biotransformation and is excreted unchanged primarily in the urine.

Therapeutic Uses The primary use of penicillamine is to eliminate excess copper in patients with Wilson's disease (hepatolenticular degeneration due to an abnormality in copper metabolism). Penicillamine has been used on an investigational basis in the treatment of lead intoxication. Though it is less effective in chelating lead than are calcium disodium edetate or dimercaprol, it has the advantage of being effective orally. With this drug it is possible to maintain the blood lead concentration within the normal range. The efficacy of penicillamine has also been established in treatment of cystinuria. By increasing the solubility and hence the excretion of cystine, the drug prevents the formation of stones in the urinary tract. The drug has also been reported to be effective in cases of rheumatoid arthritis, but its use as an antiarthritic is only in the investigational state.

Route of Administration and Dosage As mentioned above, penicillamine has the advantage of being effective following oral administration. In the treatment of lead intoxication, the drug is given at concentrations of 250 to 500 mg twice daily for 1 to 3 months. Infants and young children are given 125 mg three times daily until the lead concentration drops below 60 μg per 100 mL of plasma. In Wilson's disease, penicillamine is given at concentrations of 250 mg four times daily to adults and 250 mg/day to infants and small children. In cystinuria, the drug is given at 1 to 4 g daily in divided doses. Dosages for treatment of all these syndromes must be individualized.

Adverse Reactions The most common adverse effects are allergic reactions manifested by maculopapular or erythematous rash occasionally accompanied by fever, arthralgia, or lymphadenopathy. Urticaria has also been reported. Adrenal corticosteroids and antihistamines may be given to relieve these reactions. Cross-sensitivity to penicillin may exist; therefore, the drug is contraindicated in patients with penicillin hypersensitivity. Other adverse reactions include gastrointestinal irritation, hepatic dysfunction, thrombocytopenia, leukopenia, and purpura. Severe glomerulonephritis and intraalveolar hemorrhage has been rarely reported. Penicillamine increases the need for pyridoxine, and patients should receive this vitamin along with the drug. The patient must be closely observed to determine liver function and to prevent nephrotic syndrome and proteinuria.

Preparations

Calcium disodium edetate (Calcium Disodium Versenate) is available in a sterile concentrated solution of 200 mg/mL in 5-mL ampuls, and in tablets containing 500 mg.

Dimercaprol (BAL in Oil) is available in 3-mL ampuls containing 100 mg/mL in peanut oil with benzylbenzoate to stabilize the solution.

Penicillamine (Cuprimine) is available in capsules containing 125 and 250 mg.

OTHER METALS

Practically all metals have important toxicities when a certain exposure level is exceeded. The route of exposure is pivotal to the degree and type of toxicity. When metals are inhaled as a fine powder, lung toxicity is the dominant picture. Oral absorption may lead to rapid toxicity, as contrasted to skin absorption which usu-

ally results in chronic symptoms. The following discussions cover some of the more common metal poisonings encountered in practice. Note that iron poisoning is covered in Chap. 33, along with the use of deferoxamine.

Zinc

Source Zinc is an element for normal growth and development of plants and animals. It is omnipresent in the environment. It is found in water, air, and living organisms. It functions as an integral part of a number of enzymes and therefore is important in many types of synthesis in the body, including DNA and RNA.

Millions of tons of zinc metal are used commercially, principally to galvanize iron and to manufacture brass. Exposure to zinc fumes is the main industrial hazard (fume fever). Many zinc salts have industrial, agricultural, and medical uses. Zinc can be found in adhesive plaster (containing zinc oxide) used to prevent dialysis coils from unwinding, water used for dialysis fluid, and galvanized iron pipes or tanks. Welders, smelter workers, and solderers are exposed to aerolized zinc.

Metabolites The normal adult body zinc content is 1.5 to 3.0 g. Daily intake ranges from 5 to 35 mg. Zinc is bound to metallothionines synthesized in the liver and is excreted by both the urine and the gastrointestinal tract, choroid plexus, and prostate; substantial amounts are also found in the bone, brain, eyes, skeletal muscle, and other tissues. Zinc has a strong affinity for red blood cell and plasma proteins.

Two human zinc-deficiency syndromes have been described, *hypogonadal dwarf syndrome* and *acrodermatitis enteropathica*. Parakeratosis and impaired wound healing are also associated with zinc deficiency. The manifestations of zinc toxicity do not necessarily correlate well with plasma or whole-blood zinc levels. Nausea, vomiting, anorexia, lethargy, irritability, abdominal pain, and anemia are the most frequent manifestations. Fever may accompany zinc toxicity, along with diarrhea, muscle pain, hyperamylasemia with or without pancreatitis, intestinal bleeding, thrombocytopenia, oliguria, hypotension, and renal failure with tubular necrosis.

Toxicities caused by aerosolized zinc may be zinc fume fever, chills, myalgias, metallic taste, cough, nausea, lethargy, and, occasionally, hemoptysis. Ordinarily, all toxicities disappear after cessation of exposure. Zinc tablets are now sold in health food stores, and excessive intake may result in toxicity.

Aluminum

Source The principal ore of aluminum is bauxite. Aluminum is widely used as a building material and for other uses where light weight and corrosion resistance are important. Aluminum oxide has industrial uses as an abrasive and catalyst. Medically, various soluble salts of aluminum have been used as astringents, styptics, and antiseptics. The insoluble salts are used as antacids and as antidiarrheal agents. Inhalation of aluminum hydroxide is used as a preventive and curative agent for silicosis.

Orally, aluminum salts are converted to the phosphate salt in the gastrointestinal tract and excreted in the feces and in the milk of nursing females. Parenteral injection of aluminum salts results in excretion in both the feces and urine as well as slight increase in the concentration of aluminum in the liver and spleen.

Aluminum-induced dialysis dementia is often a fatal disease. The tap water is usually to blame because water naturally contain high concentrations of aluminum. In other cases aluminum sulfate has been added to the community water supplies to remove organic materials. Encephalopathy thought to be caused by aluminum occurs in renal dialysis patients, especially those on this therapy for several years.

Early toxic effects include malaise, memory loss, and a characteristic speech disturbance. As the disease progresses, dysarthria, asterixis, myoclonic twitches, dementia, somnolence, and seizures occur. The electroencephalogram shows slowing, together with bursts of delta activity and high voltage, symmetric spikes. Postmortem examinations show that aluminum levels are markedly increased in the gray matter.

Other toxic effects include anemia, myopathy, and severe pain caused by profound osteodystrophy. It has been suggested that Alzheimer's disease and other types of senile dementia may be related to brain aluminum deposition, possibly caused by improper use of aluminum utensils.

Although frequently lethal, in some cases encephalopathy has regressed after intake of oral aluminum is stopped or the aluminum content of the dialysis is reduced; sometimes deferoxamine, which complexes with aluminum may be beneficial.

Those involved in aluminum processing, pottery making, explosive making, or welding may be exposed to aluminum aerosols. Pulmonary granulomas, fibrosis, and postfibrosis emphysema may supervene. In bauxite smelters, this is known as *Shaver's disease*.

Cadmium

Source Cadmium ranks close to lead and mercury as a metal of current toxicologic concern. Over 10 million pounds of cadmium are used industrially every year in the United States. It is used in the manufacture of electrical conductors and in electroplating; and it is present in ceramics, pigments, dental prosthetics, plastic stabilizers, and storage batteries. It is also a by-product of zinc smelting, and it is used in the photographic, rubber, motor, and aircraft industries. Smelters, metal-processing furnaces, and the burning of coal and oil are responsible for much of the cadmium in the air.

Cadmium is used as various inorganic salts. The most important are cadmium stearate, which is used as a heat stabilizer in PVC plastics, and cadmium sulfide and cadmium sulfoselenide, used as yellow and red pigments in plastics and colors. Cadmium sulfide is also used in photocells and solar cells. Cadmium chloride is used in the production of certain photographic films.

Acute intoxication by cadmium fumes exceeding 0.1 mg/m^3 produces a characteristic clinical picture. Four to 10 h after exposure dyspnea, cough, and substernal discomfort supervene, often accompanied by prominent myalgias, fatigue, headache, and vomiting. In more severe cases wheezing, hemoptysis, and progressive dyspnea caused by pulmonary edema may occur and may be accompanied by hypotension and renal failure.

In most cases, the pulmonary manifestations resolve rapidly but pulmonary function abnormalities may not disappear for months; in these cases vital capacity is reduced and there is a restrictive defect.

Ingestion of large amounts of cadmium results in nausea, vomiting, and abdominal pain, often accompanied by weakness, prostration, and myalgias. The onset of gastroenteritis occurs 1.5 to 5 h after ingestion and lasts for less than 24 h.

Chronic exposure to aerosol for years has resulted in emphysema. The emphysema is not accompanied by bronchitis and may appear many years after industrial exposure has stopped. It is reported that workers exposed for years to workroom concentrations of respirable cadmium greater than 0.01 mg/m^3 also suffer olfactory nerve damage, which in some cases progresses to total anosmia. The most frequent systemic long-term consequence of aerosol or oral exposure is proteinuria. After prolonged and heavy contact, cadmium urinary excretion continues for years and is associated with damage to the proximal tubule. The major urinary protein is a low-molecular-weight beta microglobulin.

On occasion the proteinuria may be accompanied by glycosuria and aminoaciduria. Only infrequently are the proteinuria and tubular damage followed by progressive renal failure. An exception to the relatively benign course of renal damage is the disease in Japan known as *itai-itai* (ouch-ouch), which affected almost exclusively multiparous women of ages 40 to 70 who lived in an area contaminated by industrial cadmium waste. Manifestation included back and joint pain, a waddly gait, osteomalacia, bone deformities, and fractures, all presumably secondary to cadmium-induced renal tubular damage.

Some studies on workers exposed to cadmium have suggested an increased risk of lung or prostatic carcinoma, but the data are not convincing.

Persons who have ingested cadmium salts should be made to vomit or given gastric lavage; persons exposed to acute inhalation should be removed from exposure and given oxygen therapy as necessary. No specific treatment for chronic cadmium poisoning is available and symptomatic treatment must be relied upon. Administration of chelating agents is contraindicated, since they are nephrotoxic in combination with cadmium.

Manganese

Source Manganese is a cofactor in a number of enzymatic reactions, particularly those involved in phosphorylation, cholesterol, and fatty-acids synthesis. While it is present in urban air and in most water supplies, the principal portion of the intake is derived from food, especially vegetables, the germinal portions of grains, fruits, nuts, tea, and some spices.

Manganese and its compounds are used in making steel alloys, dry cell batteries, electrical coils, ceramics, matches, glass, dye, fertilizers, and welding rods and are used as oxidizing agents and animal food additives. The primary uses in medicine are as antiseptics and germicides. Potassium permanganate is applied dermally for these effects and for its slight astringent action. This is virtually the only manganese compound of medical use at the present time.

Pharmacokinetics

The body burden has been estimated at 20 mg. The liver, kidney, intestine, and pancreas contain the highest concentrations. No significant changes in tissue concentration occur with age, except that tissues that have low manganese amounts in adults tend to contain higher amounts in the newborn. The lungs do not accumulate manganese with age despite significant concentration in urban air. The turnover of manganese is rapid. Injected radiomanganese quickly disappears from the bloodstream; it is concentrated in the mitochondria of the liver and pancreas. Administration of stable manganese in any valence state promotes rapid excretion of radiomanganese. Serum manganese, normally 0.1 to 1.0 μg/L, increases after acute coronary occlusion and is claimed to be more accurate index of myocardial infarction than glutamic oxalacetic transaminase.

Manganese toxicity occurs primarily in miners who have been exposed to manganese dioxide aerosols for prolonged periods. The manifestions, known as *manganic madness*, concentrate primarily in the basal ganglia and cerebellum, accounting for the extrapyramidal Parkinsonism feature—the rigidity and the difficulty in walking.

One recent point of interest has been the possibility that manganese might contribute to an excess of free radicals such as superoxide and peroxide. These normal metabolites are highly toxic, but there are free-radical trapping systems that occur naturally and protect tissues from destruction by these noxious agents.

Other manifestations include compulsive behavior (including singing, dancing, fighting, and running), explosive and involuntary laughter, headache, muscular weakness, tremors, somnolence, dystonia, hypotonia, retropulsion, propulsion, dementia, speech disturbance, irritability, hypersomnia, and memory defects. In some cases psychosis may be the dominant feature.

There is no effective therapy. After removal from manganese exposure followed by attempts to reduce the body manganese load by treatment with calcium edetate, the patients are treated with L-dopa. The mental aberrations improve, but the neurologic abnormalities tend to persist.

Bismuth

Widely used in industry in the manufacture of alloys, ceramics, magnets, and radiographic contrast media, bismuth is also much in demand as a medicinal agent. Exposure to this metal is thus as common as that to lead and mercury. For example, bismuth is one of the contaminants found in urban air. Yet bismuth is not considered a serious industrial hazard, possibly because few cases of poisoning from this source are reported.

In medicine the advent of more effective agents has displaced bismuth for the systemic therapy of syphilis and amebiasis. Today it is the insoluble salts of bismuth that are widely used for gastrointestinal complaints such as nausea and diarrhea and for topical use in mild dermatitis, diaper rash, and as a general skin protective. Some topical hemorrhoidal products also contain insoluble bismuth salts.

Chemistry The element bismuth is grayish white: the salts are white, yellow, and brown crystals. Examples of bismuth salts used in medicine are shown in Table 48-4. All these salts of bismuth are virtually insoluble in water and are considered nonabsorbable by skin and mucous membranes. Herein lies their safety, and hence they are allowed to be marketed as over-the-counter preparations.

Mechanism of Action Like the other heavy metals, bismuth forms strong covalent double bonds with sulfhydryl groups of cellular proteins, including many enzymes. It also coagulates and denatures protein. Similar to gold, mercury, and lead, bismuth has an affinity for renal and central nervous tissues. Thus encephalopathy and renal damage might be expected. Actually bismuth can also cause hepatitis and various skin disorders such as a lichen planus-like lesion.

In its clinical use the insoluble salts of bismuth are considered to be mildly antiseptic, somewhat astrin-

TABLE 48-4   Examples of medicinally used bismuth compounds

Use	Agents
1. Upset stomach, indigestion, nausea, and common diarrhea	Bismuth subcarbonate Bismuth subgallate Bismuth subsalicylate
2. Relief of irritation due to hemorrhoids	Bismuth subcarbonate Bismuth subgallate Bismuth resorcinol
3. Minor skin irritations and diaper rash	Bismuth subgallate Bismuth formic iodide Bismuth subnitrate

gent, but mainly protective by forming a firm coating on skin and mucous membranes. The skin preparations often contain other ingredients such as zinc oxide.

Pharmacokinetics All the medicinal salts of bismuth are not absorbed either by skin or mucous membranes. Even the abraded skin or ulcerated mucous membrane surface is relatively resistant.

There is the possibility that intestinal bacteria might methylate bismuth and form a soluble salt. In animals, trimethyl bismuth is highly toxic, causing an encephalopathic syndrome. Blood levels of bismuth should not exceed 20 μg/L. Urinary excretion is less than 1 μmol per day.

Toxicity Fever, diarrhea, weakness, stomatitis, black oropharynx and gum line, dermatitis, jaundice, and nephritis, so often seen when soluble salts of bismuth were used, are no longer seen. The reported cases today present as encephalopathy. At higher risk are patients who chronically take insoluble bismuth salts for gastrointestinal complaints for months and years. In Europe and Australia there is an incidence of bismuth encephalopathy due to the practice of using a bismuth subgallate powder to daily dust a colostomy to control odor and stool consistency.

The subnitrate salt of bismuth can be broken down by intestinal bacteria and thus could lead to nitrite poisoning. The subsalicylate salt of bismuth can also be dissociated and cause salicylate poisoning. Aspirin should not be given with remedies containing bismuth subsalicylate.

Topical skin preparations have very rarely caused any toxicity other than allergic reactions probably due to other components than bismuth.

Therapy Therapy of bismuth encephalopathy is expectant. Once the bismuth is stopped, recovery takes place slowly over a period of months. Attempts to remove the bismuth more rapidly by use of chelates are not recommended.

BIBLIOGRAPHY

Calesnick, B., and A. Dinan: "Zinc Deficiency and Zinc Toxicity," *Am. Fam. Phys.*, **37**:267–270 (1988).

Calne, D. B., et al.: "Alzheimer's Disease, Parkinson's Disease and Motorneuron Disease: A Biotropic Interaction between Ageing and Environment? *Lancet*, **2**:1067–1070 (1986).

Charhon, S. A., et al.: "Serum Aluminum Concentrations and Aluminum Deposits in Bone in Patients Receiving Haemodialysis," *Br. Med. J.*, **290**:1613 (1985).

DiPalma, J. R.: "Bismuth Toxicity," *Am. Fam. Phys.*, **38**:244–146 (1988).

Ellenhorn, M. J., and D. G. Barcalrix: "*Medical Toxicology, Diagnosis and Treatment of Human Poisoning*," Elsevier, New York, 1988.

Friberg, L.: "Cadmium," *Ann. Rev. Public Health*, **4**:367 (1983).

Greaves, I. A., et al.: "Respiratory Effects of Two Types of Solder Flux Used in the Electronics Industry," *J. Occup. Med.*, **26**:81 (1984).

Hassan, J., et al.: "The Immunological Consequences of Gold Therapy: A Prospective Study in Patients with Rheumatoid Arthritis," *Clin. Exp. Immunol.*, **63**:614–620 (1986).

Hurst, N. P., et al.: "Studies of the Effect of D-Penicillamine and Sodium Aurothiomalate Therapy on Superoxide Anion Production by Monocytes from Patients with Rheumatoid Arthritis: Incidence for in vivo Stimulation of Monocytes," *Ann. Rheum. Dis.*, **45**:37–43 (1986).

Kark, R. A. P., D. C. Poskanzer, J. D. Bullock, et al.: "Mercury Poisoning and Its Treatment with *N*-Acetyl-DL-Penicillamine," *N. Engl. J. Med.*, **285**:10–16 (1985).

Khandelwal, S., et al.: "Influence of Metal Chelators on Metalloenzymes," *Toxicol. Lett.*, **38**:115–121 (1987).

Kruger, G. L., et al.: "The Health Effects of Aluminum Compounds in Mammals," *CRC Crit. Rev. Toxicol.*, **13**:1 (1984).

Manton, W. I.: "Total Contribution of Airborne Lead to Blood Lead," *Br. J. Ind. Med.*, **42**:168–172 (1985).

Moel, D. I., et al.: "Slow, Natural Reduction in Blood Lead Levels after Chelation Therapy for Lead Poisoning in Childhood," *Am. J. Dis. Child.*, **140**:905–908 (1986).

Nightingale, S. L.: "Oral Chelation Products," *Am. Fam. Phys.*, **33**:325 (1986).

Plunkett, E. R.: *Handbook of Industrial Toxicology*, 3d ed., Chemical Publishing, New York, 1987.

Szeliga-Cetnarska, M., et al.: Chronic Manganese Poisoning," *Med. PR*, **36**:282–286 (1985).

Tahahashi, W., et al.: "Urinary Arsenic, Chromium and Copper Levels in Workers Exposed to Arsenic-Based Wood Preservatives," *Arch. Environ. Health.*, **38**:209 (1983).

United States Pharmacopeial Convention, Inc.: *Drug Information for the Health Care Professional*, 8th ed., Rockville, Maryland, 1988.

Weigel, H. J., et al.: "Availability and Toxicological Effects of Low Levels of Biologically Bound Calcium," *Arch. Environ. Contam. Toxicol.*, **16**:85–93 (1987).

Carbon Monoxide and Cyanide Poisoning

Joseph R. DiPalma

CARBON MONOXIDE

The most common cause of accidental and suicidal poisoning in the United States is carbon monoxide (CO), which accounts for an estimated 4000 deaths annually. In addition, at least twice as many suffer from partial poisoning, resulting in disability and absence from work. Persons with preexisting heart or brain damage are more susceptible. Victims of CO poisoning of some severity who recover are subject to various and subtle neurologic sequelae.

Sources

The body itself produces an inconsequential amount of CO from hemoglobin catabolism. The normal carboxyhemoglobin (COHb) level seldom exceeds 0.4 to 0.7 percent. Hemoglobin destruction as in hemolytic anemia may raise levels of COHb to as much as 8 percent. Heavy smokers (at least a pack of cigarettes a day) have a COHb blood level of up to 6 percent.

In today's society automobile exhaust provides the greatest source of environmental CO. The average automobile emits up to 9 percent CO in its exhaust. However, catalytic converters have reduced this to about 1 percent. Nevertheless because of the large number of cars on highways, the CO air levels can reach 25 to 100 ppm, enough to cause symptoms, especially in persons with preexisting cardiovascular disease. Running the automobile engine in a closed garage is still one of the most common causes of accidental or suicidal poisoning.

The second most common source of CO is faulty heating equipment. This includes all types of stoves whether fueled by wood, coal, gas, or oil. The rise in use of kerosene space heaters has increased the incidence of CO poisoning. All combustible material gives rise to a certain amount of CO. Therefore, the space occupied by the heating equipment must be vented at all times not only to allow a fresh and adequate oxygen supply but also to eliminate the CO produced by the heating equipment.

Deaths from fire are largely caused by inhalation of CO. Levels of this gas in fires may reach as high as 10 percent. This produces an atmosphere which can kill within minutes.

Industrial causes of CO poisoning occur in the smelting of metals, welding, ceramics working, glassblowing, and in many processes using metal carbonyls. Methylene chloride (CH_2Cl), a constituent of some paint removers, is converted by the body to CO. This type of paint remover must be used in a vented room.

Mechanism of Action

CO has an affinity for hemoglobin 250 times greater than does oxygen. Structural changes in the COHb molecule cause the oxyhemoglobin curve to shift to the left. In addition, the reduction of red blood cell 2,3-diphosphoglycerate further accentuates the left shift. This causes a severe reduction in the oxygen-carrying capacity of blood. CO has an affinity for other heme compounds, including hydroperoxidase, myoglobin, cytochrome oxidase, and P-450. Although these are considerably less important, they do add to the general toxicity, and at low blood oxygen tension they assume a greater influence.

The effects of CO depend entirely on the concentration in inspired air and the duration of exposure. It turns out that a brief exposure to a high concentration is less dangerous than a long exposure to a lower concentration for a longer period of time. Another critical factor is the partial pressure of CO relative to the partial pressure of oxygen. High partial pressures of oxygen will tend to impede the uptake of CO, and vice versa. This is the basis of therapy with 100 percent oxygen and the use of the hyperbaric chamber.

Chronic exposure to low concentration of CO (as in smokers) accelerates the development of atherosclerosis. Endothelial hypertrophy, subintimal edema, and increased vessel permeability are observed in experimental animals. The cardiac output is increased along with minute ventilation. Animals dying of CO poisoning show dilated ventricles, particularly the right, which is associated with a rise in central venous pressure.

Central nervous system (CNS) lesions are mainly restricted to the white matter. Pathologic changes range from mild inflammation to myelin necrosis. In severe poisoning cerebral edema occurs. The CNS changes are not unique to CO poisoning.

Clinical Signs and Symptoms

CO is a nonirritating, colorless, odorless gas slightly lighter than air. Because of these features, the individual is not aware of poisonous concentrations of CO in inspired air.

The organ systems causing symptoms are the CNS, cardiovascular, respiratory, and musculoskeletal. The most common CNS symptoms are headache and dizziness and in severe cases convulsions and coma. Most commonly the cardiovascular disorder noted is hypertension. Shortness of breath is not often felt, but a tight feeling in the chest is experienced by some. Profound weakness and inability to perform routine tasks are a dominant symptom. Over 5 percent of victims with a concentration of 50 percent COHb who survive have permanent sequelae. Exposure to CO concentrations of COHb of over 50 percent is often fatal. The duration of exposure is of critical importance, and this is illustrated in Fig. 49-1. An exposure to 0.01 percent of CO in inspired air for as long as 9 h results in nothing more than a headache. Contrast this to exposure to a concentration of 1 percent of CO in inspired air for 10 min, which is uniformly fatal. All gradations exist in between, as shown in Fig. 49-1.

CO toxicity is increased by numerous factors. Some of these are decreased barometric pressure (high alti-

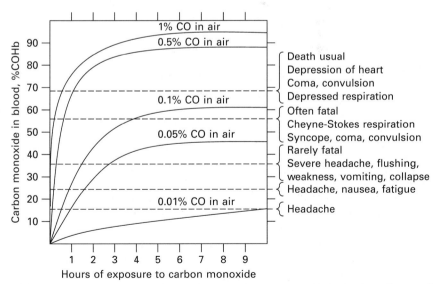

FIGURE 49-1   The effect of the concentration of carbon monoxide in the air on the rate of uptake expressed as percent of COHb. The relationship to time of exposure and the symptoms to be expected is also shown.

tude), a higher degree of alveolar ventilation such as in excitement or exercise, high metabolic rate (birds, children), preexisting cardiovascular and CNS diseases, and anemia.

Treatment

Removal of the individual from the contaminated environment is the most important step. Rescuers themselves have become intoxicated because of delay in an atmosphere of high CO concentration. Establishment of an airway and administration of 100 percent oxygen by a tight-fitting mask or an endotracheal tube, if required, is the next step.

The half-life of COHb is about 5 to 6 h under no treatment. Administration of 100 percent oxygen reduces this to ½ to 1 h. Hyperbaric oxygen (3 atm) further reduces the half-life of COHb to 20 to 30 min. This is illustrated in Fig. 49-2.

The actual value of hyperbaric oxygen is somewhat controversial. Once a degree of tissue damage has occurred, there is doubt that more rapid elimination of CO with the use of hyperbaric oxygen has a significant advantage over 100 percent oxygen. The situation is made difficult by the scarcity of hyperbaric oxygen units. Usually the patient must be transported over long distances to a suitable facility.

There is no other specific antidote. Supportive therapy especially for acidosis, cardiovascular support, and hydration, where indicated, is important.

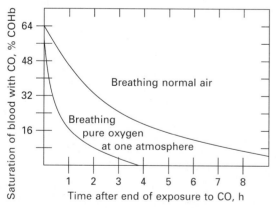

FIGURE 49-2 Rates of elimination of carbon monoxide from blood when room air, as compared to 100 percent oxygen, is respired.

CYANIDE

In recent times cyanide poisoning has achieved prime media attention because of the cyanide-Tylenol homicides. Actually cyanide ion is a fundamental building block of organic life processes and has a significant role in the metabolism of both plants and animals. In excessive amounts it is one of the deadliest and most easily available poisons.

Source

Endogenously cyanide is part of vitamin B_{12} metabolism. It is taken in as food especially in certain plants such as *Prunus* species (cherry, almonds, and peaches), bamboo sprouts, cassava, and *Sorghum* species. Tobacco smoke also contains cyanide. Ordinarily the amount of cyanide for endogenous sources is too small to cause significant toxicity. However, it is possible to ingest enough almonds or peach pits to cause poisoning. The bitter taste is attractive to some palates. Tobacco amblyopia is probably caused by the cyanide content of smoke.

Industrial sources are many and include the industries involved in electroplating, extraction of ores, photography, synthetic rubber, and manufacture of plastics. Many chemical synthetic processes utilize cyanide; thus chemists are particularly subject to accidental poisoning. Cyanide has also been used as a fumigant for rodents and insects.

Medicinally long-term nitroprusside therapy may cause cyanide toxicity. Laetrile, amygdalin, promoted as a cure for cancer produced cyanide toxicity.

Mechanism of Action

Cyanide forms a stable coordination complex with ferric iron, thus keeping this metal in a higher oxidation state (Fe^{3+}). Thus it greatly diminishes its activity as an electron carrier in reactions involving $Fe^{3+} + e \longrightarrow Fe^{2+}$ transitions. Numerous enzymes may be involved, but the main one is ferricytochrome oxidase, which is changed to ferricytochrome oxidase-cyanide. This seriously impairs cellular oxygen utilization. Consequently the many pathways which converge at the cytochrome system to utilize oxygen are arrested, and aerobic metabolism ceases. This histotoxic hypoxia results in a shift to anaerobic metabolism, which in turn causes the accumulation of lactate, pyruvate, and glucose.

Cells are unable to utilize the oxygen in oxyhemoglobin. Venous blood becomes bright red and has almost the same oxygen saturation as arterial blood. Physiologically the most sensitive cells in the body to tissue hypoxia are the carotid and aortic bodies. A small amount of cyanide injected intravenously will upon reaching the carotid body cause an inspiratory gasp. This phenomenon has been used as a measure of circulation time. By this same reflex hyperpnea is an instantaneous response to cyanide exposure.

Tissues most sensitive to hypoxia are first affected. Obviously the CNS and the heart are organs which are critically first disturbed in cyanide poisoning. All cells eventually are affected; those with the lowest metabolism tend to survive the best.

Other hematin compounds which complex with cyanide are catalase, peroxidase, cytochrome-C-peroxidase, and methemoglobin. Some metal-bearing enzymes complexing with cyanide are tyrosinase, ascorbic acid oxidase, xanthine oxidase, succinic acid, lactic acid, and formicdehydrogenase. The role of cyanide in hydroxocobalamin metabolism is described in Chap. 33.

Pharmacokinetics

Cyanides can be absorbed by all routes, although fatalities by skin absorption are rare. Most instances of poisoning are either by inhalation of HCN or oral absorption of cyanide salts such as KCN or NaCN. Distribution is very rapid, since cyanide is water-soluble and carried by blood to every organ. The concentration in blood is the highest except for the spleen, salivary glands, thyroid, and stomach. In survivors cyanide is converted to the much less toxic thiocyanate ion, which is excreted in the urine. The enzyme mitochondrial sulfurtransferase (rhodanese) catalyzes this reaction (Fig. 49-3). Other minor pathways of excretion and biotransformation are also shown in Fig. 49-3.

The liver and kidneys contain large amounts of sulfurtransferase, but a limiting factor is the amount of intracellular-reducing sulfur which can serve as a substrate. In vivo suitable sulfur is found in thiosulfate, cystine, and cysteine. To effectively combat poisoning, exogenous-reducing sulfur must be provided.

Acute Toxicity

Inhaled cyanide acts as rapidly as intravenous cyanide. Immediate symptoms are flushing, headache, dizziness, and tachypnea. This is followed by stridorous breathing, coma, and death within 10 min. Oral exposures are less rapid because of a slower rise in blood levels and some first-pass biotransformation in the liver. Death may occur in 30 min to 1 h. The absence of cyanosis despite intensive respiratory distress should suggest cyanide poisoning.

Five parts HCN per million of air (5 ppm) is the threshold limit for continual occupational exposure. One hundred ppm of HCN in air endangers life in 1-h exposure. Any higher concentration is likely to be fatal with immediate symptoms.

The minimum lethal dose of the salts of cyanide is 0.2 g for adults. Persons attempting suicide usually take a teaspoonful (2 to 6 g).

Chronic Toxicity

Headache, dizziness, nausea, sometimes vomiting, and a bitter or abnormal taste have been reported as symptoms of chronic exposure to sublethal doses of cyanide. This usually occurs in industrial occupations such as metal smelting. Certain clinical syndromes have been attributed to chronic cyanide poisoning. These include tobacco amblyopia, Leber's hereditary optic atropy, and Nigerian nutritional ataxic neuropathy. The last syndrome is associated with elevated plasma thiocyanate levels and reduced levels of sulfur-containing amino acids. It is caused by the consumption of large amounts of cassava containing cyanogenic glycoside. Thus nutritional factors and genetic defects must be considered in cases of chronic toxicity.

Treatment

The absolute necessity for immediate institution of therapy as soon as symptoms appear cannot be overemphasized. Of first importance is support of respiration and circulation. Institution of 100 percent oxygen, assistance of respiration as needed, insertion of intravenous lines, and cardiac monitoring are the first steps. Correction of metabolic acidosis (pH below 7.15) is also necessary. Hemodialysis and hemoperfusion are ineffective measures. Hyperbaric oxygen effectiveness has not been proven and should be resorted

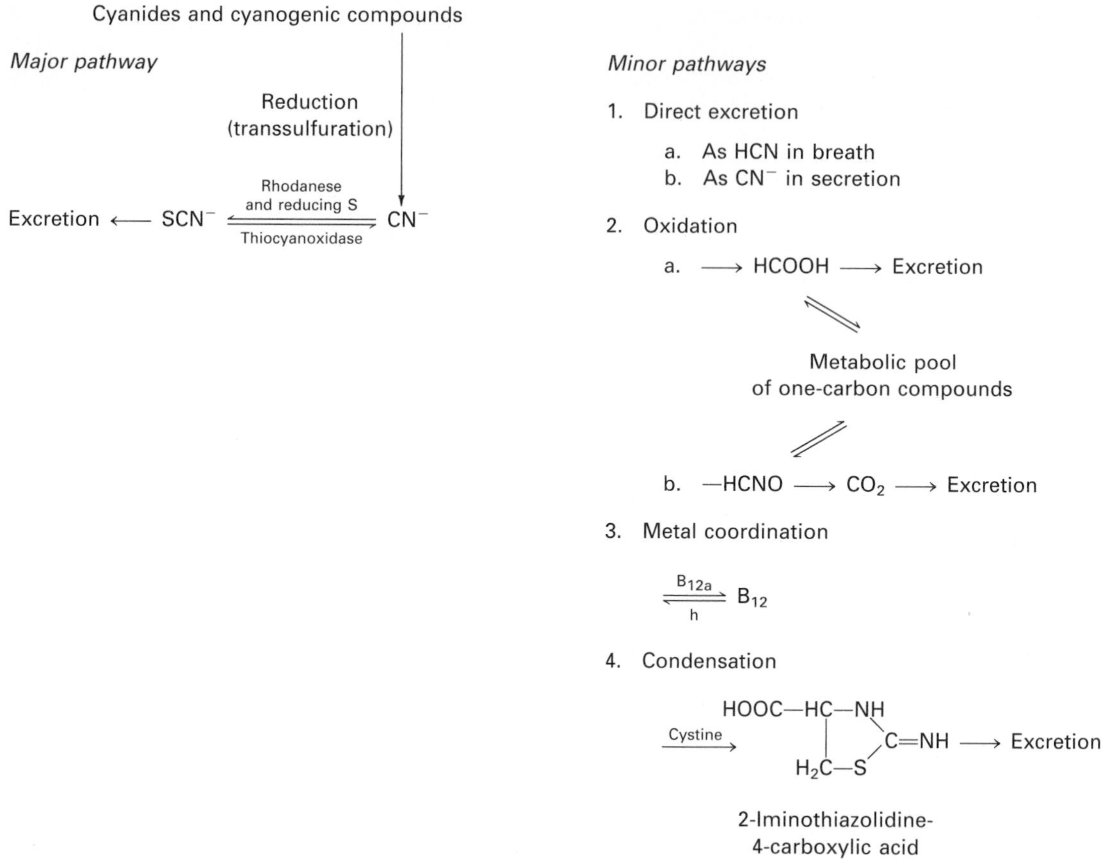

Cyanides and cyanogenic compounds

Major pathway

Reduction
(transsulfuration)

Rhodanese
and reducing S

Excretion ⟵— SCN⁻ $\rightleftharpoons$ CN⁻

Thiocyanoxidase

Minor pathways

1. Direct excretion

    a. As HCN in breath
    b. As CN⁻ in secretion

2. Oxidation

    a. $\longrightarrow$ HCOOH $\longrightarrow$ Excretion

Metabolic pool
of one-carbon compounds

    b. —HCNO $\longrightarrow$ CO_2 $\longrightarrow$ Excretion

3. Metal coordination

$\xrightarrow[h]{B_{12a}}$ B_{12}

4. Condensation

HOOC—HC—NH
$\xrightarrow{\text{Cystine}}$ C=NH $\longrightarrow$ Excretion
                      H_2C—S

2-Iminothiazolidine-
4-carboxylic acid

FIGURE 49-3   The fate of absorbed cyanide: detoxication and excretion pathways.

to only in the most extreme cases. Meanwhile, decontamination should be carried out where indicated. Removal of contaminated clothing and washing affected skin with green soap are important measures.

Institution of antidote therapy should be next; then gut decontamination should be done if less than 2 h have passed since ingestion. Gastric lavage, charcoal, and cathartics can all be used. While some patients may survive with supportive care alone, antidote therapy is usually very effective.

Antidotes

The principles of combating cyanide poisoning traditionally are, first, to encourage the formation of methemoglobin, which has a great affinity for cyanide, and, second, to provide reducing sulfur in the form of

thiosulfate so that the body can excrete cyanide as thiocyanate.

The three-step Eli-Lilly cyanide kit is the approved preparation in the United States. It contains sodium nitrite, 300 mg in 10 mL (2 amps); sodium thiosulfate 12.5 g in 50 mL (2 amps); amyl nitrite inhalant 0.3 mL (12 aspirols). In practice, amyl nitrite is given by crushing the aspirol and inhaling the vapor. This will produce a 3 to 5 percent methemoglobinemia. Sodium nitrite 300 mg is then administered IV slowly over 4 min and will produce a 20 percent methemoglobinemia. After nitrites are given, thiosulfate is administered IV as a 25 percent solution. The usual adult dose is 12.5 g IV at a rate of 3 to 5 mL/min.

Cyanide poisoning, especially that caused by nitroprusside, has been successfully treated with hydroxocobalamin (vitamin B_{12a}). This provitamin combines with cyanide to form cyanocobalamin (vitamin B_{12}), which is excreted in the urine. This is an FDA nonapproved use, and, unfortunately, the available commercial solutions are too dilute for routine therapy. A suggested dose is 50 times the estimated cyanide dose. An amount of 25 mg/h has been recommended for nitroprusside-induced cyanide toxicity. At present there is not sufficient evidence to recommend hydroxocobalamin therapy in preference to the standard nitrite-thiosulfate treatment.

BIBLIOGRAPHY

Beamer, W. C., R. M. Shealy, D. S. Prough: "Acute Cyanide Poisoning from Laetrile Ingestion," *Ann. Emerg. Med.*, **12**:449–451 (1983).

Blanc, P., M. Hogan, K. Mallin, et al.: "Cyanide Intoxication among Silver Reclaiming Workers," *JAMA*, **253**:367–371 (1985).

Caplan, Y. H., B. C. Thompson, B. Levine, et al.: "Accidental Poisonings Involving Carbon Monoxide, Heating Systems and Confined Spaces," *J. Forensic Sci.*, **31**:117–121 (1986).

Drew, R. H.: "The Use of Hydroxocobalamin in the Prophylaxis and Treatment of Nitroprusside-Induced Cyanide Toxicity," *Vet. Hum. Toxicol.*, **25**:342–345 (1983).

Ginsberg, M. D.: "Carbon Monoxide Intoxication. Clinical Features, Neuropathology and Mechanisms of Injury," *Clin. Toxicol.*, **23**:281–288 (1985).

Huber, J. A.: "Do Awake Patients with High Carboxyhemoglobin Levels Need Hyperbaric Oxygen?," *J. Emerg. Med.*, **1**:555–556 (1984).

Kizer, K. W.: "Hyperbaric Oxygen and Cyanide Poisoning," *Am. J. Emerg. Med.*, **2**:113 (1984).

Mosier, D., and R. Baldwin: "Carbon Monoxide Poisoning," South Dakota, *MMWR*, **34**:113 (1985).

Myers, R. M., S. K. Synder, and T. A. Emhoff: "Subacute Sequelae of Carbon Monoxide Poisoning," *Am. Emerg. Med.*, **14**:1163–1167 (1985).

Olson, K. R.: "Carbon Monoxide Poisoning: Mechanism, Presentation and Controversies in Management," *J. Emerg. Med.*, **1**:233–243 (1984).

O'Sullivan, B. P.: "Carbon Monoxide Poisoning in an Infant Exposed to a Kerosene Heater," *J. Pediatr.*, **103**:249–251 (1983).

Rieders, F.: "Noxious Gases and Vapors. I: Carbon Monoxide, Cyanides, Methemoglobin and Sulphemoglobin," in J. R. DiPalma (ed.) *Drill's Pharmacology in Medicine*, McGraw-Hill, New York, 1971, pp. 1180–1205.

Way, J. L.: "Cyanide Intoxication and Its Mechanism of Antagonism," *Ann. Rev. Pharmacol. Toxicol.*, **24**:451–481 (1984).

Index

I n d e x

Notes

Notes

Notes

Notes

Notes

Notes

Notes

Notes